ADVANCED EMERGENCY CARE
FOR PARAMEDIC PRACTICE

ADVANCED EMERGENCY CARE FOR PARAMEDIC PRACTICE

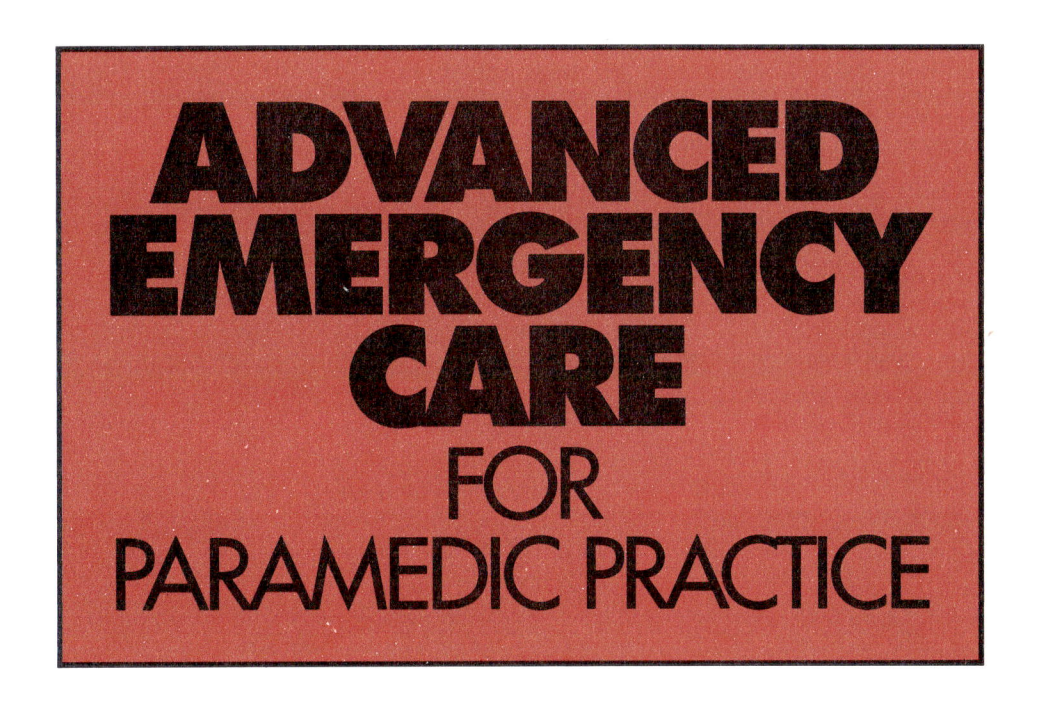

Edited by

SHIRLEY A. JONES, M.S.Ed., M.H.A., EMT–P
Allied Health Education, Program Director—EMS
Methodist Hospital of Indiana, Indianapolis, Indiana

AL WEIGEL, M.Ed., EMT–P
Laerdal Medical Corporation, Armonk, New York

ROGER D. WHITE, M.D., F.A.C.C.
Department of Anesthesiology, Mayo Clinic, Rochester, Minnesota

NORMAN E. McSWAIN, JR., M.D., F.A.C.S., NREMT–P
Professor of Surgery, Department of Surgery, Tulane University Medical Center
New Orleans, Louisiana

MARTI BREITER, R.N., B.S.N., REMT–P
Metro West EMS Quality Assurance Coordinator
Hennepin County Community Health Department—EMS, Minneapolis, Minnesota

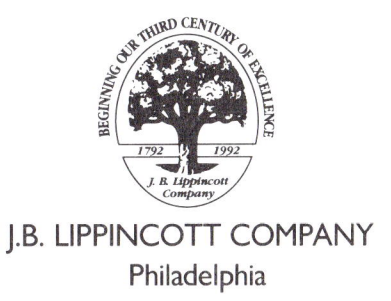

J.B. LIPPINCOTT COMPANY
Philadelphia

NEW YORK • LONDON • HAGERSTOWN

Sponsoring Editor: *Andrew Allen*
Coordinating Editorial Assistant: *Miriam Benert*
Project Editor: *Lorraine D. Smith*
Copy Editor: *Rosina Miller*
Indexer: *Alexandra Nickerson*
Designer: *Doug Smock*
Production Manager: *Helen Ewan*
Production Coordinator: *Kathryn Rule*
Compositor: *G&S Typesetters, Inc.*
Printer/Binder: *Courier Book Company/Westford*

Editorial Consultants: *Shirley A. Jones, M.S.Ed., M.H.A., EMT-P*
Indianapolis, Indiana

John A. Rasmussen, Ph.D., REMT-P
Greenville, South Carolina

Michael D. Greenberg, M.D.
Queens, New York

Copyright © 1992, by J. B. Lippincott Company
All rights reserved. No part of this book may be used or reproduced in any manner whatsoever without written permission except for brief quotations embodied in critical articles and reviews. Printed in the United States of America. For information write J. B. Lippincott Company, 227 East Washington Square, Philadelphia, Pennsylvania 19106.

Library of Congress Cataloging-in-Publication Data
Advanced emergency care for paramedic practice / edited by Shirley
   A. Jones . . . [et al.].
      p. cm.
   Includes bibliographical references and index.
   ISBN 0-397-51259-7. ISBN 0-397-54592-4 (soft cover)
   1. Emergency medicine. 2. Emergency medical technicians.
   I. Jones, Shirley A.
   [DNLM: 1. Emergencies. 2. Emergency Medical Services. WX 215
A244]
RC86.7.A3   1992
616.02'5—dc20
DNLM/DLC
for Library of Congress   91-25669
                                                    CIP

6 5 4 3 2 1

Any procedure or practice described in this book should be applied by the health-care practitioner under appropriate supervision in accordance with professional standards of care used with regard to the unique circumstances that apply in each practice situation. Care has been taken to confirm the accuracy of information presented and to describe generally accepted practices. However, the authors, editors, and publisher cannot accept any responsibility for errors or omissions or for any consequences from application of the information in this book and make no warranty, express or implied, with respect to the contents of the book.

Every effort has been made to ensure that drug selections and dosages are in accordance with current recommendations and practice. Because of ongoing research, changes in government regulations, and the constant flow of information on drug therapy, reactions, and interactions, the reader is cautioned to check the package insert for each drug for indications, dosages, warnings, and precautions, particularly if the drug is new or infrequently used.

Selected figures (illustrations) in this text were reproduced with permission from the following J. B. Lippincott sources: Brunner LS, Suddarth DS: The Lippincott Manual of Nursing Practice, 5th edition, 1991; Brunner LS, Suddarth DS: Textbook of Medical–Surgical Nursing, 6th edition, 1988; Bunting–Blake L, Parker J, Weigel A, White RD: Defibrillation: A Manual for the EMT, 1985; Chaffee EE, Greisheimer EM: Basic Physiology and Anatomy, 3rd edition, 1974; Chaffee EE, Lytle IM: Basic Physiology and Anatomy, 4th edition, 1980; Huff J, Doernbach DP, White RD: ECG Workout: Exercises in Arrhythmia Interpretation, 1985; Martin L, Reeder S: Essentials of Maternity Nursing: Family Centered Care, 1991; Memmler RL, Wood DL: The Human Body in Health and Disease, 6th edition, 1987; Reeder S, Martin L: Maternity Nursing, 16th edition, 1987; Rosdahl CB: Textbook of Basic Nursing, 5th edition, 1991; Taylor C, Lillis C, LeMone P: Fundamentals of Nursing, 1989; Timby BK: Clinical Nursing Procedures, 1989; White RD: Paramedic EKG Collection

To my father, George F. Jones, and to the memory of my mother, Vivian J. Jones
Shirley A. Jones

This book is dedicated to my parents
Al Weigel

*To my daughter, Merry, whose friendship, love, and intellectual curiosity
made my part of this book possible*
Norman E. McSwain

To my mother and the memory of my father
Roger D. White

In loving memory of my father, Al C. Breiter
Marti Breiter

About The Editors

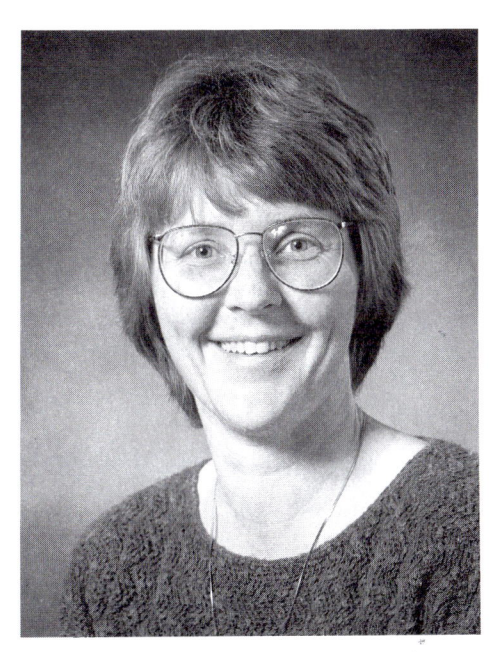

SHIRLEY A. JONES, M.S.Ed., M.H.A., EMT-P

Program director for Emergency Medical Services Education at Methodist Hospital in Indianapolis, Indiana, Shirley Jones has been an EMS educator since 1979 and an EMS manager since 1986. She received her Master of Science in Education and her Master of Health Administration degrees from Indiana University. In 1974, after completing a Bachelor of Arts degree in zoology, also from Indiana University, Shirley became the first woman to be hired as an Emergency Medical Technician in one of the largest county ambulance services in Indiana. She then became certified as a paramedic. During her career in EMS, Shirley has been awarded five first-place honors in tri-state and state-wide advanced life support ambulance competitions and has also received an award as outstanding paramedic in a tri-state area. Having served as faculty for national conferences, Shirley has also authored the *Study Guide and Examination Review* that accompanies this text.

Shirley A. Jones

AL WEIGEL, M.Ed., EMT-P

Al Weigel is currently director of marketing for Laerdal Medical Corporation, Armonk, New York. He holds a master's degree in education from the University of Arizona and completed a 1500 hour paramedic training program at the University of Kansas. He subsequently worked 5 years as a paramedic in Kansas City, Kansas, and was a paramedic instructor at the University of Arkansas. Al started the National Registry Paramedic and Intermediate Examination processes and was a member of the U.S. Department of Transportation Paramedic National Standard curriculum committee. An author of other EMS-related texts and articles, Al is a frequent guest lecturer at state and local EMS conferences.

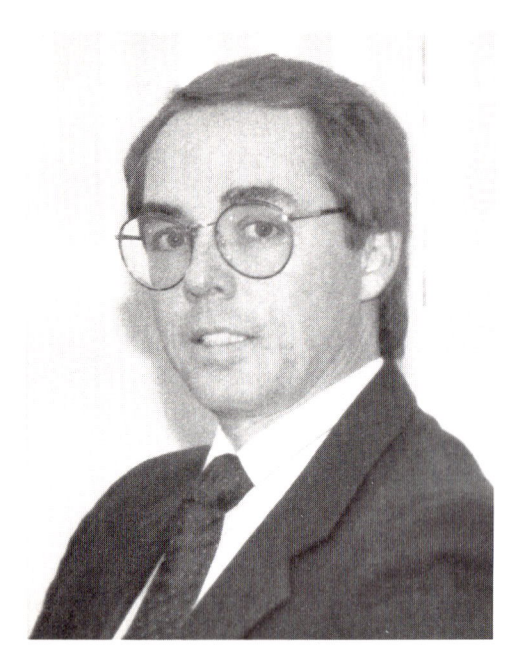

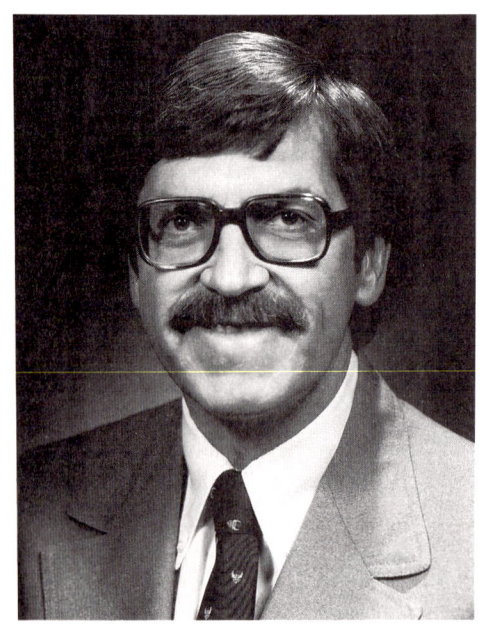

Al Weigel

ROGER D. WHITE, M.D., F.A.C.C.

Roger D. White is professor of anesthesiology at the Mayo Medical School and consultant in anesthesiology (cardiovascular) at the Mayo Clinic in Rochester, Minnesota. Roger has served on the American Heart Association's Subcommittee on Emergency Cardiac Care and has assisted in the development of the AHA Advanced Cardiac Life Support (ACLS) training program. He is a member of the ACLS national faculty and most recently served on the task force that developed the AHA Automated Defibrillation Training Program. A member of the board of directors of the National Registry of Emergency Medical Technicians, Roger is chair of the Registry's Standards and Examination Committee. He is a founding member of the National Association of Emergency Medical Technicians (NAEMT) and has served on its board of directors and as chair of its board of medical advisors. From the NAEMT he has received numerous awards for leadership, excellence, and lifetime achievement. In May of 1991, Roger received the U.S. Food and Drug Administration Commissioner's special citation "for outstanding accomplishments in development and implementation of a nationwide program to reduce problems in the use of cardiac defibrillators."

Roger D. White

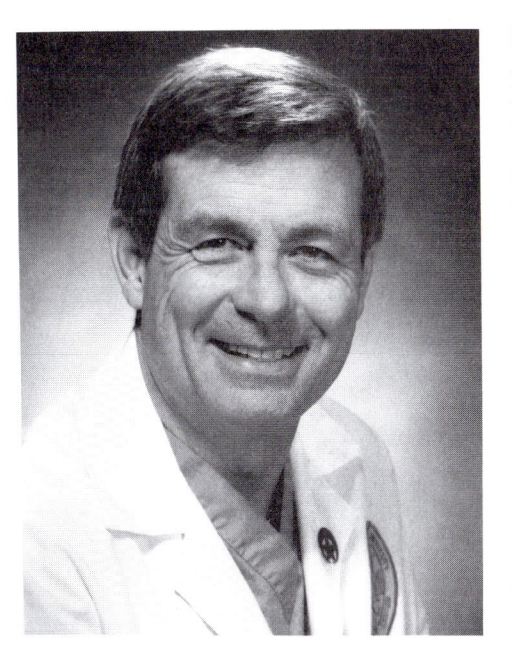

About the Editors   ix

NORMAN E. McSWAIN, JR., M.D., F.A.C.S., NREMT-P

Norman McSwain is professor of surgery at Tulane University School of Medicine in New Orleans, director of its trauma training program, and is police surgeon for the New Orleans Police Department. While finishing his trauma surgical training at Grady Hospital in Atlanta, Georgia, he was asked to create the medical organization for the new Road Atlanta Race Track and this led to the beginning of an active and close involvement with the ambulance world and its people. As assistant professor of surgery at the University of Kansas Medical Center, Norman was commissioned to develop a paramedic service for the city of Kansas City, Kansas, and later, for Johnson County, Kansas. He was also asked to develop EMT-A and EMT-P training programs for the entire state and to manage the programs, including training of all instructors-coordinators, supervising the state examination and the daily operation of the program. He has served in various capacities for the National Registry of EMTs and is its immediate past chairman. He was the first chairman of the ad hoc committee for the Advanced Trauma Life Support Course of the Committee on Trauma of the American College of Surgeons and has been active in all revisions of that course since its inception. Norman was instrumental in the development of the Prehospital Trauma Life Support Course for the National Association of EMTs and is medical director of that program.

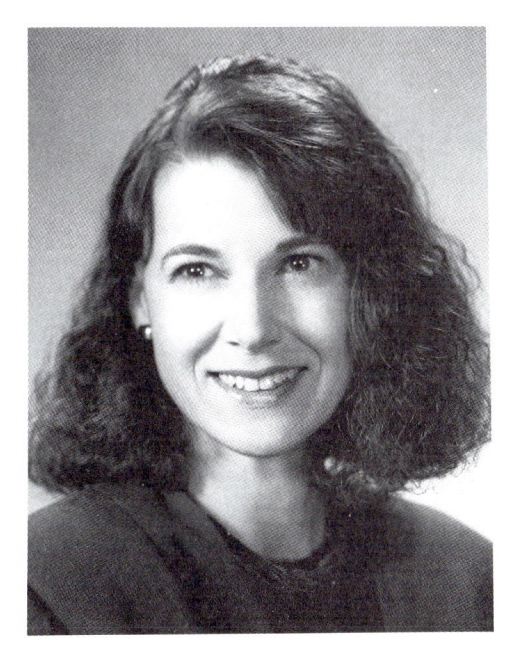

Norman E. McSwain, Jr.

MARTI BREITER, R.N., B.S.N., REMT-P

Marti Breiter received a bachelor of science degree in nursing, worked for several years as a cardiac/medical intensive care nurse, then was hired by Hennepin County (Minnesota) as its first EMS educator. Marti developed the initial paramedic curriculum and certification process for the county and coordinated its paramedic course and continuing education program for 11 years. In 1978 she was among the first in Minnesota to be certified by the National Registry as an EMT-paramedic. Marti transferred to the Hennepin County Community Health Department, Minneapolis, in 1985, where she is involved in EMS planning, quality assurance, education, and regulation of the Metro West EMS System, a four-county system with over 325 paramedics making in excess of 100,000 ALS runs per year. She has been active at both local and national levels of EMS as conference speaker, consultant, instructor-trainer and is currently an Advanced Cardiac Life Support affiliate faculty member of the American Heart Association. She was a member of the U.S. Department of Transportation's committee that developed the 1985 revision of the Paramedic National Standard Curriculum.

Marti Breiter

Contributors

Scott Bourn, R.N., M.S.N., C.E.N., REMT-P
President, Scott Bourn Associates, Lafayette, Colorado
Staff Nurse, Emergency Department, University Hospital, Emergency Medicine Course Director, Child Health Associates Program, University of Colorado Health Sciences Center, Denver, Colorado
    Chapter 10: *Airway Management and Ventilation*
    Chapter 19: *Respiratory Emergencies*

Marti Breiter, R.N., B.S.N., REMT-P
Metro West EMS Quality Assurance Coordinator, Hennepin County Community Health Department—EMS, Minneapolis, Minnesota
    Chapter 20: *Cardiovascular Emergencies*

Peter Wood Brewster, B.S.
Administrative Coordinator, Emergency Medical Preparedness Office, Department of Veteran Affairs, Indianapolis, Indiana
    Chapter 6: *Disaster Management*

Alexander Butman, B.A., EMSI, REMT-P
Executive Director, Emergency Training Institute Coordinator, Graduate Education Paramedic Training, Akron General Medical Center, Akron, Ohio
    Chapter 15: *Injuries to the Head, Neck, and Spine*

Debra Cason, M.S., R.N., EMT-P
Assistant Professor and Emergency Medical Services Program Director, The University of Texas Southwestern Medical Center at Dallas, Dallas, Texas
    Chapter 9: *Patient Assessment*
    Chapter 24: *Allergic and Anaphylactic Reactions*

Eddi Cohen, B.S., R.N., M.I.C.N., C.C.R.N.
President, EMS Network International, Santa Monica, California
    Chapter 6: *Disaster Management*

Kate Dernocoeur, B.S., EMT-P
Team Dernocoeur, Grand Rapids, Michigan
    Chapter 4: *Emergency Medical Services Communication*
    Chapter 5: *Rescue Management*

Barbara C. Eckhaus, M.A., C.H.E.S., EMT-P
EMS Consulting and Training, Derry, New Hampshire
    Chapter 2: *The Emergency Medical Services System*
    Chapter 28: *Geriatric Emergencies*

Larry S. Eckhaus, J.D., EMT
EMS Consulting and Training, Derry, New Hampshire
    Chapter 3: *Medical and Legal Considerations*

Mary Ellen Gillespie, R.N., EMT-P, I/C
Director of Education, Davenport College, Center for the Study of EMS, Grand Rapids, Michigan
    Chapter 23: *Gastrointestinal, Urinary, and Reproductive Emergencies*

John C. Goll, EMT-P
Director of Prehospital Care and Ambulance Services, The Aid Company, Inc., Indianapolis, Indiana
    Chapter 16: *Thoracic Injuries*
    Practical Skills

Carol Goodykoontz, M.S., R.N., EMT-P
Assistant Professor and Emergency Medical Services Assistant Program Director, The University of Texas Southwestern Medical Center at Dallas, Dallas, Texas
    Chapter 9: *Patient Assessment*

Alice "Twink" Gorgen, R.N., B.S.N., N.R.P.M., C.E.N., NREMT-P
Paramedic Nurse Coordinator, Omaha Fire Division Prehospital Education Program, Creighton University, Omaha, Nebraska
    Chapter 8: *Medical Terminology and Human Systems*

Michael D. Greenberg, M.D.
Attending Physician, Department of Emergency Medicine, Mary Immaculate Hospital, Queens, New York
    Chapter 17: *Abdominal Trauma*
    Chapter 21: *Endocrine Emergencies*

Jerome Hauer, M.H.S.
Director, State Emergency Management Agency, Indianapolis, Indiana
    Chapter 27: *Environmental Emergencies and Hazardous Materials*

Frank S. Impicciche, B.A., EMT-P
Emergency Medical Services Instructor, Allied Health Education Center, Methodist Hospital of Indiana, Indianapolis, Indiana
  Chapter 14: *Soft-Tissue and Burn Injuries*
  Chapter 15: *Injuries to the Head, Neck, and Spine*
  Chapter 18: *Musculoskeletal Injuries*
  Chapter 22: *Neurologic Emergencies*

Barbara Bennett Jacobs, B.S.N., M.P.H.
Education Research Consultant, Department of Education, Hartford Hospital, Hartford, Connecticut
Adjunct Faculty, St. Joseph's College School of Nursing, Hartford, Connecticut
Editor, Emergency Care Quarterly
  Chapter 30: *Gynecologic, Obstetric, and Newborn Emergencies*

Shirley A. Jones, M.S. ED., M.H.A., EMT-P
Program Director, Emergency Medical Services Education, Allied Health Education Center, Methodist Hospital of Indiana, Indianapolis, Indiana
  Chapter 8: *Medical Terminology and Human Systems*
  Chapter 11: *Pathophysiology of Shock and Fluid Management*
  Chapter 13: *Kinematics of Trauma*
  Chapter 14: *Soft-Tissue and Burn Injuries*
  Practical Skills

Lindi Kempfer, M.S., NREMT-P, ATC
Emergency Medical Services Instructor, Allied Health Education Center, Methodist Hospital of Indiana, Indianapolis, Indiana
  Chapter 7: *Stress Management*
  Chapter 31: *Behavioral and Psychiatric Emergencies*

Norman E. McSwain, Jr., M.D., F.A.C.S., NREMT-P
Department of Surgery, Tulane University Medical Center, New Orleans, Louisiana
  Chapter 11: *Pathophysiology of Shock and Fluid Management*
  Chapter 13: *Kinematics of Trauma*
  Chapter 14: *Soft-Tissue and Burn Injuries*
  Chapter 15: *Injuries to the Head, Neck, and Spine*
  Chapter 16: *Thoracic Injuries*
  Chapter 17: *Abdominal Trauma*
  Chapter 18: *Musculoskeletal Injuries*

Loren Marshall, B.A., NREMT-P
Clinical Instructor, Oregon Health Sciences University, School of Medicine
Chief of Paramedic Training, Municipality of Anchorage Fire Department, Anchorage, Alaska
  Chapter 27: *Environmental Emergencies and Hazardous Materials*

Ken Miller, M.D., PH.D.
Emergency Medicine Resident, University of California Medical Center—Irvine, Orange, California
  Chapter 25: *Toxicology and Drug and Alcohol Abuse*

Jeffrey T. Mitchell, PH.D.
Clinical Associate Professor of Emergency Health Services, University of Maryland
Vice President, American Critical Incident Stress Foundation, Baltimore, Maryland
  Chapter 7: *Stress Management*
  Chapter 31: *Behavioral and Psychiatric Emergencies*

Jeanne O'Brien, R.N., REMT-P
Education Specialist, Tacoma Fire Department, Tacoma, Washington
  Chapter 14: *Soft-Tissue and Burn Injuries*

Jonathan F. Politis, B.A., EMT-P
Director, Department of Emergency Medical Services, Town of Colonie, Colonie, New York
  Chapter 12: *General Pharmacology*

John A. Rasmussen, PH.D., REMT-P
Department Head of Emergency Medical Technology, Greenville Technical College, Greenville, South Carolina
  Chapter 28: *Geriatric Emergencies*

Carolyn S. Sanders, M.S., MT(ASCP)SM, C.I.C.
Assistant Coordinator, Department of Infection and Environmental Control, The Queens Medical Center, Honolulu, Hawaii
  Chapter 26: *Infectious Diseases*

Audrey Satterblom, M.S., EMT-P
Indianapolis, Indiana
  Practical Skills

Carol Shanaberger, J.D., EMT-P
EMS Liaison and Investigator, State of Colorado Board of Medical Examiners, Denver, Colorado
Member of Legal Affairs Committee, National Association of Emergency Medical Services Physicians
  Chapter 1: *Roles and Responsibilities*
  Chapter 2: *The Emergency Medical Services System*
  Chapter 3: *Medical and Legal Considerations*

Paul Smith, M.S., J.D., EMT
Chief Executive Officer, The Aid Company, Inc., Indianapolis, Indiana
  Chapter 3: *Medical and Legal Considerations*
  Chapter 4: *Emergency Medical Services Communication*

Kay L. Strombeck, B.A., EMT-P
Training Coordinator, State Emergency Management Agency, Indianapolis, Indiana
  Chapter 27: *Environmental Emergencies and Hazardous Materials*

Patricia L. Tritt, B.S., R.N.
Director of Prehospital Services, Swedish Medical Center, Englewood, Colorado
  Chapter 29: *Pediatric Emergencies*
  Chapter 30: *Gynecologic, Obstetric, and Newborn Emergencies*

Linda Van Scoder, ED.D., R.R.T.
Program Director—Cardiopulmonary Sciences, Allied Health Education Center, Methodist Hospital of Indiana, Indianapolis, Indiana
  Chapter 10: *Airway Management and Ventilation*
  Chapter 19: *Respiratory Emergencies*
  Chapter 20: *Cardiovascular Emergencies*

Georgia Wasnetsky, B.S.N., EMT-P
Emergency Medical Services Instructor, Allied Health Education Center, Methodist Hospital of Indiana, Indianapolis, Indiana
- Chapter 12: *General Pharmacology*
- Appendix D: *Emergency Drugs*
- Appendix E: *Common Home Medications*

Katherine H. West, B.S.N., M.S.ED., C.I.C.
Consultant, Infection Control/Emerging Concepts
Springfield, Virginia
- Chapter 26: *Infectious Diseases*

Robert L. Zickler, M.S., EMT
Deputy Chief of Special Operations, Indianapolis Fire Department, Indianapolis, Indiana
- Chapter 5: *Rescue Management*

Foreword

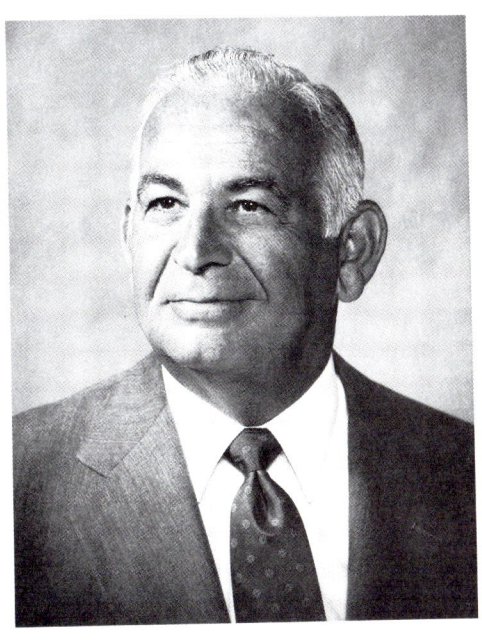

Rocco V. Morando

(Mr. Morando was the executive director of the National Registry of Emergency Medical Technicians from 1971 to 1988.)

The historical evolution of the Emergency Medical Technician–Paramedic (EMT–P) provides the basis upon which the authors have pooled their expertise and resources to develop this text. The concerns of emergency medical service pioneers and the tribulations of all who have sought and fought for quality education of this pre-hospital professional have provided a solid foundation. In 1968, the Committee on Emergency Medical Services of the National Academy of Sciences–National Research Council (NAS–NRC) published recommendations and guidelines for the training of ambulance personnel, listing the fundamentals of basic-level training. Moreover, the report stressed the need for more advanced training, so that measures could be carried out *in the field* that were, at the time, applied only by qualified personnel within the hospital setting.

In 1963 (prior to the NAS–NRC report), Dr. W. Day had developed a method of continuous monitoring and early definitive in-hospital treatment of the high-risk coronary patient. From Dr. Day's activities, it was a short step for Dr. J. F. Pantridge of Belfast, Ireland, to initiate these methods in the field. "Mobile" coronary care became an extension of Dr. Day's original in-hospital procedures. The first physician-directed "Mobile Coronary Care" units in the United States were developed by Dr. William Grace in the late 1960s at St. Vincent's Medical Center in New York City and by Dr. James Warren at the Ohio State University Hospital in Columbus, Ohio. During this same period, Dr. Eugene Nagel and Dr. J. C. Hirschman of Miami, Florida, first experimented with telemetry. It was their idea that direction of ambulance and rescue personnel could be carried out by hospital-based physicians using special communication and telemetry equipment.

During the late 1960s and early 1970s, advanced pre-hospital training programs were, for the most part, customized programs developed in concert with the local ambulance service, the local hospital, and concerned local physicians. Training programs during that period ranged from a minimum of 60 hours to those in excess of 1200 hours; the majority were geared specifically toward mobile coronary care.

The training and operational experience provided by these programs led, in 1970, to the development of guidelines and recommendations by the NAS–NRC subcommittee on ambulance services for a national uniform training program for the "Advanced Emergency Medical Technician." Calling for a minimum of 480 hours' training, the program emphasized the development of greater proficiency in emergency medical skills through advanced study in the basic sciences and management of life-threatening problems, including an understanding of the anatomic and pathophysiologic basis of a disease process and how early treatment can alter that process.

The concept of standardizing an advanced EMT training program was accepted nationally; however, controversy developed concerning topical content and method of administration. The proliferation of training programs continued, with a mixture of provincial assumptions of the "required" clinical skills.

This "home-cooking" led to additional controversy that split the country into two camps: Those advocating only the development of a "mobile coronary care" program, requiring approximately 120 hours of instruction, and those advocating the development of a program that would include advanced skills and knowledge addressing the entire range of traumatic and medical emergencies, not merely coronary care.

To overcome this dichotomy the National Registry of Emergency Medical Technicians (organized in 1970 by the American Medical Association to serve as the national certification agency for pre-hospital personnel) in April of 1974 called a national meeting of physicians and educators involved in the development and administration of existing EMT-Paramedic training programs. Its purpose was to realize a consensus regarding the required level of skill and knowledge and to schedule the development of a modular curriculum outline, including necessary behavioral objectives. The completed material was forwarded to the U.S. Department of Transportation to serve as a guide in the development of the EMT-Paramedic training package. This package included a course guide that outlined the development of other EMT levels, namely the cardiac technician, the trauma technician, the respiratory technician, and the intravenous technician. This facilitated the grouping of select modules for each of the so-called "intermediate" levels. Although the cardiac technician status was implemented in several states, the trauma technician and respiratory technician levels were acknowledged in only a few, and all three levels were short lived. The exception was the recognition and acceptance of an EMT-Intermediate, whose training included the administration of IV fluids, the application of the pneumatic anti-shock garment, and additional procedures for airway maintenance.

The EMT-Paramedic modular curriculum served as the national standard for approximately ten years, resulting in the training of thousands of EMT-Paramedics. With continued advances in teaching methods and in pre-hospital treatment protocols, the curriculum underwent a major revision. Completed in 1985, the revised curriculum was structured into "divisions," with each division being somewhat homogeneous as far as topical content of instruction was concerned.

With the continued advancement of the EMT-Paramedic in skill, knowledge, and occupational identity, it became evident that this practitioner should be recognized by the American Medical Association as an allied health professional. In seeking this recognition and stature for the EMT-Paramedic, the National Registry of Emergency Medical Technicians on January 20, 1975 submitted a brief to the secretary of the Committee on Health Manpower of the AMA, recommending that the position of Emergency Medical Technician-Paramedic be identified as a bona fide emerging health occupation. The brief was accepted by the AMA Council on Medical Education in the fall of 1975. As a result of these actions, subsequent meetings were held, leading to the development of a joint review committee through the AMA Council on Allied Health, Education and Accreditation (CAHEA) and the development of the essential processes for the accreditation of EMT-Paramedic teaching institutions.

This new text, *Advanced Emergency Care for Paramedic Practice*, is indeed a self-contained comprehensive resource for all involved in pre-hospital care, regardless of the level of current or aspired certification. The combined experience and practice of the authors have prescribed this new approach in the development of a text that takes into account the "street sense" of the EMT-P, often overlooked by educators and others involved in training and administration. The effort and concerns of the authors to offer in one volume the latest principles of advanced emergency medical care is commendable.

Utilization of the text by all pre-hospital personnel will prove beneficial not only as a study guide during training, but as an available resource manual to review the skill and knowledge necessary to minimize morbidity and mortality. It is most important that the competence of the pre-hospital provider be evaluated on the basis of observed performance in actual or simulated circumstances, rather than in terms of hours of formal training. This was the premise predicated by the authors in the preparation of this text.

Rocco V. Morando
Executive Director Emeritus
National Registry of Emergency Medical Technicians

Preface

Advanced Emergency Care for Paramedic Practice provides a foundation upon which the general concepts of advanced prehospital emergency care, including knowledge and skills, are built. Care has been taken to adhere strictly to the objectives of the 1985 U.S. Department of Transportation Emergency Medical Technician-Paramedic National Standard Curriculum. Additional updated information has been included to reflect the constantly changing nature of health care. In addressing these changes this text attempts to provide a clear vision of both current and future directions in the field.

Some General Comments

The text is geared to the student in the field of emergency medical services who is working toward a career as an Emergency Medical Technician-Intermediate or Emergency Medical Technician-Paramedic. (Herein, the latter term has been shortened to *paramedic*.) The student will find its content applicable from classroom through clinical experience and later, as a graduate practitioner. Graduates will consider this text a valuable resource tool; the text is also useful for the nursing or medical student taking course work in prehospital emergency care. Chapters on pharmacology and cardiovascular emergencies, which are wide in scope, eliminate the need for supplemental textbooks.

Overall, the authors have taken care to eliminate gender-specific nouns and pronouns whenever possible. It is common knowledge that language shapes thought. What we say and write can limit how we think and behave. This text recognizes the contributions of both men and women in the provision of emergency medical services.

Organization

Advanced Emergency Care for Paramedic Practice is organized into five units that follow the same unit and topic sequence as the U.S. Department of Transportation Emergency Medical Technician-Paramedic National Standard Curriculum.

Describing the prehospital environment, Unit One introduces the reader to the profession of advanced emergency care, the role and responsibilities of the paramedic, medical and legal issues, and other areas pertinent to the field.

Unit Two offers fundamental knowledge in the foundations of emergency care. Individual chapters describe the "tools" the reader will need to function capably (medical terminology . . . patient assessment . . . general pharmacology). Practical skills are emphasized.

A comprehensive study of trauma is provided in Unit Three, including the kinematics of trauma, soft-tissue and burn injuries, trauma to the head, neck, and spine, and detailed discussions of various body systems and how they are affected by trauma.

Unit Four focuses on a wide variety of medical emergencies. Chapters address the anatomy, physiology, and pathophysiology of body systems. Advanced Cardiac Life Support algorithms for life-threatening arrhythmias are included with 59 six-second EKG strips from actual prehospital care patients; each strip is interpreted in detail. A chapter that meets the Occupation Safety and Health Administration's (OSHA) training requirements for both the awareness and operations level hazardous materials courses is also included. The chapter on infectious diseases complies with the Centers for Disease Control guidelines for universal precautions.

The concluding Unit Five presents the foundational skills needed in caring for clients with special needs: the pediatric and geriatric patient; gynecologic, obstetric, and newborn emergencies; behavioral and psychiatric disorders.

Special Features

Special features have been developed to aid the reader. The following deserve note:

CHAPTER OUTLINES. Each chapter begins with a detailed outline of its content, allowing the reader quick reference to its topical sequence.

BEHAVIORAL OBJECTIVES. Following the chapter outline is a comprehensive list of behavioral objectives—the learning goals for the reader of the chapter.

KEY TERMS. These terms are listed at the beginning of each chapter and are defined both in the chapter itself (emphasized in the text with bold face italic type) and in a Glossary of more than 1000 terms.

INSIDE FRONT AND BACK COVERS. Full color hazardous materials charts are displayed inside the front and the back covers.

FULL COLOR PLATES.. Sixteen pages of full-color figures illustrate the anatomy of all body systems.

CHARTS AND ILLUSTRATIONS. Students learn more easily when they *see* what they are learning. This text offers a wide variety of photographs, drawings, tables and charts (more than 700) that give a visual dimension to explanations.

APPENDICES. Five appendices provide important testing and reference material. Included are the National Registry of Emergency Medical Technicians Advanced Level Practical Examinations, performance sheets for evaluation of cardiopulmonary resuscitation and foreign body airway obstruction management, an appendix displaying five trauma scoring systems, information about more than 60 emergency drugs, and an appendix listing over 350 common home medications.

PRACTICAL SKILLS. Twenty-one practical and specialized skills in step-by-step format are accompanied by easy-to-understand explanations and pertinent photographs. For each activity within a skill there is instruction on *how* and *why* it is performed, the rationale being that a student who understands the how's and why's of a routine will remember the skill and perform it safely and correctly.

IMPORTANT SYMBOLS. Three important symbols are shown in the margins of the text to alert the reader to the need for special precautions.

Blood and Body Fluids. 🅑 indicates that universal precautions should be used.

Hazards. 🅗 indicates potential hazards for the paramedic or patient.

Spinal Precautions. 🆂 indicates the need for special spinal precautions.

Supplemental Package

To facilitate mastery of this text's foundation content, a supplementary item has been developed to assist faculty and students.

STUDENT STUDY GUIDE AND EXAMINATION REVIEW MANUAL. A workbook based directly on the text is available. It can be used for review, to measure learned information, and to study for tests. Flash cards are included to assist the student in studying emergency drugs and electrocardiograms.

Our attempt to provide comprehensive coverage of advanced emergency practice is evident in the choice of our 36 contributors. Each is an expert in his or her field and we believe that they have provided a wholly new foundation text—an overview of the principles and practice of advanced emergency care. We hope our readers will find this text refreshing and pertinent to their practice, and that their satisfaction in the field of emergency medical services will be as great and as enduring as ours. The editors welcome the comments, criticisms, and ideas of the reader for the improvement of future editions.

Shirley A. Jones, M.S.Ed., M.H.A., EMT-P
Al Weigel, M.Ed., EMT-P
Roger D. White, M.D., F.A.C.C.
Norman E. McSwain, Jr., M.D., F.A.C.S., NREMT-P
Marti Breiter, R.N., B.S.N., REMT-P

Acknowledgments

Most successful accomplishments in life are in large part the result of the support and assistance received from others. This text is no different. In addition to the numerous emergency medical service professionals who dedicated their time and expertise to develop chapters for *Advanced Emergency Care for Paramedic Practice,* many more offered additional contributions essential to the success of this project. We appreciate that they shared our dream and helped to deliver the comprehensive, state-of-the-art text we envisioned.

We are grateful to the management staff of the J. B. Lippincott Company for its willingness to publish a textbook that attempts to chart new directions. Their support of our ideas was unwavering and unconditional. Our special thanks to Andrew Allen, our creative, rigorous, and sympathetic editor who was an inspiration to us all. In addition to becoming our friend, his constant belief in the project and continued ability to make things happen will always be appreciated. To Diana Intenzo, publisher, for her support and wisdom. To Miriam Benert, editorial assistant, for her close attention to detail and constant encouragement. We appreciate the professional supervision of all text material by Senior Project Editor Lorraine Smith, the painstaking copy editing of Rosina Miller, the exceptional art direction of Doug Smock, the marketing expertise of Emily Barrosse, and the help of the entire team at J. B. Lippincott.

We are grateful to the following: The many skilled reviewers who read the manuscript at all stages and who, through their advice and wisdom, helped us shape this text. The Methodist Hospital of Indiana Allied Health Education department under the direction of Mark Mattes, and Medical Media Productions, directed by Michael McKittrick, for invaluable resources. Joel Ito, for his brilliant artwork throughout the text. Michael McKittrick, photographer, for his committment to excellence in the photographs accompanying the special Skills sections. Doug Biggerstaff, photographer, of Medical Media Productions, for his exceptional cover photographs. Carol Swartz and Bill Bussell, photographers, of Medical Media Productions, for their professional assistance.

Thanks also to J. Lynn Sager for her tireless hours of wordprocessing. To the Pike Township Fire Department of Indianapolis, Indiana. To Emergency Training, a division of Educational Direction, Inc., Akron,

Ohio, for permission to reprint part of Chapter 15 (Injuries to the Head, Neck, and Spine) from McSwain NE, Butman AM, McConnell WK and Vomacka RW: Prehospital Trauma Life Support, 2nd ed. Akron, Emergency Training, 1990.

We are also grateful to Cover models John Berthiaume, Steve Cohen, Jane Mounts, Sue Overstreet, Rachel O'Brien, and Bob Spuhler, and to other models in the text: Brendan Adams, Diane Ciciora, Marsha Davison, John Goll, Anne Healey, Mae Jones, Shirley Jones, David Kelleher, Virginia Kelleher, Dale Lanham, Bill Ludwig, Stephanie Roberts, Eric Rossock, Dudley Taylor, Scott Tilev, and Georgia Wasnetsky.

Indeed, we owe a debt to all our students, past and present, for providing us with the insight and motivation to write this textbook.

Contents

UNIT ONE
The Prehospital Environment 1

1. Roles and Responsibilities — 3
- Professionalism — 4
- Ethics — 4
- Responsibilities of the Paramedic — 6
- Certification — 7
- Licensure — 7
- Reciprocity — 7
- Continuing Education — 8
- National Organizations — 8

2. The Emergency Medical Services System — 9
- Medical Control — 10
- Emergency Medical Services System Components — 12
- Vehicles and Equipment — 13
- Aeromedical Transport — 14
- Personnel — 16
- Citizen Access — 16
- Communications — 17
- Medical Standards — 17
- The Emergency Medical Services System in Operation — 17
- The Emergency Medical Services System in Retrospect — 18

3. Medical and Legal Considerations — 19
- Classifications of Law — 20
- Medical Practices Act — 21
- State Emergency Medical Services Legislation — 21
- Motor Vehicle Laws — 21
- Additional Laws That Affect the Paramedic — 21
- Good Samaritan Law — 22
- Governmental Immunity — 24

xxiii

Privilege	24	
Malpractice Actions	24	
Consent	25	
Patient Refusal	26	
Bases of Liability	26	
Problem Areas for the Paramedic	27	
Insurance and Liability Protection	28	

4. Emergency Medical Services Communication — 29
- Radio Communications — 30
- Emergency Medical Services Communications System Capabilities — 32
- Technological Components — 33
- Emergency Medical Services Communications Operator — 34
- The Emergency Medical Services Incident Sequence — 35
- Radio Technique — 37
- Equipment Maintenance — 38

5. Rescue Management — 41
- Principles of Safety — 42
- Assessment of the Scene — 46
- Gaining Access — 47
- Disentanglement — 48
- Removal — 48
- Emergency Care and Transportation — 49

6. Disaster Management — 51
- Defining Levels of Intensity — 52
- The Disaster Plan — 55

7. Stress Management — 63
- The Stress Process — 64
- Types of Stress Reactions — 65
- Specific Paramedic Stressors — 69
- Coping With Stress — 69
- The Grieving Process in Death and Dying — 71
- Dealing With Death and Dying — 72

UNIT TWO
Foundations of Emergency Care 75

8. Medical Terminology and Human Systems — 77
- Medical Terminology — 78
- Human Systems — 80

Full Color Plates of Human Body Systems

9. Patient Assessment — 89
- Scene Survey — 90
- Scene Control — 92
- Primary Survey — 92
- SKILL 9-1. PATIENT ASSESSMENT — 93
- Secondary Survey — 103
- Trauma Scoring Systems — 119
- Re-evaluation of the Patient — 121
- Communication of Patient Data — 121

10. Airway Management and Ventilation — 125
- Anatomy and Physiology — 126
- Upper Airway Obstructions — 128
- Assessment of the Airway — 129
- Management of Airway Disorders — 131
- SKILL 10-1. ENDOTRACHEAL INTUBATION, ORAL — 143
- SKILL 10-2. ENDOTRACHEAL INTUBATION, NASAL — 150
- SKILL 10-3. PHARYNGEO-TRACHEAL LUMEN AIRWAY — 156
- SKILL 10-4. ESOPHAGEAL OBTURATOR AIRWAY AND ESOPHAGEAL GASTRIC TUBE AIRWAY — 161
- SKILL 10-5. SURGICAL CRICOTHYROIDOTOMY — 165
- SKILL 10-6. TRANSLARYNGEAL JET VENTILATION — 170

11. Pathophysiology of Shock and Fluid Management — 175
- Pathophysiology of Shock — 177
- Stages of Shock — 191
- Assessment of the Patient in Shock — 193
- Management — 195
- SKILL 11-1. PNEUMATIC ANTI-SHOCK GARMENT — 197

12. General Pharmacology — 205
- General Drug Information — 207
- Drug Sources and Legislation — 207
- Drug Names — 208
- Drug References and Resources — 209
- Forms of Drugs — 209

Drug Pharmacokinetics	209	SKILL 12-6. CENTRAL LINE PLACEMENT (INTERNAL JUGULAR, ANTERIOR APPROACH)	242
Drug Pharmacodynamics	215		
Calculating Drug Dosages	219		
Drug Administration	222	SKILL 12-7. CENTRAL LINE PLACEMENT (INTERNAL JUGULAR, MIDDLE APPROACH)	245
SKILL 12-1. INTRADERMAL INJECTION	225		
SKILL 12-2. SUBCUTANEOUS INJECTION	228	SKILL 12-8. CENTRAL LINE PLACEMENT (INTERNAL JUGULAR, POSTERIOR APPROACH)	248
SKILL 12-3. INTRAMUSCULAR INJECTION	231	SKILL 12-9. CENTRAL LINE PLACEMENT (SUBCLAVIAN APPROACH)	252
SKILL 12-4. PERIPHERAL VENIPUNCTURE	235	SKILL 12-10. INTRAOSSEOUS INFUSION	256
SKILL 12-5. CENTRAL LINE PLACEMENT (FEMORAL)	239		

UNIT THREE
Trauma 261

13. Kinematics of Trauma	263	Injuries That Cause Inadequate Ventilation	327
Physics	264	SKILL 16-1. THORACENTESIS	333
Penetrating Trauma	268	Injuries That Cause Inadequate Cardiac Output	336
Blunt Trauma	273	SKILL 16-2. PERICARDIOCENTESIS	337
14. Soft-Tissue and Burn Injuries	285		
Anatomy and Physiology of the Skin	286		
Soft-Tissue Injuries	287	17. Abdominal Trauma	341
Burn Injuries	292	Mechanisms of Abdominal Trauma	342
		Complications of Abdominal Trauma	342
15. Injuries to the Head, Neck, and Spine	303	Specific Intra-abdominal Injuries	343
Injuries to the Head	304	18. Musculoskeletal Injuries	349
Soft-Tissue Injuries to the Neck	318	Anatomy and Physiology of the Muscular System	350
Injuries to the Spine	319		
16. Thoracic Injuries	325	Anatomy and Physiology of the Skeletal System	355
Assessment of Thoracic Injuries	326	Injuries to Muscle	365
Pathophysiology of Thoracic Injuries	327	Injuries to Bone	366

UNIT FOUR
Medical Emergencies 375

19. Respiratory Emergencies	377	Patient Assessment for Cardiac-Related Problems	416
Anatomy and Physiology of the Respiratory System	378	Cardiovascular Disease States: Recognition and Management	418
Assessment of the Patient in Respiratory Distress	385	Other Acquired and Congenital Diseases of the Cardiovascular System	426
Respiratory Disorders	393		
20. Cardiovascular Emergencies	405	Prehospital Interventions for Specific Cardiac Conditions	430
Anatomy and Physiology of the Cardiovascular System	407	Arrhythmias: Interpretation and Therapeutic Intervention	434

SKILL 20-1. DEFIBRILLATION AND SYNCHRONIZED CARDIOVERSION	514	

21. Endocrine Emergencies — 521
- Anatomy and Physiology of the Endocrine System — 522
- Assessment of Endocrine Emergencies — 529
- Diabetic Emergencies — 530

22. Neurologic Emergencies — 535
- Anatomy and Physiology of the Nervous System — 536
- Assessment of Nervous System Emergencies — 548
- Types of Nervous System Emergencies — 550

23. Gastrointestinal, Urinary, and Reproductive System Emergencies — 557
- Anatomy and Physiology of the Gastrointestinal System — 558
- Anatomy and Physiology of the Abdomen — 560
- Anatomy and Physiology of the Urinary System — 561
- Anatomy and Physiology of the Reproductive Systems — 562
- The Acute Abdomen — 563
- Pathophysiology of the Urinary System — 566
- Pathophysiology of Reproductive System Disorders — 568

24. Allergic and Anaphylactic Reactions — 571
- Concepts and Terminology — 572
- Common Allergens — 573
- Pathophysiology — 574
- Assessment of the Anaphylactic Patient — 575
- Management of Allergic and Anaphylactic Reactions — 576
- Prevention and Patient Education — 577

25. Toxicology and Drug and Alcohol Abuse — 579
- Poisoning and Overdose — 580
- Drug Abuse Emergencies — 593
- Alcoholism — 598

26. Infectious Diseases — 601
- Immune System — 602
- Communicable Diseases of Adults and Children — 603
- Techniques of Management — 611

27. Environmental Emergencies and Hazardous Materials — 617
- Thermoregulation — 619
- Disruptions of Thermoregulation — 622
- Water Emergencies — 627
- Hazardous Materials — 633

UNIT FIVE
Caring for Patients With Special Needs — 647

28. Geriatric Emergencies — 649
- Anatomy and Physiology of the Aging Process — 651
- Assessment of the Geriatric Patient — 653
- Respiratory Emergencies — 655
- Cardiovascular Emergencies — 656
- Neurologic Emergencies — 658
- Psychiatric Disorders in the Elderly — 659
- Musculoskeletal Problems — 660
- Gastrointestinal Emergencies — 660
- Trauma in the Elderly — 662
- Pharmacology in Geriatrics — 663
- Environmental Emergencies — 663
- Geriatric Abuse — 664

29. Pediatric Emergencies — 667
- Approach to the Pediatric Patient — 668
- Developmental Stages — 671
- Common Pediatric Problems — 672
- Problems Specific to the Pediatric Patient — 673
- Techniques of Management — 684

30. Gynecologic, Obstetric, and Newborn Emergencies — 689
- Anatomy and Physiology of the Female Reproductive System — 690
- Ovulation and the Menstrual Cycle — 692
- Pregnancy and Fetal Growth — 694

Assessment of the Gynecologic and Obstetric Patient	696
Gynecologic Emergencies	698
Complications of Pregnancy	700
Labor and Delivery	704
Care of the Newborn	714

31. Behavioral and Psychiatric Emergencies — 719

Misconceptions	720
Forms of Emotional Disorders	721
Characteristics of Emotional Disorders	722
Assessment of Behavioral Emergencies	723
Other Factors Associated With Behavioral Emergencies	726
Principles of Crisis Intervention	728

Appendices

APPENDIX A: The National Registry of Emergency Medical Technicians Advanced Level Practical Examinations	733
APPENDIX B: Performance Sheets for Cardiopulmonary Resuscitation and Foreign Body Airway Obstruction Management—American Heart Association	748
APPENDIX C: Trauma Scores	762
APPENDIX D: Emergency Drugs	765
APPENDIX E: Common Home Medications	829

Glossary — 841

Index — 861

UNIT ONE

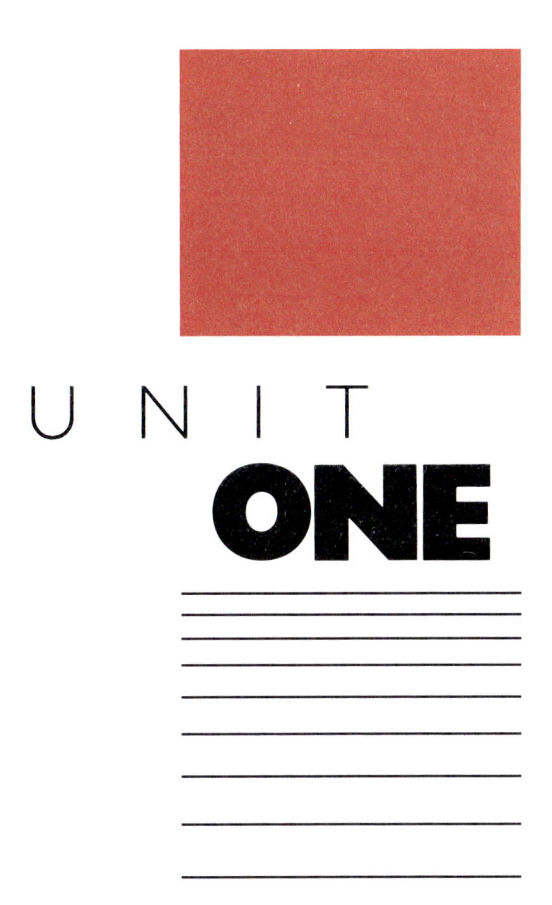

The Prehospital Environment

CHAPTER 1

Roles and Responsibilities

Professionalism
Ethics
Responsibilities of the Paramedic
    Assessment at the Scene
    Emergency Management
    Emergency Transport
    Record Keeping
    Equipment Maintenance
    Vehicle Maintenance
Certification
Licensure
Reciprocity
Continuing Education
National Organizations
Summary

BEHAVIORAL OBJECTIVES

On successful completion of this chapter, the reader will be able to:

1. Define professionalism and discuss its importance in the development of the modern emergency medical services system
2. Explain the concept of ethics
3. Identify and define six specific responsibilities of a paramedic
4. State the importance of the patient report form and what information is required for documentation
5. Differentiate between certification and licensure
6. Explain the importance of continuing education
7. List four national organizations in which paramedics may participate to benefit their profession
8. Define all of the key terms listed in this chapter

KEY TERMS

The following terms are defined in the chapter and glossary:

certification
code of ethics
continuing education
ethics
licensure
profession
professionalism
reciprocity
run report

Emergency medical services (EMS) is a well-organized system with identifiable purposes and functions that are performed by specially trained personnel. The paramedic is one of several providers of prehospital emergency care and is increasingly recognized as an accomplished contributor to EMS. The role of the *paramedic* is quite different from that of the "ambulance driver" of yesterday, and the personal fulfillment can be challenging and rewarding.

As a professional, the paramedic is affiliated with medical technologists, physical therapists, and occupational therapists, to name a few, in the allied health field. With the expansion and specialization of medicine and health care, the paramedic fills a unique role in the health care arena.

PROFESSIONALISM

A ***profession*** is characterized by the existence of a specialized body of knowledge or expertise. Additionally, a profession generally is self-regulating, through licensure or certification, educational requirements, and continued education and training to maintain competency. ***Professionalism*** denotes a position in which *integrity* and *diligence* are assumed in the fulfillment of its responsibilities. These principles of professionalism are as applicable to the allied health professionals as they are to physicians.

The paramedic, as an allied health professional, is a person with specialized training and education in prehospital emergency care. The patient's well-being is a primary responsibility, and all injuries and illnesses are managed according to the interests and needs of the patient.

Implied in the concept of professional conduct is the fact that the interests and needs of the patient form the basis of any decision or task. Personal gain or motivation is contrary to the idea of professionalism in any field. While medicine in some respects has become an economic undertaking, professionalism demands that the patient's needs remain separate and uncompromised by the paramedic. The performance of the professional cannot be affected or deterred by personal dislike of the patient or disdain for the actions of the patient. For example, the drunk driver who causes a motor vehicle accident may be unpopular to society, but the paramedic cannot allow personal judgment or anger to interfere with the patient's medical treatment. Thus, the term professional is more than just a label; it implies day-to-day methods of decision making and performance.

ETHICS

The role of the professional is complex; it involves serving the medical interests and needs of patients in a society of multiple values and customs. Many professional groups rely on the concept of ethics as a source of guidance. ***Ethics*** are a system of principles that identify conduct deemed morally desirable. Similarly, *medical ethics* for the paramedic refer to the ideal conduct in the relationship of the paramedic to the patient, as well as to the other paramedics and to the public. A code of ethics for the paramedic has

CODE OF ETHICS OF THE NATIONAL ASSOCIATION OF EMTS

Professional status as an Emergency Medical Technician and Emergency Medical Technician–Paramedic is maintained and enriched by the willingness of the individual practitioner to accept and fulfill obligations to society, other medical professionals, and the profession of Emergency Medical Technician. As an Emergency Medical Technician at the basic level or an Emergency Medical Technician–Paramedic, I solemnly pledge myself to the following code of ethics.

A fundamental responsibility of the Emergency Medical Technician is to conserve life, to alleviate suffering, to promote health, to do no harm, and to encourage the quality and equal availability of emergency medical care. The Emergency Medical Technician provides services based on human need with respect for human dignity, unrestricted by considerations of nationality, race, creed, color, or status.

The Emergency Medical Technician does not use professional knowledge and skills in any enterprise detrimental to the public well-being.

The Emergency Medical Technician respects and holds in confidence all information of a confidential nature obtained in the course of professional work unless required by law to divulge such information.

The Emergency Medical Technician, as a citizen, understands and upholds the law and performs the duties of citizenship. As a professional, the Emergency Medical Technician has the never-ending responsibility to work with concerned citizens and other health care professionals in promoting a high standard of emergency medical care to all people.

The Emergency Medical Technician assumes responsibility for individual professional actions and judgment, both in dependent and independent emergency functions, and knows and upholds the laws that affect the practice of the Emergency Medical Technician.

An Emergency Medical Technician has the responsibility to be aware of and participate in matters of legislation affecting the Emergency Medical Technician and the Emergency Medical Services System.

The Emergency Medical Technician adheres to standards of personal ethics that reflect credit upon the profession.

Emergency Medical Technicians, or groups of Emergency Medical Technicians, who advertise professional services do so in conformity with the dignity of the profession.

The Emergency Medical Technician has an obligation to protect the public by not delegating to a person, less qualified, any service that requires the professional competence of an Emergency Medical Technician. The Emergency Medical Technician will work harmoniously with, and sustain confidence in, Emergency Medical Technician associates, the nurse, the physician, and other members of the emergency medical services health care team.

The Emergency Medical Technician refuses to participate in unethical procedures, and assumes the responsibility to expose incompetence or unethical conduct of others to the appropriate authority in a proper and professional manner.

---

come from various entities. The National Association of Emergency Medical Technicians has established a code of ethics shown in the box "Code of Ethics of the National Association of EMTs." The **code of ethics** exemplifies the ethical considerations and guidelines of the paramedic. While a code is not enforceable as a law, it is a persuasive example for uniformity and expectation of members of the profession.

Ethical decisions need to be made more and more frequently in all aspects of medicine. Changing values in both the patient's interest in autonomy and the professional's role in providing treatment have caused this increased need. Conflicts often arise between what the patient wants and what society has valued. As a result, the paramedic, like other medical professionals, is more often faced with conflicts that inevitably confront personal, professional, and societal values.

The paramedic may find that the patient's preferences are not the same as the paramedic's desire to provide care that is arguably beneficial to the patient's well-being. The simple yet common problem of the patient who is ill and in need of treatment but who wants to be left alone poses ethical questions for the paramedic to resolve. For example, decisions about life support treatment, which can include the concepts "*do not resuscitate*" and "*death with dignity,*" are filled with ethical and legal dilemmas that have challenged physicians for years, and they now challenge the paramedic. Because the "*right thing to do*" is subject to different interpretation by values and laws, the paramedic may have to struggle so that a personal belief or the pleading of a family member or bystander does not compromise professional responsibilities.

Another aspect of ethical conduct is of a more personal nature. The paramedic will be confronted with negative outcomes or management errors. As a professional, the necessity to disclose such events is an ethical concern that the paramedic must address. The primary objective must always be the patient's welfare and not the possible reprimand for committing an error. The paramedic, as a professional, must always act according to the interests of the patient.

RESPONSIBILITIES OF THE PARAMEDIC

An established paramedic training curriculum was distributed on January 1, 1977 by the United States Department of Transportation. Paramedics had been functioning previously, but structure was minimal and the concept of a system not yet a reality. Today, with extensive training, testing, and physician direction, the tasks performed by the paramedic are many and multifaceted. Patient care is only one aspect in the role of the paramedic.

Assessment at the Scene

The paramedic is responsible for assessing an emergency scene to ensure the *safety* and *well-being* of the patient, manage the medical and associated emotional needs of the patient, perform extrication, or be able to coordinate the efforts of extrication. The paramedic also acts in concert with other agencies such as fire, police, or hazardous materials teams. The actual transportation of the patient may require interfacing with ground and air transport units, which the paramedic must activate at a suitable time.

The paramedic's ability to communicate with the patient is as important as the communication that takes place with family, bystanders, and other professionals involved in the EMS system. The paramedic must be aware of the patient's perception and understanding of a medical problem and must be able to gather information from patients who are frightened, hostile, or insulting. Without skills in communication, management may be inadvertently denied or misapplied. Called the "*eyes and ears of the physician*," the paramedic's communication with the receiving hospital is vital for the smooth progression of the patient through the EMS system.

Emergency Management

The ability to recognize what emergency management is and under what circumstances it is to be initiated is the essence of the professional judgment required by the paramedic. Although guidelines established by physicians provide the substance of emergency care to be provided, the paramedic must be able to assess and interpret the needs of the patient before care is rendered. Whether confronted with a cardiac emergency or a psychiatric crisis, the paramedic must be able to weigh multiple factors, such as transport time, patient stability, potential side effects and complications of care, and limitations of managing the patient in a moving ambulance. Contributing to the complexity of decisions are such distractions as hysterical family members, police directives, and language barriers. The paramedic must be able to coordinate a multitude of on-going events while rendering patient care.

Emergency Transport

On accepting a patient for transport, the paramedic accepts a wide variety of responsibilities. The patient becomes dependent on the paramedic's capabilities. Patient transport, a seemingly simple task, requires consideration of the medical specialization and of the particular needs of a patient (*e.g.*, hyperbaric chamber, burn unit, or neonatal care). In addition, with the expansion of aeromedical transport, the paramedic must also consider the mode of transportation required while assessing the patient's needs.

The use of interhospital transfers in EMS, whether emergent or nonemergent, has increased. Prescheduled transport does not relieve the paramedic of the responsibility for patient care. "*Routine*" transports have become emergent en route, and the paramedic must be prepared to deal with such untoward events.

Record Keeping

Documentation is as important a responsibility in patient care as any other skill. The patient **run report** is an integral part of the patient's medical history and management and also serves as a legal document. Documentation of the paramedic's management of the patient can affect subsequent care provided by other health care professionals. In addition, the patient run report is a resource for determining the quality of the performance of the paramedic and for court testimony. Increasingly, the paramedic is being subpoenaed to court to testify about observations at a scene, statements of witnesses, and the condition of a patient. The patient run report is factual; thus, the report should be accurate, understandable, objective, and complete. Many states or regions collect data from the patient run report. The information is compiled and used in annual reports and in studies of performance, patient populations, services, or future funding applications.

There are many styles and methods of writing a report. Regardless of individual technique, the document must be *comprehensive* and *legible* to fulfill its designed purpose, which is communication of pertinent patient information. The document should serve as a complete testimonial of the condition of the patient, emergency management, and the results of the interaction between the patient and paramedic.

The minimum amount of information required for documentation may be delineated by state regulations; however, the document should include at least the following:

- Basic identification information of the patient (*e.g.,* name, age, address or location of patient contact), EMS personnel, and level of certification and service
- Times of events (*e.g.,* responses, management technique, changes in patient condition)
- Specific emergency management techniques rendered
- Events that may have affected patient care or outcome (*e.g.,* extrication problems or combativeness)
- The reason for and effects of emergency management techniques rendered (*e.g.,* oxygen for shortness of breath or improvement of sensation after splinting)
- Reference to supporting evidence (*e.g.,* electrocardiogram (EKG) strips, glucose sticks, blood drawn)
- Observations (not subjective conclusions) of the patient's condition (*e.g.,* patient's speech was slurred, rather than "drunk"; patient unresponsive to loud verbal stimuli, rather than "lethargic")

As a *legal document,* the patient run report should be completed as soon after the event as possible. The longer the delay in writing the report, the more questionable the document's reliability, because the passage of time reduces recall of events and details. In addition, a court may conclude that if it wasn't written down, it didn't happen. Any paramedic will have trouble remembering events not in the report and even more trouble convincing a jury that pertinent events not recorded did occur.

Equipment Maintenance

The paramedic is also responsible for maintaining the equipment and supplies required in the performance of the job. The EKG monitor batteries, oxygen tubing, and syringes are as important as drug dosages, EKG interpretation, and patient history in fulfilling the role of the paramedic.

Vehicle Maintenance

The ambulance vehicle must be maintained on a regular basis. Given the type and amount of use demanded of an emergency vehicle, the paramedic must note wear and tear and potential servicing that the vehicle needs to remain operable in a *safe* and *efficient* manner. Instances of faulty equipment are almost indefensible if the defect was discoverable by a daily check. The condition and availability of the equipment (*e.g.,* tires, lights, brakes, oxygen, suction) are the responsibility of the paramedic through regular, if not daily, servicing and maintenance.

CERTIFICATION

Graduation from a training program is only the first step in the qualification of the health care professional. Usually, at the state level, a certificate is granted to a paramedic by a governmental agency after the fulfillment of prerequisites (*e.g.,* completion of training from an approved program, successful testing in Advanced Cardiac Life Support, certification by the National Registry of Emergency Medical Technicians, possession of a valid driver's license). **Certification** grants authority to an individual who has met predetermined qualifications to participate in an activity; both governmental and nongovernmental agencies or associations regulate certifications. For example, a certificate in Advanced Cardiac Life Support denotes qualification and specialized training and is granted by a national association (*e.g.,* American Heart Association). However, the certificate issued by the government denotes qualification and authority to engage in specified aspects of medical care. Thus, the certificate is an indication of competency and entitles the person to function as a paramedic, but only according to the conditions of the certification.

LICENSURE

A similar process of occupational regulation is **licensure,** in which a governmental agency, such as the State Medical Board, grants permission to an individual who meets the established qualifications to engage in the profession or occupation. Without the license, the individual is prohibited from engaging in the occupational activity. A licensed occupation is usually subject to a "*scope of practice*" that is deemed necessary to protect the public health, safety, and welfare. The state regulates the licensee through mandated training, practice standards, and registration as it deems necessary to protect the public from incompetency.

RECIPROCITY

Some states recognize other states' certification or licensure by **reciprocity**. They may also recognize the National Registry of Emergency Medical Technicians for reciprocity. If the training program and continued education requirements for maintaining certification or licensure are similar from one state to another, a state can, through reciprocity, accept the certification or licensure as qualifying for certification or licensure in that state. The paramedic, thereby, is able to move to other areas without complete retraining. The state may still have requirements such as proof of training or experience, current Advanced Cardiac Life Support certification, and a driver's license. Standardization of curriculums and qualifications has helped agencies and states offer reciprocity to paramedics, allowing them to be more mobile, vertically and horizontally, in society.

CONTINUING EDUCATION

On acquiring the *authority to act*, the paramedic must continually and actively strive to maintain competency in skills and knowledge to assure proper patient care. **Continuing education** is recognized as essential by all states because of the ever-changing body of knowledge in medicine and the problems of skill deterioration. The *quality* of patient care is dependent on continued practice and study. As a result, postgraduate training is required; the number of hours of training, however, varies considerably from state to state.

NATIONAL ORGANIZATIONS

As EMS has solidified and standardized, many national associations have developed for prehospital care providers, such as the National Association of Emergency Medical Technicians (NAEMT), and for other related areas of prehospital care, such as the American Society of Hospital Based Emergency Air Medical Services (ASHBEAMS), the American Ambulance Association, and the National Council of Instructors and Coordinators. The National Registry of Emergency Medical Technicians (NREMT) promotes a national standard in prehospital EMS certification. Those certified by the NREMT must meet entry requirements, pass a written and practical examination, and present, on a biannual basis, refresher and continuing education documentation. Many states recognize certification through the NREMT as qualifying for state certification.

The collective efforts of a national EMS organization provide several important contributions to the profession as a whole and to the individual paramedic. The organization can provide a clearinghouse of information, resource experts, program accreditation, and national representation in other health care organizations. It can encourage national standardization and reciprocity in training and testing, sponsor continuing education programs, and promote the professional status of the paramedic. There are also state, regional, and local levels of similar EMS organizations for the active paramedic to join.

As emergency medicine has become recognized as a medical specialty, research and publications in emergency medical care have proliferated. Prehospital care has benefited from the knowledge, expertise, and advances in this specialty. The many professional journals, research projects, and national organizations of physicians devoted to quality emergency medical care are invaluable resources for the paramedic. They provide information on continuing education and awareness of current trends and advancements. Also, EMS journals offer a means for the paramedic to publish and contribute to the national growth of the profession.

The paramedic is encouraged to teach courses, such as cardiopulmonary resuscitation, at schools or for civic groups and to become actively involved in educating the public about EMS. The paramedic's ability to act as a resource or liaison is essential to the growth of EMS and to the recognition of the paramedic as a professional.

SUMMARY

The role of the paramedic has evolved into a complex occupation that combines elements of medicine with interpersonal and communicative skills. As a professional, the paramedic interacts in many situations with a vast number of people. Paramedics in the modern EMS system must study, retrain, and continually practice to remain capable of rendering quality care to the patient in need of their services.

SUGGESTED READING

Ampolsk AG: Paramedics, EMTs push for licensing. J Emerg Med Serv 22(4):48, 1990

Beauchamp TL, Childress JF: Principles of Biomedical Ethics, 3rd ed. New York, Oxford University Press, 1989

Chapman CB: Physicians, Law & Ethics. New York, New York University Press, 1984

Childs BJ, Ptacnik DJ: Emergency Ambulance Driving. Englewood Cliffs, Prentice-Hall, 1986

Cotton SL: Mosby's Paramedic Study Guide: Certification, Preparation, and Review. St. Louis, CV Mosby, 1989

Eisenberg MS, MacDonald SC: The Paramedic Manual, 2nd ed. Philadelphia, WB Saunders, 1987

Greenwald J: The Paramedic Manual. Englewood, CO, Morton, 1988

US Department of Transportation, National Highway Traffic Safety Administration: Emergency Medical Technician—Paramedic: National Standards Curriculum. Washington, DC, US Government Printing Office, 1985

Veatch, RM: A Theory of Medical Ethics. New York, Basic Books, 1984

CHAPTER 2

The Emergency Medical Services System

Medical Control
   Medical Director
   Protocols
   Standing Orders
   Off-line Medical Control
   On-line Medical Control
Emergency Medical Services System Components
   Manpower
   Training
   Transportation
   Disaster Linkage and Mutual Aid Agreements
   Communications
   Facilities/Critical Care Units
   Public Safety Agencies
   Transfer of Patients
   Access to Care
   Coordinated Medical Record Keeping
   Consumer Information and Education
   Evaluation
   Systems Management
Vehicles and Equipment
Aeromedical Transport
   Application of Aeromedical Service
   Indications for Use
   Establishing a Landing Zone
   Helicopter Safety
Personnel
Citizen Access
Communications
Medical Standards
Hospital Care
The Emergency Medical Services System in Operation
The Emergency Medical Services System in Retrospect
Summary

BEHAVIORAL OBJECTIVES

On successful completion of this chapter, the reader will be able to:

1. Describe the role of medical control in emergency medical services
2. Describe the role of the medical director in an advanced life support system
3. Differentiate between protocols and standing orders
4. Explain the difference between on-line and off-line medical control
5. Discuss citizen access to emergency medical care
6. Describe the various methods of communication between the paramedic and physician from the scene of an emergency
7. Explain the components of an emergency medical services system and their importance to the daily operations of the advanced life support system
8. Discuss indications for aeromedical transport
9. Describe how to establish a landing zone and helicopter safety
10. Define the national standard levels of prehospital training
11. Review the importance of paramedic continuing education
12. Explain run reviews and their importance to prehospital care
13. Define all of the key terms listed in this chapter

> **KEY TERMS**
> *The following terms are defined in the chapter and glossary:*
>
> aeromedical transport
> duplex system
> EMT-Ambulance
>   (EMT-A)
> EMT-Intermediate
>   (EMT-I)
> EMT-Paramedic
>   (EMT-P)
> KKK standards
> medical control
>   (medical direction)
> off-line medical
>   control
> on-line medical
>   control
> protocols
> run reviews
> simplex system
> standing orders
> 911

Citizen participation in emergency medical care historically has been confined to the most basic care of the injured person. Control of hemorrhage, cardiopulmonary resuscitation, and keeping the patient immobile before the arrival of health care providers were limited but helpful efforts of citizens. The need for rapid, systematic intervention by medically trained personnel to care for the ill and injured patient was recognized by the medical community and federal government in the 1960s. In 1966, a report entitled "Accidental Death and Disability: The Neglected Disease of Modern Society" declared the need and framework for emergency medical services (EMS) systems in the United States.

The *Highway Safety Act of 1966*, in addition to requiring standards for highway safety, established standards for EMS to be used throughout the United States. The system of EMS, however, evolved slowly and unevenly, with funding from the federal level for many years. In the mid-1960s, the first paramedics to render patient care were working in Miami, Florida. Through the pioneering efforts of Dr. Eugene Nagel and many other physicians who saw the benefit of prehospital emergency medical care, EMS became a reality.

The EMS system has progressed in its capabilities, purposes, and goals, and the prehospital emergency care system is now the combined effort of many entities and individuals. Communication, transportation, training programs, hospitals, public safety agencies, consumers, and medical personnel at many levels all unite to form a network of manpower, protocols, and capabilities that provide a high quality of care for the citizens of the United States.

Research has confirmed that major trauma responds best from early transportation to the hospital and immediate medical intervention and surgery. The *rapid* and *safe* transport of major trauma victims, with resuscitative measures begun en route is a major contributing role of EMS in health care today. The EMS system also serves a unique health care function for medical conditions such as cardiac, diabetic, and seizure disorders. In many cases, early medical stabilization by trained personnel who work under medical direction and according to specific guidelines and protocols before transport is advantageous to the patient's welfare (Fig. 2-1). The paramedic must have the ability to recognize the needs of the medical and trauma patient and use the system accordingly. By doing so, patient survival increases, while complications and disability decrease.

MEDICAL CONTROL

The concept of medical control is essential to the success of an advanced life support system.

Medical Director

Medical control (medical direction) refers to the physicians' roles and responsibilities in supervising and monitoring all medical aspects of the EMS system, such as ensuring that protocols are medically sound, management and triage decisions are properly made, and medication and treatment are rendered according to

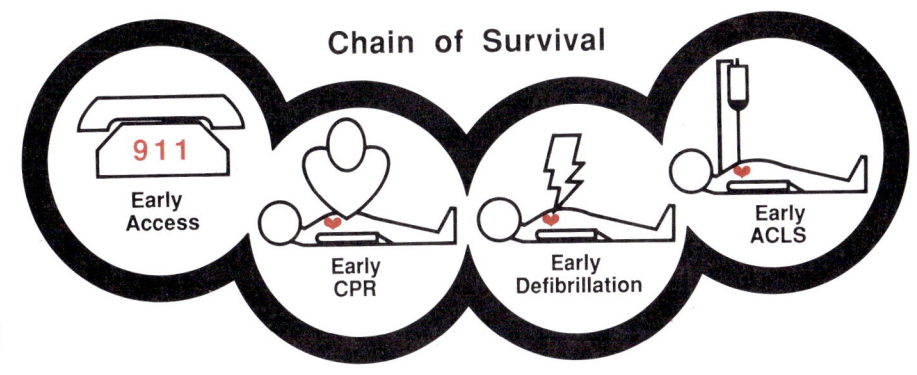

FIGURE 2–1.
Chain of survival. (Courtesy of Laerdal Medical, Armonk, New York)

protocols. Each state's regulations vary on the specific requirements and obligations; generally, however, a physician who becomes a medical director or physician advisor accepts the task of medical direction and, thereby, has the final responsibility for the quality of medical care in the prehospital EMS setting. Through protocols and standing orders, the paramedic serves as an active participant in patient care, rather than merely a transporting unit.

Protocols

Protocols are guidelines for the management of many types of medical conditions. They provide a framework for the paramedic to assess and manage the patient in the field. Protocols provide predictability and organization to the evaluation and management of these patients. *Local protocols* are based on accepted medical practice, the capabilities of the paramedics, and the needs of a given EMS system.

Standing Orders

Standing orders are authorizations for specific protocols to be initiated before or without direct voice contact with the medical control physician. Generally, standing orders are limited to treatment modalities to be performed in life-threatening situations, in which the time to contact medical control would jeopardize patient care.

Off-line Medical Control

Medical control is generally divisible into "on-line" and "off-line" supervision. ***Off-line medical control*** refers to the administrative components of medical control, including protocols and standing orders. The medical director ultimately is responsible for the total advanced life support system design and implementation, approval of participating paramedics, selection of participating physicians, content of the training curriculum, run reviews of advanced life support performance, remedial training, and continuing education for the paramedics. Off-line medical control provides the framework, standards, and protocols for the operation of the advanced life support system. Through interdisciplinary contacts with public safety and governmental agencies, medical societies, citizen groups, and health care institutions, off-line medical control serves a broad role in the total advanced life support system operation.

On-line Medical Control

On-line medical control refers to the supervision of patient care provided by the paramedic at the scene and en route to the hospital via voice communication between the paramedic and emergency physician. The emergency department staff and other designated physicians at the base hospital provide this type of medical direction. The day-to-day operations of the EMS system and personnel are monitored by the on-line medical control physician. Any on-line medical control problems encountered by hospital or prehospital emergency personnel are documented and referred to the medical director of the advanced life support system.

The paramedic is accountable to and under the direct supervision of the on-line medical control physician. This relationship is particularly important in situations in which the paramedic and another physician meet at the scene of an emergency. The paramedic may not interfere with the patient-physician relationship when a physician is attending a patient without permission of the patient or the physician. Because paramedics can only act on the authority of the on-line medical control physician or designated staff, they cannot follow orders from the attending physician that conflict with the paramedic's protocols and standing orders, unless such deviation is approved by the on-line medical control physician. If the physician at a scene attempts to interfere with the care provided at the scene by the paramedic, the on-line medical control physician should be contacted to resolve the conflict.

The paramedic should consider medical control as a valuable resource, not a guardian. The role of the paramedic is not independent or autonomous. The paramedic must work within the total system of medical control to be effective. Advanced life support care in the prehospital setting was founded on the premise of direct involvement and supervision by medical control. The role of the paramedic is no less dependent on its involvement today.

EMERGENCY MEDICAL SERVICES SYSTEM COMPONENTS

The EMS system has been defined by the federal government's Department of Health and Human Services (in the early federal EMS legislation) as: "*A system that provides for the arrangement of personnel, facilities and equipment for the effective and coordinated delivery of health care services in an appropriate geographical area under emergency conditions.*" The following sections discuss the components necessary for the development of a comprehensive EMS system (Fig. 2-2).

Manpower

This component concerns the adequate number of health professionals, allied health professionals, and other personnel with appropriate training and experience to provide EMS 24 hours a day, 7 days a week. This category includes police and fire first responders, ambulance personnel, dispatchers, and hospital emergency personnel.

Training

Training for emergency personnel must be available for initial certification and continuing education as well. The cost to each student must be kept at a reasonable amount, and the training programs must be coordinated throughout the system.

Transportation

This component concerns the adequate number and proper distribution of appropriately equipped emergency vehicles to meet the needs of the area. State and local EMS plans usually identify the minimum response times that must be met in urban and rural areas for evaluation of this component to be completed.

COMPONENT	OPERATIONAL UNIT
• Manpower • Training • Transportation • Mutual aid	INITIAL OPERATIONS
• Communications • Facilities • Critical care units • Public-safety agencies • Transfer of patients • Disaster linkage	SUPPORT SERVICES
• Consumer participation • Accessibility to care • Coordinated record keeping • Consumer information/education • Evaluation	SYSTEM EVALUATION
• System management	SYSTEM MANAGEMENT

→ EMERGENCY MEDICAL SERVICES DELIVERY SYSTEM → OUTCOME: IMPROVED EMERGENCY PATIENT CARE

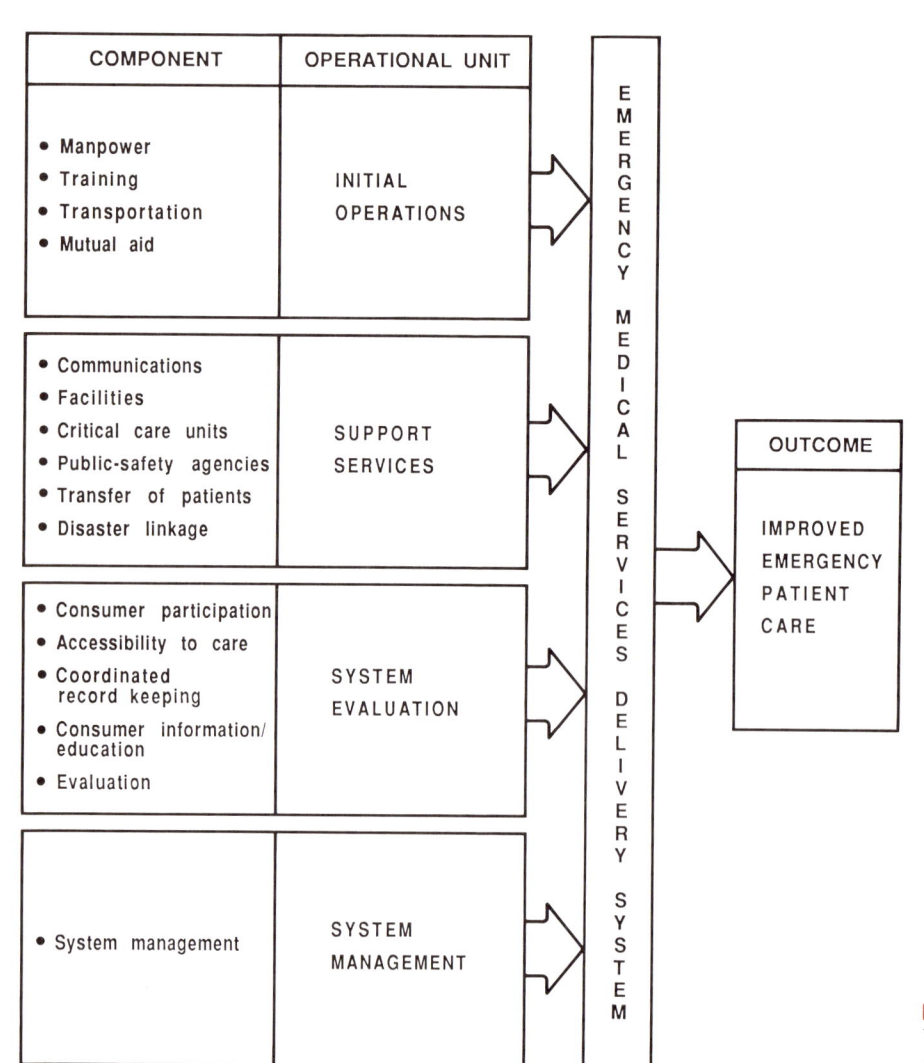

FIGURE 2–2.
The emergency medical services system concept.

Disaster Linkage and Mutual Aid Agreements

Anytime the demand for EMS exceeds the available resources to meet that demand, EMS providers and public safety agencies need to coordinate response and resources. Mutual aid may be necessary in natural disaster situations, a multiple casualty incident on a highway, or a major fire in a public building. It is important that the response of all rescue personnel be well coordinated so that the patients receive the best possible care in these situations.

Communications

The EMS system must include linkages between personnel, hospital facilities, and public safety agencies so that requests for emergency medical care are handled by a system that uses emergency phone screening, the 911 system, or an equivalent seven digit number and that has direct communications connections with all personnel within the system and with surrounding EMS systems.

Facilities/Critical Care Units

The system must include the necessary numbers and types of emergency department facilities and specialized critical care units (trauma, newborn, cardiac, poison, behavioral, burn, and spinal cord). Some systems designate specialty care facilities with prehospital transportation protocols that identify the criteria for a patient to be transported to a particular facility, for example, Trauma Centers, Level I, II, or III.

Public Safety Agencies

An EMS system must provide for the effective use of public safety agencies, including the sharing of resources and personnel in EMS and disaster operating procedures (*e.g.*, the personnel to operate helicopters and rescue boats).

Transfer of Patients

Provision must be made for the efficient transfer of patients between emergency medical care facilities and critical care units through written transfer protocols and agreements. Transfer agreements are now a part of the American Hospital Association's accreditation requirements and may be updated annually or may be standing agreements between hospitals in a particular area.

Access to Care

An EMS system must provide emergency medical care to all patients, regardless of their ability to pay. A hospital emergency department cannot refuse to provide life-saving medical aid to a patient because of a lack of insurance. An ambulance service with a contract to provide emergency ambulance service to a community cannot refuse to transport emergency patients based on their inability to pay.

Coordinated Medical Record Keeping

The record keeping system used within an EMS system helps to follow the patient's care from the scene through final discharge. This record keeping system is used to evaluate the success of the entire EMS system and individual components, such as training.

Consumer Information and Education

The EMS system must include a program to inform and educate the public about the goals and objectives of the system and the proper use of the services within the system. This component usually includes lay CPR and first aid training, presentations at schools and civic organizations, and public service announcements through the media.

Evaluation

An EMS system must provide for periodic, comprehensive review and evaluation of the extent and quality of the emergency health care services provided by the system. These evaluations are done by the systems management personnel and by personnel within each component of the system. Evaluation provides the mechanism for identifying problems within the system and for the initiation of improvements within the system.

Systems Management

Due to its complexity, an EMS system must have a formal method of management and administration to direct and maintain the system. A local EMS system must coordinate its efforts with regional and state systems to function efficiently. Every state EMS system participates in national organizations to share ideas and attempt to standardize certain components of the EMS system nationally.

VEHICLES AND EQUIPMENT

Federal design specifications for ambulances, by which they are manufactured, are known as **KKK standards**. Efficiency, comfort, and safety are incorporated into the construction of ambulances. The required design characteristics of ambulances are outlined in state EMS rules and regulations. However, greater flexibility in "extras" is provided at the local level.

The Committee on Trauma of the American College of Surgeons has outlined an "Essential Equipment List," which has been adopted by regulation or statute in most states as the minimum acceptable equipment required on all ambulances for licensure or certification. Many ambulances carry additional equipment and supplies, however, for special needs or capabilities.

AEROMEDICAL TRANSPORT

For some patients, even the best paramedic response may not be enough. An estimated 10% to 15% of all trauma patients sustain severe multiple injuries that require the specialty services of a trauma center. These injuries are often so severe that rapid transportation and surgical intervention are necessary to prevent death.

The first reported application of air transportation of trauma patients was in 1860 during the Franco-Prussian War using hot-air balloons. The military routinely used air transportation during the Korean War and the Vietnam conflict. In October 1972, St. Anthony's Hospital in Denver, Colorado, established the first civilian, hospital-based EMS flight program. Today, more than one hundred and fifty such programs have been established in the United States.

Aeromedical transport refers to the air transportation of ill or injured persons to special care facilities, either by fixed-wing (airplane) or rotor-wing (helicopter) aircraft. Fixed-wing transport typically involves a long distance transfer and poses special concerns because of the amount of time spent in the aircraft and the altitude flown. For this discussion, the main emphasis is on rotor-wing aircraft, since helicopters can be integrated into accident scenes or interhospital responses (Fig. 2-3).

Application of Aeromedical Service

Aeromedical services provide many advantages both to the patient and to the EMS system in smaller, more rural communities.

The primary role of the service is to be a tertiary care responder that transports critically injured or ill patients to a center that offers specialized care. Another common role is that of a secondary EMS responder that assists primary EMS agencies directly at the scene of accidents. Aeromedical services can provide advanced life support care in communities where land-based advanced life support units are not available or are omitted.

Indications for Use

The need for air transport is based on several factors. Included among these are the severity of the patient's condition, the time involved in getting the patient to definitive care, the specific site or location of the patient, the smoothness of transport required for the patient, and the skill level of the flight crew.

Establishing a Landing Zone

The area chosen for landing the aircraft should be as large as possible and free of any overhead obstructions. The minimum landing zone size varies depending on the individual aircraft, but generally a one hundred foot by one hundred foot area provides an adequate safety margin. In addition, the ground at the landing site must be level or at a slope of less than 15°. The landing area should be within a reasonable distance from the scene without being so close as to cause problems from the *rotor wash* (the wind generated by the main rotor blades in motion). Be-

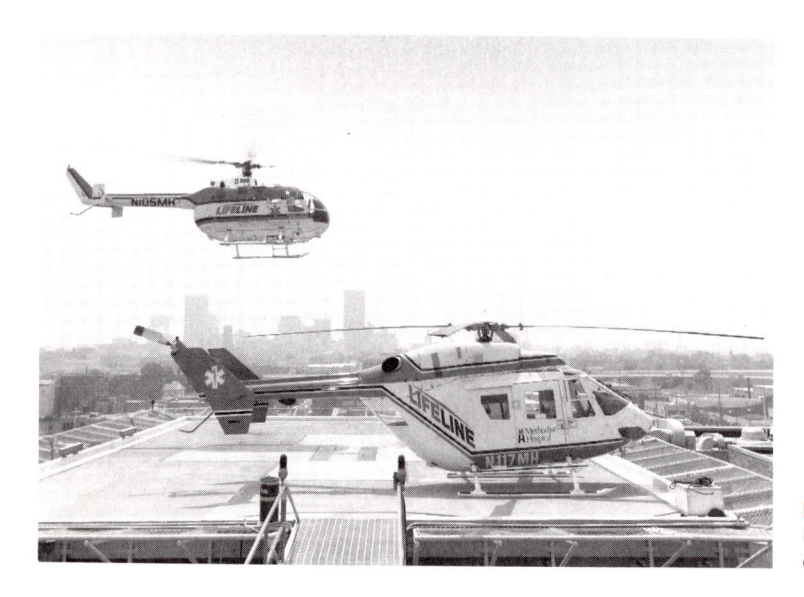

FIGURE 2-3.
Helicopters are an integral part of the emergency medical services system.

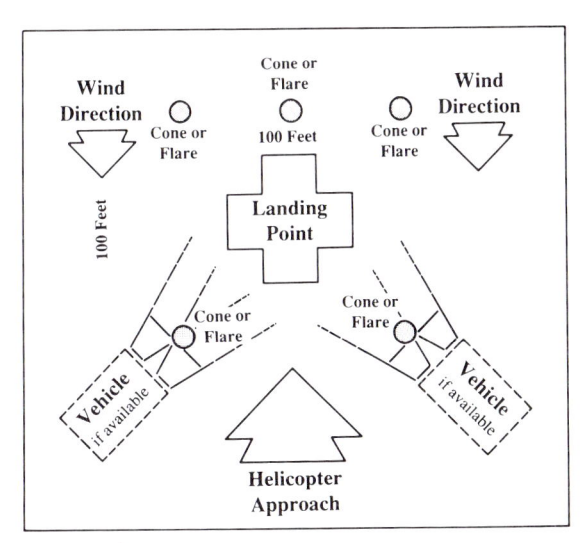

FIGURE 2-4.
Establishing a landing zone.

cause rotor wash can generate winds in excess of 60 mph, the landing zone should be relatively free of loose soil, gravel, or sand. Loose objects such as sheets, stretcher mattresses, and other light equipment should be secured to prevent injury to personnel, vehicles, and the aircraft from wind-propelled objects.

Landing zones should be marked at all four corners with weighted cones or flares. A fifth marking device should be placed on the windward side of the landing zone to alert the pilot to wind direction (Fig. 2-4); this information also can be communicated to the pilot by radio. Other information needed by the pilot before landing includes the compass location of any overhead hazards, such as power lines or guy wires. After dark, landing zones may be marked with flares or by the crossed headlights of vehicles parked at the corners of the landing area. Because the pilot is dependent on excellent night vision for safe landing, bright lights aimed in the direction of the aircraft can blind the pilot and result in disastrous consequences. For that reason, on-scene personnel should not be allowed to take flash photographs or use lighted video recorders during landing or lift off. In addition, if crossed headlights are used to mark a landing zone, the headlights should be turned off before they reach the plane of the pilot's vision. Bright lights used as search lights to guide the aircraft during landing are unnecessary and dangerous. Lights should be used to illuminate overhead obstructions, such as power lines, but should be aimed at an angle that avoids the pilot's visual plane.

Helicopter Safety

Several hazards that may be encountered by personnel who are working around emergency aircraft can easily be avoided.

Frequently, the flight crew choose not to shut down the aircraft engines to keep on-scene time to a minimum. Depending on the situation, the flight crew may ask ground personnel to help unload equipment. It is important that a minimum number of designated personnel approach the aircraft and that no one approach until given a signal to do so by the pilot. It is also helpful to designate one ground crew member to "police" the landing zone and limit or prevent other personnel from approaching the aircraft while the crew is at the accident scene.

A specific helicopter *danger zone* is shown in Figure 2-5. Hazards arise from the two helicopter rotors, the main rotor, and the tail rotor. The height of the rotors vary with the type of aircraft. The main rotor is usually 7 to 10 feet off the ground, but some aircraft have flexible rotors that may dip much lower in certain circumstances. For that reason, personnel should not approach the helicopter in an upright position. If the landing zone is on a slope, the rotor blades come much closer to the ground on the uphill side of the slope, adding to potential hazards. The tail rotor is often less than 6 feet from the ground and is virtually invisible while in motion. This fact makes the area at the rear of the aircraft extremely dangerous; it is important to prevent any ground personnel, bystanders, or members of the media from approaching the helicopter from the rear.

Flight crew members are responsible for safety as well as patient care at the accident scene, and ground personnel should follow their direction to keep hazards to a minimum.

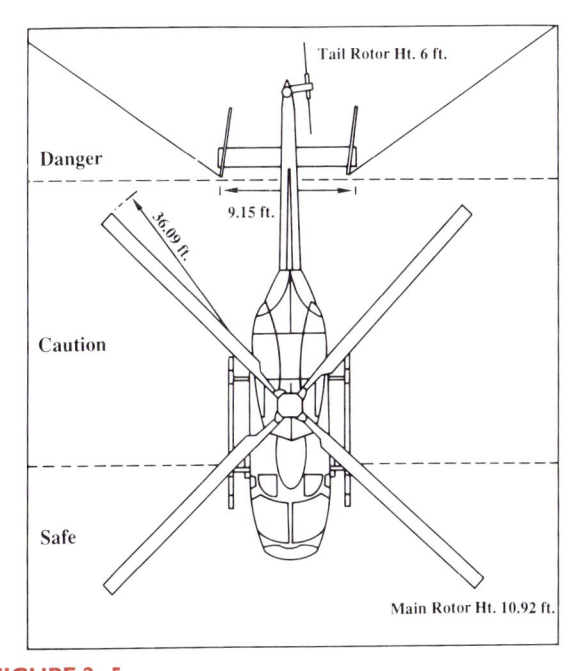

FIGURE 2-5.
Specific danger zones for the Messerschmitt–Bölkow-Blohm BK117 helicopter.

PERSONNEL

Ambulances are staffed by trained personnel who have met specific training and certification standards required by individual state EMS systems. Three levels of staffing for ambulances are nationally accepted in the United States: emergency medical technician–ambulance (EMT-A), emergency medical technician–intermediate (EMT-I), and emergency medical technician–paramedic (EMT-P). The **EMT-A** certification is considered entry level for persons who wish to work for an ambulance service. The EMT-A has completed an EMT-A Basic Training Course that meets the standards of the Department of Transportation's National Standard Curriculum for EMT-As and has passed written and practical certification examinations. The EMT-A has been trained in the following:

- Patient assessment
- Cardiopulmonary resuscitation
- Basic airway management
- Hemorrhage control
- Pneumatic anti-shock garment
- Childbirth
- Pediatric emergencies
- Medical and environmental emergencies
- Extrication
- Special rescue techniques
- Ambulance operations
- Communications skills

An optional module offered by some states is defibrillation.

An advanced life support system was developed in response to the need for emergency care beyond the scope of the EMT-A. Because of their higher level of training, EMT-Is and EMT-Ps are able to stabilize certain emergency medical patients at the scene or while en route to the hospital. The advanced life support activities of these technicians are specified and closely monitored by the hospital's medical control system. Advanced life support personnel are trained to provide all the basic life support skills and certain advanced life support skills.

The **EMT-I** is an EMT-A who has taken a course that includes as a minimum the following modules of the Department of Transportation's EMT-P curriculum:

EMT Roles and Responsibilities
Human Systems and Patient Assessment
Shock and Fluid Therapy
Respiratory System
Telemetry and Communications

The advanced life support techniques for which the EMT-I is trained are: medical and legal issues, roles and responsibilities, patient assessment and initial management of patient care, esophageal obturator airway insertion, ventilation techniques, use of the pneumatic anti-shock garment, and administration of intravenous fluids for volume replacement. Optional modules offered by some states are defibrillation and intubation.

The **EMT-P**, on completion of the Department of Transportation's curriculum for EMT-Ps and the required written and practical skills examinations for either state or national certification, is qualified to perform the following skills in addition to the skills of the EMT-A and EMT-I: advanced airway management (including endotracheal intubation), interpretation of electrocardiogram monitor strips (static and dynamic), defibrillation, cardioversion, and parenteral injections of appropriate medications. In most states, the EMT-P also is trained in the advanced management of trauma and cardiac care.

Both the EMT-I and EMT-P training programs include two phases of training: didactic classroom sessions and hospital clinical experience. The EMT-P program also provides an ambulance preceptorship program during which the EMT-P student may practice the skills learned under the direct supervision of a qualified preceptor.

CITIZEN ACCESS

The initial element of any EMS system is citizen access. Speedy access through the development of **911** as a nationally recognized emergency telephone number has heightened the capabilities of EMS to respond to an emergency. Citizens must be educated to use the seven digit numbers readily available for emergency situations where the 911 number is unavailable.

Further public education is required regarding the availability of services, the information to be communicated to a dispatcher, and the function of a 911 system.

With the centralization of information by one communications center for all public safety services, the task of communication has become more rigorous. Specialized training programs have evolved. Communications operators are a critical link in the system. They enable a network of assistance to be activated as needed, and they immediately make priorities for notification of appropriate agencies. In addition, the communications operator also has become involved in patient care. In many areas, communications operators are trained as EMT-As or as emergency medical dispatchers. The emergency medical dispatcher course is a specialized training program that teaches communications operators how to question callers to better help identify the problem and the patient's needs. Instructions in life-saving first aid measures are also provided to the caller until medical help arrives. The paramedic who responds to the call also benefits from this interdisciplinary effort. The communications operator's telephone assessment and informational gathering before arrival of the paramedic at the scene allows the paramedic to prepare appropriately.

COMMUNICATIONS

Since 1974, certain *frequencies* have been appropriated by the Federal Communications Commission (FCC) for medical emergency communications. Emergency medical services transmissions, including telemetry, are assigned to a frequency band, either *ultra-high frequency (UHF)* or *very-high frequency (VHF)*. In addition, radio communication with base hospitals and direct contact with physicians are enabled.

Several types of radio communication formats are available. The most common is the ***simplex system***. This system uses a single channel that allows communication between two points in only one direction at a time (*i.e.*, two people cannot transmit to each other simultaneously). A ***duplex system*** allows for simultaneous reception and transmission between two stations. In addition to two-way radio communications, a "phone patch" can be made. The paramedic in the ambulance can contact the centralized communications center and be linked to the telephone system of a base hospital, for example. Therefore, the physician has the ability to speak directly with the field personnel, by telephone or radio, on the assigned frequencies. This method is beneficial because the communications center can record the transmissions for future reference. The ability to communicate rapidly with field personnel is critical for medical control to be fully operational, and the paramedic should not hesitate to use this resource to benefit patient care.

MEDICAL STANDARDS

The overall operational protocols for advanced life support systems should be based on sound, established *medical standards*. Through research and practice, standards for prehospital care can be identified and evaluated. Active involvement by the medical community is imperative for the success of the advanced life support system. The local medical society should be involved in the off-line aspects of medical control to provide input and assure uniformity in on-line medical control. The medical director should explain the capabilities and functions of the advanced life support system and be receptive to the concerns of the medical community. Standards for transfers, mass casualty incidents, nursing home calls, and treatment protocols should be the collective effort of accepted medical standards and not the result of politics.

Hospital Care

Classification of hospitals regarding their capabilities to treat patients and availability of staff has implications for the capabilities of any advanced life support system. The availability of surgical staff, laboratory equipment, and consulting physicians must be considered when developing transport protocols for the advanced life support system. The transition of the patient from prehospital care to in-hospital care requires coordination through notification, communication through description of mechanism of injury or changes in patient condition, and cooperation through follow-up, auditing, and training.

The medical control or medical resource hospital usually is responsible for equipment and drug exchange. Some hospitals even provide crew lounges for paramedics to use while waiting for calls. Paramedics are sometimes allowed to help in the emergency department during this time. It is important for the paramedic to follow up on the hospital's assessment and treatment of the patients for the evaluation of prehospital performance to be complete. Paramedics and hospital emergency department staff are constantly working together. The emergency department is a valuable resource for paramedic training and critique with proper guidelines. The quality of interaction between emergency room staff and field personnel contributes directly to the quality of the field performance of the paramedic.

THE EMERGENCY MEDICAL SERVICES SYSTEM IN OPERATION

The EMS system at its most visible level is the arrival of the ambulance at the scene of the call. On arrival, the paramedic must evaluate the overall scene for safety. Information gained at this stage can minimize harm to the paramedic, be used to alert other agencies of needs and dangers, and prevent the paramedic from tunneling in on one particular site or patient. While moving to the patient's side, even before physical contact, the paramedic gains considerable information about the patient by a visual assessment. Level of consciousness, skin color, audible breathing, mechanism of injury, and access limitations are all important pieces of information to be gained in the initial scene assessment. Life-threatening injuries, of course, should be managed. The patient's state of responsiveness, airway, breathing, and circulation are always the first priority in patient care.

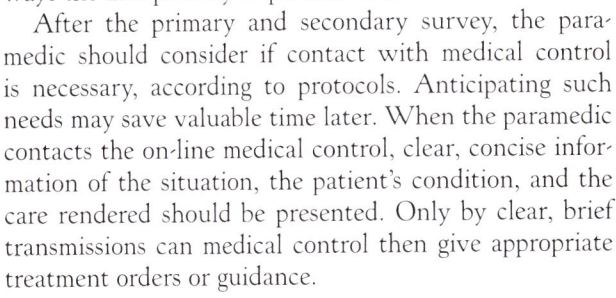

After the primary and secondary survey, the paramedic should consider if contact with medical control is necessary, according to protocols. Anticipating such needs may save valuable time later. When the paramedic contacts the on-line medical control, clear, concise information of the situation, the patient's condition, and the care rendered should be presented. Only by clear, brief transmissions can medical control then give appropriate treatment orders or guidance.

Actual management of patient care is in the hands of the paramedic. The particular medical needs of the patient, preparation for transport, stabilization, and extrication should be promptly and efficiently managed.

Rapid transport of the trauma patient to definitive medical care is imperative for patient survival. However, stabilization of the medical patient, before transport, usually is appropriate. The paramedic should become proficient at minimizing delays in stabilization at the scene and in functioning efficiently in the back of an ambulance. Excessive on-scene time can compromise patient status in both medical and trauma patients.

THE EMERGENCY MEDICAL SERVICES SYSTEM IN RETROSPECT

Mastery of skills comes with practice. The retrospective examination of an entire call is a valuable tool to improve performance, identify weaknesses, and develop solutions to problems. The adequacy of scene assessment, treatment rendered, radio communications, management of the call, and complete, accurate reports should be reviewed. This examination applies to successful calls as well as unique or troublesome calls. Both new and experienced paramedics can benefit from these critiques.

Continuing education programs should also incorporate reviews of runs. **Run reviews** can expose gaps or identify needed additions to operational and treatment protocols. In addition, run reviews may reveal weaknesses in training or on-the-job orientation that need additional attention. If a protocol has proven hazardous or ineffective, waiting for another disaster or blunder is senseless. Both medical control and paramedic personnel should continually reassess individual and system protocols vs. performance.

Medicine is constantly evolving. Theories in pharmacokinetics, pathology, and techniques are always being published, scrutinized, and modified. New methods of intubation or drug administration are studied for field use. The intraosseous route for intravenous fluid therapy is now part of field training. Automatic defibrillators are already in use by EMT-As and first responders. The paramedic must become familiar with these new developments as they evolve. Not only are medications subject to new theories of efficacy, the indications for drug use are always subject to change. As such, indications and contraindications should be reviewed regularly by the paramedic. Given the ever-changing and immense body of medical knowledge, the paramedic must consciously strive to be informed and receptive to flexibility in a profession of continually advancing technologies and potentials.

SUMMARY

The *Highway Safety Act of 1966* was the driving force that eventually established standards for EMS to be used throughout the United States. Although it evolved slowly and unevenly for many years, the EMS system today is a combined effort of many entities and people. Communication, transportation, training programs, hospitals, public safety agencies, consumers, and medical personnel form the network of manpower, protocols, and capabilities that provide a high quality of patient care.

The concept of medical control is essential to the success of an advanced life support system. Individual state EMS system regulations vary on the specific requirements and obligations for medical control. However, in all cases, the medical director of an advanced life support system has the final responsibility for the quality of that system, and the paramedic is fully accountable to and functions only under the supervision of medical control.

SUGGESTED READING

Braun O, McCallion R, Fazackerley J: Characteristics of mid-sized urban EMS systems. Ann Emerg Med 19:536, 1990

Federal Communications Commission: Report and Order. Washington PR Docket No. 87-312, 1988

Globerman M: The new KKK ambulance specs. Third Annual Emergency Vehicle Maintenance Seminar Syllabus, Conference Corporation, Sept. 7–9, 1988

Gonsalves D: Historical background of emergency medical services in the United States. Emergency Care Quarterly 4(3):73, 1988

Kaplan L, Walsh D, Burney RE: Emergency aeromedical transport of patients with acute myocardial infarction. Ann Emerg Med 16:79, 1987

Neely KW, Norton R, Bartkus E et al: The effect of base station contact on ambulance destinataion. Ann Emerg Med 19:906, 1990

Phillips JD, Peters MW: Indications and preparation for aeromedical transport. Indiana Med 80:1049, 1987

Letter to the editor: Telemetry in prehospital care. Ann Emerg Med 16:923, 1987

US Department of Transportation, National Highway Traffic Safety Administration: Emergency Medical Technician—Paramedic: National Standards Curriculum. Washington, DC, US Government Printing Office, 1985

CHAPTER 3

Medical and Legal Considerations

Classifications of Law
    Criminal Law
    Civil Law
    Administrative Law
Medical Practices Act
State Emergency Medical Services Legislation
Motor Vehicle Laws
Additional Laws That Affect the Paramedic
    Child and Adult Abuse
    Use of Force
    Living Will
    Do Not Resuscitate
    Blood Samples
    Organ Donor

Good Samaritan Law
Governmental Immunity
Privilege
Malpractice Actions
    Standard of Care
    Claim of Malpractice
Consent
    Minors and Consent
Patient Refusal

Bases of Liability
    Abandonment
    Battery
    False Imprisonment
    Libel
    Slander
    Invasion of Privacy
Problem Areas for the Paramedic
Insurance and Liability Protection
Summary

BEHAVIORAL OBJECTIVES

On successful completion of this chapter, the reader will be able to:

1. Explain the difference between criminal law and civil law actions
2. Describe the application of the medical practices act to prehospital emergency care
3. Explain the paramedic's responsibilities regarding motor vehicle laws and emergency driving
4. Review the good Samaritan law as it relates to volunteer vs. paid emergency care providers
5. Discuss standard of care and its role in medical malpractice issues
6. List three types of consent and explain the legal considerations when caring for minors
7. Discuss battery, abandonment, and false imprisonment as bases for criminal or civil liability
8. Explain the difference between slander and libel
9. Review the importance of maintaining patient confidentiality in prehospital emergency care
10. Describe three potential problem areas that may lead to legal action against the paramedic
11. Explain the role of insurance policies and the importance of understanding the terms and conditions
12. Define all of the key terms listed in this chapter

KEY TERMS

The following terms are defined in the chapter and glossary:

abandonment
administrative law
assault
battery
causation
civil law
competent
confidentiality
consent
criminal law
Do Not Resuscitate
expressed consent
false imprisonment
Good Samaritan law
implied consent

incompetent
informed consent
invasion of privacy
involuntary consent
libel
living will
malpractice
medical practices act
parens patriae
privilege
signature of release
slander
sovereign immunity
standard of care
tort

In any position of responsibility, corresponding potential liabilities are found. The position of paramedic includes numerous responsibilities that the public and the patient have a right to expect to be performed in appropriate circumstances. Moreover, paramedics do not exist in a vacuum; the impact and consequences of their decisions and actions can be exceptionally or tragically lasting. Therefore, in any given situation, paramedics should be thoroughly informed not only of their obligations but of the potential legal consequences as well.

CLASSIFICATIONS OF LAW

The American legal system contains two areas of law, criminal and civil.

Criminal Law

Criminal law refers to conduct or offenses that have been codified in statutes by the legislature as "*public wrongs*" or "*crimes against the state.*" Therefore, such conduct is prohibited as it is deemed inappropriate for the betterment of society, and the wrong is considered to have been committed against the public in general. Thus, the prosecuting party is "*the State*" or another public governmental entity. On conviction of charges of a crime, the defendant is then punished by the state, through imprisonment, fines, or both.

Civil Law

Civil law refers to private law, as between any two recognizable parties, which may include a corporation or other entity. A private party or individual, as the plaintiff, may seek recovery of money or other forms of relief from another private party, the defendant. Civil law includes actions based on contract or tort. A **tort** is a legal term that refers to any wrongful act or injury done by a private person in a negligent or willful manner against another person or property, thereby causing injury or damage. For example, a claim of personal injury or malpractice is a tort action.

The parameters of what constitutes a tort is defined by many sources, including statutes, customs, regulations, and, to some degree, policies. As society's *values* and *technologies* change, that which constitutes a tort or wrong also changes. Thus, the law is always in a condition of change. A clear example of technological change that affects the law is found in the definition of "*death.*" Medical advances have necessitated the redefinition of death and the duty of the medical profession to treat patients maintained solely on machines. Because the emergency medical services (EMS) system has changed dramatically over the past decade, most states have amended legislation to meet the modern day capabilities and technology of prehospital care.

Administrative Law

Another area of civil law is administrative law. **Administrative law** pertains to the government's authority to enforce the rules, regulations, and pertinent statutes of governmental agencies. The paramedic is granted a license by the State; any violation of the conditions and provisions of the licensure would be conducted as an administrative proceeding. Certain decisions at the administrative level can be appealed to the civil court system for final resolution.

MEDICAL PRACTICES ACT

The paramedic is a creature of statute; that is, the paramedic can only function by virtue of the statutory authority afforded by the state legislature. One of the sources of legal responsibility of the paramedic is the medical practices act. The **medical practices act** is legislation that governs the practice of medicine and may vary from state to state. Such statutes identify the aspects of medical practice that may be delegated by a physician to a paramedic. The specific "*acts allowed*" are the basis of the paramedic's ability to function. Acting beyond or in violation of these statutory provisions may constitute practicing medicine without a license. Therefore, the paramedic should be familiar with the "acts allowed" section of the state medical practices act. Violation of this act would be one source of civil liability.

STATE EMERGENCY MEDICAL SERVICES LEGISLATION

Every state has some enabling legislation that provides for the practice of prehospital emergency care by the paramedic in that state. Such legislation generally defines the scope of acts allowed to be performed by the paramedic; the acts also may be defined in rules or regulations promulgated by a council or board. The legislation usually addresses the prerequisites to licensure or certification, the basis for maintaining licensure (such as continued education requirements or retesting), and the disciplinary action that may result in loss of certification or licensure.

MOTOR VEHICLE LAWS

Another source of law that affects the paramedic is the *motor vehicle code*. As with other laws, this one varies from state to state. The operation of an emergency vehicle is fraught with dangers in the best of circumstances, and the paramedic may be liable for injury to a patient or another person if the injury is due to a violation of a state statute while the paramedic is driving on an emergency run. Lights and sirens are not a defense to liability; their use is only one factor considered in the determination of fault. Most important is the fact that paramedics who drive negligently or carelessly defeat the primary goal of prehospital care if they never get to the patient or never get the patient to the hospital. Although this fact is obvious, the frequency of accidents that involve emergency driving indicates poor observance of the motor vehicle statutes that govern emergency driving.

The need to drive with the lights and siren for any particular call will be scrutinized by the courts. In addition, while operating an ambulance, the paramedic is expected to exercise greater caution than the private citizen driver.

ADDITIONAL LAWS THAT AFFECT THE PARAMEDIC

Most states have *statutes* that mandate the reporting of certain problems, such as situations of suspected child abuse, abuse of elderly persons, communicable diseases, rape, animal bites, and gunshot wounds. Failure to report observations or knowledge of such situations may be grounds for both civil and criminal liability, depending on the state's laws. The duty to report suspected child abuse or abuse of certain adults is examined in greater detail in the following section.

Child and Adult Abuse

Among the most difficult situations encountered by EMS providers is suspected abuse of a child or helpless adult. It is common for a state to have a statute that requires a paramedic to report suspected child abuse or neglect, and some states have a similar statute that requires a report of suspected abuse or neglect of adults who are unable to protect themselves.

Typically, such a law describes the class of persons protected by the law, creates a legal duty for certain persons to report suspected cases of abuse or neglect as defined in the law, sets forth the means by which the duty may be met, establishes a penalty for failure to report, and establishes a qualified legal immunity for an individual who makes a report under the law. Paramedics should be familiar with the requirements of such a law or laws in their state.

Some states establish a *duty to report* for any person in the state, not just a health care provider, who believes or has reason to believe that a child is a victim of abuse or neglect as defined by statute. Commonly, the report is required to be made to a law enforcement department or governmental social services agency. A similar statutory duty to report exists in some states for cases of suspected abuse or neglect of adults who are incapable of caring for themselves for such reasons as insanity, mental condition, senility, old age, or similar infirmities.

A general feature of laws that mandate a report of abuse or neglect is that the person who makes the report need not be able to definitively prove that neglect or abuse has occurred, but only that there is reasonable belief under the circumstances. Another common feature is that the person who makes the report or causes the report to be made is *immune* from civil or criminal liability for making the report, provided it was made in good faith.

Failure to make a report of abuse or neglect as required by law may lead to civil or criminal penalties, depending on the law of the state. A paramedic who makes a report under the law should treat patient information as confidential and discuss suspicions only with authorized individuals from the agency or agencies to which the law requires that the report be made or as needed for medical treatment of the individual who is suspected of being abused or neglected.

Use of Force

Other legal principles and laws may affect the paramedic. *Use of force*, as defined by statute, may be a source of criminal or civil liability. In most cases, the use of force is allowed only in circumstances of reasonably perceived immediate risk of harm. The amount of force allowed is only that which is necessary to prevent such harm or to subdue the aggressor. Any greater use of force is considered excessive. The paramedic should avoid the use of force unless absolutely necessary. In addition, provocation is certainly inexcusable conduct by the paramedic.

Living Will

Another emerging source of legal involvement is the living will. In a **living will**, the patient declares in writing the desire not to receive specified forms of treatment or measures of resuscitation, in the event the patient is rendered incapable of denying consent or expressing such desires at a later date. Depending on the state the patient lives in, the document usually refers to "*extraordinary*" treatment such as respirators (although the term extraordinary is subject to varied interpretation) and in conditions in which treatment would only prolong the act of dying and in which the chance of recovery is none. Legislation that authorizes these declarations is becoming commonplace in today's society; however, because limitations and prerequisites to the validity of the document usually exist, the paramedic should be sure to know the state law before withholding treatment of a patient. A living will prepared by Concern for Dying, an educational council, is shown in Figure 3-1.

Do Not Resuscitate

The living will is not the same as a Do Not Resuscitate order, also referred to as "DNR," "no-code," and "no heroic measures." The **Do Not Resuscitate** order is an entry by the physician in the patient's medical chart. It usually means that in the event the patient has a cardiopulmonary or respiratory arrest, cardiopulmonary resuscitation is not to be commenced. A Do Not Resuscitate order does not necessarily mean that the patient does not want other forms of treatment; thus, a simple entry of DNR should be clarified. The order should be written by the patient's attending physician, only after consultation with the patient. In some situations, the physician consults with close family members if the patient is incapable of communication. Because of the possible conflicts or confusion about a Do Not Resuscitate order, the paramedic should turn to the medical control physician for guidance, both as a matter of policy or protocol and in immediate situations.

Blood Samples

Another area of legal involvement for the paramedic that has become commonplace is the drawing of blood samples for use by law enforcement. Statutes usually govern the authority of the police to order blood samples, and system regulations should dictate how, or if, the procedure is to be performed by the paramedic.

Organ Donor

Transplantation is no longer part of medical experimentation or research. Organ and tissue transplantation is a widely accepted treatment for hundreds of thousands of persons each year. With major advances in immunology, surgery, preservation, and tissue matching, transplantation achieves high success rates.

To serve as a *legal document*, the donor must sign a donor card as shown in Figure 3-2. Many states have a similar form on the back of the driver's license. The next of kin should be notified of the donor's commitment since that individual will be consulted at the time of the donor's death. All expenses related to the recovery of organs and tissue usually are paid by the recipient's coverage.

The patient who is a potential organ donor should not be managed differently by the paramedic, and maximum resuscitative measures should be instituted. The receiving hospital personnel and family carry out the patient's wishes in the event of death.

GOOD SAMARITAN LAW

Every state in the United States has passed legislation of some form that purports to grant *immunity* (i.e., bar liability) for acts performed by a person who renders care in an emergency situation. The concept of the **Good Samaritan Law** was thought to be a necessary incentive for one to provide medical assistance to the injured, uncared-for victim, such as a victim of a motor vehicle accident. So long as the Good Samaritan did not seek compensation, did not act recklessly, or did not purposefully do wrong, no liability for harm or injury caused by such assistance would be actionable.

CHAPTER 3: Medical and Legal Considerations

To My Family, My Physician, My Lawyer And All Others Whom It May Concern

Death is as much a reality as birth, growth, and aging—it is the one certainty of life. In anticipation of decisions that may have to be made about my own dying and as an expression of my right to refuse treatment, I _____ , (print name) being of sound mind, make this statement of my wishes and instructions concerning treatment.

By means of this document, which I intend to be legally binding, I direct my physician and other care providers, my family, and any surrogate designated by me or appointed by a court, to carry out my wishes. If I become unable, by reason of physical or mental incapacity, to make decisions about my medical care, let this document provide the guidance and authority needed to make any and all such decisions.

If I am permanently unconscious or there is no reasonable expectation of my recovery from a seriously incapacitating or lethal illness or condition, I do not wish to be kept alive by artificial means. I request that I be given all care necessary to keep me comfortable and free of pain, even if pain-relieving medications may hasten my death, and I direct that no life-sustaining treatment be provided except as I or my surrogate specifically authorize.

This request may appear to place a heavy responsibility upon you, but by making this decision according to my strong convictions, I intend to ease that burden. I am acting after careful consideration and with understanding of the consequences of your carrying out my wishes. *List optional specific provisions in the space below. (See other side)*

_____ **Durable Power of Attorney for Health Care Decisions** (Cross out if you do not wish to use this section) _____

To effect my wishes, I designate _____
residing at _____ (Phone #) _____ ,
(or if he or she shall for any reason fail to act,) _____ (Phone #) _____ ,
residing at _____) as my health care surrogate—
that is, my attorney-in-fact regarding any and all health care decisions to be made for me, including the decision to refuse life-sustaining treatment—if I am unable to make such decisions myself. This power shall remain effective during and not be affected by my subsequent illness, disability or incapacity. My surrogate shall have authority to interpret my Living Will, and shall make decisions about my health care as specified in my instructions or, when my wishes are not clear, as the surrogate believes to be in my best interests. I release and agree to hold harmless my health care surrogate from any and all claims whatsoever arising from decisions made in good faith in the exercise of this power.

I sign this document knowingly, voluntarily, and after careful deliberation, this _____ day of _____ , 19 _____ .

_____
(signature)

Address _____

I do hereby certify that the within document was executed and acknowledged before me by the principal this _____ day of _____ , 19 _____ .

_____
Notary Public

Witness _____
Printed Name _____
Address _____

Witness _____
Printed Name _____
Address _____

Copies of this document have been given to:

(Optional) My Living Will is registered with Concern for Dying (No. _____)
Distributed by Concern for Dying, 250 West 57th Street, New York, NY 10107 (212) 246-6962

How to Use Your Living Will

The Living Will should clearly state your preferences about life-sustaining treatment. You may wish to add specific statements to the Living Will in the space provided for that purpose. Such statements might concern:

- Cardiopulmonary resuscitation
- Mechanical or artificial respiration
- Artificial or invasive measures for providing nutrition and hydration
- Blood transfusion
- Surgery (such as amputation)
- Kidney dialysis
- Antibiotics

You may also wish to indicate any preferences you may have about such matters as dying at home.

The Durable Power of Attorney for Health Care

This optional feature permits you to name a surrogate decision maker (also known as a proxy, health agent or attorney-in-fact), someone to make health care decisions on your behalf if you lose that ability. As this person should act according to your preferences and in your best interests, you should select this person with care and make certain that he or she knows what your wishes are and about your Living Will.

You should not name someone who is a witness to your Living Will. You may want to name an alternate agent in case the first person you select is unable or unwilling to serve. If you do name a surrogate decision maker, the form must be notarized. (It is a good idea to notarize the document in any case.)

Important Points to Remember

- Sign and date your Living Will.
- Your two witnesses should not be blood relatives, your spouse, potential beneficiaries of your estate or your health care proxy.
- Discuss your Living Will with your doctors; and give them copies of your Living Will for inclusion in your medical file, so they will know whom to contact in the event something happens to you.
- Make photo copies of your Living Will and give them to anyone who may be making decisions for you if you are unable to make them yourself.
- Place the original in a safe, accessible place, so that it can be located if needed—not in a safe deposit box.
- Look over your Living Will periodically (at least every five years), initial and redate it so that it will be clear that your wishes have not changed.

FIGURE 3–1.
A living will. (Courtesy of Concern for Dying, an Educational Council)

ORGAN DONOR CARD

_____
Print or type name of donor

In the hope that I may help others, I hereby make this anatomical gift, if medically acceptable, to take effect upon my death. The words and marks below indicate my desires.

I give: (a) _____ any needed organs or parts

(b) _____ only the following organs or parts

_____
Specify the organ(s) or part(s)

for the purposes of transplantation, therapy, medical research or education;

(c) _____ my body for anatomical study if needed.

Limitations or special wishes, if any: _____

Signed by the donor and the following witnesses in the presence of each other:

_____   _____
Signature of Donor   Date of Birth of Donor

_____   _____
Date Signed   City & State

_____   _____
Witness   Witness

This is a legal document under the Uniform Anatomical Gift Act or similar laws.

Methodist Hospital. For further information, contact Methodist Hospital's Transplantation Program, 1701 North Senate Boulevard, Indianapolis, Indiana 46202, 317/929-8677.

FIGURE 3–2.
Organ donor card.

The first such law was passed in California in 1959, before the existence of the EMS system as it is known today. Originally, such laws applied only to physicians and surgeons and later were expanded to apply to any person or group of persons. Today, every state has a form of such legislation that singles out certain roles and individuals who may be immune from liability in certain circumstances. Most states have a statute of immunity that refers to emergency medical care providers in the prehospital setting, such as emergency medical technicians, paramedics, nurses, doctors, police, and rescuers.

However, before any paramedic relies on the Good Samaritan law as a basis for avoiding liability, the statutes should be carefully reviewed for wording and interpretation. Several states have expressly rejected the use of the law by one who has a pre-existing duty to provide care to the injured victim. Thus, a paramedic who is on duty and, thereby, obligated to render care, whether paid or unpaid, may not be able to use the law as a defense to a legal claim of liability for injuries. Other states have specifically limited the environment (e.g., such as outside of a hospital or doctor's office) or position (e.g., volunteer of a search and rescue unit) to which the law applies. Most, if not all, Good Samaritan statutes excuse liability only for acts done "*in good faith*," which means in a reasonable manner, without malicious intent or reckless disregard for the consequences of the action. Clearly, what constitutes good faith conduct for a paramedic at the scene of an accident is different from that of the untrained private individual. Even if the paramedic is off duty, the knowledge and experience of the paramedic are considered in evaluating good faith.

In most states, the Good Samaritan law is a defense that must be affirmatively presented in court and does not automatically bar a suit from being filed. The judge or jury decides if it is applicable under the circumstances. If the paramedic was grossly negligent, did not act in good faith, had a pre-existing duty, or created the emergency, then the paramedic would not be relieved of liability for the injury. Even if the law is applicable, the Good Samaritan's care should not render the patient in worse condition than before the Good Samaritan undertook the care.

GOVERNMENTAL IMMUNITY

The doctrine of **sovereign immunity** once was a strong protection from liability for the governmental employee. However, the principle that "*the king can do no wrong*" has been abolished in some states and stringently limited in others. If the doctrine is allowed, it relieves the governmental employee from liability for certain types of negligent acts. Because the doctrine is strictly construed against the government, the publicly employed paramedic must be careful to act appropriately and not assume that the doctrine will be a shield against liability. The doctrine does not cover the paramedic who is off-duty and generally only covers conduct within the scope of employment, if at all.

PRIVILEGE

The legal principle of **privilege** refers to a statutory restriction on testimony. Statements made by a person to a professional in certain statutorily identified relationships (e.g., patient to physician) may not be revealed in testimony without the permission of the patient. Exceptions to the restriction apply, however. For example, if the patient makes a statement to the physician that is irrelevant to the treatment or medical condition and, thus, was not necessary to advance the relationship, the information may be divulged. Another exception occurs should the patient clearly indicate an intention to harm another identifiable person; then the physician has a duty to warn that other person or take reasonable steps to prevent the harm.

Few states recognize paramedic-patient privilege. Even in the absence of the statutory restriction of privilege, the paramedic should be cautious about divulging information about a patient. The principle of **confidentiality** refers to communications made in a relationship of trust of nondisclosure and is a broader concept than the testimonial privilege. In the field of health care, the patient has a reasonable expectation of privacy as to treatment, records, and condition. The paramedic, as an allied health professional, should also recognize the patient's confidentiality.

MALPRACTICE ACTIONS

Because the patient potentially is entitled to compensation for injuries caused by the careless acts of a health care provider, the paramedic can become a defendant in a civil action. **Malpractice**, which is a claim of negligent conduct of a professional person, is the common basis of civil liability. The system of American jurisprudence allows money to be awarded for injury, pain, and loss of life in an effort to compensate the plaintiff for the loss legally attributable to the health care provider's conduct.

Standard of Care

The **standard of care** is the basis for evaluating a claim of negligence. The paramedic is expected to act within the standard of care; the deviation may be by *action* (e.g., administering the wrong medication) or *omission* (e.g., failing to administer a necessary medication). What constitutes the standard of care is determined by what the reasonably prudent paramedic, of similar training, skill, and experience, would do in like or similar circumstances.

The paramedic is not held to a standard of perfection or performance in ideal circumstances but is expected to perform in a *reasonable* and *prudent* manner, with due regard and consideration of the reasonably foreseeable consequences of the actions taken. Anything less is considered substandard.

The standard of care is determined by the recognized training programs, such as the Advanced Cardiac Life Support Provider course, curriculums approved by the Department of Transportation, state statutes, and regulations. To some degree, protocols, customs, and local policies may be considered, so long as these do not conflict with the training and content of the state and nationally recognized material.

Claim of Malpractice

A *claim of malpractice* is comprised of four elements, all of which must be proven by the plaintiff against the defendant. They are: 1) a duty to act according to the standard of care; 2) a breach of that duty; 3) **causation**, which is the cause or link between the breach; and 4) the element of injury to the patient, to which a dollar figure can be assessed.

The duty to act includes all the responsibilities for which the paramedic has been trained (*e.g.*, to assess, manage, transport, know medication dosages and contraindications). The paramedic who is employed by a private company usually does not have a duty to act unless the company agrees to provide services. The paramedic who is employed by a public agency, such a municipality, has a duty to all persons in the district and must respond to all requests for treatment to any person in the municipal or jurisdictional boundaries.

CONSENT

The law recognizes that an individual has a constitutional right to accept or refuse medical treatment. Therefore, before initiation of treatment, the paramedic must obtain permission to treat by obtaining **consent**. The principle of **informed consent** mandates that before a patient can consent to treatment, adequate information about the treatment that is to be rendered, the risks and consequences of the proposed treatment, alternative methods, if any, or no treatment must be given to the patient. If the patient is not informed of these matters, the health care professional is not authorized to render treatment and the patient's agreement, if already made, may be invalid.

Who can give or refuse consent? The conscious adult, which, according to most state statutes, means a person older than age 18, may give or refuse consent. In addition, persons younger than age 18 who are in the armed services, married, or who have been legally emancipated (and thereby live independent of family support) are considered adults and, therefore, may give or refuse consent.

Unfortunately, the issue of consent is not only determined by the age of the patient. The terms competency and incompetency are only labels and are of little value to the paramedic in making treatment decisions. It was once a simple matter to identify a person as "incompetent" by the fact that the person was declared mentally ill or confined to a psychiatric facility. In modern civil rights and medicine, a patient committed to an institution also has the right to make decisions about medical treatment. To determine if the adult has the capacity to give or refuse consent (which is presumed, but subject to rebuttal), the paramedic must assess the patient's mental status, derive sufficient information, and then make the determination whether the patient is *capable* (**competent**) or *incapable* (**incompetent**) of granting or refusing consent.

In determining if an adult patient (including a psychiatric patient) can give or refuse consent for treatment, the paramedic must consider the ability of the patient to make the decision about treatment. This decision-making capacity is based on several evaluations, which the paramedic should implement in consent-related problems. This capacity is based on the determination of whether or not the patient indicates an understanding and appreciation of the *nature of the decision* (*e.g.*, agreeing or refusing to be transported to a hospital for medical treatment) and of the *consequences of the decision* (*e.g.*, that failure to go to the hospital may result in further injury, infection, or death).

How the paramedic derives the information to establish the patient's decision-making capacity is based on the paramedic's own ability to inquire, listen, and communicate. Certainly, the paramedic should determine if the patient is alert, oriented, and functionally able to effectively communicate. The paramedic should determine if the patient understands the decision being made, that is the acceptance or refusal of medical care. It should then be determined if the patient understands the consequences of the decision.

Obviously, "yes or no" questions provide little or no information for the paramedic to evaluate the patient's comprehension; therefore, the determination of the patient's decision-making capacity is derived by the content of the paramedic's explanations and patient's response. If a patient is simply asked why a decision is being made, the answer may reveal underlying causes of fear, money, religion, or confusion that affect the decision. Moreover, if the paramedic does not communicate with the patient clearly and in nontechnical terms, communication has not taken place. Factors such as alcohol, age, medications, anxiety, hypoxia, trauma, and intelligence all must be computed into the paramedic's assessment of the patient's mental status.

Three forms of consent are recognized by law. The paramedic must have one of the three to proceed with treatment. **Expressed consent** is an unequivocal expression by the patient of a desire and willingness to be treated, made either verbally, nonverbally, or in writing. **Implied consent** to treat is created in circumstances in which a patient is unable to communicate consent. Consent is implied if the patient is an adult who is unconscious and suffering from a life-threatening injury or illness. Life-threatening injury or illness can usually be assumed if the patient is unconscious; the cause may be the tongue occluding the airway, an arrhythmia, or diabetic coma; regardless, treatment of the life-threatening injury or illness is allowed. Emergency treatment rendered in these circumstances is acceptable because delay could cause irreversible harm to the patient, and it is presumed by law that the patient would ask for treatment if able to do so. Some legal theorists believe that consent is not required in the case of the unconscious patient; because of the emergency situation, the requirement of consent essentially is waived to avoid delay in rendering treatment. The consent, however, may only permit those measures to be taken that are reasonably necessary to meet the emergency.

The third form of consent is ***involuntary consent*** in which permission to treat is granted by the authority of law, such as a court order for treatment, regardless of the patient's desire. This form of consent can be necessary in situations of involuntary mental health and is also applicable for mentally or physically incompetent persons to whom a guardian has been appointed, with alcohol treatment orders, and, in some circumstances, with prisoners in need of treatment.

Permission to treat is usually expressed by a patient to a paramedic when a request for an ambulance is made. Written permission is seldom necessary because of the specific request or conduct by the patient. However, the paramedic should be careful when a person other than the patient calls for an ambulance. Permission to treat and transport should be clarified and never assumed.

Minors and Consent

A *minor* legally lacks the capacity to grant or refuse permission to treat. Thus, the paramedic must obtain consent from other sources. Most states allow only the parent or legal guardian to grant consent on behalf of the child, although other surrogates may be authorized, such as grandparents or other close blood relatives, to give express consent if the parent is unavailable.

Implied consent to treat a minor requires only that the child is suffering from what reasonably presents as a life-threatening injury or illness. The child need not be unconscious because the child's statement of consent, generally, is not legally recognized. Courts have given consideration to a mature minor's desires in nonemergency situations.

Involuntary consent for a minor can occur in several circumstances. Under the doctrine of ***parens patriae***, the State acts in place of the parents and has the authority to protect the welfare and health of a minor. Thus, if the parents cannot be located after extensive efforts, for example, the State may intervene to authorize treatment if requested by the physician, police, or a social service. In addition, most states have legislation that prohibits a parent from denying a child emergency medical treatment and considers such conduct child abuse, child neglect, or criminal negligence. A parent's right to privacy in the care of a child is not without limitations, and a court may be petitioned for an order to treat in such situations.

PATIENT REFUSAL

A *refusal* by a patient to consent to treatment or transport is a common occurrence that blocks the paramedic's performance of the job. The competent adult has a right to refuse consent to treatment, and the paramedic must honor this right, despite charitable and honorable intentions on the part of the paramedic or possible negative outcomes for the patient, so long as the patient has the capability to make the decision. As with any patient contact, the paramedic should document the assessment and evaluation of the patient, including the need for medical care and the refusal by the patient. It should be clear from the report that the patient was capable of making the decision and was adequately informed of the consequences of refusing treatment, such as complications of infection, possible recurrent seizures, or death from intracranial bleeding. Wherever possible, the paramedic should obtain a witnessed statement in writing (***signature of release***) from the patient who refuses treatment or transport. The paramedic should use caution against reliance on a patient's signature scrawled across the bottom of a preprinted form. The release statement should be read aloud to the patient to avoid any confusion if the patient cannot read, and the paramedic should be assured that the signature is legible. *Patience* and *thoroughness* by the paramedic are imperative.

BASES OF LIABILITY

In addition to the claim of negligence or malpractice, other types of civil actions can create liability.

Abandonment

Abandonment is the unilateral termination of the relationship with the patient by the paramedic, when the patient still needs care and treatment but provision is not made for care, and, as a result, the patient is injured. The patient has the right to terminate care, thereby relieving the paramedic of further responsibility, but the paramedic is not free to abandon the patient. Anytime a gap is found in patient care, abandonment is a possible claim. Refusal to transport a patient or talking a patient out of going to the hospital is an invitation for this type of claim. While the burden is on the patient to prove abandonment occurred, the paramedic may be required to provide a basis for ceasing to provide medical care to an injured or ill person.

Battery

In honor of the patient's right to refuse treatment, a claim of **battery** may be made if the paramedic touched the patient without consent. This action can create civil and criminal liability. Physicians have faced claims of battery for performing surgery beyond that which was specifically consented to by the patient; the paramedic should be careful when starting intravenous therapy, for example, in instances in which the patient expresses unwillingness. Situations of improper use of force or restraints also have the potential for a claim of battery. **Assault** is a separate cause of action in which the patient has a reasonable apprehension of immediate bodily harm without consent being given, such as with a threat of restraints or a hypodermic injection.

Paramedics usually can avoid problems of consent and battery by making their actions and intent clear to the patient and by ascertaining with words or unequivocal conduct the willingness of the patient. Good communication skills often save the patient and the paramedic from misunderstandings and hostile encounters.

False Imprisonment

False imprisonment is a claim based on an intentional and unjustifiable detention of an unwilling, conscious person. Thus, the unconscious patient would have no claim for false imprisonment, nor would a patient who agreed to transport. However, the patient detained or transported unwillingly may make such a claim. Detention of an individual can include merely stopping someone against their will for a brief period of time.

Libel

A legal claim of **libel** is a tort action based on a written defamatory statement, falsely or inaccurately made, which damages a person's character, name, or reputation. The paramedic could encounter this type of claim if defamatory comments about a patient are made in the ambulance report, that is then read by others, causing injury to the patient's character. Statements considered libelous are, for example, derogatory entries of a patient's alcohol problems, psychiatric illness, or criminal behavior.

Slander

Slander involves similar conduct as libel but pertains to verbal defamatory statements made about a person to another person. If a patient's conduct or condition is falsely and maliciously discussed in a context that is injurious to the patient's character, name, or reputation, then a claim for damages may result against the person who made the statement. As with libel, it is important that the paramedic, as a professional, remain objective, accurate, and respectful of the patient's situation. The use of derogatory comments or criticisms should always be avoided.

Invasion of Privacy

A claim of **invasion of privacy**, or *breach of confidentiality*, is similar to libel and slander in that a disclosure about the patient is made. However, the plaintiff need not show malicious intent or falsity. Instead, the claim of invasion of privacy is based on an unauthorized release of confidential or private information that causes the plaintiff damages. Release of the ambulance trip report to a patient's employer without a subpoena or permission of the patient, for example, may give rise to such a claim.

PROBLEM AREAS FOR THE PARAMEDIC

Human error and mistakes in judgment are inevitable components of life. The point at which these meet and become actionable negligence is not always clear and is often left to the determination of a jury. Paramedics are urged to take stock of their individual capabilities and weaknesses and be willing to confront them, before a claim arises. It is worth emphasizing a few areas that create an invitation for a plaintiffs to file a claim.

The "*problem patient*" encounters may be potential claims not because of negligent treatment but because of anger, hostility, and simple misunderstanding. Patients who sue have a belief, not necessarily supported by fact, that something was done improperly. The paramedic should take the time to explain what needs to be done or what cannot be done. The paramedic's ability to dispel a patient's fear, confusion, or anger can immeasurably reduce the potential for a future adversarial relationship.

The intoxicated patient is always a challenge and a source of concern in the medical field. However, these patients have injuries and memories and require competent, professional care in every case. The patient who refuses transport should be given the time and consideration necessary to adequately explain the importance of the decision to refuse. Anything less may result in either a return response to a deteriorated patient or a claim of abandonment or negligent assessment.

The paramedic should not overlook the fact that basic life support skills are an integral part of prehospital care. If the paramedic cannot perform a quality patient assessment, the ability to interpret the EKG may be meaningless. Proficiency in advanced airway techniques, such as intubation, is not a substitute for basic airway maneuvers. Liability has been established in cases in which the paramedic either overlooked obvious signs and symptoms or failed to use basic life support skills when needed.

Poor documentation could be a fatal error for the paramedic. It is imperative that a proper run report be filled out (see Chapter 9). The report should include not only the paramedic's findings but lack of findings as well. For example, the notation "the patient is complaining of shortness of breath without chest pain" creates a clear picture of what is and what is not happening. A court of law can only replay the situation by what is written; the paramedic should remain constantly aware of the importance of documentation.

INSURANCE AND LIABILITY PROTECTION

Insurance is not a means to avoid liability itself, but rather it provides payment for legal representation and damage awards entered against a person determined to be liable. Because the EMS system is a unique and specialized aspect of medical care, it would be wise for the paramedic to have a policy for coverage with an insurance company that is familiar with emergency medical procedures.

An insurance policy is a complex legal document that establishes the responsibilities of the paramedic to ensure coverage and the responsibilities of the insurance company when a claim is filed. An insurance policy is highly recommended, but the paramedic should be sure to understand the terms and conditions of the agreement.

SUMMARY

The role of the paramedic holds numerous responsibilities, including legal obligations. Paramedics have won increasing acceptance as part of the health care team, with a corresponding increase in accountability and the potential for legal consequences that stem from their actions. These actions may lead to civil liability, involvement in administrative agency proceedings, or, less commonly, criminal prosecution.

Many different statutes and administrative regulations may affect the function of paramedics, including statutes that define the practice of medicine or the role of the paramedic, motor vehicle laws, statutes that require reporting certain types of occurrences, and Good Samaritan laws. In some instances, the law is evolving, such as with the legal implications of living wills and Do Not Resuscitate orders. Paramedics should be aware of the content of the statutes, administrative regulations, and policies that govern their performance as paramedics.

The actions or omissions of paramedics could result in liability for professional negligence or malpractice. Particularly, paramedics should obtain consent for treatment, render treatment as would be reasonable by prudent paramedics in like circumstances, and be especially wary on runs in which the patient is not transported to the hospital. No definite way to achieve immunity from lawsuits exists; but compassion, effective communication with the patient, and professional patient care may minimize the possibility.

SUGGESTED READING

Dix A, Errington M, Nicholson K, et al: Law for the Medical Professional. Boston, Butterworths, 1988

Fish RM, Ehrhardt ME: Malpractice Depositions: Avoiding the Traps. Oradell, Medical Economics Books, 1987

Frew SA: Street Law. Reston, Reston Publishing, 1983

Goldstein AS: EMS and the Law: A legal Handbook for EMS Personnel. Bowie, MD, Prentice-Hall, 1983

Page JO: Anatomy of a lawsuit. J Emerg Med Serv 14(4):36, 1989

Salomone J: Ethics in EMS: Making choices you and your patient can live with. J Emerg Med Serv 14(5):28, 1989

Shanaberger CJ: The legal file. J Emerg Med Serv 14(4),1989

Shanaberger CJ: Why releases are ineffective. J Emerg Med Serv 13(2):47, 1988

Shanaberger CJ: Running hot. J Emerg Med Serv 112(4):75, 1987

US Department of Transportation, National Highway Traffic Safety Administration: Emergency Medical Technician-Paramedic: National Standards Curriculum. Washington, DC, US Government Printing Office, 1985

CHAPTER 4

Emergency Medical Services Communication

Radio Communications
Emergency Medical Services Communications System Capabilities
  Easy Access
  Resource Coordination and Allocation
  Communications With Medical Facilities
  Trained Personnel
Technological Components
  Federal Communications Commission
  Frequencies
  Communications Center
  Repeaters and Remote Receivers
  Mobile Radio
  Portable Radio Equipment

Emergency Medical Services Communications Operator
  Receive Requests for Response
  Provide Selected Medical Instructions to Callers
  Allocate and Monitor System Resources
  Establish Communication Links
The Emergency Medical Services Incident Sequence
  Occurrence and Detection
  Notification
  Response
  On-site Treatment
  Transport
  At the Hospital
  Preparation for Next Response

Radio Technique
  Techniques for Transmitting Codes
  Communications With Medical Facilities
Equipment Maintenance
Summary

BEHAVIORAL OBJECTIVES
On successful completion of this chapter, the reader will be able to:

1. Describe early and modern emergency medical services communications systems
2. List and describe at least four capabilities of the modern emergency medical services communications system
3. Describe the functions and responsibilities of the Federal Communications Commission
4. Distinguish between UHF and VHF
5. Describe the vehicular repeater system
6. Name factors that affect the coverage of mobile transmitters/receivers
7. List four common functions of an emergency medical services communications operator
8. List four information items typically gathered from a caller by an emergency medical services communications operator
9. Describe the phases of a typical emergency medical services incident sequence
10. List three radio techniques that might improve the quality of a radio transmission
11. Demonstrate and list at least four radio techniques widely recognized as proper radio procedure
12. Present a concise, organized, and clinically complete radio report to a medical facility
13. Give a common cause of radio equipment breakdown
14. Define all of the key terms listed in this chapter

KEY TERMS

The following terms are defined in the chapter and glossary:

base station
EMS communications operator
enhanced 911
Federal Communications Commission (FCC)
frequency
mobile repeater
satellite receiver system
simplex
squelch
telemetry
ultra-high frequency (UHF)
very-high frequency (VHF)
911

The modern emergency medical services (EMS) communications system has evolved considerably since the inception of paramedic services in the late 1960s. Perhaps no technical component of the function of the paramedic has changed so much as that which relates to communications. The model EMS communications system is available around the clock, the method of access to the system is widely known, and the system is easily accessed from all geographic areas. People in the system who are especially at risk or who have special communications needs, such as the deaf, are able to access the system through dedicated devices that they wear or that are installed in their homes.

The resources of the EMS communications system are monitored continuously by computer and are shifted so as to offer optimal response times throughout the system. Computer-aided dispatch programs permit rapid dispatch of the appropriate units. Persons who operate the model EMS communications system are specially trained in monitoring the status of the system and capable of offering prearrival medical instructions. The model system takes advantage of the most modern technology. Mobile units can communicate with the communications center, with each other, and with medical facilities. Data can be freely exchanged among all providers, and the EMS communications system monitors the status of all providers within the system.

RADIO COMMUNICATIONS

The most rudimentary radio communications system consists of a fixed site **base station** and one or more vehicle-mounted mobile transmitter-receivers with a single radio channel. This system, usually conducted on low band or high band VHF frequencies, was used in many early EMS radio systems and permitted ***simplex*** communications, which allows only one party to transmit or receive at a time. This configuration gained widespread popularity for dispatching vehicles, and many ambulance dispatch systems throughout the country continue to use this or a similar system. By the addition of a base station at a hospital, or hospitals, communications between field personnel and a physician became possible; this step was important in the development of the paramedic as an allied health professional.

The EMS communications systems today continue to be oriented toward communications between a communications facility, which provides dispatch services, and mobile units and between mobile units and medical facilities. Many current systems are much more complex, because the early simplex systems were limited in their ability to provide both effective dispatch services and patient related communications. In such a simplex system, field personnel usually must be in their vehicle to make or receive a transmission, and the proliferation of agencies that require communications capabilities can overwhelm the radio system.

The development of portable radio equipment freed the paramedic from the vehicle and permitted bedside communications; however, more complex equipment configurations became necessary. Portable radio equipment necessarily had less power than vehicle radios, and portable radio equipment must deliver the radio signal through obstacles such as buildings. Initially this problem was solved by turning the vehicle-mounted radio into a **mobile repeater** for the weaker signal generated by the nearby portable radio.

Some EMS systems were unwilling to use this method or were unable to do so effectively because of geography or limitations of technology; they, therefore, turned to a technology that had been used to bring in radio signals from far away, the **satellite receiver system**. Carefully located around a given geographic area, satellite receivers can pick up the weak signals from portable units or vehicle units and then clearly relay them by dedicated telephone lines or microwave channels across comparatively great distances.

From the beginning, paramedic systems emphasized communications between a paramedic in the field and a physician usually located at a hospital; these communications usually consisted of voice contact and electrocardiogram (EKG) telemetry. **Telemetry** is defined as sending nonvoice data (*e.g.,* EKG) by radio to a medical facility. Voice contact with hospital personnel in many earlier systems was, and continues to be in many current systems, accomplished in the same manner as voice dispatch. Many states developed statewide radio networks, usually using a **frequency** or frequencies in a range of radio frequencies known as high band VHF for ambulance to hospital communications. Often such systems used an encoder device that resembled a telephone dial or a series of push buttons attached to the vehicle radio that sent pulses or tones over the radio frequency and activated the audio circuit in a medical facility.

The genesis of civilian paramedic programs included the need to provide rapid, technically advanced care to patients with acute myocardial infarction. The requirement to communicate a patient's EKG was quickly determined to be essential for prehospital care radio systems. By the mid to late 1970s, more compact portable units were available, and many EMS systems were routinely using the UHF radio frequencies that recently had been set aside by the Federal Communications Commission for coordinated medical communications. Many EMS radio systems have changed little over the past decade; fueled by the technological revolution that has enveloped society, however, EMS systems continue to seek ways to improve communications.

Computers have long been used by large EMS systems to track data about ambulance responses, but capability now exists to use computers to pinpoint the location of calls, to assist in locating units to better respond to calls, and to recommend units to send to a particular call (Fig. 4-1). Digital communications technology even permits data to be sent back and forth between computer terminals installed in the ambulance and the EMS communications center.

A variety of technologies now permit the EMS communications operator to view the movement of vehicles dispatched by the system in "*real time*" on a map display. New areas of the radio spectrum in the 800 MHz range are available that provide better coordination of emergency agencies and facilitate communications among the field personnel.

Field to medical facility communication has also benefited from the technological revolution. *Cellular telephones* have provided EMS systems with a new means for medical communications. Portable computer technology has even brought electronic interpretation of EKGs to the field.

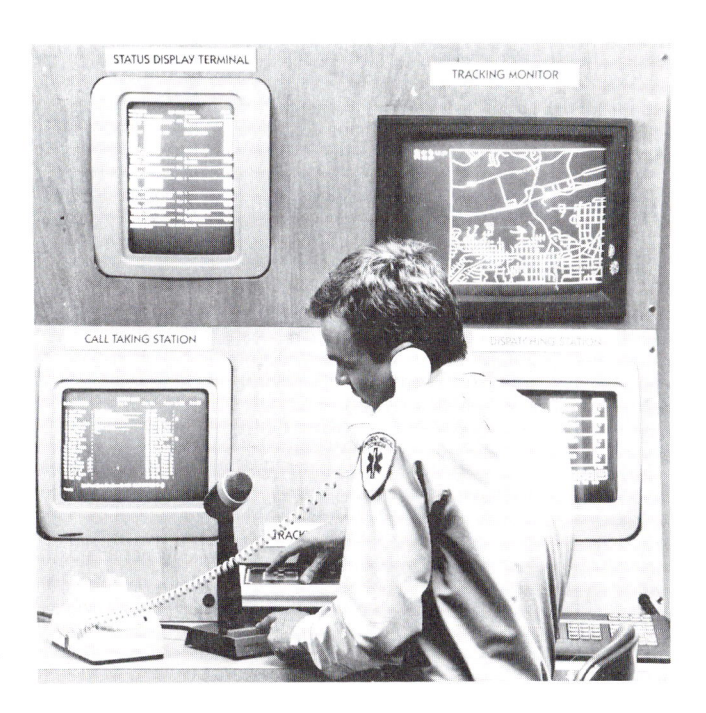

FIGURE 4-1.
Computer-aided communications system. (Courtesy of Recordata West, Inc., Burbank, California)

EMERGENCY MEDICAL SERVICES COMMUNICATIONS SYSTEM CAPABILITIES

The modern EMS communications system is more complicated than the traditional picture of the largely unseen dispatcher who communicates by radio with field units. The modern, model EMS communications system is the product of dramatic technological change and reflects an increasing appreciation of the complex role of the EMS communications operator. While it may use a single communications facility for coordination of all units in its service area, it may also consist of multiple subsystems, each with their own facilities linked by modern technology and protocols.

The modern EMS communications system should have at the minimum the general capabilities discussed in the following sections.

Easy Access

Among the most important tasks of the EMS system is the provision of around-the-clock, rapid, emergency patient access. In most cases, this access is by telephone, oftentimes from a widely publicized number such as **911**. Increasingly, communities are installing **enhanced 911**, which offers such capabilities as immediate display of the caller's telephone number (automatic number identification) and identification of the caller's location (automatic location identification), particularly important features if the geographic area is served by several different EMS providers.

Although the predominate means of access to the EMS system is by a telephone voice request, an EMS communications system should offer access to people who are hearing impaired through Teletype (TTY) or the telephone device for the deaf (TDY). Provision should also be made to receive requests from people who are especially at risk and who wear monitoring devices or have them installed in their homes.

Although the EMS communications system is often thought to be designed to respond to emergencies, not to be overlooked is the means of access to the system for people who require medical or ambulance transportation on a nonemergency basis.

Resource Coordination and Allocation

An EMS system is made up of diverse components, including public safety agencies, ambulance providers, and medical facilities. The communications system that serves the EMS system must possess the means to link these services and permit the immediate exchange of information between the components. For example, a multiple casualty auto accident requires communication between the base station that dispatches the necessary ambulances and the ambulance crews themselves. It also requires communication between the base stations that dispatch law-enforcement and fire units, if all the providers are not served by an integrated dispatch system, as well as on-the-scene communication between the ambulances, police units, and fire units. Communication is necessary between on-the-scene units and medical facilities and perhaps with helicopter ambulances as well.

Emergency medical services communications operators are charged with the responsibility of knowing the capabilities of the various components of the EMS system so that the proper units may be dispatched. They are also responsible for monitoring the status of the units directly under the control of the EMS communications center. This responsibility will be greatly aided by the increased use of automatic vehicle tracking systems that accurately display the location of each on-duty unit and display the location of the closest unit to the scene of a perceived medical emergency.

An important task of the EMS communications system is to maintain the readiness of the entire system for the next request for assistance. To achieve this purpose, the EMS communications system must shift units around so that coverage of the geographic area is maintained and response times may be kept within clinically and locally acceptable standards.

Communications With Medical Facilities

At the minimum, the EMS communications system must provide for voice communications between the field paramedic and a physician. More commonly, the system also provides for transmission of biomedical telemetry of patient data, such as transmission of an EKG.

Trained Personnel

The role of the EMS communications operator has become recognized as central to the success of any EMS systems. The EMS communications operator should be meticulously trained in the operation of all communications equipment that may be used in the systems. In addition, medical training and the use of medical protocols for questioning callers may permit the EMS communications operator to provide prearrival instructions. Training should also be available to emergency medical technicians and paramedics on how to use communications equipment necessary for field communications.

Regardless of the complexity of the system, paramedics are likely to encounter certain pieces of radio equipment in their practice. These pieces of equipment and certain technological aspects of the EMS communications system are the subject of the next section.

TECHNOLOGICAL COMPONENTS

Federal Communications Commission

The **Federal Communications Commission (FCC)** is the federal agency responsible for allocating frequencies, granting licenses, and setting certain standards for radio equipment operation. In 1974, the FCC established a bank of UHF radio frequencies for the use of EMS systems. Because these frequencies are shared by EMS radio systems throughout the nation, close coordination is required to prevent interference.

Frequencies

Emergency medical services radio communications continue to be conducted mainly in the areas of the spectrum known as **very-high frequency (VHF)** and **ultra-high frequency (UHF)**, although some EMS systems are conducting operations in the 800 MHz range.

Very-high frequency communications were used widely by pioneering EMS communications systems, and many dispatch functions continue to be provided in this area of the spectrum. Some early paramedic programs sent biomedical telemetry from field units to hospitals by using VHF frequencies; today, however, telemetry is routinely sent over UHF frequencies. In many areas of the nation, voice communications with hospital personnel continue to be conducted on VHF frequencies.

Both VHF and UHF radio bands used in EMS are basically line-of-sight communications, with their range being a function of the transmitter power, antenna height, and antenna type. Very-high frequency communications may have a greater range than UHF communications, and VHF communications are more susceptible to unpredictable "skip" interference from users far away.

The VHF frequency band is crowded with users, and frequency expansion capability is minimal. Therefore, many EMS communications systems operate in the UHF portion of the frequency spectrum. The FCC has established a series of UHF frequencies for medical communications, and communications between paramedic units and medical facilities are commonly conducted in the UHF frequency band.

Communications Center

At the hub of every EMS communications system is a site for the control of the transmitters and receivers used for dispatch purposes, communications with medical facilities, and, perhaps, for communications with other public safety agencies (Fig. 4-2). A wide variety of equipment configurations that serve those purposes is in use. In one type of system, the radio transmitter and receivers used for dispatch operate on a single frequency and are located adjacent to the communications center that provides dispatch services. In a much more complex system, transmitter and receiver sites are geographically dispersed, use many different frequencies, and are linked to several communications centers and medical facilities by dedicated telephone lines or microwave links.

System configuration for communications between mobile units and medical facilities is equally varied. In one type of system, the paramedic communicates with the desired medical facility through a preassigned radio frequency or channel used by a transmitter and receiver located at the medical facility. In a more complex system, the communication is routed through a satellite site via a regional communications center to the desired medical fa-

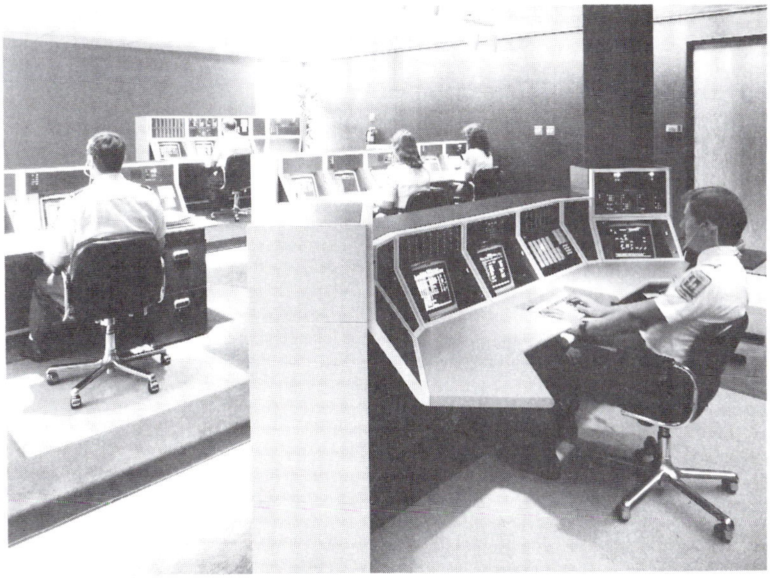

FIGURE 4–2.
Communications center. (Courtesy of Hartson Medical Services, San Diego, California)

cility. Regardless of the actual technique employed, paramedics are expected to be familiar with the operation of the system in their area.

Repeaters and Remote Receivers

The considerable distances or urban density in which paramedic field units operate often require additional means of relaying the radio signal generated by the mobile unit other than direct transmission to the base station or medical facility. One means of accomplishing this objective is to turn the radio located in the paramedic's vehicle into a vehicular repeater to repeat, typically at a higher power or by using digital technology, a transmission that originates in a portable unit carried by the paramedic. Another method is to locate mobile repeater units at fixed sites throughout the service area of the EMS system. Yet another method is to locate satellite receiver units around the geographic area and then relay the signal through dedicated telephone lines to the intended base station.

Mobile Radio

Typically, an EMS vehicle contains a transmitter/receiver permanently mounted in the vehicle to contact the EMS communications center, medical facilities, and other vehicle units. Virtually always, if the vehicle is used to provide paramedic service, the radio is capable of operation on multiple frequencies.

Common controls on the vehicle radio include the following:

- A combination on/off switch and speaker volume control
- A channel selector to choose the appropriate radio channel
- A **squelch** control to control the circuitry that suppresses the noise otherwise present between transmissions
- A transmit switch that, when depressed, or "keyed," activates the radio microphone

Paramedics should be thoroughly familiar with the controls on the radio equipment used in their EMS communications system.

Portable Radio Equipment

Portable equipment used by a paramedic varies considerably from system to system. Hand-carried units, powered by rechargeable batteries, may be used for communications between the units in the field and their communications center, between field units and a hospital or other medical facility, or for field unit to field unit communications.

The need for portability of hand-carried radio units results in a comparatively low power output. Therefore, a method is required to effectively increase the range of the portable unit through use of satellite receiver sites strategically located around the area, mobile repeater sites, or vehicle repeater systems. Important controls and features found on portable units are similar in function to those found on radios mounted in the vehicle, with the addition of a carrying case and device for recharging batteries.

Hand-carried radio equipment is typically used for communications with an EMS communications center, although in some EMS systems it may also be used for communications with medical facilities. However, additional equipment is often used for the transmission of biomedical telemetry from the scene to a physician who may be located in a hospital or elsewhere. In some cases, this radio equipment may be combined with a monitor/defibrillator, or it may be a separate unit that is connected to a portable monitor/defibrillator. Special equipment is installed in the hospital emergency department for conversion of the radio signal back to an EKG strip for viewing by hospital personnel.

EMERGENCY MEDICAL SERVICES COMMUNICATIONS OPERATOR

For a person who requests emergency medical help, the first contact with the EMS system is likely to be the voice of a telecommunications specialist. Known variously as a dispatcher, emergency medical dispatcher, controller, telecommunicator, system status manager, or, throughout this chapter, as **EMS communications operator,** this specialist occupies a pivotal role in the EMS system (Fig. 4-3).

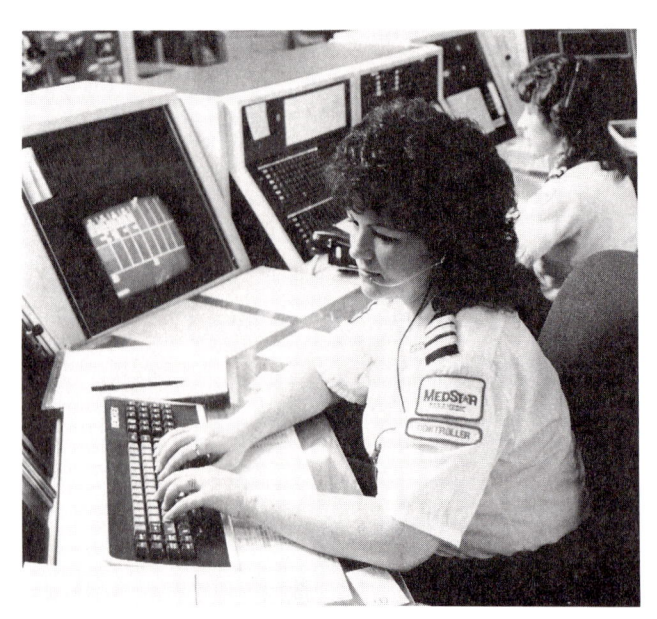

FIGURE 4–3.
Communications operators are the first contact for the patient in the emergency medical services system. (Courtesy of Hartson Medical Services, San Diego, California)

Communications operators have different duties in different EMS systems, based on the size of the system, the configuration of communications hardware used in the system, and the type of services provided in the system. However, responsibilities of communications operators in an EMS system that provides advanced life support typically include those discussed in the following sections.

Receive Requests for Response

In most cases, requests for emergency medical assistance are received by telephone. The initial goal of the medically trained EMS communications operator is to obtain sufficient information according to clinically accepted protocols to assess the urgency of the request, which units from which agencies will be needed to respond (an especially important process in multitiered systems with different medical capabilities of responding units), and what the units may expect on arrival. A system that provides emergency response as well as nonemergency transfers or a system that responds to different tiers of care, such as first responder, basic life support, or advanced life support, obviously depend on a competent initial assessment by the communications operator.

A minimum of four pieces of information is required by most systems: the location of the patient, the phone number of the caller, the caller's description and perception of the medical condition of the patient, and any hazards that may be encountered by the responding units.

Eliciting information from callers is among the most challenging aspects of the role of the communications operator. A competent communications operator is calm (regardless of the state of the caller), polite, caring, nonjudgmental, and alert.

Provide Selected Medical Instructions to Callers

Increasingly, the first response of the EMS system to a request for medical assistance comes in the form of instructions from the communications operator to the caller on what to do, or what not to do, until the arrival of responding units. Communications operators trained in the special techniques of a telephone interrogation and the issuance of prearrival instructions according to medically accepted protocols can provide life-saving advice.

Allocate and Monitor System Resources

The communications operator is the manager of the status of the EMS system. As calls are received and processed, units are dispatched, and information and instructions are given to the responding units. This task is complex in any system, but especially in an area served by multiple providers with different levels of service and, perhaps, overlapping service areas.

The readiness of the EMS system for the next request should always be an important consideration of the EMS communications operator. The modern EMS system often uses a prepared deployment plan for shifting the location of the remaining units so that coverage of all geographic areas is maintained and clinically acceptable response times are provided.

In addition to monitoring the status of field units, many EMS communications systems monitor the availability and status of medical facilities through radio or telephone links; this information is important, particularly in disaster situations.

Establish Communication Links

In some EMS communications systems, the communications operator is responsible for establishing radio or radio-telephone links between paramedic units in the field and medical facilities. This action may take the form of assigning a radio frequency for the linkage or establishing a radio-telephone patch for communication.

THE EMERGENCY MEDICAL SERVICES INCIDENT SEQUENCE

The typical emergency medical services incident progresses through sequential steps.

Occurrence and Detection

The perception of the need for assistance begins the sequence of an EMS incident response. This need may be determined by the patient, a relative, or bystander and is influenced by a variety of factors, including the perceived seriousness of the patient's condition. The chief influence of the paramedic at this stage of the EMS incident sequence takes place through involvement in public education and EMS awareness programs designed to teach the public how to detect and react to medical emergencies.

Notification

More often than not, an EMS provider is alerted to the need for medical assistance by telephone. A growing number of communities are implementing 911 for EMS, police, and fire service requests. Many communities with existing 911 systems are upgrading to enhanced 911 systems.

Many communities are served by more than one EMS provider, often with overlapping response areas. In such cases, protocol should allow for the use of all of the resources of the community to ensure that an appropriate agency is notified of the request for assistance if the agency that was initially called is unable to respond in a timely manner.

Response

Proper response to an EMS incident results from identification of the need for response and the allocation of the appropriate community EMS resources to the request. A single vehicle and its crew may be all that is warranted, or multiple agencies and multiple vehicles of a variety of capabilities may be required. For example, police, fire, and medical authorities may be required to respond to a multiple vehicle accident that involves patient entrapment. Increasingly, the EMS communications operator is also part of the response by providing instructions to the caller until the EMS units arrive.

Actual dispatch of the emergency units is usually accomplished by radio, either by direct two-way contact or by pager. The information that is gathered by questioning the caller according to established protocols, including the location of the patient and a preliminary assessment of the patient's condition, is provided to the responding units (Fig. 4-4). Special instructions about hazards that may be encountered en route or on the scene are also furnished to responding units. Some EMS systems have installed computer links in the ambulance for direct transmission of information from the communications center to the ambulance.

A significant number of EMS systems monitor the availability of EMS units and select the appropriate unit to send through computer-aided-dispatch (CAD) programs.

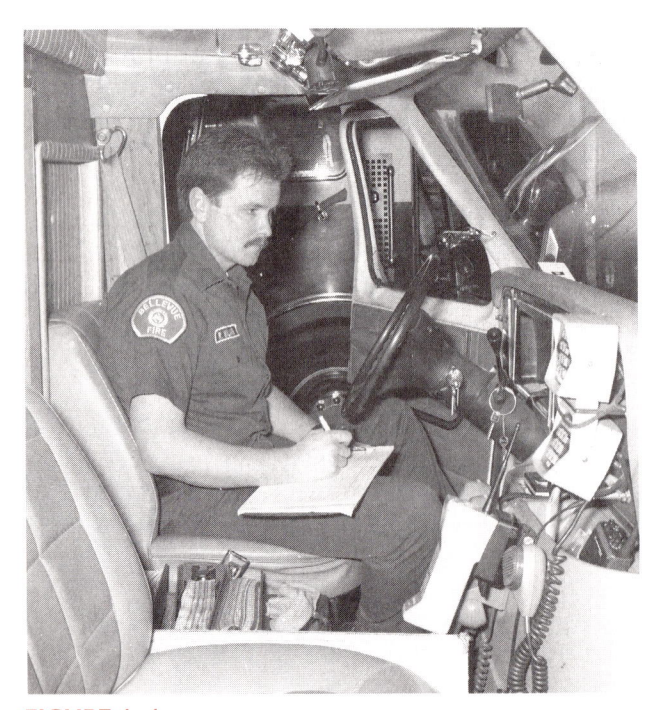

On-site Treatment

In many communities, paramedics provide care according to medically established protocols that sanction "standing orders" for treatment that may be provided by the paramedic before contacting a medical facility. Radio or telephone contact is then required for further treatment or, in some EMS systems, if the paramedic does not feel transportation to a medical facility is warranted.

Two decades ago, much of the equipment used for communications from field units to medical facilities was bulky and heavy. Today, reliable and comparatively lightweight devices permit voice contact between medical personnel at the hospital and the paramedic in the field as well as the transmission of EKG signals.

Contact between field units and medical personnel is usually accomplished either by ordinary telephone from the patient's bedside, through special EMS radio systems, often quite elaborate in design and maintained for that purpose, or through cellular telephone units. The latter is a sophisticated radio-telephone system that divides a given geographic area into "cells," with a transmitter in each cell linked to a central facility and the local telephone system. In some areas, such a system holds promise for even more use in paramedic communications as cellular telephone systems expand and the effective range of portable telephone units increases. Mobile equipment now available transmits voice and EKG signals and provides the paramedic with a computer-generated interpretation of the patient's EKG (Fig. 4-5).

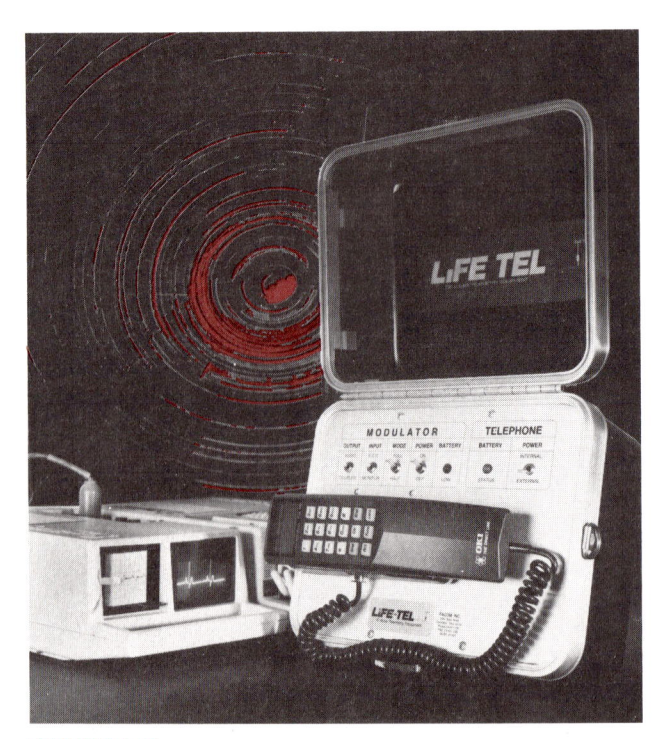

FIGURE 4–4.
The paramedic gathers information about the emergency run as it is transmitted by radio from the communications operator. (Courtesy of Laerdal Medical, Armonk, New York)

FIGURE 4–5.
Cellular phones are used to transmit voice and EKG signals. (Courtesy of Racom, Inc., Cleveland, Ohio)

Transport

Contact with the EMS communications center that initially performed the dispatch is maintained throughout transport and care of the patient. As well, medical communications initiated on the scene are often continued en route to the medical facility. Although the form and requirement for contact with the hospital vary from system to system, the hospital usually is notified of selected patients, especially critical patients, so that it may have the appropriate staff and equipment on hand for the arrival of the patient.

At the Hospital

If a hospital is notified of the impending arrival of a patient, preparations are made to continue the care begun in the field. Based on the paramedic's description of the condition of the patient, treatment rendered up to that point, and the reception of any telemetry of patient data, such as an EKG, the appropriate staff and critical care units within the hospital may be notified so as to be prepared for the arrival of the patient.

Because airwaves are easily monitored, the transmission of the patient's name by radio from the field often is discouraged out of concern for the patient's privacy. However, if contact is made by telephone or a relatively secure radio method, or if the system's protocol permits, transmission of the patient's name is advantageous because it allows the facility to research its medical records for information about the medical history of the patient.

Preparation for Next Response

Preparing for the next response is an important aspect of the practice of the paramedic and the EMS communications operator. The EMS communications operator must ensure that units are properly distributed to minimize response times to emergency scenes. Paramedics must return their units as quickly as possible to a state of readiness after a response so that the units are available for another run.

RADIO TECHNIQUE

Proper radio technique increases the effectiveness of a communications system. While procedures vary from system to system, certain conventions have emerged.

1. Pronounce each word clearly and at an understandable rate. A loud voice can be just as unintelligible as a soft voice.

2. Use an emotionless voice. A calm, deliberate voice enhances the intelligibility of the communications and establishes the impression that the speaker is a professional. A tone of voice that conveys impatience, anger, sarcasm, an attempt at humor, or the use of slang is never justified, regardless of the circumstances.

3. Use unit identifiers rather than proper names when referring to other persons or units in the system.

4. Be brief, but clear and accurate. Superfluous words should be avoided. Words such as "sir," "please," and "thank you" are unnecessary because politeness should be understood from a proper radio voice.

5. Confine radio transmissions to those related to dispatch functions or patient care. Personal messages and announcements not related to the immediate readiness and status of the EMS system should be relayed over the telephone.

Techniques for Transmitting

Instructions provided by the manufacturer of the radio equipment should be followed. However, certain general techniques for use with field or vehicle radios may enhance the effectiveness of radio communications.

1. Listen for other radio traffic before transmitting. This step prevents one unit from canceling out the transmission of another unit. A momentary depression of the transmit switch on the radio before beginning to speak helps to prevent the first part of the transmission from being cut off.

2. If a poor quality radio reception is encountered at the EMS communications center, in the hospital, or by the unit in the field, quality may be improved by movement of the field radio unit, sometimes by movement of only a few feet. This fact can be particularly true inside buildings, near energy sources such as power lines, or in dense urban areas, where the airwaves are crowded with radio transmissions of many kinds.

3. The higher the antenna, the greater the clarity of transmission, usually. The paramedic should ensure that the antenna on any portable equipment is pointed straight up and is elevated as much as is reasonable. Movement of a portable radio unit from the floor up to a table can occasionally make a dramatic difference.

4. Speak directly into the microphone or at a slight angle to the face of the microphone. A distance of 2 or 3 inches from the face of the microphone usually is optimal. Finding the optimal distance is important; a distance too close leads to distortion and noise from exhaled breath, while one too far results in a voice too weak to hear and interference from background noise.

5. Repeat back, or "echo," directions received from the communications operator or medical facility personnel to minimize the possibility of misunderstandings.

Codes

Many EMS systems use a *code system* as a form of radio shorthand; 10-Code systems are the most predominant. Common examples are 10-4 to signify "affirmative" or "message understood" and 10-9 to signify "repeat your message." Properly used, such codes can improve the accuracy of communications and decrease the amount of time required for a radio transmission. A further advantage is that codes can be used to avoid terms that could be unsettling to people on the scene, such as codes to signify that a coroner is needed or that the police are required because of the mental state of a patient.

Associated Public-Safety Communication Officers, Inc. (APCO), an association of public safety communications professionals, has developed a standard set of codes; however, the codes are far from universally used. In neighboring systems, the same code may stand for something different, and the opportunity for confusion is great, particularly when a paramedic is communicating with people who may not be familiar with the codes, such as hospital personnel. As such, many EMS systems have come to question the use of codes for all but a few select conditions. The paramedic should be aware of the local meanings for any codes used; however, if there is any doubt that the listener will understand, or if the listener infrequently uses the codes, brief, plain English should be used to enhance communications.

Communications With Medical Facilities

The general principles of good radio technique apply to communications with medical facilities. However, some special aspects exist for reporting patient information.

A good radio report depends not only on good radio technique but excellent patient assessment skills and the ability to "*paint a picture*" of the patient for the person who is receiving the report, usually a nurse or doctor many miles away.

In general, codes and specialized terminology used in dispatching should be avoided in communications with a medical facility because personnel at the medical facility are often less familiar with the terminology and the possibility for misunderstanding is great. Use of plain English and standard medical terminology, free of potentially misunderstood abbreviations, is usually the best practice. It is always a good idea to take a minute to mentally compose the report that will go to the hospital so that the appropriate information is conveyed. Local protocols should be carefully followed so that the paramedic has gathered all the pertinent information and performed all the appropriate procedures before contacting the medical facility. These actions prevent interruptions in the communications process while the paramedic returns to the patient to gather more information or perform a procedure that could have been initiated before contact with the hospital.

The paramedic should make every effort to avoid labeling the patient. The role of the paramedic is not to determine the precise diagnosis of the patient but rather to accurately and concisely describe how the patient presents to the paramedic.

Especially in systems in which multiple units may use the same frequencies, paramedics should identify their units in each transmission to prevent confusion with other units that may also be on the radio channel.

The format for presenting patient medical information to a medical facility varies among EMS systems. One such format is found in Chapter 9. Paramedics should be intimately familiar with the procedure used in their area and follow that procedure. Faithful adherence to a single procedure helps organize the care given to the patient and, with practice, ensures that the pertinent information is communicated.

EQUIPMENT MAINTENANCE

Among the most critical equipment used by a paramedic, certainly among the most expensive, is radio equipment. The harsh environment in which the paramedic must operate can take its toll on equipment, but a few common sense precautions can help ensure that radio equipment will function properly.

Rough handling is a common cause of radio equipment failure. For example, dropping a radio, exposing it unnecessarily to the elements, or abusing it, such as lifting or carrying a portable radio by its antenna, can shorten the life of the radio and increase the likelihood that it will fail at a crucial time. Cleaning a radio by use of a damp rag and mild detergent and taking care not to allow water to enter the radio mechanisms can improve the appearance of the equipment and perhaps prevent contaminants from getting inside the radio.

Radio equipment should be checked regularly to ensure that it functions properly, especially radio equipment that is used infrequently. Many paramedics make it a practice to check all their radio equipment at the beginning of their shift.

SUMMARY

Communications with EMS communications operators at a dispatch base station and with medical personnel at a hospital are important functions of a paramedic. The EMS communications system has grown in complexity and certainly will continue to evolve, and paramedics are expected to be familiar with the field communications equipment that is necessary to provide care in a modern EMS system.

A paramedic is part of a medical team that includes the EMS communications operator, who takes the initial call for assistance, and the medical staff, who assume responsibility for the care of a patient on arrival at the hospital. Recognition of the importance of the roles of other members of the team, including effective communications with the other team members, proper use of communications equipment, and excellent radio technique, are expected of the professional paramedic.

SUGGESTED READING

Clawson JJ: The hysteria threshold: Gaining control of the emergency caller. J Emerg Med Serv 11(8):40, 1986

Dernocoeur KB: Street Sense Communication, Safety and Control. Bowie, MD, Prentice-Hall, 1985

Garza MA: Cellular technology: Revolutionizing EMS communications. J Emerg Med Serv 15(5):46, 1990

Johnson M: Is EMS communicating with the FCC? J Emerg Med Serv 14(7):50, 1989

Ullman K: Dispatcher CPR saves lives in King County, WA. American Fire Journal 40(2):24, 1988

US Department of Transportation, National Highway Traffic Safety Administration: Emergency Medical Technician-Paramedic: National Standards Curriculum. Washington, DC, US Government Printing Office, 1985

Vines T: What future MSS (Mobile Satellite Services)? Clogging the prospects for more efficient communication? Response. Journal of the National Search and Rescue Association 5(3):19, 1986

Yvorra JG: Mosby's Emergency Dictionary: Quick Reference for Emergency Responders. St. Louis, CV Mosby, 1989

Zydlo S: EMS solutions. Chief Fire Executive 3(4):31, 1988

CHAPTER 5

Rescue Management

Principles of Safety
  Personal Safety
    Gloves
    Turnout Gear
    Eye Protection
    Respiratory Protection
    Footwear
  Patient Safety
  On-scene Hazards

Assessment of the Scene
Gaining Access
Disentanglement
Removal
Emergency Care and Transportation
Summary

BEHAVIORAL OBJECTIVES

On successful completion of this chapter, the reader will be able to:

1. Identify the protective gear worn by rescue personnel
2. Explain how environmental factors can complicate rescue operations and jeopardize the condition of the patient
3. Identify several safety hazards that may exist at the scene of an accident
4. Describe the elements involved in the assessment phase of rescue
5. Explain the role of the communications operator in the coordination of an efficient rescue operation
6. Describe the mechanism of gaining access to the patient
7. Explain the paramedic's patient assessment and emergency management responsibilities during a rescue operation
8. Give four examples of specialized rescue teams
9. Identify the difficulties that may be encountered during the removal phase
10. Discuss several considerations in the selection of the appropriate mode of transportation of a trauma patient
11. Define all of the key terms listed in this chapter

KEY TERMS

The following terms are defined in the chapter and glossary:

bunker coat
disentanglement
extrication
hazards
self-contained breathing apparatus (SCBA)
self-contained underwater breathing apparatus (SCUBA)
turnout gear

The delivery of emergency medical services (EMS) often occurs in diverse rescue situations. The rescue situation may be as simple as removing a child's finger from a bottle or as complex as extricating a person trapped in an industrial machine. This chapter presents general insights and basic concepts of rescue operations.

Important concerns of the paramedic who works rescue incidents include a knowledge of local rescue resources, a working relationship with specially trained area rescue teams, a knowledge of safety hazards associated with rescue incident operations, and experience in how to best assess and manage the patient in these situations. It is important that the paramedic keep a clear focus on the patient's needs during the rescue to help maintain patient safety and care as a key element in the rescue operation.

Complex rescue incidents often generate tension among rescuers. Tension may stem from a strong sense of drama and urgency. This tension may be compounded by the shear numbers of personnel who are participating in the rescue. The more personnel and the larger the number of agencies present, the greater the need for the paramedic to take a strong and authoritative role in patient advocacy.

No two rescues may be alike, but the basic principles of incident management still apply. Rescue is best thought of as a process of options and not absolutes. To be an effective participant in the rescue process, the paramedic needs to continually gather data (e.g., about the environment, rescue operations, patient status, hazards, risk) and adapt medical care to best fit the patient given the current restrictions. Each time a patient needs more than the standard, hands-on approach to care, the rescue effort must be custom designed for that situation. This need requires the leadership of creative, open-minded and clear thinking professionals, paramedics who think of options and not absolutes. The safe and effective management of the rescue incident requires rescuers to be able to assess and stabilize the scene, select the best method to reach the patient, provide the essential medical care, then extricate, package, and remove the patient. Rescue is a team effort that choreographs all of the available resources to accomplish these tasks.

PRINCIPLES OF SAFETY

Personal Safety

Personal safety is a matter of professional responsibility. It is the responsibility of the paramedic to anticipate and prepare for the hazards to be found in rescue environments. Failure to provide oneself with appropriate protective equipment and garments may result in unnecessary injury and further jeopardize the care and safety of the patient.

It is easy for rescuers to develop a false sense of security about personal safety. For example, it may seem obvious that the site of a motor vehicle accident should generate extra caution to on-coming drivers. However, scene safety should be a constant concern, since many drivers are likely to be blinded or distracted by the emergency lights and the rescue operations. Paramedics must always keep a watchful eye for moving vehicles when working around any vehicular accident scene.

Personal protective clothing and equipment should be selected and worn to minimize the adverse effects of the rescue environment and reduce the chances of injury.

Gloves

One item of protective apparel needed for all rescue incidents is gloves. The types of gloves required at a given rescue may vary, depending on the working environment and hazards present. Gloves that are primarily designed to protect against the cold are different from gloves designed for structural fire fighting.

The rescue environment may dictate that all personnel who are working the incident wear gloves that protect against such hazards as extreme heat, cold, sharp objects, open flame, chemicals, or communicable disease. No one glove can provide protection against all of these hazards. The glove selected should provide the maximum protection while minimizing interference with the handling and operation of essential tools and equipment. It is likely that more than one type of glove will be needed to obtain maximum protection. For example, it is appropriate to replace heavier gloves necessary for vehicle extrication with thin, light-weight protective latex gloves when patient care is initiated.

Turnout Gear

Turnout gear is a fire service term. It denotes protective clothing designed for structural fire fighting. The general trend in the design of this protective clothing is to provide layers of material so that the chance of injury is reduced while the performance potential of the user is increased. The exterior layer of material and fabric for structural fire fighting is designed to minimize the effects of heat, open flame, sharp objects, and sometimes impact trauma for the user. The inner layer's design supports the barrier protection of the outer layer while providing for personal comforts. For example, structural fire-fighting helmets have inner layers that help distribute the forces of an impact, while providing a comfortable material to fit tightly against the head.

The coat worn for structural fire fighting, sometimes called a **bunker coat**, provides environmental protection and guards against smoke and fire, but not against hazardous chemical spills or radiation. The bunker coat is but one part of the total envelope of protection needed to carry out rescue in the structural fire environment. The total envelope includes equipment and clothing that encompass the paramedic rescuer from head to toe (Fig. 5-1).

The best helmets for rescue provide protection from penetrating objects, are able to minimize the effects of blows to the head from the sides, front, back, and top,

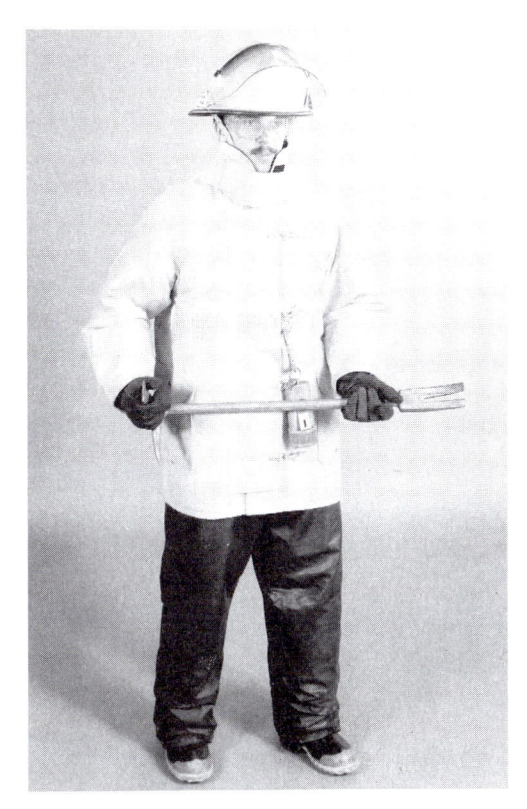

FIGURE 5–1.
Turnout gear for heavy rescue and extrication.

have secure nonelastic straps, and do not impair vision to the top or sides. Many of the helmets designed for rock climbing, caving, fire fighting, and industrial work are suitable for the paramedic rescuer to use (Fig. 5-2). Figure 5-3 shows typical "hard" hats worn at construction sites. These helmets are used for protection against scalp lacerations but are not durable enough for rock climbing.

Eye Protection

Eye protection is essential in all rescue situations. Eye protection must be selected according to the rescue environment. The concern at vehicle accidents is for flying debris, equipment, hydraulic oil, and possibly body fluids. The concern in mountain rescue situations might be from loose rock, dirt, and sun reflected off the snow. Even a slight irritation or injury to an eye of the paramedic rescuer will likely cause a reduced or impaired ability to carry out needed patient care.

Respiratory Protection

Many rescue environments present respiratory hazards, including fires, hazardous materials, confined space, and radiologic-biologic incidents. Two well-known respiratory protection devices are the **self-contained breathing apparatus (SCBA)**, the term used by the fire service, and

44 UNIT ONE: THE PREHOSPITAL ENVIRONMENT

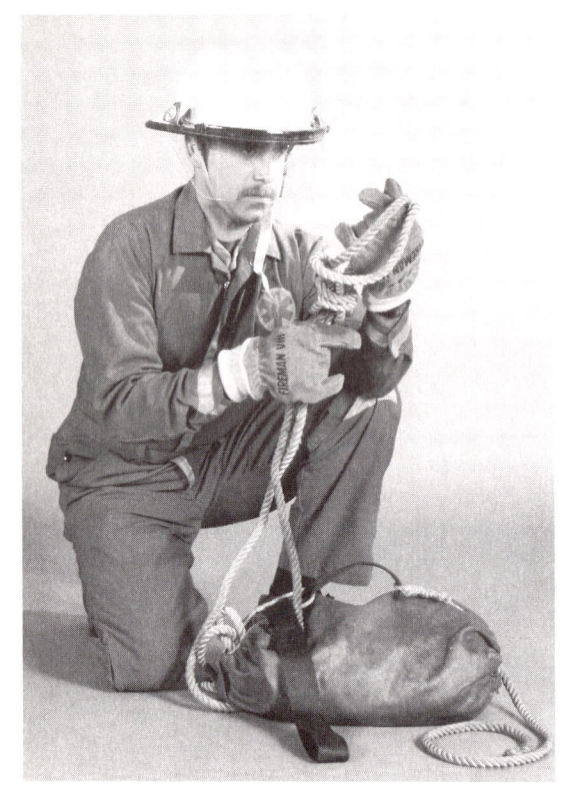

FIGURE 5-2.
Protective helmet designed for fire fighting is suitable for other forms of rescue work.

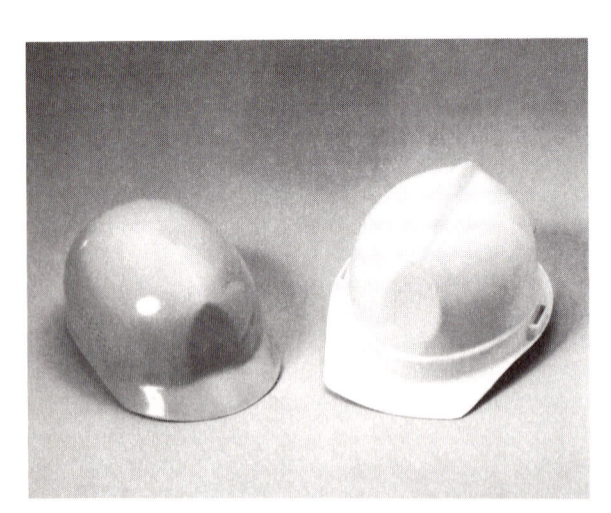

FIGURE 5-3.
"Hard" hats protect against scalp lacerations. (Courtesy of Parr Emergency Sales, Inc., Galloway, Ohio)

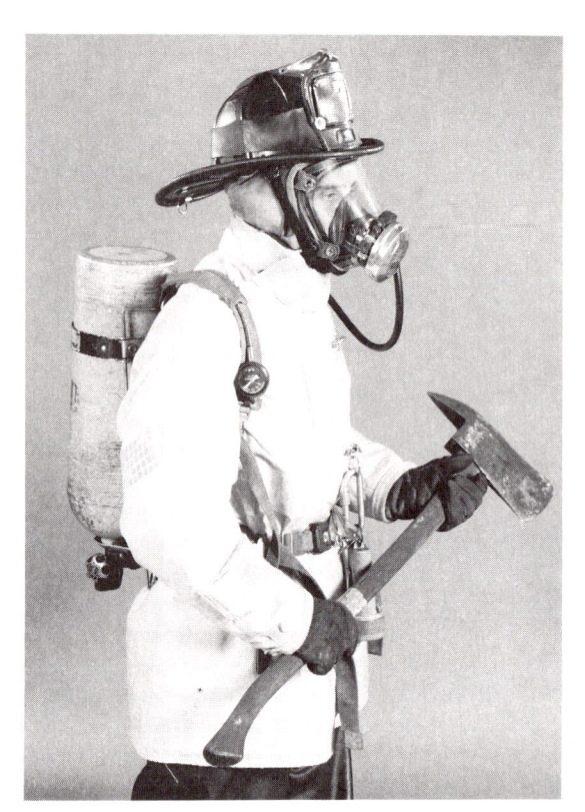

FIGURE 5-4.
The self-contained breathing apparatus (SCBA).

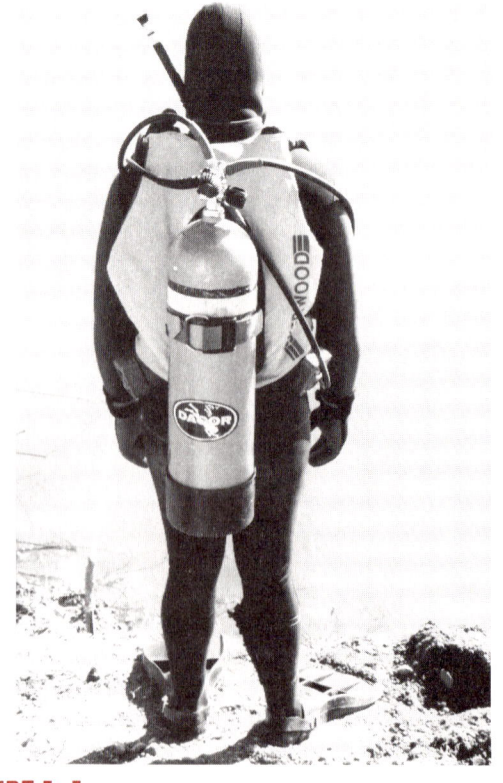

FIGURE 5-5.
The self-contained underwater breathing apparatus (SCUBA). (Courtesy of Indianapolis Fire Department)

the *self-contained underwater breathing apparatus (SCUBA)*, the term used by divers (Figs. 5-4 and 5-5).

Both the SCBA and SCUBA provide a totally enclosed system of air for use in a hazardous environment. The air is carried on the back of the rescuer in a tank under high pressure. The system includes control valves, pressure regulation, and air flow controls. Some systems for underwater and confined space or hazardous material situations permit the user to receive air through an attached hose line. This type of system reduces the weight and size of the compressed air cylinder carried by the user (the small air tank is used for escape or entry and is not the primary source of air) and at the same time gives an extended or unlimited supply of compressed air.

Working with respiratory protection in place requires practice. Paramedic rescuers need to know how to cope with the stress of restricted breathing, added weight, and confined visual space. They must become accustomed even to the filter and canister types of mask worn in certain industrial work settings.

Footwear

Rescue incidents expose the paramedic rescuer's feet to chemicals, biologic agents, pathogens, sharp objects, water, and unstable footing. Protective footwear must be selected to minimize the adverse effects of these hazards. One source of good protective footwear is from manufacturers that meet the specifications of footwear for structural fire fighting. These boots provide puncture-resistant barriers for the foot, crush resistance for the toes, cut resistance for the foot and ankle, and water penetration protection (Fig. 5-6). This type of boot is not the best for rugged terrain or mountain rescue; for most rural and urban rescue, however, these boots help minimize adverse effects on the feet and ankles.

Personal safety is a *professional obligation*. The medical professional must learn to anticipate and take actions that minimize the risk associated with the delivery of medical care in the rescue environment. An injured paramedic is a patient and not a care giver. A paramedic handicapped by heat or cold is not able to provide a sustained high level of care to the patient. Paramedics should review rescue incidents in their service areas, anticipate problems, and equip themselves with appropriate protective clothing to optimize their ability to provide quality patient care.

Patient Safety

Many hazards at the scene of a rescue must be considered regarding the safety and welfare of the patient. Initially and throughout the rescue process, patients must be protected from the environment in which they are found to prevent additional injury, heat loss, or inoculation of toxic products.

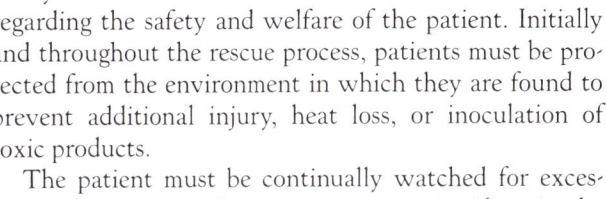

The patient must be continually watched for excessive heat loss. On almost every rescue incident in the winter, and even in summer when it is rainy and cool, heat loss can be a major problem. To prevent excessive heat loss (hypothermia), wet clothing should be removed as soon as safely possible and replaced by dry blankets. The head and trunk areas are of particular importance in the management of excessive heat loss. Waterproof protection to prevent additional evaporative and conductive heat losses must be provided, and the patient should be moved to a warm environment as soon as possible.

Hyperthermia can also be a serious threat to the health of a trapped patient in the extreme heat of a desert or a long hot spell in the inner city. Maintaining a near normal body temperature should be an important consideration during a rescue in all environments.

During rescue maneuvers, the patient and the paramedic must be covered and well protected against flying and falling debris and against the potential of injury from breaking or dislodged rescue equipment in the area. The barrier protection selected might be a wooden backboard or a thick blanket that protects from small, lightweight, flying particles such as glass, but also from sparks, fire, and pieces of metal. In many cases, it is helpful if the patient barrier protection is waterproof.

With smoke and toxic chemicals in the air, the patient's respiratory system must also be protected. In some cases, this protection necessitates the full exclusion of outside air by the use of a SCBA. An oxygen mask alone does not suffice because the oxygen promotes combustion in a fire, and oxygen masks do not provide facial protection, particularly protection of the eyes.

On-scene Hazards

It is easy to become wrapped up in the demands of a particular call so that personal safety is forgotten or ignored. Many types of on-scene **hazards** may be encountered by

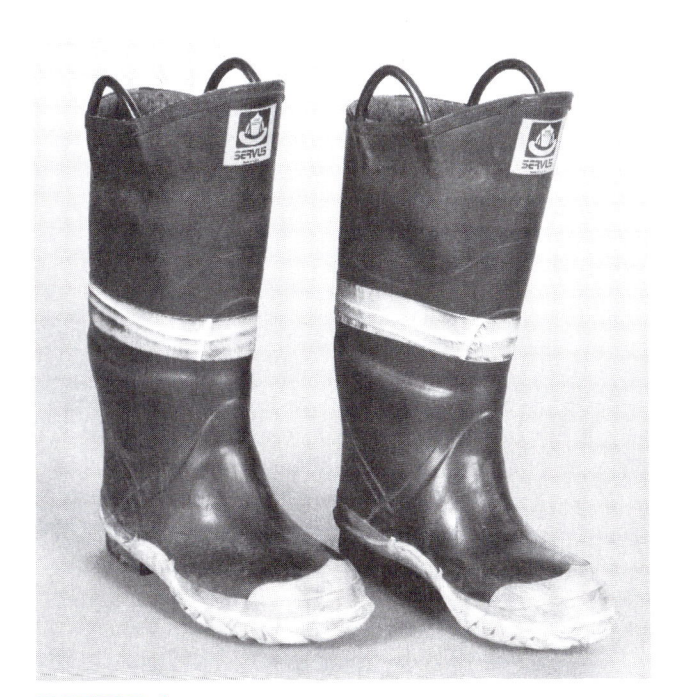

FIGURE 5-6.
Steel-toed, steel-shanked boots used in conjunction with bunker pants.

the paramedic. Chemicals and other hazardous agents are either in liquid or gas form and can present toxicity or burn problems. It is impossible to learn all of the various types of agents that may be encountered in a situation, and it is impossible to carry a book in every ambulance that describes all of these products. It is important for every paramedic to understand the general principles of management of chemicals and protection from them and to know how to access the poison control center from the scene to determine the management techniques to be used for specific hazardous materials at the scene.

Radiation produces a different set of problems for which general rules are easily learned. The specifics of any given situation, however, should be handled according to the peculiarities of the radiation source present. A local protocol must be developed, and each paramedic should become familiar with this protocol in regions where the possibility of radiation accidents exists.

Other environmental hazards include smoke, fire, and the threat of explosion. Vehicle ignitions, including those of motorcycles, should be turned off and fuel sources checked for leaks before any rescue operations are begun. While it is uncommon for vehicles to explode, it does happen. Caution should also be used when operating or working around power hydraulic rescue tools, pneumatic rescue tools, and any chain or cable under load. It is possible for sparks to ignite gasoline fumes that have leaked into the area. Bystanders with cigarettes in hand should be asked to put them out carefully and completely. All rescue personnel must be careful about the potential for fire when deploying flares at vehicular accident scenes. Explosions may also be caused by natural and manufactured gas, and patients must be quickly removed from the scene if this hazard is possible.

Electrical hazards must be handled only by personnel with specific expertise in this area. If a paramedic is not trained in the management of electrical equipment, the rescue must be delayed until properly trained assistance arrives. This procedure may be frustrating to follow, especially when the initial instinct is to get to the patient quickly. However, it can be disastrous for a paramedic to make ill-informed and foolhardy rescue efforts because a sense of urgency overwhelmed good judgment and reasoning.

Hazards such as broken or rotten stairways, unstable buildings, or dirt walls of a ditch can create difficult rescue situations. If, for example, a vehicle is found balanced on the edge of a precipice, the first priority must be to protect all rescuers from the risk of tumbling over the edge if the vehicle moves. The stabilization of vehicles and structures requires specific equipment and specially trained rescue teams.

In temperature extremes, the environment plays a critical role in the safety of both the patient and the rescuer. In cold temperatures, the patient must be protected from the temperature, the ice or snow, and from conditions such as an avalanche or icy lake. In the heat, a patient who is trapped or who must stay in the environment for a period of time should be cooled or at least protected from overheating. Heat stroke, with its associated dehydration and loss of temperature control, must be of concern to the paramedic. In hot weather, paramedics must drink large quantities of water and seek protection for themselves from the sun.

The bystander who wants to be helpful, but who does not know what to do, also creates a hazard at the scene of an accident. Bystanders may be given a passive role by having them provide psychological assistance to minimally injured patients. Uniformed bystanders can be given a more active role at the scene by allowing them to assist with crowd control, in some instances. It is important to remember that lay people are unaccustomed to emergency situations. Their safety must be guarded as well. Specific instructions must be given and their actions monitored at all times. Never expect too much of bystanders. If they perform well, it should be regarded as a bonus.

Occasionally, a situation may become hostile, and the paramedic must either request that law enforcement assist or must quickly move a patient to prevent a volatile situation from injuring the patient further.

ASSESSMENT OF THE SCENE

Assessment of the scene begins when the call is initially received. The communications operator should be able to provide the exact location and a general description for each call. The communications operator should also be encouraged to get an estimate of the number of patients, known hazards, and which rescue operations may be needed. Obtaining a relatively precise nature of the call helps minimize unnecessary surprises and gives responders time to consider options while en route.

Even though the initial call for help indicates a scenario that requires rescue, some systems have the first arriving team confirm the need for additional resources before having them sent. This procedure depends on the response time. The response time may be so long that the communications operator is forced to make an educated guess and send additional help based on the caller's perception of the situation. However, it saves system resources to wait whenever possible until trained personnel can judge the needs of the scene firsthand.

Assessment also includes the need to decide if a mass casualty situation will overstress the capabilities of the local EMS system. In some areas, a mass casualty incident exists when more than two stretchers are needed for patients, because only one ambulance is available. Rescue options may include mutual aid response from a nearby community or air evacuation. If so, these resources must be requested quickly so they can arrive at the scene as soon as possible.

On arrival at the scene, before exiting the vehicle, the paramedic has an opportunity to reassess the information received and the capabilities of managing the situation without additional help. Requests for additional help should be placed before leaving the vehicle if it is likely that they will be needed. Other factors that must be considered include the following:

- Time of day
- Traffic conditions
- Time and distance to the hospital
- Number of people expected on the scene
- Possible hostile nature of the scene
- Lighting expectations on the scene

When backup crews have been requested, the paramedic must establish the best route into the scene. This depends on the nature of the situation as well as such factors as rush hour traffic. The best entrance may not be the front door or the street where the paramedics first arrived. It should be kept in mind that backup ambulances must also leave. Therefore, it is best to have them all come from the same direction so they can exit efficiently.

The final decision that must be made at the scene, before exiting the vehicle, is the possible need for specialized transportation, such as a helicopter. Traffic conditions, weather, and driving time to the medical facility are factors that must be considered when this decision is being made. If it is determined that helicopter transportation may be required, helicopter dispatch should be alerted so that initial steps to mobilize the helicopter crew can be taken early.

Failure to take these steps before leaving the vehicle can put the paramedic in a precarious situation. If patient assessment is begun before the request for backup is made, patient care will suffer. It is as great a mistake in priorities of patient care to not call for backup on arrival at the scene if it is needed as it is to splint a fractured leg before initiating airway management.

The paramedic should be careful not to develop *tunnel vision* directed only at the medical aspects of patient care. Total medical evaluation of the patient includes caring for the whole patient, not just one component. The EMS system takes into consideration not only the medical care needed, but extrication, rescue, patient protection, and all factors necessary to assure that the patient is transported to the correct hospital as rapidly as possible.

Paramedics are not required to be heroes. They must recognize personal limitations, both in physical ability and in knowledge. Not everyone can be hazardous materials experts, and everyone cannot always handle a lifting problem. Paramedics should never try to bluff when providing care to people who depend on them for their lives and well-being.

GAINING ACCESS

When the scene evaluation has been completed and steps have been taken to assure its management and control, attention can be turned to the specific medical needs of the patient. This procedure begins, as does all other initial management of patient care, with the primary survey of responsiveness, airway, breathing, and circulation. To provide such evaluation, access to the patient must be gained. Gaining access depends on the situation in which the patient is found and the impediments that exist between the rescuer and patient. These must be analyzed, and a quick pathway to the patient must be created, not for removal of the patient, but for the rescuer to gain access to the patient and begin initial medical care. Creating a small portal of entry, which is perhaps even tortuous, is often easier and quicker than creating a large hole through which a patient can be removed.

Mechanisms to gain access to the patient and the use of special techniques and equipment when dealing with structural collapse and wilderness or underwater rescue are subjects of technical training courses within themselves and are not included in this chapter. The reader is referred to specialty courses for specific education in the individual areas required by the potential working environment.

At times, it is necessary for the paramedic to stand by while access to the patient is achieved. If the paramedic does not have the necessary skills, such as technical rock climbing expertise, to allow safe access to the patient, the wisest approach is to wait for those with the appropriate technical skills to access, manage, and transport the patient out (Fig. 5-7). Special rescuers may lose sight of patient care because of the demands of the rescue operation. It may be appropriate for the paramedic to ask for frequent updates on patient status and management to help balance the priorities of the rescuers.

Rescue operations proceed more smoothly if the people involved with each specialty team know one another before an emergency. Cross continuing education is a good way to enhance relations between groups. Paramedics should investigate the special resources in their service area and build a rapport with these personnel ahead of time. In this manner, unrealistic expectations on all sides can be reduced, and respect for the expertise of all parties can be built.

After the primary assessment has been completed, unless the environment or rescue tactics dictate otherwise, oxygen should be started with an appropriate device to maintain adequate oxygenation. The ability to totally evaluate the patient at this point is limited. Therefore,

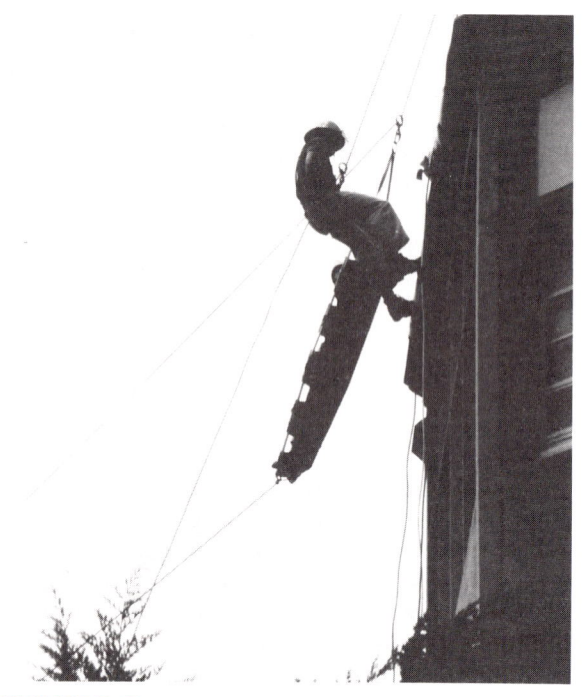

FIGURE 5–7.
Technical skills may be required for specialized forms of rescue.

adequate oxygenation should be used prophylactically. Patient assessment during the secondary survey is carried out while steps for disentanglement are started. Two jobs must now be accomplished simultaneously: packaging for identified fractures and packaging for extrication.

Extrication preparation is accomplished by one team, while disentanglement is accomplished by another. The types of splints and immobilization devices used must be dictated by the specific problems of patient removal and disentanglement. A typical rescue litter for high-rise, confined-space, or steep-terrain rescue is shown in Figure 5-8. It can be hoisted or lowered in either a vertical or

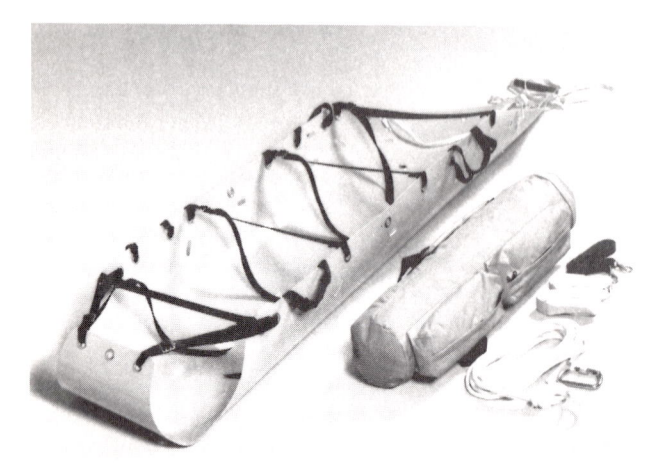

FIGURE 5–8.
A rescue litter. (Courtesy of Parr Emergency Sales, Inc., Galloway, Ohio)

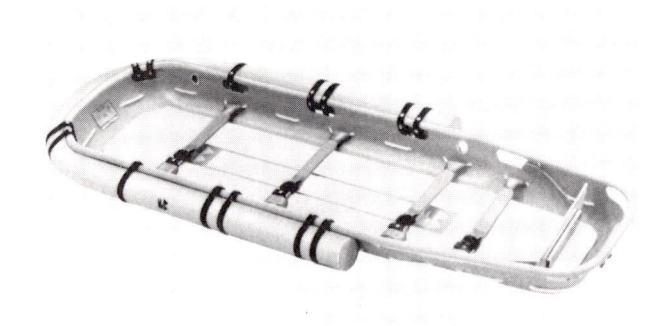

FIGURE 5–9.
A floating rescue litter. (Courtesy of Parr Emergency Sales, Inc., Galloway, Ohio)

horizontal position. The rescue litter shown in Figure 5-9 accommodates a backboard and floats.

DISENTANGLEMENT

The ***disentanglement*** phase of a rescue, whether it is needed for an automobile accident, collapsed building, cave-in, or airplane accident, is the most technical of the phases of rescue and requires a great deal of training for the specific types of rescue. Preplanning is required for disentanglement to be conducted smoothly and efficiently. Technical expertise available in the paramedic's local area includes some or all of the following:

Mountain Search and Rescue (Fig. 5-10)
Extrication Units
Dive Teams
Cave and Mine Rescue Teams
National Ski Patrol (Fig. 5-11)

Whenever possible, the constraining forces on the patient must be removed, rather than the patient removed from these forces. Using the automobile as an example, the door of the car can be removed from the patient's side, seat pulled back toward the rear of the car, and the dash or steering column bent out of the way if necessary to remove a patient safely. Disentanglement in this example means that the car is removed from the patient. The techniques and problems of disentanglement vary widely with the existing situation, location of the emergency, and the surrounding environment. Unique individual situations cannot be covered in this chapter. The reader is referred to appropriate works and courses that teach specialized rescue techniques.

REMOVAL

After the patient has been adequately immobilized and devices have been placed around the patient for stabilization, a final evaluation of the patient's condition must

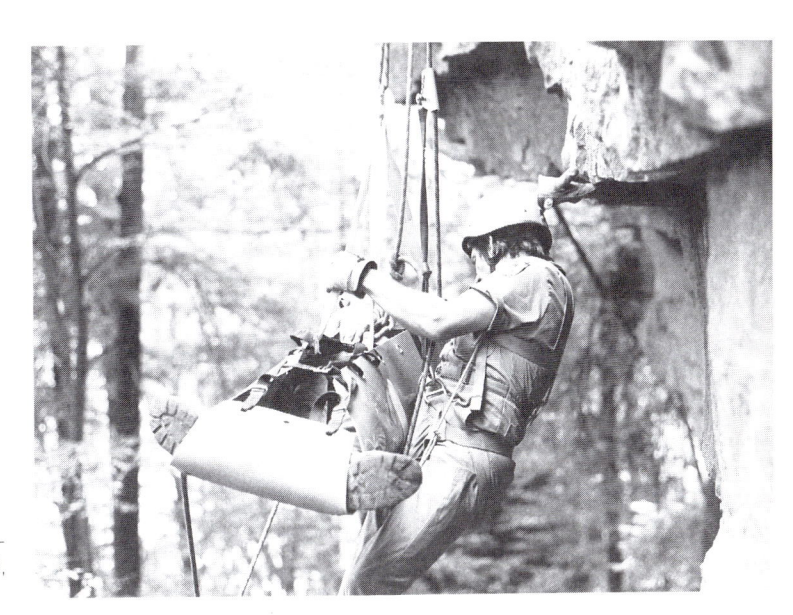

FIGURE 5-10.
An example of a mountain search and rescue team delivering patient care. (Courtesy of Skedco, Inc., Portland, Oregon)

be made by the rescuer. The patient is then removed and loaded into an ambulance for transportation to the hospital. The type of packaging required, technique of removal (**extrication**), and patient protection during the removal vary according to the conditions that prevail.

At times, rapid extrication from an automobile is necessitated by the patient's initial condition or deterioration. Manual techniques, without immobilization devices, become the priority. Rapid extrication from an automobile can be accomplished safely by using three or four rescuers to provide stabilization of the spine and other parts of the body while the patient is rotated and moved onto a long backboard. Paramedics should become familiar with this and other accepted techniques of patient handling.

EMERGENCY CARE AND TRANSPORTATION

Once a patient has been removed, time must not be wasted at the scene to provide comprehensive medical care. The airway must be secured, and it is acceptable to apply the anti-shock garment at the scene. Other prehospital care of the severely traumatized patient, including intravenous lines, splinting, and so on, must be provided during transport. Patients with injuries not of a life-threatening nature should be splinted and packaged appropriately before removal and transport.

The type of transportation to the appropriate trauma center or other hospital is dictated by the availability of transportation, time and distance from the medical facility, environmental conditions, and other factors. In the wilderness and remote areas, helicopter transportation frequently is beneficial. For specifics of patient care, the use of helicopters, and the requirements of setting up such a system, see Chapter 2.

SUMMARY

Rescue and extrication activities are an adjunctive part of prehospital care. Some EMS systems provide these specialized services themselves, others do not. In some areas, first responders are the rescue experts, in others, it may

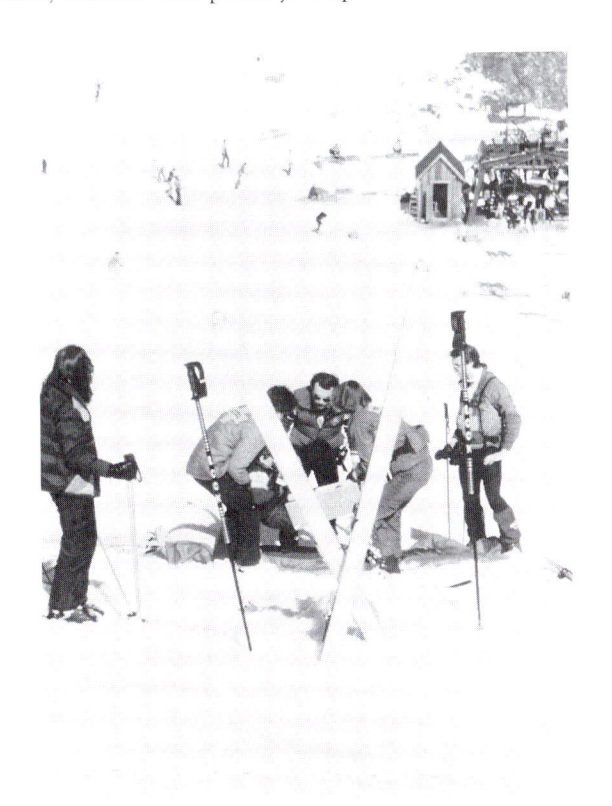

FIGURE 5-11.
An example of a National Ski Patrol delivering patient care.

be the police. It is vital to investigate the availability of these services and to have a good working relationship with those personnel who provide rescue services.

If a particular scene is outside the usual resources of a paramedic's system, these limitations must be acknowledged. Appropriate personnel must be summoned and allowed to do their job. In many cases, the paramedic may be able to gain access to the patient while disentanglement is being accomplished, so that assessment and emergency management procedures may be started as soon as possible. If this action is impossible, the paramedic should stand back and trust that the rescue team is doing its best to provide appropriate and timely rescue.

SUGGESTED READING

Abrid WW: Managing rescue tools. Chief Fire Executive 3(2):46, 1988

Bronstein AC, Currance PL: Emergency Care for Hazardous Materials Exposure. St. Louis, CV Mosby, 1988

Dextras PA: Daring rescue from grain elevator. Fire Command 55(12):20, 1988

Donelan S: The rescue trainer. Rescue 3(3):28, 1990

Gordon D: High-rise fire rescue: Lesson from Las Vegas. Emergency Medical Services 15(5):20, 1986

Henky M: Alert 3: A 727 in the dirt. Fire Command 55(12):26, 1988

Kidd JS, Czajkowski JD: Commanding the extrication scene. J Emerg Med Serv 12(2):30, 1987

Occupational Safety and Health Administration: NFPA firefighter rules require equipment that saves lives. Occup Health Saf 56(9):30, 1987

Smith MG, Andrews R: Rural rescue: Tractor rollovers. J Emerg Med Serv 11(1):27, 1986

Sullivan J: Fire and rescue operations at the terrorist incident. American Fire Journal 40(9):22, 1989

Sundberg C: Mass casualty response: A case study. J Emerg Med Serv 2(9):33, 1986

US Department of Transportation, National Highway Traffic Safety Administration: Emergency Medical Technician-Paramedic: National Standards Curriculum. Washington, DC, US Government Printing Office, 1985

CHAPTER 6

Disaster Management

Defining Levels of Intensity
   Emergency
   Major Incident
   Disaster
The Disaster Plan
   Phase I: The Preplan
      Hazard Analysis
      Resource Inventory
   Triage

Phase II: The Response Plan
   Scene Management Considerations
      Patient Care Areas
      Morgue
      Ambulance Staging
      Ambulance Loading
      Medical Supply Pool
      Manpower Staging and Canteen
      Command Post
   Analysis of Actual Disaster Incidents
      Communication
      Control and Command
      Congestion
      Collection of Resources
      Coordination of Triage and Transportation

Phase III: The Postdisaster Plan
Summary

BEHAVIORAL OBJECTIVES
On successful completion of this chapter, the reader will be able to:
1. List the characteristics of an emergency, major incident, and disaster
2. Explain the preplanning process in a disaster
3. Describe hazard analysis and the components of a resource inventory
4. Describe the different types of triage systems
5. Explain the importance of triage tagging systems
6. Explain the response plan in a disaster
7. Describe the issues to consider when establishing command sites
8. Explain scene management considerations in a disaster
9. List the five common problems generic to all incidents
10. Describe the postdisaster plan
11. Define all of the key terms listed in this chapter

KEY TERMS

The following terms are defined in the chapter and glossary:

critical incidents
Critical Incident Stress Debriefing (CISD)
disaster
emergency
Incident Command System (ICS)
major incident
triage

Historically, medical disaster management has referred to the coordination and prioritization of the medical treatment and transportation of large numbers of victims during times of natural and man-made catastrophes. Disasters offer the supreme test and challenge to emergency medical services (EMS) capabilities. Commonly, new relationships must quickly be established, often between agencies that do not routinely work together. By nature, disasters are complex events that are constantly changing, requiring management plans that are flexible and adaptive to any and all situations. Most important, agencies must constantly learn from local and national incidents and update and adjust their plans accordingly. Lessons learned by other agencies provide valuable information about mistakes and problems encountered by others during similar events. Ultimately, local providers must avoid complacency and realize that disasters can and do happen in their communities.

DEFINING LEVELS OF INTENSITY

The application of disaster management principles must begin with the operational definition of disaster and its levels of intensity. A **disaster** is any event that overwhelms existing manpower, facilities, equipment, and capabilities of a responding agency or institution. It is important to note that a particular level of intensity for one community may not be the same for another. For instance, what may be a routine incident for one agency may be a major incident for another if the number of victims overwhelms existing and available resources. This example is best illustrated by comparing the response capabilities of a rural area to that of a large urban community. In addition, the availability of hospitals and trauma centers ultimately affects patient survival rates.

The following sections describe types of intensity levels that involve EMS response. These levels involve routine incidents (emergencies), major incident situations (often described as disasters), and disasters.

Emergency

An **emergency** is defined as a situation that could not have been reasonably foreseen, threatens public health, welfare, or safety, and requires immediate action. Examples are victims of accidents, shootings, stabbings, and fires. Characteristics of emergencies include the following:

- Single incident site with one, clear jurisdictional authority
- Multi-casualty incident (MCI) and fatalities
- Involves normal agency chain of command
- No mutual aid is required from outside agencies

Priorities in managing an emergency include controlling any on-going hazards, creating a safety zone, locating, accessing, triaging, and transporting victims, and documenting the operation per local protocols.

Major Incident

A ***major incident*** is an event that causes injury or death and damage to property or environment to a degree greater than that which occurs on a routine basis. These events can be natural, as in floods, hurricanes, tornadoes (Fig. 6-1), or earthquakes, or man-made, as in fires, accidents (Fig. 6-2, 6-3), or explosions. The term major incident is sometimes used interchangeably with the term disaster. The fine line between the definitions of a major incident and a disaster is often related to the specific numbers of victims. Unfortunately, this variable is vague and specific to local jurisdictions and not applicable in a generic sense. Each agency must determine what is a major incident based on its own resources, including manpower, equipment, facilities, and communications capabilities. However, the general characteristics of a major incident are the following:

- A single event that involves one or more incident sites that have overlapping jurisdictional boundaries
- Local prehospital care response system is taxed and overloaded
- More patients exist than can be handled by responding units
- Mutual aid required from outside agencies
- Specific situations, such as hazardous materials and chemical spills, need for special resources, such as dog search and rescue teams, specialized rescue teams that deal in mine and trench situations, and one or more helicopters for transportation

The management priorities used in handling a major incident are similar to those used in an emergency. However, priorities are met through mutual aid with other EMS providers and fire agencies, law enforcement, and other resources, such as construction companies, public

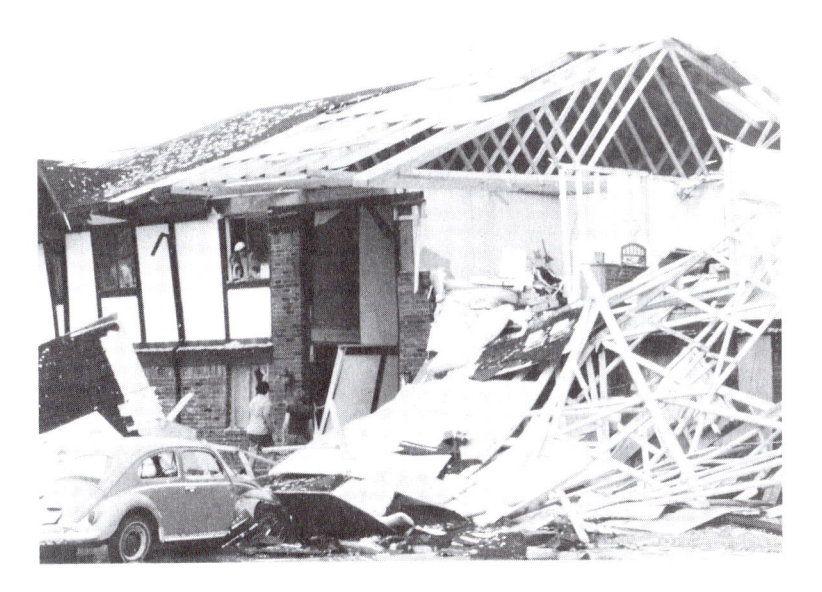

FIGURE 6-1.
Tornado damage of a 150-unit apartment complex.

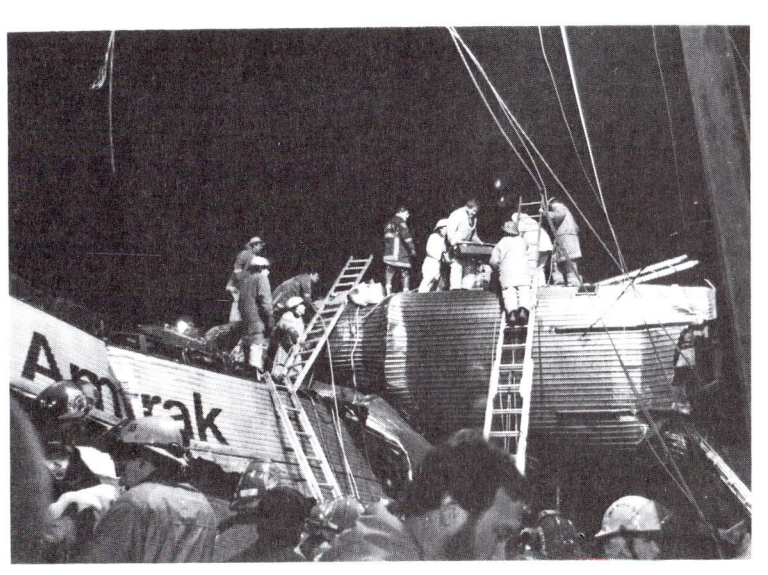

FIGURE 6-2.
Amtrak derailment. (Courtesy of Maryland Institute for Emergency Medical Services Systems)

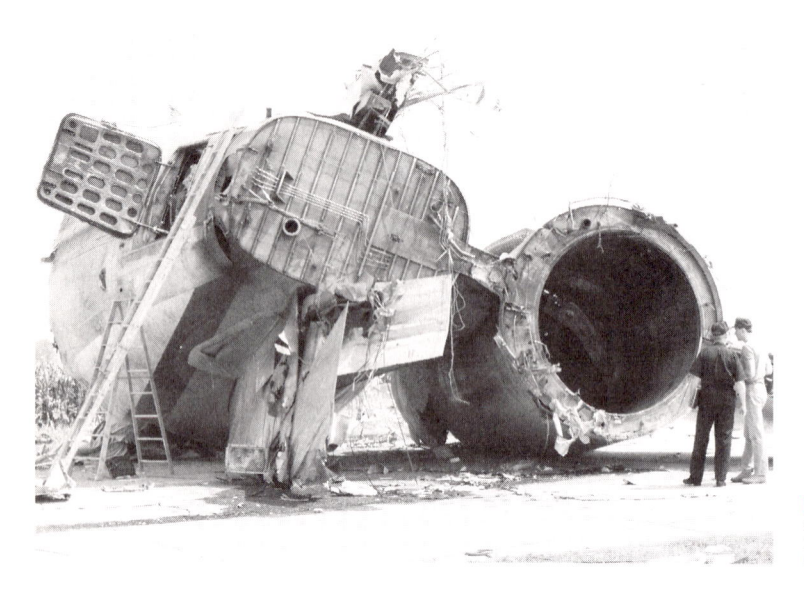

FIGURE 6-3.
Sioux City, Iowa, plane crash. (Courtesy of James J. McCue)

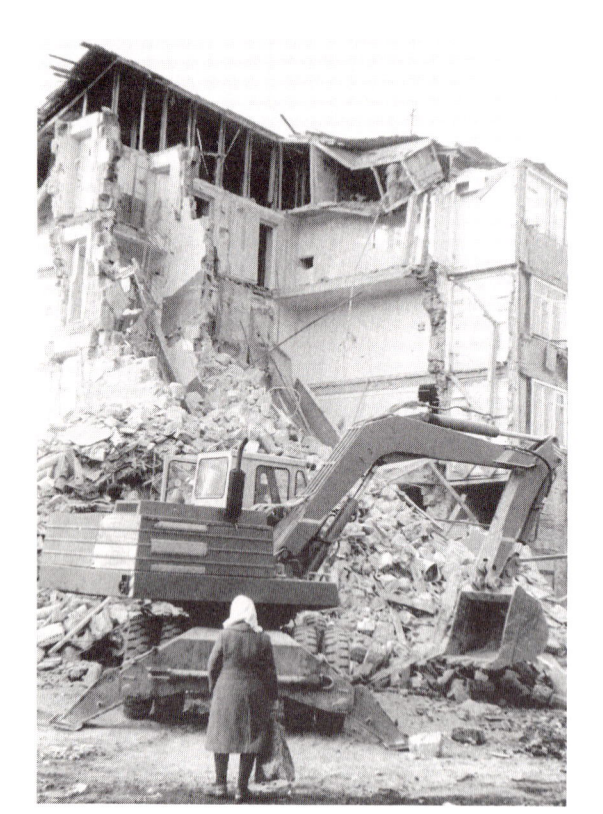

utilities, architects, mass transit agencies, and experts from different fields.

Disaster

A disaster may disrupt both the structure and function of a community and, many times, requires the assistance of outside agencies, usually state and federal, to manage the incident and its aftermath. Damage, injury, and loss of life or property, generally, are widespread. Classically, these incidents include hurricanes, earthquakes (Fig. 6-4), tornadoes, and large destructive explosions or accidents, such as airplane crashes into residential communities. Some agencies define disasters purely on a numeric level. For instance, in one area of the country, local operational definitions include the following:

Expanded medical emergency: 5 to 15 patients, 5 with critical injuries
Major medical emergency: 16 to 50 patients
Medical disaster: more than 51 patients

It is often difficult to accurately count the number of victims present at the scene. Estimates are always part of the initial size-up, but accuracy is usually in doubt and must constantly be updated.

The characteristics of a disaster are the following:

- Multiple or widespread incident sites that may overlap multiple jurisdictions and boundaries
- Usually involves mass casualties and fatalities
- Requires interagency coordination and management; secondary levels of management, such as emergency operation centers, are instituted by local, county, state, and federal agencies as necessary
- Mutual aid response necessary to cover the incident site and normal community services; mutual aid to involve local jurisdictions, county, state, and federal re-

FIGURE 6-4.
An earthquake that registered 6.9 on the Richter scale tore through the Iron Curtain at 11:41 AM Armenian standard time, December 7, 1988. An estimated 100,000 people were injured, dead, or missing. The all-volunteer Seattle–King County (Washington) Disaster Team and Alaska's SEADOGS joined with search and rescue experts from the Soviet Union, Armenia, Belgium, France, Greece, United Kingdom, Austria, and Yugoslavia in an unprecedented international effort. A woman is shown with belongings from her apartment as a back hoe moves rubble. (Courtesy of Judith Reid Graves)

sources; in some extraordinary situations foreign aid may be offered

Management principles and priorities in a disaster are similar to those of major incidents. However, disasters involve a massive effort of multiple coordinating agencies and jurisdictions. Operations may last several days, weeks, or months. Usually, traditional public safety services are unable to meet the demands for service. Basic first aid, search, and rescue are provided by citizens during the first 12 to 72 hours or longer, depending on the incident. In situations such as earthquakes, additional tremors may generate more victims and threaten the safety of rescuers.

THE DISASTER PLAN

The real concern for disaster management is not the controversy over the different terminology but rather the development and implementation of a well-researched and prepared disaster plan. The development of the plan can be divided into three phases. Phase I is known as the preplan, Phase II, the response plan, and Phase III, the postdisaster plan. Local disaster preparedness involves a variety of agencies, organizations, and individuals working together. It is through this preparedness process that the community is guaranteed a fully articulated plan that includes all possible providers of services.

Phase I: The Preplan

Disaster planning begins with an honest and unbiased evaluation of existing resources and capabilities of public safety providers and local emergency facilities. The committee that gathers and evaluates resources should consider all types of services available in the community. These include representatives of local public service agencies (law, fire, and EMS), public health agencies, hospitals, local Red Cross and Salvation Army, volunteer search and rescue groups, amateur radio operators (RACES), and other concerned groups. Also included may be church groups in rural areas, housing authority, school districts, local media, general contractors capable of supplying heavy rescue tools and vehicles, public utilities, state or federal agencies, and local military units.

The committee must take into consideration the specific resources and capabilities of an agency or group available during daylight vs. nighttime hours, weekday vs. weekend periods, and holidays. Most important, they must look at realistic response times. In particular, they must avoid the pitfall of tabulating all available resources in one community, including those on a "reserve" or on-call basis. These resources are usually the last to be available. Consideration should be given to the possibility of simultaneous events. It is indefensible to commit all resources to an individual incident. Other resources and staffing must be left available to respond to routine events and simultaneous and multiple site situations.

Preplanning includes an analysis of how a major incident or disaster may be defined for a particular region or community. Other factors to consider are incidents that also include areas of minimal lighting, difficulties in extrication and accessing of victims, secondary explosions, large scale evacuations, hazardous materials and chemicals, and extreme adverse weather conditions. It is crucial that the response plan take into account a variety of incident types and be broad enough to allow for adaptation to any and all events.

The preplanning process should provide an analysis of the conditions discussed in the following sections.

Hazard Analysis

Local hazards to the community must be identified as potential disaster risks. These include the transit, manufacturing, and storage of hazardous materials; mass transit vehicles, airports, and railroad systems; local fire threats and other potential natural phenomena, such as tornadoes, hurricanes, floods, and earthquakes; and local violent elements, such as gangs and drug labs. Each community presents its own unique profile for disaster risks, no matter how small or large.

Resource Inventory

Resource inventory takes many forms and includes manpower, equipment, facilities, and communications availability. Special resources need to be identified during the preplan to guarantee their availability and access during an actual event. Realistic response times and manpower mobilization must be scrutinized and acknowledged. The resources to inventory include the following:

- Air evacuation
- Aeronautical evacuation and rescue
- Shelter and mass feeding
- Hazardous materials management
- Search and rescue
- Heavy rescue equipment
- Lighting and adverse weather equipment
- Medical equipment and supplies
- Mental health services
- Communications network

Triage

Triage is a process of prioritization of medical care, treatment, and transportation. Its purpose is to sort large numbers of victims and maximize limited resources to do the most good for those best able to survive serious injuries. It is not meant for emergency personnel to perform heroics and save those who have obvious life-threatening injuries that are considered lethal and nonviable. Triage can be performed both by those with minimal medical training and those with advanced degrees. However, it is imperative that all on-scene personnel practice the same form of triage, or they may find themselves in conflict.

A number of *triage systems* have been developed over the years. Most were influenced by the military numeric system. Types of numeric systems of triage included numbering of patients (based on severity of injuries) from 1 to 5, 1 to 4, or 0 to 3. Numeric and color-coded (black, yellow, green, red) systems present problems since there is little free association for the rescuer, and colors and numbers become confusing during the stress of an incident. In addition, different agencies may use various color systems for triage that are not compatible during an incident.

Recently, a system of "*common language*" has become more popular. Examples of this system are the easily understood terms "urgent" vs. "nonurgent" and "immediate" vs. "delayed." The benefit of this system is the free association or memory triggers of the words themselves. Most important, untrained or uninitiated personnel can more easily understand the intent of the words when suddenly put into the situation of assisting with triage or transportation.

Historically, triage categorization was based on specific injuries and assumed diagnosis of injuries. For example, a victim with a tension pneumothorax or ruptured spleen would be considered a high-priority patient. The problem with categorization by injury (or anatomical assessment) is the inability of both field and hospital personnel to diagnose without in-depth medical assessment and evaluation. In the past few years, triage has turned away from an injury evaluation format to an evaluation of the patient's clinical presentation, regardless of the injuries seen. This system is known as Simple Triage and Rapid Treatment (START). It categorizes patients based on the evaluation of three parameters: level of consciousness, respiratory status, and perfusion status (Fig. 6-5). A patient who displays an abnormal status in any one or more of the three parameters is designated as a high-priority patient (*immediate*). A patient who displays no abnormal findings in any of the three assessment parameters becomes a lower-priority patient (*delayed*). However, one pitfall to avoid with START is the classification of all unconscious patients as "immediate." Pupils first must be assessed for signs of neurologic death. Only patients who have altered mental status or who are unconscious without evidence of brain death would be triaged as "immediate care." The following are examples of patients triaged under START:

Patient 1: Unconscious with unequal pupils, normal respiratory status, delayed capillary refill with tachycardia
Decision: Immediate care category
Patient 2: Normal mental status with anxiety, normal respiratory status, normal capillary refill with slight tachycardia (pulse 100)
Decision: Delayed care category
Patient 3: Unconscious, fixed and dilated pupils, abnormal respiratory status, delayed capillary refill
Decision: Delayed care category (nonviable with massive neurologic injuries)

Notice that the START system makes no mention of the victim's specific or assumed injuries. Therefore, START triage is based solely on the patient's presenting clinical condition (or physical response to the injuries incurred). START is not meant as a secondary triage system but rather as a method for initial triage during the early phases of an incident. Secondary triage and evaluation can take into consideration the types of injuries and hemodynamic status. Triage should be based on the potential for survival, without the immediate availability of heroic medical management, and the need for expeditious medical management. Triage should assess the patient's clinical condition, determine the urgency (priority) of that condition as it relates to other victims, assign priority of field treatment, and determine the disposition of the patient.

Once a triage system has been established and training programs developed, a *triage tagging system* must also be considered and planned. Many triage tags have been developed over the years. The most popular is the "Mettag" (Fig. 6-6). However, this tag uses the number-color system for triage. Controversy over triage tags exists because the need and use for the tag are unclear. Some tags are simply "filing" systems so that patients are "filed" or triaged into the appropriate category; others are used as mini medical records in addition to tags for sorting victims. Determine which tags are most efficient for your particular system. No triage system is complete unless an analogous triage tag is included in the development and training. Triage tags are necessary to document the destination of the victim (category), identify the victim by a number and not a name, and provide, if desired, a brief description of injuries and treatment rendered at the scene.

Phase II: The Response Plan

Once the preplan phase has been completed, a response plan or disaster management plan can be developed. Standard operation plans are constantly evaluated and updated. They are reworked based on drills, both table top and practical, critiques of actual incidents, and lessons learned and shared by other agencies. The response plan should never be considered static. It should always be evolving and updated. A good plan allows for flexibility and coordination with other agencies and jurisdictions. Its application should be practical and should adhere to present standards of practice.

The immediate priority of first on-scene personnel is to communicate a "size-up" to the dispatch center. The ad-

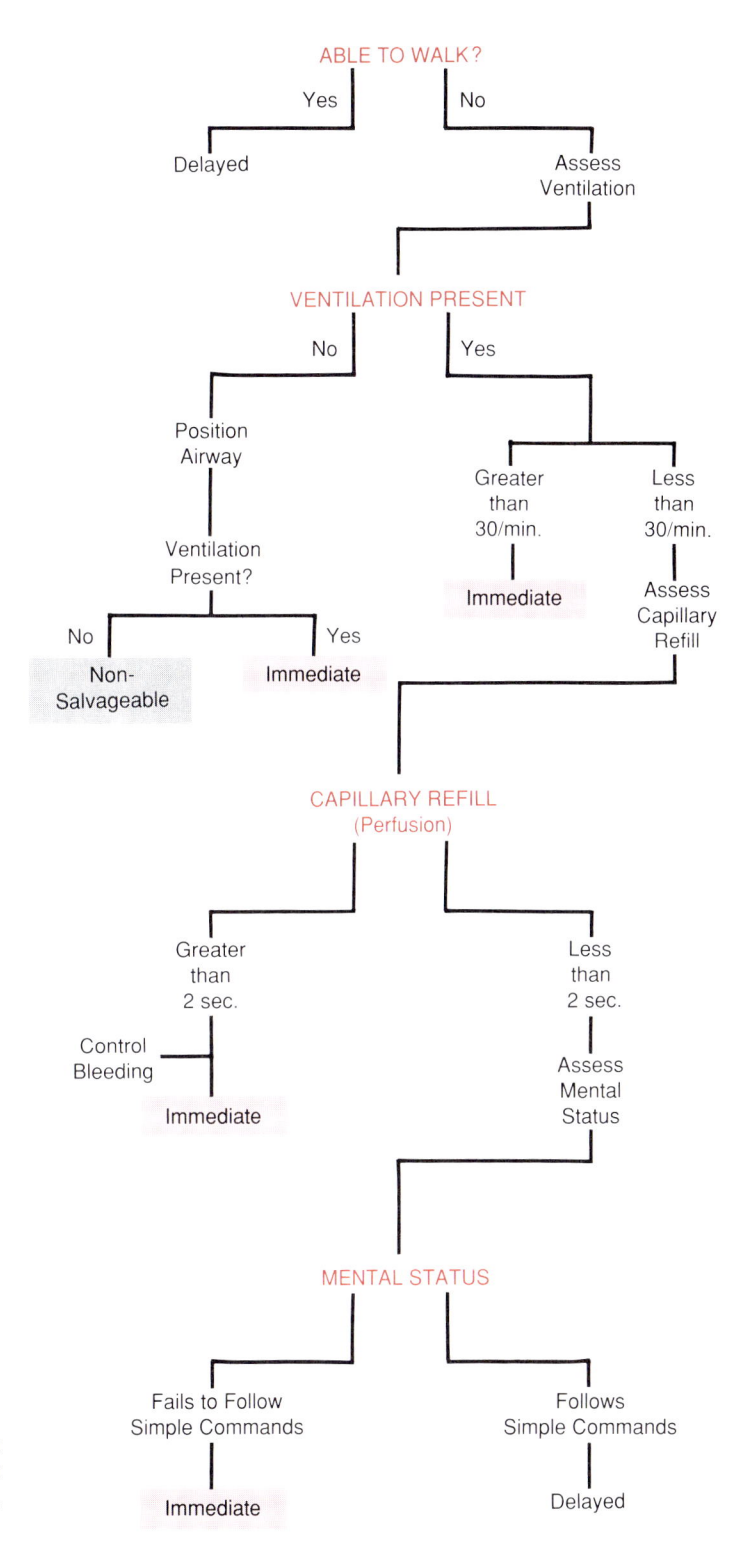

FIGURE 6–5.
The START triage system. (Adapted from Cleary V, Hewett M, Schmehl A: START Instructor's Manual, 2nd ed. Newport Beach, California, Hoag Memorial Hospital Presbyterian, 1984)

age of "scoop and run" no longer applies. Communications must take priority over patient care and triage. The initial size-up must include the following:

WHAT happened: A concise, accurate account of what the incident is and what has happened. This would include the possibility of hazardous materials, secondary explosions, additional dangers to arriving units, and making the incident clear to the dispatcher.

WHAT resources are needed: Concise, accurate directive of what type of fire, EMS, and law enforcement units and other specialty resources for rescue, shelter, and transportation are needed.

WHERE it happened: Concise and accurate location of

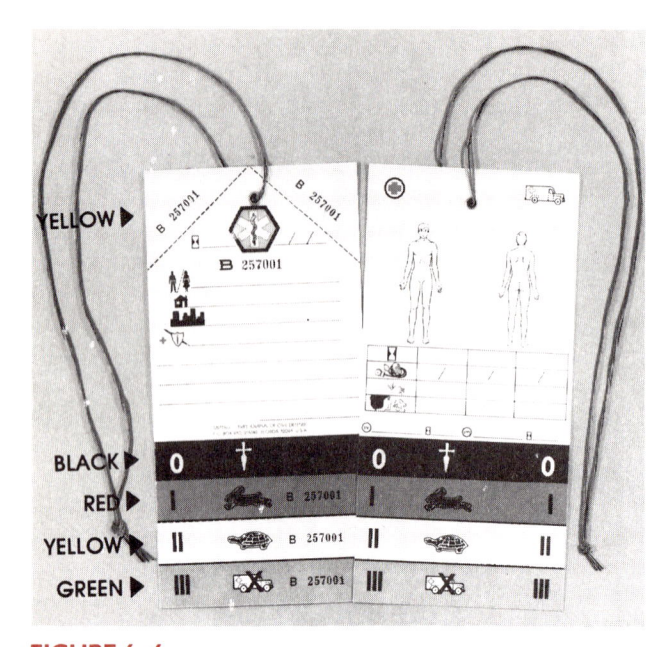

FIGURE 6–6.
Mettag triage tagging system. (Courtesy of Mettag, Starke, Florida)

the incident site, including cross streets, floor location, and major geographic landmarks. This information is crucial for a timely response from first and secondary responders.

HOW many victims are involved: This information does not have to be concise or even accurate. Estimate real and potential victims. If applicable, specify victim types, such as children (e.g., school bus incident), elderly, or handicapped.

Activation for disaster response is the primary responsibility of the first responding units. If units first attempt triage or rescue, they lose valuable time in mobilizing desperately needed resources. Once the priority of calling for additional units has been completed, first arriving units can initiate the process of fire suppression, search and rescue, extrication, and triage. Concurrently, command is established under the agency's standards of operation. Most popular with public service agencies is a process of command called the **Incident Command System (ICS)**. The highest ranking officer for each agency is designated as the incident commander (IC), and each share responsibility for scene management. Depending on the situation, one IC manages overall command, and the other ICs assist and facilitate coordination between the agencies. Within the ICS, a medical division operates and functions under its own unit leader. In this chapter, the general principles that guide command or leadership positions during the medical operations of a disaster are discussed.

The medical unit leader (or in some areas known as medical commander or supervisor) is responsible for managing the delivery of EMS and coordinating efforts between various prehospital care personnel and hospital facilities. The medical unit leader works directly with the incident commander and advises and updates command on EMS activities, manpower needs, and equipment. The medical component of the ICS is responsible for setting up medical command, triage, staging, and transportation. The following issues must be considered when establishing command sites:

1. The command post should be in an area that is not directly involved or near the incident site. The area must be remote enough not to be influenced or affected by the disaster site but close enough to maintain communications and control.

2. Access to land lines, secure and accessible roadways, and safety from potential hazards of falling debris, flooding, toxic material, and fire are essential.

Areas for staging of patient care and triage should be established using the following guidelines:

1. Area should be large enough to adequately handle the number of victims involved and capable of being expanded as needed to accommodate additional victims not previously anticipated.

2. Area should be free from further danger of falling debris, flooding, toxic material and smoke, and fire.

3. Area should be easily accessible to transport vehicles and personnel.

4. Psychological impact of the disaster should be minimized by placing the staging area away from morgue area and other disturbing sights. While this positioning is not always feasible or even realistic, the psychological impact should be taken into consideration when establishing staging areas.

5. Nonambulatory victims should be placed side by side, approximately 3 feet apart, in designated areas (immediate, delay). This linear approach allows for a more organized and systemic method for triage treatment.

Crucial to the establishment of *command posts* and *staging areas* is the clear identification of these areas and designated personnel. Areas may be established in an appropriate manner; however, if they are not clearly designated and identified, they become less effective and efficient. It is imperative that the medical unit leader take a manager's perspective and step back, assess the situation, avoid tunnel vision, and look at the "*big picture.*" The manager is not necessarily the doer but is the organizer and leader. If managers get involved in direct patient care, then they stop being managers.

Scene Management Considerations

The size of a specific incident (number of victims involved and the surrounding geography) determines the size of the management structure needed to organize the scene. In a large-scale incident, the management structure is more involved and diverse. However, no matter the size of an incident, the ICS is applicable, particularly the medical management component. In disaster operations, the medical manager must establish the sites discussed in the following sections.

PATIENT CARE AREAS. The following patient care areas must be established: immediate (life-threatened, but salvable patients), delayed (not immediately life-threatened or life-threatened and nonsalvable patients; can wait for treatment and transportation), and ambulatory holding (minor-injured and noninjured patients). Triage officers manage each individual area and coordinate teams for triage and treatment. *Retriage* of victims, optimally, is done every 15 minutes. Treatment personnel include paramedics and emergency medical technicians; hospitals may send physicians and nurses to assist on-scene. They should never be in charge of triage, unless they have been thoroughly trained and planned for as part of the EMS operations.

MORGUE. Rescue personnel should not remove bodies from an incident site. However, if body removal is necessary to rescue other live victims, then a morgue must be established. Security must be arranged to prevent looting and desecration of bodies.

AMBULANCE STAGING. Ambulances should not respond directly into the incident site for the purposes of transportation. Once key personnel have responded, ambulances are held at a distance from the patient care area until needed for actual transportation. Ambulances need to be available, but they should not be in the middle of the action, as they may become blocked in or create their own obstacles. Staging areas for ambulances are best located a block or so away from the patient care areas and loading zones. Some ambulances, if not all, are also stripped of equipment and supplies before use for transportation. Use of an ambulance staging or holding area maintains control of the transportation of victims to various medical facilities and reduces the chances of arbitrary use of ambulances to transport nontriaged victims or those not designated for priority transportation. An ambulance control officer records all arriving units and assigns them destinations when they pick up patients.

AMBULANCE LOADING. The ambulance loading zone should be centrally located near the patient care areas. Included in this area is a designated landing zone for helicopters. As patients are brought to the area for transport, their triage tag numbers are noted and their destination is recorded before they are loaded in the ambulance. The ambulance control officer documents which ambulance took the patient and logs the time out. Optimally, ambulances should follow a traffic flow that maximizes the transport process and prevents gridlock. Ideally, the ambulance should pull into the ambulance loading area, load the patient, and pull forward to exit the area without impeding incoming traffic. For the large-scale movement of minor-injured patients, buses can be used.

MEDICAL SUPPLY POOL. In a large-scale incident, it is advisable to strip ambulances of supplies and place them in a specific storage area. Additional large inventories of supplies can then be funneled into the supply area as they are delivered to the scene. Resupply of the staging areas comes from the supply pool only. The supply officer keeps abreast of needs and inventory and advises the medical unit leader of needed resources. Returning ambulances can bring supplies back into the area from supplies given by hospital emergency departments or other suppliers.

MANPOWER STAGING AND CANTEEN. It is imperative that an area be established to which responding personnel can report. This area can serve as a rest area or "*rehabilitation*" area for those being relieved and rotated from the "hot zone" (area surrounding a hazardous materials incident that is dangerous to life and health). The added benefit is that an accurate count of available manpower and resources can be tabulated and tracked at all times. Those personnel who respond out of uniform (in areas that may use a call back or volunteer system) can be given appropriate identification and safety equipment.

COMMAND POST. This area includes the Incident Command Post managed by the highest ranking public service officer and the Medical Command Post run by the medical unit leader. The medical unit leader works with the ambulance control (or transportation) officer to determine the destination of patients to available medical facilities. The medical unit leader is advised through local communications networks of the capabilities of local medical facilities. This information is then passed on to the ambulance control officer. In some systems, it is the responsibility of the ambulance control officer to be in contact with the hospitals directly or a central communications center to ascertain bed availability. An additional concern for the command post is to determine the best access routes to and from the incident site. Aerial support may assist in locating roads that are open and passable vs. those that are blocked. This information is then passed to the ambulance control officer.

Figure 6-7 shows the components of the EMS organization in a disaster.

Analysis of Actual Disaster Incidents

The best lessons in response planning for disaster management can be learned in the analysis of actual disaster incidents and simulations. Research has exposed five common problems (known as the "Five C's") generic to all incidents, small and large. They are discussed in the following sections.

60 UNIT ONE: THE PREHOSPITAL ENVIRONMENT

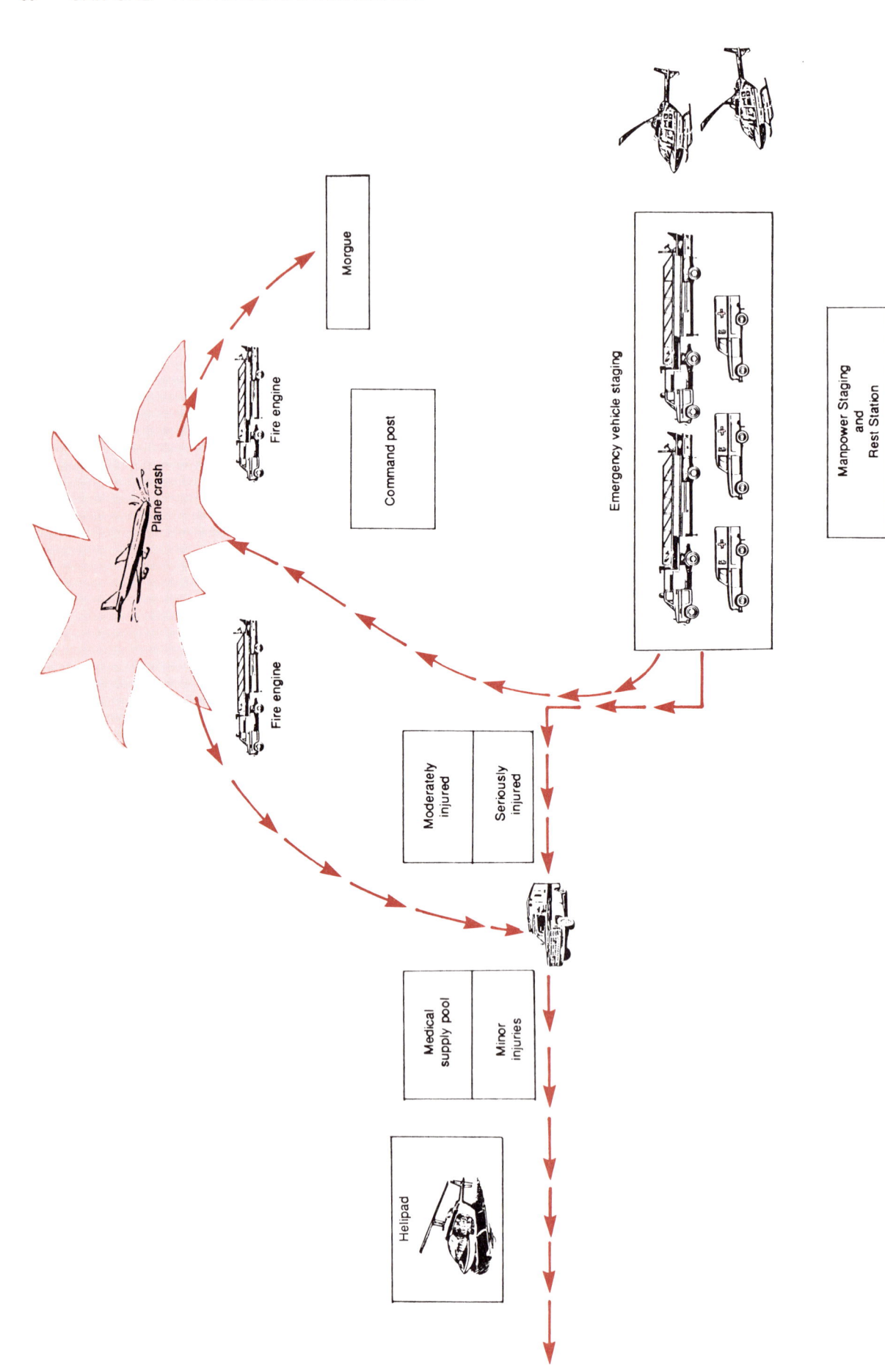

FIGURE 6–7. Components of the Emergency Medical Services organization in a disaster.

COMMUNICATION. Communications fail, in part, because of communications hardware or poor communications techniques by field and hospital personnel. Complicated "ten" codes should be avoided, and simple language should be used to accurately convey a picture of the incident and its victims. Problems exist when response agencies cannot communicate with each other because of incompatible frequencies and systems. In addition, necessary resources are often not alerted in a timely manner. Historically, 10- to 20-minute delays in dispatching appropriate resources have been caused by delays in activating a disaster plan.

CONTROL AND COMMAND. Control and command are only as effective as those assigned to command positions and those responsible for following their orders. If the command position is not recognized or acknowledged by all involved, then the commander/leader becomes ineffective. Often it may be unclear who is in charge, particularly when a jurisdictional dispute exists among different agencies and their respective leaders. Often there are too many command level positions. Command decisions and management fail when personnel and their specific skill levels are not properly used. Specialized resources may not be used. Unplanned negative media relations may also increase problems during and after the incident.

CONGESTION. A given in any disaster is pedestrian and vehicular congestion. This problem is caused by the physical congestion and traffic impedance of civilian and rescue vehicles, onlookers, media personnel, and rescuers themselves. This congestion becomes a management problem for the control of ambulance and rescue vehicle flow and the movement of victims from one area to another. A great mistake of command is to retain excess personnel who are not needed for scene management. Too often, excess personnel create a problem rather than a solution to scene control and command.

COLLECTION OF RESOURCES. Resources, both manpower and equipment, may become a problem because they are either limited or overabundant. Anticipated resources may or may not materialize. If unrequested or unauthorized personnel appear on-scene or at the hospital, they may become a physical impedance to both traffic flow and command and coordination. It is a great error for command personnel to make judgments based on anticipated resources, rather than those that exist at the moment.

COORDINATION OF TRIAGE AND TRANSPORTATION. Triage is effective only if those who are involved in triage coordinate their activities. Most important, transportation of victims must not be an independent decision of field personnel. Communications must be established with local hospitals to determine their patient care capacity and capabilities. Field personnel must avoid the tendency to "relocate the disaster" by overloading one local facility with victims. Victims must be spread out among available facilities. Obviously, all on-scene personnel must have identical training and continuing education in disaster management.

Awareness of problems encountered by other EMS agencies in disaster management helps to avoid the same problems. Though problems may not be eliminated entirely, they can be minimized.

Phase III: The Postdisaster Plan

No disaster plan is complete unless a postdisaster management plan is instituted. Too often the psychological effects of a disaster are ignored, particularly its effects on rescuers and hospital personnel. The effect of post-traumatic stress on rescuers is potentially the most long-term impact of a disaster situation. As the veterans of Vietnam and victims of violence have done, EMS planners must address the issues of post-traumatic stress and its prevention and treatment. Otherwise, disaster planning is incomplete and, ultimately, counterproductive.

Equally important is the effect of stress on rescue efforts and manpower performance. Signs and symptoms that occur during times of maximum stress, such as disasters, include palpitations, tremors, cramps, sweating, chills, headache, muffled hearing, and decreased concentration and perception abilities. These reactions are important when noting the communications difficulties encountered in disaster management. If the rescuer has physiologic and psychological reactions of decreased concentration, perception, and muffled hearing, then the communication problems become easy to understand. Therefore, it is imperative to use simple, concise language when giving directions to peers, patients, and others. To better understand why rescuers and medical personnel are affected, the unique stressors that influence care givers need to be examined.

Personal loss and injury: The disaster situation is dangerous, fatiguing, and decreases one's ability to function.
Traumatic stimuli: The rescuer is bombarded with the grotesque via the senses of sight, smell, hearing, and touch.
Mission failure: Care givers are highly motivated to complete their tasks successfully, to be perfect. The media will document success or failure of the mission.

Essentially, the care giver experiences the same terror as the victim, while operating at an increased energy level. This fact increases the potential for personal injury.

Disaster operations are a type of situation labeled "***critical incidents***" by Jeffrey T. Mitchell. Critical incidents are those situations or events that evoke a profound emotional response and have the potential to interfere with the rescuers ability to function either on-scene or later. Examples of critical incidents include the following:

- Serious injury or death of a coworker during line of duty activities
- Suicide of a coworker
- Unusually tragic deaths of children
- Events in which victims are known to rescuers
- Events that attract excessive media attention
- Events that seriously threaten the lives of the responders

Postincident symptoms may include depression, sleep disturbances (e.g., nightmares, repetitive dreams usually violent in nature, insomnia), cold sweats, decreased appetite, nausea, cramps, sexual dysfunction, fatigue, and an array of somatic (physical) complaints.

Mitchell has devised a method for postdisaster psychological care known as **Critical Incident Stress Debriefing (CISD).** This debriefing process allows for timely intervention to lessen the psychological effects of the incident and prevent long-term problems. In addition, onsite debriefing teams trained in CISD can monitor rescuers for signs of undue stress and intervene and advise command as needed.

It is imperative to recognize that rescue and medical personnel are not immune from the stressors and aftermath of disasters. *Cumulative stress* from nondisaster incidents can have an impact as severe as a sudden devastating incident. Intervention and debriefing become mandatory and cost effective in salvaging experienced personnel.

SUMMARY

Disaster planning, whether for rural or urban responders, must include an honest and unbiased evaluation of existing and proposed resources. Disaster simulations and drills must reflect the same goals and objectives of the actual event. Exercises can test the effectiveness of the plan only after adequate training has been instituted. Initial response to a major emergency or disaster involves confusion, shortage of manpower, supplies, and equipment, and inadequate radio communications. However, effective and efficient disaster operations are possible if all responding agencies regularly discuss, train, and drill on an interagency basis.

SUGGESTED READING

Auf der Heide E: Disaster Response: Principles of Preparation and Coordination. St. Louis, CV Mosby, 1989

Comfort LK: Managing Disaster: Strategies and Rating Perspectives. Durham, Duke University Press, 1988

Mitchell JT: Teaming up against critical incident stress. Chief Fire Executive 1:24, 36:84, 1986

Noji EK, Kelen GD, Armenian HK et al: The 1988 earthquake in Soviet Armenia: A case study. Ann Emerg Med 19:891, 1990

Raphael B: When Disaster Strikes: How Individuals and Communities Cope With Catastrophe. New York, Basic Books, 1986

START: A Triage Method. Newport Beach, CA, Hoag Memorial Hospital Presbyterian, 1989

US Department of Transportation, National Highway Traffic Safety Administration: Emergency Medical Technician–Paramedic: National Standards Curriculum. Washington, DC, US Government Printing Office, 1985

CHAPTER 7

Stress Management

The Stress Process
   Fight or Flight
Types of Stress Reactions
   Acute Stress Reaction
   Delayed Stress Reaction
   Cumulative Stress Reaction
Specific Paramedic Stressors
Coping With Stress
   Defense Mechanisms
      Repression
      Denial
      Rationalization
      Humor
   Coping Strategies

The Grieving Process in Death and Dying
   Stage One: Denial and Isolation
   Stage Two: Anger
   Stage Three: Bargaining
   Stage Four: Depression
   Stage Five: Acceptance
Dealing With Death and Dying
   Management of Death and Dying
Summary

BEHAVIORAL OBJECTIVES
On successful completion of this chapter, the reader will be able to:

1. Describe the effects of stress reactions on body processes
2. List the three types of stress reactions and identify characteristics of each
3. Identify specific events that are stressful to the paramedic
4. Describe four defense mechanisms
5. Discuss coping strategies that can be practiced to reduce stress
6. Discuss the five stages of the grieving process
7. Describe common needs of the patient, family, and paramedic in dealing with death and dying
8. Discuss how the paramedic can manage situations that involve death and dying
9. Define all of the key terms listed in this chapter

KEY TERMS

The following terms are defined in the chapter and glossary:

acceptance
acute stress reaction
anger
bargaining
coping
cumulative stress reactions
defense mechanisms
delayed stress reaction
denial
depression
fight or flight
general adaptation syndrome
humor
isolation
rationalization
repression
stress
stressor

For centuries human behavior under battle conditions has been observed, studied, and written about. Severe stress has equally influenced both acts of cowardice and heroism, fear and bravery, self-focus and selflessness, precision and carelessness.

The study of stress experienced by the emergency care provider, specifically by paramedics, has barely passed its first decade. Yet, the similarities between combat stress and paramedic stress are notable. Stress experienced by both soldiers and paramedics may be a driving, protective, and even productive force. Adversely, stress may also act as a destructive, debilitating process that inhibits actions, corrodes individual confidence, and deteriorates one's personal health and the total enjoyment of life.

The study of stress in paramedic personnel may be new, but problems with stress management have been in existence since the development of the first paramedic. In 1981 Graham noted that, by the late 1970s, emergency medical researchers were noticing "a significant and growing number of professionals in emergency medicine who, after two to five years, had already opted out of the system being done-in, fed up, burned out, and calling it quits."

To control the destructive elements of stress and to enhance the positive factors, it is important to understand the stress process. This chapter provides information to give the paramedic an understanding of the stress process and provides strategies to help ease the stress impact and allow for a fuller, healthier life experience.

THE STRESS PROCESS

The word **stress** comes directly from Latin to mean a hardship, force, or pressure. Stress is thought of as a cluster of physiologic and psychological signs and symptoms that appear as a response to some external stimulus (**stressor**). The simplest and best working definition of stress is that stress is a state of physiologic and psychological arousal.

For a stress reaction to take place, a *stressor event* must first be present. The stressor event may be the death or injury of a coworker, death or injury of a child, or a mass casualty incident. The stressor is received by the person's senses and then interpreted by the brain. The brain, in turn, in a complex but rapid manner, causes the body to respond to the stressor. Because of this reaction, stress is described as a state of physiologic and psychological arousal. The brain and body are tied together in an intricate network that responds to both internal and external stressors.

In brief, the *stress reaction* works in the following manner. The person's senses are first stimulated by the stressor. The cerebral cortex of the brain then categorizes the stressor and picks out important elements from stored memory that may be helpful to the person in understanding and dealing with the current stressor. The information processed by the cortex of the brain is instantaneously interpreted and the stressor is assigned an emotion (e.g., fear, terror, anger, joy, excitement). Within a fraction of a second, the brain stem or midbrain is stimulated. Signals are sent to the adrenal glands to release adrenaline and other substances, which circulate to the brain and throughout the body. The pituitary gland, stimulated by the above events, signals the adrenal cortex to discharge a variety of chemicals that activate many body systems and cause a full stress reaction, that is, a hyperalert state of readiness.

Fight or Flight

The overall stress reaction is commonly called the **fight or flight** response. Once the mind and body are sufficiently aroused, the person usually attempts to work through (i.e., fight) the problem. If the situation is overwhelming, running away from it (i.e., flight) occurs. The fight or flight response is a primitive response. Our earliest ancestors, when confronted by a stressor such as a large animal, had the choice of fighting or fleeing. Their bodies responded with appropriate physiologic means, such as increased heart rate and blood pressure, dilated pupils, and increased blood sugar. These responses enabled the individual to fight or run away.

Hans Selye, a famous stress researcher, called the fight or flight reaction the **general adaptation syndrome** because he noticed that the stress reaction was present in all forms of demand on the brain or body and in all types of people. The stress reaction was much the same even when the stimuli were different. The general adaptation syndrome or stress response works in the following manner. The stressful event occurs, and the senses perceive it. The brain rapidly interprets the stimuli, and a state of alarm is aroused. The brain arouses the body instantly, and the person is ready for action. The resistance phase of the general adaptation syndrome includes all of the actions the person takes to attempt to deal with the stressful circumstance. The efforts to cope may be right or wrong, good or bad, effective or noneffective. What matters most is that some action occurs. Sooner or later the person enters the final phase of the stress response, the exhaustion phase. Whether successful or not, efforts to cope with stress drain off energy, and eventually the person is unable to maintain further efforts to cope with the stress. Selye suggests that Figure 7-1 describes the general adaptation syndrome.

Stress comes in various degrees. It can be mild, moderate, or severe. The degree of the stress reaction depends on the seriousness of the stimulus. A minor event generally produces little stress, and a major incident produces a much stronger stress reaction. The amount of stress encountered also depends on a person's perception of the event. People may react in totally different manners when exposed to the same stressful event. Almost any stimulus can produce stress. Delays, shortages of supplies and equipment, failures, losses, restrictions, obligations, illnesses, conflicts, and pressures all produce stress. Among paramedic personnel, the work shift, loud noises, poor lighting, working around the dead, system abuse, boredom, excessive workloads, and the responsibility for the life and safety of others may contribute substantially to the degree of stress encountered.

Stress has many causes, and it is difficult to discuss each one individually. The four main areas that contribute to the causes of stress are social, personal, occupational, and environmental factors in one's life. Within each of these areas, several influences may play a critical role in the level of stress encountered. The box "Contributing Causes of Stress" lists specific examples of influences that may create stress.

TYPES OF STRESS REACTIONS

Three major types of stress reactions are found: acute, delayed, and cumulative. Delayed stress reactions are called post-traumatic stress disorders. The complete recovery of a person who suffers from post-traumatic stress

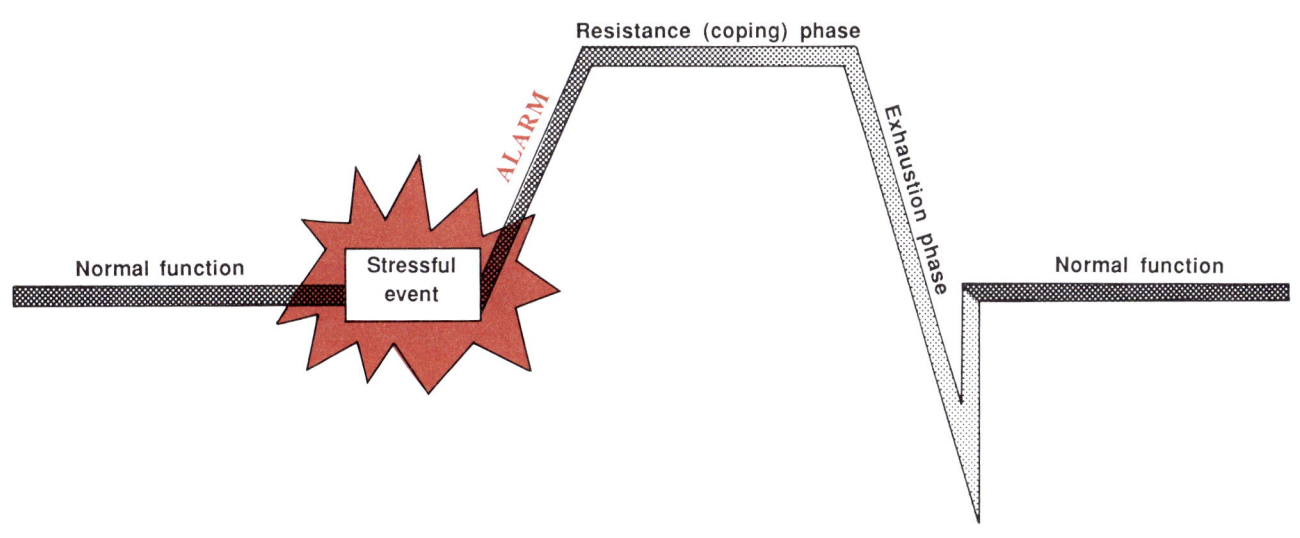

FIGURE 7-1.
General adaptation syndrome.

CONTRIBUTING CAUSES OF STRESS

Social

- Cultural differences
- Discrimination
- Prejudice
- Social conflict
- Politics
- Male vs. female roles
- Lack of public support or open rejection
- Family
- Poor social network
- Economic pressure

Personal

- Emotions
- Self-image
- Values
- Personal needs
- Personality
- Need to be needed
- Mental outlook
- Fantasy
- Life changes
- Failures
- Personal losses
- Illness
- Embarrassment
- Frustration
- Fear
- Decision making

Occupational

- Shift work
- Direct work with people
- Poor supervision
- Poor leadership
- Boredom
- Excessive activity obligations
- Lack of proper training
- Night work
- Two or more jobs
- Responsibility for life of others
- Job ambiguity

Environmental

- Noise
- Dirt
- Dust
- Lack of privacy
- Poor lighting
- Poor ventilation
- Cramped space
- Smoking
- Poor diet
- Inadequate equipment
- Alcohol abuse
- Time pressures

---

disorders may require professional mental health assistance.

Acute Stress Reaction

An *acute stress reaction* is sometimes called "catastrophic stress" or "critical incident stress," and, as the name implies, it is generally a powerful experience. An acute stress reaction is incident specific. That is, it only begins after a person has been exposed to an upsetting, frightening, disgusting, or threatening event or any situation that, for whatever reason, has a powerful emotional impact. These kinds of highly emotional events are called "critical incidents."

People can also have significant stress reactions from relatively mild stressors. When the stressor triggers unconscious or forgotten stress reactions, for example in the case of a person sensitized by a previous incident, the present stressor reignites the old stress reaction.

An acute stress reaction usually begins either immediately at the emergency scene or shortly after the event (usually within the first 24 hours). The signs and symptoms of an acute stress reaction can be grouped into four categories: cognitive, physical, emotional, and behavioral. Although normal, they can be quite alarming to the unsuspecting person involved. The box "Signs and Symptoms of an Acute Stress Reaction" lists several signs and symptoms in each of the four categories that may be experienced by a person during acute stress reactions.

In addition to the initial effects, an acute stress reaction can produce other more serious effects, including the following:

- Stress-related illness
- Job dysfunction
- Psychological dysfunction
- Change in usual behaviors
- Death (under unusually stressful circumstances)

SIGNS AND SYMPTOMS OF AN ACUTE STRESS REACTION

Cognitive
- Blaming someone
- Confusion
- Memory problems
- Poor attention span
- Difficulties with decision making
- Heightened or lowered alertness
- Difficulties with problem solving
- Disorientation
- Slowed thinking
- Poor calculations
- Poor concentration
- Difficulty naming familiar objects
- Seeing event over and over

Physical
- Nausea
- Vomiting
- Tremors (lips, hands)
- Feeling uncoordinated
- Profuse sweating
- Chills
- Diarrhea
- Dizziness
- Chest pain
- Difficulty breathing
- Shock symptoms
- Rapid heart beat
- Rapid breathing
- Excessively elevated blood pressure
- Headaches
- Muscle aches
- Fatigue

Emotional
- Anxiety
- Fear
- Guilt
- Grief
- Anger
- Depression
- Sadness
- Feeling lost
- Feeling abandoned
- Feeling isolated
- Worrying about others
- Wanting to hide
- Wanting to limit contact with others
- Irritability
- Feeling numb
- Startled
- Shocked

Behavioral
- Change in activity
- Change in speech
- Withdrawal
- Angry outbursts
- Suspiciousness
- Change in communications
- Change in interactions with others
- Increased or decreased food consumption
- Increased alcohol consumption
- Intense fatigue
- Antisocial acts
- Hyperalert

Fortunately, most people recover within a few weeks after a critical incident stress and do not experience the more profound stress reactions.

Delayed Stress Reaction

A ***delayed stress reaction*** is similar to the acute stress reaction except that it occurs in the days and weeks after the event. Occasionally, a delayed stress reaction may occur months or even years after the critical incident. It too is incident specific. Without a specific disturbing event, the stress reaction would not exist. Delayed stress reactions are characterized by the following effects:

- Obsessive thoughts about the event
- Distressing dreams or nightmares
- Daytime flashbacks of the event
- Fear of recurrence of the event
- Emotional numbing
- Lowered interest in important activities
- Loss of emotional control
- Inability to express appropriate emotions
- Sleep disturbance
- Excessive guilt related to surviving
- High anxiety
- Trouble concentrating
- Avoidance of any activity associated with the event

Cumulative Stress Reaction

Cumulative stress reactions have often been called "*burnout*" in the past, but this term has been so overused and misapplied that the more precise term cumulative stress is now being used. A cumulative stress reaction is not associated with a single recognized critical incident. Instead, it is caused by a destructive stress process that has occurred over many years. A cumulative stress reaction usually has many interrelated causes, including home and personal life, experiences of one's childhood, frustrations, losses, problems with one's administrators, and a variety of demanding emergency events combined with minor everyday job situations. A cumulative stress reaction is characterized by a growing emotional exhaustion and negative attitude shift. It is also characterized by a decline in job performance and signs of physical as well as emotional deterioration.

SIGNS AND SYMPTOMS OF A CUMULATIVE STRESS REACTION

Stage 1: The early warning signs

- Vague anxiety (feeling of impending doom)
- Excessive and constant fatigue
- Feelings of depression
- Boredom with one's job or home life
- Apathy

Stage 2: Mild cumulative stress reaction

- Lowered emotional control
- Increased anxiety
- Sleep disturbance
- Headaches
- Irritability
- Muscle aches and pains
- Loss of energy
- Hyperactivity and restlessness
- Excessive fatigue
- The beginnings of withdrawal from friends, family, and coworkers
- Nausea
- Increased depression

Stage 3: Moderate cumulative stress reaction

- Skin rashes
- Generalized physical weakness
- Strong feelings of depression
- Increased alcohol abuse
- Increased smoking
- High blood pressure
- Migraine headaches
- Loss of appetite for eating
- Angry outbursts
- Marital conflict
- Loss of sexual appetite
- Ulcers
- Severe withdrawal from friends, family, and coworkers
- Constantly feeling angry
- Crying spells
- Serious depression
- Serious anxiety
- Problems with clear thinking and decision making
- Problems with memory
- Rigid thinking patterns

Stage 4: Cumulative stress reaction

- Severe depression
- Severe anxiety
- Low self-confidence
- Inability to appropriately manage one's job or personal affairs
- Severe withdrawal
- Excessive alcohol abuse
- Uncontrolled emotions
- Suicidal thoughts
- Muscle tremors
- Feeling desperate and out of control
- Severe fatigue
- Overreaction to minor events
- Agitation
- Constant tension
- Hostile feelings
- Homicidal thoughts
- Chronic state of anger
- Accident prone
- Carelessness
- Development of moderate to severe thought disturbance
- Hallucinations
- Sleep disturbance

Signs and symptoms that may occur in a cumulative stress reaction are divided into four stages according to the severity of the cumulative reaction. A person may experience early warning signs in stage one of the cumulative reaction and, if unattended, may progress through stages two and three, mild and moderate cumulative stress reactions, finally to stage four, the severe stress reaction. The box "Signs and Symptoms of a Cumulative Stress Reaction" lists specific signs and symptoms that may be seen within each of these four stages.

SPECIFIC PARAMEDIC STRESSORS

Many stress-producing situations that occur in the emergency medical services work environment are either not found in other types of work or do not occur with the same intensity or frequency. The paramedic's responsibility for the lives and well-being of others can often be overwhelming. Working with the acutely ill or injured and being exposed to their sometimes hostile, panicky, and depressed states, in an atmosphere in which even small mistakes are potentially catastrophic, are anxiety-producing and stressful experiences for the paramedic. Paramedics routinely list infant deaths, child abuse, mass casualties, disasters, and high-rise fires as their most stressful calls. Personal, organizational, and operational influences are three common categories within which paramedic stressors are included. The box "Common Paramedic Stressors" lists several of the most common stressors routinely identified by paramedic personnel.

COPING WITH STRESS

Hundreds of books and thousands of articles have been written on the topic of stress. However, a more in-depth review of the subject of stress is not likely to be helpful to the practicing paramedic. Rather, a discussion of what

---

COMMON PARAMEDIC STRESSORS
Personal
- Marital conflict
- Need to be needed
- Self-blame for mistakes
- Excessive expectations
- Responsibility for life of others
- Fatigue
- Anxiety
- Fear of personal injury and illness
- Lack of time with families
- Lack of self-confidence
- Sleep interruptions
- Mental load
- Continuous state of alertness
- Getting sick after a call

Organizational
- Poor supervision
- Administrative hassles
- Lack of training
- Poor equipment
- Low morale
- Poor conflict resolution
- Poor acceptance by hospital
- Multiple bosses
- Poor career ladder
- Budget cuts
- Politics
- Poorly defined policies
- Lack of feedback
- Lack of recognition
- Low pay
- Work overload

Operational
- Death of children
- Concern for battered children
- Well-being of coworkers
- Boredom
- Gory sights and sounds
- Work with acutely ill or injured
- Intoxicated patients
- Psychiatric patients
- Suicide cases
- Communications
- High call volume
- Abusive patients
- Public view
- Shift work
- Night work
- Paperwork
- Unnecessary calls
- Surprises

can be done to lessen stress and to protect paramedics from illness, marital problems, job dysfunction, and other ill effects related to acute and chronic stress is preferable. The remainder of this chapter, therefore, focuses on defense mechanisms and coping strategies, both areas intimately related to effective stress management.

Coping is any behavior that protects an individual from both internal and external stressors. The word "coping" implies adaptation, defense, and mastery over stressors. Coping is an active, assertive process, during which the stressed paramedic takes charge of the circumstances and attempts to control them.

Defense Mechanisms

Coping efforts, collectively known as **defense mechanisms**, may be internal, unnoticed, and sometimes unconscious and automatic efforts to adjust to stressful situations. Defense mechanisms help to relieve anxiety, minimize conflict, and allow the person to carry out required activities. Some of the more common defense mechanisms discussed are repression, denial, rationalization, and humor.

Repression

Repression is one of the most commonly used defense mechanisms. Repression refers to the banishment of painful ideas from the conscious into the unconscious mind in an attempt to alleviate anxiety and conflict. The fact that people so easily "*forget*" the details of distressing events is testimony to the effectiveness of this process.

Denial

Denial is another frequently encountered defense mechanism. As its name implies, denial is generally an unconscious reaction in which the person denies the reality of the situation. Denial is often used to ignore the signs and symptoms of a stress reaction. For instance, paramedics commonly deny sleeplessness as a stress reaction and explain that the work shift was busy and their adrenaline level too high to sleep. In reality, the paramedic is suffering from a mild stress reaction. The work shift was busy, a fact which caused countless signals to be sent to the adrenal cortex to release a variety of chemicals, leaving the body in a hyperalert state of readiness.

Rationalization

Rationalization is a defense mechanism in which the person attempts to justify unacceptable actions by using excuses or reasonings that are objectively incorrect. For example, toward the end of a long work shift, a paramedic decides not to start an intravenous line on a patient who presents with chest pain and low blood pressure, because, he/she states, they are just 5 minutes away from the hospital. While this statement may be correct in some instances, rationalization was used to justify a lack of desire to carry out what the paramedic knows is the correct management procedure.

Humor

Humor is a defense mechanism often used. Humor can reduce tension by providing an outlet or escape valve for the person faced with a distressing situation. Although helpful in many instances, humor must be cautiously monitored by the paramedic so that it is not used inappropriately. It can cause serious and negative reactions in family members and others when it is badly timed and poorly used.

Coping Strategies

There is virtually no end to the types of coping strategies that can be used to reduce stress by changing the situation or by managing the physiologic or psychological reactions so they do not become overwhelming. Some of the most helpful strategies are discussed below.

Recognize the existence of stress. *Awareness* of the problem is essential for the management of stress. Ignoring the problem only produces psychological exhaustion. Believe that something can be done to reduce stress. Failure to believe that stress can be reduced results in a sense of helplessness. Remember that stress management is a personal responsibility. No one person can do it for another. Every person has to be a prime mover to manage stress as an individual. Know when to fight, run, or not exert energy to control stress. Do not waste energy to control unimportant and minor stresses. Keep in mind that a positive mental attitude is essential in stress management. Stress is a situational problem that does have an ending.

Preincident education can help reduce stress. Learn about stress before living it. Paramedics should take advantage of courses in stress management, human communications, crisis intervention, time management, and other courses and workshops that contain good ideas for decreasing stress.

Rest, relaxation, and physical exercise are important in the control of stress. Most articles about controlling stress suggest rest as an important part of stress management. Paramedics need to slow down between calls and between work shifts. Frequent time off from the job is helpful, especially when two or three days are worked in a row. Relaxation is important to evoke the quieting response, an emotional and physical state of relaxation that is brought about by such strategies as progressive muscle relaxation, deep breathing, and a quiet room away from the hassle of everyday activity. Hand in hand with rest and relaxation is physical exercise. Physical exercise is perhaps the most significant method of stress reduction available and is fast, inexpensive, and effective. If paramedics stay physically fit, they have a far greater chance of surviving their stressful job environment. Physical exercise should be performed within a 24-hour period after experiencing a critical incident of stress. This period is important because the stress reaction is most intense during the 24 hours that follow a stressful incident.

Having a life outside of the job is also important in reducing stress. Paramedics need family support, friendships, and support from their colleagues. Without this emotional support, they are left feeling isolated and empty. Paramedics should spend time socializing with people who are not paramedics. They can, therefore, leave the stress of the job behind them when they leave work.

Since good health goes hand in hand with decreased stress, important recommendations include not smoking and watching what one eats. Nicotine enhances the stress response, in addition to its many other adverse effects on body function. A good diet with attention to decreasing sugar intake, caffeine, and excessive salt is advisable. It is important to include a warning against alcohol or street drugs, because some people see alcohol or marijuana as a way to reduce stress.

At the supervisory level, administrators should attempt, whenever possible, to keep work shifts to a normal level without excessive overtime to ensure that their employees are well rested. Enhanced administrative support does much for a paramedic service. It has been shown that, in places where administrators meet frequently with their personnel, attempt to understand and support them, and stand behind them when the personnel are right, the staff turnover is lower and a much happier atmosphere is created. If feasible, employee assistance programs should be developed to handle such areas as the following:

- Counseling for employees with personal problems
- Family support programs
- Spouse support programs
- Marital counseling
- Clergy support
- Stress education for the employee's family
- Vocational counseling
- Alcohol and drug abuse counseling
- Disaster planning and intervention programs
- Life-enhancement programs

THE GRIEVING PROCESS IN DEATH AND DYING

Emergency medical personnel encounter death and dying patients on a frequent basis. The paramedic must understand the grieving process of those who are experiencing death or those who are closely associated with someone who is dying or may have recently died.

Most patients go through five stages or levels of the grieving process in either experiencing their own death or the death of a loved one. The grieving process is a normal, healthy emotional outlet and is necessary to come to terms with the upcoming death or recent death of a loved one. The characteristics of each stage are more closely defined below.

Stage One: Denial and Isolation

Stage one, or the denial and **isolation** stage in the grieving process, is common to patients who are suffering from a terminal illness. This stage is normal and is needed to act as a buffer between the shock of finding that death is imminent and dealing with death itself. The denial stage is temporary and aids in partial acceptance of the death. Terminally ill patients re-enter this stage periodically throughout their illness.

Stage Two: Anger

The second stage in the grieving process is **anger**. Often, the patient or family asks "why me?" This anger can be projected toward anything or anyone. The paramedic should recognize that this displaced anger has little to do with those who become the targets of it.

Stage Three: Bargaining

As the person progresses through the grieving process, they enter stage three, the **bargaining** stage. In bargaining stage, the patient enters into some type of agreement in an attempt to postpone the inevitable. For example, a terminally ill patient might bargain "to stay alive" to attend the upcoming wedding of his or her youngest child. When the period of time that was "bargained for" has passed, the patient may enter into yet another bargain or, if they can no longer deny their illness, may advance into the fourth stage of grieving.

Stage Four: Depression

When the patient or family is no longer able to deny the illness, **depression** and a great sense of loss become evident. Often financial burdens become overpowering and force some patients to sell their most precious possessions. The financial burdens along with the extensive treatment and hospitalizations are only a few of the many losses that are realized during the depression stage of the grieving process.

Stage Five: Acceptance

The final stage in the grieving process is the **acceptance** stage. This is not a happy stage, but rather one of disengagement or disassociation. In the acceptance stage, the patient or family has accepted the inevitable and is without fear or despair and void of feelings. The patient usually becomes less involved with people, preparing to face the death alone. During the acceptance stage, the family of the terminally ill patient is in greater need of understanding and support than the patient. Once the patient and the family have passed through the acceptance stage, they are prepared for the death and are able to face it with less difficulty.

DEALING WITH DEATH AND DYING

The patient, family, and, occasionally, the paramedic have specific needs that must be met to assist with the dying process. The patient may need sharing and communication, hope, privacy, respect and dignity, and control of the situation. The paramedic must realize what the patient's needs are and attempt to meet those needs when appropriate.

In addition, the family may exhibit needs as well. They progress through the same stages of the grieving process as the patient, but individual family members may progress through the stages at varying rates. Reactions by individual family members are appropriate to their present stage of grieving. These people may express feelings of despair, anger, and rage that are often displaced toward the paramedic.

The paramedic may experience the same grief processes as the patient, particularly when contact with the patient is frequent. The average person uses a lot of energy to cover feelings without ventilating thoughts and emotions about the situation. The paramedic can reduce the stress reaction and prevent a more serious reaction by making a conscious attempt to ventilate thoughts and emotions after experiencing situations that involve death.

Management of Death and Dying

The manner in which the paramedic deals with the death of other people reflects personal thought processes and the activities performed immediately after the death. The paramedic may feel uncomfortable interacting with the dying patient or family members of the patient, but the use of nonverbal communication is helpful during these situations. The tone of voice, facial expressions, and appropriate use of touch are all ways to make the situation more comfortable for the family and the paramedic.

Dealing with terminally ill patients and their families can be difficult. The patient and family should not be falsely reassured about the patient's condition. Many times a terminally ill patient welcomes someone to talk with who is open and honest. The patient may be reluctant to speak openly with family members for fear of upsetting them but will speak openly about the illness with the paramedic. Occasionally, terminally ill patients may ask if they are dying. The paramedic should not be afraid to answer the patients honestly, as this helps them work through their own grieving process.

When a terminally ill patient has died, the family then becomes the patient. The paramedic should use the word "dead" in referring to the patient rather than "passed away" or "expired" so that the family can pass through the grieving process and accept the death more readily. The paramedic should offer to call neighbors, family, or clergy to support the family in a time of need.

Initial reactions from the family concerning a terminally ill patient's death may vary from relief to hysteria. The paramedic should be aware that family members will cope with the death the same way they cope with everyday stresses and, thus, may exhibit several different reactions.

Several issues become involved when the paramedic deals with death and the dying patient. Before actual patient care, the paramedic should be aware of personal feelings toward issues such as resuscitation of the terminally ill patient, resuscitation of the patient for training purposes, and the existence and use of "do not resuscitate" orders. The paramedic should be familiar with local policies and protocols that address these situations and perform patient care accordingly.

Coping with death and dying is perhaps one of the most difficult aspects of the paramedic's occupation. A thorough understanding of the death and grieving process helps the paramedic support the family and terminally ill patient without becoming emotionally involved. Paramedics who provide patient care for the dying may experience strong emotions in certain situations. It should be emphasized again that paramedics must avoid becoming emotionally involved with the patient or family, causing a lose of objectivity. If paramedics have trouble with this detachment, they may need to explore, with a trained professional, their own feelings about death and dying.

SUMMARY

Paramedics suffer from a great deal of stress as a normal by-product of their jobs. This fact does not mean, however, that paramedics need to experience stress without some relief or without the possibility of turning stress into a productive, driving, creative force. Cumulative stress reactions and post-traumatic stress disorders that become so severe that the paramedic is unable to continue in the emergency medical services profession might be avoided, or the effects lessened, if the paramedic is aware of the signs and symptoms of stress.

Coping with stress through defense mechanisms helps to relieve anxiety, minimize conflict, and allow the person to continue to function in required activities. Recognition of stress and the use of coping mechanisms can help with stress management. Stress management must be internally initiated by the individual. The paramedic should remember that a positive mental attitude is essential in the management of stress.

Rest, relaxation, and physical exercise also help to control stress. Physical exercise is particularly helpful during the 24-hour period following the stressor event, since this period is the most intense time of the stress reaction.

Dealing with death and dying is one of the more stressful situations encountered by the paramedic. An understanding of the grieving process that the patient and family pass through helps the paramedic deal with these situations. The grieving process is a normal, healthy emotional outlet and is necessary to allow the patient and family to come to terms with the upcoming death.

The paramedic may also experience stages of the grieving process when caring for the terminally ill. Recognition and early ventilation of thoughts and emotions help the paramedic through the grieving process and allow energy to be devoted to the family of the deceased or dying.

SUGGESTED READING

Cydulka RK, Lyon J, Moy A et al: A follow-up report of occupational stress in urban EMT-Paramedics. Ann Emerg Med 18: 1151, 1989

Drabek TE: System Responses to Disaster: An Inventory of Sociological Finndings. New York, Springer-Verlag, 1986

Everly GS: A Clinical Guide to the Treatment of Human Stress. New York, Plenum, 1989

Grady GP, Mitchell JT: Emergency Services Stress. Baltimore, Chevron Publishing, 1989

Graham NK:Done in, fed up, burned out: Too much attrition in EMS. J Emerg Med Serv 6:24, 1981

Garza MA: For crying out loud! J Emerg Med Serv 14(3):52, 1989

Kennedy-Ewing L: Delaware County Critical Incident Stress Management Program: Operational Guidelines. Media, PA, Delaware County Department of Human Resources, 1988

Mitchell JT: The history, status and future of critical incident stress debriefings. J Emerg Med Serv 13:47, 1988

Mitchell JT: Effective stress control at major incidents. Maryland Fire and Rescue Bulletin 15:3, 1987

Selye H: Stress Without Distress. Philadelphia, JB Lippincott, 1974

US Department of Transportation, National Highway Traffic Safety Administration: Emergency Medical Technician-Paramedic: National Standards Curriculum. Washington, DC, US Government Printing Office, 1985

UNIT TWO

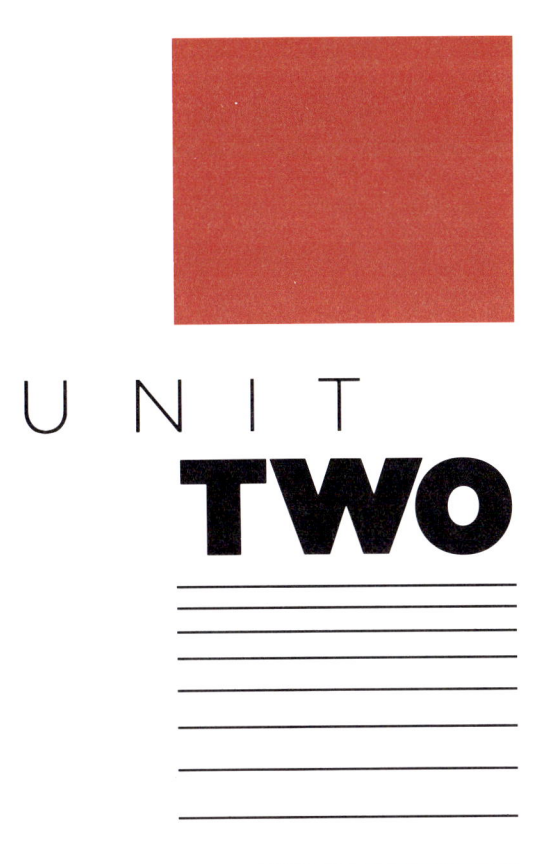

Foundations of Emergency Care

CHAPTER 8

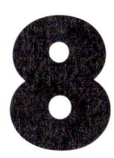

Medical Terminology and Human Systems

Medical Terminology
   Pronunciation and Spelling
   Word Building
      Word Roots
      Prefixes
      Suffixes
      Combining Vowels
      Combining Forms
   Abbreviations
Human Systems
   Body Orientation
      Directions
      Planes
      Movements
      Postures
      Cavities

   Body Systems
      Skeletal
      Muscular
      Nervous
      Cardiovascular
      Respiratory
      Digestive
      Urinary
      Reproductive
      Endocrine
      Integumentary
Summary

BEHAVIORAL OBJECTIVES

On successful completion of this chapter, the reader will be able to:

1. Describe the importance of proper pronunciation and spelling in medical terminology
2. Differentiate between word root, prefix, suffix, combining vowel, and combining form
3. List twenty commonly used abbreviations and define their meanings
4. Describe the normal anatomical position
5. Describe the eight anatomical directions
6. Describe the four planes of the body
7. Describe the eight normal body movements
8. Describe the two major and five smaller body cavities
9. Identify the components and functions of the ten body systems
10. Define all of the key terms listed in this chapter

KEY TERMS

The following terms are defined in the chapter and glossary:

abduction	*laterally recumbent*
adduction	*medial*
anterior	*posterior*
circumduction	*prefix*
combining form	*prone*
combining vowel	*proximal*
distal	*rotation*
erect	*sagittal*
extension	*suffix*
flexion	*superior*
frontal	*supine*
inferior	*transverse*
lateral	*word root*

This chapter opens with a discussion of the basic building blocks of medical terminology. Explanations of how terms came to be used and how they are formed follow. The second part of this chapter reviews human systems. The direct relationship of medical terminology to human systems is readily apparent. An introduction to human systems presents information on the body's orientation with discussion of body directions, planes, movements, positions, and cavities. A brief discussion of the ten systems of the body concludes the chapter.

MEDICAL TERMINOLOGY

In any field of knowledge, a special vocabulary is necessary to speak or write exactly. Medical terminology is the foundation of the language of medicine. It is the goal of this section to make medical terminology understandable as well as easy to learn. Words are divided into basic elements: roots, prefixes, suffixes, combining vowels, and combining forms. With the knowledge of word building and the meanings of specific word elements, even the longest and most complicated terms can be understood. A medical dictionary is a useful tool to have at hand in the initial stages of learning medical terminology.

Pronunciation and Spelling

Since medical terminology is a technically exact vocabulary used by professionals, it is important for the paramedic to *speak* and *write* the words correctly. Learn to *pronounce* each term correctly and say it aloud several times. Spelling is especially critical because many words are pronounced alike but spelled differently and have entirely different meanings. For example:

ileum (il'e‑um) is a part of the small intestine

and

ilium (il'e‑um) is a part of the pelvic, or hip, bone

A misspelled word may also completely alter the meaning of a term. For example:

hyperglycemia (hi'per‑gli‑se'me‑ah) is too much blood sugar

and

hypoglycemia (hi'po‑gli‑se'me‑ah) is too little blood sugar

Words spelled correctly but pronounced incorrectly may be easily misunderstood. For example:

urethra (u‑re'thrah) is the urinary bladder to the external surface

and

ureter (u‑re'ter) is one of two tubes that leads from the kidney to the urinary bladder

The above examples illustrate the importance of learning the correct spelling and pronunciation of medical terms.

Word Building

Word building is the construction of medical terms. Most terms are compound words consisting of word parts. These word parts are Greek or Latin word roots, prefixes, suffixes, combining vowels, and combining forms. To interpret the meaning of a medical term, it is best to start at the end of the word, by defining the suffix back to the first part of the word. For example:

HEMAT- + -OMA = HEMATOMA
blood   swelling   swelling containing blood

and

PERI- + CARD- + -ITIS = PERICARDITIS
around heart   inflammation   inflammation of the membrane that surrounds the heart

Word Roots

All words have a word root that serves as the foundation of the word. The **word root** of a medical term usually indicates the tissue, organ or body system that is involved, such as derma- (skin), nephro- (kidney), and neuro- (nerve). The box "Common Word Roots" illustrates some of these roots.

Many medical words are compound words that are made up of more than one root, such as the term cardiopulmonary. This term combines two word roots to make one word: cardio, which means heart, and pulmonary, which means lungs. Word roots may also be combined with prefixes, suffixes, and combining vowels. For example:

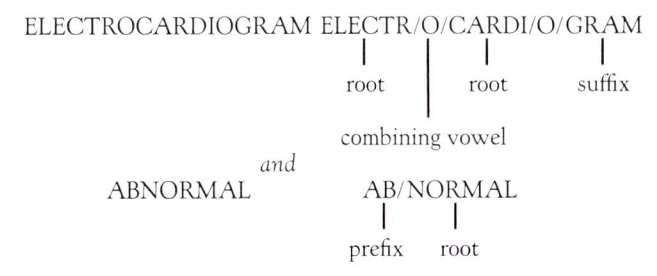

ELECTROCARDIOGRAM ELECTR/O/CARDI/O/GRAM
root root suffix
combining vowel

and

ABNORMAL   AB/NORMAL
prefix root

Prefixes

The **prefix** is attached to the beginning of a word and can never stand alone. It is placed before verbs, nouns, and adjectives to change or modify their meanings. The box "Common Prefixes" illustrates some of these prefixes. Prefixes often denote in what direction, how, or how much. Some prefixes change their spelling depending on the word root, but the meaning remains the same. For instance, the "d" in the prefix "ad-," which means to or toward, becomes "s" if the stem begins with "s," as in the term "assimilation."

AS (to) SIMULATION (simulate or make like)

COMMON WORD ROOTS

Root	Meaning
brachi-	arm
carp-	wrist
cephal-	head
chondr-	cartilage
cyst-	bladder
encephal-	brain
fibr-	fibers
gastr-	stomach
gloss-	tongue
later-	side
my-	muscle
mel-	limb
nas-	nose
nephr-	kidney
oss-	bone
ot-	ear
phleb-	vein
somat-	body
thorac-	chest
ventr-	front
viscer-	viscera

COMMON PREFIXES

Prefix	Meaning
a-, an-	not, without
ab-	away from
ad-	to, toward
ana-	up, toward
anti-	against
auto-	self
bi-	two, double
brady-	slow
circum-	around
co-, con-	with, together
contra-	opposed, against
de-	down, from
di-	two, twice
dis-	apart
ec-, ecto-	outer
ep-, epi-	on, upon
hyper-	excessive
hypo-	under
inter-	between
para-	beside
retro-	backward
super-	above
trans-	across

Suffixes

The **suffix** is sometimes referred to as the terminal element or word ending. The suffix attaches to the end of a word and, like the prefix, can never stand alone. A word can have its entire meaning changed by replacing one suffix with another. The suffix is added to the word root to change or modify its meaning. The box "Common Suffixes" illustrates some of these suffixes. Suffixes often indicate what is happening in relation to the word root. For example, in the term cystitis, the root "cyst-" means bladder, and the suffix "-itis" means inflammation. Therefore, cystitis is inflammation of (what is happening to) the bladder.

COMMON SUFFIXES

Suffix	Meaning
-ac, -al	pertaining to
-algia	pain
-ate, -ize	use, subject to
-cle, -cule	small
-cyte	cell
-emesis	vomit
-emia	blood condition
-gram, -graphy	recording
-ites, itis	inflammation
-phobia	abnormal fear
-pnea	breathing
-rrhage	excessive flow
-rrhea	flow or discharge
-stomy	surgical opening
-scope	instrument to examine
-tomy	cutting, incision

Combining Vowels

The **combining vowel** (usually "o") links the root to the suffix or to another root to ease pronunciation. For example:

ONCOGENIC   ONC/O/GEN/IC
             root | root suffix
             combining vowel

Word parts that begin or end with a vowel may drop the vowel of the prefix or suffix when combined. The "i" in "anti" is dropped before words that begin with a vowel, making the prefix "ant-."

Combining Forms

A **combining form** is a word root followed by a vowel to facilitate pronunciation. It combines a word root with a suffix or other root. The combining form is used to build compound words. For example:

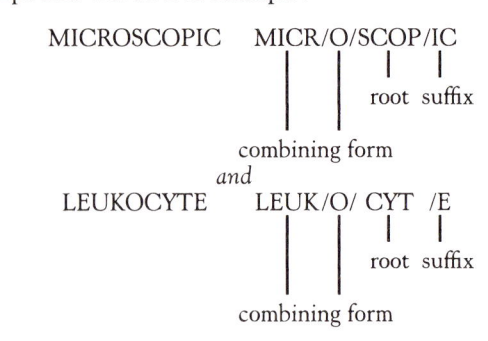

MICROSCOPIC   MICR/O/SCOP/IC
                    root suffix
               combining form

and

LEUKOCYTE   LEUK/O/ CYT /E
                   root suffix
             combining form

The box "Common Combining Forms" illustrates some of these forms.

COMMON COMBINING FORMS

Combining Form	Meaning
brachi/o-	arm
cervic/o-	neck
derm/a-	skin
dors/i-	posterior
occipit/o-	back of head
ophthalm/o-	eye, eyes
ot/o-	ear
tal/o-	ankle
thorac/o-	chest
ventr/o-	anterior

Abbreviations

Abbreviations are used to shorten words for ease of writing. Abbreviations may vary for each medical institution. Most institutions have an approved list of abbreviations. The box "Common Medical Abbreviations for the Paramedic" presents a list of the most common abbreviations that the paramedic may encounter.

HUMAN SYSTEMS

This section has a direct correlation with medical terminology. Medical terms are used to describe body orientation: the directions, planes, movements, postures, and cavities within the body. Body systems are described so that the paramedic has an initial orientation to the functioning of the body. This orientation allows the paramedic to process information on what is happening to the patient in relation to normal body functions. More explicit detail on each body system is described in later chapters.

COMMON MEDICAL ABBREVIATIONS FOR THE PARAMEDIC

Abbreviation	Meaning	Abbreviation	Meaning
AIDS	acquired immune deficiency syndrome	LLQ	left lower quadrant
		LMP	last menstrual period
A & P	auscultation and percussion	LUQ	lower upper quadrant
ASAP	as soon as possible	mcg	microgram
AX	axillary	mg	milligram
BM	bowel movement	MI	myocardial infarction
BP	blood pressure	ml	milliliter
BSA	body surface area	mm	millimeter
c̄	with	MVA	motor vehicle accident
CA	cancer	NaHCO$_3$	sodium bicarbonate
CAD	coronary artery disease	NaCl	sodium chloride
CC	chief complaint	NG	nasogastric
CCU	cardiac care unit	NS	normal saline
CHF	congestive heart failure	NSR	normal sinus rhythm
CNS	central nervous system	O$_2$	oxygen
C/O	complains of	OB	obstetrics
COPD	chronic obstructive pulmonary disease	OD	overdose
		OR	operating room
CPR	cardiopulmonary resuscitation	PDR	Physicians' Desk Reference
		PE	physical exam
CSF	cerebrospinal fluid	PH	past history
CVA	cerebrovascular accident	PI	present illness
DC	discontinue	PO	by mouth
DOA	dead on arrival	PRN	when necessary
DT	delirium tremens	Pt	patient
Dx	diagnosis	q	every
EKG or ECG	electrocardiogram	qd	every day
ED	emergency department	qh	every hour
EMS	emergency medical services	qid	four times a day
ETT	endotracheal tube	RLQ	right lower quadrant
ETOH	ethyl alcohol	RUQ	right upper quadrant
Fx	fracture	Rx	prescription
GI	gastrointestinal	SQ	subcutaneous
g or gm	gram	SIDS	sudden infant death syndrome
gtt	drops		
GSW	gunshot wound	stat	immediately
Gyn	gynecologic	s̄	without
H & P	history and physical	T	temperature
HR	heart rate	TID	three times a day
Hx	history	TKO	to keep open
ICU	intensive care unit	TPR	temperature, pulse, and respiration
IM	intramuscular		
IUD	intrauterine device	VD	venereal disease
IV	intravenous	V/S	vital signs
Kg	kilogram	WD	well developed
KUB	kidney, ureter, bladder	y.o.	year old

Body Orientation

An understanding of certain anatomical directions, planes, movements, postures, and cavities is essential for orientation to the human body. Communication of this information is an important factor in patient care. Locations of injuries can be better identified and reported. For descriptive purposes, the normal anatomical position of the human body is in the erect position with eyes directed straight ahead, arms hanging by the side, feet together, and the palms of the hands facing forward, as shown in Figure 8-1. Regardless of the position in which the body is found, the description of information should always refer to the normal anatomical position.

Directions

Parts of the body are described in relation to one another by anatomical directions (Fig. 8-2). *Superior* or cranial denotes direction upward or toward the head of the body. In contrast, *inferior* or caudal means downward or away from the head. The chest is superior to the abdomen, and the mouth is inferior to the nose. *Anterior* or ventral describes the front surface of the body in contrast to the term *posterior* or dorsal, which means the back surface of the body. *Medial* is the term that defines reference toward the midline of the body, as opposed to *lateral*, which is a direction away from the midline. The arm lies lateral to the chest wall, and the sternum is medial to the ribs. *Proximal* means nearest the point of origin or nearer to the attachment of an extremity to the trunk or a structure. *Distal* means away from the point of origin or further from the attachment of an extremity to the trunk or a structure. The hand is distal to the elbow, and the elbow is proximal to the wrist.

Planes

The planes of the body represent imaginary divisions that cut through the body in different directions (Fig. 8-3). *Sagittal* is an imaginary plane that passes vertically from front through back, dividing the body into right and left portions. If the sagittal plane divides the body into equal parts, right down the midline, it is called a midsagittal plane. The *frontal* plane passes vertically through the body at a right angle to the sagittal plane and divides the body into anterior and posterior portions. The *transverse* plane divides the body or any of its parts horizontally into superior and inferior portions. This division is sometimes referred to as a cross section.

Movements

Movements produce changes in the relative positions of the body. Most commonly these are described as movements at the joints. *Flexion* is a bending motion that decreases the angle at a joint, whereas *extension* straightens or increases the angle. *Abduction* reflects movement of a part away from the midline of the body, while *adduction* is movement of the part toward the midline. *Rotation* involves the turning of a part on its own axis. Lateral rotation means to rotate outward away from the body's midline. Medial rotation means to rotate inward toward the body's midline. *Circumduction* is the swinging of a part in a circle; it involves displacement of the axis. Figure 8-4 illustrates normal body movements.

Postures

The anatomical postures of the body are erect, supine, prone, and laterally recumbent. The *erect* posture holds the body standing upright in a vertical position. The *supine* position places the body horizontally, lying flat on the back; *prone* places the body horizontally, lying flat, but face down. *Laterally recumbent* positions the body lying flat on either the left or right side.

Cavities

The human body contains two sets of cavities, ventral and dorsal. Each of these contains yet smaller cavities. The ventral cavity consists of the thoracic and abdominopelvic cavity. The thoracic cavity houses the heart and lungs and is separated from the abdominopelvic cavity by the diaphragm. The abdominopelvic cavity consists of an upper portion, the abdominal cavity that contains the stomach, intestines, liver, and other organs, and a lower portion, the pelvic cavity, that contains the reproductive organs, bladder, and rectum. The dorsal cavity is subdi-

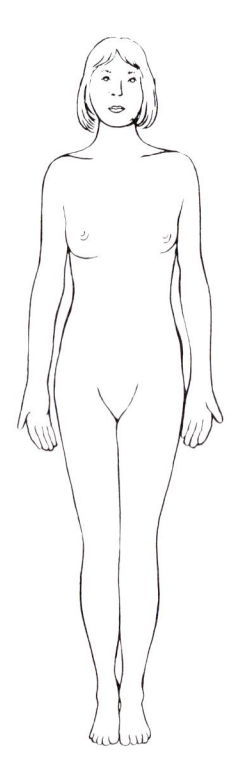

FIGURE 8-1.
The normal anatomical position.

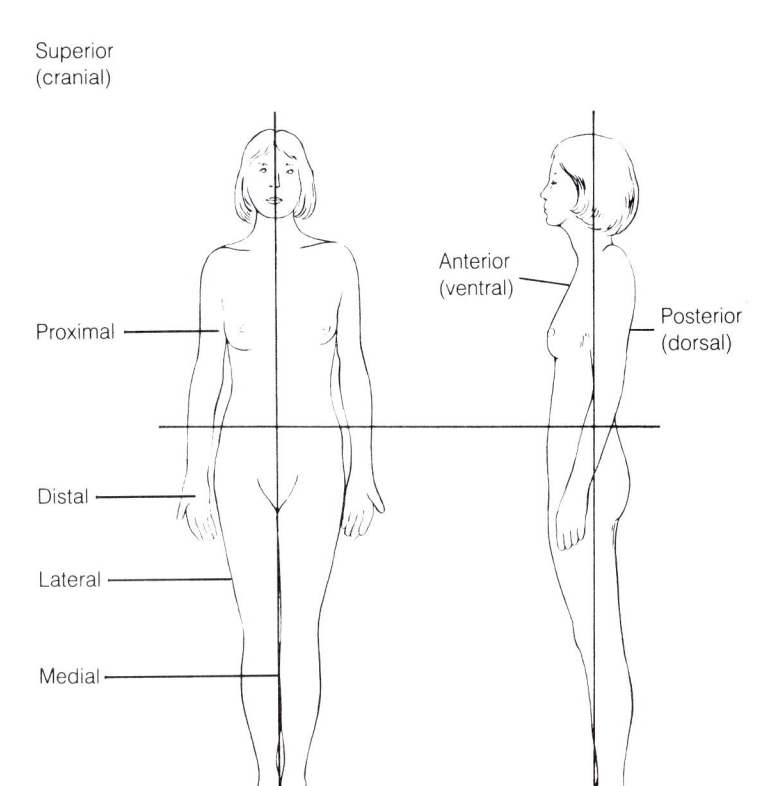

CHAPTER 8: Medical Terminology and Human Systems 83

FIGURE 8–2. Anatomical directions.

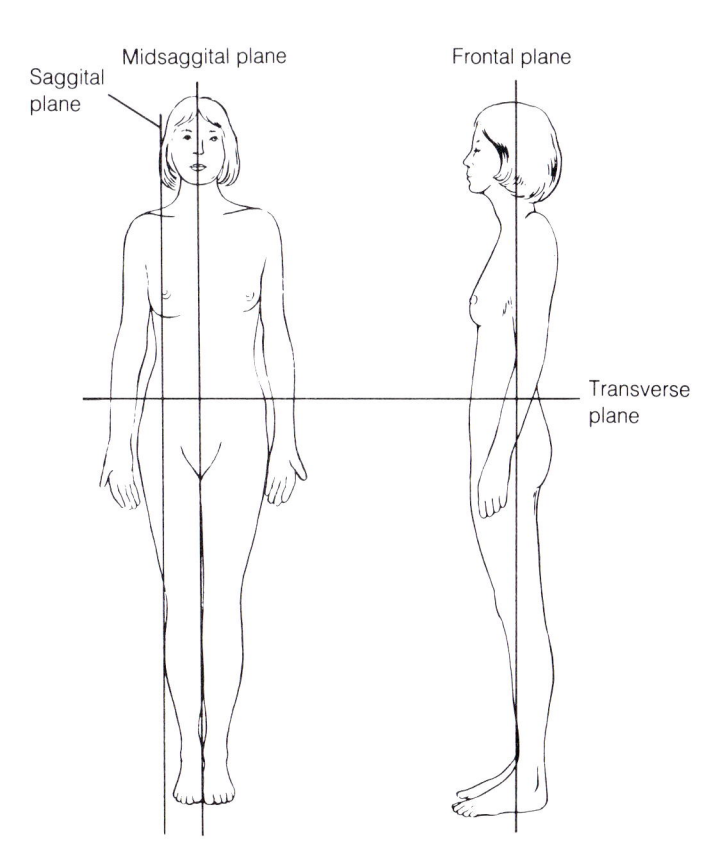

FIGURE 8–3. Planes of the body.

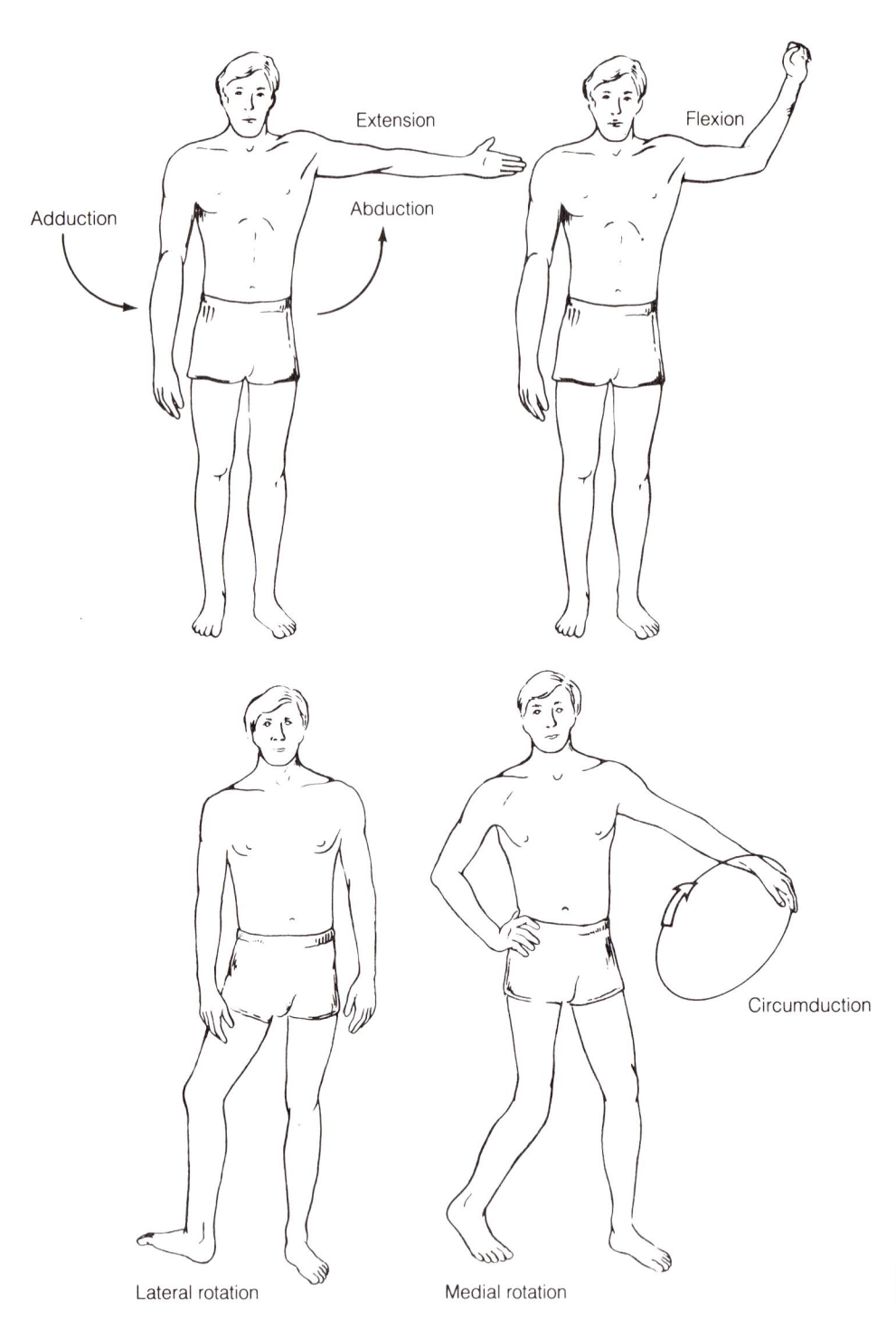

FIGURE 8–4.
Normal body movements.

vided into the cranial and spinal cavities. The cranial cavity lies in the skull and houses the brain. The spinal cavity lies in the spinal column and houses the spinal cord. Figure 8-5 illustrates the cavities of the body.

Body Systems

The human body is organized from the simplest unit of living matter to complex units that work together to maintain life. The smallest structural units in the body are called cells. Specialized groups of cells form tissues, and tissues may function together as organs. A system is composed of a number of organs that work together to perform complex functions for the body. Each body system is explained independently in more detail in the following chapters. A brief introduction to each system, however, is given in this section.

Textbooks list from nine to twelve systems, depending on how they are divided and subdivided. The ten most common systems have been selected for this discussion.

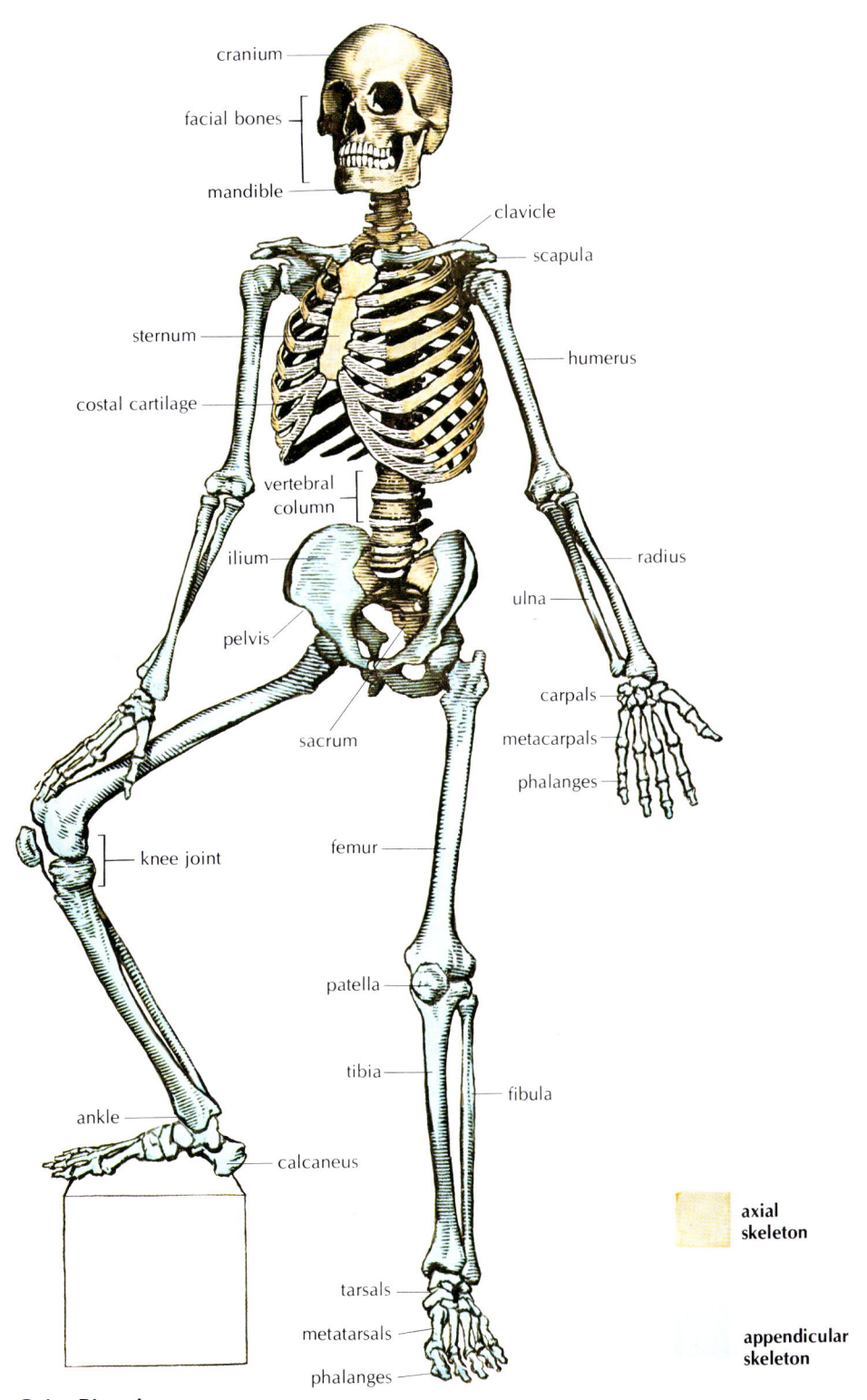

Color Plate 1.
The bones of the human skeleton. (Memmler RL, Wood DL)

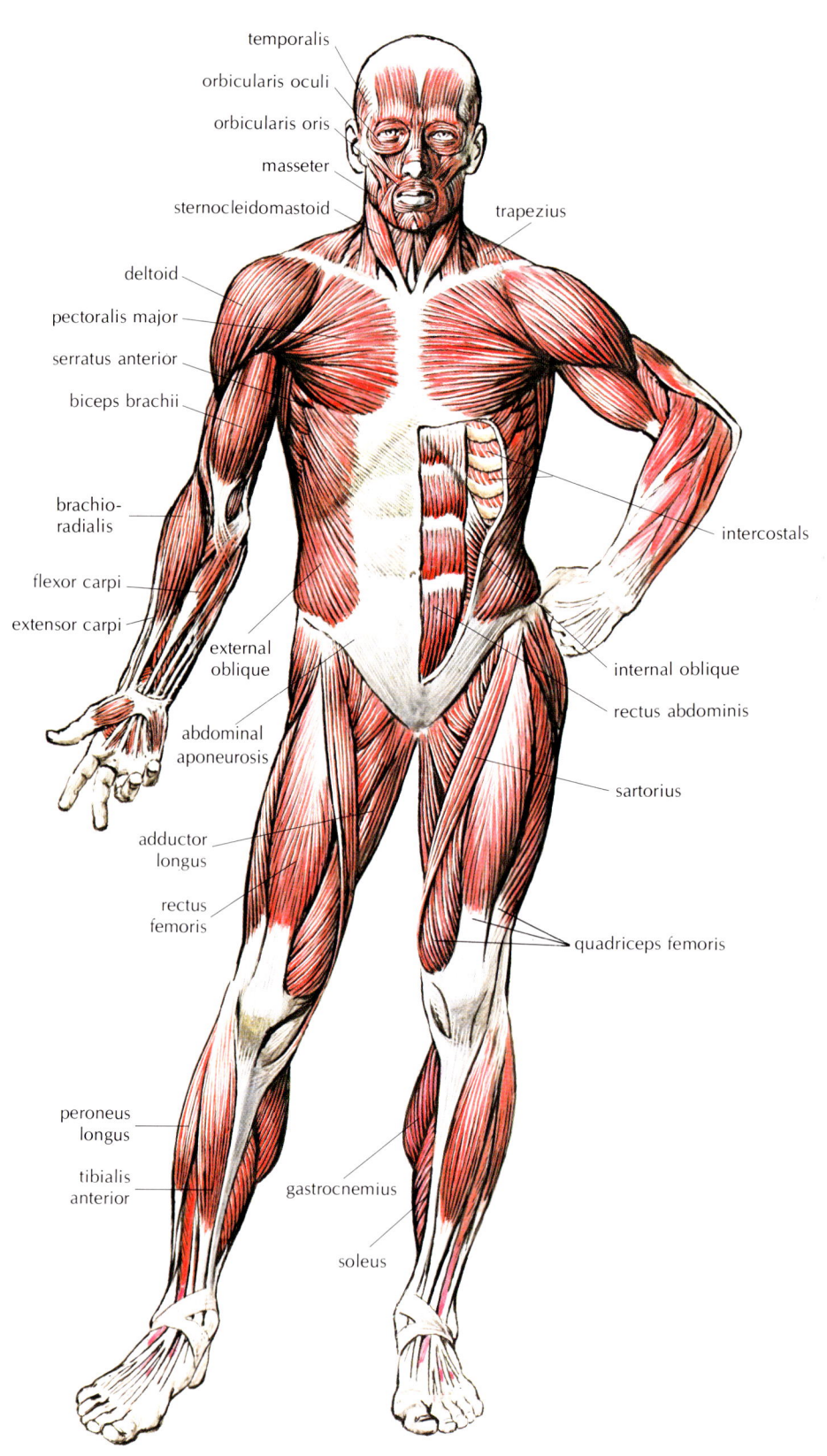

Color Plate 2.
Muscles of the body from an anterior (front) view. (Memmler RL, Wood DL)

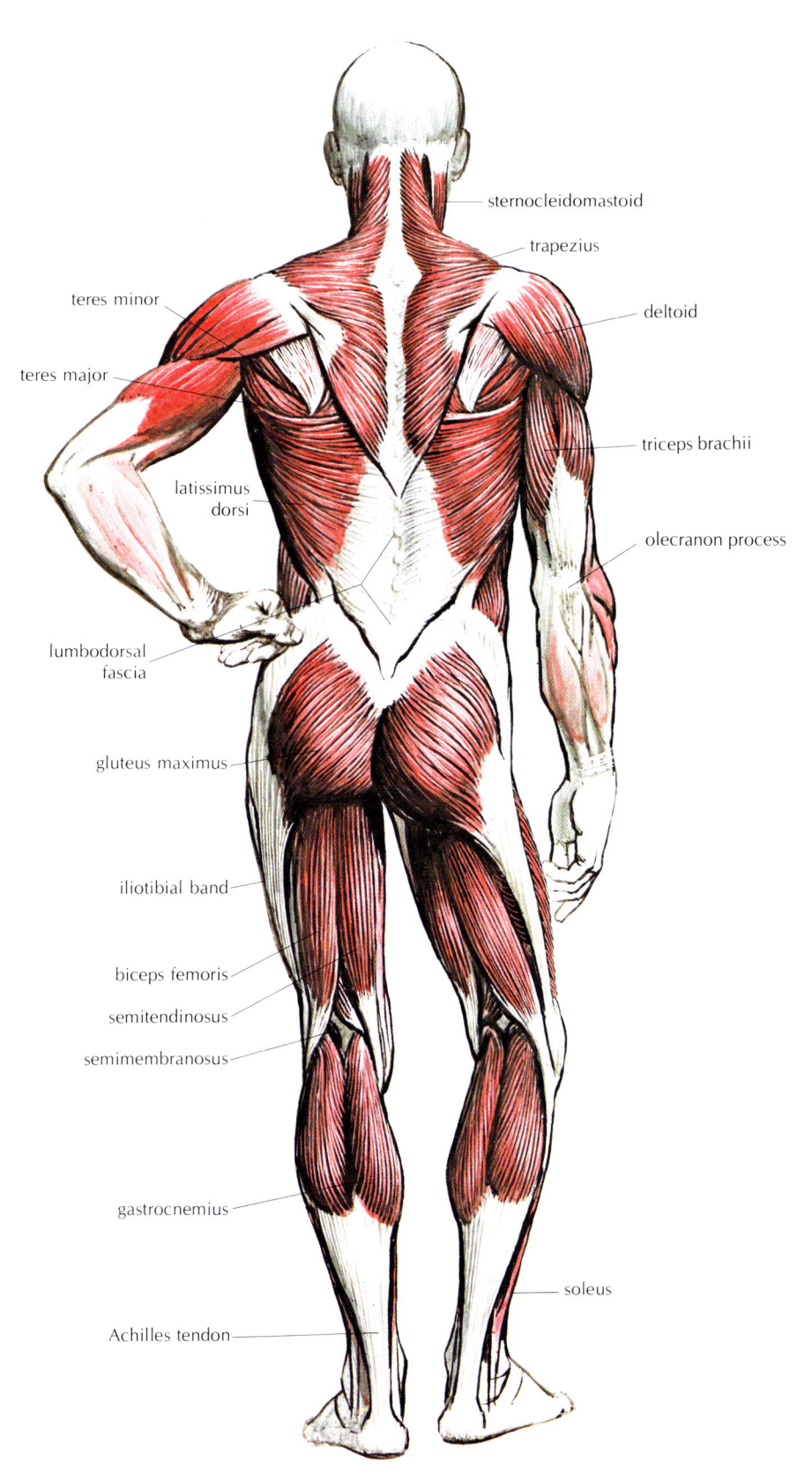

Color Plate 3.
Muscles of the body from a posterior (back) view. (Memmler RL, Wood DL)

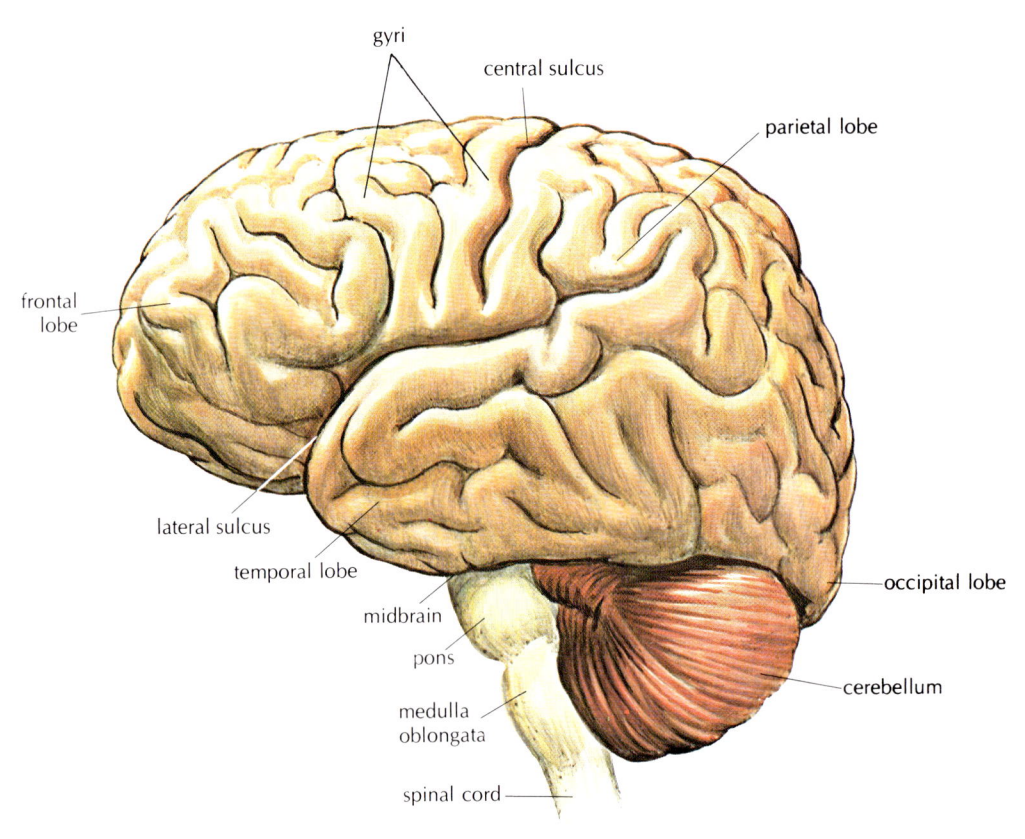

Color Plate 4.
The external surface of the brain shows the main parts and some of the lobes and sulci of the cerebrum. (Memmler RL, Wood DL)

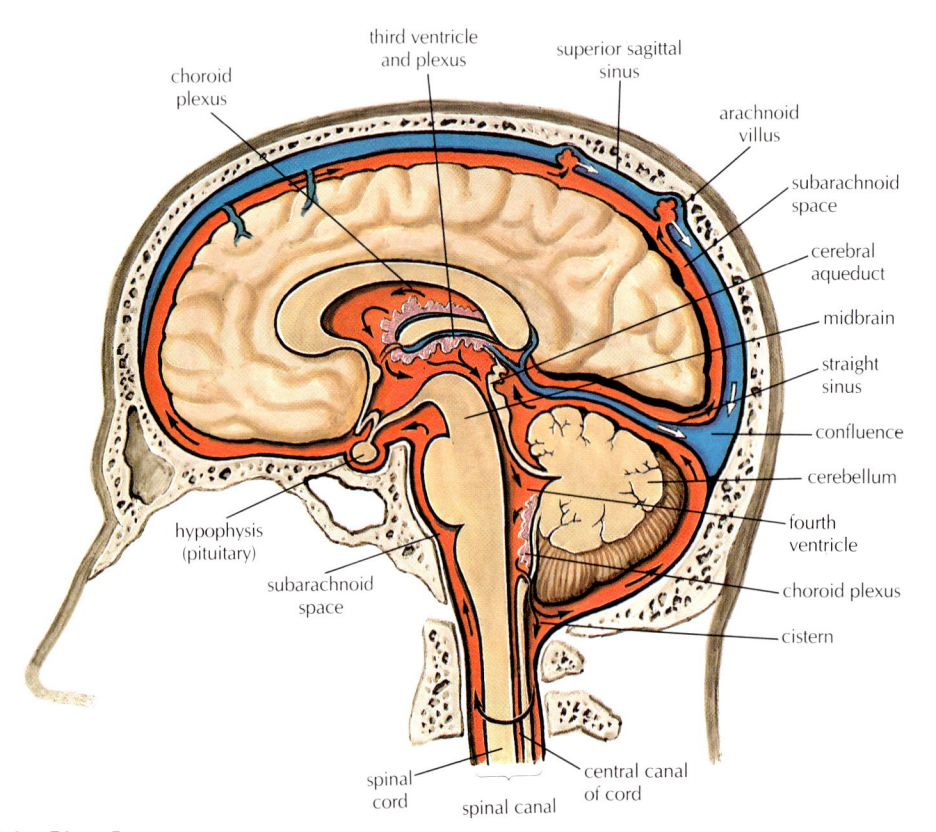

Color Plate 5.
Flow of cerebrospinal fluid from choroid plexuses back to blood in venous sinuses is shown by the black arrows; flow of blood is shown by the white arrows. (Memmler RL, Wood DL)

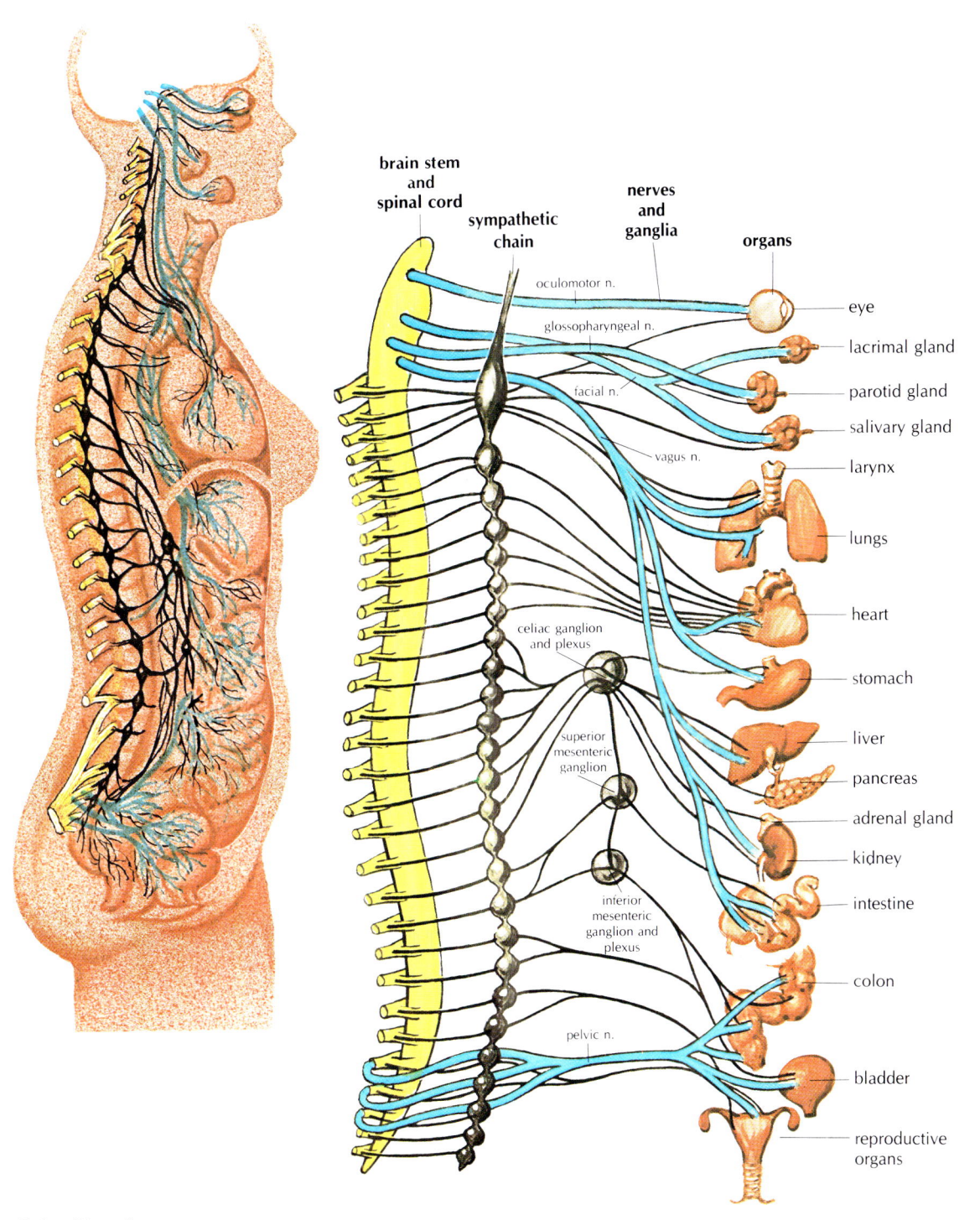

Color Plate 6.
Anatomy of the autonomic nervous system. (Memmler RL, Wood DL)

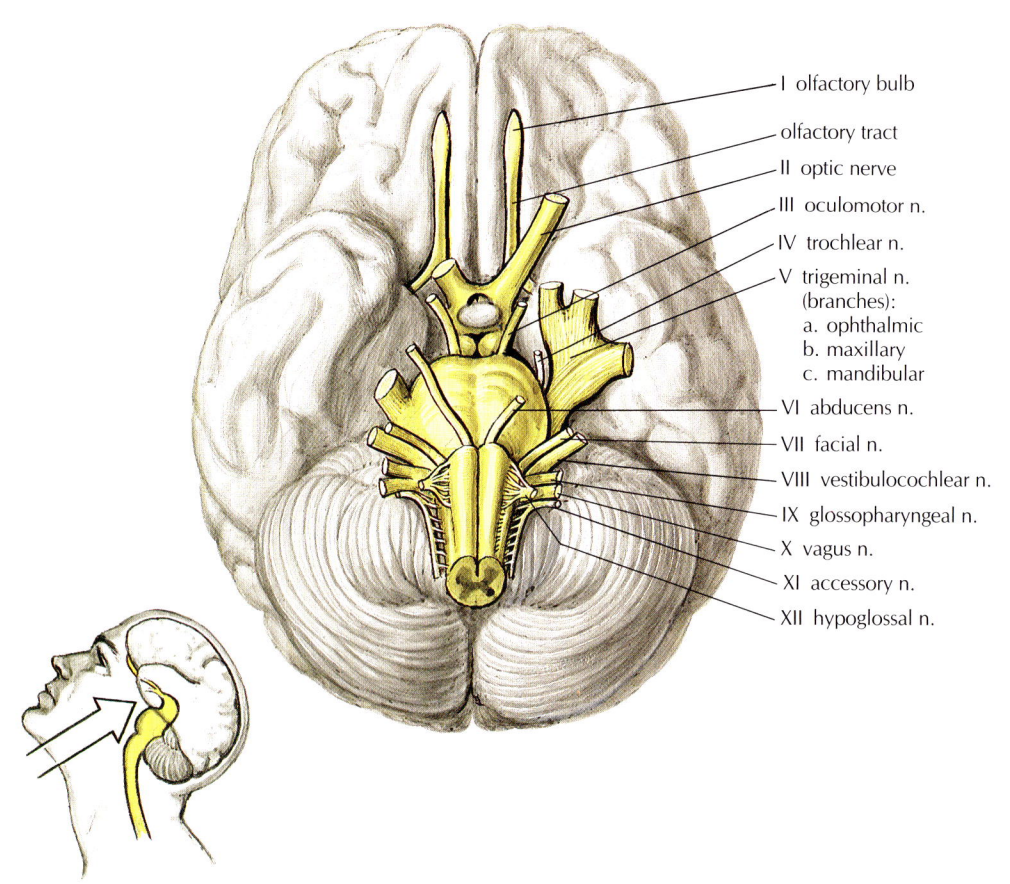

Color Plate 7.
The base of the brain, which shows cranial nerves. (Memmler RL, Wood DL)

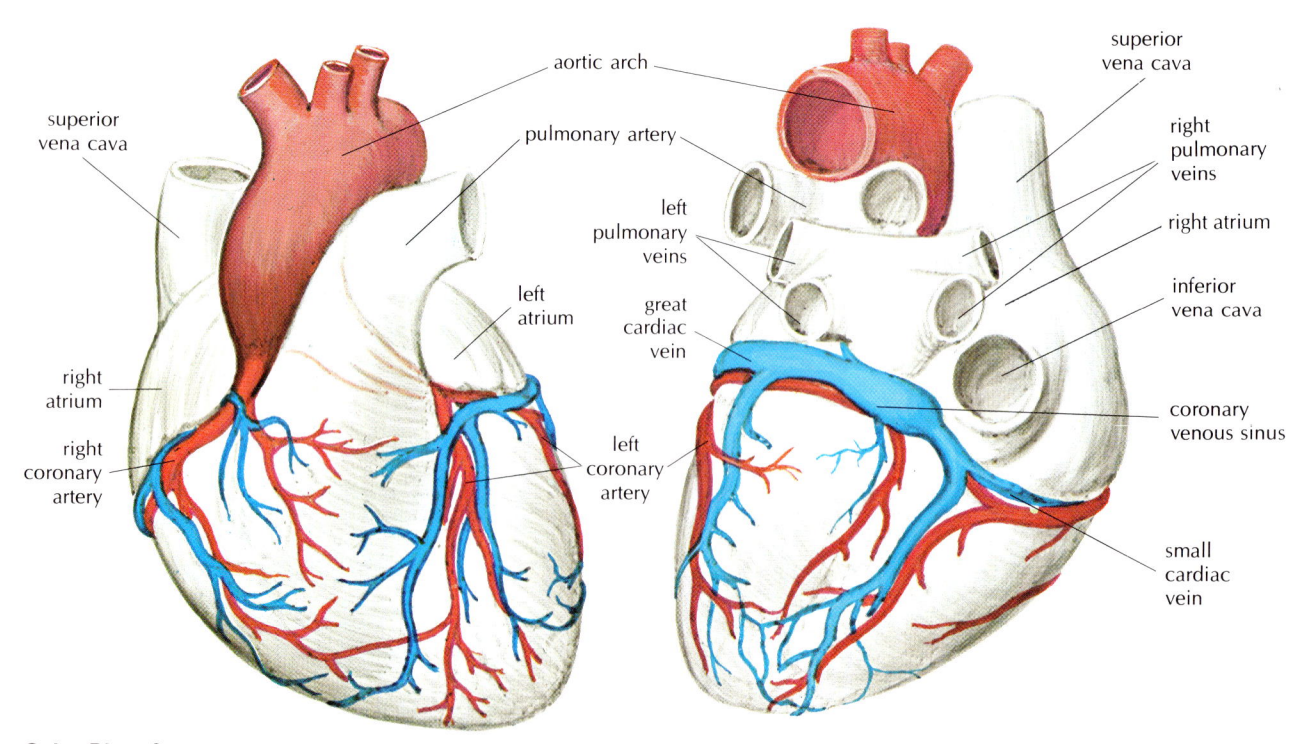

Color Plate 8.
Coronary arteries and cardiac veins, shown from the anterior (left) and posterior (right) views. (Memmler RL, Wood DL)

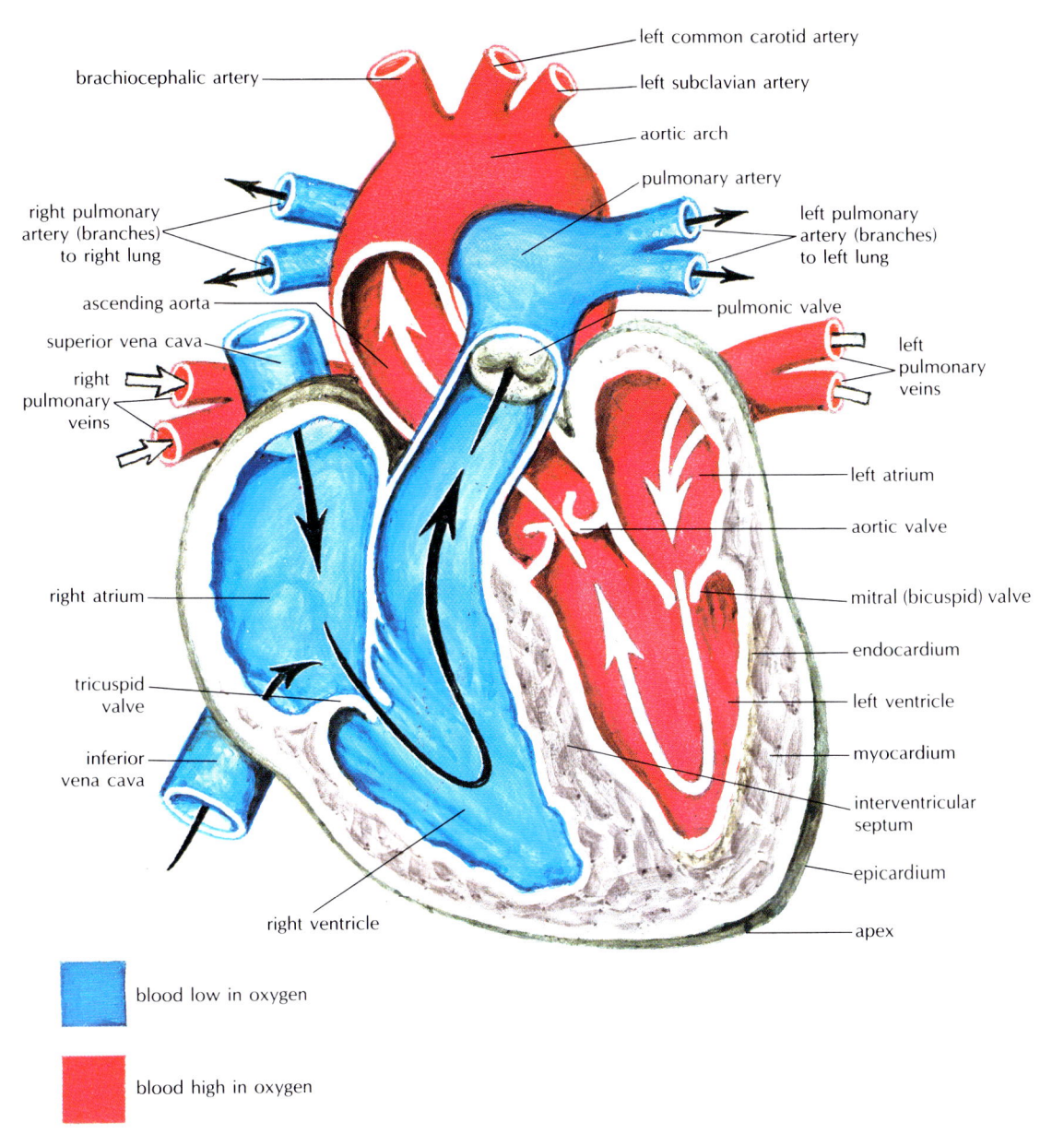

Color Plate 9.
The heart and great vessels. (Memmler RL, Wood DL)

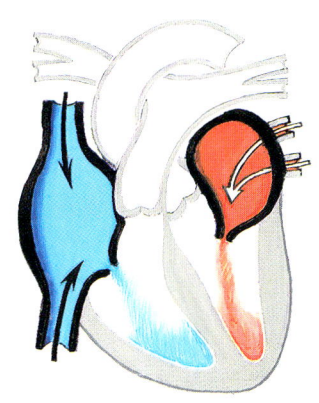

Diastole
Atria fill with blood which begins to flow into ventricles as soon as their walls relax.

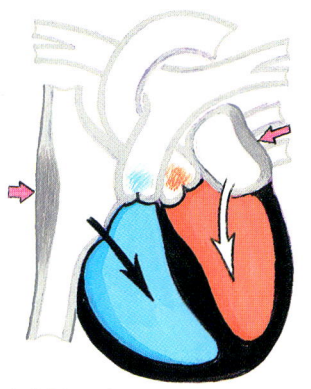

Atrial Systole
Contraction of atria pumps blood into the ventricles.

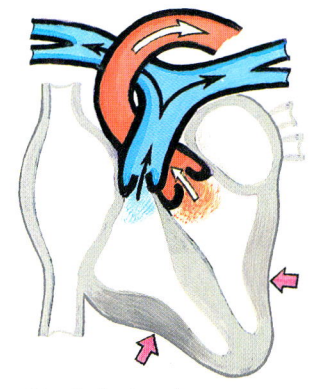

Ventricular Systole
Contraction of ventricles pumps blood into aorta and pulmonary arteries.

Color Plate 10.
The pumping cycle of the heart. (Memmler RL, Wood DL)

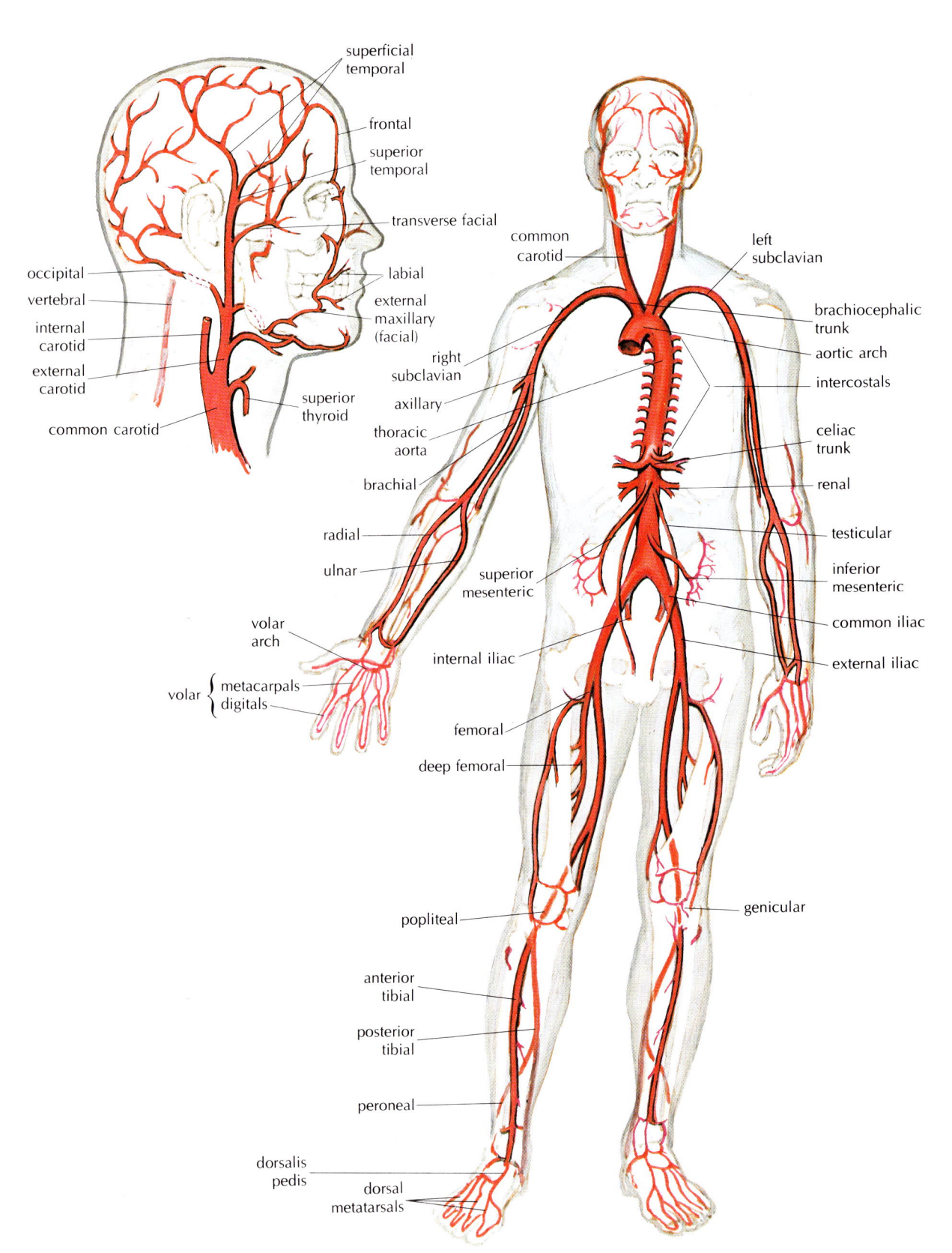

Color Plate 11.
The principal arteries. (Memmler RL, Wood DL)

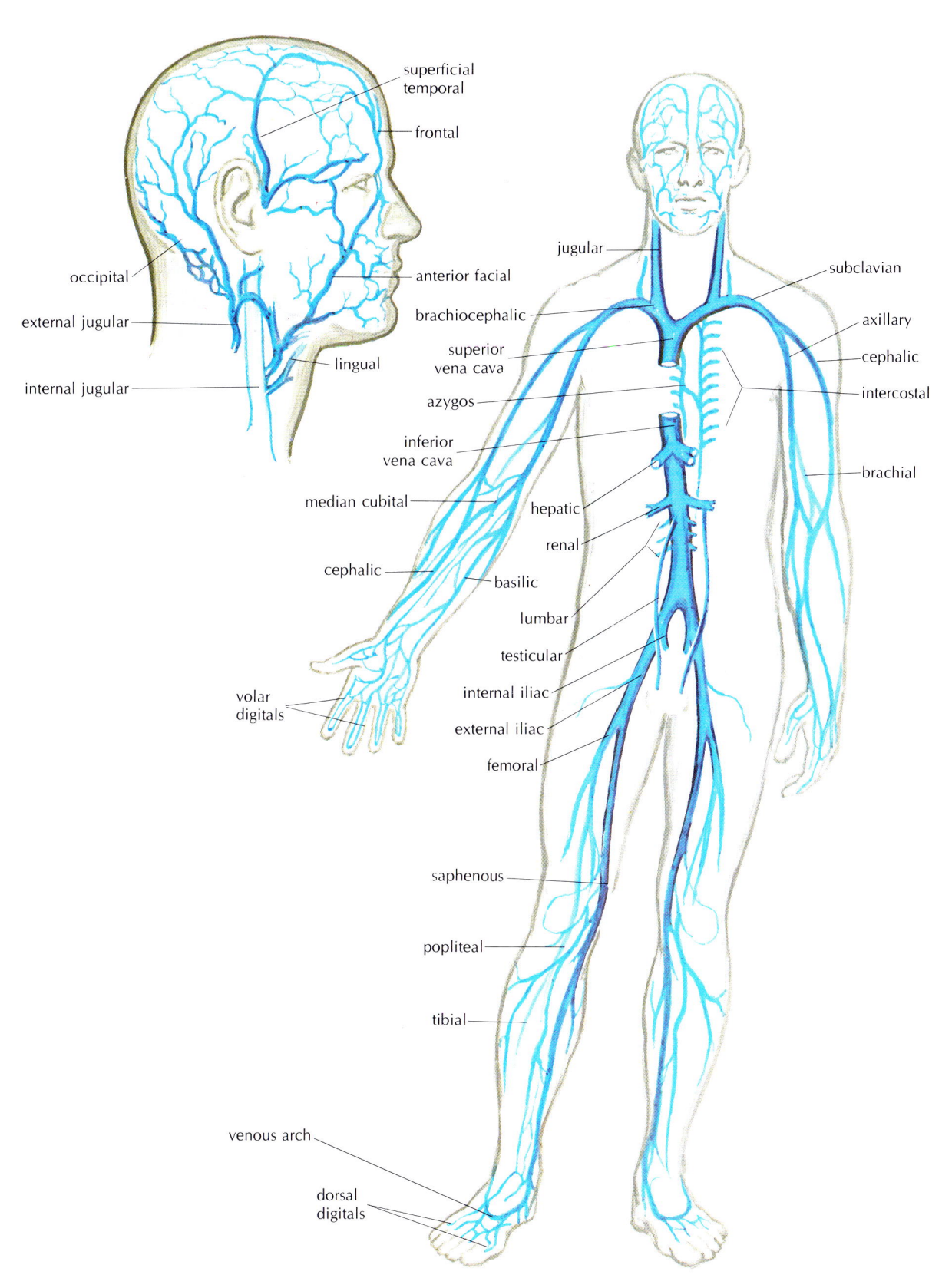

Color Plate 12.
The principal veins. (Memmler RL, Wood DL)

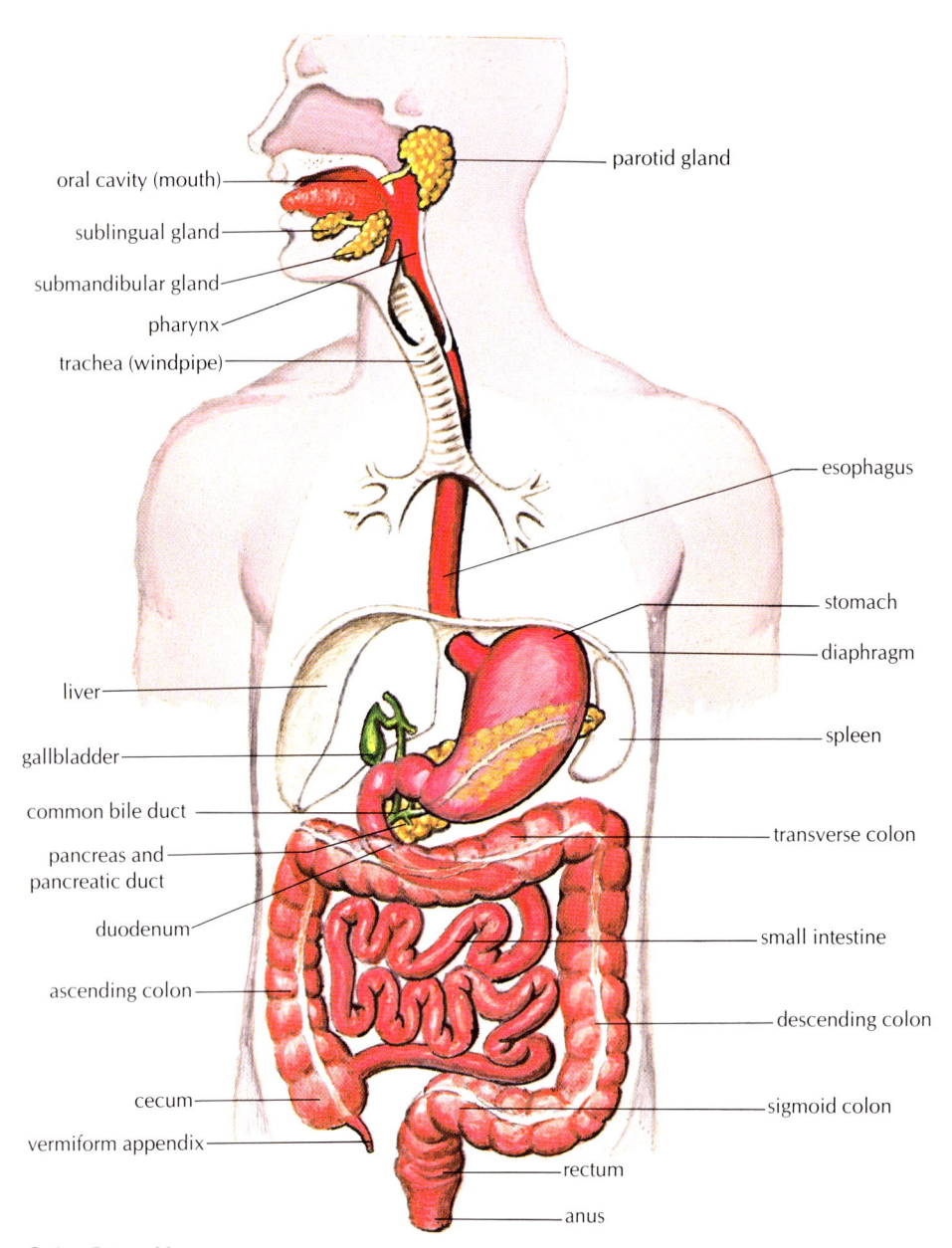

Color Plate 13.
The digestive system. (Memmler RL, Wood DL)

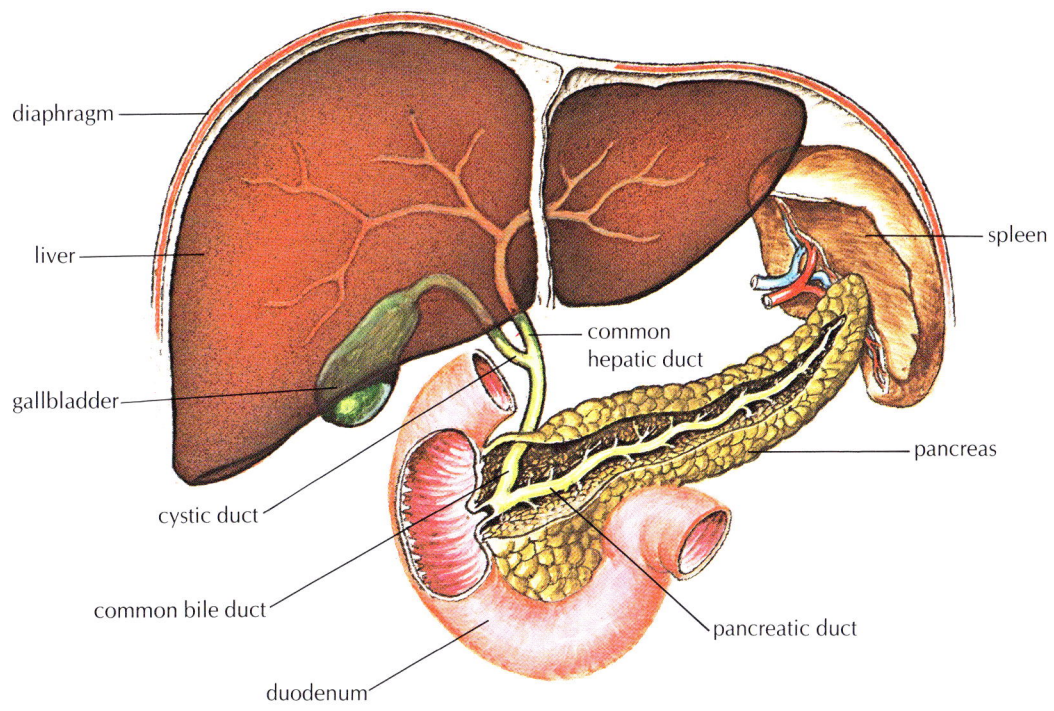

Color Plate 14.
The accessory organs of digestion. (Memmler RL, Wood DL)

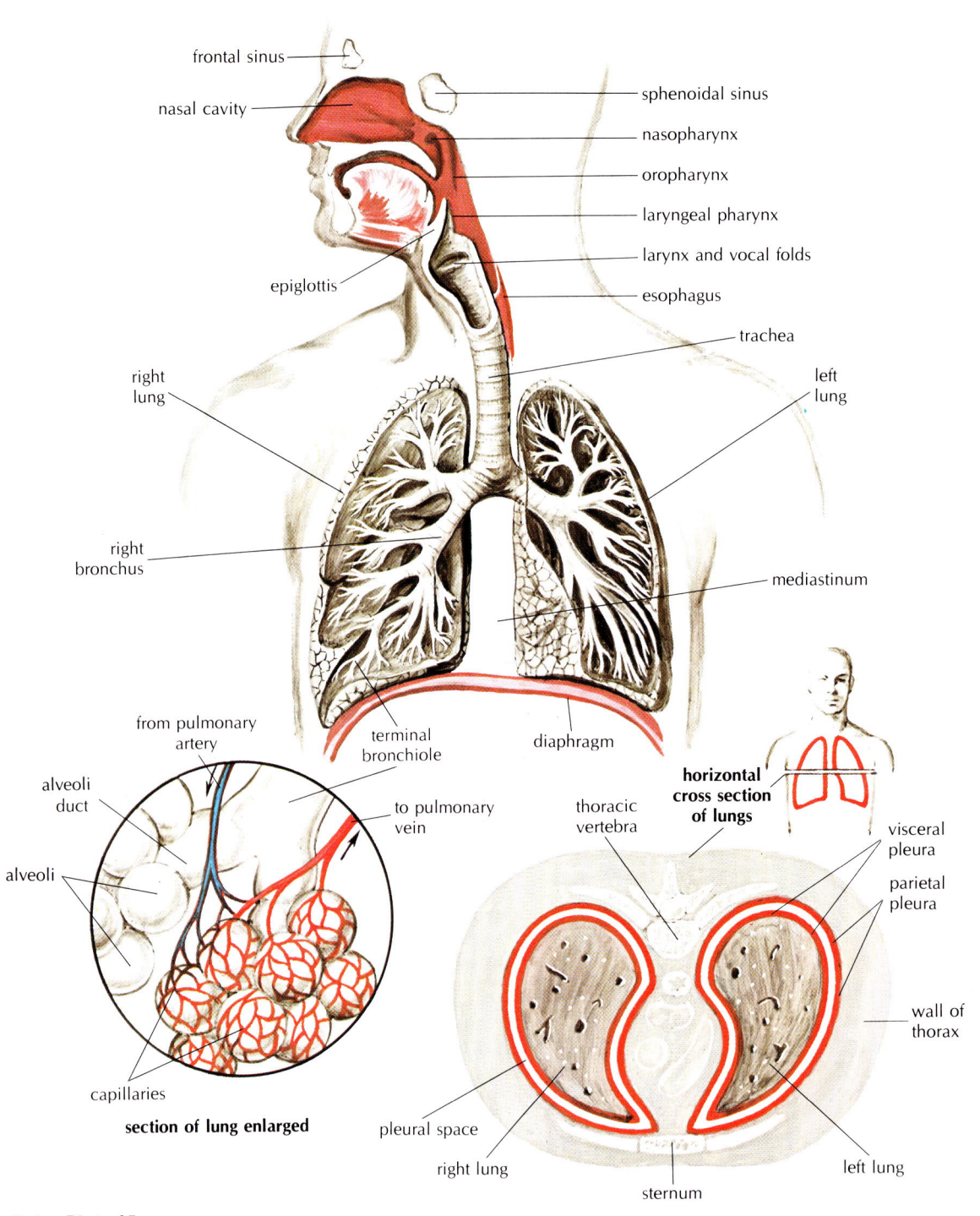

Color Plate 15.
The respiratory system. (Memmler RL, Wood DL)

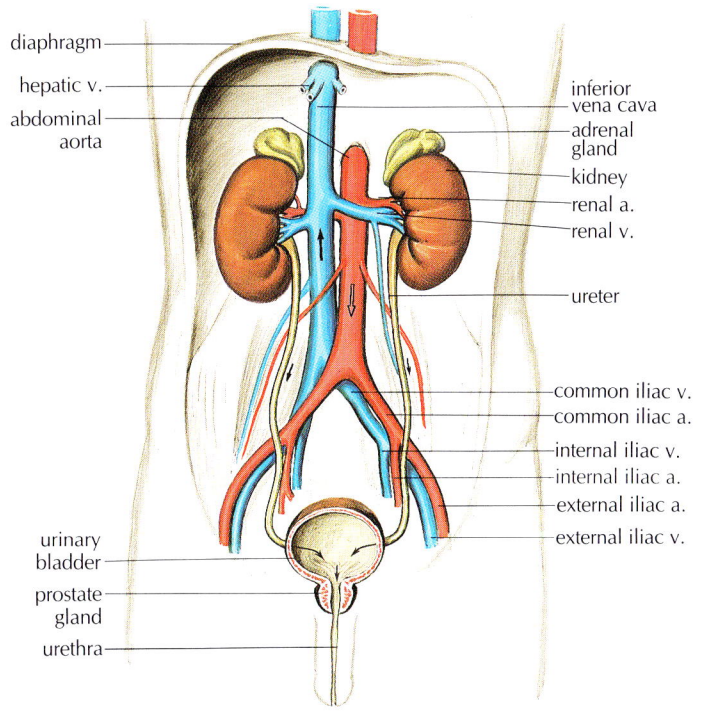

Color Plate 16.
The urinary system, with blood vessels. (Memmler RL, Wood DL)

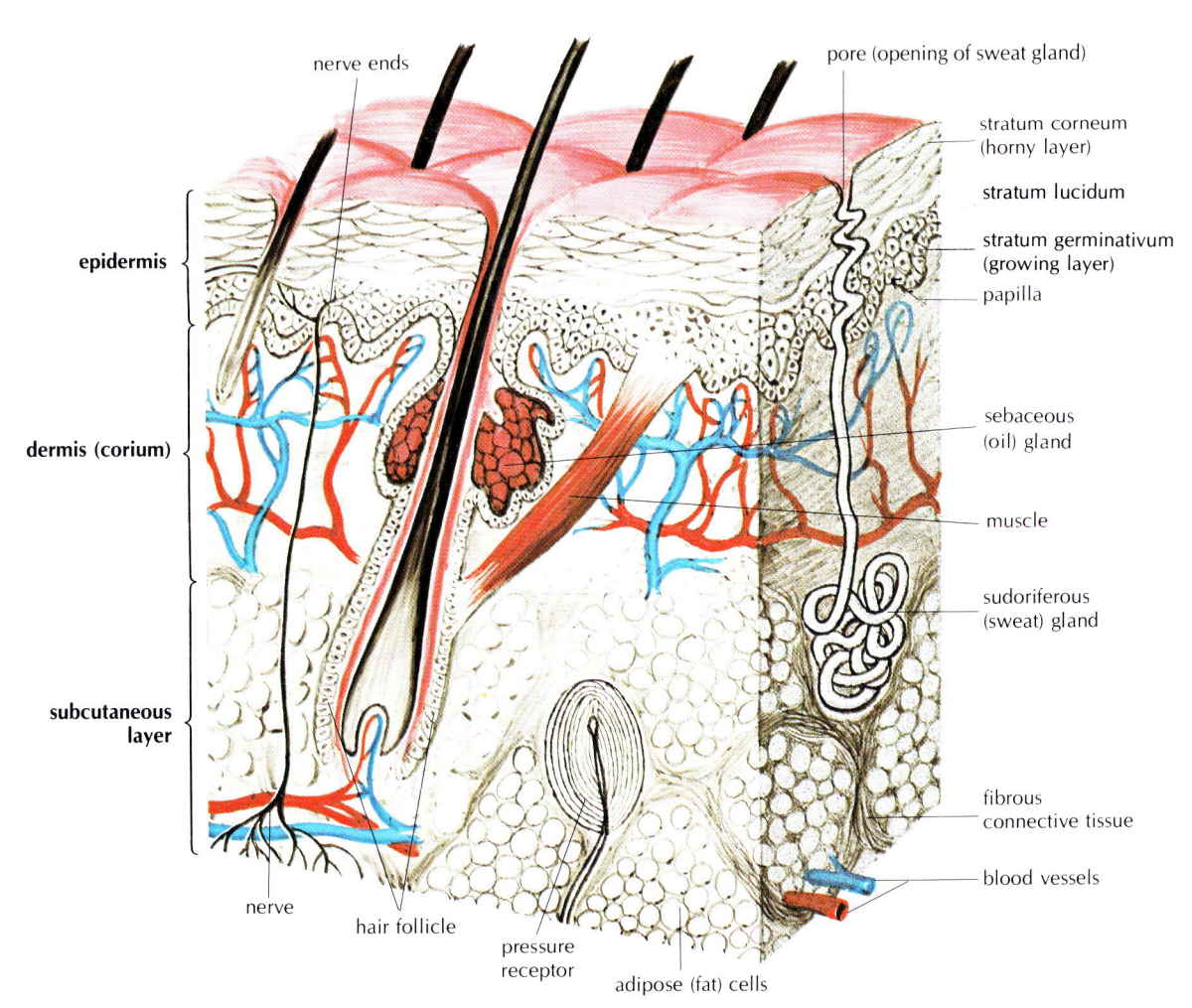

Color Plate 17.
A cross section of the skin. (Memmler RL, Wood DL)

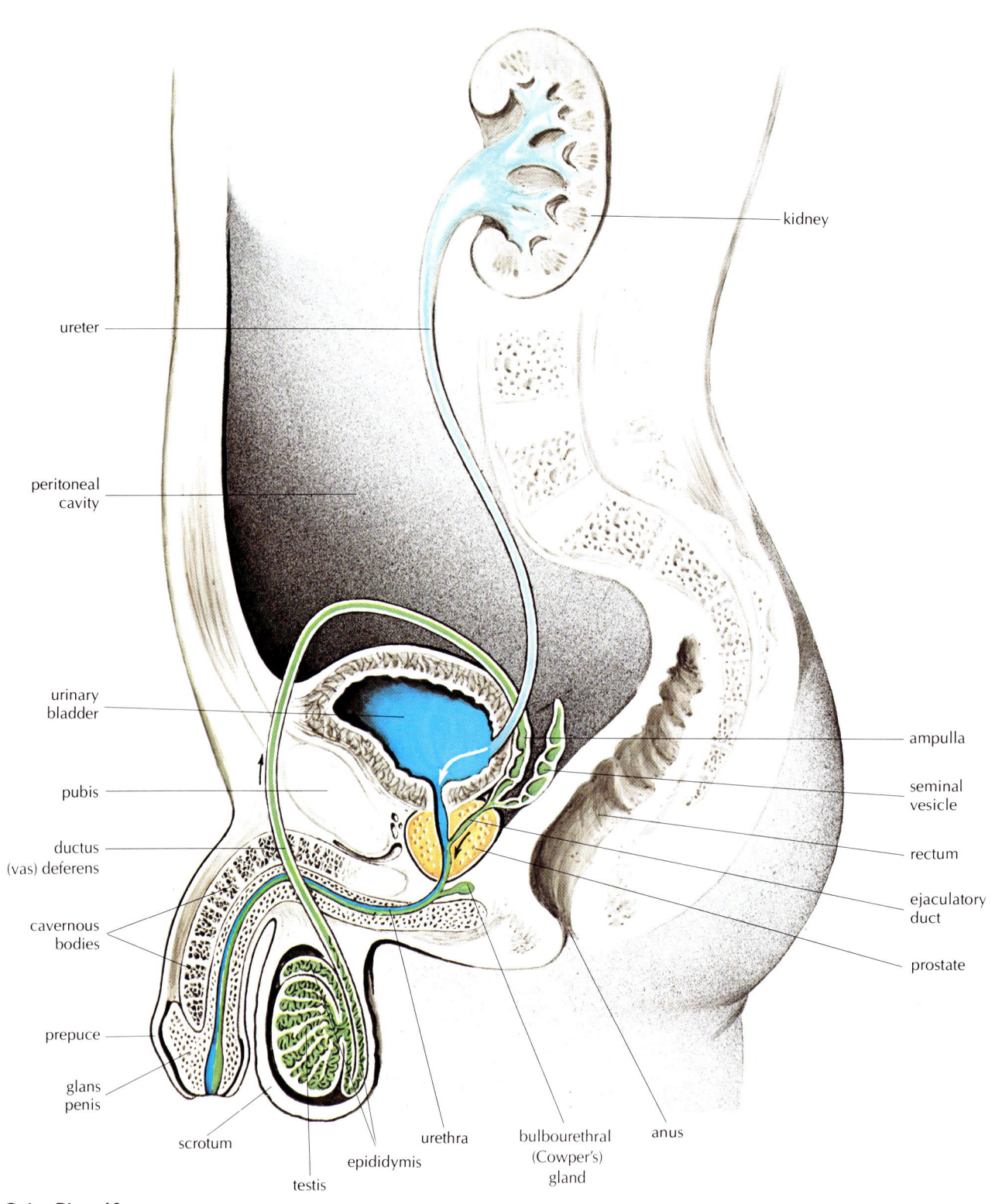

Color Plate 18.
The male genitourinary system. The black arrows indicate the course of spermatozoa through the duct system; the single white arrow indicates the course of urine. (Memmler RL, Wood DL)

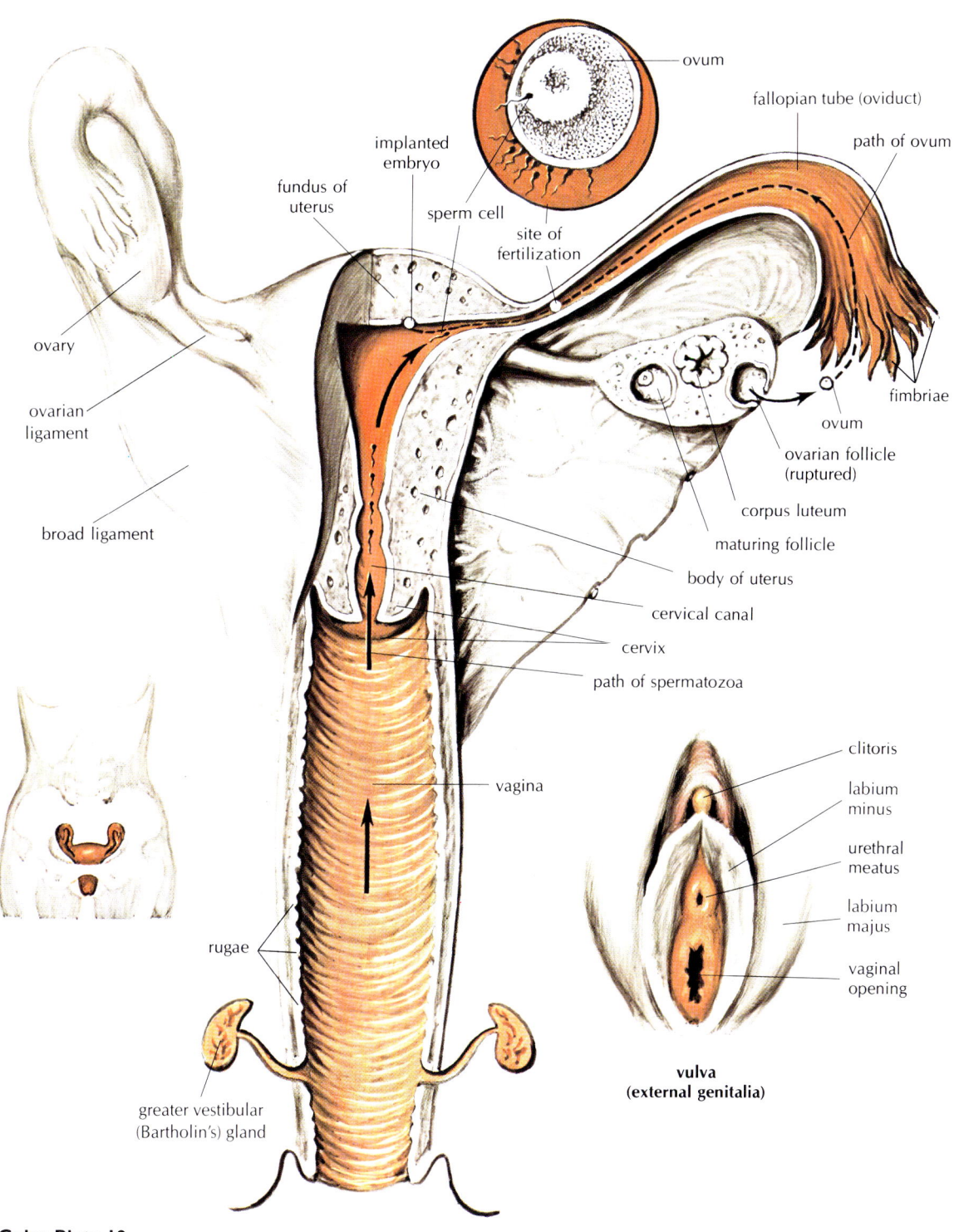

Color Plate 19.
The female reproductive system. (Memmler RL, Wood DL)

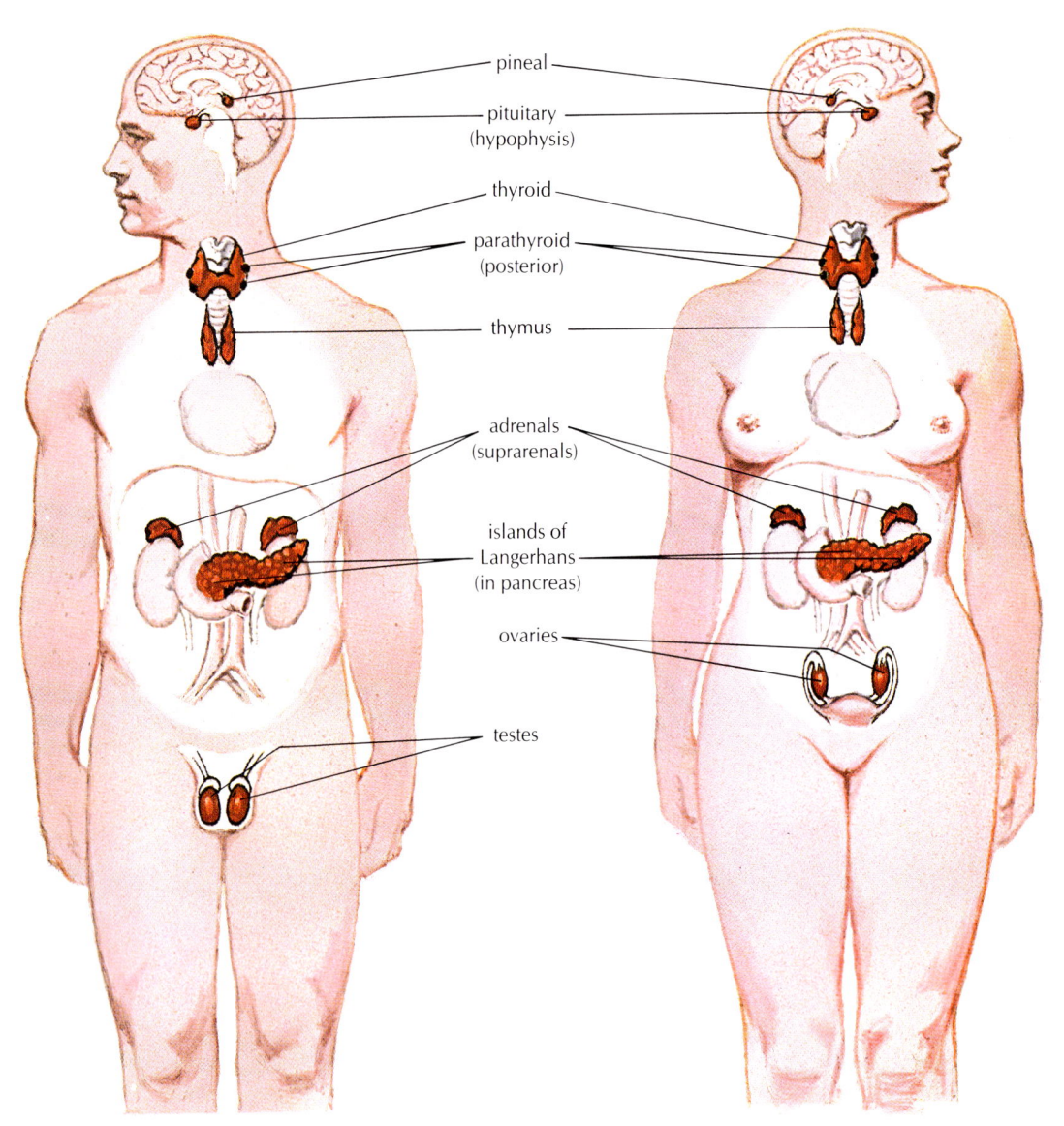

Color Plate 20.
The glands of the endocrine system. (Memmler RL, Wood DL)

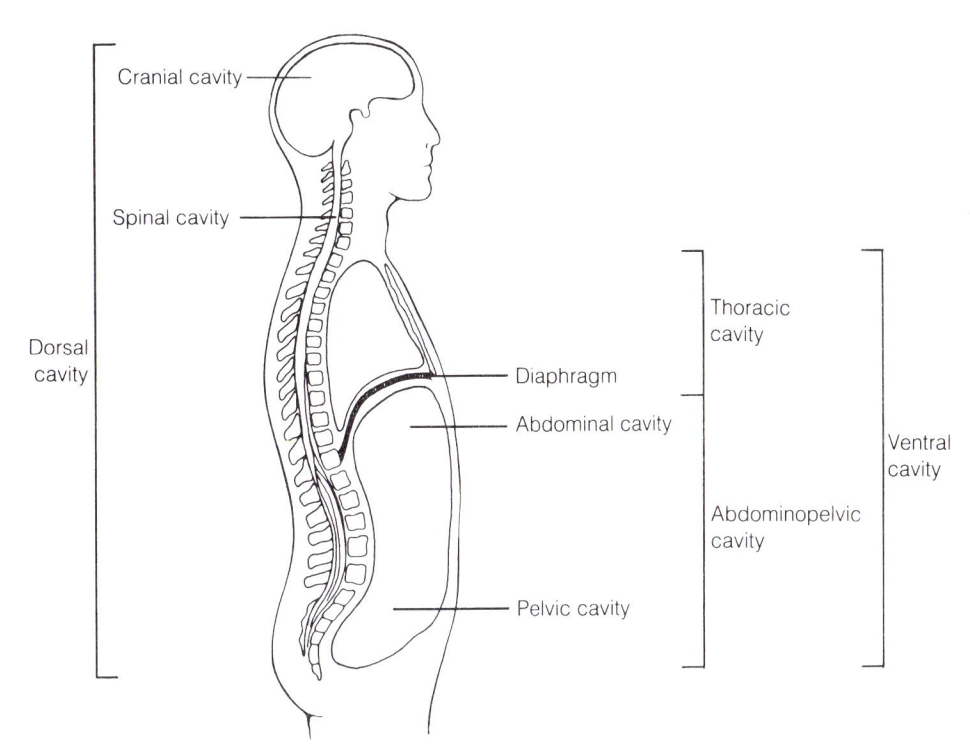

FIGURE 8–5.
The cavities of the body.

Skeletal

The skeletal system consists of bones, cartilage, and connective ligaments. The adult skeleton is composed of 206 separate bones. The functions of the skeletal system are to form a framework for the body, protect vital organs, and produce red blood cells. The human skeleton consists of two main divisions, the axial and appendicular skeleton. The axial skeleton includes 74 bones that form the upright axis of the body and 6 tiny ear bones. The appendicular skeleton consists of 126 bones that form the appendages to the axial skeleton, that is, the shoulders and upper extremities and hips and lower extremities. Color Plate 1 illustrates the bones of the human skeleton.

Muscular

The muscular system includes the muscles, fascia, tendons, and ligaments. The human body contains more than 600 individual muscles that are divided into three types: smooth, skeletal, and cardiac. Smooth muscle is also called involuntary muscle because we normally have no control over its contractions. Smooth muscle is found in the walls of the blood vessels and in organs of the ventral body cavities, with the exception of the heart. Skeletal muscle attaches to bones and is sometimes called voluntary muscle since it is usually under conscious control. Cardiac muscle is unique since it composes the bulk of one organ, the heart. Cardiac muscle is also called involuntary muscle since we normally have no control over its contractions. In addition to movement and the formation of many of the internal organs, the muscular system supports and maintains posture and produces body heat. Color Plate 2 illustrates the muscular system from an anterior view and Color Plate 3 illustrates the system from a posterior view.

Nervous

The nervous system includes the brain and spinal cord as well as other nerves of the body. The nervous system maintains and controls all body functions by voluntary and automatic responses. The three large divisions of the nervous system are the central nervous system, which consists of the brain and spinal cord; the peripheral nervous system, which consists of motor and sensory nerves that carry information to and from the central nervous system—this system includes the cranial and spinal nerves; and the autonomic nervous system, which regulates the internal environment of the body. The autonomic nervous system consists of specialized peripheral nerves that control activities automatically. The autonomic nervous system is further subdivided into the sympathetic and parasympathetic nervous systems. The sympathetic part of the autonomic nervous system tends to act as an accelerator of body functions, and the parasympathetic part acts as a balance for the body. Color Plates 4 through 7 illustrate various parts of the nervous system.

Cardiovascular

The cardiovascular system includes the heart, blood vessels, blood, and the spleen. The heart is a muscular pump that drives the blood through the blood vessels. The heart has its own specialized conduction system, which generates an electrical impulse that begins the heartbeat. The blood vessels, working with the heart, act to carry blood throughout the body. The cardiovascular system is a closed system; blood escapes only by an injury to some part of the system. The blood has several functions: it transports nutrients and carries waste products away from the cells, regulates proper pH, temperature, and osmotic pressure, and finally carries defenders against pathogens. The spleen is an organ that, as part of the cardiovascular system, filters bacteria and other foreign particles from the blood. Color Plates 8 through 12 illustrate various parts of the cardiovascular system.

Respiratory

The respiratory system includes the nose, pharynx, larynx, trachea, bronchi, lungs, thorax, and diaphragm. The respiratory system acts as a transporter of oxygen and carbon dioxide. Oxygen is supplied to individual tissue cells, and the gaseous waste product, carbon dioxide, is removed through the process of respiration. The actual act of breathing involves the use of several muscle groups that include the diaphragm. As air is taken into the body through inspiration, the respiratory muscles contract to enlarge the thoracic cavity. Air is expelled by expiration, which is a passive process that causes the respiratory muscles to relax, allowing the ribs and diaphragm to return to their original positions. Through this air exchange, the respiratory system functions to filter, warm, and humidify the air we breathe. Color Plate 13 illustrates the respiratory system.

Digestive

The digestive system includes the mouth, esophagus, stomach, and small and large intestine. Accessory organs of the digestive system are the salivary glands, liver, gallbladder, and pancreas. As food is taken into the body, it must be broken down into particles small enough to pass through the cell membrane to provide needed nutrients for the cell. Waste products from the cells and food that is not fully digested are eliminated from the body. The digestive system functions to break down and carry food for digestion, prepare it for absorption, and carry waste material for elimination. Color Plates 14 and 15 illustrate the digestive system.

Urinary

The urinary system consists of the kidneys, ureters, urinary bladder, and urethra. The kidneys play an important role in the regulation of the water and acid-base balance in the body, and they act to excrete waste products from cell metabolism. Urine is produced in the kidneys and travels through the ureters to the urinary bladder. The bladder acts as a temporary reservoir for urine. The urethra differs in the male and female but serves the same function in the urinary system by emptying the bladder of urine. Color Plate 16 illustrates the urinary system.

Reproductive

The reproductive system includes the male reproductive system: penis, testicles, epididymides, scrotum, prostate gland, and seminal vesicles; and the female reproductive system: mons pubis, labia majora and minora, clitoris, vestibular glands, vagina, fallopian tubes, and uterus. The male reproductive system functions to produce, transfer, and, ultimately, introduce mature sperm onto the female reproductive tract. The female reproductive system functions to allow fertilization of the sperm and egg cell and serves as an environment for the developing embryo. Although the male and female systems differ in structure, they serve one common purpose, to ensure survival of the species. Color Plate 17 illustrates the male reproductive system, and Color Plate 18 represents the female reproductive system.

Endocrine

The endocrine system is made up of the ductless glands of the body, that is, those glands that secrete their hormones directly into the blood instead of a duct. Endocrine glands include the pituitary, thyroid, parathyroids, adrenals, pineal body, pancreas, ovaries, and testes. Some of the glands included in this system, such as the pancreas, ovaries, and testes, have other nonendocrine functions as well. Even with the nonendocrine functions, hormone secretion is one of their main functions. The endocrine system functions to circulate hormones to maintain homeostasis or stability of the body's internal environment. In addition, hormones are the main regulators of growth and development and reproduction. Color Plate 19 illustrates the endocrine system.

Integumentary

The integumentary system includes the skin and its appendages, the hair, nails, sweat, and sebaceous glands. The skin is the largest, thinnest, and one of the most important organs of the human body. The skin has a total surface area of roughly 17 to 20 square feet (1.6–1.9 m^2) in an average-size adult. This area forms a protective barrier between the body and the external environment. In addition to protection, the skin plays a part in temperature regulation and acts as a sophisticated sense organ. The skin has two main layers, the epidermis and dermis. The epidermis is the outer, thinner layer, which constantly sheds and replaces cells. It has the ability to repair itself after injury or disease. The dermis lies underneath the epidermis and is a much thicker layer. The dermis is well supplied with blood vessels and nerves. The appendages to the skin, including the hair, nails, sweat and sebaceous glands, are located in the dermis. Color Plate 20 illustrates the anatomy of the skin.

SUMMARY

Use a medical dictionary when a term is not recognized and cannot be defined by analysis or when the meaning is unclear. Learning the meanings of word parts will make most of the medical words that appear in the following chapters easy to define. Medical words potentially can have five parts, with the word deriving its meaning from the combination of these parts. The terminology found within human systems is directly related to word building. Various terms that describe body orientation must be learned to report patient information correctly. The description of the ten most common body systems acts as an introduction to more explicit detail in further chapters.

SUGGESTED READING

Austrin MG, Austrin HR: Learning Medical Terminology, 6th ed. St. Louis, CV Mosby, 1987

Cohen BJ: Medical Terminology: An Illustrated Guide. Philadelphia, JB Lippincott, 1989

Dox I, Melloni BJ, Eisner GM: Melloni's Illustrated Medical Dictionary, 2nd ed. Baltimore, Williams & Wilkins, 1985

Logan C, Rice MK: Logan's Medical and Scientific Abbreviations. Philadelphia, JB Lippincott, 1987

Memmler RL, Wood DL: The Human Body in Health and Disease, 6th ed. Philadelphia, JB Lippincott, 1987

Tortora GJ, Anagnostakos NP: Principles of Anatomy and Physiology, 6th ed. New York, Harper and Row, 1990

CHAPTER 9

Patient Assessment

Scene Survey
    Potential Hazards
    Mechanism of Injury
    Clues to Medical Illness
Scene Control
    Removing Distractions
    Dealing With People on the Scene
Primary Survey
Skill 9-1. Patient Assessment
    Responsiveness
    Airway
    Breathing
    Circulation
    Simultaneous Evaluation
Secondary Survey
    Patient History
        General Communication Principles
            Establishing Rapport With the Patient
            Practicing Good Listening Skills
            Communicating Through Body Language and Touch
            Managing Communication Barriers

        Interview Techniques
            Open-ended Questions
            Direct Questions
        Components of Patient History
            Chief Complaint
            History of Present Illness
            Medical History
            Medications and Allergies
    Collecting Data
        Sight
        Hearing
        Touch
        Smell
        Equipment Needs
    Diagnostic Signs
        General Appearance
        Level of Consciousness
            Arousability
            Content of Consciousness
        Vital Signs
            Respiration
            Pulse
            Blood Pressure

        Tilt Test
        Temperature
        Skin
        Capillary Refill Test
    Physical Examination
        Head and Neck
        Chest and Back
        Abdomen
        Extremities
Trauma Scoring Systems
    Adult Trauma Score
    Pediatric Trauma Score
    Adult Glasgow Coma Scale
    Pediatric Glasgow Coma Scale
    CRAMS Scale
Re-evaluation of the Patient
Communication of Patient Data
    Patient and Family
    Base Station or Hospital
    Written Record
Summary

BEHAVIORAL OBJECTIVES
On successful completion of this chapter, the reader will be able to:

1. Identify and describe the components of patient assessment: scene survey, scene control, primary survey, secondary survey, and communication of patient data
2. Describe the proper elements of communication and interview techniques
3. Explain the four components of taking a patient history
4. Describe the importance of a secondary survey
5. Describe five diagnostic signs used in gathering patient data
6. Explain and list all components of a head-to-toe survey
7. Given the proper equipment, demonstrate the procedure for taking vital signs, including pulse, respiration, and blood pressure, of a patient
8. Define and explain the tilt test
9. Given five patient situations, correctly use the five trauma scores to interpret the severity of injury
10. Given the proper equipment, demonstrate the procedure for conducting a primary and secondary survey on a patient
11. Explain the importance of re-evaluating the patient
12. Describe the three components of communication of patient data
13. Define all of the key terms listed in this chapter

KEY TERMS

The following terms are defined in the chapter and glossary:

- Adult Glasgow Coma Scale
- Adult Trauma Score
- arousability
- auscultation
- AVPU system
- blood pressure
- capillary refill test
- chief complaint
- content of consciousness
- CRAMS Scale
- cyanosis
- diastolic pressure
- direct questions
- dopplers
- head-to-toe survey
- hypertension
- hypotension
- Korotkoff's sounds
- level of consciousness
- mechanism of injury
- medical history
- open-ended questions
- palpation
- Pediatric Glasgow Coma Scale
- Pediatric Trauma Score
- percussion
- present illness
- primary survey
- pulse
- rapport
- re-evaluation
- respiration
- scene control
- scene survey
- secondary survey
- surname
- systolic pressure
- tilt test
- vital signs
- written record

The concept of patient assessment is best described, perhaps, as the foundation for providing quality patient care. Throughout a paramedic course, the student learns a vast amount of information. Technical skills are learned, practiced, and perfected. This sound knowledge base and skill proficiency are critical elements in the development of competency as a paramedic. However, correct use of these critical elements is impossible without keen patient assessment skills.

Patient assessment is the link that enables a paramedic to properly care for the patient. The two primary objectives in patient assessment are to *identify* and *correct* any life-threatening problems and to identify any associated problems, providing necessary care. The order of patient assessment, typically, is systematic: scene control, scene survey, primary survey, secondary survey, management, communication, and transportation.

As a result of information gained from the patient assessment, each step must be managed effectively before proceeding to the next. For example, the scene must be free from life-threatening hazards before proceeding to the primary survey. Airway, breathing, and circulation must be intact before taking a patient history, and the patient's history guides the secondary survey. The components of patient assessment are diagrammed in a flow chart shown in Figure 9-1.

The patient assessment process changes frequently, as does the patient and the environment. The paramedic must quickly evaluate a multitude of variables, integrate the information, and respond promptly and appropriately. Patient assessment is, at best, a difficult skill that requires practice, experience, and patience. Some elements may be learned in the course of a paramedic program; however, the mastery of this skill is most effectively acquired through field experience. The purpose of this chapter is to provide a general overview of the facets of patient assessment. Specific system assessments are detailed in later chapters.

SCENE SURVEY

The **scene survey** is the quick, yet observant, evaluation of potential hazards, mechanism of injury, and clues to medical illness that are provided by the patient's environment. The initial size-up may alter the normal priorities as well as provide helpful information. For example, a quick glance at a high scaffold at a construction site may compel the paramedic to include a cervical collar and backboard in the equipment taken to the patient's side. Coffee ground-like emesis in the basin next to the patient's bed may be a clue to identify peptic ulcer disease and gastrointestinal hemorrhage.

Potential Hazards

An important aspect of scene survey is the assessment of potential hazards to the paramedic and the patient. The presence of environmental hazards, such as a downed power line, toxic substances, or hazardous chemical spills, should all be quickly evaluated. Intervention may be necessary before further patient assessment. A busy highway with fast-moving traffic is a potential hazard frequently encountered by the paramedic and the patient. In addi-

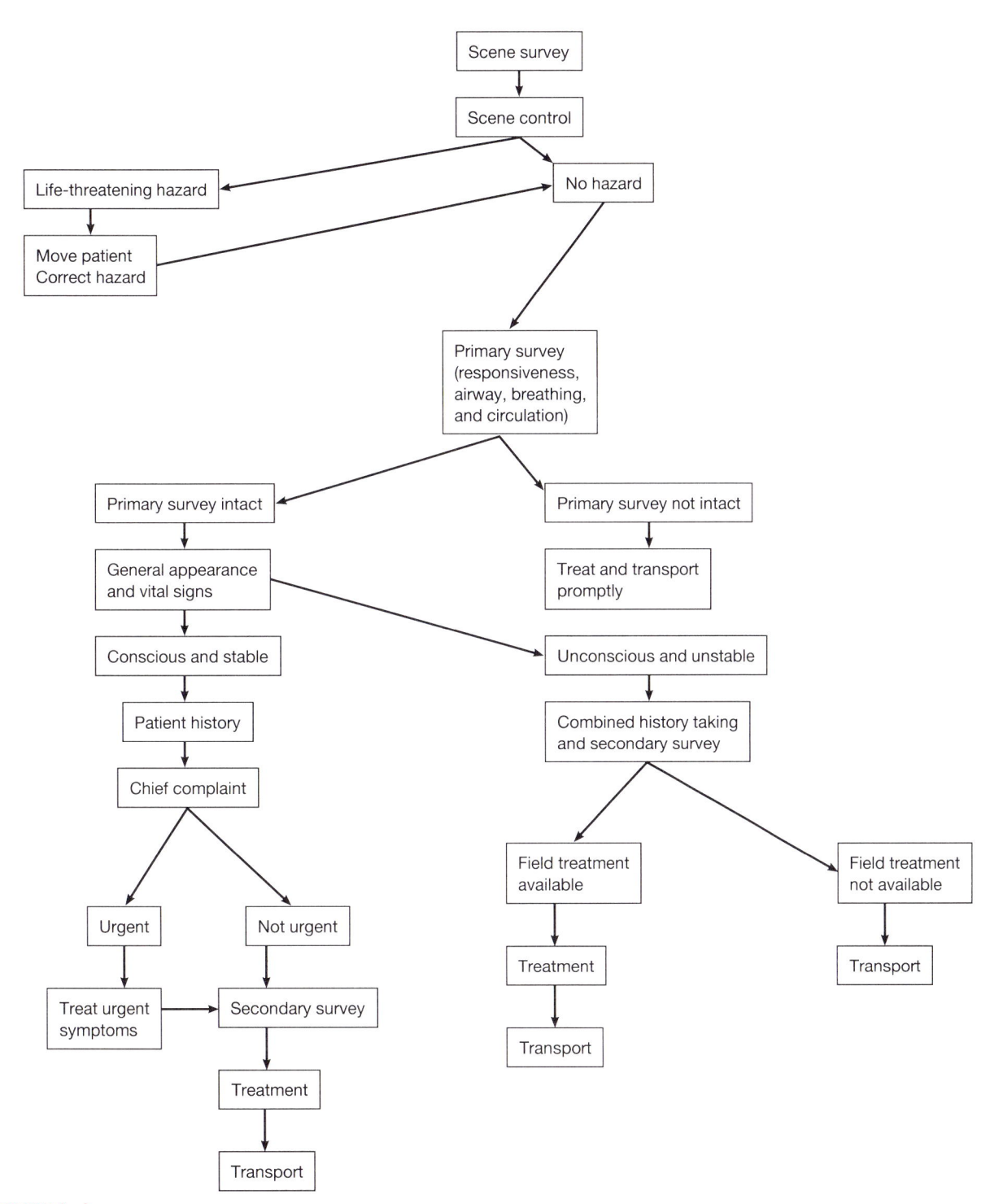

FIGURE 9–1.
Components of patient assessment.

tion, an angry crowd, a dark alley, or information given by the dispatcher, such as "assailant still possibly on the scene," should alert the paramedic to potential dangers. Necessary assistance, such as the police, additional ambulances, fire units, or the utility company, should be mobilized immediately. When necessary, time is well spent putting on protective equipment, such as a hard hat, fluorescent vest, or other protective clothing.

Mechanism of Injury

A key aspect of initial scene survey in the trauma call is the evaluation of the **mechanism of injury**. Such information enables the paramedic, and eventually the physician, to anticipate potential injuries, particularly those that are not readily apparent. Frequently, in the prehospital setting, a patient may look stable initially yet deteriorate in transit due to hidden injuries. Evaluation of the mechanism of injury may help manage the injury before it becomes a life- or limb-threatening problem.

In a motor vehicle accident, different injuries can be anticipated for the driver and passengers depending on whether the collision was a frontal, rear end, or lateral impact accident. A cracked windshield may indicate a head or neck injury, and a bent steering wheel should lead the paramedic to anticipate chest or abdominal injuries. Information, such as sudden deceleration, the speed of the vehicle, and whether or not the occupants were wearing seat belts, helps determine injury potential. For the victim of a fall, relevant information obtained from the scene would be an approximation of the distance that the patient fell and how the patient landed. The mechanism of injury is explained in detail in Chapter 13.

Clues to Medical Illness

When responding to the scene of a medical call, paramedics have a number of *valuable clues* at their disposal. The temperature of the patient's environment may be significant to note, particularly in heat emergencies or cold exposure. A call to a low economic neighborhood may alert the paramedic to the possibility of a lack of preventative health care. Indications of alcohol or drug abuse, empty pill bottles, or other medications may help identify pertinent medical history.

In the process of scene survey, however, the paramedic should be careful not to jump to conclusions. No two emergencies are exactly the same. What is initially observed at the scene may not always be associated with the patient's current problem. An empty bottle of sleeping pills next to an unconscious patient does not eliminate the possibility of a head injury or other cause of unconsciousness. An auto accident victim may have chest pain from a myocardial infarction rather than from a steering wheel injury. Syncope from an arrhythmia may have produced a fall. Diabetic ketoacidosis may be the etiology of vomiting.

Access to definitive care as soon as possible varies between the trauma patient and the medical patient. In the latter, definitive care can be started on the scene (e.g., defibrillation, cardiac drugs). In the trauma patient, the blood loss must be stopped, the injury repaired, and whole blood replaced. Except for controlling external bleeding, these actions cannot be taken at the scene. Unnecessary delays in transporting the trauma patient could result in serious complications.

SCENE CONTROL

Once the paramedic arrives at the location of the emergency, *scene control* becomes important. Scene control takes special expertise, and even the best paramedics encounter many different situations before this skill is mastered. The paramedic must quickly take control of the scene to insure personal safety and to be able to properly assess and manage the patient.

Removing Distractions

The first step in taking control of the scene is to remove distractions. This step enhances concentration on the patient and the circumstances surrounding the patient's illness or injury. Eliminating noise from a television or radio, providing an adequate work space, and turning on additional lights can also benefit patient assessment and management. Pets may need to be restrained or removed.

Dealing With People on the Scene

Another element of scene control is dealing with emergency medical technicians, first responders, bystanders, and concerned family members. Tact, diplomacy, and self-control are often necessary to deal with these individuals, who are sometimes considered distractions. First responders may provide valuable clues about the initial scene or condition of the patient. They should be thanked for their assistance, no matter how insignificant it may seem. Emergency medical technicians, if available, should be used as assistants for patient care. Family and bystanders can be a benefit at the scene if properly directed. Simple tasks, such as holding the intravenous container or flashlight, can help the paramedic and at the same time enhance patient care and give bystanders something to do to make them feel important in the outcome of the situation.

PRIMARY SURVEY

The *primary survey* is always the first step once the paramedic is at the patient's side. The primary survey is a rapid evaluation, less than 45 seconds, to determine the patient's status in the following areas:

- Responsiveness
- Airway
- Breathing
- Circulation

The purpose of the primary survey is to *identify* and *correct* any life-threatening problems. The primary survey is shown as part of Skill 9-1. It is not the purpose of this text to teach cardiopulmonary resuscitation. The reader is referred to Appendix B on performance sheets for cardiopulmonary resuscitation and foreign body airway obstruction management.

SKILL 9-1
PATIENT ASSESSMENT

ACTIVITY	HOW PERFORMED	WHY PERFORMED
1. Visually observe the patient and the surrounding area	Perform a quick look over the patient's whole body and the area around the patient. Note the patient's position and the condition of the scene or environment where the patient is found.	The patient's position and surroundings frequently provide clues about mechanism of injury and patient history.
2. Assemble and check: Primary equipment (Activity 2): • Blood pressure cuff • Stethoscope • Penlight Accessory equipment and supplies: • Gloves • Watch • Scissors	Check to make sure equipment is in working order. Place all equipment within easy reach.	Having equipment ready and in working order reduces time delays during the procedure.

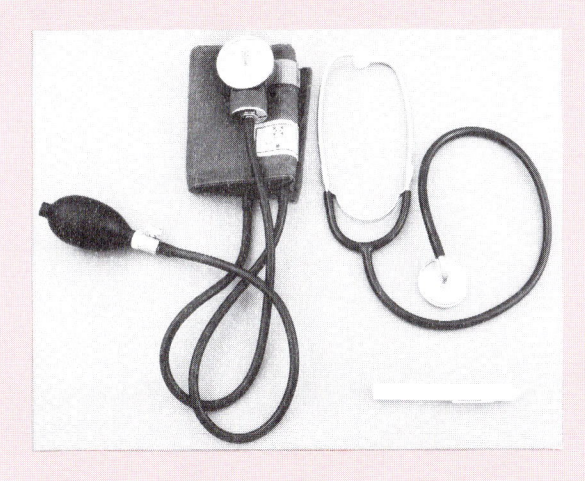

Activity 2. Primary equipment.

3. Check responsiveness	Gently tap the patient on the shoulders and ask, "Are you okay?" Note the patient's response to verbal stimuli (Activity 3). If responsive to verbal stimuli, question patient to determine orientation to person, place, and time. If unresponsive to verbal stimuli, note response to mild noxious stimuli.	The type of response to various stimuli is important to provide a baseline for later comparisons.

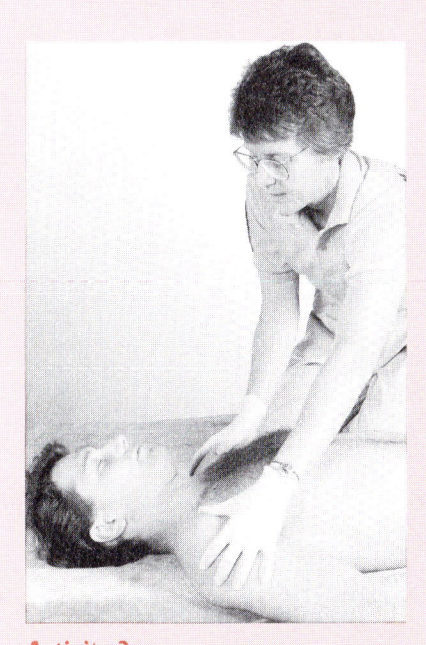

Activity 3. Check responsiveness.

(*continued*)

SKILL 9-1
PATIENT ASSESSMENT (continued)

ACTIVITY	HOW PERFORMED	WHY PERFORMED
4. Check airway	Open the airway with the head-tilt/chin-lift method (Activity 4A). If a cervical spine injury is suspected, however, do not tilt the head. Instead, keep the neck in a neutral position and use the jaw-thrust method (Activity 4B). Suction and insert an oropharyngeal or nasopharyngeal airway as required.	An open airway is the most essential first step in patient assessment and treatment. All other assessment and treatment efforts are futile until an open airway is established and maintained.

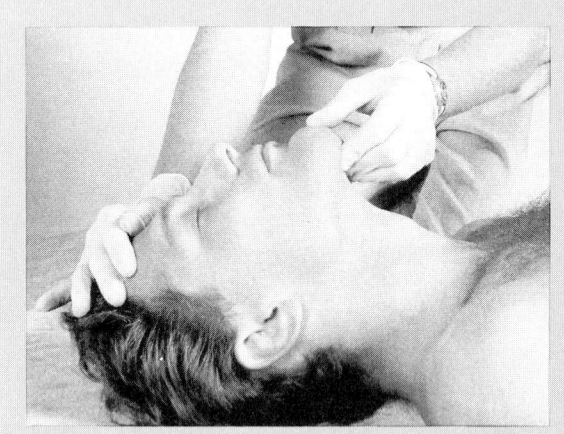

Activity 4A.
Check airway: Head-tilt/chin-lift method.

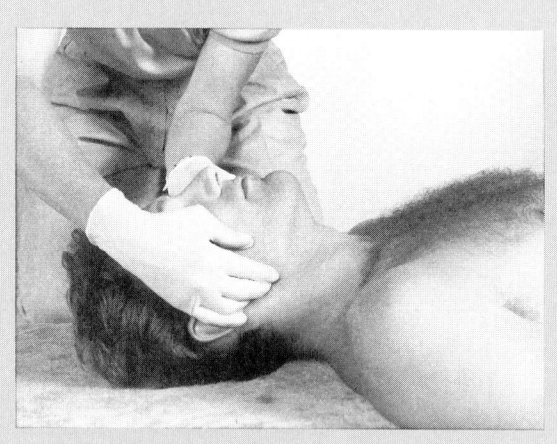

Activity 4B.
Check airway: Jaw-thrust method.

5. Check breathing	With the airway open, position your ear over the patient's mouth, while looking down across the surface of the patient's chest. *Look* for chest movement, *listen* for sounds of air movement, and *feel* for the flow or air from the patient's nose and mouth on the side of your face (Activity 5). Start rescue breathing or mechanical ventilation immediately if breathing is absent.	Weak or shallow respiration may be difficult to detect by a single means. The careful use of looking, listening, and feeling will detect nearly any respiratory effort. Absence of breathing requires immediate resuscitative efforts before any other assessment or treatment is done.

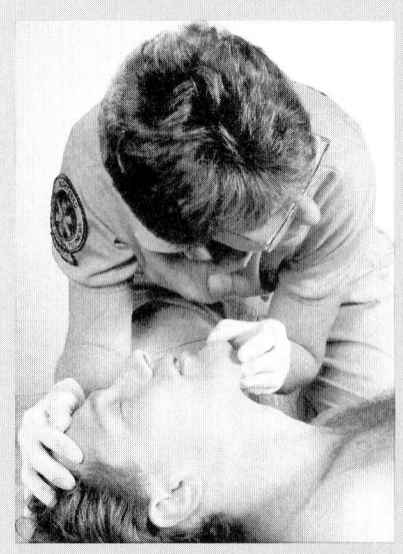

Activity 5.
Check breathing.

(continued)

SKILL 9–1
PATIENT ASSESSMENT (continued)

ACTIVITY	HOW PERFORMED	WHY PERFORMED
6. Check circulation	Feel for a carotid pulse on the side of the patient's neck closest to you. Allow 5 to 10 seconds for accuracy in determining presence or absence of a pulse (Activity 6). If pulse is absent, start CPR immediately.	The pulse may be weak, rapid, or slow and difficult to assess. Absence of a pulse requires immediate resuscitative efforts before any other assessment or treatment is done.

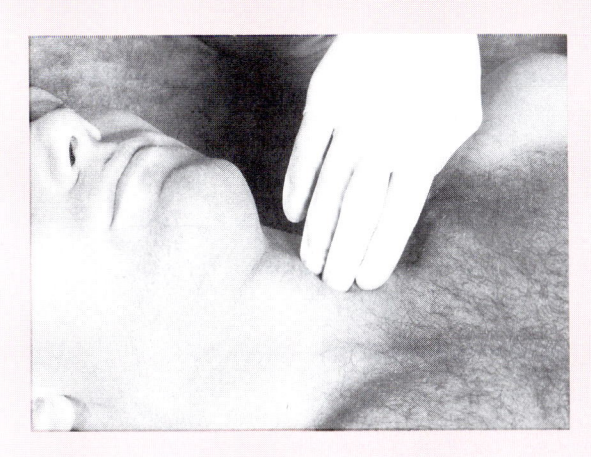

Activity 6. Check pulse.

7. Check for obvious external hemorrhage	Visualize patient for potentially life-threatening hemorrhage (Activity 7). If such bleeding is found, immediately control the bleeding with direct pressure.	Profuse bleeding may lead to exsanguination and must be controlled immediately before any other assessment or treatment is done.

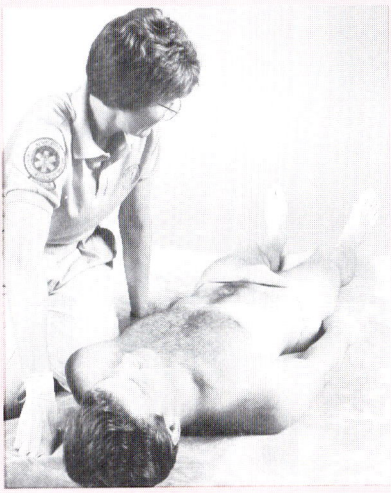

Activity 7. Check for obvious external hemorrhage.

(continued)

SKILL 9–1
PATIENT ASSESSMENT (continued)

ACTIVITY	HOW PERFORMED	WHY PERFORMED
8. Evaluate and document vital signs. (May be performed by partner during exam or after patient assessment)	Record: • Respirations • Pulse (Activity 8A) • Blood pressure (Activity 8B)	A baseline set of vital signs is essential for comparison throughout the course of transport and treatment to allow early detection of changes in the patient's condition

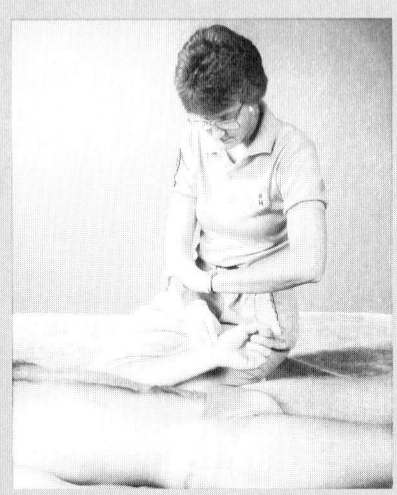

Activity 8A.
Evaluate and document vital signs—pulse.

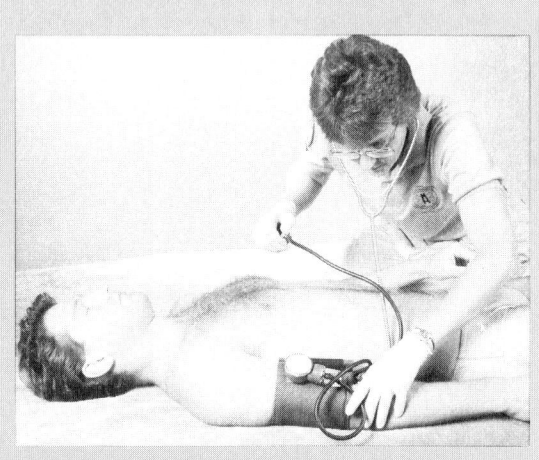

Activity 8B.
Evaluate and document vital signs—blood pressure.

9. Inspect and palpate scalp	Palpate all areas, looking for deformity, swelling, laceration, discoloration, hemorrhage (Activity 9).	Provides clues to possible head injuries.

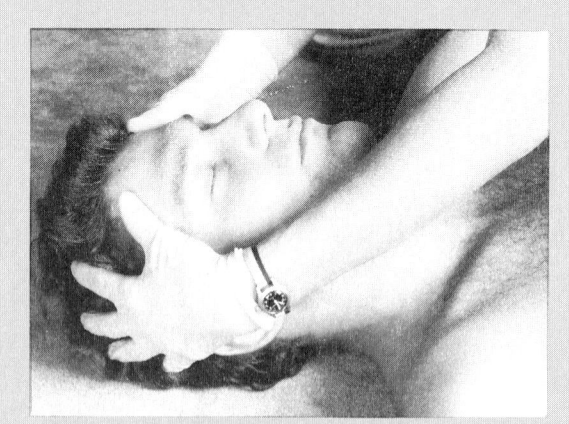

Activity 9.
Inspect and palpate scalp.

(continued)

SKILL 9–1
PATIENT ASSESSMENT (continued)

ACTIVITY	HOW PERFORMED	WHY PERFORMED
10. Inspect eyes	Observe for purposeful movement and pupillary response. Look for swelling, discoloration, or deformity on orbits and eye lids (Activity 10).	Provides clues to possible problems such as head injuries, eye injuries, drug use, and stroke.

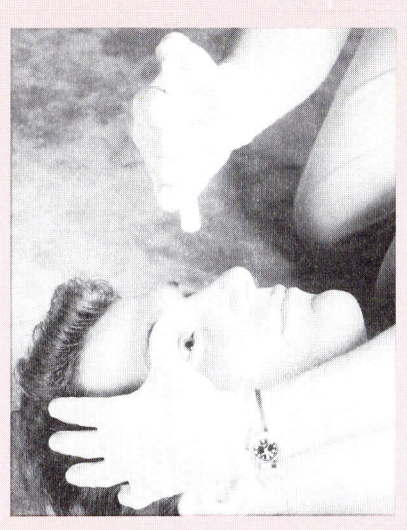

Activity 10.
Inspect eyes.

11. Inspect and palpate face, nose, and mouth	Palpate the facial bones (Activity 11A) and nose (Activity 11B). Look for deformity, swelling, lacerations, and discoloration, or hemorrhage. Observe for cerebral spinal fluid coming from nose. Inspect mouth for loose teeth or dentures (Activity 11C). Smell for unusual odor on patient's breath. Feel skin for temperature and moisture.	Provides clues to possible problems such as head injuries, facial bone fractures, skull fractures, dental injuries, diabetic problems, alcohol ingestion, and the presence of shock.

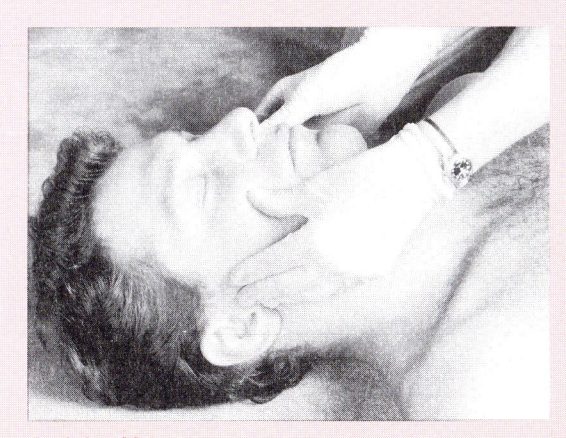

Activity 11A.
Inspect and palpate facial bones.

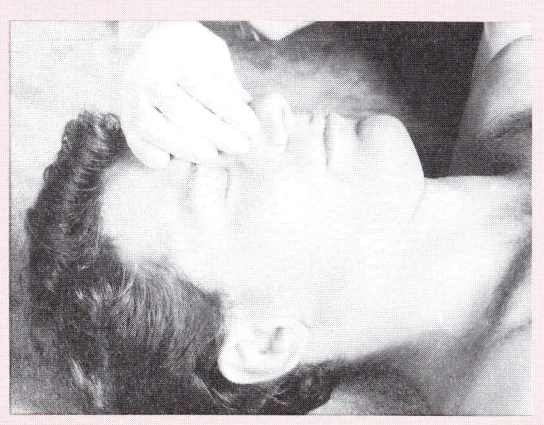

Activity 11B.
Inspect and palpate nose.

(continued)

SKILL 9–1
PATIENT ASSESSMENT (continued)

ACTIVITY	HOW PERFORMED	WHY PERFORMED

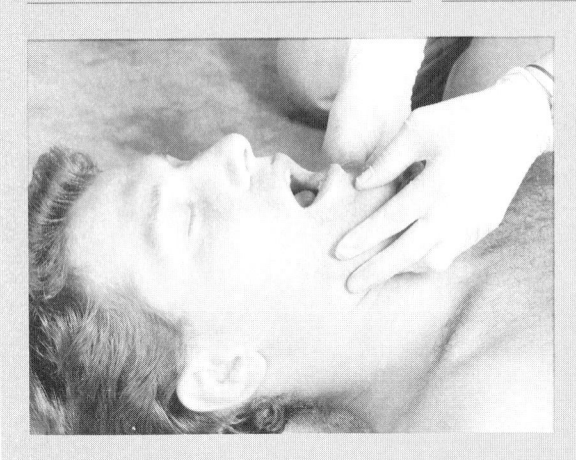

Activity 11C.
Inspect mouth for loose teeth and dentures.

12. Inspect and palpate ears.	Look for cerebral spinal fluid or blood coming from ears (Activity 12A). Assess if patient can hear normally. Look behind ears for bruising, swelling, or discoloration (Activity 12B).	Provides clues to possible problems such as hearing loss or impairment, skull fracture, and head injury.

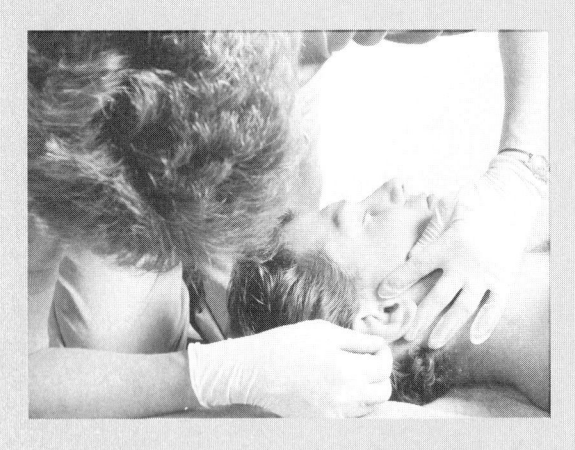

Activity 12A.
Inspect and palpate ears. Look for cerebral spinal fluid or blood coming from the ears.

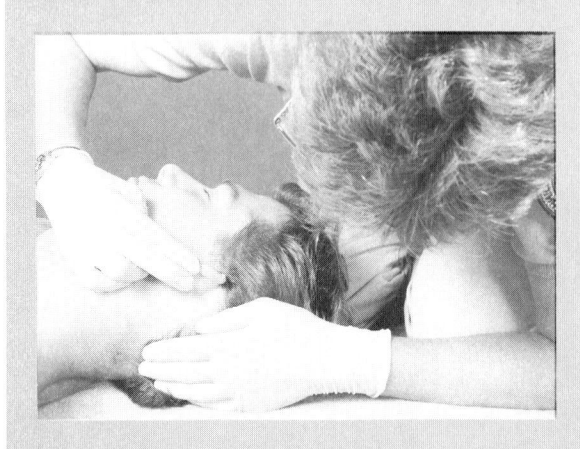

Activity 12B.
Inspect and palpate ears. Look behind ears for bruising, swelling, or discoloration.

(continued)

SKILL 9-1
PATIENT ASSESSMENT (continued)

ACTIVITY	HOW PERFORMED	WHY PERFORMED
13. Inspect and palpate neck	Look for neck vein distention, lacerations, bruises, and deformity. Note if trachea is in midline (Activity 13). Cervical spine should be palpated, without moving the head, for tenderness, swelling, or deformity.	Provides clues to possible problems such as congestive heart failure, cardiac tamponade, tension pneumothorax, and cervical spine injuries.

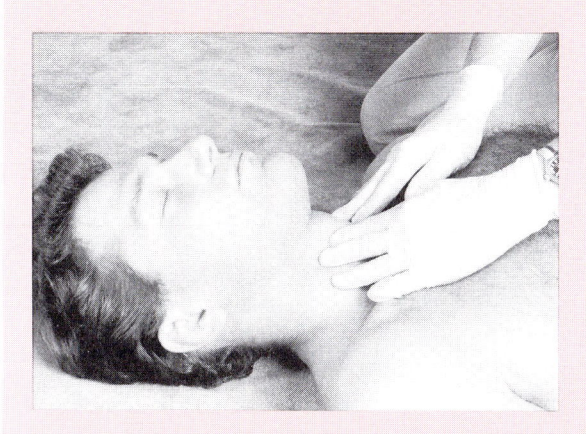

Activity 13. Inspect and palpate neck.

14. Inspect and palpate the chest	Observe chest movements. Palpate entire chest surface. Note bruising, fractures, swelling, deformity, abnormal or uneven movement, and subcutaneous emphysema (Activity 14).	Provides clues to possible problems such as impaired breathing, pneumothorax, and flail chest.

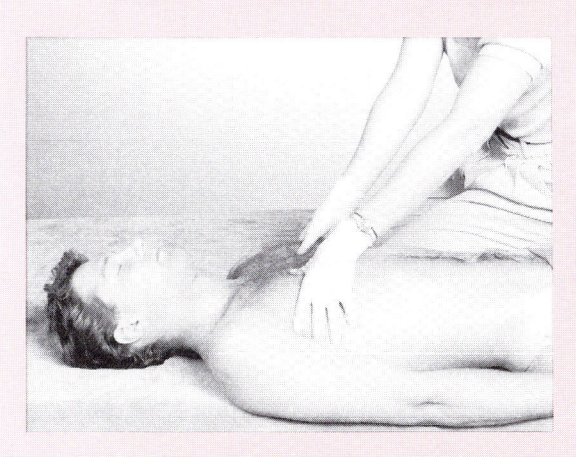

Activity 14. Inspect and palpate chest.

(continued)

SKILL 9-1
PATIENT ASSESSMENT (continued)

ACTIVITY	HOW PERFORMED	WHY PERFORMED
15. Evaluate breath sounds	Auscultate breath sounds bilaterally (Activity 15A, Activity 15B) in all four quadrants of the chest both anteriorly and posteriorly. Listen for presence, equality, and abnormal sounds in all areas.	Provides clues to possible problems such as congestive heart failure, pulmonary edema, asthma, and pneumothorax.

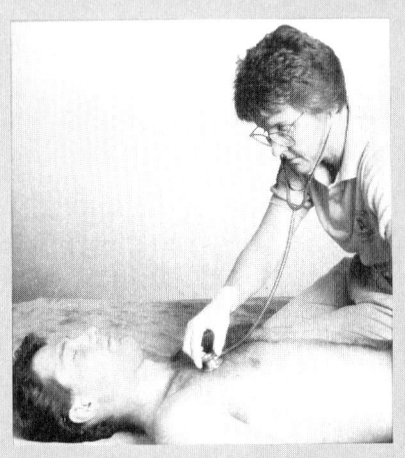

Activity 15A.
Evaluate breath sounds bilaterally.

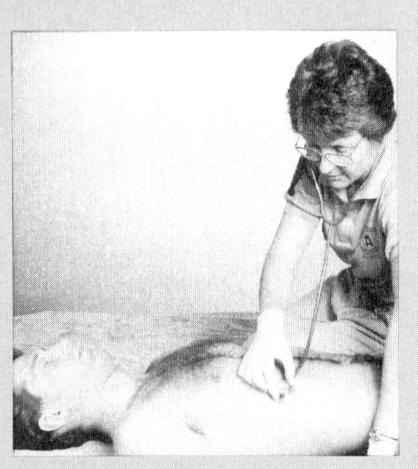

Activity 15B.
Evaluate breath sounds bilaterally.

16. Inspect and palpate abdomen	Look for distention, contusions, wounds, deformity, hemorrhage, evisceration, and pulsating masses. Note tenderness or rigidity. Palpate all four quadrants individually (Activity 16).	Provides clues to possible problems such as intra-abdominal bleeding, peritonitis, appendicitis, and abdominal aortic aneuryism.

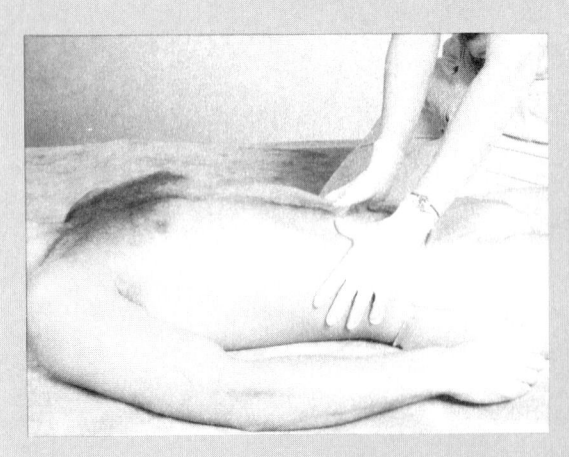

Activity 16.
Inspect and palpate abdomen.

(continued)

SKILL 9–1
PATIENT ASSESSMENT (continued)

ACTIVITY	HOW PERFORMED	WHY PERFORMED
17. Inspect and palpate pelvic region	Apply gentle pressure on the iliac crests posteriorly, medially, laterally, and posteriorly on the symphysis pubis. Note tenderness, instability, crepitus, or deformity (Activity 17).	Provides clues to possible problems such as pelvic fractures.

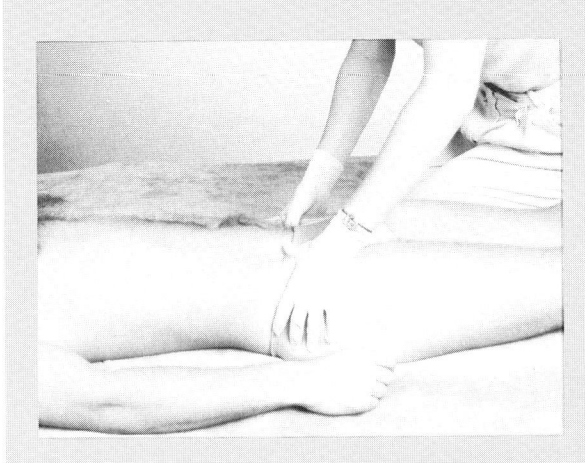

Activity 17.
Inspect and palpate pelvic region.

18. Inspect and palpate extremities	Look for lacerations, contusions, edema, deformity, and movement (Activity 18A, Activity 18B). Palpate for tenderness, pitting edema, pulses, and sensation (Activity 18C). Pinch the fingernails to assess capillary refill (Activity 18D). Grip strength as well as voluntary movements of fingers should be noted in both hands and compared (Activity 18E).	Provides clues to possible problems such as fractures, dislocations, spinal injury, head injury, stroke, impending shock, and congestive heart failure.

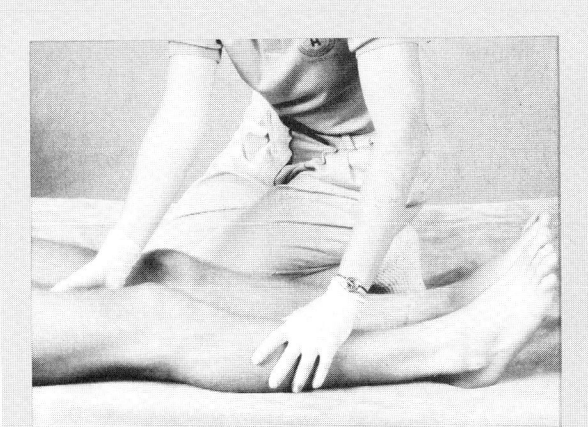

Activity 18A.
Inspect and palpate extremities.

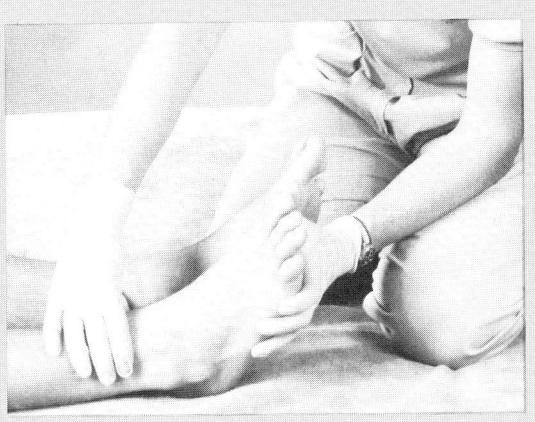

Activity 18B.
Inspect and palpate extremities.

(continued)

SKILL 9–1
PATIENT ASSESSMENT (continued)

ACTIVITY	HOW PERFORMED	WHY PERFORMED

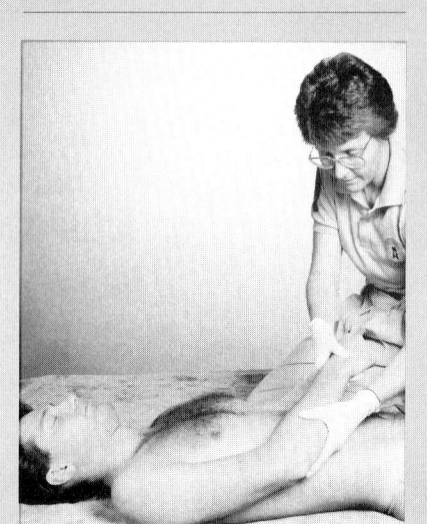

Activity 18C.
Palpate extremities for tenderness, pitting edema, pulses, and sensation.

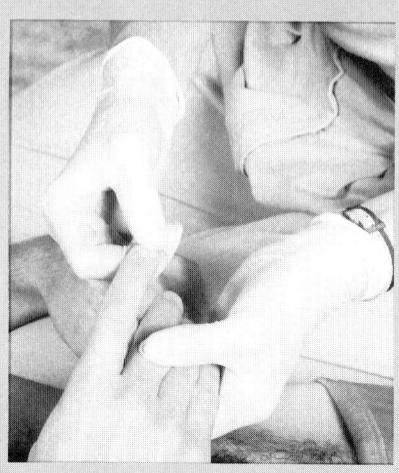

Activity 18D.
Pinch the fingernails to assess for capillary refill.

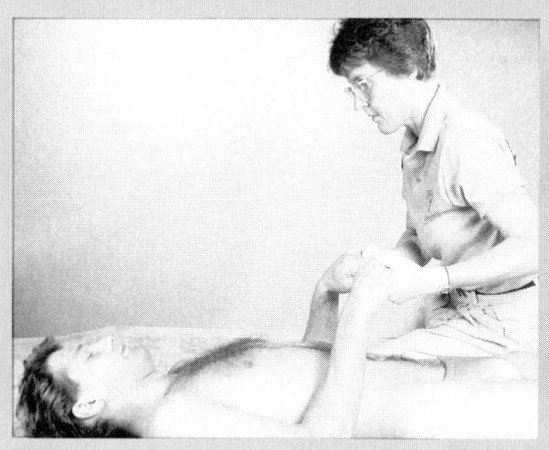

Activity 18E.
Grip strength and voluntary movement of fingers should be noted in both hands and compared.

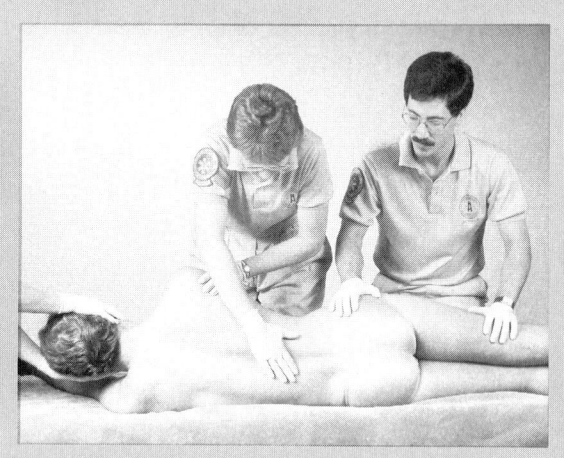

Activity 19.
Inspect and palpate back.

19. Inspect and palpate back	As patient is log-rolled on the backboard, the spinal area should be inspected and palpated for tenderness, deformity, contusions, or hemorrhage. Evaluate the cervical, thoracic, lumbar, and sacral areas of the spine (Activity 19).	Provides clues to possible problems such as spinal injuries and internal injuries.

Responsiveness

The performance of the primary survey begins with attempts to awaken the patient by verbal and physical stimulation. Checking the patient's responsiveness is the initial determination of the patient's overall level of cerebral function. The *cerebrum* is the seat of conscious mental processes, and deterioration in this status is one of the earliest signs of hypoxia. Checking the patient's responsiveness should not be confused with the more specific level of consciousness, which is part of the more thorough secondary survey. State of responsiveness is quickly noting whether the patient is conscious or unconscious.

Airway

Depending on the circumstances, the airway should be opened by using the head-tilt/chin-lift or jaw-thrust method as described in Chapter 10. Special precautions are employed with the trauma patient. The possibility of a cervical injury must be known before opening the airway. If a cervical spine injury is suspected, the neck must be kept in the neutral position, neither tilted backward nor forward. Excessive movement, such as the head-tilt/chin-lift maneuver, could cause neurologic damage to an already injured spine. The mouth should be quickly inspected for any obvious obstruction, and prompt removal is essential before continuing the patient survey. The tongue that has fallen back into the oropharynx is the most common cause of airway obstruction and should be assessed first.

Breathing

Once the airway is clear and secure, the patient's breathing is evaluated. The paramedic should watch the patient's chest while listening and feeling over the mouth and nose for adequate ventilation. If the patient is not breathing, artificial ventilatory support is given immediately. Any labored breathing is evaluated for the degree of distress involved.

Ventilation that is too slow, irregular, or too fast, requires immediate intervention. The quality and pattern of breathing is simultaneously evaluated. Any obvious noises, such as stridor or wheezes, should be noted. Special conditions need to be considered for the trauma patient, such as pulmonary contusion or flail chest (see Chapter 16).

Circulation

Circulation is evaluated in either the adult or child by a check of the carotid pulse and the capillary refilling time. The brachial pulse is used to evaluate circulation in the infant. If the patient has no pulse, external chest compressions should be performed. Any *hemorrhage* (profuse bleeding) should be observed and controlled.

If the pulse is present, the rate and quality are quickly noted. *Perfusion* (flow of blood through tissues) is evaluated by skin temperature, moisture, and capillary refilling. Findings that indicate the presence of shock affect the steps of the secondary survey and ultimate patient management.

Simultaneous Evaluation

Several components of the primary survey can be evaluated at the same time. A simple example of a simultaneous evaluation is found in the conscious, alert patient who is sitting in a chair conversing with family members when the paramedic arrives. As the paramedic approaches this patient, it can easily be seen that the patient is responsive, that the patient's airway and breathing are intact since movement of air is displayed by speech, and that circulation is present since the patient is shown to be in a state of alertness. Although the paramedic has evaluated the complete primary survey in less than 5 seconds, each step was mentally performed.

Another example is that the paramedic can hold the patient's wrist and ask, "What happened today?" The patient's response indicates the status of responsiveness, airway, and breathing. The paramedic is also simultaneously checking the patient's pulse, noting skin color and temperature, and taking a quick look to make these first few seconds with the patient serve as an overall scene survey of the patient and an evaluation of life-threatening conditions.

The overall circumstances of each patient situation dictate the order of patient assessment and management once the primary survey has been performed. For example, a patient who is experiencing severe chest pain, appears distressed, and has a weak, slow pulse would have an immediate priority of oxygen and electrocardiogram (EKG) evaluation. Taking a thorough history or secondary survey would be a secondary priority for that patient. A patient who has called paramedics for an extremity fracture sustained in a fall may need a thorough history and secondary survey before management. The reason for the fall must be found. The ability to set priorities is a key element in proper patient assessment.

SECONDARY SURVEY

The **secondary survey** is an assessment tool that is a necessary component to make correct decisions regarding patient care. The secondary survey includes a patient interview, is a more thorough physical evaluation, and proposes to find less obvious and less acute problems than those evaluated in the primary survey. Ideally, management follows as a logical extension of the examination. The degree of thoroughness and the evaluation method are dependent on the acuteness and specific circumstances of each patient situation.

The secondary survey should be conducted in an organized, systematic manner so as not to omit a step and, consequently, miss an injury or important clue to a medical or trauma problem. While being organized and systematic, the survey should be flexible enough to allow for the variation in patient situations. Typically, the physical assessment of an adult is performed in a *head-to-toe* manner. Children are frequently upset when strangers, or others, have anything to do with their face or head, and a *toe-to-head* assessment is most appropriate for them. An evaluation of the patient's general appearance and vital signs should precede the physical assessment. Visualization, listening, and palpation should be conducted in a region-by-region manner.

Touching another person's body is not a normal practice in our society, unless the other person happens to be a family member or close friend. New paramedics often express anxiety with this practice initially. Patients may also experience anxiety about being touched and examined. Expressing concern for the patient's problem demonstrates compassion and helps to reassure the patient. Describe each step of the examination before it is begun, even if the patient appears unconscious and unresponsive.

During the secondary survey, the paramedic should be sensitive to the patient's anxiety, physical comfort, and privacy. For example, in the absence of more acute injuries, splinting an obvious fracture may provide enough pain relief to complete a secondary survey. Removing clothes to properly examine a patient with multiple trauma is appropriate, but this should be done in private if at all possible. A sheet or blanket should be used to drape the patient. The paramedic should not convey surprise or dismay at abnormal discoveries. There is an appropriate time at the end of the assessment to communicate impressions of the patient's illness or injury and to explain to the patient what may be done concerning the situation.

Patient History

The information obtained in the patient history is vitally important in determining the patient's problems. A patient history is obtained for two primary purposes:

- To develop a database of information
- To guide the physical examination

The patient is the primary source of information for obtaining the patient history. If the patient is able to communicate, the initial questions should be directed to the patient and not to a family member or bystander. Children older than age 5 or 6 can often provide much information about their illness. Once the patient has been questioned, relatives or bystanders may provide additional information that is both valuable and informative. An effective technique of interviewing may be to have one paramedic interview the patient, while the other paramedic interviews the family. Information must then be exchanged so that interpretation of data is based on the complete picture.

The reliability of the patient history obtained should be evaluated to properly interpret the data. For example, a teenage girl should not be asked about the possibility of pregnancy in the presence of others. Another patient may relay inaccurate information about a medical history because of limited understanding of medical facts or procedures. History taking is both a skill and an art. A paramedic does not develop good history taking techniques easily or quickly. Proficiency is best achieved by observation of instructors and peers, diligent practice, and the ability to learn from mistakes. The key elements in effective history taking are to develop good communication skills and proper interview techniques.

General Communication Principles

A patient interview is only as successful as the interviewer. Important aspects of the interview process include the following:

- Establishing rapport with the patient
- Practicing good listening skills
- Communicating through body language and touch
- Managing communication barriers

ESTABLISHING RAPPORT WITH THE PATIENT. **Rapport** is defined as a harmonious or sympathetic relationship. While methods of establishing rapport may vary depending on the circumstances of the emergency, in every situation, a calm, nonjudgmental, and open attitude toward the patient is essential. A brief introduction of the paramedic's name and organization is appropriate in all circumstances when the patient is conscious. Calling the patient by name also helps establish rapport. First names may be used for patients who are close to the questioner's age or younger. Older patients should be given respect by using "ma'am" or "sir," or the appropriate title (Ms., Mrs., Mr.) before their **surname** (last name).

Rapport with the patient and the confidence the patient has in the paramedic are further established by the paramedic's appearance. A neat, clean professional look demonstrates a sense of pride in the paramedic's work and concern for the patient. Simple measures taken to establish rapport with the patient help gain the patient's confidence and communicate concern for the patient as an individual.

PRACTICING GOOD LISTENING SKILLS. An additional component of becoming a successful interviewer is to be a good listener. The development of this skill requires both practice and patience. The patient should be given time to answer each question, while the paramedic concentrates on the answer. Two errors commonly made by the interviewer are becoming distracted or concentrating on what to ask next, instead of listening to the patient. Good eye contact enhances listening and effective communication.

COMMUNICATING THROUGH BODY LANGUAGE AND TOUCH. Communication also occurs through body language and the use of touch. The use of touch is frequently beneficial to communicate concern and empathy. Typically, the paramedic should stand or kneel close to the patient, at the patient's eye level. Reassurance may be given to the patient by the paramedic touching the patient's arm or holding a patient's hand. Even though touch is an important aspect of patient care, the paramedic should not get close to or touch hostile, paranoid, or belligerent patients.

MANAGING COMMUNICATION BARRIERS. For effective communication to take place, the patient must understand the paramedic's questions, and the paramedic must understand the patient's responses. The patient may not understand the question, "How often do you urinate?" but may provide the correct answer to, "How often do you pass water?" The paramedic should avoid the use of medical terminology unless the patient has a medical background. The paramedic's communication may be enhanced by the use of local cultural colloquialisms, providing they are not used in a judgmental manner. Patients of a foreign background who speak English poorly may misuse words and distort their meaning. Translators are usually helpful but tend to summarize or interpret the patient's words, thus accidentally altering the content. Cultural differences may alter the patient's willingness to communicate important information. Anytime a communication barrier is present, the paramedic is obligated to provide conservative care and transportation.

Communication barriers also exist when dealing with the patient who is sensorially handicapped. Medical personnel often have limited skills in these special circumstances and may be uncomfortable or even intimidated by the situation. Also, the paramedic often views the patient as "helpless," even though the patient has adapted to individual limitations and developed independence. Simply asking the patient "how can I best help you?" is a safe and sensitive approach.

Deaf patients adapt to their quiet world by employing alternative communication methods, such as sign language or lip reading. The paramedic can begin the interview by writing the patient a note to determine which communication method should be used. A reliable translator for sign language may or may not be available, thus requiring an alternative approach. If the patient is able to read lips, the interviewer should face the patient directly in a well-lit room. Slow and clear speech is helpful. Lip reading may only serve to frustrate the patient who is in severe pain or distress; therefore, writing questions or messages is a more practical approach.

Blind patients require a different orientation. The patient should be kept informed throughout the assessment in regard to procedures or anticipated environmental changes. If the patient is walking to the ambulance, assistance may be necessary.

A common error made when communicating with deaf or blind patients is to raise the voice unnecessarily. Maintaining a consistent voice and using the sense of touch throughout the call is especially reassuring for sensorially impaired patients.

Interview Techniques

Two types of questions are usually employed in the interview process: open-ended and direct.

Both types of questions have benefits and are appropriate to use in the prehospital setting. The open-ended question allows an elaborate answer, while direct questioning requires only a simple "yes" or "no" response. For example, history questions for the patient with abdominal pain are shown in Table 9-1.

OPEN-ENDED QUESTIONS. **Open-ended questions** allow patients to tell the story in their own words. The responses are usually more accurate and complete. The interviewer is able to obtain a larger amount of information with fewer questions asked. The open-ended format may, however, require more time than is available, depending on the acuteness of the patient's situation.

DIRECT QUESTIONS. **Direct questions** are appropriate to use when the patient has an altered level of consciousness, or when time does not permit open-ended responses. In addition, more specific information can be obtained toward the end of the interview with direct questions. A hazard to this technique is that patients can be led inadvertently to answer "yes" to every question. This direct interview technique may also contribute to "tunnel vision" on the part of the interviewer. Tunnel vision refers to the narrow perspective and premature conclusion that is made about the patient's illness before adequate evaluation.

TABLE 9-1.
HISTORY QUESTIONS FOR THE PATIENT WITH ABDOMINAL PAIN

Open-ended	Direct
1. Describe or tell me about your pain.	1. Does the pain radiate to your back?
2. Tell me how your pain feels.	2. Does the pain feel knifelike? Generalized?
3. If there has been any vomiting with this, tell me how it looks.	3. Are you vomiting blood?

Both techniques, open-ended and direct, are necessary to obtain the needed information for accurate patient assessment. The circumstances of each situation determine how and when each method is used.

Components of Patient History

The basic principles of communication and interview techniques should be applied to each component of the patient history. The four components are the following:

- Chief complaint
- History of present illness
- Medical history
- Medications and allergies

CHIEF COMPLAINT. Inquiries about the **chief complaint** should be the first step after appropriate introductions. The chief complaint is the answer to the question, "Why did you call us today?" The chief complaint should be recorded in the patient's own words and not in the way the call was dispatched or with the medical conclusions of the paramedic. Examples of chief complaints are "chest pain," "coughing up blood," "dizzy spells," "fell and injured my arm," and "trouble breathing." A chief complaint of "unconscious" can be used for patients who are unresponsive for an unknown reason. Of course, if the patient is unconscious due to an observed gunshot wound to the head, then "gunshot wound to the head" would be used as the chief complaint.

HISTORY OF PRESENT ILLNESS. The history of **present illness** logically follows the chief complaint because it is an elaboration of the chief complaint. The purpose of the history of present illness is to determine the chronology, nature, and severity of the patient's current illness or injury. The greatest factor in making a correct assessment is taking a complete and accurate history. This fact applies to prehospital as well as in-hospital situations. A history of chest pain separates cardiac from gastrointestinal disease. A description of the collision provides clues to most of the injuries present. Components may include the following:

- Patient's age
- Date and time of onset
- Gradual or sudden onset
- Duration
- Precipitating factors
- Course since onset (including remissions and aggravations)
- Location
- Quality
- Quantity
- Associated symptoms
- Alleviating or aggravating factors

The open-ended type of questioning is particularly important and beneficial in this phase of the history. For example, if the problem is an accident, appropriate questions are "what happened?" or "how were you hurt?" For a medical complaint, the paramedic may ask, "describe your pain," "tell me more about it," or "how did this begin?"

Direct questions may be helpful to obtain more specific information about an element of the history of present illness. For example, when a patient reveals an associated symptom of nausea, the paramedic may specifically inquire, "Have you been vomiting?" or "Were you vomiting blood?" or a specific open-ended question, "What did the vomitus (or similar word the patient understands) look like?"

Other history of the present illness should be determined. Inquire about associated symptoms the patient may have, such as shortness of breath, dizziness, nausea, vomiting, or diarrhea. In addition, history information about the mechanism of injury should be obtained. For the patient who has been involved in a motor vehicle accident, helpful information might include the approximate speed and path of the vehicle, the location of the patient in the vehicle, whether or not the patient was wearing a seat belt, and where the patient may have impacted the vehicle. For the patient with a penetrating injury, the length and type of weapon is helpful information, if available. Evaluating the cause of a fall may lead to key information about a syncopal episode or dizzy spell that preceded the injury. A patient who cannot recall the details of an accident was clinically unconscious or has retrograde amnesia.

The series of questions that the paramedic asks the patient should follow a logical format. When obtaining the history of present illness in the patient with a chief complaint of pain, the paramedic should determine certain information about the pain itself. One method frequently used to systematically evaluate pain is the PQRST method, shown in Table 9-2.

TABLE 9–2.
EVALUATION OF PAIN BY THE **PQRST** METHOD

P =	PROVOKING OR PALLIATIVE	What brought the pain on? How did the pain start? Is there anything that makes it better or worse?
Q =	QUALITY	How does it feel? Describe the pain.
R =	REGION OR RADIATION	Where is the pain? Do you have pain in any other place?
S =	SEVERITY	How bad is your pain? Can you compare it to anything?
T =	TIMING	How long have you had the pain? Does it occur constantly? Intermittently?

MEDICAL HISTORY. The purpose of the **medical history** is to identify the patient's past health problems that may affect the current illness or injury. In the prehospital setting, a thorough evaluation of the medical history may not be necessary. The information gathered from the following questions generally helps evaluate the patient's problem:

1. Has this ever happened before?
2. Do you have any major medical problems (e.g., heart disease, diabetes, hypertension, epilepsy)?
3. Have you ever been in the hospital as a patient?
4. Are you under a physician's care for any reason?
5. Have you ever had surgery?
6. Do you smoke, drink, or use recreational or intravenous drugs? (This question could be stated in easier terms for the patient to understand.)
7. Is there any history in your family of similar problems?

One of the most common errors made in the field is that paramedics bypass the history of present illness and go directly to the patient's medical history. For example, a patient with a chief complaint of epigastric pain and dizziness may be asked a question such as, "Have you ever had a heart attack before?" If the answer is "yes," the assumption may be made prematurely that the same problem is occurring, rather than considering the possibility of acute gastrointestinal bleeding. The present pain may be in the same region but different in character. A better line of questioning would be, "Have you ever had pain like this before?" and "What was the diagnosis then?" and "How is this pain different?"

Information from the medical history may not be relevant to the patient's current problem. For the patient who is 55 years and complaining of chest pain, an appendectomy at age 16 is not pertinent information. Throughout the interview, the current problem should be the focus, and information from the medical history should be used as it applies to the patient's condition.

MEDICATIONS AND ALLERGIES. After questions about the patient's medical history, questions about any prescribed or over-the-counter medications should be asked. Information gained about these medications may provide additional clues to the patient's history and condition. Inquiry should determine the patient's compliance in prescription drug use. Patient allergies are also important to note for both field and hospital personnel. Patients who are allergic to iodine should not be exposed to Betadine solutions, since they have an iodine base. The medical control physician can help evaluate the potential allergy vs. the need to administer drugs.

A description of the type of reaction is important. For example, if the patient claims to be allergic to Novocaine, the paramedic may ask, "How do you know that?" If the patient answers, "I got real shaky and passed out in the dental chair," the condition may not be an allergy to Novocaine but a response to the epinephrine in the anesthetic agent used by the dentist. No evidence of cross sensitivity has been found, however, among the ester-type local anesthetics, such as procaine (Novocaine), and the drugs with an amide linkage, the most common of which is lidocaine.

A sample patient interview is shown in Table 9-3, which demonstrates how to use the components of a patient history.

Collecting Data

Four of the five senses should be used to collect data during the secondary survey. These are the following:

- Sight (observation and inspection)
- Hearing (auscultation)
- Touch (palpation)
- Smell

Sight

Inspection, the skill of visual observation, is one of the most important techniques used to collect patient information. Inspection begins the moment the patient is seen. Scrutiny of the patient as a whole should take place, as well as inspection of involved body systems. Any variation from normal should be noted. Observation of the entire scene should be included. The patient's living quarters, people with the patient, condition or cleanliness of the bed, room, or house, and any medication at the bedside offer important clues.

Hearing

During the secondary survey, the sense of *hearing* is used directly or is aided by the stethoscope. **Auscultation**, listening to sounds, can provide important information about the patient, particularly concerning the respiratory system. Since a wide variety of breath sounds constitutes "normal," the skill of auscultation is difficult and requires practice.

Touch

Palpation makes use of the sense of *touch* and provides clues to moisture, temperature, vibrations, and altered textures or contours on the body. Palpation may confirm observations made during inspection.

Smell

The sense of *smell* can also provide helpful data, such as possible alcohol intake or the acetone breath of a patient in diabetic ketoacidosis. Patients with uremia may smell like ammonia or stale urine.

Equipment Needs

In addition to the use of the human senses, other tools are necessary for proper patient assessment. A watch with a

TABLE 9–3.
SAMPLE PATIENT INTERVIEW

Call dispatched: Possible heart attack. A 55-year-old alert male is sitting in a chair clutching his chest.

History Component	Paramedic Question	Patient Response
1. Chief complaint	Why did you call us today?	My chest hurts. I'm having chest pain.
2. History of present illness (Apply PQRST for complaint of pain)	Tell me more about your pain and what you were doing when it started.	I was reading the paper and it just hit me all of a sudden. ($P = provoking$) It feels like a squeezing sensation right here in the center of my chest. ($Q = quality$) ($R = region$)
	Does the pain go anywhere else?	NO ($R = radiation$)
	Does anything make it better or worse?	I took two nitroglycerin and it didn't help. Nothing seems to help. I'm short of breath too. ($P = Palliative$)
	How bad is the pain?	It's the worse pain I've had in my life. ($S = Severity$)
3. Medical history	How long have you had the pain?	About 30 minutes. ($T = Timing$)
	Do you have any other problems associated with it now?	Just shortness of breath.
	Has this ever happened before?	No, I've had pain in my chest, but not like this.
4. Medications and allergies	Tell me about your other pain, and have you seen a doctor for it?	The pains would come and go; I had a stress test and the doctor just had me lose weight, quit smoking and take these pills.
	Any other major medical illnesses or problems?	No.
	Are you on any other medications?	Aldomet for my blood pressure.
	Do you have any allergies?	Penicillin.

second hand is important for counting the pulse and respirations. A pen light is necessary to examine the patient's pupils and to inspect wounds. A flashlight is helpful in poorly lit circumstances. A sphygmomanometer, gloves, scissors, and stethoscope are also required.

The stethoscope does not need to be expensive, yet it must enable the paramedic to hear and isolate noises made by the patient. The diaphragm end-piece of the stethoscope is used most often since it best transmits high-pitched sounds such as breath sounds (Fig. 9-2). The diaphragm is properly used by firmly holding it in place (usually with one or two fingers) against the patient's skin. The bell end-piece of the stethoscope is primarily used for low-pitched sounds, such as heart murmurs and bruits, and is, therefore, not usually necessary in the field. The stethoscope ear piece should slope toward the paramedic's nose and should fit snugly but not uncomfortably in the ear. Long tubing (more than 14–16 inches) in the neck of the stethoscope may distort the sound, as can movement of the end-piece.

During examination of the patient, it is important for the paramedic to employ the principles of *universal precautions* as described in Chapter 26. The correct ap-

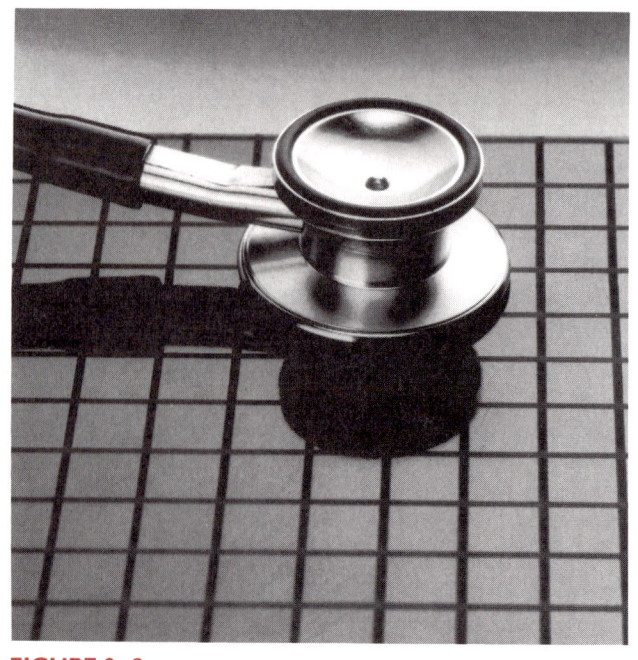

FIGURE 9–2.
Diaphragm (bottom) and bell (top) of a stethoscope are used for auscultating sounds. (Courtesy of © Dixie USA Inc., Houston, Texas)

proach advocates the use of gloves on all patients. Protective eye wear and masks should be worn to prevent exposure of the examiner's mouth, nose, and eyes to blood droplets or other body fluids. Gowns are indicated when splashes of blood or body fluids may occur. Extreme caution is exercised when handling needles or other sharp instruments. Careful attention to hand washing is equally important. Caution should be used in all patient situations.

Diagnostic Signs

Six diagnostic signs are necessary to gain an accurate impression during the secondary survey. They are the following:

- General appearance
- Level of consciousness
- Vital signs
- Tilt test
- Temperature
- Skin

General Appearance

The first step in the secondary survey is to evaluate the patient's general appearance. This step begins when the patient is first seen and continues throughout the time with the patient. The patient's skin color and moisture, facial expression, posture, motor activity, speech, and state of awareness give the paramedic important clues about the patient's condition. Quick observation of the patient's dress, grooming, weight, and odors can also provide data. Medical alert bracelets or medicine bottles in pockets can prove to be helpful. Pain, respiratory distress, restlessness, and a drawn, emaciated appearance are examples of information that may be gathered initially. An infant or child who cries or smiles can indicate a better condition than one who makes no attempt to respond to a stranger or who is listless and lethargic. The continuation of the secondary survey may confirm or deny initial suspicions seen by the patient's general appearance.

Level of Consciousness

The *level of consciousness* is further evaluated in the secondary survey. By the time the paramedic has completed the primary survey and noted the patient's general appearance, the level of consciousness may be apparent. A thorough neurologic assessment is obtained as information is gathered throughout the secondary survey. The paramedic evaluates four key areas of the neurologic exam: the level of consciousness, pupils, pattern of breathing, and motor status. This exam, sometimes called the "DERM" method, is shown as follows:

D = Depth of consciousness
Is the patient awake or unresponsive?

E = Eye signs
Are the pupils equal or unequal? Do they respond to light?

R = Respiratory status
Are respirations normal, abnormal (labored, shallow), or absent?

M = Motor status
Does the patient respond to command or painful stimulus?
Does the patient move all extremities and have sensation in each extremity?

AROUSABILITY. **Arousability** or wakefulness is described according to the patient's response to various types of verbal or painful stimuli. Various descriptions for these responses are used, including lethargic, drowsy, stuporous, semicomatose, or comatose. Since interpretation of a single term can vary from one practitioner to another, it is preferable to describe the observed patient responses and what type of stimulus was used to elicit them.

The *"AVPU" system* is one example that uses a common language to describe the patient's level of consciousness. AVPU is an acronym that represents the following:

A = Awake and alert
The patient's eyes open spontaneously, and the patient is oriented to person, time, place, and situation.

V = Responds to voice
The patient responds when spoken to but may not be oriented to person, time, and place.

P = Responds only to pain
The patient does not respond when spoken to but reacts to a painful stimulus.

U = Unresponsive or unconscious
The patient does not react to a painful stimulus.

Another tool used to precisely describe the patient's neurologic behavior is the Glasgow Coma Scale (see Appendix C). The patient's eye opening, verbal response, and motor response are given numeric values. The numbers are added, and the score reflects the patient's neurologic status. The Glasgow Coma Scale is particularly helpful when the patient's level of consciousness must be evaluated at frequent intervals and compared to the previous findings. The Glasgow Coma Scale should be performed on all patients with a decreased level of consciousness and is explained in further detail for both the adult and pediatric patient in the section on trauma scoring systems.

CONTENT OF CONSCIOUSNESS. **Content of consciousness**, or mentation, evaluates the patient's ability to respond to simple commands, general orientation, and mental ability. Responses to simple commands, such as "wiggle your toes" or "squeeze my hand," can be elicited during the physical examination. Orientation to time, place, and person may be obtained easily while asking questions to complete the run record. Patients in motor vehicle accidents often exhibit disorientated behavior as they repeat the question, "What time is it?" A complete mental status examination may be important in some patients and includes the following:

- Appearance
- Behavior and mood
- Thought content
- Orientation
- Attention and concentration
- Memory
- Judgment

Retrograde memory loss can be determined by asking the question, "What happened?" Further neurologic evaluation is conducted when the paramedic examines the patient's pupils, respirations, and extremities during the physical examination.

Vital Signs

The next step in the secondary survey is assessment of **vital signs**. Vital signs should be determined before further assessment in most patients. Every patient should have this basic but informative assessment. In some situations, for example, uncooperative patients are important to include in this rule, as they have a great potential for alterations in their vital signs. Infants sometimes require more patience and time to assess; yet respiratory rate, pulse rate, and blood pressure are important assessment clues that should not be omitted.

The secondary survey of vital signs includes proper measurement techniques of each vital sign as well as appropriate interpretation of the readings. This interpretation should be based on both the initial reading and on serial measurements of each vital sign. In addition, the vital signs must be evaluated together, relative to each other, to make accurate interpretations. The following vital signs are discussed: respiration, pulse, and blood pressure.

RESPIRATION. Since the presence of **respiration** has been established in the primary survey, the secondary survey involves the more thorough evaluation of respirations to include rate, depth, and rhythm.

Although breathing is typically thought of as an involuntary process, one can consciously or unconsciously control respirations. Consequently, the most accurate way to observe respirations is to do so without the patient's awareness. Bulky clothes, such as a coat or jacket, should be removed before vital sign determination. In infants and small children, observing the abdomen (due to diaphragmatic breathing) or use of the stethoscope may help determine respirations.

Respiratory rate refers to the number of breaths taken in a minute. The *respiratory rhythm* refers to the subjective evaluation of the pattern of breathing, and the *depth* refers to an estimate of the amount of air (tidal volume) in a respiration. These determinations can be evaluated by observing and counting the rise and fall of the chest. A regular pattern of respirations may not require observation for a full minute and can be counted in 30 seconds and multiplied by two. An irregular pattern of breathing requires further evaluation (a full minute) to accurately count respiratory rate and to determine a pattern and depth.

Normal breathing has a regular pattern; medium depth (about 500 ml tidal volume) is effortless and almost silent. The normal adult respiratory rate is 12 to 20 breaths a minute, and more rapid rates are normal in infants and children. Table 9-4 illustrates average respiratory rates by age. Further assessment of the respiratory system is done during the examination of the chest and back.

PULSE. The presence of a **pulse** is determined in the primary survey. The secondary survey allows the paramedic to evaluate the patient's pulse to include rate, rhythm, and strength.

The *pulse rate* is number of pulses in a minute, the *rhythm* refers to the pattern, and the *strength* refers to the subjective assessment of the force of pulsation. The radial pulse is normally used to make these determinations, since it usually is easily accessible. In infants, auscultating the brachial pulse is preferred, especially if the rate is rapid. Figure 9-3 shows other locations to palpate for a pulse.

Pulse rate of a patient with a regular rate is determined by counting pulsations for 30 seconds and multiplying by two. When the patient's condition is urgent, counting for 15 seconds and multiplying by four provides a slightly less accurate pulse rate yet saves important seconds. An irregular rate requires counting for a full minute. The pads of the paramedic's first two or three fingers should be used to palpate the patient's artery. The paramedic's thumb should not be used to palpate a pulse. A normal pulse rate is between 60 and 80 pulses per minute in the adult. An infant or child's pulse rate is faster. Table 9-5 illustrates average pulse rates by age. A normal pulse has a regular rhythm, and the quality should not be bounding, thready, or weak.

TABLE 9–4.
AVERAGE RESPIRATORY RATES BY AGE

Age	Respiratory Rate (breaths/minute)
Infant	25–36
Child	18–26
Adult	12–20

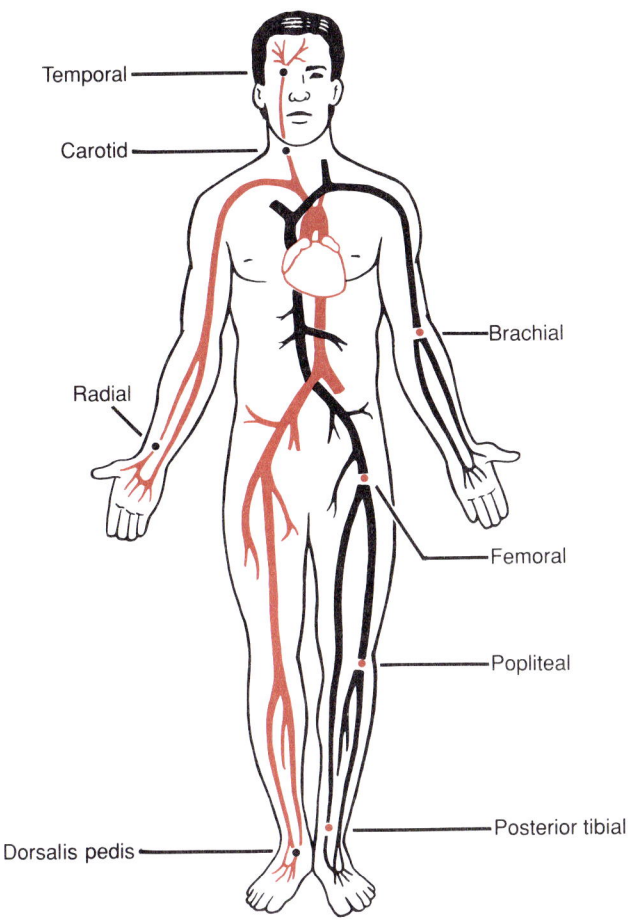

FIGURE 9-3.
Sites of peripheral pulses. (Earnest VV. Clinical Skills and Assessment Techniques in Nursing Practice. Glenview, IL, Scott Foresman/Little, Brown College Division, 1989)

The paramedic will likely encounter some *normal* and *abnormal* deviations in the regularity of a pulse. In the patient with sinus arrhythmia, the pulse rate may speed up with inspiration and slow down with expiration. This pattern is a normal deviation in the pulse rate and occurs with some frequency in children and young adults. Some irregular pulse rates may be from dangerous, premature heart beats. Chapter 20 explains irregular pulse rates and underlying arrhythmias in detail.

The causes of a fast pulse rate are numerous. Pain, anxiety, fear, and anger are all emotions that stimulate the sympathetic nervous system and, therefore, cause a tachycardia, or fast pulse. Exercise requires additional oxygenation and consequently increases the pulse rate. During early shock, the body attempts to compensate for inadequate perfusion, and the pulse rate speeds up. Tachycardia is a heralding sign of early shock.

Bradycardia, a slow pulse rate, can occur abnormally, as in a life-threatening incident, or normally, as in the fit athlete. In the latter, the heart muscle pumps so efficiently with each stroke that it does not need to pump as many times per minute to perfuse adequately. Drugs, such as digitalis, and conditions, such as increasing intracranial pressure, can cause a slow pulse rate. Stimulation of the vagus nerve by carotid massage or *Valsalva's maneuver* (see Chapter 20) also slows the pulse. Bradycardia can occur with a myocardial infarction or some other significant cardiac dysfunction. Bradycardia is also the onset of the terminal phase of hypovolemia.

The pulse rate in infants and children can vary more dramatically and is more responsive to the effects of exercise, emotion, and illness than in adults. Table 9-6 illustrates common causes of fast and slow pulse rates in both adults and children.

BLOOD PRESSURE. The **blood pressure** measurement is the next vital sign to be assessed. This measurement provides information about the patient's blood volume, heart, peripheral vascular integrity, and arterial elasticity.

A single low blood pressure measurement may be all the paramedic needs to confirm strong suspicions of late shock, yet a single normal measurement does not confirm or deny any specific condition or problem. Reassessment of the blood pressure is often necessary to interpret findings as well as to keep track of such a dynamic physiologic function.

The **systolic pressure**, which is recorded as the top number in the blood pressure measurement, represents the maximum pressure against the arteries when the heart contracts. The **diastolic pressure**, which is the bottom number, represents the constant force of blood on the arteries when the heart is resting and, as such, is an estimate of systemic vascular resistance. The difference between the systolic and diastolic pressures is called the pulse pressure.

TABLE 9-5.
AVERAGE PULSE RATES BY AGE

Age	Pulse Rate (beats/minute)
Infant	80–160
Child	80–100
Adult	60–80

TABLE 9-6.
CAUSES OF ABNORMAL PULSE RATES

Causes of Fast Pulse Rates	Causes of Slow Pulse Rates
Exercise	Well-conditioned athletes
Anxiety	Medications (digitalis)
Shock	Myocardial infarction
Fever	Hypothermia
Hyperthyroidism	Hypothyroidism
Medications	Cardiac dysfunction
Cardiac dysfunction	Myocardial ischemia

The measurement of the patient's blood pressure warrants discussion. False high and false low blood pressure readings can distort the perception of the actual condition of the patient; accuracy is imperative to provide correct intervention.

The blood pressure cuff has a bladder inside of it that should be long enough to encircle completely the patient's extremity. The width of the bladder should be at least 20% wider than the diameter of the patient's extremity that is being used. If the blood pressure is taken on the patient's arm, the standard 12 cm wide cuff may yield false high pressures in obese or very muscular arms. The same cuff may give a lower than accurate pressure on a child or small woman with slender arms. The blood pressure measurement may also be taken in the patient's thigh using an extra wide cuff. Sizes of blood pressure cuffs are shown in Figure 9-4.

When blood pressure is measured, the patient should be lying on the stretcher or sitting as comfortably as possible, since pain and discomfort elevate the blood pressure. If the patient's arm is used, the arm should be free of clothing and the forearm should be relaxed and at the level of the patient's heart. The following procedure should be used:

1. The cuff should be totally deflated before being wrapped snugly around the upper arm, with the lower edge approximately 1 inch above the antecubital space.
2. The cuff and bladder should be placed directly over the brachial artery and rapidly inflated to well above the suspected systolic level.
3. The bladder should be deflated smoothly at a rate of approximately 2 mm Hg per second, while listening with the diaphragm of the stethoscope over the brachial artery.
4. When the bladder is deflated, tapping sounds are heard as blood surges into the previously collapsed artery. The systolic pressure is read at that first sound.

As the bladder continues to be deflated, the tapping sounds become muffled and develop a soft blowing quality. This muffling of sound is the point that is generally accepted as the diastolic reading.

A recheck of the patient's blood pressure should not be attempted during deflation of the bladder, as this act causes an inaccurate reading. When a recheck is necessary, the bladder should be completely deflated for at least 30 seconds for venous blood to return before reinflating the bladder. Common errors in blood pressure assessment, shown in Table 9-7, can be avoided by following the proper procedures.

Korotkoff's sounds are a series of sounds sometimes used to record blood pressure (Fig. 9-5). If careful attention is paid to listening for Korotkoff's sounds, errors of underestimating systolic pressure or overestimating diastolic pressure may be avoided. The American Heart Association has recommended that the first sound recorded be the systolic pressure (e.g., 120). The second sound recorded should correspond to the diastolic number that occurs at the onset of phase IV (e.g., 80), and the last number recorded is the second diastolic number (e.g., 74), which is the last sound heard just before a period of continuous silence. The recording for this example would be 120/80/74. If the last sound is heard down to zero, the recording would be 120/80/0.

Paramedics may encounter situations in which obtaining an accurate blood pressure measurement is difficult. The ability to hear blood pressure sounds is hampered frequently in the prehospital environment. Under these conditions, an approximation of blood pressure can be ob-

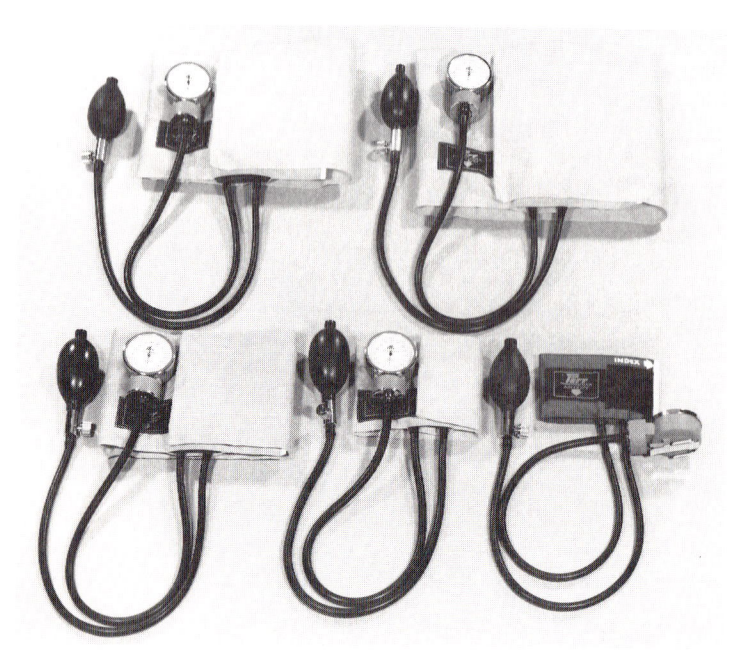

FIGURE 9-4.

Sizes of blood pressure cuffs. (Courtesy of Parr Emergency Sales, Inc., Galloway, Ohio)

TABLE 9–7.
COMMON ERRORS IN BLOOD PRESSURE ASSESSMENT

Error	Contributing Causes	Error	Contributing Causes
Falsely low assessments	• Hearing deficit • Noise in the environment • Applying too wide a cuff • Inserting eartips of stethoscope incorrectly • Using cracked or kinked tubing • Releasing the valve rapidly • Misplacing the bell beyond the direct area of the artery • Failing to pump the cuff 20 to 30 mm Hg above the disappearance of the pulse	Falsely high assessments	• Using a manometer not calibrated at the zero mark • Assessing the blood pressure immediately after exercise • Applying a cuff that is too narrow • Releasing the valve too slowly • Reinflating the bladder during auscultation

(Modified from Taylor C, Lillis C, LeMone P: Fundamentals of Nursing, p 428. Philadephia. JB Lippincott. 1989)

Phase	Description
Phase I	Characterized by the first appearance of faint but clear tapping sounds which gradually increase in intensity. The first tapping sound is the systolic pressure.
Phase II	Characterized by muffled or swishing sounds. These sounds may temporarily disappear, especially in hypertensive persons. The disappearance of the sound during the latter part of phase I and during phase II is called the auscultatory gap and may cover a range of as much as 40 mm Hg. Failing to recognize this gap may cause serious errors of underestimating systolic pressure or overestimating diastolic pressure.
Phase III	Characterized by distinct, loud sounds as the blood flows relatively freely through an increasingly open artery.
Phase IV	Characterized by a distinct, abrupt, muffling sound with a soft, blowing quality. In adults the onset of this phase is considered to be the first diastolic figure.
Phase V	The last sound heard prior to a period of continuous silence. The pressure at which the last sound is heard is the second diastolic measurement.

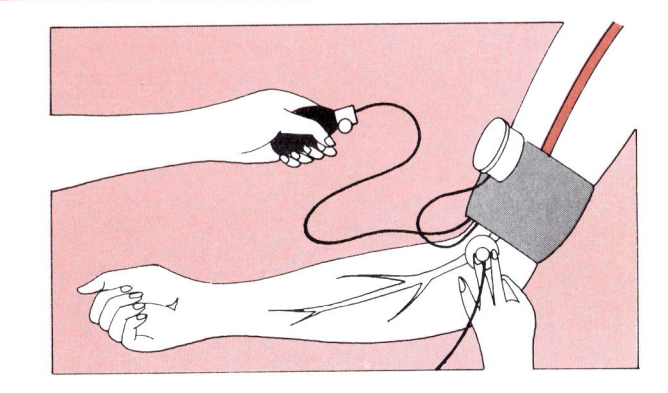

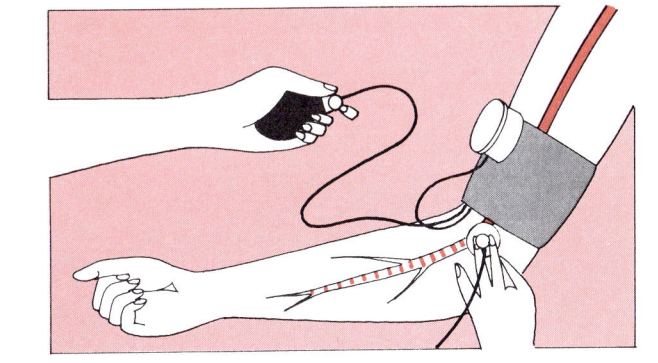

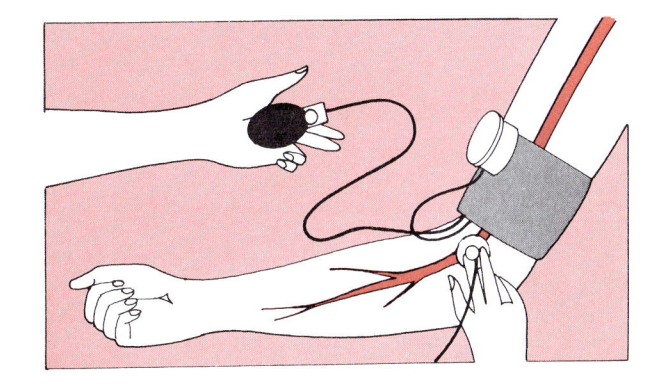

FIGURE 9–5.
Korotkoff's sounds. (Taylor C, Lillis C, LeMone P)

tained by palpating the patient's radial or brachial pulse instead of auscultating the brachial artery. As the bladder is deflated, the return of pulsation approximates the systolic pressure. Additionally, pulsation of the needle in an aneroid manometer can sometimes be used as an estimate of systolic pressure. The estimation of this blood pressure measurement should be noted in the patient's record.

An initial estimate of the patient's blood pressure can be obtained by the evaluation of pulses as shown in Table 9-8. The paramedic should remember that the evaluation of pulses is not reliable in all situations and is a rough estimate. This approximation should be followed by normal blood pressure determination as soon as possible.

Small, effective noise amplifiers, **dopplers,** are available for prehospital personnel and make blood pressure measurement easy and accurate under difficult circumstances. The dopplers enable a better evaluation of distal pulses in an injured extremity.

Any infant or child involved in trauma and all children beyond the age of 3 or 4 years should have their blood pressure measured. The proper cuff should be selected and the procedure explained. Crying and anxiety usually increase the blood pressure as well as make the paramedic's task more difficult.

Interpretation of a single blood pressure measurement may be difficult unless the reading is very low (below 90 systolic in the adult) and accompanied by clinical signs and symptoms of shock. The other vital signs, especially the pulse, are necessary for accurate interpretation, as are other clinical indicators. Normal blood pressure measurements vary from one individual to another, just as considerable variation is found within each person from moment to moment. Factors such as age, gender, time of day, fear, physical discomfort, a full bladder, and body position can alter the blood pressure.

Although no formula can apply to all patients, the adult patient's age plus 100 is a frequently used formula to approximate a normal systolic blood pressure measurement in the male. The diastolic pressure ranges in the male from 65 to 90 mm Hg. A female has a systolic and diastolic blood pressure 8 to 10 mm Hg less than the male. In children, normal systolic pressures can be roughly estimated by doubling the patient's age and adding 80. A normal pediatric diastolic pressure is typically estimated

TABLE 9–8.
ESTIMATE OF SYSTOLIC BLOOD PRESSURE BY PALPATION

Pulses Present	Estimate of Minimal Systolic Pressure
Radial	80 mm Hg
Brachial	70 mm Hg
Femoral	60 mm Hg
Carotid	50 mm Hg

TABLE 9–9.
AVERAGE BLOOD PRESSURE BY AGE

Age	Blood Pressure
Adult man	Systolic: 100 + age = mm Hg (up to 150) Diastolic: 65–90 mm Hg
Adult woman	Systolic and diastolic 8–10 mm Hg lower than in man of same age
Child	Systolic: Age × 2 + 80 = mm Hg Diastolic: Systolic (mm Hg) × 2/3 = mm Hg

to be two thirds of the systolic reading. Table 9-9 illustrates normal systolic and diastolic blood pressures by age.

The World Health Organization defines **hypertension** as a consistent finding, in the adult, with a blood pressure measurement higher than 140/90. Hypertension is seen in the prehospital setting as a result of heart disease, kidney disease, head injury, or increasing intracranial pressure. Also the use of coffee, tobacco, or certain drugs can increase blood pressure. An acute hypertensive crisis constitutes a serious medical emergency.

Hypotension is a systolic reading below 90 mm Hg in the adult. Clinical signs and symptoms of shock, including measurements of other vital signs, should be evaluated to make a determination of hypotension. The paramedic must be aware, however, that a blood pressure of 110/80 may indicate hypotension if the patient's normal reading is 170/110. Hypotension indicates shock caused by low blood or fluid volume, poor peripheral vascular integrity, or inadequate pumping ability of the heart.

Normal pulse pressure is approximately 30 to 40 mm Hg in the adult. The pulse pressure may be widened with fever, arteriosclerosis of the aorta, vigorous exercise, or increasing intracranial pressure. Cardiac tamponade and heart failure may cause a narrowed pulse pressure.

Tilt Test

In some patients, an important assessment tool to measure vital signs is the **tilt test**. The tilt test is indicated in patients with suspected blood or fluid volume loss. Patients who complain mostly of dizziness, fainting, abdominal pain, or persistent vomiting are appropriate candidates. The tilt test should never be performed if the patient is suspected of having any kind of spinal injury.

The tilt test is performed by first taking the pulse and blood pressure with the patient in the supine position and then sitting the patient up with the feet dangling to obtain a second set of measurements. Approximately 30 to 60 seconds should lapse between supine and sitting measurements. The difference in the measurements is then evaluated. An increase in the pulse rate and a decrease in the blood pressure in the sitting position is a positive tilt test and indicates the early stages of shock. Patients in shock for other reasons, such as cardiogenic or anaphylactic shock, may also have a positive tilt test. Their conditions, however, are usually apparent and do not require evaluation for hidden or subtle volume loss.

The patient is able to compensate for an early state of shock when the supine position and gravity help even the fluid distribution. On sitting, however, the patient's system no longer efficiently compensates, and the patient demonstrates some signs and symptoms of shock. Usually, an increase in the pulse rate of 10 to 20 beats per minute or a decrease in the systolic blood pressure of 10 to 20 mm Hg indicates a positive tilt test. Insignificant alterations indicate a negative tilt test. In healthy individuals, the blood pressure actually rises somewhat with the exertion of sitting.

Temperature

Temperature determination is important for patients with altered skin temperature or patients who have been exposed to environmental temperature extremes. Patients with a history of infection, chills, or fever and children with seizures should have their temperatures taken. Transport should not be delayed, however; the patient's temperature should be taken en route to the hospital.

Rectal, rather than *oral*, temperatures should be taken on infants and children up to age 6. Also, patients who are unconscious, restless, confused, or who have or may have seizure activity should not have oral temperatures performed. Glass rectal thermometers should be left in place for 2½ minutes. They should be lubricated before insertion and should be inserted 1½ inches into the anal canal. The paramedic or the parent should hold the rectal thermometer in place for an infant or small child or for any adult who may move.

Oral temperature readings may not be accurate for patients who have recently swallowed liquids or smoked in the previous 15 to 30 minutes. The glass oral thermometer should be left in place under the patient's tongue for 3 to 4 minutes for maximum accuracy. Rectal and oral thermometers are shown in Figure 9-6.

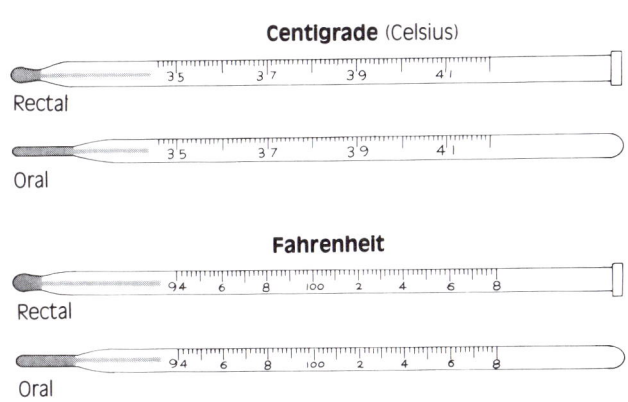

FIGURE 9–6.
Rectal and oral glass thermometers show centigrade and Fahrenheit temperature scales. (Taylor C, Lillis C, LeMone P)

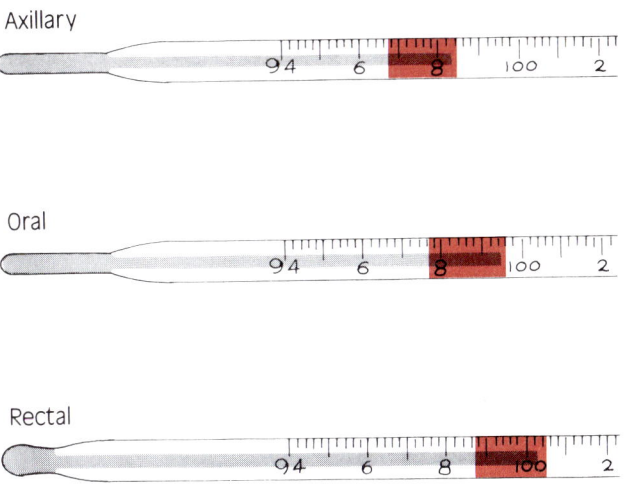

FIGURE 9–7.
Comparison of normal adult axillary, oral, and rectal temperature ranges in Fahrenheit. (Taylor C, Lillis C, LeMone P)

An *axillary temperature*, which is measured by placing the thermometer in the patient's axilla (between the junction of the arm and chest), is the least accurate temperature measurement. It may be helpful, however, in some situations, since it can be measured en route to the hospital. Approximately 10 minutes are required to assess an axillary temperature. The paramedic should not make a definite determination that the patient does not have a fever or has a lowered body temperature based on an axillary temperature reading alone. A comparison of the normal adult axillary, oral, and rectal temperature ranges is shown in Figure 9-7.

Electric thermometers are convenient devices that significantly shorten the necessary time to obtain an accurate temperature reading to 10 seconds. These devices measure rectal, oral, and axillary temperatures and are available with disposable probe covers.

An adult's temperature may fluctuate normally during the course of a day. Normal oral temperatures may be as low as 35.8°C (96.4°F) in the early morning and as high as 37.2°C (99°F) in the evening. Rectal temperatures average 1° higher than oral temperatures. Oral temperatures may vary based on the patient's respiratory rate. Axillary temperatures average 1° less than oral readings. Children's temperatures fluctuate more within the same day than adult's and may rise normally to 38.3°C (101°F) rectally in the evening after an active day. Infants may sometimes be erroneously bundled with excessive clothes and blankets, an act which can cause their temperatures to rise unnecessarily.

Skin

The next step in the secondary survey is to evaluate the patient's skin. An initial evaluation of the skin that included both *temperature* and *moisture* should have been noted during the primary survey or assessment of vital signs. A more thorough look should now be taken, preferably under good light. Skin is normally dry and somewhat warm. Moist, cool skin may indicate poor perfusion and possible shock and should alert the paramedic to act quickly.

The *color* of the skin should also be noted as an indication of the circulation near the surface of the body and of oxygenation. Normal skin tones vary greatly from one person to another. The patient or family member may be more likely to notice any skin color changes. Pale skin (or pale mucous membranes in a dark-skinned individual) may indicate anemia or constriction of the vasculature that supplies the skin. This constriction occurs in very low environmental temperatures and in shock from any cause.

Cyanosis, a bluish discoloration observed in the skin and mucous membranes, indicates a decrease in adequate tissue perfusion of oxygenated blood. Central cyanosis is due to heart or lung disease and is observable in the lips, mouth, and nail beds. Peripheral cyanosis occurs from anxiety or from a very cold environment and is usually noticed in the nail beds.

A pink skin color is present if increased blood flow or vasodilatation occurs, such as in the case of high environmental temperatures, alcohol intake, or fever. A localized pink or red area may indicate an inflammation or allergic reaction. Also, acute blunt trauma may cause the injured area to be pink or red. Severe acute blunt trauma usually results in bruised, reddish blue skin at the site of the injury. An increase in the number of red blood cells causes a reddish blue skin color in the emphysema patient. Carbon monoxide poisoning sometimes results in red skin, although associated cyanosis may mask the redness.

A yellow hue (jaundice) to the skin or sclera of the eye (usually caused by an elevated bilirubin) may indicate liver disease. This yellow hue may be present normally in the newborn with physiologic jaundice from the second to tenth day. Table 9-10 summarizes abnormal skin colors.

Skin turgor should also be evaluated in patients in which dehydration is suspected. Skin turgor or tenting refers to the speed that a lifted fold of skin returns to place. The return normally occurs quickly, unless the patient is elderly and the skin has lost much elasticity.

Any other variations in the skin should be noted. These may include scars or "tracks" from intravenous drug abuse, a rash or whelps in the allergic patient, petechia (small, flat, reddish purple lesions) in the patient with a bleeding disorder or meningococcal meningitis, or bruising in the victim of trauma or child abuse.

Capillary Refill Test

Adequacy of circulation to the extremities is gauged by the **capillary refill test**. To perform this test, gentle pressure is exerted on the patient's nail bed. The pressure should be sufficient to *blanch* (whiten) the underlying cutaneous tissue. If circulation to the extremity is good, the nail bed should become pink again when pressure is released within 1 to 2 seconds. The length of time that the underlying cutaneous tissue takes to become pink is dependent on adequacy of perfusion to that area.

Physical Examination

The **head-to-toe survey** is organized as follows: head and neck, chest and back, abdomen, and extremities. The procedure for conducting a physical examination is shown in Skill 9-1.

Head and Neck

The examination of the patient's head and neck begins the head-to-toe survey. The head should be inspected and

TABLE 9-10.
ABNORMAL SKIN COLORS AND CAUSES

Color	Possible Cause	Possible Conditions
Pink	Vasodilation	Heat illness
		Hot environment
	Increased blood flow	Exertion
		Fever
		Alcohol consumption
White, pale	Decreased blood flow	Shock
		Fainting
	Decreased red blood cells	Anemia
	Vasoconstriction	Cold exposure (can also cause pink skin due to decreased O_2 use in the skin)
Blue	Inadequate oxygenation	Airway obstruction
		Congestive heart failure
		Chronic bronchitis
Yellow	Increased bilirubin	Liver disease
	Retention of urinary elements	Renal disease

palpated. If a cervical spine injury is suspected, the spine should be immobilized immediately and the neck should not be manipulated while the head is being evaluated. The face should be examined for edema, bruising, bleeding, asymmetry, or fluid from the nose or ears. The mastoid process behind the ear should be inspected for ecchymosis. The mouth should be examined for loose teeth or dentures. In infants, the condition of the anterior fontanel should be noted.

The pupils can provide important clues for the paramedic in certain patients. All trauma patients and every patient with an altered level of consciousness or a neurologic complaint or finding should have their pupils checked. The pupils should be examined for several items:

- Equal size
- Dilation in both eyes caused by darkness
- Constriction in both eyes caused by light
- Constriction that occurs rapidly
- Reaction to light that is equal

To evaluate these items, both pupils should be observed in a somewhat dark area or with the light shaded from both eyes. The clipboard with the patient information form can be used to shield light. Pupillary reactions are exaggerated in darkness. The pupils should be the same size and somewhat dilated, depending on the amount of light. With the eyes still shaded, the paramedic should quickly shine a flashlight at one eye from an angle about 6 to 8 inches from the eye. The patient should not look directly into the light. Both pupils should quickly constrict.

About 5% of the population normally have a measurable (greater than 1 mm) difference in pupil size. A patient who is blind in one eye has a normal reaction in both eyes when the sighted eye is examined, with both eyes constricting to light. The same patient does not have a response in either eye when the blind eye is illuminated. No pupillary reaction occurs in the patient with a prosthetic eye.

Bilateral dilated and fixed pupils can result from profound hypoxia or severely increased intracranial pressure. This finding should cause the paramedic to act quickly. Drugs, such as atropine and glutethimide (Doriden), also cause this reaction. Bilateral constricted and fixed pupils may be due to narcotic poisoning, some eye drops given for glaucoma (*miotics*), and an unusual type of cerebral hemorrhage (*pontine*). A single dilated, fixed pupil is of concern and may signify a subdural or epidural hematoma, early intracranial pressure, a stroke, or history of surgery on that eye.

Any other abnormality of the eyes should be noted. Red or bloodshot sclera may indicate allergy, trauma, or infection. Jaundice may first appear as yellow sclera before being noticeable in the skin. Nystagmus, rhythmic oscillation of the eyes, is commonly associated with drug toxicity or cerebral dysfunction. The doll's eyes exam, which requires turning the patient's head rapidly to one side, should never be performed in the prehospital assessment of a patient who is suspected of having cervical spine trauma.

The patient's neck should be examined for the presence of jugular vein distention and for tracheal deviation. The trachea can normally be seen or palpated in the midline of the neck during inspiration. A deviation of the trachea during inspiration could indicate a pneumothorax, which should be further assessed by evaluating breath sounds. The presence of bruising, swelling, or subcutaneous emphysema should also be noted. Subcutaneous emphysema occurs when air escapes into the tissues and may be felt by the paramedic's finger pads as a crackling sensation. When subcutaneous emphysema is present in the neck of a trauma patient, a major injury to the esophagus or large airway may be present.

Chest and Back

The examination of the patient's chest is the next step of the secondary survey. This area is important because the chest yields information about the respiratory and cardiovascular systems. The chest is evaluated to some degree when the patient's respirations are evaluated. A further inspection of the chest is necessary, especially in the trauma patient or in any patient with abnormal vital signs. The patient with a cardiac or respiratory complaint, finding, or history is also a candidate for a more thorough chest evaluation.

Auscultation of breath sounds is an important aspect of the physical assessment of the chest and back. Breath sounds are evaluated with a stethoscope while the patient, if able, breathes deeply with the mouth open. The paramedic's familiarity with underlying anatomy aids in a thorough lung evaluation. All four quadrants of the anterior and posterior chest should be auscultated (see Chapter 19). The breath sounds are evaluated for presence, equality of one side to another, and abnormal sounds.

Normally, breath sounds are present and heard equally on each side of the chest. Inspiration usually creates a longer and louder sound as the air flows into the bronchioles and alveoli. Expiration is usually quiet or silent. No additional sounds are usually present. Decreased breath sounds may be heard when fluid or air is in the pleural space and, consequently, interferes with the sound. Bronchial obstruction also causes diminished or absent breath sounds since there is no air flow.

Abnormal sounds can sometimes be heard along with the normal breath sounds. Abnormal sounds include rales, rhonchi, and wheezes. Rales are sounds caused by fluid either in the alveoli (*fine rales*) or larger airway (*coarse rales*). Rales are heard during inspiration and can be simulated by rolling hair between the thumb and forefinger close to one's ear. Rhonchi are typically more coarse, or similar to snoring in character, and are also heard on inspiration. Rhonchi are heard in breath sounds when mucus or fluid narrows the air passages. Wheezing is caused by air that flows through narrowed airways, but it is typically heard at the end of expiration.

Auscultation of the heart may occasionally provide helpful information in the prehospital environment if the setting is quiet. The examiner should listen with the bell or diaphragm of the stethoscope at the patient's left sternal border, in the fourth intercostal space. The primary purpose of prehospital auscultation of heart sounds is to establish presence and regularity.

The paramedic may hear additional heart sounds over the usual "*lub-dub*," indicating possible congestive heart failure or other acute or chronic heart conditions. Extra heart sounds may be normal and benign in some individuals. Distant or muffled heart sounds refer to the decreased volume of the sounds, as in cardiac tamponade. Detection of this finding is difficult even in the quieter hospital environment.

Percussion is an evaluation tool that involves striking or tapping the patient's skin to determine the size, location, and density of an underlying structure. Since a quiet environment and skilled examiner are necessary to perform this procedure, it is not practical to use in the field.

In the trauma patient, inspection of the chest and back should be made for rib or tracheal retractions, abdominal breathing, a barrel chest, bruising, asymmetry, or paradoxical chest movement. The paramedic may best evaluate paradoxical chest movement by watching the chest motion from the patient's side at eye level. Palpation of the chest may reveal tender areas that possibly indicate rib fractures. Subcutaneous emphysema palpated in the chest may be a clue to rib fractures, a pneumothorax, or a penetrating wound of the chest or neck.

Auscultation of breath sounds for their presence and equality is the most important aspect of auscultation of the chest in trauma patients. Absent or diminished breath sounds on one side could indicate a pneumothorax or hemothorax. Evaluation for abnormal breath sounds in the trauma patient helps to determine pulmonary status before administration of large amounts of intravenous fluids that are sometimes required for shock resuscitation.

In the nontrauma patient, inspection of the chest and back should evaluate the possibility of a barrel chest (the increased anterior-posterior diameter associated with emphysema), any abnormal breathing patterns, rib or tracheal retractions, surgical scars, or restricted chest expansion. Palpation of the chest, particularly in the posterior kidney area, may reveal tenderness, indicating inflammation or infection that involves the kidney. The presence of abnormal breath sounds, such as rales, could indicate congestive heart failure and pulmonary edema.

Abdomen

The abdomen should be evaluated on all patients but particularly those with gastrointestinal symptoms or suspicion of volume loss as seen in dizziness, fainting, vaginal bleeding, vomiting, or *melena* (blood in the stool). The evaluation of the abdomen on a trauma patient should be limited to inspection and rapid palpation. This trauma exam should not delay transportation.

Nontrauma patients should be examined while they are comfortably lying on their backs, usually with knees up. Conversation or questions may be helpful during the exam as they can distract and relax the patient. This relaxation may prevent voluntary guarding of the abdomen and may help obtain accurate information. Keeping the patient warm and preserving the patient's modesty while still performing an adequate exam are important.

Inspection of the abdomen should be performed to observe for scars, bruises, masses, or localized bulging. A distended abdomen may indicate intra-abdominal hemorrhage or an accumulation of fluid in the peritoneum (*ascites*). Pulsation of the abdominal wall in the epigastric area may be a normal observation in the thin person and is due to aortic pulsations. Otherwise, a pulsating mass may indicate an aneurysm, which should prompt immediate action. The umbilicus is normally inverted but may become extruded normally or with pregnancy, ascites, or an abdominal mass.

Auscultation of bowel sounds requires a quiet environment, a fact which makes this evaluation tool difficult in the prehospital environment. The diaphragm of the stethoscope is lightly held against the skin of the patient's abdomen while all four quadrants are auscultated. Normal bowel sounds occur as a result of air and fluid moving through the small intestine. The sounds are normally high-pitched and gurgling. Findings of five to thirty sounds a minute are normal, related to the time of the last ingestion of food. Frequent high-pitched, loud, tinkling bowel sounds may indicate gastroenteritis and early bowel obstruction. Diminished or absent bowel sounds may occur with abdominal trauma, inflammation, or peritonitis. Auscultation must take place for about 2 to 5 minutes before the accurate determination of diminished or absent bowel sounds can be made. For this additional reason, auscultation of bowel sounds is not practical in the field. Transportation should not be delayed in the trauma patient to evaluate bowel sounds.

Palpation of all four quadrants of the abdomen can provide important information for the paramedic. If the patient has abdominal pain, care should be taken to examine the painful area last, as involuntary muscle guarding impedes further evaluation. Fear and ticklishness may cause abdominal muscles to tense. This type of tenseness is of concern. True abdominal muscle guarding is an involuntary reflex that occurs when the peritoneum is inflamed by blood, pus, or other irritants. The patient should be encouraged to breathe deeply and slowly to relax the muscles as the paramedic gently depresses the abdomen with the finger pads. Masses, tender areas, or rigidity of muscle guarding should be noted.

Examination of the external genitalia is appropriate under some circumstances. Trauma to the genitals requires a discreet inspection. A woman in labor or with her "bag of waters" ruptured should be visually examined for crowning or a prolapsed cord. Priapism, sustained penile erection, may be an ominous sign of spinal cord injury.

Extremities

The examination of the extremities is the last step of the head-to-toe survey. The musculoskeletal system is inspected and palpated for swelling, temperature, deformity, or tenderness. Tremors in the hands should be noted. Comparing one side to another is necessary. Pain, pallor, paraesthesia, paralysis, peripheral pulses, and capillary refill should be assessed in any injured extremity to evaluate the integrity of the peripheral vascular system.

Neurologic status of the extremities is evaluated and tested for strength, movement, range of motion, and sensation. Muscle strength is checked by having the patient squeeze both of the paramedic's hands. Lower extremity strength may be determined by having the patient push the feet against the paramedic's hand. The ability to move each extremity is simultaneously evaluated. Sensation is assessed by using a safety pin or other tool to determine the patient's response to pain. Throughout the exam, a comparison of both sides is again essential.

In the unconscious patient, the manner in which the extremities react to painful or noxious (e.g., an ammonia capsule) stimuli is important to note. The appropriateness of the response is also evaluated. Hemiparesis, or one-sided weakness and decreased sensation to pain, is commonly observed in the stroke patient. Decorticate posturing is termed the "*flexor*" response, as any or all four extremities may flex and rotate inward. In decerebrate posturing, called the "*extensor*" response, all four extremities are rigid and fully extended. In some cases, a combination of decorticate and decerebrate posturing may be seen. These abnormal postures are primitive responses that indicate severe intracranial pressure and possible brain stem involvement.

The lower extremities often provide important information about peripheral edema; this finding should be evaluated in any cardiac or respiratory patient. Testing for peripheral edema can be done by pushing one's thumb firmly on the skin behind the patient's ankle or over the tibia. Edema related to the heart typically is present in both lower extremities and stays indented for several seconds. This reaction is called pitting edema. Unilateral edema that is not pitting may be due to occlusion of a deep vein or artery.

Tenderness and warmth in the calf muscle may indicate an irritated deep vein due to a blood clot (thrombophlebitis). Pain that occurs when the foot is sharply dorsiflexed is also an indication of thrombophlebitis.

TRAUMA SCORING SYSTEMS

Several systems have been developed to help accurately determine injury severity in the trauma patient. These systems are used to gather statistics and determine which patients should be transported directly to a trauma center. These systems do not replace a thorough patient assessment. The trauma scoring should occur only after a complete patient assessment has been performed and should not delay patient management.

The five trauma scoring systems to be discussed are the following:

Adult Trauma Score
Pediatric Trauma Score
Adult Glasgow Coma Scale
Pediatric Glasgow Coma Scale
CRAMS Scale

The purposes of these trauma scoring systems are to determine the severity of injuries, identify changes in patient status, and determine the need for urgent transport to a trauma center. None of these systems has proven to be an effective triage device for the adult. The triage decision scheme (developed by Dr. Champion) shown in Figure 9-8, which is based on general condition and mechanism of injury, has proven to be the best device to decide which patients should be transported directly to a trauma center.

Adult Trauma Score

The **Adult Trauma Score** places a numerical value on the assessment of the patient in several categories. Categories include the following:

- Respiratory rate
- Respiratory expansion
- Systolic blood pressure
- Capillary refill

The total numerical value of these categories is added to an adjusted Adult Glasgow Coma Scale value (which is reduced to approximately one third of total value). The combination of the category total and adjusted Adult Glasgow Coma Scale value gives the total trauma score points. More severe injuries generate a lower trauma score for the patient. The Adult Trauma Score shown in Appendix C is a revised and updated version of the original Trauma Score developed by Drs. Champion, Sacco, and Carnazzo.

Pediatric Trauma Score

The **Pediatric Trauma Score** is a variation of the Adult Trauma Score and assesses six components commonly

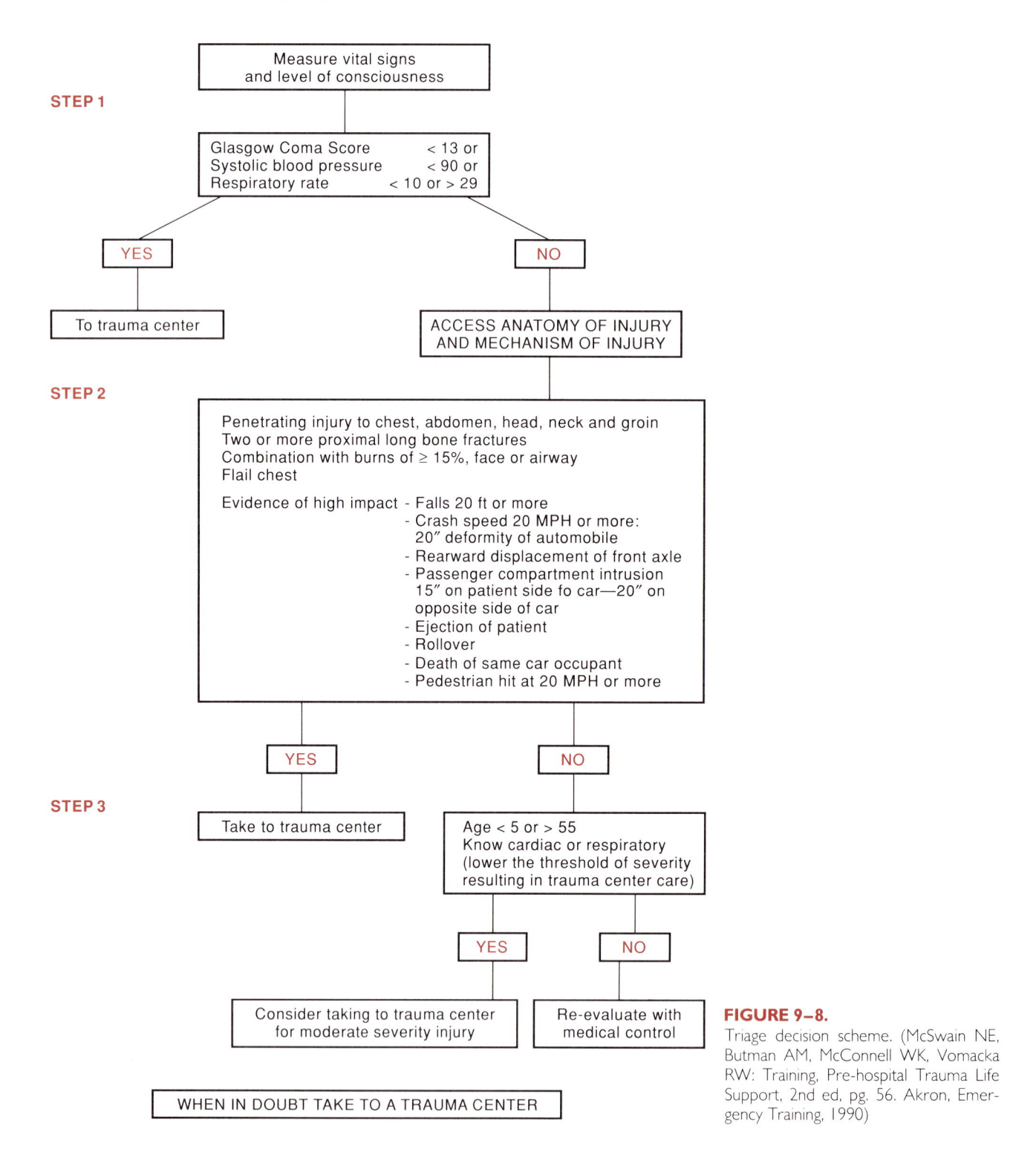

```
                    ┌─────────────────────────────┐
                    │   Measure vital signs       │
                    │   and level of consciousness│
STEP 1              └──────────────┬──────────────┘
                                   │
                    ┌──────────────┴──────────────┐
                    │ Glasgow Coma Score  < 13 or │
                    │ Systolic blood pressure < 90 or │
                    │ Respiratory rate  < 10 or > 29 │
                    └──────────────┬──────────────┘
                    ┌──────────────┴──────────────┐
                  YES                             NO
```

STEP 1

- Glasgow Coma Score < 13 or
- Systolic blood pressure < 90 or
- Respiratory rate < 10 or > 29

YES → To trauma center

NO → ACCESS ANATOMY OF INJURY AND MECHANISM OF INJURY

STEP 2

- Penetrating injury to chest, abdomen, head, neck and groin
- Two or more proximal long bone fractures
- Combination with burns of ≥ 15%, face or airway
- Flail chest

Evidence of high impact
- Falls 20 ft or more
- Crash speed 20 MPH or more: 20" deformity of automobile
- Rearward displacement of front axle
- Passenger compartment intrusion 15" on patient side fo car—20" on opposite side of car
- Ejection of patient
- Rollover
- Death of same car occupant
- Pedestrian hit at 20 MPH or more

YES → Take to trauma center

NO →

STEP 3

Age < 5 or > 55
Know cardiac or respiratory (lower the threshold of severity resulting in trauma center care)

YES → Consider taking to trauma center for moderate severity injury

NO → Re-evaluate with medical control

WHEN IN DOUBT TAKE TO A TRAUMA CENTER

FIGURE 9–8.
Triage decision scheme. (McSwain NE, Butman AM, McConnell WK, Vomacka RW: Training, Pre-hospital Trauma Life Support, 2nd ed, pg. 56. Akron, Emergency Training, 1990)

evaluated in pediatric trauma and grades them into three categories. The six components are the following:
- Weight
- Airway
- Level of consciousness
- Systolic blood pressure
- Open wounds
- Fractures

Each component is assigned a grade of either +2 (minimal or no injury), +1 (minor or potentially major injury), and −1 (major or immediate life-threatening injury). The sum of the grades assigned to the six components is the Pediatric Trauma Score. The total can range between −6 and +12, with the lower scores indicating severe injuries. The Pediatric Trauma Score is shown in Appendix C.

Adult Glasgow Coma Scale

The **Adult Glasgow Coma Scale** is accepted worldwide and is particularly helpful when the patient's level of consciousness must be evaluated at frequent intervals and compared to previous findings. Numeric values are given to the following categories:

- Eyes opening
- Motor response
- Verbal response

The numbers are added, and the score reflects the patient's neurologic status. Lower scores indicate severe injury. The Adult Glasgow Coma Scale may be adjusted to be used with the Adult Trauma Score as previously shown. The Glasgow Coma Scale is shown in Appendix C.

Pediatric Glasgow Coma Scale

The **Pediatric Glasgow Coma Scale** is similar to the Adult Glasgow Coma Scale except that the pediatric patient is evaluated by age ranges. Categories included in the Pediatric Glasgow Coma Scale are the following:

- Eyes opening
- Motor response
- Verbal response

Numeric values are given to each category, and the numbers are added depending on the age of the patient. The total score reflects the patient's neurologic status. The Pediatric Glasgow Coma Scale is shown in Appendix C.

CRAMS Scale

The **CRAMS Scale** is concerned with the following categories:

- Respiratory rate
- Respiratory expansion
- Systolic blood pressure
- Capillary return

As with the Adult Trauma Score, the CRAMS Scale total is added to a number that grades the score of the Adult Glasgow Coma Scale. Once again, as with the other trauma scores, more severe injuries generate lower scores. The CRAMS Scale is shown in Appendix C.

RE-EVALUATION OF THE PATIENT

Re-evaluation of the patient is as important an assessment tool as the initial patient assessment. Serial measurements of the vital signs give clues to improvement or deterioration of the patient's condition. Missed injuries can be caught in the re-evaluation process. Many times the patient's environment is not conducive to an appropriate initial patient assessment. The room may be dark with little or no lighting. Further investigation can reveal problems that may require the paramedic to change or modify patient management.

Re-evaluation should be done periodically, depending on the severity of the patient's condition. Vital signs should be measured about every 10 minutes, if not sooner, if the patient's condition is deteriorating. Constant observation of the patient's appearance, level of consciousness, EKG, and overall body system functions alerts the paramedic to problems that need attention.

COMMUNICATION OF PATIENT DATA

Communication of patient data involves the following components: patient and family, base station or hospital, and the written record.

Patient and Family

The amount of information given to any patient about a condition is usually determined by how much the patient wants to know, how serious the patient's condition is, and how confident the paramedic is about the findings. A careful balance of common sense and good judgment should be employed. If specific information is requested by the patient, an honest approach is probably best. For example, if the patient asks, "Am I having a heart attack?" an appropriate response could be as follows: "It is hard to establish such a diagnosis in the field, but the chest pain and symptoms you're experiencing are concerning. As a precaution, we are contacting a doctor and starting an intravenous infusion in your arm. We will watch your electrocardiogram carefully on the way to the hospital." A calm, honest response of this type reassures the patient that the paramedic is knowledgeable of the situation. On the contrary, omitting pertinent findings and falsely reassuring the patient by saying "everything is just fine" when it is not is inappropriate. In addition, this false reassurance may create suspicion and cause the patient to question the paramedic's ability.

The patient's family or significant others should be handled with honesty and sensitivity. Patient confidentiality should also be maintained. Having limited medical knowledge, the family member frequently feels anxious, frightened, or hysterical. The family's response to stress may not correspond to the actual seriousness of the emergency. The paramedic's conscious effort to empathize with the family provides motivation to spend a few moments reassuring the family. If the patient's condition precludes the paramedic from talking to the family, the paramedic should designate this task to an auxiliary rescue worker. The paramedic who omits this interaction with the family may find a family member anxious and demanding. The family member then becomes a distraction and consequently increases the paramedic's stress as the situation slips out of control.

Base Station or Hospital

Radio communication of patient data in the prehospital setting is aimed at providing a clear visual image of the patient to the physician. Without a mental picture, the physician is handicapped at helping the paramedic provide optimal management.

Patient data should be presented in a standard, orderly format. This consistent sequence not only helps the nurse or physician on the other end of the radio, but also assists the paramedic in remembering details. When reporting to the base station or hospital, appropriate medical terminology should be used and unclear radio jargon avoided. Information need not be lengthy but must be meaningful. A standard report protocol follows:

- Paramedic unit calling
- Patient's age and sex
- Chief complaint
- General patient condition, including level of consciousness, vital signs, and other information that relates to the urgency of the situation
- Pertinent history of present condition: illness or accident
- Pertinent medical history
- Physical examination findings and EKG
- Management initiated and further orders desired
- Estimated time of arrival

Communication of patient data to the physician includes the use of "*pertinent positives*" and "*pertinent negatives.*" These terms describe history or physical exam findings that relate positively or negatively to the chief complaint. For example, in the patient with abdominal pain, pertinent positives would be nausea, vomiting, and a rigid or tender abdomen. Pertinent negatives would be the absence of melena (blood in the stool), no diarrhea, and a negative tilt test. Negative as well as positive findings help form a mental picture of the patient for the physician. If negative findings are not relayed to the physician, unnecessary radio time may be expended as the physician asks for additional signs and symptoms. A sample radio report is included in the box "Communication of Patient Information to Hospital or Base Station."

After the physician gives the orders, the paramedic should repeat the orders back to the base station or hospital for verification. This step is necessary to reduce the possibility of errors. If an order seems inappropriate or unreasonable, the paramedic should ask for clarification or should re-explain patient assessment information before carrying out the order.

COMMUNICATION OF PATIENT INFORMATION TO HOSPITAL OR BASE STATION

Medic One to Memorial Hospital. We have an 83-year-old female who is complaining of chest pain. She is awake and alert. Her blood pressure is 100/60, pulse 120 and thready, respirations 24 and shallow, and her skin is cool and clammy. The pain started while she was gardening and lasted 2 hours before she called for an ambulance. She had taken five nitroglycerin tablets without relief. She describes the pain as an intense pressure and denies radiation. She is nauseated, short of breath, and dizzy. She has a history of hypertension and is on Aldomet, but denies cardiac history or other medication. On physical exam, we find rales in both lungs, no cyanosis or edema in her feet. Her EKG is sinus tachycardia, we have her on 8 liters of oxygen by Venturi mask at 40% FiO_2, and have initiated an IV of D_5W. Our ETA to your facility is 8 minutes. What further treatment would you like us to carry out?

If further orders are required, the paramedic should request these from the physician. While en route, the *estimated time of arrival* (ETA) should be communicated to the hospital.

Once the patient and paramedic arrive at the hospital, patient information is communicated to the receiving nurse or physician. After the patient is introduced, the same logical format of presentation used for radio communication should be used to present relevant patient findings. This presentation normally should be done out of the hearing range of the patient. The physician or nurse will likely take another history from the patient. This action does not signify mistrust of the paramedic but serves as an appropriate safeguard to verify accurate patient history and determine the level of consciousness of the patient. The clear, organized, and concise report of patient information that is communicated to the base station and the hospital greatly helps to establish respect and confidence in prehospital care providers.

Written Record

Completing the **written record** of the call is the final, important step in communicating patient data. The importance of this record cannot be over emphasized, since it serves as the legal medical record of the incident. The report should include complete, accurate, and legible information that is pertinent to the call.

A written record that includes check lists and blanks to be filled in is a desirable type of form to use in the prehospital setting. The form must also include adequate space to document other relevant information and de-

CHAPTER 9: Patient Assessment 123

EMS
REPORT #

EMS REGION II
STATE OF NEW HAMPSHIRE
STANDARD PATIENT RECORD   DATE

EMS

Resp. Unit:	Attendants:		Age:	Dispatched:
				Time Out:
Pt's Name:			D.O.B.	On Scene:
Address:			Sex: M F	Enroute-
			MD:	@ Hosp.-
Incident Loc:			**STATUS:**	In Service-
Next of Kin:			Amb. Srv:	Hosp.

CHIEF COMPLAINT, HISTORY & DETAILED OBSERVATIONS: _____

MEDS: _____   MEDIC ALERT: _____
Allergies: _____

MENTAL STATUS
___ A-Alert
___ V-Verbal Stim.
___ P-Painful Stim.
___ U-Unresponsive

PULSE: _____
Rhym: ___ Reg.
          ___ Irreg.
Strength ___ Weak
             ___ Strong

Blood Pressure:
____ / ____

RESP: _____
Rhym: ___ Reg.
          ___ Irreg.
Cond ___ Norm.
          ___ Lab.

Breath Sounds
L: ___ R: ___
___ CLEAR
___ RALES
___ RHONCHI
___ WHEEZES
___ STRIDOR
___ OTHER

Type of Illness / Injury
☐ 1. Trauma
☐ 2. Burn
☐ 3. Cardiac
☐ 4. Neonate
☐ 5. Behavioral
☐ 6. Poison
☐ 7. Spinal Cord
☐ 8. Head
☐ 9. Respiratory
☐ 10. M/V
☐ 11. OD
☐ 12. CVA

SKIN
COLOR
___ Cyanotic
___ Pale
___ Flushed
___ Normal

TEMP.
___ Hot
___ Cold
___ Normal
Body Temp. ___°
Oral ___

MOISTURE
___ Dry
___ Moist
___ Normal

Rectal ___

PUPILS
___ Equal
___ Unequal
___ Fixed Dilated
___ Constricted
___ Responsive
___ Unresponsive

EOM's
___ Full &
     Conjugate
___ Disconjugate
___ Fixed Gaze
___ Nystagmus

CRAMS SCORE ___

TIME	OBSERVATIONS				TIME	TREATMENT		
	P	R	BP	EKG. RHYM & OTHER		IV'S	MEDICATIONS	OTHER

ATTENDANT: _____   Base Physician: _____

FIGURE 9–9.
Run sheet.

scribe the sequence of events if the patient's condition changes. The middle of a busy emergency, when patient care is the priority, is an impractical time to complete the form. However, the paramedic benefits in the long run by completing this task once the patient is delivered to the hospital. After the run report has been filled out, it should be signed by the paramedic and checked for completeness. Typical written records include the standard information shown in Figure 9-9.

Like radio communication, a frequent error in written documentation is the omission of findings, particularly pertinent negatives. This information is essential to record when the patient refuses or is not transported for some reason. The paramedic is unlikely to recall the justification for actions taken if it is not reflected on the written record. For example, consider a question on the lack of cervical immobilization. Documentation that reflects no indication for spinal immobilization based on the mechanism of injury and other pertinent negatives could prevent a costly lawsuit.

Statements on the report should be limited to the facts. Assumptions or judgments must not be included in the written record. For example, if a female patient's history revealed low abdominal pain and heavy discharge, an assumption that she has gonorrhea should not be included on the written record.

Abbreviations are useful in efficient record keeping (see Chapter 8). Time and space can be saved. Every ambulance organization or emergency medical services provider should keep a list of acceptable abbreviations or symbols for personnel to use so that interpretation of information can be consistent and undisputed. If errors occur in writing on the patient record, they should be crossed out with a single line and initialed or signed. The written record should be recorded in black ink so it can be copied clearly or filmed for conserving space if necessary.

Written records also provide the opportunity to collect data for the emergency medical services system. For example, information about average response time may demonstrate the need for an additional ambulance. The average time spent on the scene for serious trauma patients is helpful data for quality assurance. Unsuccessful endotracheal intubations may indicate a need for additional clinical training or continuing education. The retrieval of such data can impact system effectiveness and quality patient care.

SUMMARY

As the paramedic collects clues from the scene, the patient history, and the physical examination, a particular illness or injury usually becomes apparent. Even if the evidence does not lead the paramedic to an exact illness or injury, at least a specific body system can usually be identified as the source of the problem. This conclusion forms the basis for patient management.

Advanced life support protocols typically require communication of patient data to the base station or hospital. In addition, a few minutes communicating findings to the patient and family are well spent. During transport to the hospital, the patient should be re-evaluated periodically for vital signs, appearance, level of consciousness, and general patient assessment.

SUGGESTED READING

Arneson DJ, Bruce ML: The EMT Handbook of Emergency Care. Philadelphia, JB Lippincott, 1987

Ball RA: Documentation: The overlooked aspect of emergency care. J Emerg Med Serv 15(5):31, 1990

Bates B: A Guide to Physical Examination, 5th ed. Philadelphia, JB Lipppincott, 1991

Campbell JE: Basic Trauma Life Support for Advanced Prehospital Care, 2nd ed. Englewood Cliffs, Prentice-Hall, 1988

Copes WS, Champion HR, Sacco WJ et al: The injury severity score revisited. J Trauma 28:69, 1988

Dernocoeur K, Thurnher O: Total patient care: Treating your patient as a person. J Emerg Med Serv 14(5):50, 1989

Eichelberger MR, Gotschall CS, Sacco WJ et al: A comparison of the trauma score, the revised trauma score, and the pediatric trauma score. Ann Emerg Med 18:1053, 1989

Kennedy WC: Vital signs: Reading the essentials. J Emerg Med Serv 15(5):26, 1990

McSwain NE, Butman AM, McConnell WK et al: Prehospital Trauma Life Support, 2nd ed. Akron, Emergency Training, 1990

McSwain NE, Kerstein MD: Evaluation and Management of Trauma. Norwalk, Appleton-Century-Crofts, 1987

Taylor C, Lillis C, LeMone P: Fundamentals of Nursing. Philadelphia, JB Lippincott, 1989

US Department of Transportation, National Highway Traffic Safety Administration: Emergency Medical Technician-Paramedic: National Standards Curriculum. Washington, DC, US Government Printing Office, 1985

CHAPTER 10

Airway Management and Ventilation

Anatomy and Physiology
   Structures and Functions of the Upper Airway
      Nose
      Pharynx
      Larynx
Upper Airway Obstructions
   Obstruction by the Tongue
   Foreign Body Aspiration
   Laryngeal Spasm
   Laryngeal Edema
   Fractured Larynx and Airway Trauma
Assessment of the Airway
   Mechanism of Injury
   Primary Survey
      Head-tilt/chin-lift
      Jaw-thrust
      Airway Obstruction
      Evaluation
   Secondary Survey
      History
      Physical Examination
         Inspection
         Palpation
         Auscultation
         Overall Assessment

Management of Airway Disorders
   Oxygen
      Oxygen Delivery Devices
   Oropharyngeal and Nasopharyngeal Airways
      Oropharyngeal Airway
      Nasopharyngeal Airway
   Suction
   Positive-pressure Ventilation
   Airway Management
      Endotracheal Intubation
         Oral Intubation
            Equipment
            Procedure
Skill 10-1. Endotracheal Intubation, Oral
         Nasal Intubation
            Procedure
Skill 10-2. Endotracheal Intubation, Nasal
      Pharyngeo-tracheal Lumen Airway and the Esophageal Airways
         Pharyngeo-tracheal Lumen Airway
            Equipment
            Procedure

Skill 10-3. Pharyngeo-Tracheal Lumen Airway
      Esophageal Airways
         Equipment
         Procedure
Skill 10-4. Esophageal Obturator Airway and Esophageal Gastric Tube Airway
      Cricothyroidotomy
         Surgical Cricothyroidotomy
Skill 10-5. Surgical Cricothyroidotomy
         Translaryngeal Jet Ventilation
Skill 10-6. Translaryngeal Jet Ventilation
Summary

BEHAVIORAL OBJECTIVES

On successful completion of this chapter, the reader will be able to:

1. Identify the anatomy of the upper airway
2. Describe the functions of the upper airway
3. Describe the various ways in which the upper airway may be obstructed
4. List the steps required in assessment of the airway
5. Describe the head-tilt/chin-lift and jaw-thrust methods for opening the airway
6. Given a patient disorder, choose an appropriate oxygen delivery device
7. Describe and demonstrate the correct techniques for oral and nasal intubation, pharyngeo-tracheal lumen airway, esophageal airways, surgical cricothyroidotomy, and translaryngeal jet ventilation
8. Describe the indications and contraindications for each of the above airways
9. Define all of the key terms listed in this chapter

KEY TERMS

The following terms are defined in the chapter and glossary:

- aspiration
- auscultation
- bactericidals
- bag-valve-mask device
- central cyanosis
- ciliated epithelium
- coughing
- cricothyroidotomy
- cyanosis
- dyspnea
- endotracheal intubation
- endotracheal tube
- epiglottis
- esophageal gastric tube airway (EGTA)
- esophageal obturator airway (EOA)
- finger sweep
- FiO_2
- flowmeters
- glottis
- head-tilt/chin-lift
- hypercarbia
- hypoxemia
- inspection
- jaw-thrust
- laryngeal edema
- laryngeal spasm
- laryngopharynx
- laryngoscope
- larynx
- Magill forceps
- nasal cannula
- nasal intubation
- nasopharyngeal airway
- nasopharynx
- nonrebreathing mask
- nose
- oral intubation
- oropharyngeal airways
- oropharynx
- oxygen
- oxygen pressure regulator
- oxygen-powered demand valve
- palpation
- partial rebreathing mask
- peripheral cyanosis
- pharyngeo-tracheal lumen (PtL) airway
- pharynx
- phonation
- pin-indexing system
- pocket face mask
- positive-pressure ventilation
- pulsus paradoxus
- retractions
- simple mask
- stridor
- stylet
- subcutaneous emphysema
- suction
- suction catheters
- surgical cricothyroidotomy
- tachypnea
- tongue
- tonsil tip
- translaryngeal jet ventilation
- universal precautions
- upper airway
- vallecula
- Venturi mask
- vocal cords
- Yankauer

This chapter discusses the importance of adequate airway management. The anatomy and physiology of the upper airway are presented, as are the techniques of assessment of airway patency. Management of airway and ventilatory insufficiency are presented, including the use of oxygen, oropharyngeal and nasopharyngeal airways, suction, bag-valve-mask devices, endotracheal intubation, pharyngeo-tracheal lumen airway, esophageal obturator and esophageal gastric tube airways, and cricothyroidotomy. Along with the use of these devices, it is imperative that the paramedic follow **universal precautions** (see Chapter 26). These include the use of protective eye wear, mask, and gloves.

Few, if any, responsibilities of prehospital care are as important as management of the airway. The human body is composed of 100 trillion cells. Each of these cells is serviced by a capillary that delivers nutrients and removes waste. Oxygen serves as the principle nutrient and is required for cellular metabolism. The amount of oxygen delivered to each cell is a function of three factors: oxygen exchange in the lungs, circulation to the cells, and the presence of enough red blood cells to transport oxygen. Considered together, these factors play a major role in determining the patient's clinical status. The consequences of inadequate oxygenation and ventilation include cellular hypoxia, acidosis, and cell death.

ANATOMY AND PHYSIOLOGY

The respiratory system serves two vital functions: to remove carbon dioxide from the blood and to transfer oxygen from the environment into the blood. The respiratory system is divided into four subsystems: the upper airway, lower airway, alveolar-capillary interface, and the chest wall and diaphragm, which move air through the first three subsystems. The role of the upper airway is the topic of this chapter; lower airway, alveolar, and chest wall disorders are discussed in Chapter 19.

Structures and Functions of the Upper Airway

The **upper airway**, which includes the structures shown in Figure 10-1, begins at the nose and ends, by definition, at the cricoid cartilage located just below the vocal cords. In addition to being a conduit through which air flows into the lower airways and alveoli, the upper airway warms, humidifies, and filters inspired air. The tissues of the nasal cavity, nasopharynx, oropharynx, and laryngopharynx warm air through conduction. In addition, the air is humidified through these same tissues, imparting a minimum of 0.75 L of water per day to the inhaled air. The amount of water that is required for humidification

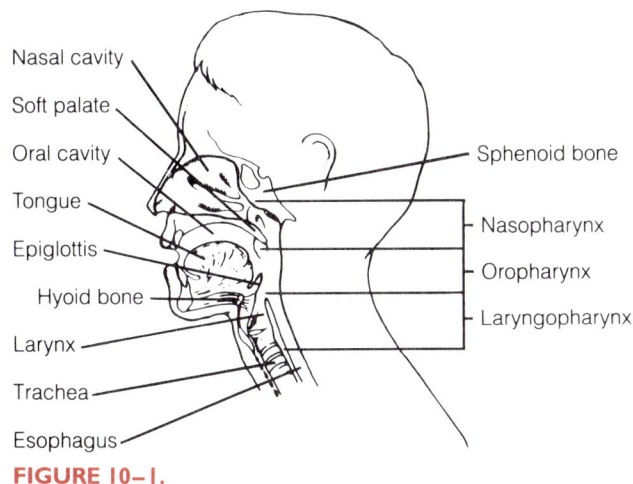

FIGURE 10–1.
Structures of the upper airway.

way. To initiate a cough, the lungs are quickly filled to capacity by a deep, rapid breath. After the lungs are full, the glottis closes and the intercostal muscles and diaphragm contract, increasing the intrathoracic pressure. When the pressure reaches a maximum, the glottis opens and the air that has been held under pressure in the thorax is allowed to rush out through the larynx and upper airway. Foreign bodies and mucus are swept out simultaneously.

Nose

The **nose** serves principally as a conduit for inspired air, moving the air from the outside into the posterior pharynx. The nasal mucosa is **ciliated epithelium,** which means that cilia are present on the surface. Also found is a thick mucous layer which, in conjunction with the nasal hairs, plays a major role in filtration of inspired air, another function of the nose. The mucous layer also helps prevent infection; the mucus contains **bactericidals** that engulf and kill bacteria that enter through the nose. In addition, air flow over the nasal cavities allows maximum contact between inspired air and the nasal mucosa, thus providing heat and humidification. The nasal mucosa requires approximately 1 L of water a day under normal conditions to humidify incoming air. Hyperventilation requires greater amounts of water, a fact which explains the dehydration that is common in hyperventilating patients.

Paramedics seldom deal with patients who have major diseases of the nose. However, patients who have tracheostomies or who have been intubated have lost the functions of the nose. When caring for these patients, especially during long transports, the paramedic must be aware of the need to provide warmed, humidified air and should realize that the patient has a distinctly impaired ability to protect the lower airway from foreign particles and infection.

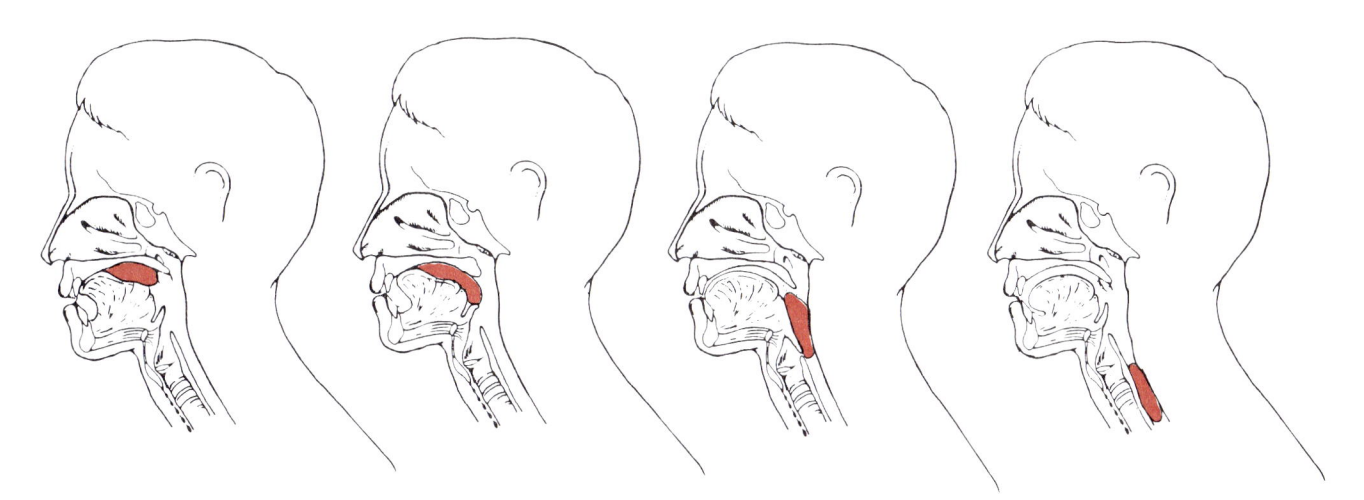

increases with respiratory rate, a fact which explains the dehydration that may result from hyperventilation. Air is filtered through the nasal hairs. **Phonation,** or the ability to speak, is another function of the upper airway, with the vocal cords located in the larynx.

A final function of the upper airway, which is critical in the prehospital arena, is protection of the lower airway from foreign matter. This protection is exerted mostly by the epiglottis, located within the larynx at the juncture of the larynx and esophagus. The **epiglottis** functions as a sort of trap door that prevents food and fluid from entering the larynx. Figure 10-2 shows how the epiglottis operates as food moves through the oropharynx into the esophagus. The **glottis,** which is the opening between the vocal cords, plays a major role in the cough reflex. **Coughing** is a modified form of respiration that serves to remove foreign bodies that inadvertently enter the larynx. In addition, coughing is effective in removing mucus from the lower air-

FIGURE 10–2.
The epiglottis functions as a trap door. As food moves into the esophagus, the epiglottis closes, securing the airway.

Pharynx

The **pharynx** provides a passageway for air between the nose or mouth and the larynx. The pharynx is subdivided into the **nasopharynx,** located posterior to the nose, the **oropharynx,** which is located behind the mouth, and the **laryngopharynx,** which leads to the larynx and esophagus. The pharynx primarily serves as a passageway for air, although some warming and humidification are provided. A number of lymphatic glands, including the nasopharyngeal tonsils (more commonly called the adenoids), lingual tonsils, and palatine tonsils, are present in the pharynx. Also present is the eustachian tube, which connects the middle ear with the nasopharynx. This connection allows for equalization of pressure between the middle ear and the pharynx, which is important for the function of the tympanic membrane (eardrum). Finally, the **tongue,** located in the oropharynx, assists with speech and the swallowing of food.

A number of disorders that originate in the pharynx may confront the paramedic. The first, and most common, is airway obstruction by the tongue. When patients are in the supine position, gravity often forces the tongue back into the oropharynx, effectively obstructing the airway. This condition is amplified in patients who are under the effect of central nervous system depressants or who have an alteration in the function of the 10th cranial nerve (from a stroke or head injury), which innervates the pharynx. Another problem that may develop in the pharynx is airway obstruction caused by inflammation of the tonsils. This condition, which is generally due to a streptococcal infection, may create a significant partial or even total obstruction of the upper airway.

Larynx

The **larynx** serves as a transition between the upper and lower airway. Located at the level of the fourth to sixth cervical vertebrae (it is somewhat higher in females and children), the larynx serves several functions. In addition to providing a passageway for air, the larynx protects the lower airway by using the epiglottis and the cough reflex. The **vocal cords,** which are in the larynx, allow for voice production.

The larynx is an important structure in prehospital care. Endotracheal intubation requires a thorough understanding of laryngeal structure and function. Identifying landmarks for endotracheal intubation are shown in Figure 10-3. Blunt trauma to the neck may cause a crushing injury to the larynx, leading to airway obstruction. Airway obstruction may also be caused by foreign bodies, which frequently lodge in the larynx because of its small diameter.

UPPER AIRWAY OBSTRUCTIONS

Because of its essential function in filtering and transporting air, the upper airway plays a major role in providing respiration. Damage, injury, or bypass of the upper airway may have significant consequences. For example, the patient who has a tracheostomy cannot filter air adequately, nor can inhaled air be humidified and warmed. Because the larynx has been bypassed, the cough reflex is also diminished, making the lower airway more vulnerable to foreign matter and mucus buildup. A number of other conditions exist that can interfere with the functions of the upper airway.

Obstruction by the Tongue

An unconscious patient who is in a supine position frequently has a partial or total airway obstruction due to the tongue falling back into the oropharynx. In addition, the epiglottis occludes the airway by falling back over the laryngeal opening when its muscular attachments become

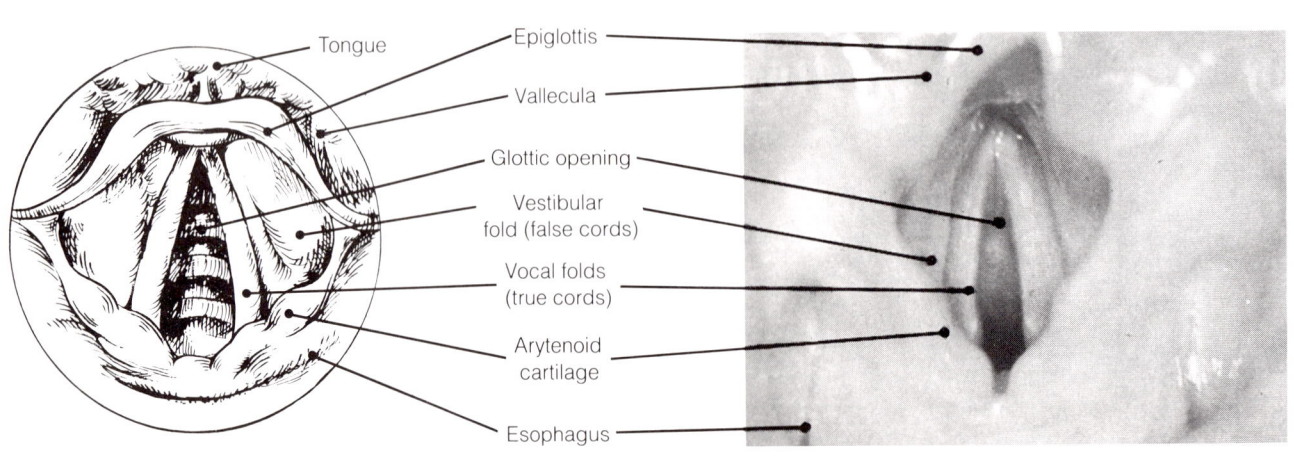

FIGURE 10-3.
Illustration (left) and photograph (right) of identifying landmarks of the larynx for endotracheal intubation.

flaccid. Patients with central nervous system depression from drugs, alcohol, or disease processes are more prone to this disorder because of poor tone in the facial muscles. Clinical signs include snoring respiration or total airway obstruction.

Foreign Body Aspiration

Aspiration of foreign bodies has two effects on the airways. First, aspiration of any foreign material, including fluid, initiates a protective response that consists of sudden coughing and spasm of the airways from the larynx to the bronchioles. This spasm frequently causes **dyspnea** (air hunger resulting in labored or difficult breathing) as well as wheezing; in severe cases, such as near drowning, it can produce partial or total airway obstruction. In addition, if the aspirated material is large enough, a foreign body obstruction ensues. Frequently, the object lodges in the larynx at the vocal cords because the adult airway is narrowest at this point. As with obstruction by the tongue, foreign body aspiration in adults is associated most frequently with drug and alcohol ingestion or altered mental states, such as retardation or Alzheimer's disease. Often these patients have a decreased ability to feed themselves and a diminished *gag reflex*.

Laryngeal Spasm

Laryngeal spasm is a nonspecific response of the larynx to a variety of stimuli. The response includes spasm of the vocal cords as well as the smooth muscles that line the larynx. The condition can be caused by such stimuli as near drowning or exposure to irritating gases as well as blood, secretions, and vomitus. Some cases also seem to be related to psychiatric phenomena, although the physiology of these cases is poorly understood. Laryngospasm can also be induced by physical manipulation, such as tracheal suctioning or tracheal intubation.

Laryngeal Edema

Laryngeal edema, which is swelling in the larynx due to fluid in the interstitial spaces, may be caused by both traumatic and medical conditions. Traumatic causes include blunt trauma to the larynx, in which the structures of the larynx are intact, but the airway is compromised by edema of adjacent tissues. Tracheal intubation may also result in laryngeal edema. Medical causes of laryngeal edema include epiglottitis and anaphylaxis; in both cases, inflammation of the tissues of the upper airway causes respiratory compromise.

Fractured Larynx and Airway Trauma

Fracture of the larynx is a rare but extremely serious condition associated with trauma. Most frequently, the cause is a motor vehicle accident in which the front seat occupants are unrestrained. With rapid deceleration, the head impacts the windshield, causing forward flexion of the neck. This forward flexion exposes the anterior neck to impact on the steering wheel or dashboard. Other common causes are motorcycle and snowmobile accidents in which the anterior neck impacts the windshield. In addition to blunt trauma, penetrating trauma can cause fracture of the larynx. Regardless of the cause, disruption of the larynx decreases the volume of air that can pass into the trachea. The air may leak into the surrounding tissues of the neck, resulting in subcutaneous emphysema.

Far more common is trauma to the other structures of the upper airway. Fractures of the nose, mandible, maxilla, and teeth cause swelling, bleeding, and loose teeth that may obstruct the airway and cause respiratory compromise.

ASSESSMENT OF THE AIRWAY

Assessment of airway patency and ventilation is particularly important because a patient's condition may deteriorate rapidly when the airway is compromised. Assessment of the patient with possible airway compromise may be divided into recognition of the mechanism of injury and the primary and the secondary survey. The following section describes this assessment as it pertains to airway-related problems. However, it is important to note that this assessment is only part of the total patient assessment presented in Chapter 9.

Mechanism of Injury

In the trauma patient, the initial scene survey should include the *mechanism of injury*. A history of hyperflexion of the neck or of actually striking the neck is suggestive of upper airway trauma. Injuries that involve bicycles or motorcycles, and those that involve striking a fixed object, such as a fence or clothesline, should increase the index of suspicion of laryngeal trauma.

Primary Survey

The purpose of the primary survey is to identify life-threatening conditions during the first 45 seconds of contact with the patient. This rapid assessment includes checking for patency of the airway and adequacy of breathing. In the breathing patient, airway patency is confirmed by the absence of snoring or gurgling sounds. Included in the assessment of adequacy of ventilation are the rate and depth of breathing and observation of chest wall movement. In the nonbreathing patient, several steps should take place. First, the airway should be opened by using the head-tilt/chin-lift or jaw-thrust method.

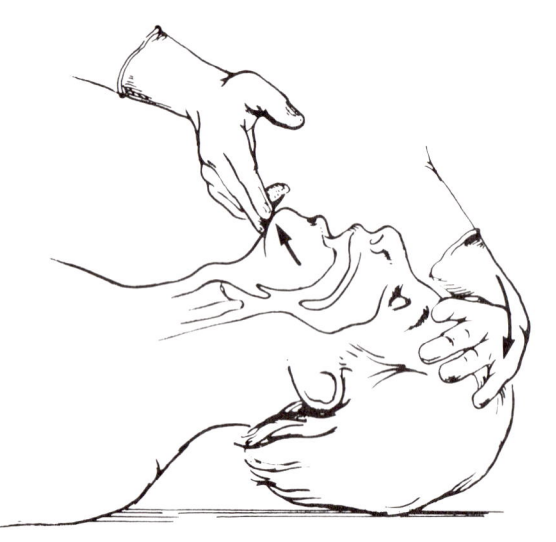

FIGURE 10–4.
The head-tilt/chin-lift technique. The head is tilted backward with one hand (downward arrow), while the fingers of the other hand lift the chin forward (upward arrow).

Head-tilt/Chin-lift

The **head-tilt/chin-lift** method of opening the airway should be used on the nontrauma patient who is not suspected of having cervical spine injury. The patient's head should first be tilted back by placing one hand on the forehead and applying firm backward pressure. The other hand should be placed with the fingers under the bony part of the patient's lower jaw, near the chin, thus lifting the mandible and helping to tilt the head back (Fig. 10-4).

Jaw-thrust

The *jaw-thrust* method requires forward displacement of the jaw without any tilting of the head. It is the safest method of opening the airway and should always be used on a patient suspected of having cervical spine injury. The angles of the patient's jaw should be grasped with both hands, one on each side, displacing the mandible forward (Fig. 10-5). The head should be supported without tilting it backward or turning it from side to side.

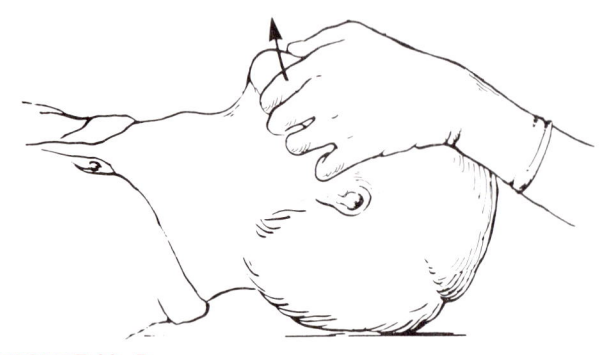

FIGURE 10–5.
The jaw-thrust technique. The hands are placed on either side of the head. The fingers grasp behind the angle of the jaw, bringing it upward, as shown by the arrow.

Airway Obstruction

If a foreign body is seen in the patient's mouth, it should be removed with gloved fingers. A *finger sweep* should only be performed in the unconscious patient. If a foreign body is not seen but strongly suspected, abdominal thrusts may be used to move or dislodge it. It is not the purpose of this chapter to teach the basic method of cardiopulmonary resuscitation (CPR) that includes foreign body airway management. See Appendix B for appropriate guidelines.

Evaluation

Evaluation for circulatory compromise, neurologic deficiency, and major visible injuries is the final stage in the primary survey. If gross abnormalities are identified during the primary survey, management must be instituted immediately to correct the defects.

Secondary Survey

After the primary survey is completed, the more detailed secondary survey should be started. The secondary survey for patients with suspected airway problems should focus on the history and physical examination.

History

History-taking in the patient with possible airway compromise is necessarily short. For the patient who is unable to answer questions because of airway obstruction, a history is impossible. However, some information helps the paramedic discover the cause of the obstruction and the seriousness of the patient's condition. The history of the current episode enables the paramedic to determine how long the particular problem has been present. This determination allows differentiation of the patient with a chronic or slowly developing condition from the patient with an acute onset. The information should include a history of recent trauma as well as details of the patient's actions when the condition developed. A recent history of eating or drinking frequently contributes to the diagnosis of foreign body obstruction.

The medical history does not always help diagnose the cause of an acute airway obstruction. However, a history of allergies or anaphylactic episodes may be helpful. As discussed previously, a history of mental impairment or alcohol ingestion may also contribute to the diagnosis.

Physical Examination

The physical examination can be separated into the three phases of inspection, palpation, and auscultation. Each may contribute information to the diagnosis of airway compromise.

INSPECTION. **Inspection** begins with simply observing the patient. A look of panic on the patient's face along with sitting or standing while leaning forward are indicative of respiratory distress. Obvious trauma to the face, neck, or chest increases the likelihood of airway compromise. Restlessness, combativeness, or drowsiness is often indicative of profound **hypoxemia** (insufficient oxygenation of the blood) or **hypercarbia** (increased amount of carbon dioxide in the blood). Grasping at the throat may suggest foreign body obstruction. Skin color is also a valuable clue. **Cyanosis** is a bluish or dark purple discoloration of the skin due to the presence of abnormal amounts of reduced hemoglobin in the blood. **Central cyanosis,** which is discoloration around the mouth or in the cheek mucosa, is useful in the assessment of dark-pigmented patients and is indicative of hypoxemia. **Peripheral cyanosis** in the extremities may indicate hypoxemia, although it may also be caused by poor circulation, hypothermia, or orthopaedic disorders. Pallor and diaphoresis are caused by sympathetic nervous system discharge and indicate a compensatory response to a crisis, frequently hypoxemia.

In addition to inspecting the skin, the paramedic should observe the patient for signs of respiratory distress. **Tachypnea** (abnormally rapid respiration) may indicate hypoxemia. The use of the accessory muscles of respiration (the sternocleidomastoid and trapezius muscles in the neck) is an indication of respiratory obstruction, either acute or chronic. **Retractions,** caused by excessive negative intrathoracic pressures generated by breathing against obstruction, help diagnose airway obstruction. Retractions may be observed as the skin retracting between the ribs (intercostal), under the clavicle (subclavicular), above the clavicle (supraclavicular), and under the sternum (substernal) on inspiration. A tracheal tug, which is retraction above the suprasternal notch, may also be observed. Chapter 19 describes and illustrates a patient with retractions. The presence of jugular venous distension may be indicative of airway obstruction as well as congestive heart failure. Finally, the upper airway should be inspected briefly for the presence of mucus, blood, vomitus, teeth, or foreign bodies that could be responsible for the obstruction.

PALPATION. **Palpation** follows inspection. Palpation includes evaluating the pulse; tachycardia is one of the early signs of hypoxemia. In addition, the neck and anterior chest should be palpated for evidence of subcutaneous emphysema, a common physical finding in cases of traumatic disruption of the upper airway. **Subcutaneous emphysema** can be recognized as a "*popping*" sensation under the fingertips on mild to moderate palpation and is caused by air that has leaked from the airways into the subcutaneous tissue. Broken ribs and tracheal deviation can also be found through palpation.

AUSCULTATION. The final step in examining the patient with a suspected airway disorder is **auscultation.** Before using the stethoscope, the paramedic should simply listen to the patient. Patients who are attempting to speak but make no noise have total airway obstruction. Patients who are able to speak give an indication of their respiratory impairment by their ability to speak in single words, short phrases, or full sentences without needing to take a breath. Patients with "*one word*" dyspnea are clearly in great distress. In addition, audible stridor or wheezing may be heard without a stethoscope.

A number of important observations can be made with the stethoscope. First, the patient's breath sounds should be assessed (see Chapter 19 for technique of auscultation). **Stridor,** which is a harsh, brassy sound, is indicative of upper airway obstruction caused by, for example, foreign body, spasm, or inflammation. Stridor may be heard throughout the chest, although it is loudest directly over the larynx. *Silence* is another "breath sound" that has particular significance in the patient with an airway obstruction. If the chest wall is moving but no sound is heard through the stethoscope, so-called silent breath sounds are present; these are clearly ominous, as they indicate little or no air movement. Several other breath sounds that may be heard in the assessment process originate from constriction, obstruction, and spasm in the lower airways. These are discussed in Chapter 19.

In addition to auscultating breath sounds, the paramedic can auscultate pulsus paradoxus while taking the blood pressure. **Pulsus paradoxus** is an accentuated decrease in systolic blood pressure on inspiration. It may be caused by significantly increased intrathoracic pressures created by breathing against obstruction. Pulsus paradoxus may indicate severe airway obstruction, although it is also present in a number of other disorders. A more thorough discussion of pulsus paradoxus can be found in Chapter 19.

Overall Assessment

A rapid, accurate assessment of the patient with a possible airway disorder is essential. The primary survey must be completed initially to locate and control life-threatening problems. The secondary survey follows and begins with a brief history of the current episode. A medical history of similar problems is also elicited. After the history is taken, the physical examination is performed. Particularly significant findings on the exam include an altered level of consciousness, cyanosis, tachycardia (or bradycardia in the case of severe hypoxemia), retractions, use of accessory muscles, stridor, and pulsus paradoxus.

MANAGEMENT OF AIRWAY DISORDERS

After rapid assessment of the patient with airway compromise, immediate management must be started to establish and maintain an open airway. Because of the importance of correct airway management, constant assessment and reassessment is vital to insure that the airway is maintained adequately.

A variety of devices are available to assist in airway maintenance. It is imperative that the paramedic follow universal precautions when performing airway maintenance (see Chapter 26). These include the use of protective eye wear, mask, and gloves. Oropharyngeal and nasopharyngeal airways are used to open the upper airway and prevent the tongue from serving as an obstruction. Suction may be required to remove blood, mucus, or vomitus from the oropharynx. Endotracheal intubation is the definitive technique for protecting the lower airway and providing ventilatory assistance or control. Use of the pharyngeo-tracheal lumen airway, esophageal tracheal combitube (ETC), or esophageal obturator and esophageal gastric tube airways prevents the ventilating gas from entering the stomach and prevents vomitus from entering the lower airway. A cricothyroidotomy may be required in the patient whose upper airway damage, from edema or crushing injury, makes placement of other types of airways impossible. After any type of airway is in place and secured, the patient may require positive-pressure ventilation with a bag-valve-mask device, oxygen-powered demand valve, or similar device.

Oxygen

Increasing the concentration of **oxygen** in the inspired gas is one of the simplest respiratory therapies available. Assuming that the patient is ventilating adequately, increasing the fraction of inspired oxygen (**FiO$_2$**) above that present in room air (21%) increases the amount of oxygen in the alveoli. Since movement of oxygen into the pulmonary capillary bed is governed by simple diffusion, increasing the amount of oxygen in the alveoli improves oxygen concentration in the blood, unless a severe diffusion disorder, such as pulmonary edema, is present.

Oxygen is supplied as a compressed gas and is stored in lightweight aluminum or steel cylinders. Aluminum is only used for smaller-sized cylinders and helps to decrease the weight. Oxygen is usually contained at a pressure between 2,000 and 2,300 pounds per square inch (psi). The size of the cylinder determines the number of liters of oxygen that can be compressed (Fig. 10-6).

Oxygen cylinders of E size or smaller contain a **pin-indexing system** on their yoke to allow only the attachment of an **oxygen pressure regulator**. This system serves as a safety mechanism, since other gases have their own pin-indexing system and cannot be administered without the appropriate regulator. Pressure regulators are used to reduce the pressure to a level suitable for oxygen administration under medical conditions, usually 40 to 70 psi. **Flowmeters** usually are permanently attached to pressure regulators and permit the regulated release of oxygen in liters per minute. The female fitting on the flowmeter is for attachment to a male plug from a pres-

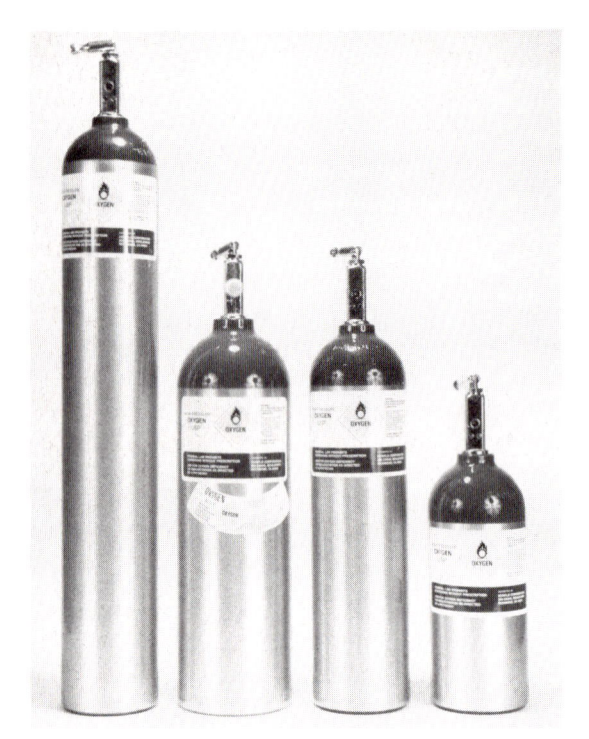

FIGURE 10-6.
Aluminum oxygen cylinders (from left to right): E cylinder, Jumbo D cylinder, D cylinder, and C cylinder. (Courtesy of © Dixie USA Inc., Houston, Texas)

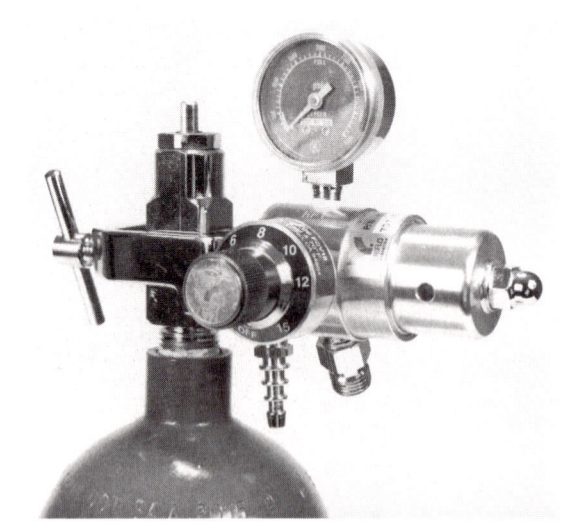

FIGURE 10-7.
Oxygen regulator with flowmeter. (Courtesy of © Dixie USA Inc., Houston, Texas)

sure hose or oxygen tubing. Figure 10-7 shows an oxygen pressure regulator with a flowmeter attached.

Oxygen Delivery Devices

Several types of *oxygen delivery devices* are available. Selection of which device to use is based on the concentration of oxygen required, adequacy of the patient's ven-

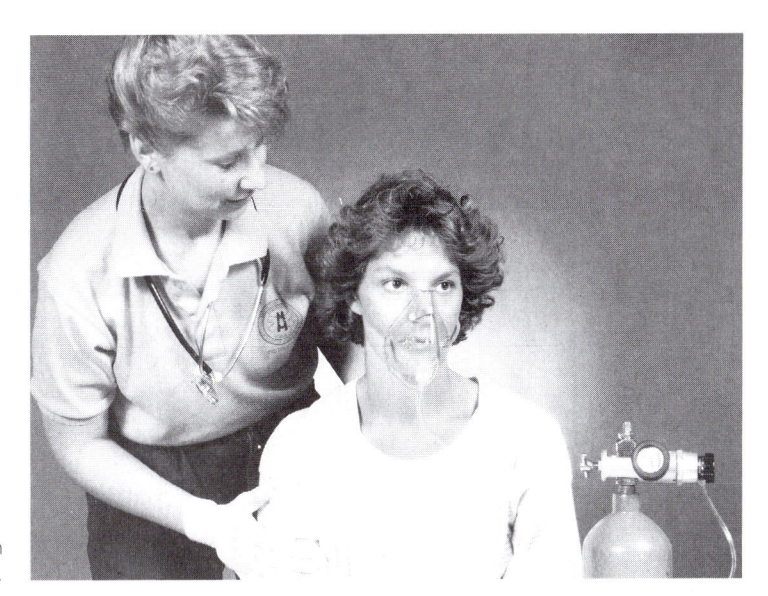

CHAPTER 10: Airway Management and Ventilation 133

FIGURE 10–8.
Reassure patients and let them know what to expect when using an oxygen delivery device, such as a simple face mask.

tilation, and patient tolerance. The procedure and device to be used should be explained to the patient. Patients who are experiencing respiratory distress may feel anxious at first about having a mask placed over their face. Calm reassurance by the paramedic helps to lessen this anxiety (Fig 10-8).

For most applications, the **nasal cannula** is appropriate (Fig. 10-9). It is capable of delivering up to 44% oxygen when operated at a maximum of 6 L/min. It is well tolerated by most patients and may be used in all cases except when the patient's nostrils are obstructed. Because dead air space in the nasopharynx acts as a reservoir for oxygen, the patient does not need to breathe through the nose; oxygen is entrained through the device even with mouth breathing (Fig. 10-10).

Face masks are used when a higher oxygen concentration is required or when the nostrils are obstructed. A **simple mask** may deliver as much as 60% oxygen at 7 to 8 L/min, while a **partial rebreathing mask** delivers a somewhat higher concentration at 10 L/min. Simple masks contain an inlet for oxygen delivery and small vents on either side of the mask to allow escape of exhaled gas. A

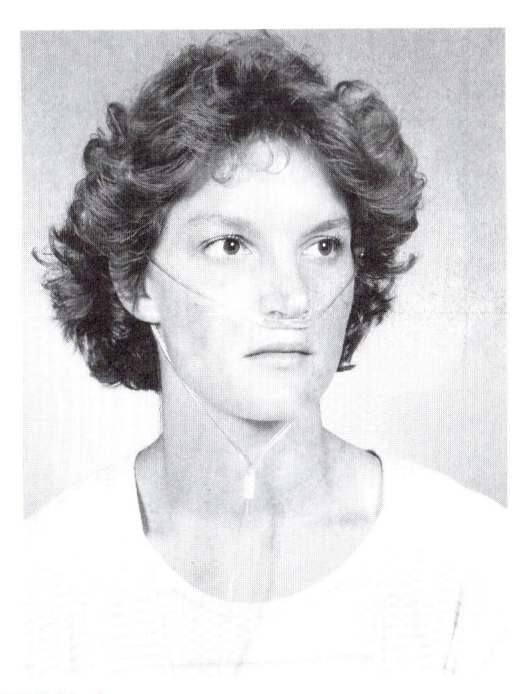

FIGURE 10–9.
Nasal cannula.

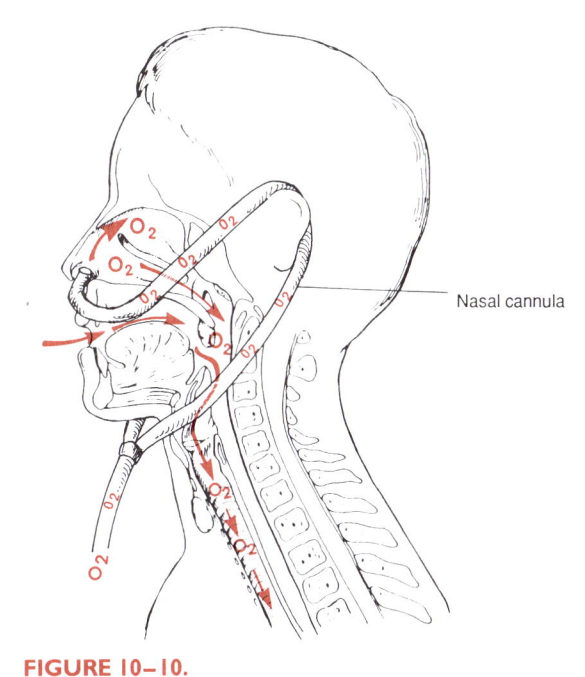

FIGURE 10–10.
When using a nasal cannula, oxygen is transported through the nasopharynx into the lungs even if the patient is breathing through the mouth.

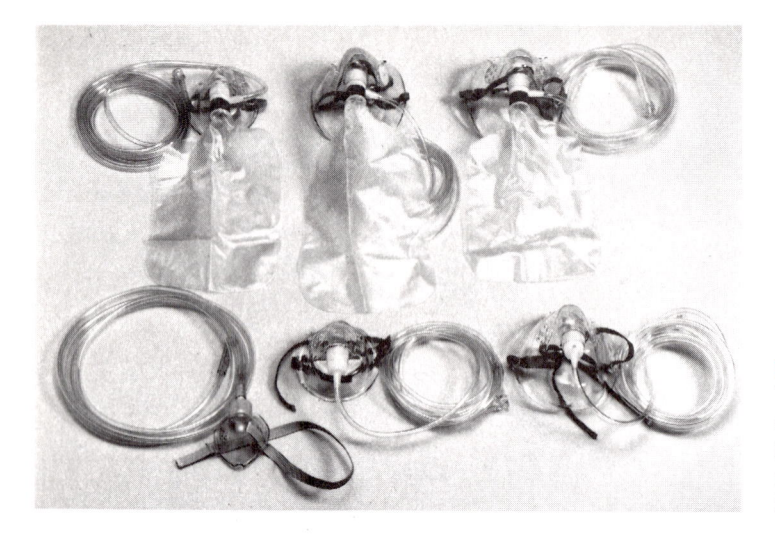

FIGURE 10–11.
Types of oxygen masks (top, left to right): Pediatric partial rebreathing, adult nonrebreathing, adult partial rebreathing; (bottom left to right): Infant simple mask, pediatric simple mask, adult simple mask. (Courtesy of Parr Emergency Sales, Inc., Galloway, Ohio)

partial rebreathing mask directs the flow of oxygen into a bag that is attached to the mask. As the patient inhales, oxygen is drawn up from the bag into the mask. Since small vents are on either side of the mask, the partial rebreathing mask does not deliver the near 100% oxygen concentrations of a nonrebreathing mask.

A **nonrebreathing mask** with a good seal delivers close to 100% with the oxygen flow at 10 to 15 L/min. A nonrebreathing mask has the same bag device as a partial rebreathing one, but a one-way valve directs oxygen into the face mask when the patient inhales. This one-way valve prevents other gases from accumulating in the bag when the patient exhales. One other factor in the near 100% oxygen concentration is the flapper valves that cover the air vents on the face mask. When the patient inhales, the flapper valves close, allowing for oxygen to be drawn up through the one-way valve. On expiration, since air cannot pass through the one-way valve, it is forced out through the air vents in the face mask. Unfortunately, many patients find masks confining and think that they accentuate feelings of dyspnea. The mask is of little use if the patient continually removes it; a cannula may be a better choice, even if higher concentrations of oxygen are desired.

When using a partial or nonrebreathing mask, a special note of caution is required. The patient inhales air from the oxygen reservoir (bag) that is attached to the mask. If the bag is not kept full, the patient is unable to breathe. For this reason, it is essential to turn the oxygen flow rate high and fill the bag completely before placing the mask on the patient. Then, titrate the flow rate so that the bag does not collapse during inspiration. If the patient completely evacuates the bag on inspiration the flow rate is too low. Usually 10 to 15 L/min is required to maintain this device. The described oxygen masks are shown in Figure 10-11.

A specialized mask called the **Venturi mask** enables delivery of precise concentrations of oxygen between 24% and 50% (Fig. 10-12). This precise delivery is valuable during transport of patients who are sensitive to oxygen, such as those with chronic obstructive pulmonary disease.

Each of the oxygen delivery devices described is useful if the patient is ventilating adequately. However, none is effective if the patient's ventilation is not of adequate rate and depth. In this situation, supplemental oxygen must be delivered in tandem with supplemental ventilation, using a pocket face mask, bag-valve-mask device, or oxygen-powered demand valve. These are discussed below. Table 10-1 summarizes the devices available for supplemental oxygen administration.

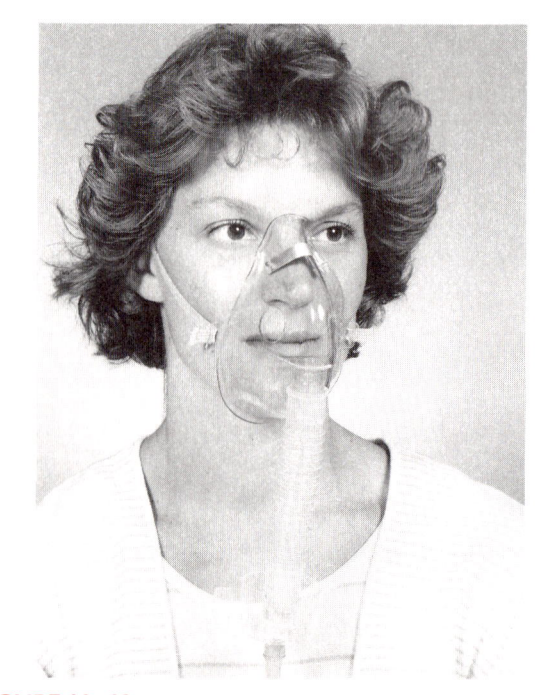

FIGURE 10–12.
Venturi mask.

TABLE 10–1.
OXYGEN DELIVERY DEVICES AND Fi_2 (%)

O_2 Flow Rate in Liters per Minute	FiO_2 (%)
NASAL CANNULA:	
1	.24
2	.28
3	.32
4	.36
5	.40
6	.44
SIMPLE MASK:	
5–6	.40
6–7	.50
7–8	.60
PARTIAL REBREATHING MASK:	
6	.35
10–15	.60
NONREBREATHING MASK	
6	.60
10–15	.90+
VENTURI MASK:	
4–8 (variable according to manufacturer)	.24–.40
POCKET FACE MASK WITH OXYGEN INLET:	
6	.40
POCKET FACE MASK WITHOUT OXYGEN INLET:	
0	.19
BAG-VALVE-MASK DEVICE WITH OXYGEN RESERVOIR:	
10–15 (variable according to manufacturer)	.90+
OXYGEN-POWERED DEMAND VALVE:	
Full flush	.100

Note: Room air is 21% oxygen.

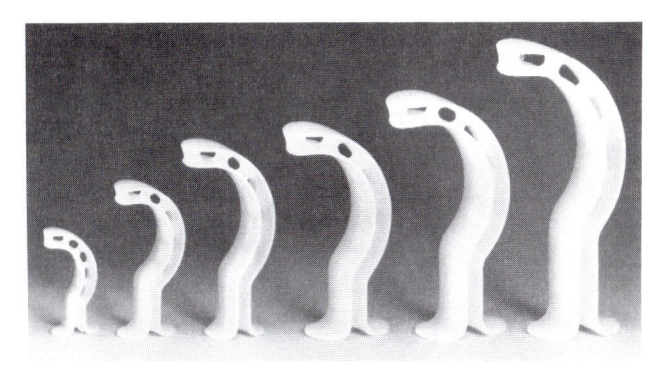

FIGURE 10–13.
Various sizes of oropharyngeal airways. (Courtesy of © Dixie USA Inc., Houston, Texas)

pharyngeal wall. Figure 10-14 shows the oropharyngeal airway in position with its tip resting at the base of the tongue. Selection of the proper sized airway is important for best results. One technique for selecting the right size is to place the airway on the patient's cheek with the flange at the lips. Proper sizing is achieved when the tip reaches the angle of the jaw (Fig. 10-15). The airway must be inserted carefully to prevent pushing the tongue into the posterior pharynx. Insertion with the airway turned upside down (tip running along the roof of the mouth) or sideways prevents the tip from forcing the tongue backward. After the airway has been inserted, it is rotated until the tip slides into place.

Use of the oropharyngeal airway is often diagnostic as well as therapeutic. Patients who are deeply unconscious

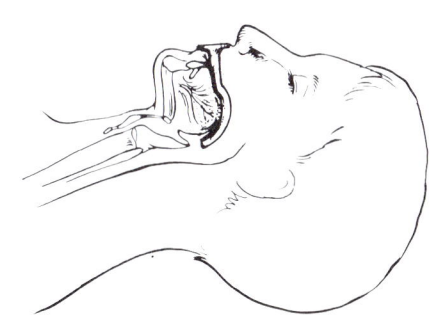

FIGURE 10–14.
Oropharyngeal airway in place.

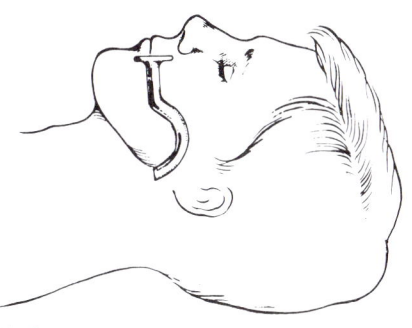

FIGURE 10–15.
Sizing an oropharyngeal airway.

Oropharyngeal and Nasopharyngeal Airways

The use of an oropharyngeal or nasopharyngeal airway is a simple procedure that is effective in preventing the tongue from obstructing the airway. Because of their simplicity and few complications, these devices are ideal for use in a patient whose airway requires maintenance for only a short period of time.

Oropharyngeal Airway

The **oropharyngeal airways,** shown in Figure 10-13, essentially serve as a tongue hook, holding the tongue at its base to prevent it from falling back against the posterior

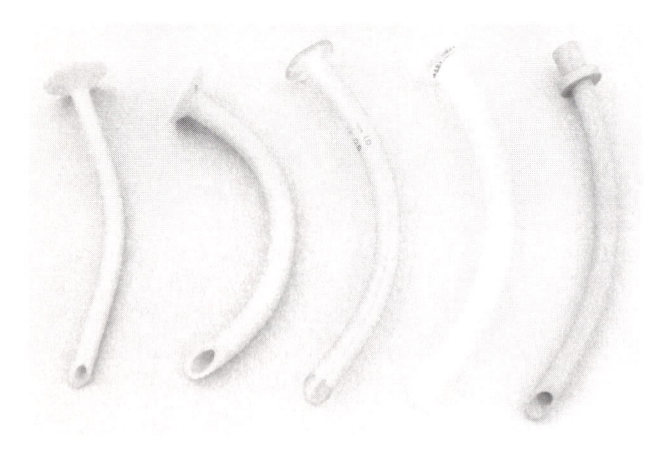

FIGURE 10–16.
Various sizes of nasopharyngeal airways.

tolerate an oropharyngeal airway because their gag reflex is no longer intact. If the patient accepts an oropharyngeal airway without gagging, placement of an endotracheal tube should be considered.

Nasopharyngeal Airway

For patients who do not tolerate an oropharyngeal airway but who still require airway maintenance, the **nasopharyngeal airway,** sometimes referred to as a nasal trumpet, is ideal. Figure 10-16 shows various sizes of nasopharyngeal airways. Like the oropharyngeal airway, the purpose of the nasopharyngeal airway is to maintain an open upper airway by preventing the tongue from obstructing the posterior pharynx. This purpose is accomplished by the nasopharyngeal airway's position posterior to the tongue in the pharynx, effectively providing a conduit for air between the nose and the larynx. Figure 10-17 shows the nasopharyngeal airway in place.

Selection of the correct size is done by nostril size; the largest airway that can comfortably fit through the nostril should be selected. Because of the delicacy of the nasal mucosa, care must be taken during insertion. A nonpetroleum base lubricant should be liberally applied to the exterior of the tube before insertion. The larger nostril should be selected, and insertion should follow the natural curve of the tube. In this fashion, the curve of the tube naturally directs it down toward the posterior pharynx rather than up into the sinuses. The tube should be advanced until the flange is flush with the nostril.

Suction

Protection of the airway from blood, mucus, and vomitus is important regardless of the type of airway used. **Suction,** when coupled with body position, provides a valuable tool for airway management. Suction employs negative pressure to withdraw foreign material from the posterior pharynx. Suction also can be used to remove blood and mucus from an endotracheal tube. Suction devices that are powered by batteries (Fig. 10-18) or manually operated (Fig. 10-19) are available.

The suction device is attached to the suction tip by the connecting tubing. Suction may be performed by using either a tonsil tip or suction catheter. Each has a slightly different purpose and use. The **tonsil tip (Yankauer)** is rigid, allowing it to be placed in the posterior pharynx easily (Fig. 10-20). The larger diameter enables it to aspirate larger or thicker substances. Notice the hole on the tonsil tip handle and the numerous vents near the tip. When the hole in the handle is left open, little or no suction is exerted at the end of the tip. When the hole is occluded by the thumb or finger, suction is initiated. The

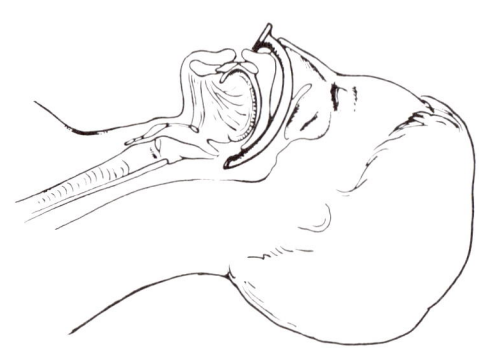

FIGURE 10–17.
Nasopharyngeal airway in place.

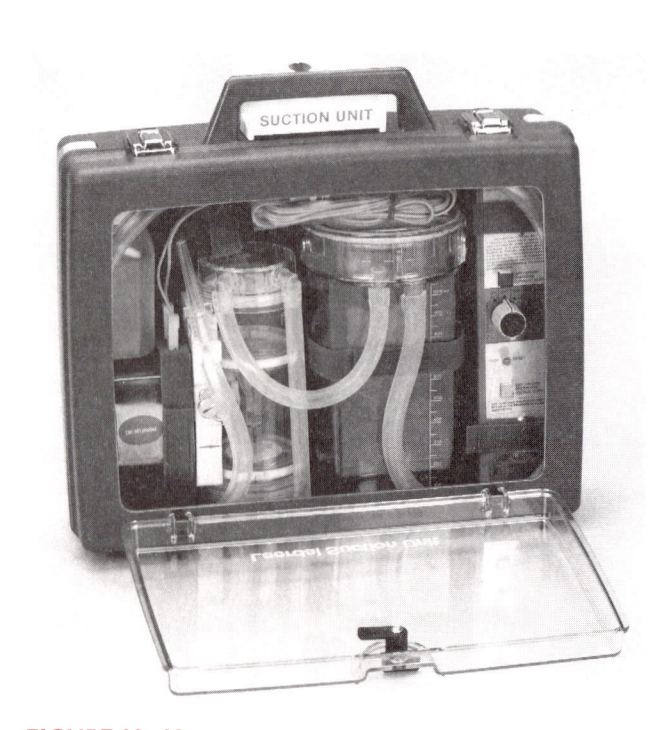

FIGURE 10–18.
Battery-powered suction unit. (Courtesy of Parr Emergency Sales, Inc., Galloway, Ohio)

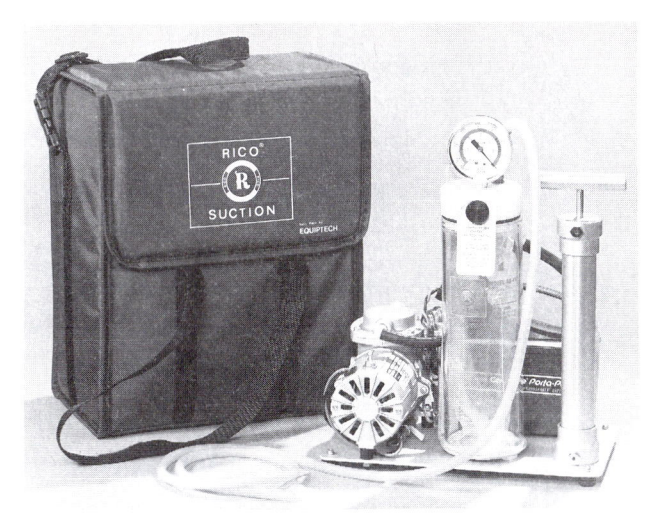

FIGURE 10–19.
Manually operated suction unit. (Courtesy of Rico Suction Labs, Inc., Burlington, North Carolina)

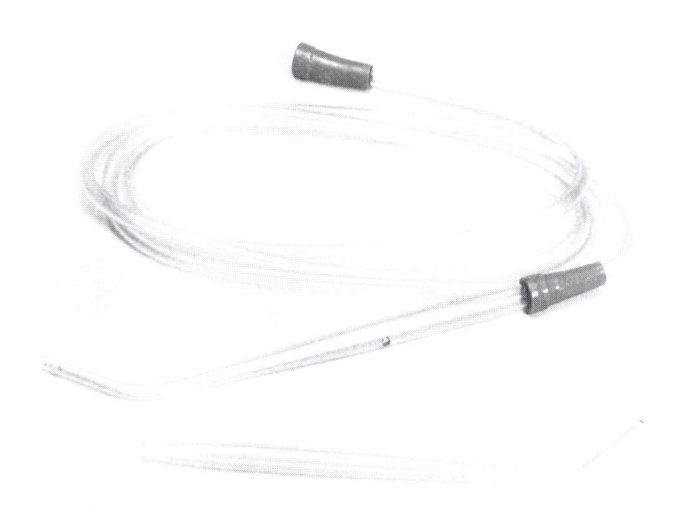

FIGURE 10–20.
Tonsil tip suction catheter with vent control attached to suction tubing (top). Tonsil tip without vent control (bottom). (Courtesy of Parr Emergency Sales, Inc., Galloway, Ohio)

FIGURE 10–21.
Various sizes of suction catheters with vent control. (Courtesy of Parr Emergency Sales, Inc., Galloway, Ohio)

vents are placed near the tip to prevent tissue destruction should the tip be inadvertently placed directly against the delicate mucosa. Because of the importance of these vents in preventing damage to the posterior pharynx, the suction connecting tubing is never used alone as a suction tip, since it has no vents.

The **suction catheters** are shown in Figure 10-21. Because of their flexibility, suction catheters are difficult to maneuver into the posterior pharynx where secretions accumulate. Their smaller diameter causes them to become clogged more easily. Their primary use is to suction blood or mucus from endotracheal tubes. Suction catheters are also useful in children whose mouth and pharynx are too small to accommodate a tonsil tip.

After the correct suction device is selected and the equipment is assembled, suctioning should be performed. Patients who are being ventilated should be briefly hyperventilated before suctioning. Oxygen should already be in place if time allows. After the suction unit is turned on, the tip of the suction device is advanced into the posterior pharynx. When the tip is in place, the thumb hole is blocked with the thumb or forefinger and the suction device slowly removed. Suctioning should not be done for more than 5 seconds; it removes air from the lungs as well as fluid from the airway. If more material must be suctioned, allow the patient to breathe oxygen (or assist ventilation as appropriate) for 15 to 30 seconds before repeating the procedure.

A number of complications may accompany suctioning. The first, and most common, is the plugging of suction tips by thick secretions. A vial of water can be used to rinse the tip by placing the tip in the water and activating the suction. The water flow carries the offending matter with it. Frequently, the fluid being suctioned contains large particles and the suction tip plugs repeatedly. In some cases, manual removal of the obstruction, using gloved fingers and a gauze square, may be the best technique. However, the fingers should not be placed in the mouth of a patient who is conscious or semiconscious.

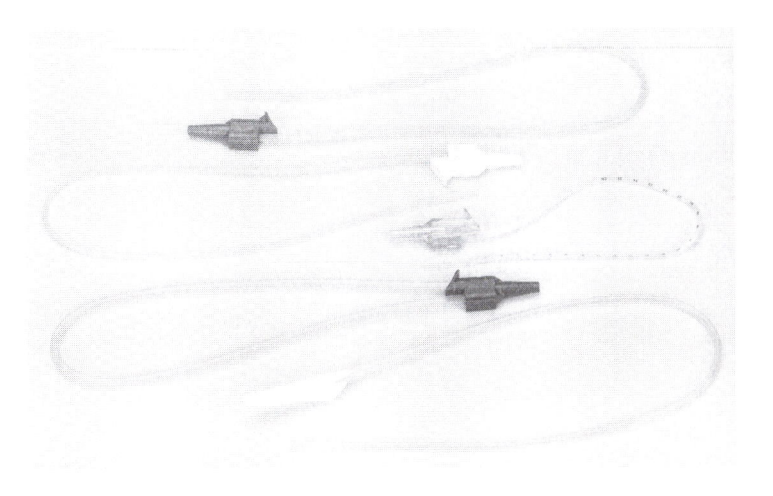

Positive-pressure Ventilation

Patients who are not ventilating adequately require ventilatory assistance or control (***positive-pressure ventilation***). Ventilation should be maintained at a rate of 12 to 20 breaths per minute for the adult, unless hyperventilation is desired (as with head injury), for which a rate of 24 to 30 breaths is required.

Several devices are available to assist or control ventilation. Each device has advantages and disadvantages. The ***bag-valve-mask device*** (Fig. 10-22) is simple to operate, once the mask seal is assured. When attached to a reservoir bag and with adequate oxygen flow rates, the device can deliver inspired oxygen concentrations as high as 100%. The ***pocket face mask*** (Fig. 10-23) is capable of providing

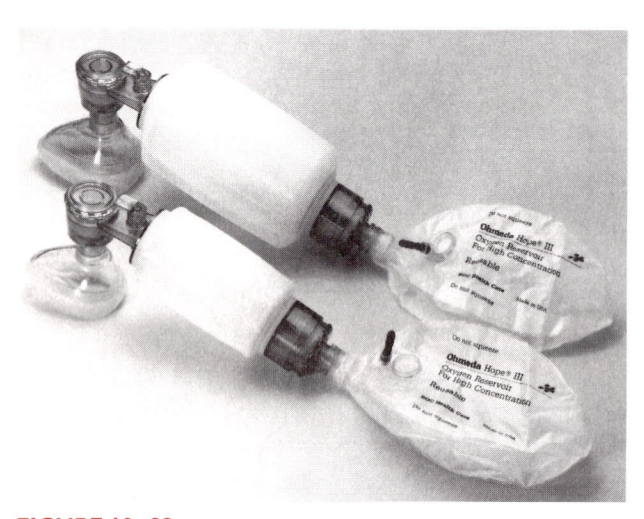

FIGURE 10–22.
Adult (top) and pediatric (bottom) bag-valve-mask devices with oxygen reservoirs. (Courtesy of Parr Emergency Sales, Inc., Galloway, Ohio)

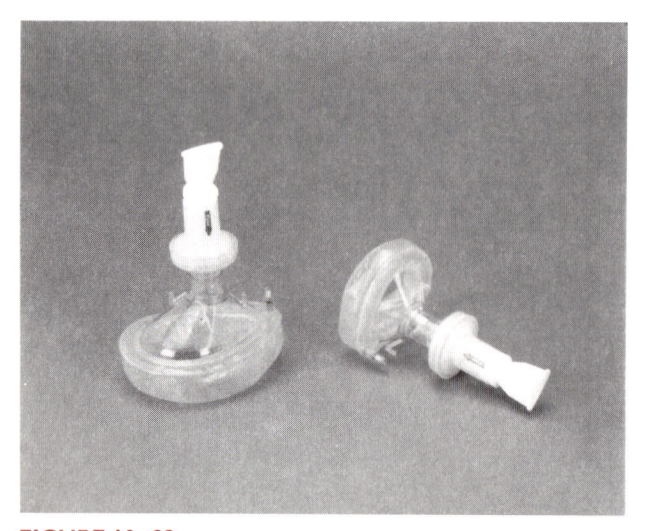

FIGURE 10–23.
Adult (left) and pediatric (right) pocket face masks. (Courtesy of Parr Emergency Sales, Inc., Galloway, Ohio)

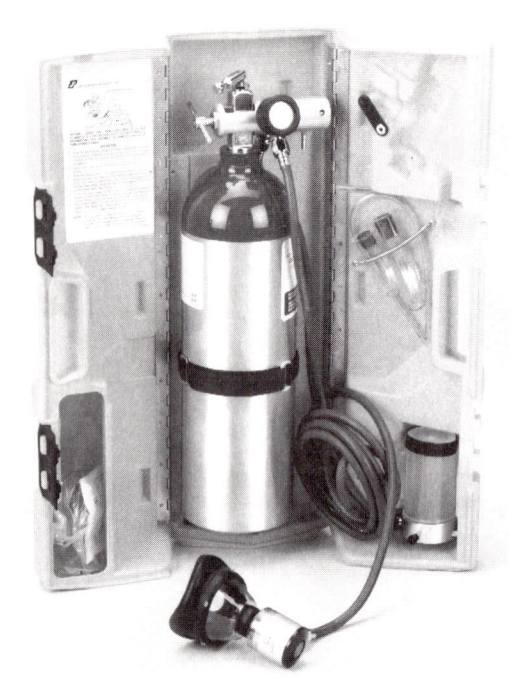

FIGURE 10–24.
Manually cycled oxygen-powered demand valve. (Courtesy of Parr Emergency Sales, Inc., Galloway, Ohio)

adequate volumes but usually cannot deliver more than 40% inspired oxygen concentration. The manually cycled ***oxygen-powered demand valve*** (Fig. 10-24) delivers both large volumes and 100% oxygen, but its use may be associated with pressure-related complications, including pneumothorax and gastric rupture. These complications generally preclude the use of these ventilators in children and make proper use and maintenance of the devices important in adults. Time-cycled, oxygen-powered ventilators that deliver preset minute volumes accurately are available for field use. These devices are ideally suited for controlled ventilation in the field, for example, for patients in cardiac arrest whose tracheas have been intubated.

Regardless of which device is used, the limiting factor until the patient is intubated is the seal of the mask. When the seal is inadequate, ventilation is poor because of the escape of ventilatory volume around the mask. It must be recognized that, frequently, only one paramedic is available to ventilate the patient. The mask should be sealed and head position maintained with one hand and the bag-valve-mask operated with the other hand. Figure 10-25 shows the technique for ventilation by one paramedic.

To provide maximum ventilation with these devices, it is best to employ two people. One team member uses both hands to seal the mask to the patient's face while the other team member operates the ventilator or squeezes the bag. Figure 10-26 shows the optimal hand placement for operating a bag-valve-mask with two people. It is also important that the person who holds the mask watch for vomiting. To make this observation easier, devices that have a clear mask are preferred.

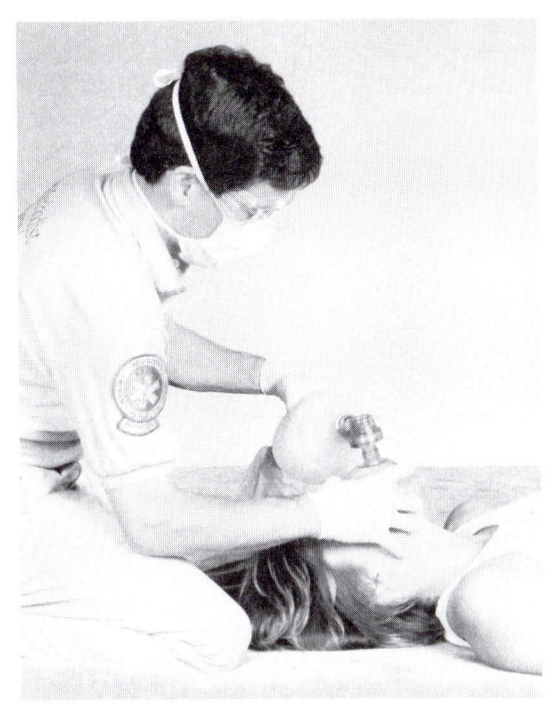

FIGURE 10–25.
Technique for bag-valve-mask ventilation with one paramedic.

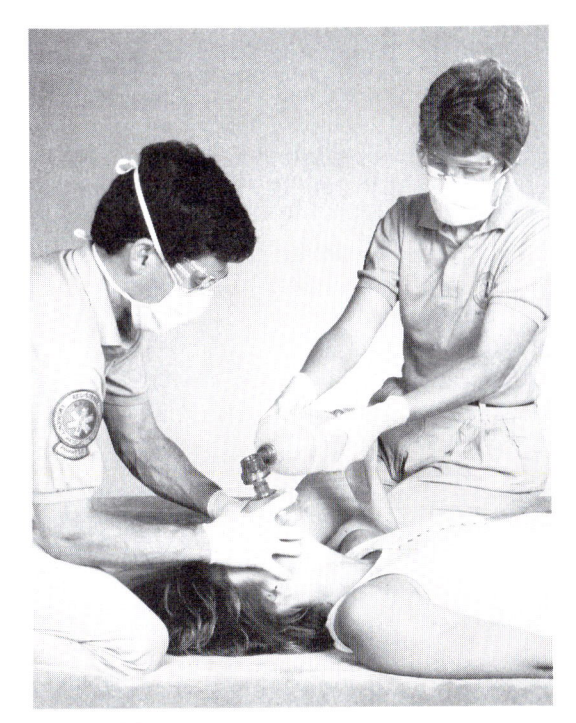

FIGURE 10–26.
Technique for bag-valve-mask ventilation with two paramedics.

Airway Management

Many patients require more definitive airway management. Deep coma, copious vomitus or secretions in the posterior pharynx, and the need for prolonged ventilation are three examples of situations in which a more secure airway is required. The definitive means of airway management is endotracheal intubation. **Endotracheal intubation,** which involves passing a cuffed tube from the mouth (or nose) directly into the trachea, allows direct ventilation of the lungs without problems of gastric distension. The cuff on the tube prevents vomitus and other substances from entering the lungs from the posterior pharynx.

Another device is the ***pharyngeo-tracheal lumen (PtL) airway***. This double-lumen airway consists of a long, cuffed tube, which may pass into either the trachea or the esophagus, and a short, cuffed tube, which is positioned just above the epiglottis. When the long tube of the device is inserted in the esophagus and both cuffs are inflated, ventilation is through the short tube. The cuff on the long tube occludes the esophagus, while the cuff on the short tube seals the oropharynx. Because the oropharynx is sealed off, a mask is not required.

Another option is the ***esophageal obturator airway (EOA)*** or ***esophageal gastric tube airway (EGTA)***. These cuffed airways are passed from the mouth into the esophagus. The patient, subsequently, is ventilated by a mask that is sealed around the nose and mouth. While the presence of the cuffed tube in the esophagus should prevent gastric contents from being regurgitated into the posterior pharynx, the lungs are not protected from blood or fluid present in the posterior pharynx. In addition, ventilation remains critically dependent on a good seal with the mask.

The esophageal tracheal combitube (ETC) has been evaluated in a variety of clinical settings, including cardiopulmonary arrest. It appears to function very effectively and thus provides still another option when endotracheal intubation cannot be accomplished. The ETC is a double-lumen airway similar to the PtL airway.

Endotracheal Intubation

Endotracheal intubation involves the placement of a tube into the patient's trachea to provide a direct route for ventilation as well as for suctioning of the trachea and upper bronchial tree. Endotracheal intubation is performed most often by passing an **endotracheal tube** through the mouth and into the trachea. A **laryngoscope** is used to facilitate alignment of the upper airway structures and allows direct visualization of the vocal cords. Another method, nasal intubation, involves passing the endotracheal tube through the nose into the trachea. Both techniques require alignment of the planes of the pharynx and trachea (Fig. 10-27). The patient is placed supine with the head in the "*sniffing*" position. This position can best be described as moderate backward flexion of the neck, similar to that assumed by a person who is sniffing the air for a slight odor of smoke. If a cervical injury is suspected, however, the neck must be kept in a neutral position, neither flexed backward or forward.

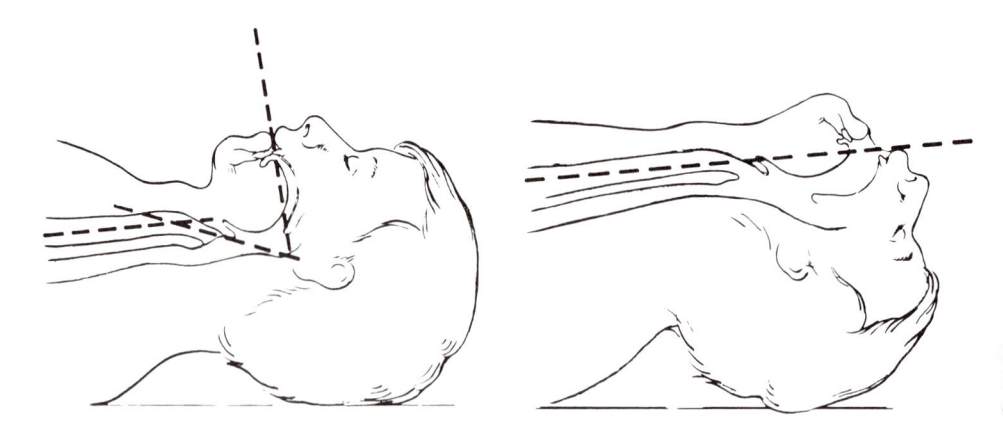

FIGURE 10-27.
Planes of the pharynx and trachea aligned for intubation.

ORAL INTUBATION. **Oral intubation** provides the most secure and reliable airway control without surgical techniques. For this technique to be accomplished, however, the patient must be sufficiently unconscious so as not to gag on the laryngoscope or tube.

Indications for endotracheal intubation include the following:

- Cardiac or respiratory arrest
- Unconscious patient in need of airway support and protection
- Potential for rapidly developing airway obstruction due to tissue swelling, as in anaphylactic reactions or damage from respiratory burns
- Need for direct tracheal suctioning or positive-pressure ventilation

Complications of several types may result from endotracheal intubation. These include the following:

- Trauma to soft tissues of the upper airway from too forceful manipulation of the laryngoscope blade
- Trauma to teeth, lips, or gums from prying backwards with the laryngoscope rather than lifting
- Increased hypoxia from prolonged attempts at intubation without pauses to hyperventilate the patient
- Laryngospasm and resulting airway obstruction caused by stimulation of the epiglottis or larynx (patients with epiglottitis are particularly prone to this problem)
- Intubation of the esophagus instead of the trachea, eliminating any possibility of effective ventilation
- Intubation of a main-stem bronchus, usually the right, caused by inserting the tube too far down the trachea and resulting in effective ventilation in only one lung
- Stimulation of the gag reflex with risk of vomiting, potential aspiration, and further airway compromise
- Accidental removal of the tube or displacement of the tube from the trachea to the esophagus during patient handling or transportation

Conditions may present relative contraindications to endotracheal intubation such as the following:

- Patients with an intact gag reflex. Although most patients who are conscious enough to have a gag reflex do not need the airway support of an endotracheal tube, situations do exist in which the patient's hypoventilation is so profound that intubation is necessary to allow positive-pressure ventilation or suction. In these cases, the patient may have to be sedated to suppress the gag reflex.
- Patients who require intubation with severe airway infections, such as croup or epiglottitis, in which unnecessary stimulation of the oropharynx or larynx may cause sudden laryngospasm and complete airway obstruction.

If the patient who requires endotracheal intubation is suspected of having a cervical spine injury, particular caution must be observed when performing intubation with a laryngoscope. Although the usual intubation method involves some backward flexion of the patient's neck, the neck must be held manually in a neutral position if a cervical spine injury is suspected. The limitation of neck flexion may make oral intubation sufficiently difficult so that nasal intubation is preferred. The technique for nasal intubation is discussed in the next section.

Equipment. To correctly perform endotracheal intubation, the proper equipment must be available and in working order. The paramedic should take personal precautions by wearing protective eye wear, mask, and gloves during the procedure. The endotracheal tube is a plastic tube available in sizes that range from 2.0 to 11.0 mm in internal diameter. The tube has a beveled distal tip, which enters the airway, and a fitting, which is compatible with the fitting of a bag-valve device at the proximal end. Figure 10-28 shows a variety of endotracheal tubes. Tubes that are larger than 5.0 mm in diameter have a cuff on the distal end that is inflated after insertion to provide protection of the lower airway from aspirates, such as vomitus, and to prevent an air leak during positive-pressure ventilation. Selection of an endotracheal tube size is based on patient size. Adult women generally tolerate a 7.0 to 7.5 mm tube, while adult men may require

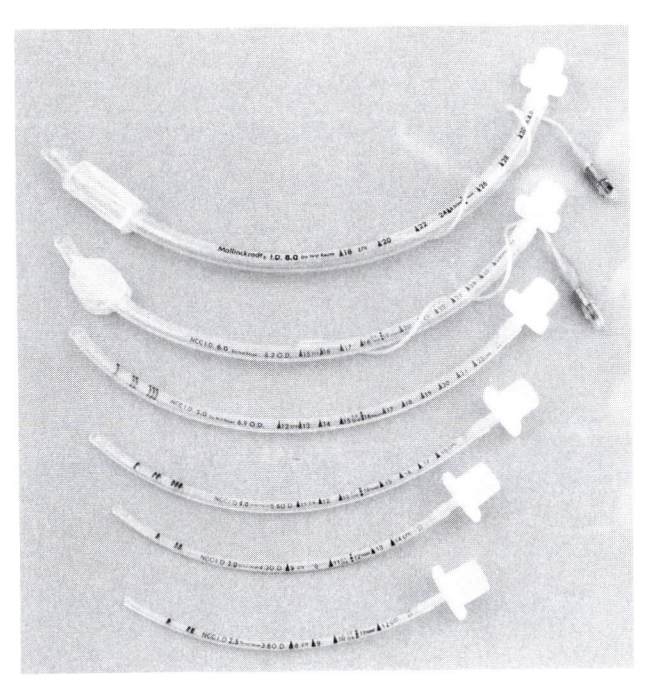

FIGURE 10–28.
Sizes of endotracheal tubes.

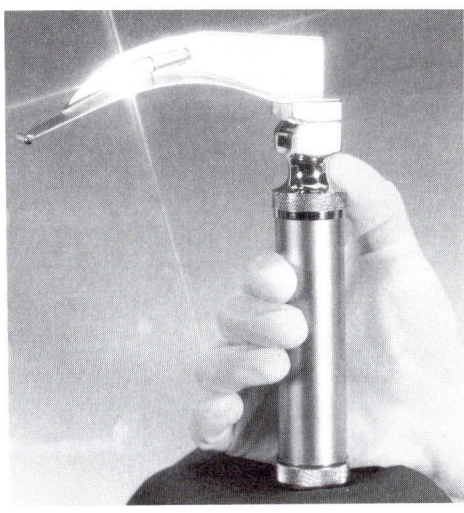

FIGURE 10–29.
Laryngoscope handle and blade. (Courtesy © Dixie USA Inc., Houston, Texas)

an 8.0 to 9.0 mm tube. Tube size for children and infants can be estimated by approximating the tube diameter to the child's small finger or nostril. A more precise guide for the pediatric patient is shown in Chapter 29.

A *stylet,* generally made of soft metal, may be placed inside the endotracheal tube to help guide it into the trachea. While not always necessary, a stylet should always be available. Some tube placements are difficult because of the anterior position of the larynx. In these cases, the stylet may provide the only means to guide the tube into the trachea. It is essential that the stylet be carefully fitted into the endotracheal tube so that the distal end does not protrude beyond the end of the tube. Protrusion of the stylet may cause it to traumatize the larynx and trachea as the tube is advanced. An alternative to the conventional stylet is the lighted stylet, which uses fiber optics to allow the tip of the stylet to be illuminated.

Besides the endotracheal tube and stylet, intubation requires a laryngoscope and blades for most endotracheal tube insertions. These items perform two important functions during intubation. The first function of the laryngoscope is to align the structures of the upper and lower airway to enable the endotracheal tube to pass through them into the trachea. The second function is to provide direct visualization of the larynx and vocal cords, through which the endotracheal tube is passed. The lighted laryngoscope allows the paramedic to see the endotracheal tube pass through the cords, assuring correct placement (Fig. 10-29).

Laryngoscope blades come in three shapes and a variety of sizes (Fig. 10-30). The curved blade, also known as the MacIntosh blade, is inserted so that the tip rests in the *vallecula* (depression between the epiglottis and the root of the tongue), from which position the epiglottis is raised to visualize the vocal cords. The straight blade, also known as the Wisconsin or Magill blade, is used to pick up the epiglottis so that the vocal cords are visible. The Miller blade is essentially straight but has a slight curve at the distal end. It is used in the same manner as the straight blade. Figure 10-31 shows the two techniques to lift up the epiglottis and expose the vocal cords.

Laryngoscope blades come in a variety of sizes to fit the airways of premature infants through large adults. Selection of blade shape is largely a matter of personal preference, although the curved blade may cause less laryngospasm and cough because it does not come into contact with the undersurface of the epiglottis, which is innervated by the vagus nerve.

A number of other supporting items should be assembled before intubation. **Magill forceps** (Fig. 10-32) may be required to remove a foreign body or assist in a difficult tube placement. A syringe (10 mL or larger) must be available to inflate the cuff on adult-size endotracheal tubes. Tape or a commercial tie device is required to secure the endotracheal tube to the patient. An oropharyngeal airway is often inserted after intubation to prevent a combative patient from biting the tube. Another important requirement is suction. Many patients who require endotracheal intubation may have vomited or have otherwise accumulated fluids or blood in the posterior pharynx that must be removed to allow visualization during the intubation process. Suction should be ready before starting the procedure. A bag-valve-mask device and oxygen should also be ready for use. The necessary equipment must be at the patient's side and ready before intubation.

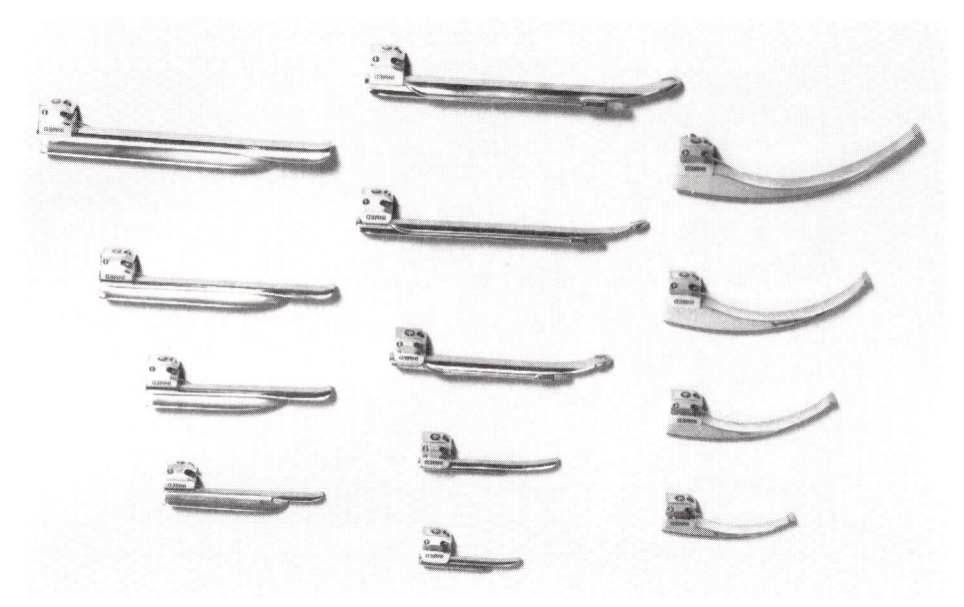

FIGURE 10–30.
Sizes and types of laryngoscope blades: Wisconsin (left), Miller (middle), MacIntosh (right). (Courtesy of Parr Emergency Sales, Inc., Galloway, Ohio)

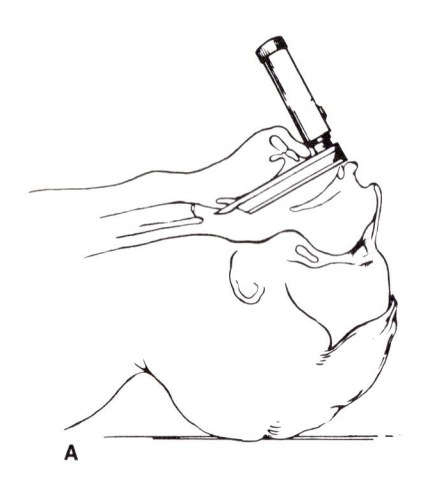

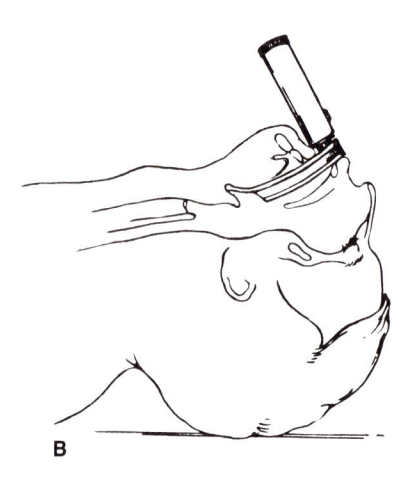

FIGURE 10–31.
A, The tip of the straight blade is placed below and lifts up the epiglottis. **B**, The curved blade lifts the epiglottis by placing the tip of the blade into the vallecula while slightly lifting upward.

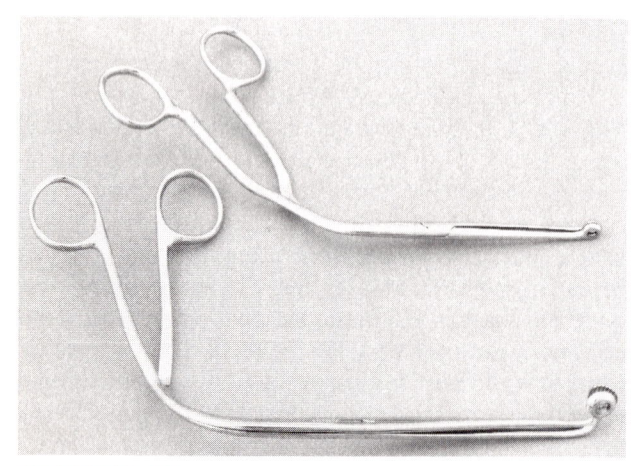

FIGURE 10–32.
Magill forceps; pediatric (top), adult (bottom).

Procedure. After determining that the patient requires intubation and after assembling the appropriate equipment, intubation is performed. The first step, and one that must be continued before and after intubation, is to establish and maintain ventilation. Intubation is not a first-line airway control technique. If respirations are absent or inadequate, ventilation with supplemental oxygen and a less sophisticated airway device should be initiated. The airway must also be cleared of foreign substances. The procedure for oral intubation is shown in Skill 10-1.

NASAL INTUBATION. **Nasal intubation** is a technique in which an endotracheal tube is passed through the nose and pharynx into the trachea without using a laryngoscope to directly visualize the vocal cords. The fact that

(*text continues on page 148*)

SKILL 10-1
ENDOTRACHEAL INTUBATION, ORAL

ACTIVITY	HOW PERFORMED	WHY PERFORMED
1. Check: • Responsiveness • Airway • Breathing • Circulation	Establish responsiveness Stabilize neck, open the airway Assess breathing Check for a pulse Check for hemorrhage	The primary survey is a rapid evaluation, less than 45 seconds, to identify and correct any life-threatening problems.
2. Assemble and check: Primary equipment (Activity 2): • Laryngoscope handle • Laryngoscope blade • Endotracheal (ET) tube • Stylet • 10 mL syringe	Select propor size of laryngoscope blade. Attach blade to laryngoscope handle. Check bulb operation. Select proper size of ET tube. Insert stylet in ET tube. Attach 10 mL syringe to pilot balloon and check cuff for leaks. Have suction unit ready.	Intubation must be accomplished rapidly. Having all equipment prechecked and ready reduces time delays during the procedure.

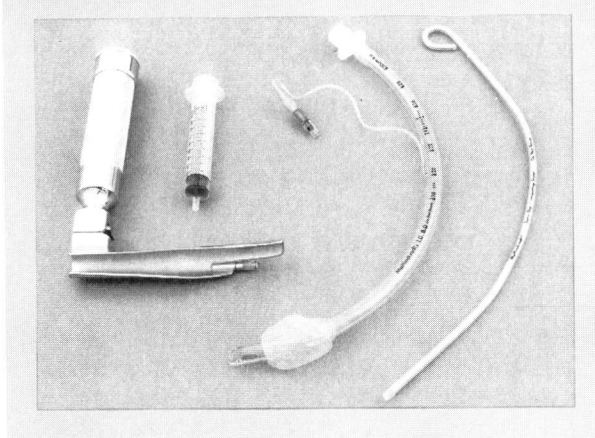

Activity 2.
Primary equipment.

Accessory equipment and supplies: • Suction unit • Suction catheter • Bag-valve-mask device • Oxygen • Stethoscope • Magill forceps • Tape or tube securing device • Protective eye wear • Mask • Gloves	Put on protective eye wear, mask, and gloves	Prevents blood or body fluid contact with nonintact skin or mucous membranes.
3. Remove potential airway obstructions	Remove the patient's dental bridgework and plates or broken teeth.	May interfere with insertion of ET tube and cause airway obstruction. Obstructions cannot be removed easily from the patient once intubated.
4. Position patient's head	Position patient supine with the head in the "sniffing" position (Activity 4). This position can best be described as moderate backward flexion of the neck, similar to that assumed by a person sniffing the air for a slight odor of smoke.	The "sniffing" position helps align the planes of the pharynx and trachea and positions these structures for easiest intubation.

(continued)

SKILL 10-1
ENDOTRACHEAL INTUBATION, ORAL (continued)

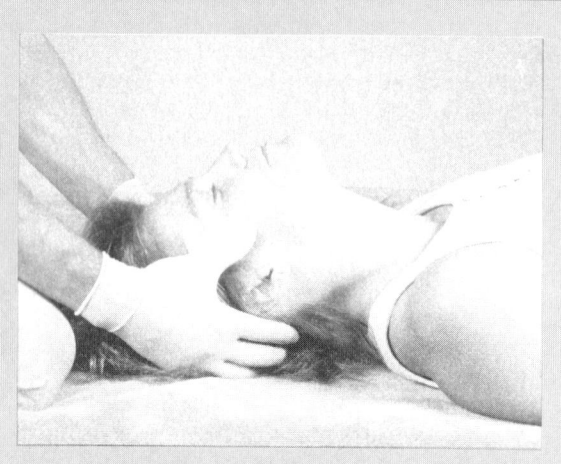

ACTIVITY	HOW PERFORMED	WHY PERFORMED
	Activity 4. Position patient's head.	
	If a cervical injury is suspected, however, keep the neck in a neutral position, neither flexed backward nor forward.	*Even moderate flexion may aggravate a cervical injury.*
5. Hyperventilate patient	With oropharyngeal or nasopharyngeal airway in place, patient should be hyperventilated with 100% O_2 (bag-valve-mask device or oxygen-powered demand valve) about 12 times in a 30-second period.	Hyperventilation before intubating lessens the detrimental effect of the short period of no ventilation while the intubation is performed.
Reventilate as needed	*Anytime the intubation procedure causes more than 30 seconds without ventilation, the procedure must be stopped and the patient hyperventilated for 30 to 60 seconds before intubation is reattempted.*	*After hyperventilation, delays in ventilation of more than 30 seconds risk worsening hypoxia and may jeopardize the patient.*
6. Insert blade	Hold laryngoscope handle in left hand (Activity 6).	All laryngoscopes are made to be held in the left hand.
	Insert the blade an inch or so into the right side of the mouth and move to the midline.	The tongue is moved out of the way for visualization.
	Insert the blade further with the tip of the blade following the roof of the mouth until the tip reaches the area of the soft palate.	Proper blade position before lifting eases visualization.
	Activity 6. Insert blade.	

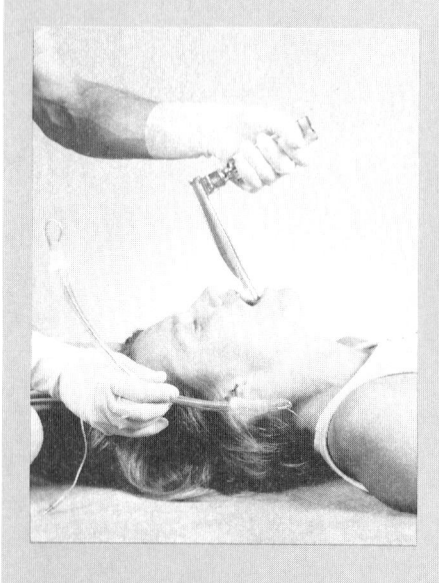

(continued)

SKILL 10-1
ENDOTRACHEAL INTUBATION, ORAL (continued)

ACTIVITY	HOW PERFORMED	WHY PERFORMED
7. Lift blade	Lift the laryngoscope straight up and slightly toward the patient's feet (Activity 7). Do not pry the blade back against the lips, teeth, or gums.	Lifting displaces the mandible forward to allow a clear view. Prying back may damage lips, teeth, or gums and may not allow a clear view.

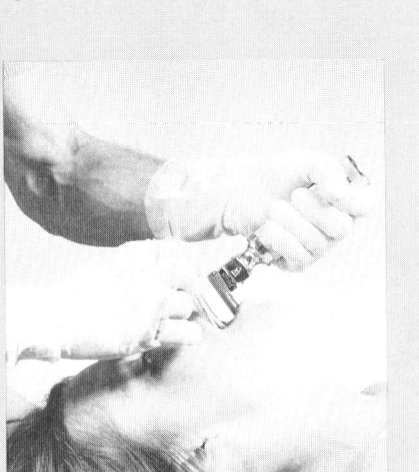

Activity 7.
Lift blade.

8. Expose and visualize: • Epiglottis • Vocal cords	Straight blade (Miller, Wisconsin): insert blade top to lift the bottom edge of the epiglottis to expose the vocal cords. Curved blade (MacIntosh): insert blade tip into the vallecula just above the epiglottis. Lifting then indirectly raises the epiglottis and exposes the vocal cords. If no identifiable structures are seen, slowly withdraw the blade. If slight withdrawal of the blade fails to produce a view of identifiable structures, try to elevate the patient's head slightly. If head elevation also fails, have an assistant place slight downward pressure on the patient's cricoid cartilage (Sellick maneuver) (Activity 8).	Each method provides direct and controlled lifting of the epiglottis and clear exposure of the vocal cords. Inserting the blade too far causes it to enter the esophagus. Gently pulling back will allow the epiglottis and vocal cords to drop into view as soon as the blade comes out of the esophagus. If the patient's larynx is positioned more anterior than normal, slight head elevation may bring the larynx into view. *Do not use this maneuver if cervical spine injury is suspected.* A very anterior larynx may be brought into view by the Sellick maneuver.

(continued)

SKILL 10-1
ENDOTRACHEAL INTUBATION, ORAL (continued)

ACTIVITY	HOW PERFORMED	WHY PERFORMED
	If exposure of vocal cords is not readily attained, withdraw the laryngoscope and hyperventilate the patient before making another attempt.	*Without a clear exposure of the vocal cords, correct placement of the ET tube cannot be assured. Delays in ventilation more than 30 seconds while intubation is attempted increase hypoxia.*

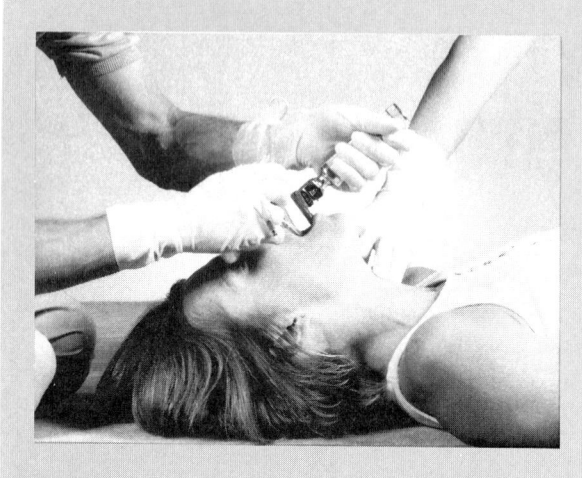

Activity 8.
Have an assistant place slight downward pressure on the patient's cricoid cartilage.

9. Insert ET tube	With the vocal cords visualized, pass the tip of the ET tube between the vocal cords. Insert the ET tube until the tube cuff is beyond the vocal cords. On a non-cuffed ET tube (usually size 5.0 mm or smaller), the distal tip of the tube should be passed about 2 cm beyond the vocal cords. Magill forceps may be used to direct the tip of the ET tube between vocal cords if needed. Hold ET tube securely in place and remove the laryngoscope. Remove the stylet (Activity 9).	Watching the ET tube go between the vocal cords is the best assurance of proper placement. With the cuff just behond the cords and no further, full ventilation of both lungs is assured. Inserting too far risks intubation of the right main-stem bronchus with little or no ventilation of the left lung.

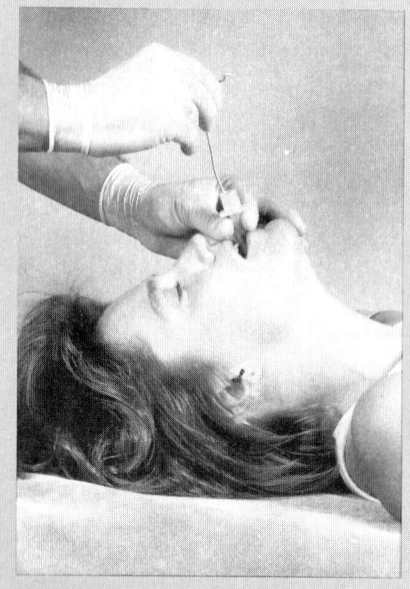

Activity 9.
Remove the stylet.

(continued)

146

SKILL 10-1
ENDOTRACHEAL INTUBATION, ORAL (continued)

ACTIVITY	HOW PERFORMED	WHY PERFORMED
10. Inflate cuff	Inflate the cuff with 8 to 10 mL of air using the syringe (Activity 10). Feel the pilot balloon for tautness.	Inflating the cuff secures the ET tube in place and provides a seal that protects the trachea from foreign material and allows each ventilation to enter the lungs.

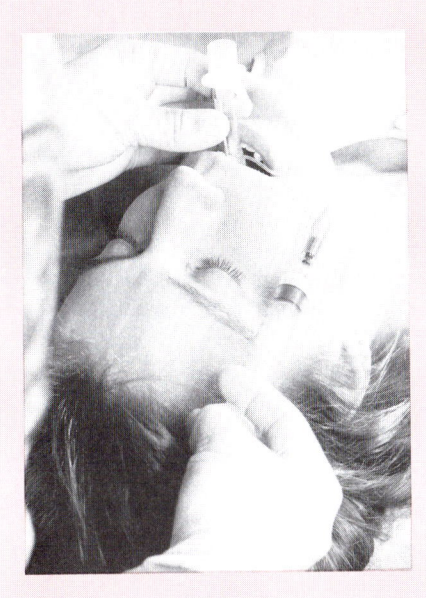

Activity 10.
Inflate cuff.

11. Assess breath sounds	Ventilate with 100% O_2 (bag-valve-mask device or oxygen-powered demand valve). Auscultate breath sounds bilaterally, starting with the upper anterior chest (Activity 11A) followed by the other lung fields. If an end-tidal CO_2 detector is available it should be used to help confirm proper tube position. Qualitative or semi-quantitative devices are very useful in non-arrested patients.	The presence of breath sounds, equal in strength on both sides, indicates proper ET tube placement.
	Auscultate over the stomach in the left upper abdominal quadrant (Activity 11B).	The absence of sounds in the stomach further verifies proper ET tube placement.

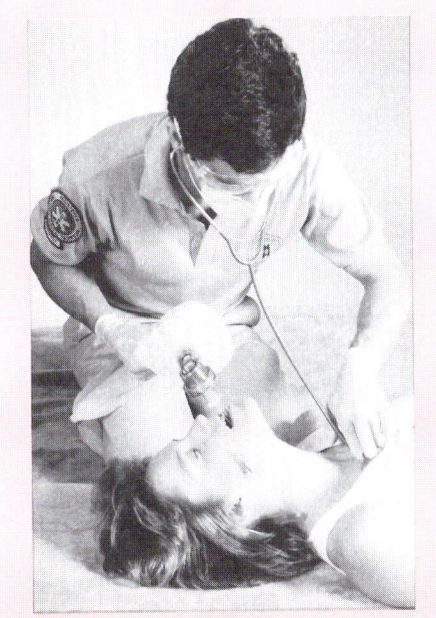

Activity 11A.
Assess breath sounds, lung fields.

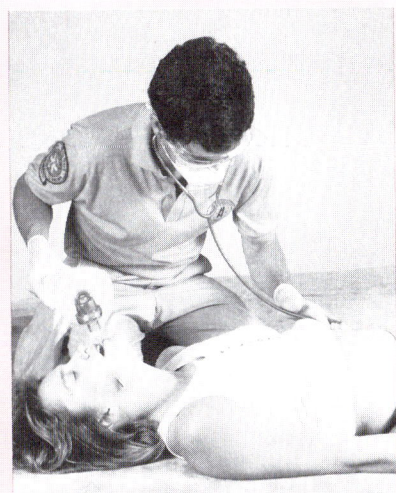

Activity 11B.
Assess breath sounds in the left upper abdominal quadrant.

(continued)

SKILL 10-1
ENDOTRACHEAL INTUBATION, ORAL (continued)

ACTIVITY	HOW PERFORMED	WHY PERFORMED
12. Correct improperly placed ET tube	If breath sounds are absent, or sounds are heard in stomach only, deflate cuff, remove ET tube and hyperventilate patient before reattempting intubation. If sounds are heard in both lungs and stomach, recheck ET tube cuff. Remove ET tube if it cannot be corrected. If sounds are softer or absent in the left lung, gently pull ET tube out until equal sounds are heard.	Sounds in stomach and none in lungs indicate esophagus was intubated, not trachea. A broken or under-inflated cuff may allow sounds in lungs and stomach due to inadequate seal. An ET tube inserted too far may enter the right main-stem bronchus, resulting in reduced or no ventilation of the left lung.
13. Stabilize ET tube	Use tape or other device to secure ET tube to avoid pulling out or pushing tube in too far (Activity 13).	Proper ET tube position is critical for optimum ventilation. Patient handling and transport may easily displace an unsecured ET tube.
14. Reassess breath sounds and correct ET tube placement as indicated	Auscultate breath sounds bilaterally as well as over the stomach.	The process of securing the ET tube may displace the tube slightly.

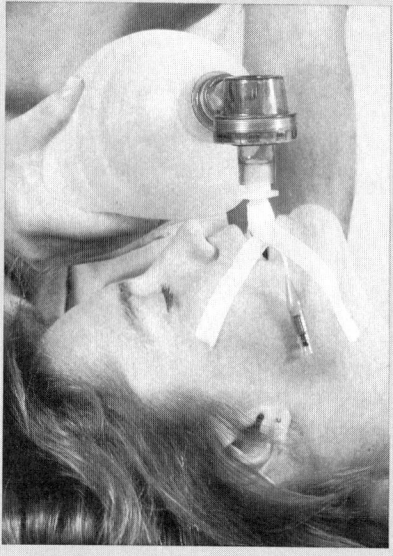

Activity 13.
Stabilize endotracheal tube.

---

it is a "*blind*" procedure generally limits the use of nasal intubation to patients who are breathing, because insertion of the tube into the trachea is timed and guided by the patient's respiration. The nasal route is preferable, however, in circumstances that may make oral intubation difficult or dangerous, such as in the following conditions:

- Severe trauma to the mouth and lower jaw that would complicate use of a laryngoscope
- Suspected cervical spine injury
- Head injury or severe, prolonged seizures in which the teeth and jaw are clamped shut and the mouth cannot be opened
- Conscious or semiconscious patients who are hypoventilating severely and need positive-pressure ventilation or tracheal suctioning

Nasal intubation may be complicated by several factors in addition to those applicable to oral intubation, such as the following:

- Fighting either the tube or the procedure by a conscious or semiconscious patient. This problem may be lessened by sedation before the procedure.
- Induced bleeding in the nasopharynx due to trauma from passage of the tube. Application of a lubricant may ease passage of the tube and minimize damage.

Contraindications to nasal intubation include those applicable to oral intubation as well as severe nasal trauma or swelling of nasal tissues that make passage of the tube through the nasopharynx difficult.

Procedure. Preparation for nasal intubation is identical to that for oral intubation. The patient must be oxygenated and, when appropriate, given supplemental ventilation before intubation. Suction must be on hand, along with the bag-valve-mask or other ventilatory device. The patient is placed supine in a "sniffing" position unless cervical trauma is suspected. The endotracheal tube selected should be slightly smaller than the patient's largest nostril. As a general rule, most patients accept a nasal tube that is one full size smaller than the tube that would be used for oral intubation. The procedure for nasal intubation is shown in Skill 10-2.

Pharyngeo-Tracheal Lumen Airway and the Esophageal Airways

Given the relative difficulty of performing endotracheal intubation and its potential danger to patients with cervical spine injuries, several alternative airway devices have been developed, including the pharyngeo-tracheal lumen airway and the esophageal airways.

PHARYNGEO-TRACHEAL LUMEN AIRWAY. The pharyngeo-tracheal lumen airway is essentially a *tube within a tube*, with a long endotracheal-type tube inside of a shorter, large bore tube. Both of the tubes are cuffed and may be inflated at the same time through one inflation valve. When the airway is inserted, the long tube may enter either the esophagus or the trachea (Figs. 10-33 and 10-34). While a tracheal placement may be preferred, the airway is effective whether it is placed in the trachea or the esophagus.

When placed, the opening of the short, large bore tube lies in the pharynx, just above the epiglottis. The long tube comes with a stylet in place, which helps guide the tube and also serves to seal the tube when it enters the esophagus. When the airway is in place, both the cuff on the long tube and the cuff on the short tube are inflated. The cuff on the short tube is large enough to fill the oropharynx, eliminating the need for a face-mask seal.

By listening for breath sounds over the chest when the short tube is ventilated, the paramedic can easily determine where the long tube is placed. If breath sounds are heard when the short tube is ventilated, then the trachea must be open and the esophagus sealed by the long tube.

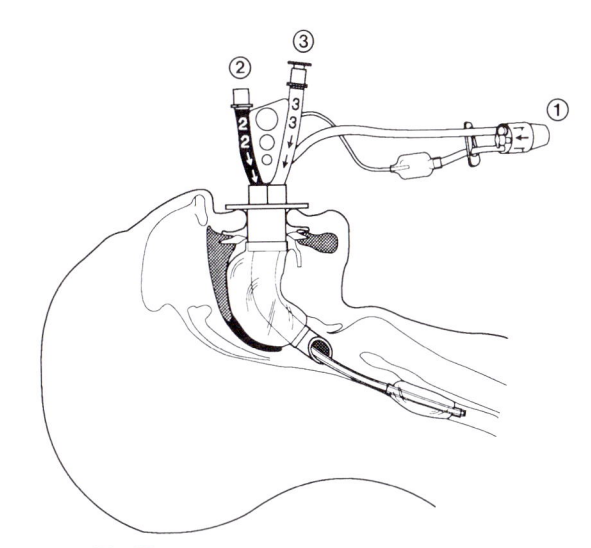

FIGURE 10-33.
Pharyngeo-tracheal lumen airway inserted into the esophagus. (Courtesy of Respironics Inc., Monroeville, Pennsylvania)

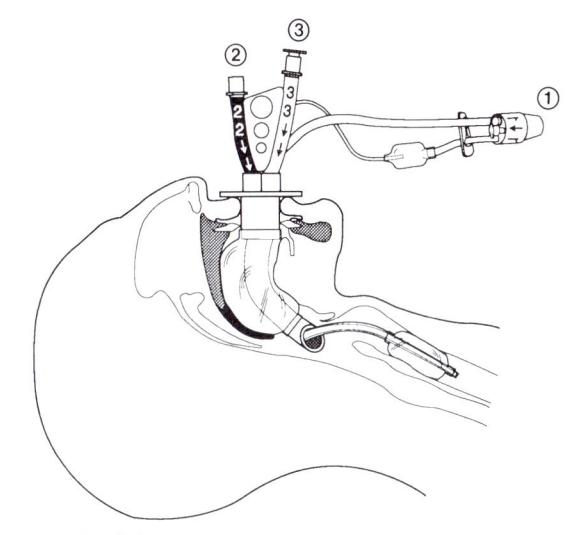

FIGURE 10-34.
Pharyngeo-tracheal lumen airway inserted into the trachea. (Courtesy of Respironics Inc., Monroeville, Pennsylvania)

If no breath sounds are heard when the short tube is ventilated, then the trachea must be blocked by the long tube. In that case, the stylet is simply removed from the long tube, opening it to serve as a regular endotracheal tube.

Indications for use of the pharyngeo-tracheal lumen airway include the following:

- Cardiac or respiratory arrest
- Unconscious patient in need of airway support or protection
- Unconscious patient in whom endotracheal intubation has been unsuccessful

(text continues on page 154)

SKILL 10-2.
ENDOTRACHEAL INTUBATION, NASAL

ACTIVITY	HOW PERFORMED	WHY PERFORMED
1. Check: • Responsiveness • Airway • Breathing • Circulation	Establish responsiveness Stabilize neck, open the airway Assess breathing Check for a pulse Check for hemorrhage	The primary survey is a rapid evaluation, less than 45 seconds, to identify and correct any life-threatening problems.
2. Assemble and check: Primary equipment (Activity 2): • Endotracheal (ET) tube • 10 mL syringe Accessory equipment and supplies: • Water soluble lubricant • Suction unit • Suction catheter • Bag-valve-mask device • Oxygen • Stethoscope • Tape or tube securing device • Protective eye wear • Mask • Gloves	Select proper size of ET tube. Attach 10 mL syringe to pilot balloon and check cuff for leaks. Lubricate the distal end of ET tube with water soluble lubricant. Have suction unit ready. Put on protective eye wear, mask, and gloves.	Intubation must be accomplished rapidly. Having all equipment prechecked and ready reduces time delays during the procedure. To prevent blood or body fluid contact with nonintact skin or mucous membrane.

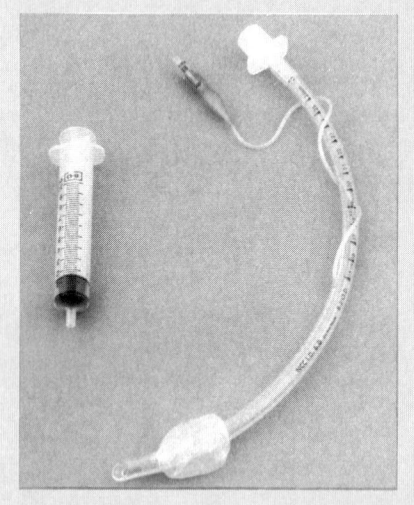

Activity 2.
Primary equipment.

3. Remove potential airway obstructions	Remove the patient's dental bridgework and plates or broken teeth.	May interfere with insertion of ET tube and cause airway obstruction. Obstructions cannot be removed easily from the patient once intubated.
4. Position patient's head	Position patient supine with the head in the "sniffing" position (Activity 4). This position can best be described as moderate backward flexion of the neck, similar to that assumed by a person sniffing the air for a slight odor of smoke.	The "sniffing" position helps align the planes of the pharynx and trachea and positions these structures for easiest intubation.

(continued)

SKILL 10–2
ENDOTRACHEAL INTUBATION, NASAL (continued)

ACTIVITY	HOW PERFORMED	WHY PERFORMED
	If a cervical injury is suspected, however, keep neck in a neutral position, neither flexed backward nor forward.	*Even moderate flexion may aggravate a cervical injury.*

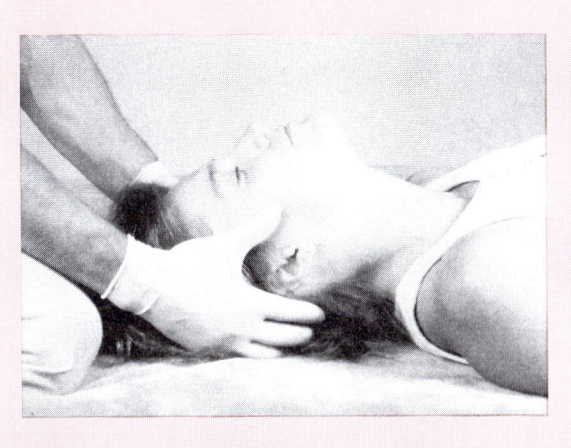

Activity 4.
Position patient's head.

5. Hyperventilate patient

Reventilate as needed

With oropharyngeal or nasopharyngeal airway in place, patient should be hyperventilated with 100% O_2 (bag-valve-mask device or oxygen-powered demand valve) about 12 times in a 30-second period.

Anytime the intubation procedure causes more than 30 seconds without ventilation, the procedure must be stopped and the patient hyperventilated for 30 to 60 seconds before intubation is reattempted.

Hyperventilation before intubating lessens the detrimental effect of the short period of no ventilation while the intubation is performed.

After hyperventilation, delays in ventilation of more than 30 seconds risk worsening hypoxia and may jeopardize the patient.

6. Choose a naris

Inspect both nares for visible obstructions or swollen membranes. Select the larger or least obstructed (Activity 6).

The right naris may be chosen because it is often larger and the bevel of the ET tube passes along the nasal septum.

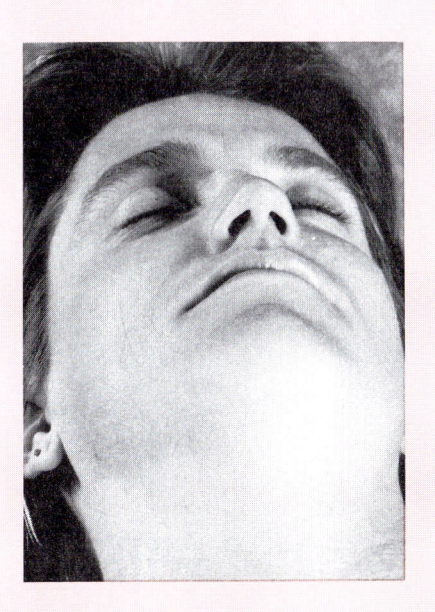

Activity 6.
Choose a naris.

(continued)

SKILL 10-2
ENDOTRACHEAL INTUBATION, NASAL (continued)

ACTIVITY	HOW PERFORMED	WHY PERFORMED
7. Insert ET tube	Advance the ET tube through the naris and along the floor of the nasal passage through the nasopharynx (Activity 7A). Forcing the ET tube in spite of resistance may damage soft tissue and further compromise the airway. If resistance is encountered, gently retry to advance the ET tube. If resistance persists, abandon the procedure.	Passing the ET tube along the floor of the nasal passage avoids the nasal turbinates, which are easily damaged and may block passage of the ET tube.
	As the ET tube approaches the glottic opening, pause to listen for exhaled air coming from the proximal end of the ET tube (Activity 7B). During inhalation, the ET tube should be passed through the glottic opening.	The glottic opening enlarges during inhalation. Passing the ET tube at this point reduces trauma to the vocal cords.
	Listen for air movement at the proximal end of the ET tube. If none is heard, withdraw the ET tube until air movement is heard, and reattempt passage into the trachea.	Absence of air movement indicates that the esophagus was entered. Presence of air movement verifies intubation of the trachea.

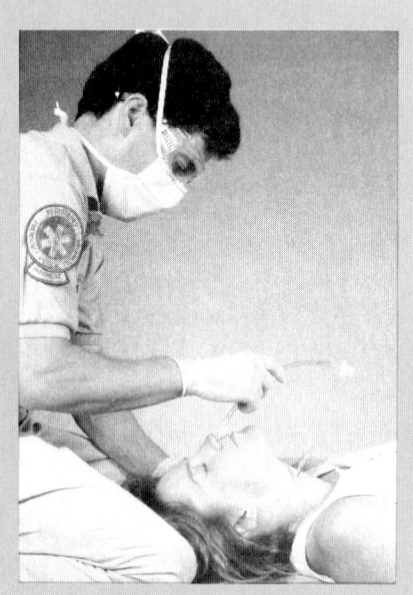

Activity 7A.
Insert endotracheal tube.

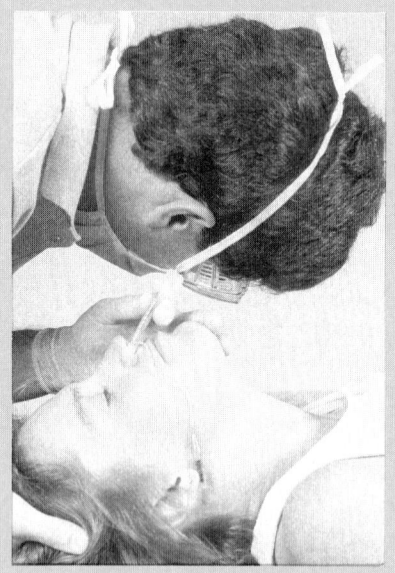

Activity 7B.
Listen for exhaled air.

(continued)

SKILL 10–2
ENDOTRACHEAL INTUBATION, NASAL (continued)

ACTIVITY	HOW PERFORMED	WHY PERFORMED
8. Inflate cuff	Inflate the cuff with 8 to 10 mL of air using the syringe (Activity 8). Feel the pilot balloon for tautness.	Inflating the cuff secures the ET tube in place and provides a seal that protects the trachea from foreign material and allows each ventilation to enter the lungs.
9. Assess breath sounds	Ventilate with 100% O_2 (bag-valve-mask device or oxygen-powered demand valve). Auscultate breath sounds bilaterally, starting with the upper anterior chest (Activity 9A) followed by the other lung fields. Auscultate over the stomach in the left upper abdominal quadrant (Activity 9B).	The presence of breath sounds, equal in strength on both sides, indicates proper ET tube placement. The absence of sounds in the stomach further verifies proper ET tube placement.

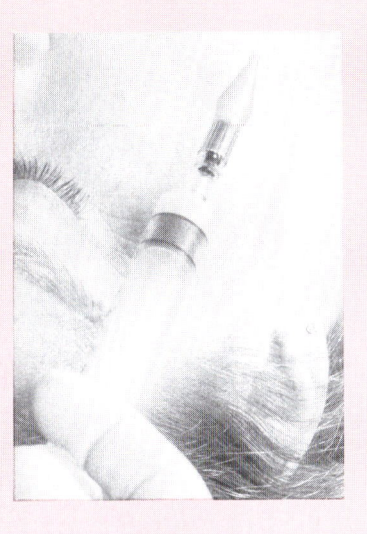

Activity 8.
Inflate cuff, using syringe.

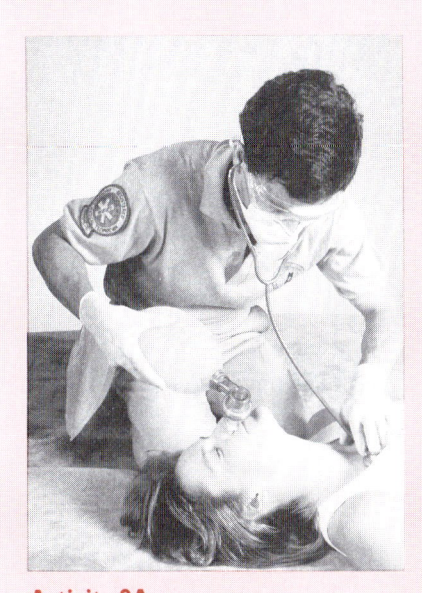

Activity 9A.
Assess breath sounds, lung fields.

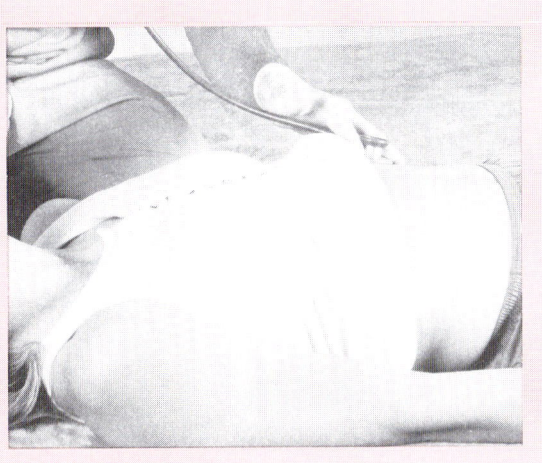

Activity 9B.
Assess breath sounds in left upper abdominal quadrant.

(continued)

SKILL 10-2
ENDOTRACHEAL INTUBATION, NASAL (continued)

ACTIVITY	HOW PERFORMED	WHY PERFORMED
10. Correct improperly placed ET tube	If breath sounds are absent, or sounds are heard in stomach only, deflate cuff, remove ET tube and hyperventilate patient before reattempting intubation. If sounds are heard in both lungs and stomach, recheck ET tube cuff. Remove ET tube if it cannot be corrected. If sounds are softer or absent in the left lung, gently pull ET tube out until equal sounds are heard.	Sounds in stomach and none in lungs indicate esophagus was intubated, not trachea. A broken or under-inflated cuff may allow sounds in lungs and stomach due to inadequate seal. An ET tube inserted too far may enter the right main-stem bronchus, resulting in reduced or no ventilation of the left lung.
11. Stabilize ET tube	Use tape or other device to secure ET tube to avoid pulling it out or pushing it in too far (Activity 11).	Proper ET tube position is critical for optimum ventilation. Patient handling and transport may easily displace an unsecured ET tube.

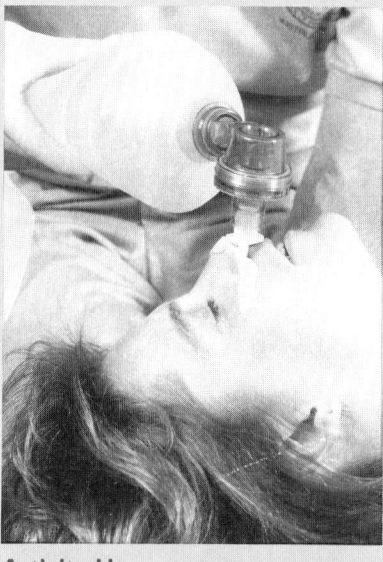

Activity 11.
Stabilize endotracheal tube.

12. Reassess breath sounds and correct ET tube placement as indicated	Auscultate breath sounds bilaterally as well as over the stomach.	The process of securing the ET tube may displace the tube slightly.

- Unconscious patient with suspected cervical spine injury

Complications associated with the pharyngeo-tracheal lumen airway include the following:

- Misinterpretation of the location of the long tube, resulting in no lung ventilation
- Soft tissue damage to airways or esophagus from high cuff pressure
- Stimulation of gag reflex with possible vomiting

The pharyngeo-tracheal lumen airway is contraindicated in the following conditions:

- Conscious or semiconscious patients with an active gag reflex
- Patients younger than age 14, because of the availability of only one adult size
- Patients with known or suspected esophageal disease or injury, such as ingestion of caustic substances

Equipment. The pharyngeo-tracheal lumen airway consists of a long, endotracheal-type tube placed within a shorter, large bore tube. A plastic bite block with a flange at its top is built into the airway. When the airway is properly inserted, the flange rests against the patient's teeth. An adjustable neck strap is provided to secure the airway. Additional equipment required includes that for suction in case of vomiting.

Procedure. Placement of the pharyngeo-tracheal lumen airway is similar to that of the esophageal obturator airway and the esophageal gastric tube airway in that it does not require the use of a laryngoscope. The paramedic should take personal protection by wearing protective eye wear, mask, and gloves. The procedure for using the pharyngeo-tracheal lumen airway is shown in Skill 10-3.

ESOPHAGEAL AIRWAYS. The esophageal obturator airway consists of a cuffed tube similar to an endotracheal tube with the distal end sealed (Fig. 10-35). In addition, the tube is fitted with a face mask and has a series of openings a few centimeters below the mask. When the esophageal obturator airway is placed in the esophagus, with the cuff inflated and the mask sealed over the patient's face, positive-pressure ventilation can be provided through the proximal end of the tube at the mask. With the esophagus sealed, air is forced through the openings in the tube in the region of the oropharynx and into the trachea, provided the face mask is also well sealed.

The esophageal gastric tube airway is similar to the esophageal obturator airway. The tube of the esophageal gastric tube airway, however, has an opening down its length for a gastric suction tube (Fig. 10-36). The tube has one-way valves to prevent gastric contents from coming up it. With the lumen for gastric suction in the main tube, ventilation with the esophageal gastric tube airway is accomplished through a second opening in the face mask. Through that opening, positive-pressure ventilation is directed into the trachea, provided the face mask is well sealed and the esophageal tube cuff is inflated.

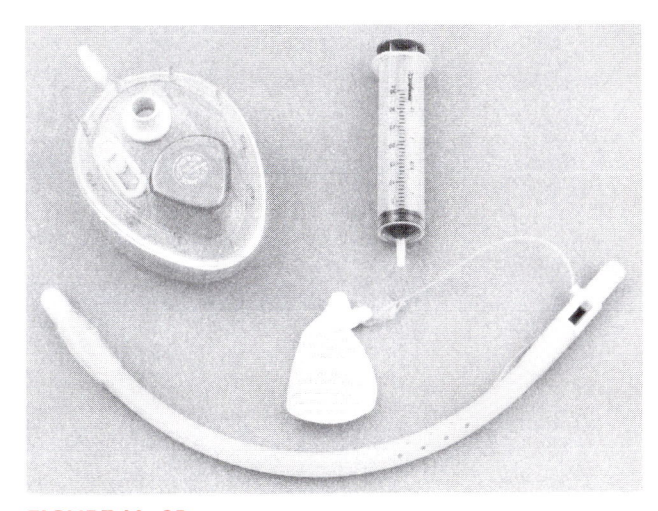

FIGURE 10-35.
Esophageal obturator airway.

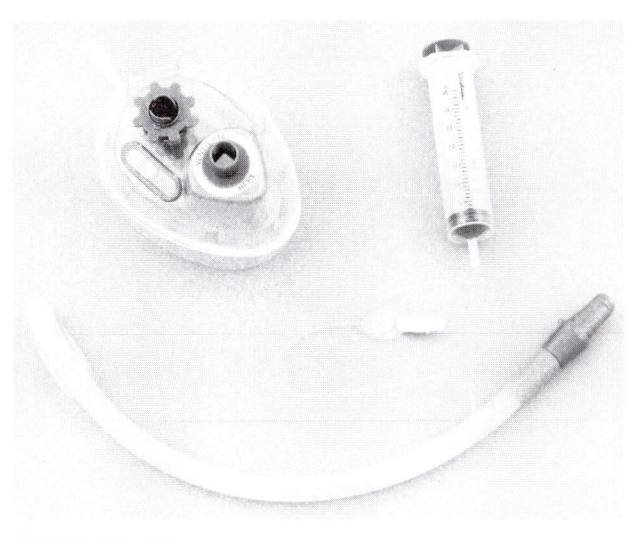

FIGURE 10-36.
Esophageal gastric tube airway.

Indications for the esophageal obturator airway and the esophageal gastric tube airway are limited to adult patients in situations such as the following:

- Cardiac or respiratory arrest
- Unconscious patient in need of airway support or protection
- Unconscious patient in whom endotracheal intubation has been unsuccessful, particularly if copious vomiting is present
- Unconscious patient with suspected cervical spine injury

Complications of the esophageal obturator airway and the esophageal gastric tube airway include the following:

- Inadvertent placement into the trachea, thus sealing it off from any ventilation
- Esophageal damage or even rupture from prolonged high cuff pressure or pressure from accumulated air and food in the stomach
- Stimulation of the gag reflex and possible vomiting
- Inadequate face-mask seal, resulting in hypoventilation

The esophageal obturator airway and esophageal gastric tube airway are contraindicated in the following conditions:

- Patients younger than age 16, because of the availability of only one adult size of tube
- Conscious or semiconscious patients with an active gag reflex
- Patients with known or suspected esophageal disease or injury, such as ingestion of caustic substances

Equipment. Two different devices are available for use when placing an esophageal airway. The esophageal obturator airway is a large bore, cuffed tube that has an occluded distal tip. The esophageal gastric tube airway

(text continues on page 160)

SKILL 10-3.
PHARYNGEO-TRACHEAL LUMEN AIRWAY

ACTIVITY	HOW PERFORMED	WHY PERFORMED
1. Check: • Responsiveness • Airway • Breathing • Circulation	Establish responsiveness Stabilize neck, open the airway Assess breathing Check for a pulse Check for hemorrhage	The primary survey is a rapid evaluation, less than 45 seconds, to identify and correct any life-threatening problems.
2. Assemble and check: Primary equipment (Activity 2): • Pharyngeo-tracheal lumen (PtL) airway Accessory equipment and supplies: • Suction unit • Suction catheter • Bag-valve-mask device • Oxygen • Stethoscope • Protective eye wear • Mask • Gloves	Both cuffs, proximal and distal, should be completely deflated. Have suction unit ready. Put on protective eye wear, mask, and gloves.	Intubation must be accomplished rapidly. Having all equipment prechecked and ready reduces time delays during the procedure. To prevent blood or body fluid contact with nonintact skin or mucous membranes.
3. Remove potential airway obstructions	Remove the patient's dental bridgework and plates or broken teeth.	May interfere with insertion of PtL airway and cause airway obstruction. Obstructions cannot be removed easily from the patient once intubated.
4. Position patient's head	Position patient supine with the head in the "sniffing" position (Activity 4). This position can best be described as a moderate backward flexion of the neck, similar to that assumed by a person sniffing the air for a slight odor of smoke.	The "sniffing" position helps align the planes of the pharynx and trachea and positions these structures for easiest intubation.

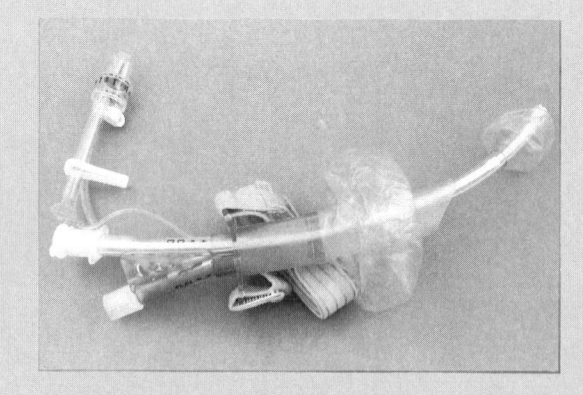

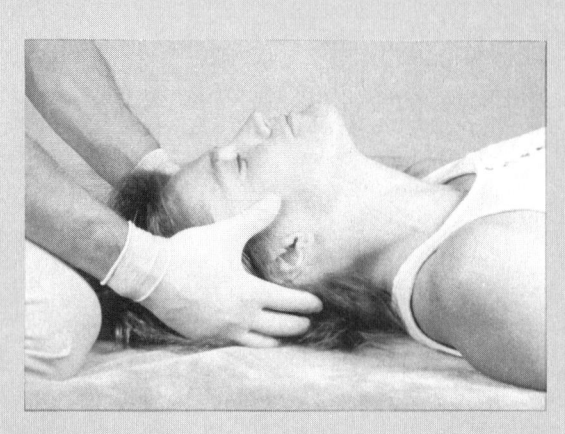

Activity 2.
Primary equipment.

Activity 4.
Position patient's head.

(continued)

SKILL 10–3
PHARYNGEO-TRACHEAL LUMEN AIRWAY (continued)

ACTIVITY	HOW PERFORMED	WHY PERFORMED
	If a cervical injury is suspected, however, keep the neck in a neutral position, neither flexed backward nor forward.	*Even moderate flexion may aggravate a cervical injury.*
5. Hyperventilate patient	With oropharyngeal or nasopharyngeal airway in place, patient should be hyperventilated with 100% O_2 (bag-valve-mask device or oxygen-powered demand valve) about 12 times in a 30-second period.	Hyperventilation before intubating lessens the detrimental effect of the short period of no ventilation while the intubation is performed.
Reventilate as needed	*Anytime the intubation procedure causes more than 30 seconds without ventilation, the procedure must be stopped and the patient hyperventilated for 30 to 60 seconds before intubation is reattempted.*	*After hyperventilation, delays in ventilation of more than 30 seconds risk worsening hypoxia and may jeopardize the patient.*
6. Insert PtL airway	Grasp the patient's tongue and lower jaw between the index finger and thumb and lift upward. Advance the tube gently along the natural curve of the upper airway until the bite block flange touches the patient's teeth (Activity 6).	Lifting the lower jaw opens the airway for easy passage of the tube.
	If tube does not advance easily, withdraw slightly, emphasize the jaw lift, and reattempt insertion.	*Difficult passage or resistance indicates the airway is somehow obstructed, probably by the tongue.*

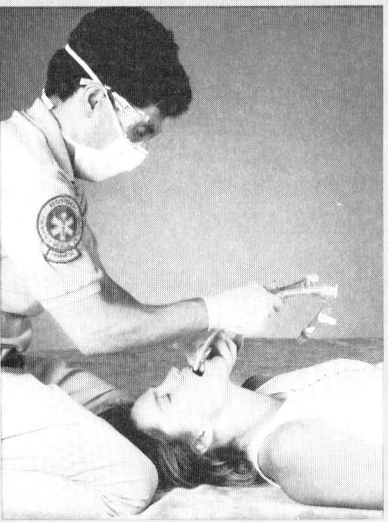

Activity 6.
Insert pharyngeo-tracheal lumen airway.

(continued)

SKILL 10-3
PHARYNGEO-TRACHEAL LUMEN AIRWAY (continued)

ACTIVITY	HOW PERFORMED	WHY PERFORMED
7. Stabilize the tube	Quickly place head strap around patient's head and attach velcro (Activity 7).	The strap prevents the tube from becoming dislodged during cuff inflation.

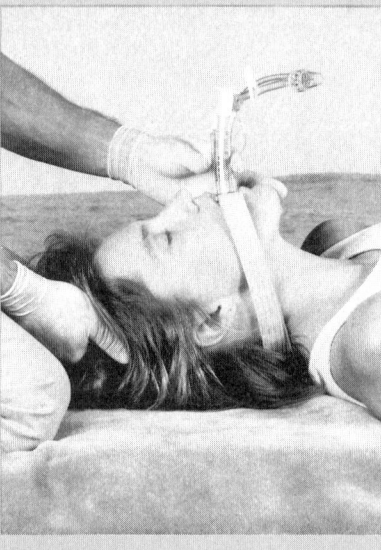

Activity 7.
Stabilize the tube.

8. Close white port cap	Push cap over opening under the #1 inflation valve (Activity 8).	Cap prevents air from escaping from the proximal and distal cuffs during and after cuff inflation.

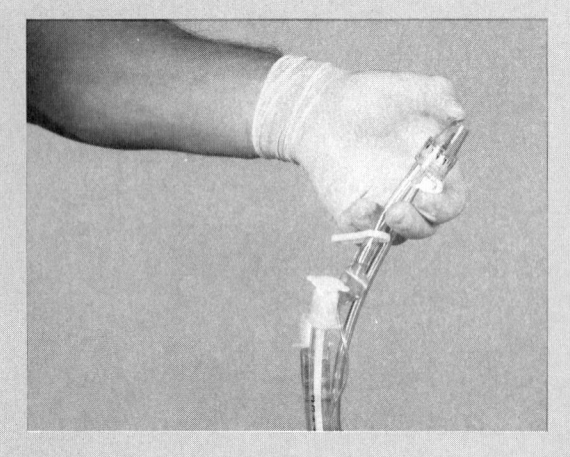

Activity 8.
Close white port cap.

9. Ventilate into the #1 inflation valve	Inflate proximal and distal cuffs simultaneously with a bag-valve-mask device or oxygen-powered demand valve attached to the #1 inflation valve (Activity 9).	Inflating both cuffs seals the oropharynx and the trachea or esophagus and allows effective ventilation.
	Inflate just until pilot balloon is firm. Secure slide clamp.	The pilot balloon indicates the inflation pressure in the cuffs.

(continued)

CHAPTER 10: Airway Management and Ventilation 159

SKILL 10-3
PHARYNGEO-TRACHEAL LUMEN AIRWAY (continued)

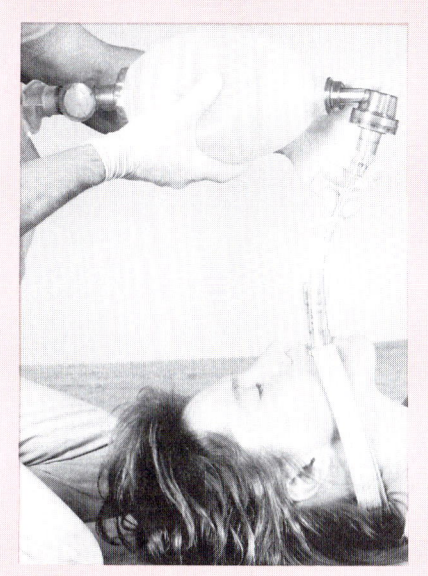

ACTIVITY	HOW PERFORMED	WHY PERFORMED
	Activity 9. Ventilate into the #1 inflation valve.	
10. Determine #3 long clear tube location	Ventilate through the #2 short green tube. Auscultate breath sounds bilaterally (Activity 10A). If breath sounds are present, continue ventilation through the #2 green tube. If no breath sounds are present, pull the stylet from the #3 long clear tube and attempt to ventilate through it (Activity 10B). If breath sounds are present, continue ventilation through the #3 long clear tube.	If breath sounds are heard while ventilating through the #2 short green tube, the #3 long clear tube is in the esophagus. If breath sounds are heard while ventilating through the #3 long clear tube, then the clear tube is in the trachea.

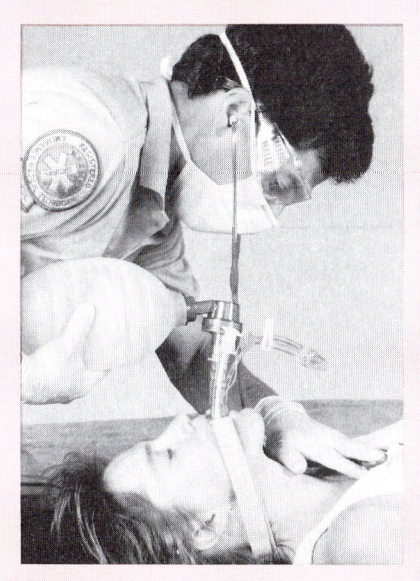

Activity 10A. Determine #3 long clear tube location; auscultate breath sounds.

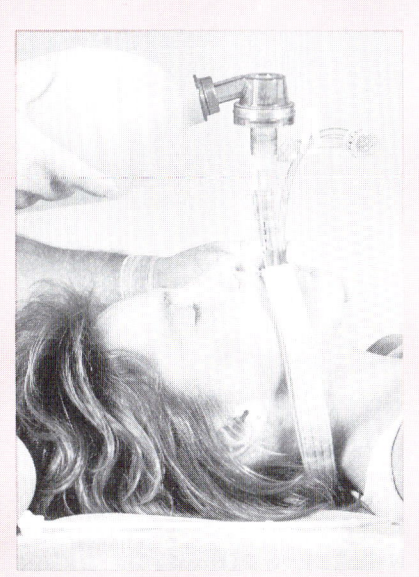

Activity 10B. Ventilate through #3 long clear tube.

(continued)

SKILL 10-3
PHARYNGEO-TRACHEAL LUMEN AIRWAY (continued)

ACTIVITY	HOW PERFORMED	WHY PERFORMED
11. Reassess breath sounds periodically and correct tube placement as indicated	Auscultate breath sounds bilaterally (Activity 11A) as well as over the stomach (Activity 11B).	The process of patient handling may displace the tube slightly.

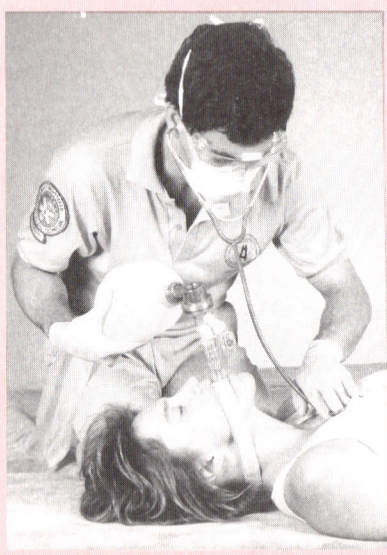

Activity 11A. Reassess breath sounds periodically; auscultate breath sounds bilaterally.

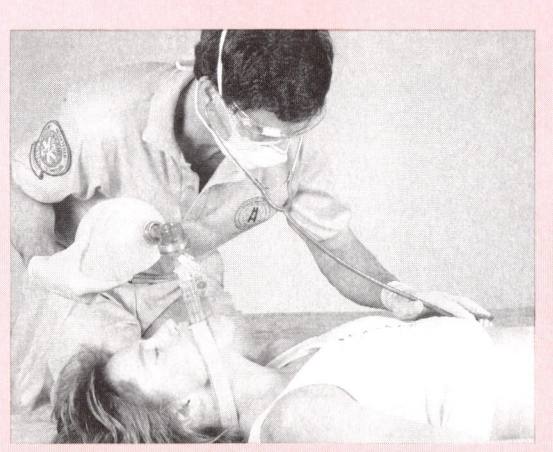

Activity 11B. Auscultate breath sounds over stomach.

---

consists of a large bore, cuffed tube of which the distal end is open. Both airways come with a mask that snaps onto the proximal end of the tube. Additional equipment required includes that for suction in case vomiting occurs and a 30 mL syringe to inflate the cuff on the airway.

Procedure. Placement of the esophageal obturator airway or esophageal gastric tube airway is a relatively simple process. Initially, the patient must be placed supine with the head in a neutral position. Ventilation should be instituted while the equipment is prepared. The paramedic should take personal protection by wearing protective eye wear, mask, and gloves. The esophageal obturator airway or esophageal gastric tube airway is checked for flaws, the mask is attached, and the cuff tested for leaks. The cuff on either airway is larger than that on an endotracheal tube; it should be tested by being inflated with 20 to 30 mL of air, then deflated. A nonpetroleum base lubricant should be applied to the tube and the suction turned on and placed near the patient's head with the tonsil tip attached. The procedure for the placement of the esophageal obturator airway and the esophageal gastric tube airway is shown in Skill 10-4.

Cricothyroidotomy

Cricothyroidotomy is an emergency airway technique that involves either a needle puncture (for translaryngeal jet ventilation) or a surgical incision through the cricothyroid membrane in the anterior larynx. Technically, insertion of a needle into the cricothyroid membrane is called a cricothyroid membrane puncture, while cricothyroidotomy is an incision, with a surgical knife, of the membrane. Cricothyroidotomy is used here in either context. Cricothyroidotomy is a last-resort technique in the prehospital setting, reserved for life-threatening situations in which no other technique can establish an airway.

Indications for cricothyroidotomy include the following:

- Complete airway obstruction that cannot be removed by abdominal thrusts or direct visualization with a laryngoscope

(text continues on page 164)

CHAPTER 10: Airway Management and Ventilation

SKILL 10-4
ESOPHAGEAL OBTURATOR AIRWAY AND ESOPHAGEAL GASTRIC TUBE AIRWAY

ACTIVITY	HOW PERFORMED	WHY PERFORMED
1. Check: • Responsiveness • Airway • Breathing • Circulation	Establish responsiveness Stabilize neck, open the airway Assess breathing Check for a pulse Check for hemorrhage	The primary survey is a rapid evaluation, less than 45 seconds, to identify and correct any life-threatening problems.
2. Assemble and check: Primary equipment: • Esophageal obturator airway (EOA) (Activity 2A) or esophageal gastric tube airway (EGTA) (Activity 2B) • 35 mL syringe	Attach face mask to tube. Lubricate the distal end of the tube. Have suction unit ready.	Intubation must be accomplished rapidly. Having all equipment prechecked and ready reduces time delays during the procedure.

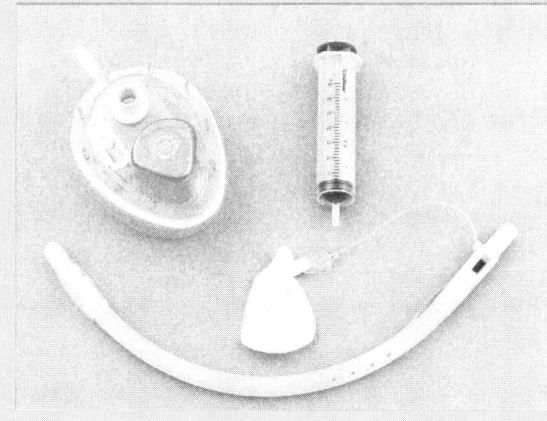

Activity 2A.
Primary equipment: Esophageal obturator airway (EOA).

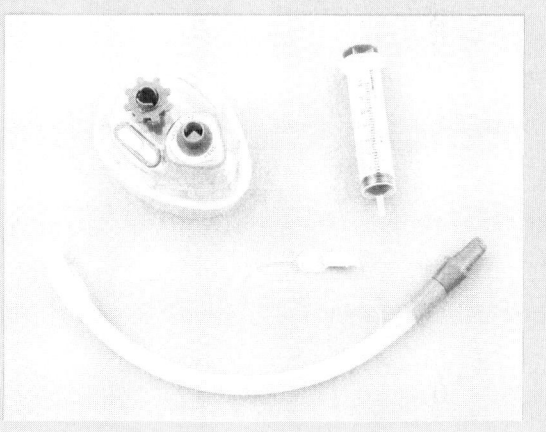

Activity 2B.
Primary equipment: Esophageal gastric tube airway (EGTA).

Accessory equipment and supplies: • Water soluble lubricant • Suction unit • Suction catheter • Bag-valve-mask device • Oxygen • Stethoscope • Protective eye wear • Mask • Gloves	Put on protective eye wear, mask, and gloves.	To prevent blood or body fluid contact with nonintact skin or mucous membranes.
3. Remove potential airway obstructions	Remove the patient's dental bridgework and plates or broken teeth.	May interfere with insertion of EOA/EGTA and cause airway obstruction. Obstructions cannot be removed easily from the patient once intubated.

(continued)

SKILL 10-4
ESOPHAGEAL OBTURATOR AIRWAY AND ESOPHAGEAL GASTRIC TUBE AIRWAY (continued)

ACTIVITY	HOW PERFORMED	WHY PERFORMED
4. Position patient's head	Keep neck in a neutral position, neither flexed backward nor forward (Activity 4).	This position allows for easy insertion of the EOA or EGTA without movement of the cervical spine.

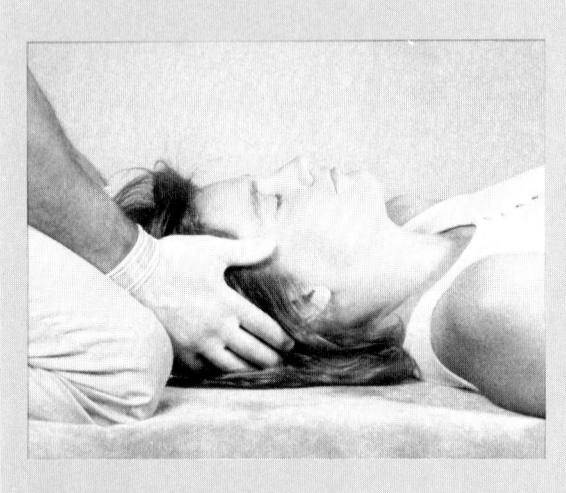

Activity 4.
Position patient's head.

5. Hyperventilate patient	With oropharyngeal or nasopharyngeal airway in place, patient should be hyperventilated with 100% O_2 (bag-valve-mask device or oxygen-powered demand valve) about 12 times in a 30-second period	Hyperventilation before intubating lessens the detrimental effect of the short period of no ventilation while the intubation is performed.
Reventilate as needed	*Anytime the intubation procedure causes more than 30 seconds without ventilation, the procedure must be stopped and the patient hyperventilated for 30 to 60 seconds before intubation is reattempted.*	*After hyperventilation, delays in ventilation of more than 30 seconds risk worsening hypoxia and may jeopardize the patient.*
6. Insert EOA or EGTA	Grasp the patient's tongue and lower jaw between the index finger and thumb and lift upward. Advance the tube gently along the natural curve of the upper airway until the face mask touches the patient's face (Activity 6). If the tube does not advance easily, withdraw slightly, emphasize the jaw lift, and reattempt insertion.	Lifting the lower jaw opens the airway for easy passage of the tube. Difficult passage or resistance indicates that the airway is somehow obstructed, probably by the tongue.

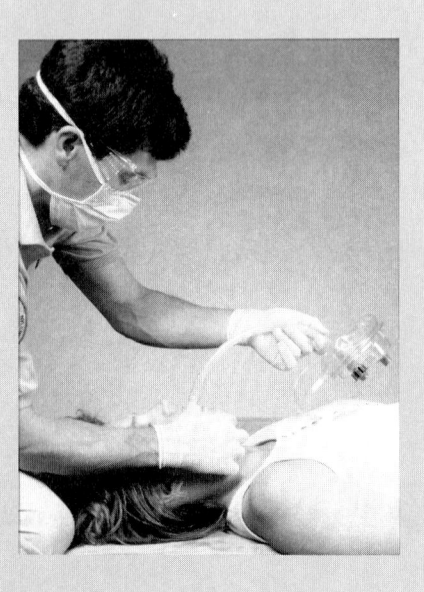

Activity 6.
Insert EOA or EGTA.

(continued)

SKILL 10-4
ESOPHAGEAL OBTURATOR AIRWAY AND ESOPHAGEAL GASTRIC TUBE AIRWAY (continued)

ACTIVITY	HOW PERFORMED	WHY PERFORMED
7. Determine tube position	Seal face mask on the patient's face and ventilate with bag-valve-mask device or oxygen-powered demand valve (Activity 7A).	A good seal prevents leakage of air around the face mask.
	Auscultate breath sounds bilaterally (Activity 7B) and over the stomach (Activity 7C). If sounds are heard over the stomach, immediately remove the tube and hyperventilate the patient before reattempting intubation.	Sounds over the stomach indicate the tube may be in the trachea.

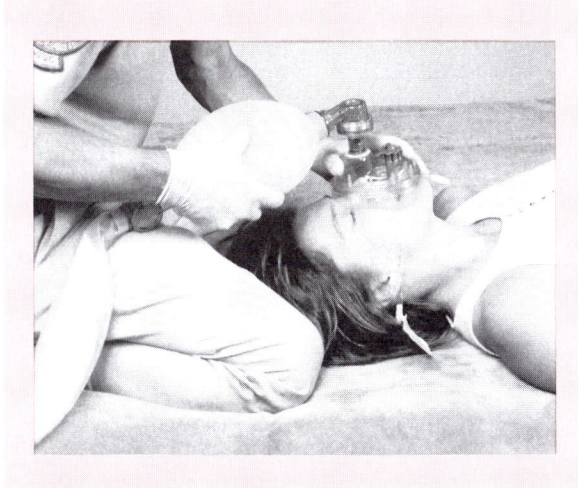

Activity 7A.
Seal face mask on patient's face and ventilate.

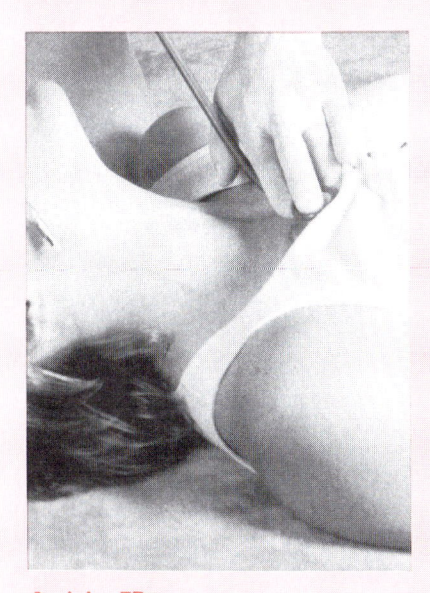

Activity 7B.
Auscultate breath sounds bilaterally.

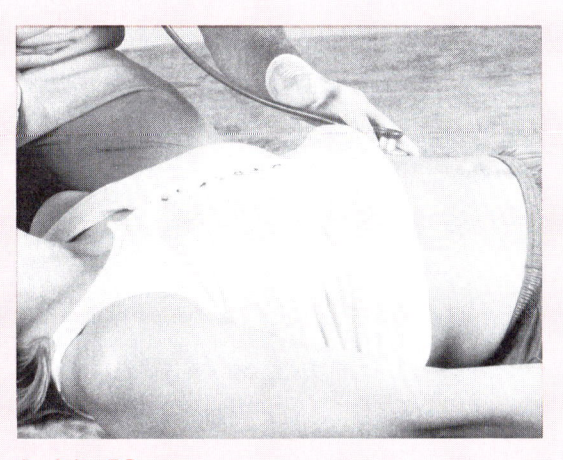

Activity 7C.
Auscultate breath sounds over the stomach.

(continued)

SKILL 10-4
ESOPHAGEAL OBTURATOR AIRWAY AND ESOPHAGEAL GASTRIC TUBE AIRWAY (continued)

ACTIVITY	HOW PERFORMED	WHY PERFORMED
	If sounds are heard only in both lungs, inflate the tube cuff with 30 to 35 mL of air using the syringe (Activity 7D). Feel the pilot balloon for tautness.	Breath sounds in the lungs indicate the tube is in the esophagus and the cuff may be inflated to seal the esophagus.

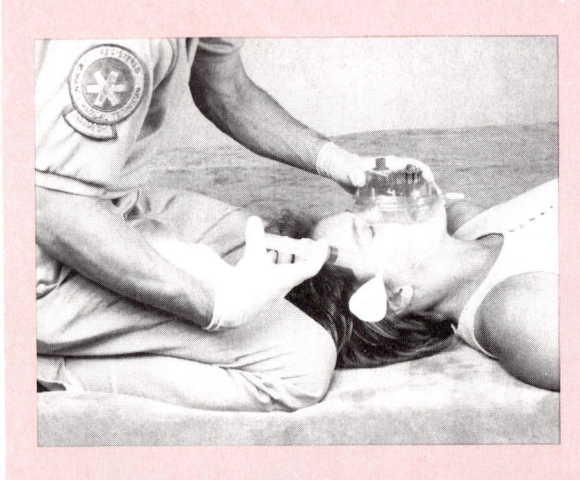

Activity 7D. Inflate tube cuff using syringe.

8. Reassess breath sounds periodically and correct tube placement as indicated	Auscultate breath sounds bilaterally as well as over the stomach.	The process of patient handling may displace the tube slightly.

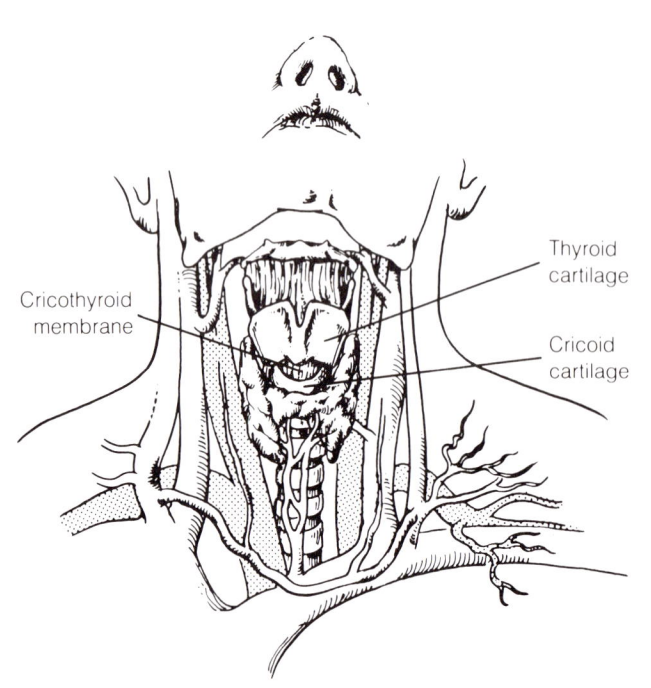

FIGURE 10-37.
Landmarks for locating the cricothyroid membrane.

- Facial or upper airway trauma, hemorrhage, or swelling so severe as to make intubation or other airway techniques impossible

The cricothyroid membrane lies in the anterior larynx below the thyroid cartilage (Adam's apple) and above the cricoid cartilage (Fig. 10-37). The membrane may be readily found by running the tip of the finger down the midline of the thyroid cartilage until a slightly softer depression is felt that is just about the size of a fingertip. That soft depression is the cricothyroid membrane.

The cricothyroid membrane is a good location for emergency airway access for several reasons:

1. The landmark is fairly easy to locate in most patients.
2. The skin over the membrane is relatively avascular, so needle insertion or a surgical incision may be performed with minimal blood loss.
3. A needle or incision through the membrane accesses the larynx just below the level of the vocal cords, which is often the site of airway obstruction.
4. The use of the cricothyroid membrane avoids damage to the area usually used for a long-term tracheostomy,

(text continues on page 169)

CHAPTER 10: Airway Management and Ventilation 165

SKILL 10–5
SURGICAL CRICOTHYROIDOTOMY

ACTIVITY	HOW PERFORMED	WHY PERFORMED
1. Check: • Responsiveness • Airway • Breathing • Circulation	Establish responsiveness Stabilize neck, open the airway Assess breathing Check for a pulse Check for hemorrhage	The primary survey is a rapid evaluation, less than 45 seconds, to identify and correct any life-threatening problems.
2. Assemble and check: Primary equipment (Activity 2): • #10 Scalpel blade and handle • 5.0 mm or 6.0 mm endotracheal (ET) tube • 10 mL syringe • Hemostat Accessory equipment and supplies: • Sterile gauze pads • Antiseptic swabs • Suction unit • Suction catheter • Bag-valve-mask device • Oxygen • Stethoscope • Tape • Protective eye wear • Mask • Sterile gloves	Prepare scalpel and blade, maintaining sterility. Place scalpel, hemostat, gauze squares, and ET tube within easy reach. Put on protective eye wear, mask, and sterile gloves.	Cricothyroidotomy must be accomplished rapidly. Having all equipment prepared and ready reduces time delays during the procedure. To prevent blood or body fluid contact with nonintact skin or mucous membranes.

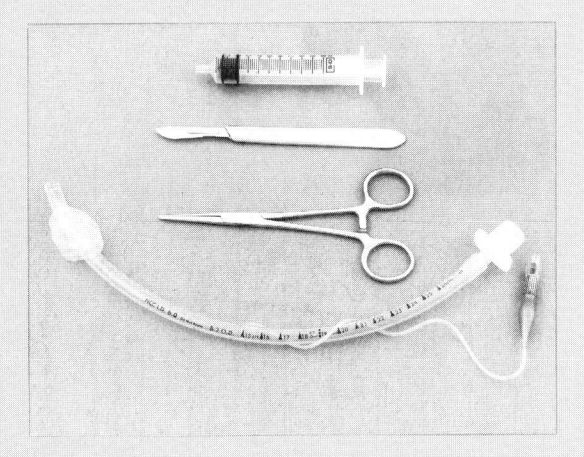

Activity 2.
Primary equipment.

3. Position patient	Position patient supine with neck in a neutral, midline position (Activity 3).	The neutral position with no rotation of the neck allows easier identification of landmarks and stabilization of the trachea during the procedure.

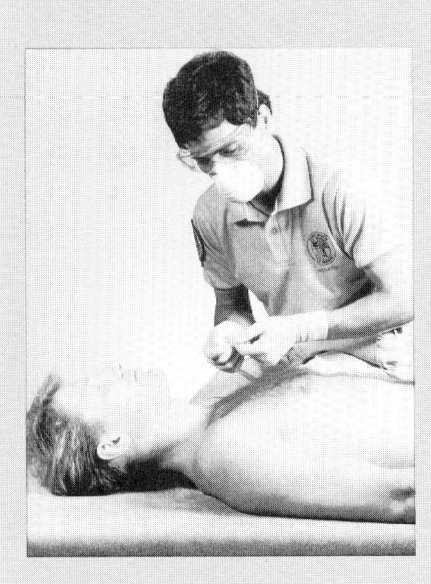

Activity 3.
Position patient with neck in a neutral, midline position.

(*continued*)

SKILL 10-5
SURGICAL CRICOTHYROIDOTOMY (continued)

ACTIVITY	HOW PERFORMED	WHY PERFORMED
4. Hyperventilate patient	If any ability to ventilate the patient exists, hyperventilate with 100% O_2 (bag-valve-mask device or oxygen-powered demand valve) about 12 times in a 30-second period.	Hyperventilation lessens the detrimental effect of the short period of no ventilation while cricothyroidotomy is performed.
5. Prepare the area	Cleanse the anterior neck with antiseptic swabs (Activity 5).	Cleaning the area helps minimize the possibility of infection.

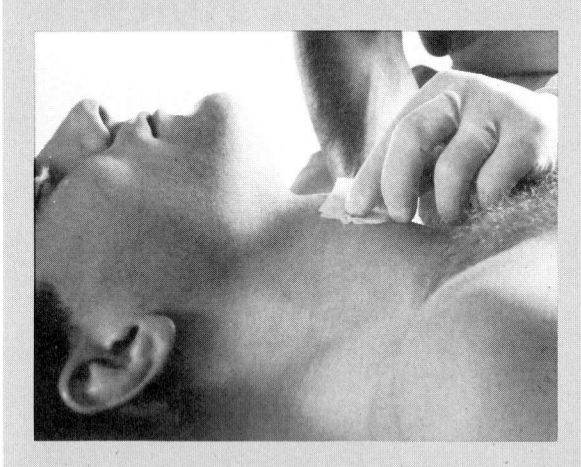

Activity 5.
Prepare the area.

6. Locate the cricothyroid membrane	Place the index finger of the nondominant hand on the patient's thyroid cartilage (Adam's apple) (Activity 6A) and run the tip of the finger down the midline until the soft depression of the cricothyroid membrane is felt between the thyroid and cricoid cartilages (Activity 6B). Keep the index finger in place on the cricothyroid membrane to positively mark the location.	Accurate location of the cricothyroid membrane is essential for the success of cricothyroidotomy.

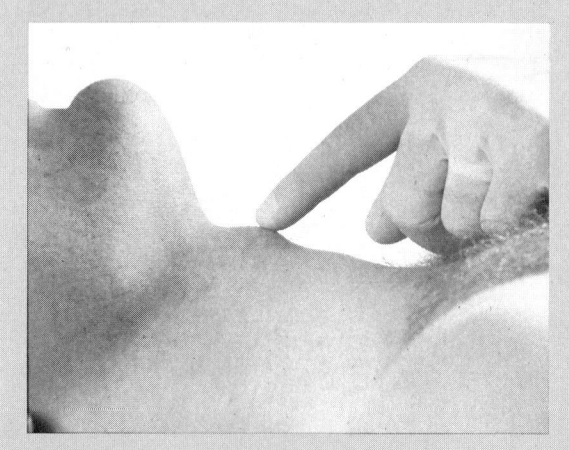

Activity 6A.
Locate cricothyroid membrane—start at thyroid cartilage.

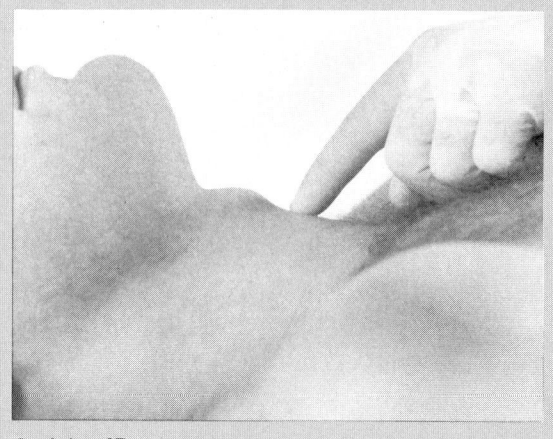

Activity 6B.
Run tip of finger down to soft depression between thyroid and cricoid cartilages.

(continued)

SKILL 10–5
SURGICAL CRICOTHYROIDOTOMY (continued)

ACTIVITY	HOW PERFORMED	WHY PERFORMED
7. Perform incision	With the index finger in place on the cricothyroid membrane, use the thumb and middle finger of the same hand to stabilize each side of the trachea from lateral movement. Move the tip of the index finger just enough to place the point of the scalpel directly over the cricothyroid membrane (Activity 7A). Holding the scalpel perpendicular to the neck, make a horizontal stab incision through the cricothyroid membrane—about 1 cm (Activity 7B). Do not withdraw the scalpel.	A single, horizontal stab incision reduces chance of damage to blood vessels lateral to the cricothyroid membrane.
	Rotate the scalpel 90° to slightly widen the opening of the incision.	Once entry into the trachea is accomplished, it must be maintained by holding the scalpel in position. Withdrawing the scalpel would allow the mobile skin of the neck to move over the incision, requiring a second incision. Rotating the scalpel widens the opening just enough to insert the hemostat.

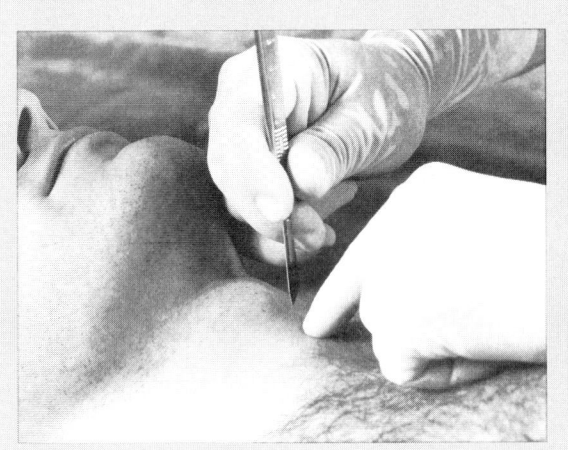

Activity 7A.
Perform incision; place tip of scalpel directly over cricothyroid membrane.

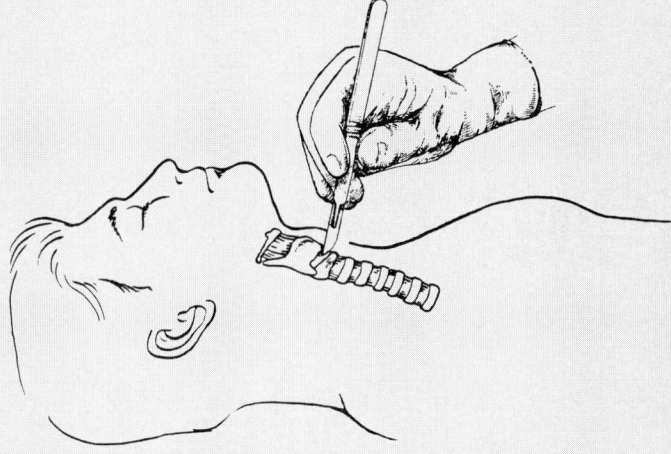

Activity 7B.
With scalpel perpendicular to neck, make a horizontal stab incision through cricothyroid membrane.

8. Insert hemostat	With the nondominant hand, grasp the curved hemostat with the jaws closed, and insert the tip of the hemostat into the trachea, through the small opening beside the scalpel (Activity 8). Open the jaws of the hemostat widely to create a workable opening into the trachea. Hold the hemostat jaws firmly open. Remove the scalpel.	The hemostat widens the opening as well as provides a secure "hold" on the trachea to allow easy insertion of the ET tube.

(continued)

SKILL 10-5
SURGICAL CRICOTHYROIDOTOMY (continued)

ACTIVITY	HOW PERFORMED	WHY PERFORMED

Activity 8.
Insert tip of hemostat into trachea, through small opening beside the scalpel.

9. Insert ET tube

Insert the ET tube between the jaws of the hemostat, directing the tip down the trachea (Activity 9). Insert just far enough for the cuff to be completely in the trachea.
When the ET tube is placed, inflate the cuff and remove the hemostat.

Inserting just far enough for the cuff to enter the trachea keeps the end of the ET tube above the bifurcation of the trachea and ensures full ventilation of both lungs.
Inflating the cuff secures the ET tube and protects the trachea from blood and other foreign material.

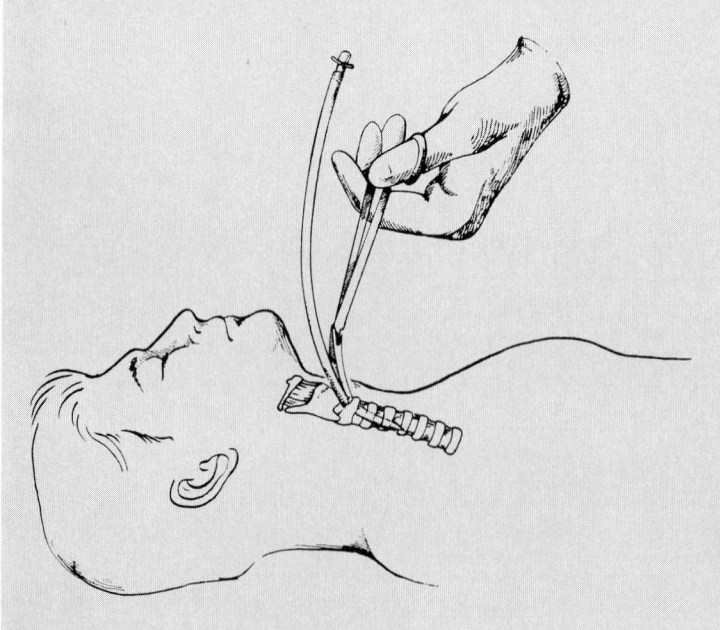

Activity 9.
Insert ET tube between jaws of hemostat, directing tip down the trachea.

(continued)

CHAPTER 10: Airway Management and Ventilation 169

SKILL 10-5
SURGICAL CRICOTHYROIDOTOMY (continued)

ACTIVITY	HOW PERFORMED	WHY PERFORMED
10. Ventilate patient	Ventilate patient with 100% O_2 (bag-valve-mask device or oxygen-powered demand valve). Observe chest expansion and auscultate breath sounds bilaterally. If breath sounds are absent or unequal check and correct placement of ET tube as needed.	Verifying proper ET tube placement is essential to ensure proper ventilation and to rapidly detect misplacement.
11. Stabilize ET tube	Control any bleeding with direct pressure. Place sterile gauze around incision and secure ET tube with tape (Activity 11).	Excess bleeding should be controlled to minimize chance of aspiration, and the ET tube must be secured to prevent accidental extubation during transport and other procedures.
12. Dispose of scalpel blade	Place contaminated blade in proper container.	Eliminates the possibility of injury or infection by contact with the contaminated blade.

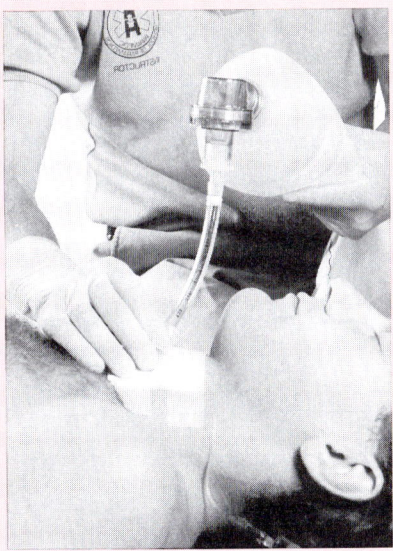

Activity 11.
Place sterile gauze around incision and secure tube with tape.

---

which lies a few centimeters farther down the trachea.

In spite of the factors above, the cricothyroidotomy technique may be severely complicated by a number of potential hazards:

- Misplacement of the puncture or incision
- Damage to nearby large blood vessels, causing severe hemorrhage
- Damage to the soft posterior tracheal wall and possible esophageal perforation
- Subcutaneous emphysema

The primary contraindication to cricothyroidotomy is if an airway can be opened and maintained by any other means. The potential risks of cricothyroidotomy are too great to accept if any other alternative is available.

As mentioned previously, cricothyroidotomy may be performed with a simple needle puncture and placement of a large-bore, over-the-needle catheter into the trachea or with a surgical incision and placement of a small cuffed endotracheal tube (usually size 5 or 5.5 mm) into the trachea.

The surgical placement of an endotracheal tube is usually preferred because it allows much greater volume ventilation than does a large-bore intravenous catheter. The over-the-needle catheter method, however, is somewhat safer and easier to perform. Because of the smaller airway

(text continues on page 173)

SKILL 10–6
TRANSLARYNGEAL JET VENTILATION

ACTIVITY	HOW PERFORMED	WHY PERFORMED
1. Check: • Responsiveness • Airway • Breathing • Circulation	Establish responsiveness Stabilize neck, open the airway Assess breathing Check for a pulse Check for hemorrhage	The primary survey is a rapid evaluation, less than 45 seconds, to identify and correct any life-threatening problems.
2. Assemble and check: Primary equipment (Activity 2): • 12 or 14 gauge over-the-needle catheter Accessory equipment and supplies: • Antiseptic swabs • Suction unit • Suction catheter • Jet ventilator • Oxygen • Stethoscope • Tape • Protective eye wear • Mask • Sterile gloves	Place over-the-needle catheter, swabs, jet ventilator, and other equipment in easy reach. Put on protective eye wear, mask, and sterile gloves.	Translaryngeal jet ventilation must be accomplished rapidly. Having all equipment prepared and ready reduces time delays during the procedure. To prevent blood or body fluid contact with nonintact skin or mucous membranes.

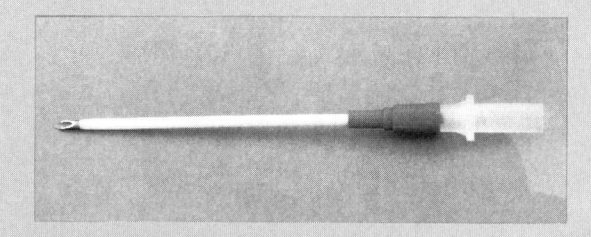

Activity 2. Primary equipment.

3. Position patient	Position patient supine with neck in a neutral, midline position (Activity 3).	The neutral position with no rotation of the neck allows easier identification of landmarks and stabilization of the trachea during the procedure.

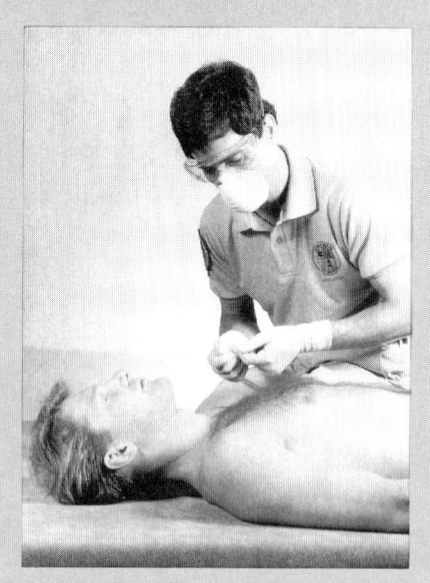

Activity 3. Position patient supine, with neck in neutral, midline position.

4. Hyperventilate patient	If any ability to ventilate the patient exists, hyperventilate with 100% O_2 several times.	Hyperventilation reduces the detrimental effect of the period of no ventilation while the procedure is performed.

(continued)

SKILL 10-6
TRANSLARYNGEAL JET VENTILATION (continued)

ACTIVITY	HOW PERFORMED	WHY PERFORMED
5. Prepare the area	Cleanse the anterior neck with antiseptic swabs (Activity 5).	Cleaning the area helps minimize the possibility of infection.

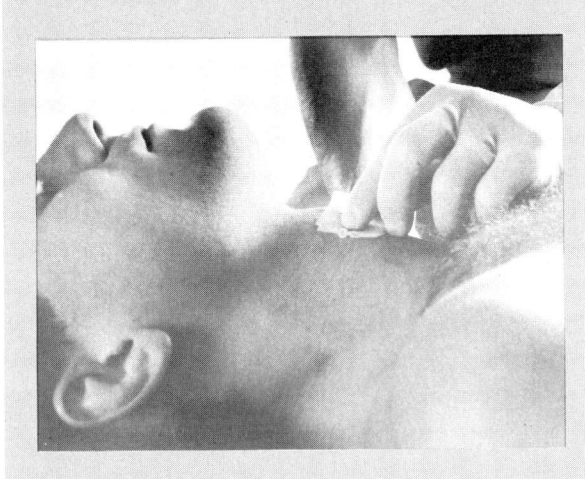

Activity 5.
Prepare the area.

6. Locate the cricothyroid membrane	Place the index finger of the nondominant hand on the patient's thyroid cartilage (Adam's apple) (Activity 6A) and run the tip of the finger down the midline until the soft depression of the cricothyroid membrane is felt between the thyroid and cricoid cartilages (Activity 6B). Keep the index finger in place on the cricothyroid membrane to positively mark the location.	Accurate location of the cricothyroid membrane is essential for the success of the procedure.

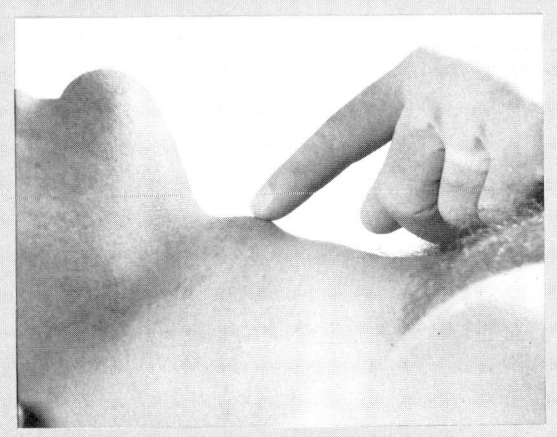

Activity 6A.
Locate cricothyroid membrane—start at thyroid cartilage.

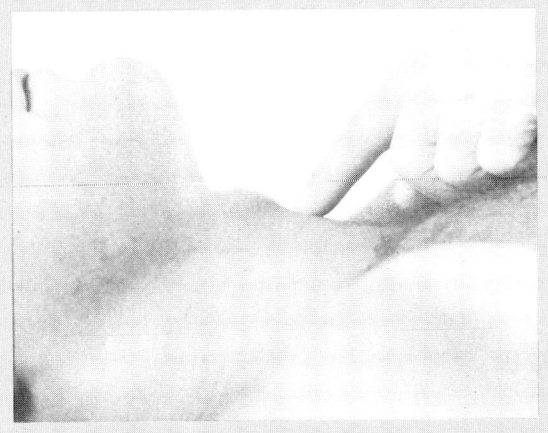

Activity 6B.
Run finger down to soft depression between thyroid and cricoid cartilage.

(continued)

UNIT TWO: FOUNDATIONS OF EMERGENCY CARE

SKILL 10-6
TRANSLARYNGEAL JET VENTILATION (continued)

ACTIVITY	HOW PERFORMED	WHY PERFORMED
7. Insert the needle	With the index finger in place on the cricothyroid membrane, use the thumb and middle finger of the same hand to stabilize the trachea from lateral movement. Move the tip of the index finger just enough to place the point of the needle directly over the cricothyroid membrane.	
	Angle the needle about 45° pointing toward the patient's feet (Activity 7). Advance the needle through the cricothyroid membrane while aspirating the syringe. Aspiration of air indicates entry into the trachea.	The angle toward the patient's feet directs the needle down the trachea.
	Stop advancing the needle as soon as air is aspirated.	Stopping as soon as air is aspirated prevents damage or puncture of the posterior tracheal wall.

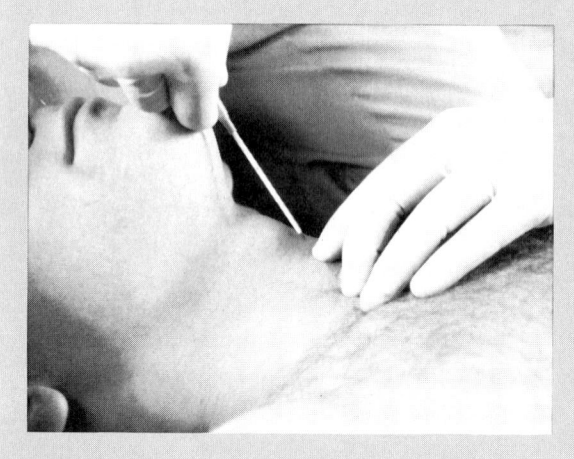

Activity 7.
Insert needle.

8. Advance catheter	Advance the catheter over the needle, placing the catheter well into the trachea and angled downward (Activity 8). Withdraw the needle.	Placement of the catheter allows safe ventilation with the jet ventilator.

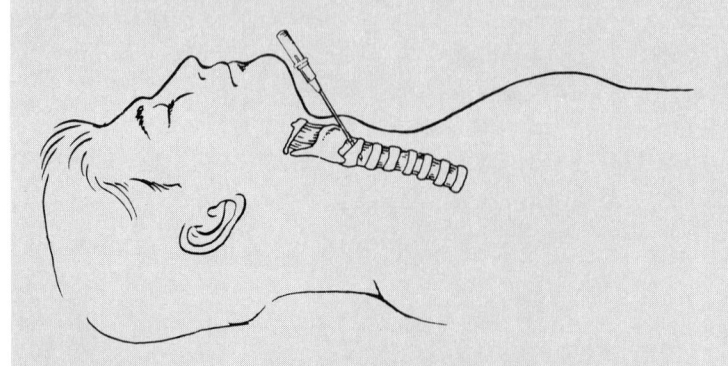

Activity 8.
Advance catheter.

(continued)

SKILL 10-6
TRANSLARYNGEAL JET VENTILATION (continued)

ACTIVITY	HOW PERFORMED	WHY PERFORMED
9. Ventilate patient	Attach the jet ventilator to the catheter and ventilate (Activity 9).	Ventilation through a catheter requires substantial pressure (40–60 psi) to move a significant volume of air. This fact necessitates the use of a jet ventilation device. Bag-valve-mask devices and oxygen-powered demand valves do not permit generation of adequate pressures.
	Carefully observe for chest expansion and auscultate the chest bilaterally.	The minimal tidal volume may make chest expansion and breath sounds difficult to verify.
10. Stabilize the catheter	Use tape to secure the catheter to the neck (Activity 10).	This action secures the catheter to help prevent accidental dislodging of the catheter.
11. Dispose of needle	Place contaminated needle in proper container.	Eliminates the possibility of injury or infection by contact with the contaminated needle.

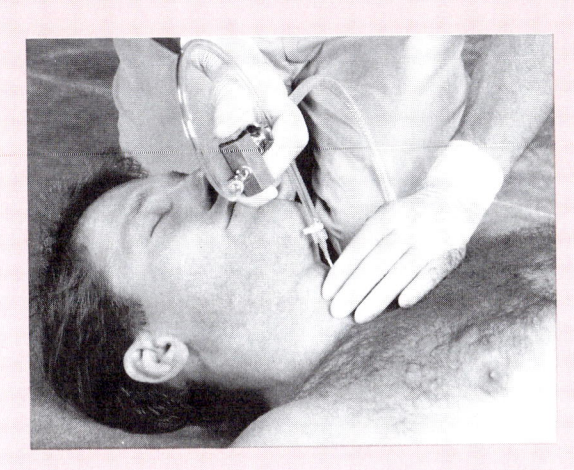

Activity 9. Ventilate patient.

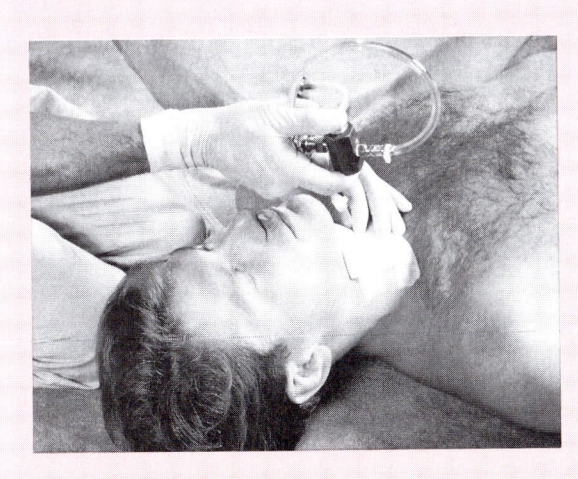

Activity 10. Stabilize the catheter.

---

structures in children, only the over-the-needle catheter method is used in patients younger than age 16.

SURGICAL CRICOTHYROIDOTOMY. Equipment for performing a **surgical cricothyroidotomy** includes a #11 scalpel, a curved hemostat, and a small cuffed endotracheal tube, usually size 5 or 5.5 mm. Sterile gauze squares, antiseptic prep swabs, a syringe to inflate the endotracheal tube cuff, tape, and a bag-valve-mask device with supplemental oxygen are also needed.

Contact with blood and body fluids while performing a cricothyroidotomy calls for appropriate precautions for the paramedic, including protective eye wear, mask, and sterile gloves.

Several surgical techniques for performing a cricothyroidotomy may be used, depending on local protocols and preference. Perhaps the simplest technique to learn and the easiest to perform reliably after minimal practice involves a single stab incision through the cricothyroid membrane, rotation of the scalpel, and insertion of the hemostat to dilate the opening, followed by immediate insertion of the endotracheal tube. This technique often can be successfully completed by paramedic students within 30 to 45 seconds on the first attempt. The procedure for surgical cricothyroidotomy is shown in Skill 10-5.

TRANSLARYNGEAL JET VENTILATION. Equipment for performing **translaryngeal jet ventilation** (*needle cricothyroidotomy*) includes a large-bore, over-the-needle catheter (usually 10, 12, or 14 gauge for adults or 14–16 gauge for children), 10 mL syringe, and a jet ventilation device. Sterile gauze squares, antiseptic swabs, and tape to secure the catheter are also needed. Contact with blood and body fluids while performing this procedure calls for appropriate precautions, including protective eye wear, mask, and sterile gloves.

It must be emphasized that adequate ventilation through a needle in the cricothyroid membrane can be accomplished only with a high-pressure oxygen source (30–50 psi). Compact equipment, including a pressure-regulating valve, pressure gauge, manually operated valve, and high-pressure tubing, is available for this purpose. Bag-valve-mask devices and oxygen-powered ventilators are inadequate for this ventilating function. They do not generate sufficient pressure when 12 or 14 gauge needles are being used. A disadvantage of this high-pressure system is that, while it can provide oxygenation, it does not allow for the efficient elimination of carbon dioxide. The procedure for translaryngeal jet ventilation is shown in Skill 10-6.

SUMMARY

Maintaining a patent airway and assuring adequate ventilation are two of the most important duties of the paramedic. They require a skilled paramedic to make the rapid, accurate assessment that is needed to insure that the vital supply of oxygen to the patient's tissues is not interrupted. However, assessment skills are not enough; the paramedic must also be proficient in the various procedures required to maintain and protect the airway. In conjunction with an appropriate assessment, the airway techniques described in this chapter are some of the most powerful life-saving tools at the paramedic's disposal.

Paramedics must be well versed in airway anatomy and the physiology of respiration. They must be able to identify the various forms of airway compromise quickly and accurately and choose the correct intervention. They must then carry out that intervention with all of the skill that their training affords them. To do any less could be fatal to the patient.

SUGGESTED READING

American Heart Association: Textbook of Advanced Cardiac Life Support, 2nd ed. Dallas, American Heart Association, 1987

Bivins G, Ford S, Bezmalinovic Z, Price H, Williams JL: The effect of axial traction during orotracheal intubation of the trauma victim with an unstable cervical spine. Ann Emerg Med 17:25, 1988

Bodai BI, Walton CB, Briggs S, Goldstein M: A clinical evaluation of an oxygen insufflation/suction catheter. Heart Lung 16:39, 1987

Finucane BT, Santora AH: Principles of Airway Management. Philadelphia, FA Davis, 1988

Frass M, Frenzer R, Rauscha F et al: Ventilation with the esophageal tracheal combitube in cardiopulmonary resuscitation. Chest 93:781, 1988

Janson-Bjerklie S, Carrieri VK, Hudes M: The sensations of pulmonary dyspnea. Nurs Res 35:154, 1986

Kleiber C, Kreuzfield N, Rose EF: Acute histologic changes in the tracheobronchial tree associated with different suction catheter insertion techniques. Heart Lung 17:10, 1988

Little CM, Parker MG, Tarnopolsky R: The incidence of vasculature at risk during cricothyrotomy. Ann Emerg Med 15:805, 1986

Rund DA: Airway management. Emerg Med Serv 19(1):19, 1990

Spaite DW, Joseph M: Prehospital cricothyrotomy: An investigation of indications, technique, complications, and patient outcome. Ann Emerg Med 19:279, 1990

Taggart JA, Dorinsky NL, Sheahan JS: Airway pressures during closed system suctioning. Heart Lung 17:536, 1988

US Department of Transportation, National Highway Traffic Safety Administration: Emergency Medical Technician-Paramedic: National Standards Curriculum. Washington, DC, US Government Printing Office, 1985

Yearly DM, Stewart RD, Kaplan RM: Myths and pitfalls in emergency translaryngeal ventilation: Correcting misimpressions. Ann Emerg Med 17:690, 1988

CHAPTER 11

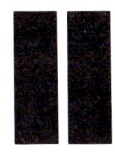

Pathophysiology of Shock and Fluid Management

Pathophysiology of Shock
  Heart
  Blood Vessels
  Fluid
    Diffusion
    Osmosis
    Active Transport
    Osmotic Pressure
    Fluid and Electrolytes
    Blood and its Components
      Blood Typing
      Blood Preparations and Substitutes
  Acid-base Balance
    Compensation Mechanisms
      Buffer Systems
      Respiration
      Kidney Function
    Clinical Abnormalities of Acid-base Balance
      Respiratory Acidosis
      Respiratory Alkalosis
      Metabolic Acidosis
      Metabolic Alkalosis
    Management of Acid-base States

Pressure Changes
Stages of Shock
  Compensated Shock
  Uncompensated Shock
  Irreversible Shock
    Cellular Pathophysiology
      Ischemic Phase
      Stagnant Phase
      Washout Phase
      Staged Death
Assessment of the Patient in Shock
  Primary Survey
    Responsiveness
    Airway
    Perfusion
      Pulse
      Skin Color
      Skin Temperature
      Capillary Refill

Secondary Survey
  Level of Consciousness
  Blood Pressure
Management
  Resuscitation
    Perfusion
      Pneumatic Anti-shock Garment
  Skill 11-1. Pneumatic Anti-shock Garment
    Intravenous Fluids
      Intravenous Access
      Fluid Replacement
      Medication
Summary

BEHAVIORAL OBJECTIVES
On successful completion of this chapter, the reader will be able to:

1. Describe the relationship of the heart, the blood vessels, and fluid in the pathophysiology of shock
2. Explain the process of diffusion, osmosis, and active transport
3. Describe the process of osmotic pressure
4. Define isotonic, hypertonic, and hypotonic solutions and list the intravenous fluids for each
5. Describe the function of blood and its components

(continued)

BEHAVIORAL OBJECTIVES (continued)

6. Describe the four types of blood
7. Explain the importance and function of acid-base balance in the body
8. Describe the four clinical abnormalities of acid-base balance and the management of each
9. Describe the four stages of shock on the cellular level
10. Explain the overall assessment and management of the patient in shock
11. Discuss the indications and contraindications for use of the pneumatic anti-shock garment
12. Given the proper equipment, demonstrate the procedure for applying the pneumatic anti-shock garment to a patient
13. Describe the use of intravenous fluids in a patient in shock
14. Define all of the key terms listed in this chapter

KEY TERMS
The following terms are defined in the chapter and glossary:

acid	*cardiac output*	*hydrostatic pressure*	*osmosis*	*respiratory alkalosis*
active transport	*cations*	*hypertonic*	*osmotic pressure*	*semipermeable membrane*
aerobic	*diffusion*	*hypotonic*	*peripheral vascular resistance*	
anaerobic	*edema*	*interstitial*		*shock—compensated, uncompensated, irreversible*
antibody	*electrolytes*	*intracellular*	*pH*	
antigen	*erythrocytes*	*intravascular*	*plasma*	*sickle cell anemia*
anions	*extracellular*	*isotonic*	*platelets*	*sodium*
base	*extravascular*	*leukocytes*	*pneumatic anti-shock garment (PASG)*	*stroke volume*
blood	*Fick principle*	*lymphocyte*		*systemic vascular resistance*
buffer	*hematocrit*	*metabolic acidosis*	*potassium*	
capillary refill test	*hemoglobin*	*metabolic alkalosis*	*respiratory acidosis*	

Shock, reduced to its simplest common denominator is a lack of tissue oxygenation of the individual cell, leading to a change from **aerobic** (with oxygen) to **anaerobic** (without oxygen) metabolism within the cell. The cells of the body still have the ability to continue to make energy, although significantly less, by switching from the use of oxygen as a nutritional source to the use of other materials. An understanding of the complicated Krebs cycle, which describes that change and the basis of it, is not required to appreciate and manage the problems of shock. The important fact is that oxygen is good; lack of oxygen is bad. This fact pertains to all tissue in the body, not just those, such as the heart and the brain, that receive publicity because of their more immediate and obvious response to lack of oxygenation, but also the intestines, kidneys, and skin.

The Fick principle accurately defines this metabolic change. The **Fick principle** describes shock as anaerobic metabolism at the cellular level; in other words, shock is prevented by maintaining aerobic metabolism. Aerobic metabolism is maintained by providing the cells of the tissue with adequate oxygen. The Fick principle has three components:

- On-loading of oxygen by red blood cells in the lung
- Delivery of oxygenated red blood cells to the tissue cells
- Off-loading of oxygen by the red blood cells at the cellular level

This principle presumes, however, that enough red blood cells are present in the system to deliver oxygen. Replacing an acute loss of red cell mass that occurs in hemorrhage with lactated Ringer's solution (or other crystalloid, non-oxygen-carrying solution) dilutes the red cells to the point that, although they can be oxygenated well, they cannot provide enough of the needed oxygen to all tissue cells.

Disruption of the normal oxygen-carrying capacity of the blood can occur if not enough oxygen is in the lungs or if not enough red blood cells are present to carry the oxygen. Management of shock requires understanding its pathophysiology so that steps can be taken to overcome the causes and allow aerobic metabolism to continue.

PATHOPHYSIOLOGY OF SHOCK

To understand shock, it is necessary to understand the cardiovascular system, which is concerned with the second component of the Fick principle, delivery of oxygenated red blood cells to tissue cells. Off-loading and on-loading of oxygen is an important component of this system. The cardiovascular system is broken down into the *pump* (heart) to move blood around the system, the *container* (blood vessels) through which the red blood cells travel, and the *blood* itself (fluid), which acts as a medium for conducting the red blood cells throughout the body. All three components are a necessary part of the delivery scheme. The failure or partial failure of any component has dramatic effects on the other two. Nothing in the system can function alone. This chapter emphasizes the delivery of red blood cells and the off-loading of oxygen. On-loading of oxygen is discussed in Chapter 19.

Heart

The pumping action of the heart is not unlike filling and emptying a syringe with a three-way stopcock attached to it. Just as the plunger of the syringe, when pulled out, creates a vacuum inside the barrel and sucks fluid into the syringe, so the heart creates a condition that allows filling of the ventricle as the cardiac muscle relaxes during the diastolic phase. During the systolic phase, the plunger is pushed down, building up pressure within the barrel that corresponds to the contraction of the heart. The position of the handle of the three-way stopcock directs fluid out and away from the syringe and along its course. The three-way stopcock is similar to the one-way valves in the heart; once fluid is directed through a valve, it cannot return to the area from which it came. If a system was set up to contain a syringe, a long, flexible rubber tube, and a three-way stopcock, it would not be unlike the system of the heart and its mechanism for pumping blood (Fig. 11-1A). When the plunger is depressed, the three-way stopcock is switched to the downstream direction and fluid from the syringe is forced out, into the tubing (Fig. 11-1B). When the plunger reaches its fullest extension and is withdrawn, the stopcock is switched to allow fluid to come in from the upstream direction (Fig. 11-1C). The continued to-and-fro motion pumps fluid in a circular fashion throughout the system.

If a partially occluding clamp is placed half-way around the tube and the system continues to operate, the resistance along the pathway of the fluid produces a build-up of pressure on the downstream side of the pump (Fig. 11-2). If the clamp is only a partially occluding one, because the expansion of the tube (blood vessels) allows variable volume determined by the pressure, some of this pressure is maintained even though the syringe is filling and no longer is applying pressure. If the system were modified even more, by using a series of smaller tubes that connected to the one large tube on each end, the system would be similar to a partially occluding clamp, except that the fluid would be able to circulate through numerous smaller areas, each of which would produce its own resistance (Fig. 11-3).

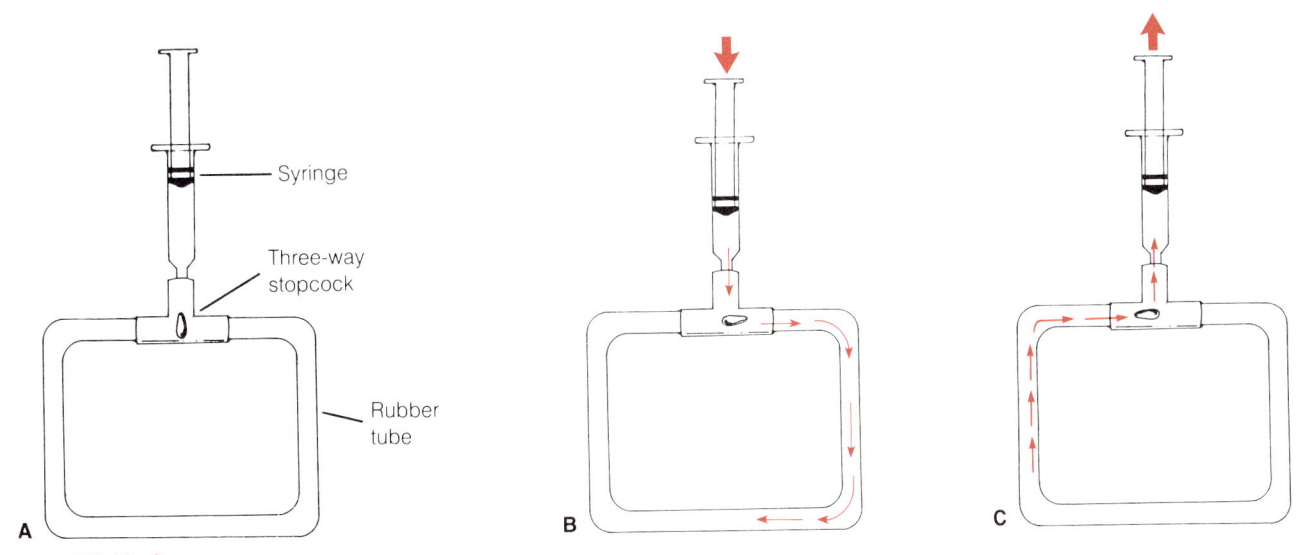

FIGURE 11-1.
Schematic drawing of the circulatory system. (**A**) The syringe is the heart, with the rubber tubing acting as the blood vessels. (**B**) Depressing the plunger forces fluid out and into the system. (**C**) Withdrawing the plunger fills the syringe from the system.

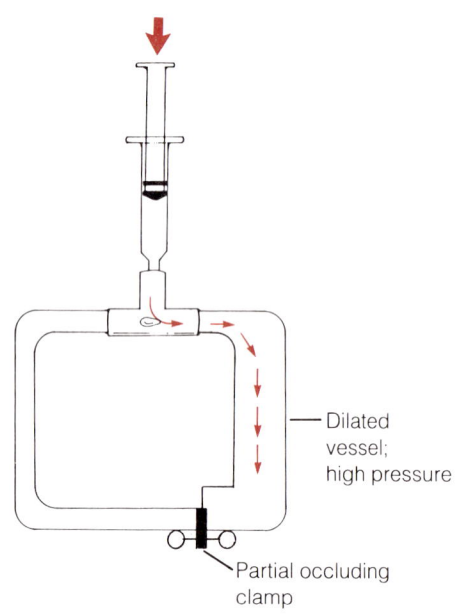

FIGURE 11-2.
A partial occluding clamp restricts fluid flow, producing a distended tube (vessel) with an increased pressure.

The tubular system described in Figure 11-3 can be compared to the heart and vascular system. The large outflow tube could be called the aorta, the large inflow tube called the vena cava, and the small tubes called capillaries. It can then be seen that the pressure inside the aortic side is higher when the plunger is depressed, but, because it bleeds off slowly, it never reaches zero, and it pulsates (expands and contracts rhythmically). The venous side is a continuous low pressure system, does not pulsate, and is driven by fluid coming from the multiple capillaries.

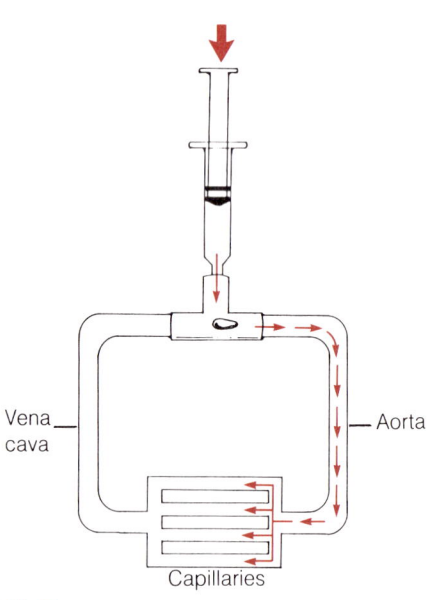

The capillaries are an extremely low pressure system that has minimal pulsation but continuous flow. If partially occluding clamps are attached to the inflow and outflow tubes at each of the capillaries, by varying the amount of occlusion, blood flow can be shunted from one capillary system to the other without altering the overall pressure in the entire system (Fig. 11-4). However, if the partially occluding clamps on the capillaries are all tightened simultaneously, or if most are tightened simultaneously, the build-up of pressure on the arterial side is greatly enhanced, whereas, the flow and, therefore, the pressure on the venous side is greatly decreased. In the body, this process is called **peripheral vascular resistance** or **systemic vascular resistance**. It is used not only to shunt blood from one inactive capillary bed to one that is more active (or needs more blood flow), but it is also used as a mechanism to maintain pressure when it is decreased in the arterial side.

If the flow or pressure on the venous side is not enough to fill the syringe each time the plunger is withdrawn, less blood is pushed into the arterial side (Fig. 11-5). Such a decreased preload affects both pressure and flow in the arterial side. *Hypovolemia* (diminished blood volume) is the major cause of such a condition. If an obstruction prevents complete withdrawal of the plunger in the syringe, the barrel could not be filled entirely (Fig. 11-6). This state also affects the pressure on the arterial side, since the volume with each downstroke of the plunger is severely restricted. Such a condition exists with constrictive pericarditis or acute cardiac tamponade.

The amount of fluid pushed out of the syringe on each stroke is called the **stroke volume**. If the volume is mea-

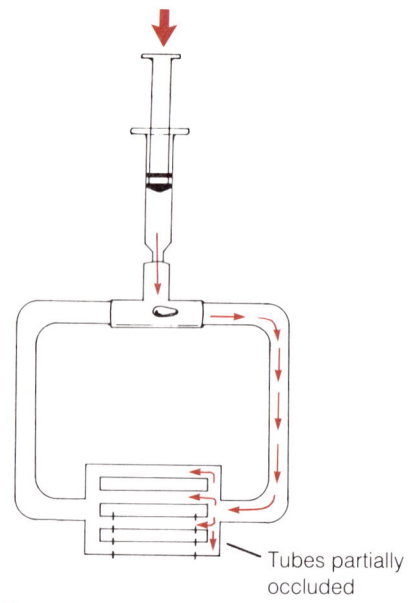

FIGURE 11-3.
Multiple smaller tubes produce more resistance than one large tube.

FIGURE 11-4.
Partially occluding some of the tubes shunts blood to those not occluded as well as increases the resistance to flow.

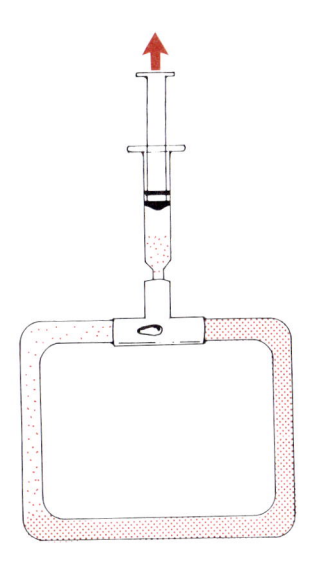

FIGURE 11-5.
If fluid is inadequate to fill syringe when withdrawn, output is decreased from the only partially filled syringe.

sured over a period of time, it is considered the syringe output. Translated into the human body, the volume of each stroke multiplied by the number of strokes per minute is known as the *cardiac output*.

Blood Vessels

The blood vessels through which the fluid from the heart is circulated are elastic; that is, they respond by changing size with each thrust of the heart. This pulsatile volume change has advantages in patient assessment. The strength of each thrust of the plunger or the contraction of the heart can be appreciated by palpating the amount of lateral expansion and the strength of each lateral expansion in the blood vessel. In addition to this method, the number of times that the plunger is pushed per minute, or the number of times that the heart contracts per minute, can be counted simply by measuring the number of pulsations per minute. This amount usually is reported in beats per minute or, simply, pulse. The body can control the size of these blood vessels by controlling the tone or contractility of the smooth muscle in their lining. Both epinephrine and norepinephrine can affect this muscle tone by constricting the vessels. If a shock condition produces dilated blood vessels, the volume within their boundaries is radically affected. Since blood vessels are essentially cylinders, the formula for the volume of a cylinder applies. The formula is: volume is equal to the height times the radius squared times pi (3.14).

$$V = h \times r^2 \times pi (3.14)$$

Since, in this system, both pi and the length of the blood vessel (height) are constants, then the volume varies directly with the square of the radius. Doubling the radius of a blood vessel increases its volume by four times:

where the radius equals 1

$[1^2 = 1]$ while $[(1 \times 2)^2$ (doubling the radius) $= 4]$

where the radius equals 2

$[2^2 = 4]$ while $[(2 \times 2)^2$ (doubling the radius) $= 16]$

As was seen in Figures 11-5 and 11-6, the output of the syringe is directly proportional to the amount of fluid presented to it, or the preload. If a container has 6 L of fluid in it with a pump situated at the top, then the pump always has adequate fluid if the system has no leaks in (Fig. 11-7A). However, if 2 L of the fluid are allowed to run off, but the volume of the container is still 6 L, then the 6-L container with only 4 L of fluid in it is not full. The pump cannot get an adequate amount of fluid (decreased preload) (Fig. 11-7B). If the same container was made smaller, either by pressure from the outside or by its own intrinsic ability to become smaller, its volume would be less and, therefore, more fluid would be available to the pump (adequate preload) (Fig. 11-7C).

If this same 6-L container, which had 6 L of fluid in it, were suddenly expanded to 8 L in size, and if no additional fluid were added, the situation would be the same as in Figure 11-7B; the amount of fluid available to the pump (preload), only 6 L of fluid in an 8-L container, would constitute inadequate preload. The latter is an example of conditions that occur with septic, neurogenic, and spinal shock. Adding fluid to the 6-L container that has lost 2 L of fluid, or the 8 L container that has lost an equal amount, restores the preload and allows the actions of the heart to continue.

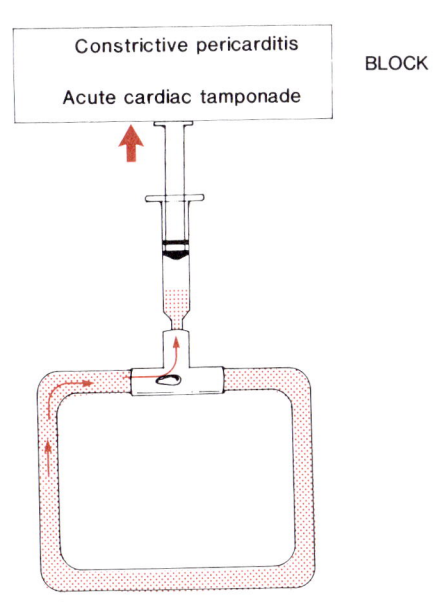

FIGURE 11-6.
Obstruction prevents plunger from being completely withdrawn. This block results in incomplete filling of syringe and thus decreased output.

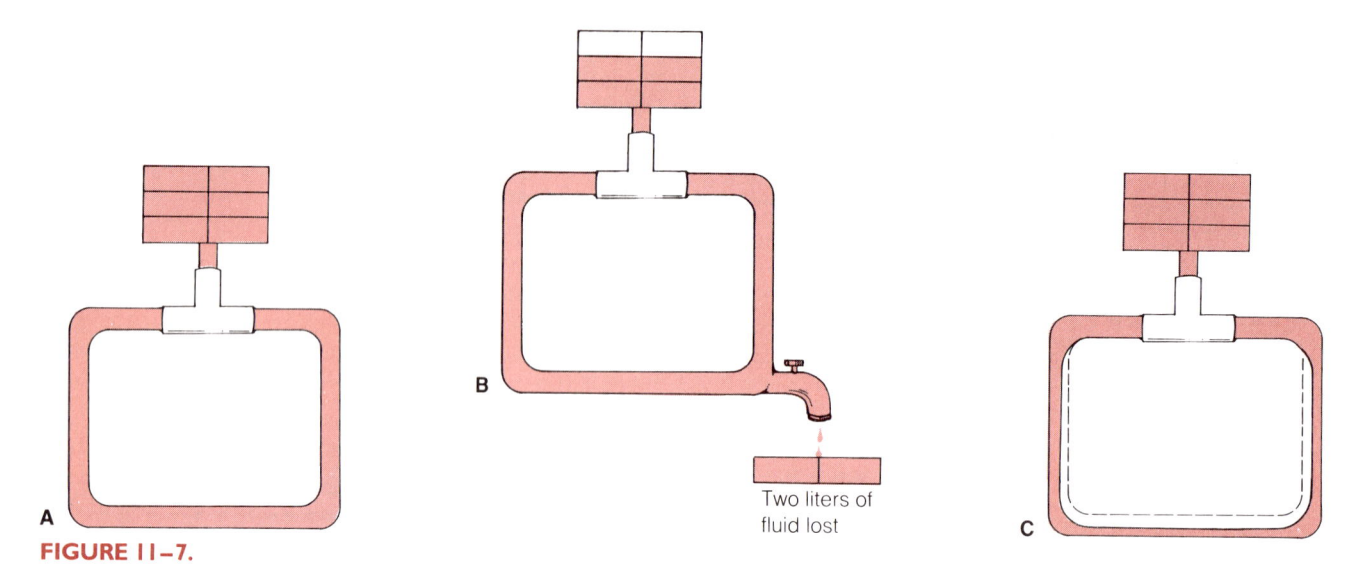

FIGURE 11-7.
(**A**) A 6-L container with 6 L of fluid provides adequate preload for the pump to move fluid around.
(**B**) A 6-L container with 2 L of fluid lost does not have adequate preload for the pump. Output is poor.
(**C**) A 6-L container with only 4 L of fluid, reduced in size to a 4-L container, would have adequate preload for the pump to produce good output.

Fluid

It is obvious that the fluid container-volume ratio should match. Acute blood loss from a hole in the container occurs in trauma. Bleeding from some portion of the gastrointestinal tract, such as a duodenal ulcer or diverticulitis, contributes significantly to loss of fluid from the container. Diarrhea, vomiting, sweating, and pulmonary water loss all produce fluid depletions, which, if not replaced, reduce preload. However, what about the internal fluid losses within the system that do not go to the outside of the body, such as *edema* (collection of fluid between the cells of the tissue) that develops in the legs or lungs of a patient with congestive heart failure, swelling that occurs around a bruise, cellulitis (the edema of an infection)? What is the origin of the edema fluid? What problems does it cause and how can it be controlled?

The cardiovascular system is not a plastic tube that keeps all of the fluid on the inside. As a matter of fact, it is composed of a membrane classified as "semipermeable." This ***semipermeable membrane*** permits some substances to pass through it freely but hinders or prevents entirely the passage of others. Various physical processes, discussed below, are responsible for exchanges through the membrane and contribute to the accumulation of edema fluid.

Classifications of shock in relationship to the heart, blood vessels, and fluid are shown in Table 11-1, together with examples.

TABLE 11-1.
CLASSIFICATIONS OF SHOCK

Organ	Classification	Example
Heart	Cardiogenic	Acute myocardial infarction
	Decreased return	Tension pneumothorax
	Decreased output	Cardiac tamponade
		Pulmonary emboli
Blood vessels	Neurogenic (spinal)	Severed spinal cord
	Septic	Severe infection
	Anaphylactic	Severe allergy
Fluid	Hypovolemic	Dehydration
	Hemorrhagic	Bleeding
	Third space	Burns, peritonitis

Diffusion

Electrolytes and other particles allowed to pass freely through the semipermeable membrane obey the law of diffusion. **Diffusion** is the constant movement of molecules from an area of higher concentration to an area of lower concentration. The molecules eventually reach an equilibrium on both sides of the membrane. For example, suppose a 25% sodium chloride (NaCl) solution was separated by a semipermeable membrane from a 15% NaCl solution. Suppose that both sodium and chloride are able to pass through the membrane, and water, a tiny molecule, is always able to penetrate the membrane. Eventually, the solutions reach equilibrium by passing from an area where they are in a higher concentration to an area where they are in a lower concentration. In other words, both solutions rapidly diffuse through the membrane until an equal number of sodium, chloride, and water molecules are on each side. The result is a 20% NaCl solution on both sides of the membrane. Figure 11-8 illustrates the law of diffusion.

Osmosis

The diffusion of water through a semipermeable membrane is known as osmosis. **Osmosis** is the physical property that allows water to proceed from one side of the membrane to another. Using the above example with the NaCl solutions, suppose this time that the membrane is impermeable to sodium and chloride but still permeable to water. Because more water molecules are in 15% NaCl than in 25% NaCl, water molecules pass through the membrane to dilute the more concentrated 25% NaCl solution. The net direction of osmosis is toward the more concentrated solution (remember the more concentrated solution has less water). *Net osmosis* produces several changes in the solutions: a equilibrium of the concentrations, an increase in the volume and pressure of the original 25% NaCl solution, with the volume and pressure of the original 15% NaCl solution decreasing proportionately.

Figure 11-9 illustrates the process of osmosis.

Active Transport

Active transport uses energy to move molecules (*other than water*) through a semipermeable membrane in an opposite direction from the way in which they would normally flow by diffusion. That is, they move from an area of lower concentration to an area of higher concentration. Since this movement is against the natural flow, energy must be present to transport molecules through the membrane. Proteins in the membrane also act as carriers to assist in this process.

Osmotic Pressure

It has been shown from the NaCl experiments that net osmosis occurs from water moving through a membrane from a less concentrated NaCl solution to one with a greater concentration. By definition, then, **osmotic pressure** is the pressure that develops in a solution as a result of net osmosis into that solution. The two NaCl solutions in Figure 11-9 show that both sodium and chloride were unable to pass through the membrane. The result was that water passing through the membrane increased the pressure of the original 25% NaCl solution. Since neither the sodium nor chloride could pass through the membrane, pressure developed from water being pulled through in an attempt to create equilibrium. Equilibrium resulted when the solutions on both sides of the membrane reached 20% NaCl. The difference in the height of each side of the container is known as the osmotic pressure.

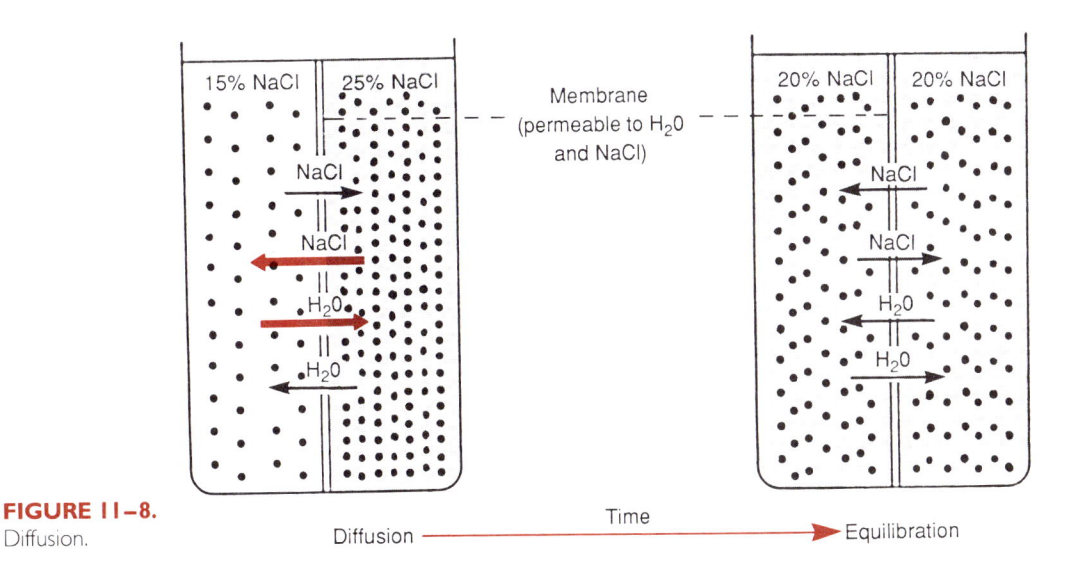

FIGURE 11-8.
Diffusion.

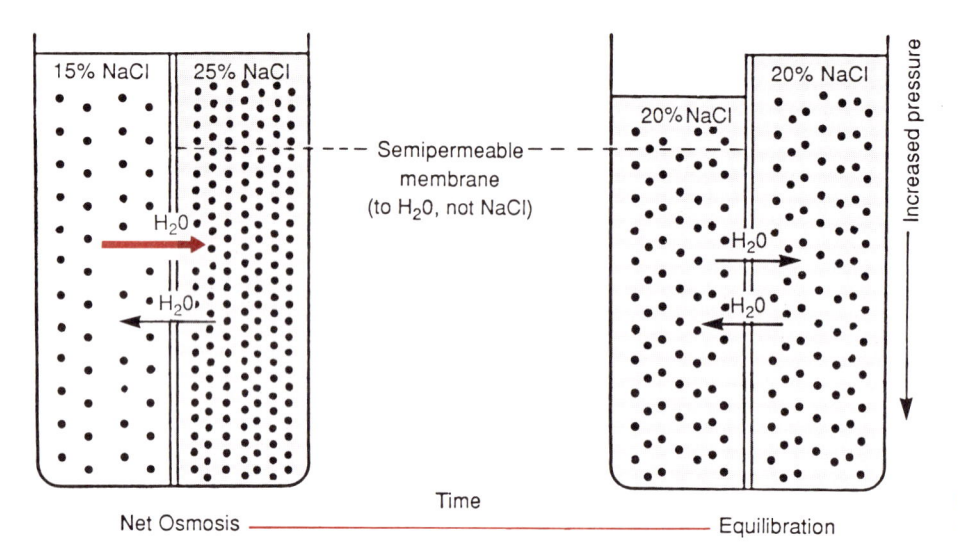

FIGURE 11-9.
Osmosis.

Solutions that have equal osmotic pressure to that of the body are known as **isotonic** solutions. Since isotonic solutions have the same osmotic pressure as body fluids, water moves in both directions freely across a semipermeable membrane without building up osmotic pressure. Therefore, if an isotonic solution is infused into human tissues or blood, no net osmosis occurs into or out of the cells. The cells neither lose nor gain water. Examples of isotonic solutions are 0.9% sodium chloride (normal saline or 0.9% NaCl), lactated Ringer's (LR) solution, and 5% dextrose in water (D_5W). Solutions that have a higher osmotic pressure than that of body cells are called **hypertonic**, and those with lower pressure are called **hypotonic**. A hypertonic solution is one into which net osmosis occurs; water is pulled from tissues or blood into the hypertonic solution. If a red blood cell is placed in a hypertonic solution, it loses water to the surrounding solution and shrinks. A hypotonic solution has the opposite effect. In the human body, water is pulled from a hypotonic solution into the tissues or blood. When this process occurs to a red blood cell, the cell swells and bursts. Figure 11-10 illustrates the process of osmotic pressure on a red blood cell. Hypertonic solutions include 5% dextrose in 0.9% sodium chloride ($D_5$0.9%NaCl, D_5NS), 5% dextrose in 0.45% sodium chloride ($D_5$0.45%NaCl, $D_5$1/2NS), 10% dextrose in water ($D_{10}W$), and 5% dextrose in lactated Ringer's (D_5LR). Examples of hypotonic solutions are distilled water and 0.45% sodium chloride (half-normal saline or 0.45% NaCl). These solutions are listed in Table 11-2. As a note, D_5W becomes hypotonic when it enters the body. The glucose is metabolized and only free water exists.

Fluid and Electrolytes

The total amount of water in an adult is approximately 50% to 60% of total body weight. In a newborn, this percentage may be as high as 75% to 80% of the body weight. Fluid outside of the cells (**extracellular**) makes up 15% to 20% of the total body water; the rest, 35% to 40%, is within the cells (**intracellular**). The normal intake of fluid in an adult averages about 2300 mL per day. Table 11-3 shows routes by which water is lost under different conditions.

Within the body, fluid is compartmentalized into **intravascular** fluid, which is inside the vascular space or blood vessels, and **extravascular** fluid, which is outside the vascular space, such as in the tissues. Intravascular fluid is subdivided into **plasma**, which is the fluid outside the cells, and "intracellular" fluid, found within the red blood cell membranes. Extravascular fluid is subdivided into **interstitial** fluid, found between the cells, and "in-

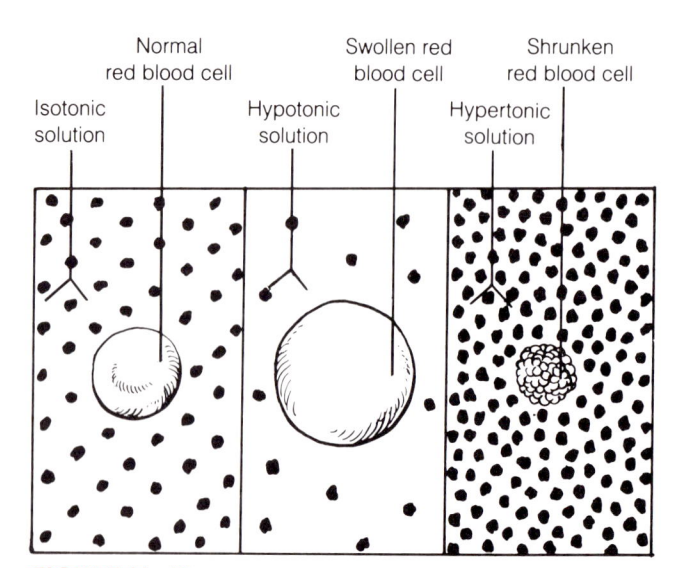

FIGURE 11-10.
Osmosis. *Left,* Isotonic solution has almost the same concentration as that of a red blood cell. Water freely moves in and out of the cell. *Center,* Hypotonic solution causes red blood cell to swell and eventually burst. *Right,* Hypertonic solution causes the water molecules to move out of the red blood cell, leaving it shrunken.

TABLE 11–2.
INTRAVENOUS SOLUTIONS

Solution	Abbreviation	Type
normal saline	0.9% NaCl, NS	isotonic
lactated Ringer's	LR	isotonic
5% dextrose in water	D_5W	isotonic
half-normal saline	0.45% NaCl, ½ NS	hypotonic
distilled water	H_2O	hypotonic
10% dextrose in water	$D_{10}W$	hypertonic
5% dextrose in half-normal saline	D_5 0.45% NaCl, D_5½ NS	hypertonic
5% dextrose in normal saline	D_5 0.9% NaCl, D_5NS	hypertonic
5% dextrose in lactated Ringer's	D_5LR	hypertonic

TABLE 11–3.
DAILY WATER LOSS (IN ML)

Mechanism of Loss	Normal Temperature	Hot Weather	Heavy Exercise
Sweat	100	1400	5000
Feces	100	100	100
Skin	350	350	350
Respiratory tract	350	250	650
Urine	1400	1200	500
Total	2300	3300	6600

tracellular" fluid, located within cell membranes. A general term for fluid outside of the cell membrane, whether it lies in or out of the vascular space, is "extracellular" fluid. A semipermeable membrane separates all of these compartments (Fig. 11-11). Water transfers between the compartments freely, electrolytes may or may not. Electrolytes respond to active transport and diffusion based on the permeability of the membranes to these materials.

Electrolytes are substances that separate into ions when in solution and conduct a weak electrical current. Electrolytes must be balanced to maintain an adequate environment for cells to function. That is, the number of positively charged ions (*cations*) must equal the number of negatively charged ions (*anions*). Although the number of electrolytes varies depending on which fluid compartment they are in, the overall charge to the body

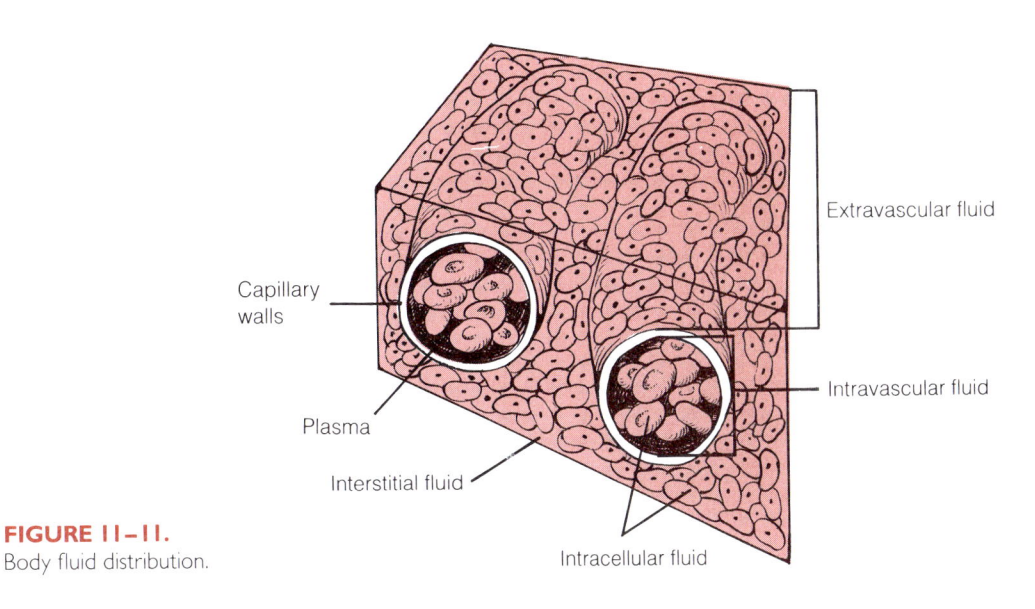

FIGURE 11-11.
Body fluid distribution.

TABLE 11-4.
CHEMICAL COMPOSITION OF BLOOD PLASMA AND INTRACELLULAR FLUID

Components	Blood Plasma	Intracellular Fluid
CATIONS		
Na+ (sodium)	142 mEq/L	10 mEq/L
K+ (potassium)	5 mEq/L	150 mEq/L
Ca++ (calcium)	5 mEq/L	<1 mEq/L
Mg++ (magnesium)	2 mEq/L	40 mEq/L
ANIONS		
Cl- (chloride)	103 mEq/L	4 mEq/L
HCO3- (bicarbonate)	26 mEq/L	10 mEq/L
HPO4-- (phosphate)	2 mEq/L	75 mEq/L
SO4-- (sulfate)	1 mEq/L	75 mEq/L
protein	17 mEq/L	40 mEq/L
OTHER VALUES		
Glucose	90 mg %	0–20 mg/dl
Cholesterol	0.5 g %	2–95 g/dl
PaO2	35 mm Hg	20 mm Hg
PaCO2	46 mm Hg	50 mm Hg
pH	7.4	7.0
Albumin	2 g %	16 g/dl

should equal zero; the number of cations should cancel out the number of anions. Electrolytes affect water distribution, osmolality, acid-base balance, and neuromuscular irritability. Normally, the body maintains fluid volume and electrolyte concentrations within a narrow range. When this balance is disturbed, it causes a profound change in the cells' ability to function. Table 11-4 shows the normal composition of blood plasma and intracellular fluid. These values are important to determine normal ranges within the body. The chief extracellular ion in the blood plasma is **sodium** (Na+), and the chief intracellular ion is **potassium** (K+).

The other component of body fluid that influences fluid movement is protein. Protein is contained in albumin, plasma, and lymph and is generally restricted to the fluid compartment in which it lies. Because of the larger size of protein, it usually does not cross a cellular membrane. However, when capillary walls become more permeable or "leaky," the larger protein molecules can transfer from the intravascular space to the interstitial space. If trapped here by closing of the leaky capillaries, water flows toward the area of protein concentration, and the increased osmotic pressure that is produced holds fluid in the interstitial space without allowing it to diffuse easily back into the intravascular space. This condition can result in tissue edema.

Osmotic pressure is one of the major forces that produces edema. Edema is defined as the presence of abnormally large amounts of fluid in the interstitial space. Osmotic pressure combined with **hydrostatic pressure** (the force or weight of a fluid pushing against a surface, in this case, the semipermeable membrane) account for almost all of the edema that develops in the body. The presence of protein in the interstitial space increases the osmotic pressure of this space. Increased hydrostatic pressure in the vascular system (hypertension) forces water into the interstitial space. Retention of electrolytes, especially sodium, increases osmotic pressure in the interstitial space. The end result of any of these are the same: the increased interstitial fluid separates the cells from each other and the cells from the capillaries. This separation produces oxygen diffusion (off-loading) problems.

Blood and Its Components

Blood is a thick fluid that lies within the intravascular space. It varies in color from bright to dark red, depending on how much oxygen it is carrying. Arterial blood is brighter red due to increased oxygen content. Venous blood carries less oxygen, a fact which contributes to its darker color. The quantity of blood carried in the human body differs depending on the size of the person, but, in general, the average adult male who weighs 70 kg (154 lbs) has about 5 L (5.2 qt) of blood. Blood accounts for about 8% of total body weight.

The blood is carried through a closed system of vessels pumped by the heart. The blood has three functions: transportation, regulation, and protection. Chapter 19 discusses how oxygen is diffused through the alveolar-capillary membrane into the blood. Carbon dioxide is a

FIGURE 11-12. Composition of normal adult blood.

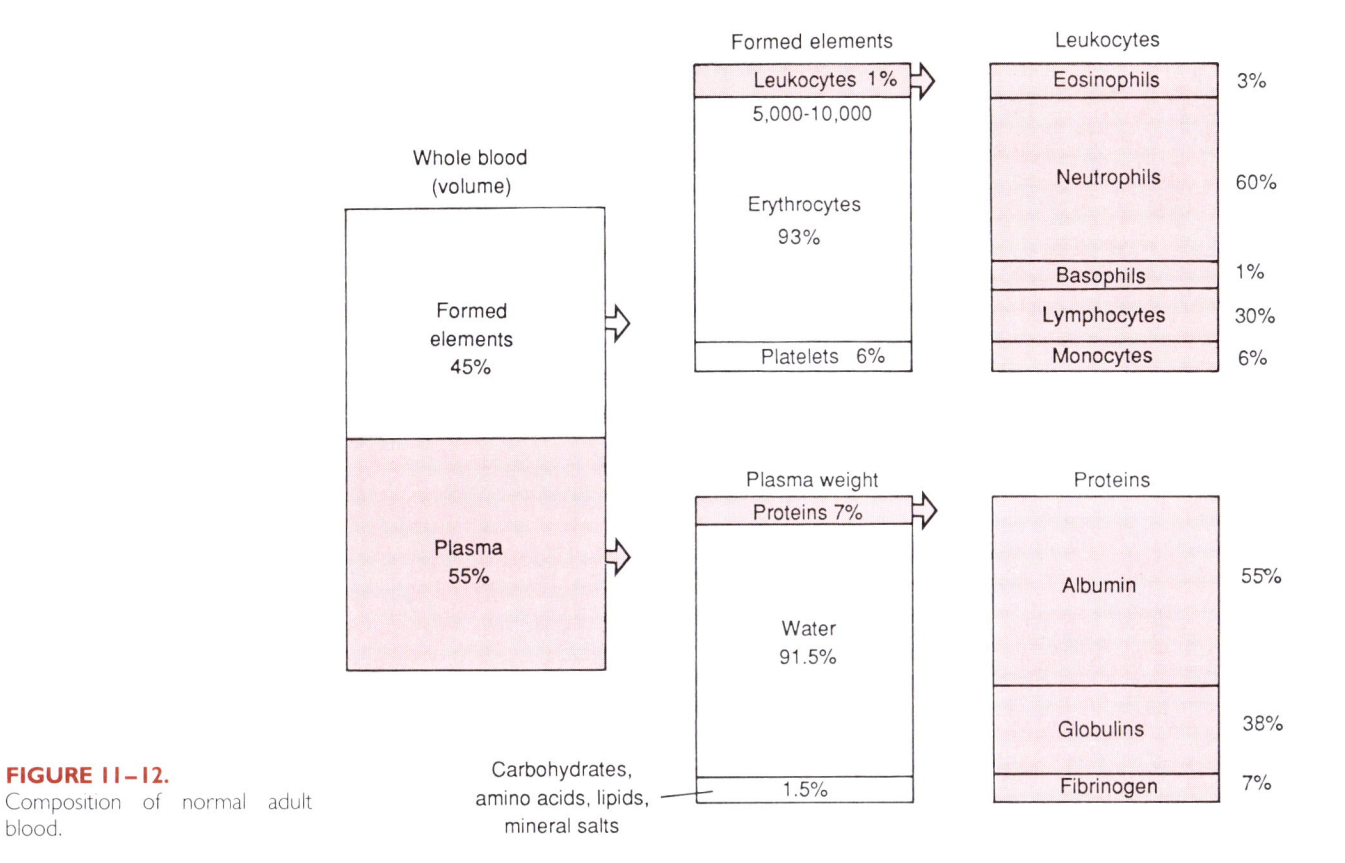

waste product of cell metabolism. It is dissolved in the plasma by the buffer system and carried out of the tissues into the lungs, where it is exhaled. The blood also delivers nutrients to the cells and picks up waste products and delivers them to excretory organs. It picks up hormones from endocrine glands and delivers them to target organs (see Chapter 21). Buffers in the blood act to regulate the pH of the body. The blood serves to regulate the amount of fluid in the tissues by means of proteins that maintain the proper osmotic pressure. Blood transports heat and aids in the regulation of body temperature. Finally, the blood contains certain factors and cells that protect the body against injury and disease.

The blood is composed of a liquid element, the plasma, and cells (Fig. 11-12). More than half of the total volume of blood is plasma. Plasma contains proteins, carbohydrates, amino acids, lipids, and mineral salts. The formed elements or cells include erythrocytes (red blood cells), leukocytes (white blood cells), and platelets, which are suspended in the plasma.

Erythrocytes, or red blood cells, are the most numerous of the formed elements in the blood. They are disk-shaped with a center depression that creates a thin center and thick edge (Fig. 11-13). Red blood cell deformity can result in "sickle cells," so-called because of an abnormal ability of the red cell to form a crescent-shape if subjected to low levels of oxygen (Fig. 11-14). A clinical condition known as **sickle cell anemia** is most commonly found in people with African or Mediterranean ethnic backgrounds. The sickle-shaped cells break down more rapidly than normal-shaped red blood cells, and the sickle shape can prevent the cells from moving through the smaller vessels in the body. Carriers of this disease can be identified by a blood test.

The red blood cells have the ability to carry oxygen. The oxygen is bound in red cells to **hemoglobin,** a protein that contains iron. Hemoglobin combined with oxy-

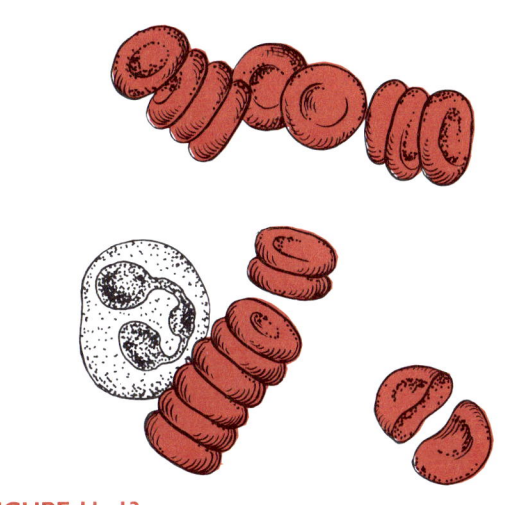

FIGURE 11-13. Red blood cells grouped in rouleaux formation. One white blood cell is also shown.

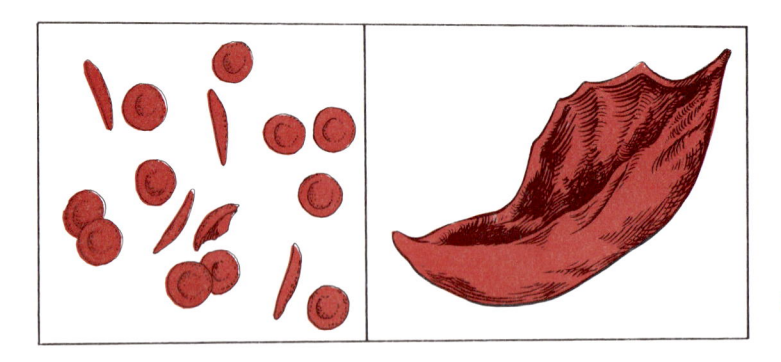

FIGURE 11-14.
Sickle cell.

gen gives blood its characteristic red color. The more oxygen carried, the brighter red the blood. **Hematocrit** is a term used to identify the volume percentage of red blood cells in whole blood. To be more specific, a hematocrit of 45 means that every 100 mL of whole blood has 45 mL of red cells and 55 mL of plasma. The average hematocrit for a man is 45 ($\pm$ 7) and for a woman 42 ($\pm$ 5).

Leukocytes are the second most predominant cells in the formed elements of blood. The leukocytes, or white blood cells, are outnumbered by red cells 700 to 1 and tend to be colorless. The most important function of leukocytes is to destroy foreign organisms. Several types of leukocytes are found in the body. One type engulfs and destroys invaders. This leukocyte can actually squeeze through the capillary wall to migrate toward microorganisms that may have invaded the tissues. Another type of white blood cell, called the **lymphocyte,** is largely responsible in providing immunity to infectious disease. Lymphocytes destroy foreign invaders either by attacking the cells directly or by producing antibodies that circulate in the blood and help destroy cells.

The third of the formed elements in the blood are called **platelets**. These are the smallest and are actually not cells in themselves, but fragments of cells. Platelets are essential to blood coagulation (clotting). When blood is put in contact with tissue other than the inside of the blood vessels, as in an injury, the platelets stick together and form a plug that seals the wound.

BLOOD TYPING. A person's blood type is determined by heredity. The term blood type refers to the type of antigen present on red blood cell membranes. An **antigen** is a substance that causes the formation of antibodies. An **antibody** is a protein developed in the body in response to the presence of an antigen that has in some way gained access to the body. Formation of antibodies can cause the red blood cells of the donor's blood to become clumped. Proper blood typing before blood transfusions is very important. Antigens A, B, and Rh are the most important antigens when dealing with blood transfusions. Blood types are named according to the antigens present on the red blood cell membranes Table 11-5.

Persons with blood type O are said to be universal donors because, in an emergency, their blood can be given to anyone. Type AB individuals are called universal recipients since they can receive blood from most donors. The Rh antigen is either *positive* (present) or *negative* (absent) from the red blood cell membrane. A person must receive the same Rh factor from a donor to be compatible. The Rh antigen is of special importance during pregnancy because Rh incompatibility between mother and fetus is often the problem when an infant has hemolytic disease. A patient's blood is tested for compatibility with the donor's blood, if time permits, before any transfusion is begun. If they are not compatible, clumping and destruction of the recipient's blood or the transfused results.

BLOOD PREPARATIONS AND SUBSTITUTES. Blood for transfusion can be processed into packed red blood cells, plasma, and other products, such as platelets, or used as whole blood. Red blood cells can be stored for about 35 days before deterioration, depending on the type of preservative used. Blood is administered to restore circulating red cell volume due to an acute loss of blood from trauma or internal hemorrhage. Plasma, the fluid portion of the blood, is transfused in patients who suffer from massive burns or in trauma where large volumes of red cell replacement is required. In this instance, the loss of protein and fluid must be replaced, not the cellular portion. Packed red blood cells used for transfusion are red blood cells that have been separated from the plasma. Packed red blood cell transfusion is indicated to improve the oxygen carrying capacity of the blood in various types of anemia.

Red blood cells have no substitutes. Therefore, once the oxygen-carrying capacity is diminished by a massive

TABLE 11-5.
BLOOD TYPES

Blood Type	Red Blood Cell Antigen	Can Donate To	Can Receive From
A	A	A,AB	A,O
B	B	AB,B	B,O
AB	A,B	AB	A,B,AB,O
O	None	A,B,AB,O	O

loss of red blood cells, only the infusion of additional red blood cells replenishes the oxygen supply to the body.

Acid-Base Balance

An *acid* is a chemical compound that gives up or donates a hydrogen [H^+] ion. A *base* is a chemical compound that accepts or receives a hydrogen [H^+] ion. The body must maintain the level of hydrogen ions within a narrow range for the body's cells to function properly. Monitoring the acid-base balance is usually accomplished through the measurement of arterial blood gases. While paramedics typically do not have access to the technology required to measure arterial blood gases, there are many important prehospital implications to understanding acid-base status. For instance, a condition of excessive acid [H^+] causes the body to increase its ventilatory rate to eliminate the acid. This effect is a sensitive diagnostic indicator for the prehospital provider. Ventilation therapy and the use of sodium bicarbonate are both guided by the patient's pH. Analysis of arterial blood gases after therapy helps the paramedic and physician evaluate the effectiveness of field management of both ventilation and perfusion.

Maintenance of a normal acid-base balance is extremely important, since chemical states outside of this narrow normal range result in rapid cellular demise and may lead to death. The overall blood pH measurement is a function of the concentration of hydrogen ions [H^+]. Because this concentration is so high, calculations using the hydrogen ion are difficult to handle. To make working with this measurement easier, *pH* is used; pH is the inverse logarithm of the hydrogen ion concentration. Therefore, the less the hydrogen ion concentration, the greater the pH. pH is an accurate indicator of the acid-base condition of the arterial blood.

The pH scale ranges from 1 to 14. A solution is neutral at a pH of 7; one example is pure water. As shown in Figure 11-15, the pH becomes more acidotic as it moves closer to zero. Conversely, the closer the pH moves to 14, the more alkalotic the solution becomes. As the pH moves toward either end of the scale, a substance becomes increasingly caustic. Examples of this fact are hydrochloric acid, with a pH of 1, which is used to etch designs in glass, and ammonia, with a pH of 12, which is used for industrial cleaning. In the human body, gastric secretions are strongly acidic and have a pH of 1 to 1.3, while strongly alkaline pancreatic secretions have a pH of 10. Normal pH of blood plasma is slightly alkaline and has a normal range from 7.35 to 7.45; any value within this range is considered a neutral state for blood. When the pH is less than normal, hydrogen ions are in excess (remember, the pH is the inverse of the hydrogen ion concentration), and the blood becomes acidotic; a pH greater than normal signals alkalosis (or decreased hydrogen ions). Therefore, a blood pH of 7.30 equals acidosis, and a blood pH of 7.50 equals alkalosis. The lower limit at which a person can live more than a few hours is about 6.8, and the upper limit is about 8.0.

The pH of the blood is very dynamic since acid is a normal waste product of the body's cells. The pH at any given moment is a balance between this acid production and acid elimination from the body. Normal metabolism results in the production of acid [H^+], which is converted to carbon dioxide (CO_2) into the blood. This CO_2 dissolves in the blood and produces pressure within the blood, much as dissolved CO_2 produces pressure and "fizz" in a can of carbonated beverage. This pressure is measured in the arterial blood as the partial pressure of CO_2, abbreviated $PaCO_2$; normal $PaCO_2$ is 35 to 45 mm Hg (pressure) at sea level. The hydrogen ions [H^+] produced by cellular metabolism are converted by this buffer system (weak acid) into water (H_2O) and carbon dioxide. The H_2O is eliminated by the kidneys and the CO_2 by the lungs.

Carbonic acid is produced as follows:

$$[H^+] \;+\; \underset{\text{bicarbonate ions}}{HCO_3^-} \;\rightleftharpoons\; \underset{\text{carbonic acid}}{H_2CO_3}$$

hydrogen ions

The breakdown of carbonic acid occurs as follows:

$$[H^+] + HCO_3^- \;\rightleftharpoons\; \underset{\text{carbonic acid}}{H_2CO_3} \;\rightleftharpoons\; \underset{\text{water}}{H_2O} + \underset{\text{carbon dioxide}}{CO_2}$$

Carbon dioxide and water are easily removed from the body when circulation, renal function, and ventilation are normal. When these functions are impaired or when the production of CO_2 is increased, acidosis can result.

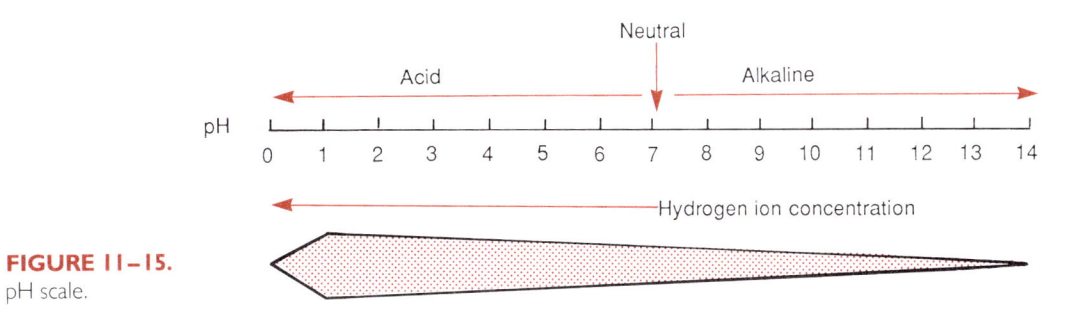

FIGURE 11-15. pH scale.

Other important acids in the body are acetic acid, sodium acid phosphate, uric acid, and acetoacetic acid.

Bases that are important in maintaining a normal acid-base balance are HCO_3^-, the bicarbonate ion, HPO_4^-, hydrogen phosphate ion, and several proteins in the body's cells. These bases combine with hydrogen ions to remove them from solutions. They are referred to as weak bases since they form weaker bonds with hydrogen ions.

An alkali is the combination of one of the alkaline metals, such as sodium or potassium, with a highly basic ion, such as the hydroxyl ion (OH^-). The basic portion, the hydroxyl ion, reacts vigorously with hydrogen ions to remove them from solutions and, therefore, is considered a strong base. Frequently the term alkali is used synonymously with the term base.

Most of the acids and bases that are involved in homeostasis are weak acids and bases, the most important of which are the carbonic acid and bicarbonate base. The term alkalosis is used to describe too few hydrogen ions in the solution. In contrast, acidosis refers to the excess addition of hydrogen ions in a solution.

COMPENSATION MECHANISMS. Because of the importance of a normal pH to cellular function, the body has three elaborate and effective mechanisms to control acid-base balance.

Buffer Systems. The first and most rapidly acting of the three is the buffer system. A **buffer** is a chemical system set up in the body to respond to changes in the hydrogen ion concentration to maintain a normal pH. Chemical reactions occur constantly in the body, releasing acids or bases into the blood. A buffer is a weak acid or base that combines with a stronger acid or base (it combines with its opposite) to form a weaker compound and water. For instance, mixing baking soda (a weak base) with vinegar (a stronger acid) results in a weaker acid and water; the baking soda is acting as the buffer. The body has a number of buffers, which circulate constantly through the bloodstream. For example, carbonic acid and phosphoric acid are buffers that mix with excess base in the bloodstream. The three major buffer systems of the body fluids are bicarbonate buffer (HCO_3^-), phosphate buffer (HPO_4^-), and protein buffer. Hemoglobin is one of the protein buffers, but it is only minimally important during resuscitation.

The body's major buffer system is the bicarbonate-carbonic acid (HCO_3^- — H_2CO_3) buffer system. Normally, there are twenty parts of bicarbonate to one part of carbonic acid. This ratio is important, since normal cellular metabolism produces an excess of acid. As long as this ratio is maintained, the pH is normal. As with all buffering systems, it requires normal functioning of the blood, renal, and pulmonary systems.

When a pathologic condition leads to an excess of acid or base, the buffer combines with the excess substance to weaken it and produce water. This process is instant and is only limited by the sheer number of buffers available. Herein lies one of the constraints of the buffer system: it is much more capable of dealing with acidosis than with alkalosis. Twenty buffers are available to combine with excess acid for every one buffer for bases. For this reason, patients who have an alkalosis are more likely to overwhelm the buffer system's ability to compensate.

Respiration. Buffer systems continuously work to maintain homeostasis. As acid is produced by the cells, it is absorbed into the buffer system, then eliminated by respiration. Respiration is slow, requiring 1 to 3 minutes to effectively eliminate the CO_2. Ventilation is controlled by the brain stem. The brain stem, in turn, is influenced by the pH of the cerebrospinal fluid in which it floats. Because cerebrospinal fluid is made continuously by the filtration of blood through the choroid plexus in the brain, changes in blood pH produce rapid changes in the pH of cerebrospinal fluid. This change then causes the respiratory system to compensate with a change in the ventilatory pattern. The ability of ventilation to alter pH is based on a simple principle presented earlier: carbon dioxide converts to carbonic acid in the bloodstream. The slower the patient breathes, the less carbon dioxide is exhaled and the more carbon dioxide in the blood is converted to carbonic acid, which helps decrease the blood pH.

$$\downarrow \text{breathing} \rightarrow \uparrow CO_2 \rightarrow \uparrow H_2CO_3 \rightarrow \uparrow H^+ \rightarrow \downarrow pH$$

Decreased ventilation increases carbon dioxide and carbonic acid (and therefore hydrogen ions) in the blood, thereby decreasing blood pH.

This additional carbonic acid may provide additional buffering power in the face of alkalosis by lowering the pH. On the other hand, hyperventilation increases the amount of CO_2 that is exhaled, thereby decreasing the amount of carbonic acid in the blood (increasing the pH).

$$\uparrow \text{breathing} \rightarrow \downarrow CO_2 \rightarrow \downarrow H_2CO_3 \rightarrow \downarrow H^+ \rightarrow \uparrow pH$$

Increased ventilation decreases carbon dioxide and carbonic acid (and therefore hydrogen ions) in the blood, thereby increasing blood pH.

This decreased carbonic acid helps restore normal pH in the patient who is acidotic.

Acids are normally produced by body metabolism and normally removed by ventilation. When compensating for acid-base abnormalities, the respiratory system alters the ventilation to either increase or decrease the amount of carbonic acid in the bloodstream. However, like buffers, the respiratory response is severely limited in its ability to compensate for alkalosis. The natural response to alkalosis is for the brain stem to slow ventilation to retain CO_2 and carbonic acid to bind with excess base. Unfortunately, profound hypoventilation leads to hypoxia, a condition that is as incompatible with normal body function as is alkalosis. The result is an inability to compensate for alkalosis.

TABLE 11–6.
KIDNEYS' RESPONSE TO ACID–BASE IMBALANCE

Imbalance	Response
Respiratory acidosis	Increased $PaCO_2$ causes increased [H^+] excretion by the kidneys. This increase adds base to the blood.
Respiratory alkalosis	Decreased $PaCO_2$ causes decreased [H^+] excretion by the kidneys. This decrease adds less base to the blood.
Metabolic acidosis	Decreased plasma HCO_3^- causes the kidneys to excrete more [H^+], thus adding more HCO_3^- to the blood.
Metabolic alkalosis	Increased plasma HCO_3^- levels cause some HCO_3^- to be excreted by the kidneys.

Understanding how the respiratory system contributes to acid-base status has many applications in the field. Patients who are not ventilating, or who are ventilating poorly, are likely to be acidotic due to inadequate removal of CO_2. In these cases, the treatment must focus on improving ventilation. On the other hand, patients who have metabolic acidosis, such as in diabetic ketoacidosis, often hyperventilate to remove CO_2 from the bloodstream and decrease the acidosis. This case is particularly true for the trauma patient. The metabolic acidosis produced by anaerobic metabolism is identified by the brain as described above. The brain tells the thoracic muscles and diaphragm to ventilate faster and eliminate more CO_2. The astute paramedic uses this effect as an early sign of shock and institutes proper treatment.

Kidney Function. The buffer system and the respiratory system are both activated immediately and provide powerful tools for returning the pH to normal. However, each has limitations (number of buffers, ventilatory rate), and neither copes well with alkalosis. Kidney function, the third system of acid-base regulation, is a slow mechanism for handling changes in the hydrogen ion concentration, requiring several hours to days to respond. The kidneys control blood pH directly by selectively reabsorbing and excreting acids or bases. When the blood is too acidotic, acids are excreted and bases reabsorbed; when the blood is too alkalotic, bases are excreted and acids reabsorbed. The kidneys are equally able to deal with alkalosis or acidosis but also have a limitation. Since it takes at least 10 to 20 hours for kidney function to respond to an alteration in pH, the kidneys are excellent for long-term compensation but are unable to stabilize pH in critical, rapidly developing conditions. Table 11-6 summarizes the kidneys' response to acid-base imbalance.

CLINICAL ABNORMALITIES OF ACID-BASE BALANCE.

Respiratory Acidosis. Any factor that decreases the rate of ventilation causes an increase in the amount of dissolved carbon dioxide in the extracellular fluid. This leads to increased amounts of carbonic acid and hydrogen ions, thus resulting in acidosis. Since this type of acidosis is a result of impaired respiration, it is referred to as ***respiratory acidosis***. Figure 11-16 illustrates the inverse relationship (seesaw effect) between pH and $PaCO_2$.

$\downarrow$ pH $\uparrow$ $PaCO_2$ $\downarrow$ H^+ = respiratory acidosis

Respiratory acidosis may occur as a result of some pathologic condition. Head injuries may cause damage to the respiratory center of the brain stem, resulting in reduced breathing states. Obstruction of the respiratory tract, pneumonia, asthma, or other conditions that interfere with the normal exchange of gases between the blood and alveolar air can result in respiratory acidosis. Hypoventilation caused by the administration of narcotics, drug overdose, or respiratory arrest decreases the body's ability to eliminate acids from the bloodstream and results in respiratory acidosis.

The major clinical effect of acidosis is depression of the central nervous system. If the pH of the blood falls below 7.0, the person may be disoriented and, later, comatose.

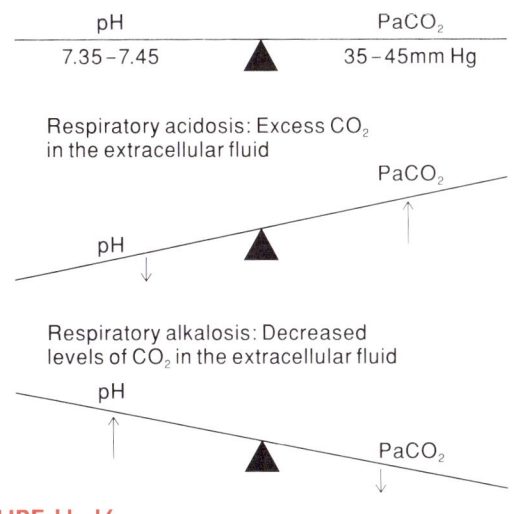

FIGURE 11-16.
Relationship between pH and $PaCO_2$.

Respiratory Alkalosis. In contrast, **respiratory alkalosis** can occur with excessive ventilation, which increases the amount of carbon dioxide elimination. This increase results in a decreased concentration of hydrogen ions in the extracellular fluid and, therefore, an elevated pH. Figure 11-16 illustrates the inverse relationship between pH and $PaCO_2$ in respiratory alkalosis.

$$\uparrow pH \downarrow PaCO_2 \downarrow H^+ = \text{respiratory alkalosis}$$

Only rarely do pathologic conditions cause respiratory alkalosis, such as in overbreathing states. A common psychologically driven respiratory alkalosis is the hyperventilation syndrome. The anxious, frightened, or disturbed patient ventilates more rapidly than normal. An excess elimination of CO_2 results. A physiologic type of respiratory alkalosis occurs when a person ascends to a high altitude. The low oxygen content of the air stimulates respiration, resulting in an excess loss of carbon dioxide and mild respiratory alkalosis.

A major clinical effect of alkalosis on the body is overexcitability of the nervous system. This may affect the peripheral nervous system before the central nervous system. The nerves may become excitable even without stimulation, which may result in muscle spasms referred to as tetany. This clinical sign may be seen first in the peripheral limbs, such as the forearm, and later in the face and trunk of the body.

Metabolic Acidosis. Several conditions can lead to an excess amount of acids in the body, referred to as **metabolic acidosis**. This accumulation of acids can be the result of renal failure, excess formation of metabolic acids in the body, loss of base from body fluids, or increased intake of metabolic acids in intravenous fluids or absorption from the gastrointestinal tract. Diarrhea and excessive vomiting of contents deeper in the gastrointestinal tract can result in metabolic acidosis due to the loss of sodium bicarbonate (base). Severe diarrhea or vomiting in young children can result in serious acidosis and subsequent death. Uremia, or uremic acidosis, can occur in severe renal disease when the kidneys fail to remove the normal amounts of acids formed each day by the metabolic processes of the body.

One of the more common conditions that cause metabolic acidosis in the patient found in the field is cardiac arrest. When the heart stops and respiration fails, a critical shortage of oxygen develops. Cells in the body shift to a less efficient form of energy production known as anaerobic (without oxygen) metabolism. This form of metabolism increases the production of lactic acid, a source of hydrogen ions.

Diabetes mellitus can cause increased amounts of acetoacetic acid (ketones) to be formed for use by the tissues as energy in place of glucose. The increased concentration of acetoacetic acid in the extracellular fluids (diabetic ketoacidosis) can lead to metabolic acidosis. If not controlled, this condition can lead to diabetic coma and death. Metabolic acidosis can also occur from overdoses of aspirin. One of the diagnostic signs of metabolic acidosis is increased pulmonary ventilation. This is the body's respiratory compensation mechanism to remove excess acid in the form of CO_2. Figure 11-17 illustrates the rela-

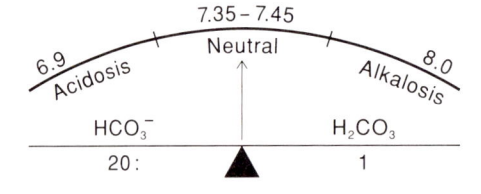

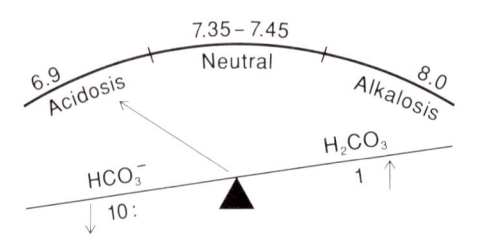

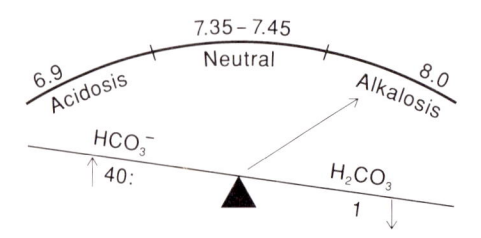

FIGURE 11-17.
Relationship between pH, HCO_3^-, and H_2CO_3.

tionship between pH, bicarbonate (HCO_3^-), and carbonic acid (H_2CO_3).

Metabolic Alkalosis. **Metabolic alkalosis** does not occur as frequently as metabolic acidosis. Excessive ingestion of alkaline drugs, such as sodium bicarbonate, for the treatment of gastritis or peptic ulcer can increase the amount of alkali or base in the body. Diuretics can also contribute to metabolic alkalosis by enhancing loss of hydrogen ions and reabsorption of sodium ions in the renal tubules. Excessive vomiting of gastric contents without vomiting of lower gastrointestinal contents leads to excessive loss of hydrochloric acid from the stomach. This type of alkalosis may occur in newborns with pyloric obstruction. Occasionally, an alkalotic person develops severe signs or symptoms, such as convulsions or extreme nervousness. Figure 11-17 illustrates the effect of excess bicarbonate on pH. The box, "Mechanisms for Alteration of Acid–Base Status," lists the various conditions and body's mechanisms that alter the acid-base balance of the body.

MANAGEMENT OF ACID-BASE STATES. Field therapy for acid-base states is largely supplemental to the body's own defenses. Ventilation is exceedingly important to prevent and treat respiratory acidosis. Assisted ventilation is the most important therapeutic maneuver available to the paramedic. Sodium bicarbonate, which is covered in Chapter 20, may be used as an adjunct to treat metabolic acidosis until the kidneys can compensate. One important point must be remembered when giving sodium bicarbonate: the body tolerates alkalosis poorly. For this reason, caution should be exercised in determining dosage of sodium bicarbonate. While overventilation can be easily reversed, alkalosis caused by excess sodium bicarbonate administration cannot be compensated for by the body and may prove fatal. Until arterial blood gases can confirm the patient's status, it is best to attempt to leave the patient slightly acidotic. It is hard to measure acidosis in the field; instead, the paramedic must use the clinical signs and symptoms of the patient as indicators of acidosis.

It is important for the paramedic to understand the body's mechanisms for maintaining pH, as well as the consequences of acidosis or alkalosis, to treat or prevent pH imbalance. Proper field management may help to stabilize the patient's condition. It is important to get the patient to the hospital quickly to treat the pathologic process that is causing the abnormality and to monitor accurately the absolute acid-base balance in the patient.

Pressure Changes

Baroreceptors, located in the carotid artery and other portions of the arterial system, identify fluctuations in pressure. These changes are relayed to the central nervous system, and adjustments in blood pressure are mediated by the sympathetic nervous system via norepinephrine and epinephrine from the adrenal gland. These changes affect the cardiovascular system, both centrally on the heart and peripherally on the vessels. Although they are to a certain extent simultaneous in occurrence, to think of them in a stepwise fashion simplifies the assessment and the management of a patient in shock.

STAGES OF SHOCK

Compensated Shock

In **compensated shock,** the body adjusts for shock in three ways: the first step is an increase in the strength of the contractions of the heart itself; the second step is increased rate of contractions; and the last step is increased peripheral vascular resistance. Increased peripheral vascular resistance frequently can be appreciated in a dete-

---

MECHANISMS FOR ALTERATION OF ACID–BASE STATUS

Acidosis

INCREASED ACID PRODUCTION
Cardiac arrest → production of lactic acid
Fever → increased CO_2 production
Diabetic ketoacidosis → production of ketoacids
Overdose of acidic substances (such as aspirin or methanol)

DECREASED ACID ELIMINATION
Respiratory arrest → retention of CO_2 in bloodstream
Acute attack of asthma/COPD → decreased ventilation
Acute pulmonary edema → decreased ventilation and diffusion

Alkalosis

DECREASED ACID/INCREASED BASE
Vomiting, nasogastric suction → excessive removal of acids
Some diuretics → increased acid elimination
Overdose of alkaline compounds (such as antacids, lye)
Renal failure → decreased acid elimination

INCREASED ACID ELIMINATION
Hyperventilation
  Anxiety
  Hypermetabolism
  Endocrine disorders
  Sepsis
  Mechanical ventilation

riorating patient by an increase in diastolic blood pressure above normal and narrowing of the pulse pressure. Recall from Chapter 9 that pulse pressure is the difference between the systolic and diastolic blood pressure. Normal pulse pressure is approximately 30 to 40 mm Hg in the adult. This process compensates partially for the decreased cardiac output by reducing the volume of the cardiovascular system (making the container smaller).

A significant portion of the blood volume under normal circumstances exists not in the capillaries and not in the arterial system but in the large capacitance vessels on the venous side. Making these vessels smaller increases the blood volume to the arterial system. This additional blood volume can act to improve pressure and perfusion by increasing preload. The change also affects the volume of blood in the system. Reducing the size of the container also reduces the amount of fluid required to provide circulation and adequate perfusion. The combination of these two effects provides a relative autotransfusion to the patient.

Another benefit of making the cardiovascular space smaller is to increase the resistance against which the heart must pump. This effect increases the blood pressure in the arterial side of circulation. As demonstrated earlier (Fig. 11-4), reduction of flow through the capillary beds increases both the systolic and diastolic pressures. If some of the capillary beds are open while others are closed, blood flow is greater in the open beds than in the closed ones. This increased pressure tends to better perfuse those critical components of the circulation that are sensitive to decreased blood flow, such as the heart and brain.

If any of these changes fail to adequately compensate for the patient's hypovolemia, relative hypovolemia, or cardiac pump failure, the systolic and diastolic pressure both begin to decline.

Cells that have been deprived of circulation may continue to function for a variable length of time, despite the fact that their metabolism has been so altered that ultimate survival is not possible. There is a period during which extreme cellular compromise has occurred because of the ischemia; however, if reversed, the organ and, ultimately, the patient will survive; restoration of oxygenation has occurred before cellular death. If cellular death has proceeded to the point that the organ will not survive, despite restoration of adequate perfusion and oxygenation, then shock has become "irreversible." The ultimate outcome of patient death may not be apparent, however, for several days, depending on the organ system that is involved in this irreversible failure.

Uncompensated Shock

Uncompensated shock is when these compensatory mechanisms are no longer able to maintain systolic pressure. Organs in which the flow has been reduced by decreasing the lumen of its supply vessels have even less blood flow, and, therefore, less oxygen is available. The anaerobic metabolism increases, and metabolic acidosis becomes more severe. The driving pressure through the already narrowed vessels has been reduced. The identifiable point of uncompensated shock is a drop in the systolic pressure.

Irreversible Shock

At some point in the ischemic process of anaerobic metabolism, the metabolism of the cells has become so compromised that they can no longer respond to the body's demands for their specialized function (**irreversible shock**). This fact is true whether the specialized function is propagation of electrical stimulation through the nerve cells, contraction of the myocardium to pump blood throughout the cardiovascular system, filtration of blood to remove toxic particles in the kidney, breakdown of metabolic particles into necessary glucose and essential amino acids by the liver, or oxygenation of red cells by the lungs. The end result of such irreversible shock may not be initially apparent, however, until the organs begin to fail several hours or several days later.

A trauma patient may not develop acute renal failure until 5 to 10 days after the ischemic event. This same patient may not develop adult respiratory syndrome for 2 to 3 days after the episode, or acute hepatic failure for 10 days. The patient with compromised myocardium from coronary artery disease or acute spasm that produces reduced blood flow or even occlusion of the coronary artery may survive but develop congestive heart failure 12 to 36 hours after the event. Perhaps congestive heart failure may not even become apparent until several weeks or months later. This organ has suffered irreversible shock. The patient who has a cardiac arrest that requires prolonged cardiopulmonary resuscitation, but eventual conversion to a normal sinus rhythm, and whose cerebral function does not return also had irreversible shock to the brain, although it did not immediately affect the body as a whole.

Irreversible shock is an organ-by-organ phenomenon, depending on that individual organ's sensitivity to ischemia. A patient with a stroke, paraplegia from a spinal injury, or on renal dialysis from chronic renal failure provides another example of the same process. A major side effect can be observed in the acutely ill patient, who has borderline function of several organs, who then develops total failure of one organ. The final "straw" produces failure of all the borderline organs. This multi-system organ failure eventually can lead to patient death. These conditions are all, in one extreme or another, examples of shock-related organ failure that was produced by irreversible changes. The initial cause in all instances was an organ without adequate oxygenation for a long enough period of time for the cells to become irreversibly damaged.

Cellular Pathophysiology

On a cellular basis, the ischemic damage that occurs is a function of the hydrostatic and arterial pressure and the ischemic vessel walls that produce the "leaky" capillary. As was described earlier, sympathetic nervous system discharge mediated through norepinephrine release and epinephrine from the adrenal gland is the first step in decreasing blood flow through regional or organ capillary beds. A model that includes precapillary and postcapillary sphincters is an ideal way to describe the pathophysiologic changes that occur on a cellular level.

On initial stimulation from the sympathetic nervous system, both the precapillary and postcapillary sphincters close, creating significantly increased peripheral resistance and decreasing flow through the specific capillary bed involved.

ISCHEMIC PHASE. The cells, which are perfused by this capillary bed, change from aerobic to anaerobic metabolism and produce increased amounts of pyruvic and lactic acids and potassium. These toxic by-products migrate by diffusion into the capillaries.

The ischemic process affects the vessels by shrinking the cells that line the vessels, allowing diffusion of protein that contains serum into the interstitial space. Before the onset of this *"leaky capillary syndrome,"* the proteins remained within the intravascular space, creating an osmotic pressure to retain fluid in the intravascular space. Loss of the protein to the interstitial space increases the osmotic pressure and subsequently the fluid in this space.

STAGNANT PHASE. As the condition is prolonged, the precapillary sphincters begin to relax and allow blood from the arterial side into this capillary system. The postcapillary sphincters do not relax. This discrepancy increases the capillary hydrostatic (blood) pressure. This pressure increase forces more protein-rich serum into the interstitial space. The increased volume of interstitial fluid increases the distance between the capillaries and the cells, so that the little oxygen that is available has a greater distance to diffuse across to reach the individual cells for metabolism. The condition in the lungs produces a reverse effect, and less oxygen can diffuse from the capillaries to the red blood cells. In addition, concentration and clumping of the red blood cells because of serum loss and increased hydrostatic pressure begins to stack the red cells into *"rouleaux formation."* This formation arranges the red blood cells like a roll of coins.

WASHOUT PHASE. As the process continues, or as the patient is resuscitated, postcapillary sphincters open and allow "washout" into the general circulation of the blood in these capillary beds. This blood contains clumps of red cells, which form microemboli to the lung, increased potassium, which produces systemic hyperkalemia, and pyruvic and lactic acids, which produce generalized systemic metabolic acidosis.

STAGED DEATH. Shock is nothing more than a progression of these ischemic changes of anaerobic metabolism throughout the body. The first step is anaerobic metabolism in each individual cell. If this anaerobic metabolism continues long enough, cellular death ensues. If enough cells die to compromise function of an individual organ, the organ may either itself be dead or noncontributory to functional metabolism and, therefore, as far as the body is concerned, relatively dead. If critical organs die or become nonfunctional, the patient will die. Therefore, shock is staged death, beginning with anaerobic metabolism at the cellular level due to hypoprofusion and ending in total body failure and patient death. Only if the process can be reversed early, does the patient survive intact.

The stages of shock and this dying process may not be immediate, since the ischemic changes that occur initially may not be manifested for several days to a week or more. Therefore, the paramedic may not realize that the patient who died 2 days or even 3 weeks after hospital admission may have died because of incorrect or incomplete management of shock and its ischemic manifestations during the first few minutes when the paramedic had charge of the patient.

Because decisions made in this critical period that result in inadequate resuscitation, including inadequate oxygenation and perfusion, can affect the ultimate outcome of the patient, an understanding of shock, anaerobic metabolism, cellular oxygenation, and the process of perfusion of the cells is critical in patient survival.

ASSESSMENT OF THE PATIENT IN SHOCK

Primary Survey

Evaluation of the patient who presents with the potential for shock begins with visually observing the patient and the surrounding area. This step is done by performing a quick look over the patient's whole body and the area around the patient. Note the patient's position and the condition of the scene or environment in which the patient is found. The patient's position and surroundings frequently provide clues about mechanism of injury and patient history.

Responsiveness

Checking the patient's responsiveness is the initial determination of the patient's gross level of cerebral function. The unconscious patient should be placed in a horizontal, supine position if cardiopulmonary resuscitation is required. Precaution must be exercised in moving the patient if any type of cervical or lower spinal injury is suspected.

Airway

Oxygenation is the first critical point in management of the patient in shock. Lack of adequate oxygenation is one of the most common reasons for early death in the trauma patient and a major cause of death or lack of response to management in patients with medical problems such as diabetes, myocardial infarction, drug overdose, and stroke. Airway management includes adequate ventilation with high-flow oxygen delivered correctly to assure adequate oxygen available to the red blood cells. The next step is to assure that the ventilatory volume is 800 to 1200 mL with each breath.

A patient with *tachypnea* (greater than 20 breaths/min), shallow respirations, or cyanosis must be assumed to have an oxygenation or perfusion problem that is producing anaerobic metabolism as the major factor or at least a major contributing factor to the patient's shocklike condition. Tachypnea identifies, in the patient with an adequate FiO_2, a respiratory rate increase produced by the need to compensate for systemic metabolic acidosis.

Perfusion

Evaluation of perfusion begins with assessment of pulse, skin color, skin temperature, and capillary refill.

PULSE. The pulse in a primary survey is not counted specifically, but a general range is taken; whether or not the pulse is felt at the wrist and the pulse strength (weak or strong) are quickly evaluated. This general impression alerts the paramedic when the patient is responding to a hypovolemic, relative volemic, or pump failure condition.

The location at which the pulse is felt is a good field indication of the amount of peripheral vascular resistance and how much of the cardiovascular system the body is able to perfuse. If the radial pulse is not palpable at the wrist, the systolic pressure is probably below 80. If not palpable at the femoral artery in the groin, the systolic pressure is probably below 70, and if the carotid is not palpable, it is probably below 60.

SKIN COLOR. Skin color is another important mechanism of evaluating perfusion, since it indicates the blood flow in the capillaries. Pink skin is well perfused and well oxygenated. If the skin is pale, perfusion is lacking and the capillary bed is probably in its ischemic phase. Cyanotic skin is one with unsaturated blood. The skin may be unsaturated because of inadequate pulmonary oxygenation of the blood or stagnant phase of capillary shock. A mottled appearance to the skin is both the stagnant and ischemic phases of capillary perfusion side by side. This appearance is an indication of severe shock, markedly decreased peripheral perfusion, and systemic metabolic acidosis.

SKIN TEMPERATURE. Skin temperature is warmer with perfusion and colder with lack of perfusion.

CAPILLARY REFILL. The body differentially shuts down the distal most parts of the circulation to try to preserve perfusion through the proximal components. The hands and feet, therefore, would be the most likely areas to have early circulatory changes. The **capillary refill test** is a way to judge the rate of blood flow through these peripheral capillary beds. The test is accomplished by compressing the nail beds of the thumb or the great toe or the skin over the hypothenar eminence to squeeze blood out of this capillary bed. When the pressure is released, the speed of return of blood into the capillary bed is an estimate of perfusion. Two seconds or less, about the time it takes to say "capillary refill," is normal; longer than this is abnormal.

Lord Kelvin said, "if you speak of something in numbers your knowledge is of the greatest kind; if you cannot speak of something in numbers, your knowledge is very meager." To manage a patient in shock, numbers must be obtained beyond the simple identification of a shocklike state in the primary survey. Those numbers begin with a pulse rate. A rapid pulse is an early indicator that hypovolemia or some type of shock and lack of oxygenation exists. Slowing of the pulse is indicative of patient response to resuscitation. Slowing below normal is an indication of severe cardiac ischemia. Pulse rate is a much earlier sign of shock than hypotension. Usually the blood pressure is maintained until 30% to 40% of the blood volume has been lost. Using various reserve mechanisms, such as increased strength of cardiac contractions and peripheral vascular resistance, the patient can maintain blood pressure in the face of decreased cardiac output.

The younger the person, the stronger the defense mechanisms and the longer blood pressure is maintained before it starts to decrease. When the blood pressure does suddenly drop, especially in a young patient, blood loss may have been so great that survivability is no longer possible. For this reason, evaluation of other indicators, such as pulse, neurologic function, and capillary refill time are important assessment criteria. One does not wish to await the arrival of hypotension before recognizing the existence of shock. Nor does one wish to stop resuscitation when the blood pressure returns to within normal range but other indicators are still outside of normal limits.

Secondary Survey
Level of Consciousness

Four conditions can alter the patient's neurologic status. These are hypoglycemia or hyperglycemia, decreased cerebral oxygenation, brain injury, and drug or alcohol overdose. Since such an altered status can be a major indication of decreased cerebral perfusion, until other etiologies can be identified, it should be assumed that shock exists. Decreased cerebral perfusion produces combativeness, anxiety, disorientation, and frank loss of consciousness. Any patient who presents these symptoms or any other indication of decreased cerebral oxygenation should be managed with 100% oxygen and assisted or controlled ventilation. Bradycardia indicates decreased cardiac oxygenation, just as decreased cerebral function indicates decreased cerebral oxygenation. Changes in level of consciousness, including anxiety and combativeness, as stated, may have several causes; however, when combined with evidence of severe cardiac ischemia (bradycardia), decreased oxygenation of both organs is critical and only immediate aggressive action prevents death.

Since brain injury and drug or alcohol overdose are conditions that do not necessarily need to be treated within the first few seconds of arrival of medical care, and even blood glucose abnormalities can be delayed for a few minutes, the person who presents with these signs and symptoms must initially be presumed to have decreased oxygenation. First, reestablish oxygenation (FiO_2 greater than 0.85) and assist or control ventilation. Then the other conditions can be addressed.

Blood Pressure

Checking the blood pressure is an important step in the secondary survey. Although it is not part of the primary survey, the information it provides should be obtained as soon as life-threatening problems are handled.

Blood pressure has two components. The systolic pressure reflects indirectly the strength of cardiac contractions, while the diastolic pressure is an indicator of peripheral vascular resistance and coronary artery perfusion. Diastolic pressure increases slightly as peripheral vascular resistance reaches its maximum and before systolic and diastolic pressure drop together. Mean arterial pressure, which is a truer indicator of organ perfusion, is diastolic pressure plus one third of pulse pressure. Pulse pressure is the difference between systolic and diastolic pressure. Therefore, a patient with blood pressure of 120/80 has a mean arterial pressure of 94 [80 + (120 − 80)/3 = 94].

After arrival in the hospital, numeric values of urinary output, central venous pressure, pulmonary wedge pressure, and arterial blood gases all provide additional information, which is important in the continued management of the patient.

MANAGEMENT

Resuscitation

Resuscitation of the patient in shock begins first and foremost with airway management, including 85% or greater oxygen, assisted or controlled ventilation to assure adequate volume of air movement, and additional airway management as necessary. As has already been emphasized, this component is extremely important in the management of the patient in shock. Inadequate airway control and ventilation produce more deaths in shock than any other one incompletely managed component.

See Chapter 10 for a full discussion of airway management.

Perfusion

PNEUMATIC ANTI-SHOCK GARMENT. Establishing adequate perfusion begins with the simplest management first, proceeding to more complicated ones. The simplest is the **pneumatic anti-shock garment (PASG)**. The paramedic should spend no longer than 60 seconds in its application. The PASG should be on the long backboard when the patient is moved from the car, bed, ground, or whatever other position in which the patient is found, and the patient placed on top of the garment. After removing the patient's clothes and evaluating the abdomen and legs, the garment is folded around the patient and the Velcro fasteners engaged. At this point, the paramedic can evaluate the patient to identify the need for the inflation of the PASG.

The PASG is a pneumatic garment that fits around the abdomen, from below the ribs to just above the ankles. The ones currently available are the three-compartment type. One compartment encircles the abdomen and one encircles each leg. Each of the compartments can be inflated individually and can be deflated the same way. This flexibility allows for inflation of the legs segment only, when an impaled object, pregnancy, or evisceration would be a relative contraindication to inflation of the abdominal compartment. Velcro fasteners are used for rapid approximation of the two sides. Although gauges are available to determine the pressure in each compartment individually, this determination is not required, since exact compartment pressure has not been shown to coincide with changes in systolic blood pressure. Many studies have shown that, unless the compartment pressure is in the range of 60 mm Hg or higher, the blood pressure is only minimally influenced by inflation of PASG. It is the patient who is in shock, therefore, whose blood pressure must be monitored, and the PASG should be maximally inflated.

If the patient is flying in a helicopter or a fixed-wing aircraft at a high altitude, or if the temperature changes significantly once the garment has been inflated, the patient's pressure should be closely monitored. Any blood pressure change would warrant investigation of its etiology. If the etiology was leakage from the device, ambient pressure, or temperature changes that changed the garment pressure and, thus, that of the patient, appropriate steps to restore inflation to a point of stabilizing the patient's blood pressure are warranted. If blood pressure changes were of another source, that source must also be found.

Much discussion has appeared in the literature about

the manner in which the PASG works. It is indisputable throughout the literature that the device does elevate blood pressure. Exactly how pressure is elevated is controversial. Initial research indicated that blood volume displacement from the lower extremities and abdomen into the heart-brain-lung circulation produced the response. Later work has indicated that is a significant increase in systemic vascular resistance and afterload is found. Either mechanism, or both mechanisms, could account for an increase in systemic blood pressure. Much of the controversy and debate about the PASG centers on its mechanism of action and whether its application is warranted in all emergency medical services settings for patients in shock. Further clinical experiences as well as investigation will help to clarify much of this controversy.

External pressure on the extremity is transmitted into the center of the enclosed body part. Since this pressure is equally distributed throughout the body part, those hollow structures or fluid-filled structures, such as blood vessels, would tend to collapse, while solid structures do not.

The formula for the volume of a cylinder is $V = hr^2 pi$, in which V equals volume, h equals height (length), r equals radius, and pi equals 3.14. Since halving the radius makes the volume four times as small, it is logical to assume that the vessels with a reduced volume would experience three effects. Because the vessels are smaller, more pressure would be required to move blood through them, thus, the first effect would be to increase peripheral vascular resistance. The smaller volume vessels would require less fluid for filling. This volume can then be used in other portions of the circulation, which were not reduced in size (step two). Thirdly, as the vessels become smaller, the fluid within them would be moved to that portion of the circulation that is not enclosed, and, therefore, some autotransfusion would take place. The result is increased afterload, increased preload, and reduced volume required to fill the vascular space.

Hypovolemic shock, spinal shock, severe blood loss, fractured pelvis, intra-abdominal hemorrhage, and a fractured femur are all indications for the application of PASG. The exact conditions that indicate inflation of the garment vary somewhat but, in general, include a blood pressure of less than 90 systolic with tachycardia, overt blood loss or other signs of existing hypovolemia, stabilization of fractured femur or pelvis, and intra-abdominal hemorrhage. As more information is gathered on the mechanism of action of this device, these indications may become more specifically defined.

A contraindication is thoracic trauma associated with hemorrhage and pulmonary edema. A ruptured diaphragm with translocation of abdominal contents into the thoracic cavity followed by decreased respiratory function is the only consistent indication for field deflation of the PASG.

Relative contraindications include impaled abdominal object, pregnancy, and evisceration. These relative contraindications may well be handled by inflation of the leg segments only unless uterine or other intra-abdominal hemorrhage is present. In this situation, inflation under medical control of the abdominal segment is appropriate.

Deflation is not a technique usually carried out in the field but is carried out either in the operating room just as surgery is about to begin (to maintain tamponade of intra-abdominal hemorrhage) or in the emergency department after evaluation of the patient has not identified significant indications for continued use (such as presence of intra-abdominal hemorrhage). Indications for field deflation would include the onset of pulmonary edema, decrease in respiratory function associated with mechanism of injury, which would indicate the possibility of diaphragmatic hernia.

Deflation is carried out gradually, first deflating the abdominal segment and then each leg segment individually. The segment valve is opened to let out a small amount of air, starting with the abdomen. The patient's blood pressure is checked and the procedure repeated until that compartment is completely deflated. The next compartment is then deflated in the same manner. Should the blood pressure drop as much as 5 mm Hg systolic, deflation should be stopped until the etiology of the blood pressure drop is identified or adequate fluid replacement has been accomplished so that the blood pressure returns to its predeflation state. At that point, deflation is continued while adequate intravenous (IV) fluid replacement is carried out.

The procedure for applying the pneumatic anti-shock garment is shown in Skill 11-1.

INTRAVENOUS FLUIDS. The next step in resuscitation is fluid replacement. The patient needs definitive management as soon as possible. An *IV line* should be started as soon as possible but should not delay transport in a critically injured patient. For example, a diabetic in hypoglycemic shock is treated most quickly and easily by IV glucose. This treatment can be given on the scene. A cardiac arrest patient is treated by defibrillation, intubation, and IV medications.

The trauma patient is hypovolemic from blood loss. The problem is hemorrhage, which cannot be controlled in the field, although PASG may decrease abdominal, pelvic, and upper leg hemorrhage. Most severe intra-abdominal or thoracic hemorrhage cannot be stopped in the emergency department, therefore, this patient needs transportation as quickly as possible to the operating room. The paramedic has the responsibility not only of beginning transportation and starting the IV as soon as practical but also of transporting the patient to a hospital that has trauma surgeons and an operating room staff available when the patient arrives, if such a prepared hospital is available in the community.

CHAPTER 11: Pathophysiology of Shock and Fluid Management

SKILL 11-1.
PNEUMATIC ANTI-SHOCK GARMENT

ACTIVITY	HOW PERFORMED	WHY PERFORMED
1. Check: • Responsiveness • Airway • Breathing • Circulation	Establish responsiveness Stabilize neck, open the airway Assess breathing Check for a pulse Check for hemorrhage	The primary survey is a rapid evaluation, less than 45 seconds, to identify and correct any life-threatening problems.
2. Assemble and check: Primary equipment (Activity 2A): • Pneumatic anti-shock garment (PASG) • Inflation device Accessory equipment and supplies: • Long backboard • Cervical collar • Gloves • Stethoscope • Blood pressure cuff	Put on gloves. Unroll the PASG face up on the long backboard, release Velcro or zipper closures. Roll down the top layer of the abdominal portion (Activity 2B) (in some models the abdominal section is rolled to each side) and roll the top layer of each leg section to the center (Activity 2C) *Remove the patient's clothing and check for sharp objects on the ground.*	The use of a long backboard is helpful in moving the patient after the PASG is applied. Rolling the top layers back opens the garment, allowing easy placement of the patient in the garment. *Patient's clothing should be removed to observe for injuries. Sharp objects are removed from the area to prevent damage to the PASG.*

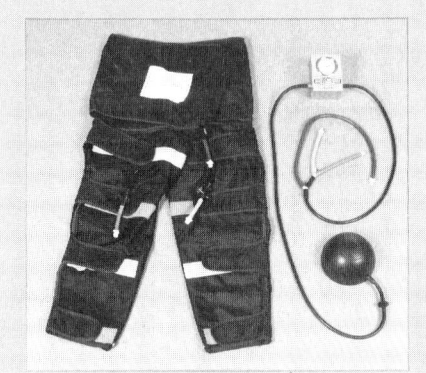

Activity 2A.
Primary equipment.

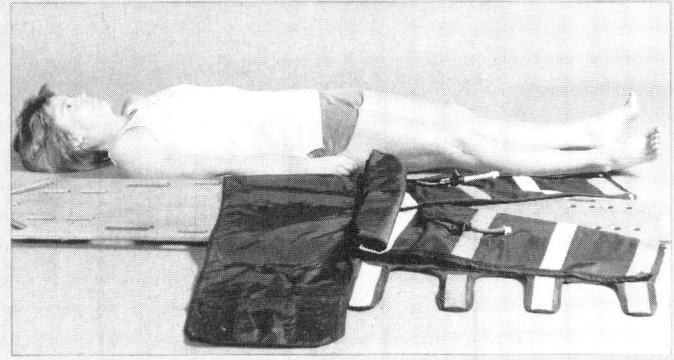

Activity 2B.
Roll down top layer of abdominal portion of PASG.

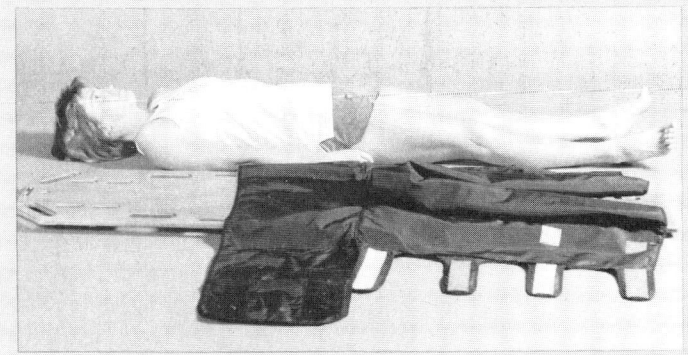

Activity 2C.
Roll top layer of each leg section of PASG to center.

(continued)

SKILL 11-1.
PNEUMATIC ANTI-SHOCK GARMENT (continued)

ACTIVITY	HOW PERFORMED	WHY PERFORMED
3. Apply cervical immobilization as indicated	If the mechanism of injury or patient assessment reveals a need for cervical immobilization, apply a cervical collar and maintain cervical immobilization (Activity 3).	Spinal injuries commonly occur along with other injuries that may require treatment with the PASG. Immobilization reduces the possibility of spinal cord damage as patient is moved onto the PASG.
4. Log-roll patient onto long backboard and PASG	With one person at the patient's head, and several assistants along one side of the patient, log-roll the patient toward the rescuer's knees as a single unit (Activity 4). Place the backboard with PASG alongside the patient and roll the patient as a unit down onto the board and the PASG.	Log rolling as a unit avoids unnecessary movement of the patient's spine. This log rolling places the patient both on the backboard and PASG in one movement.

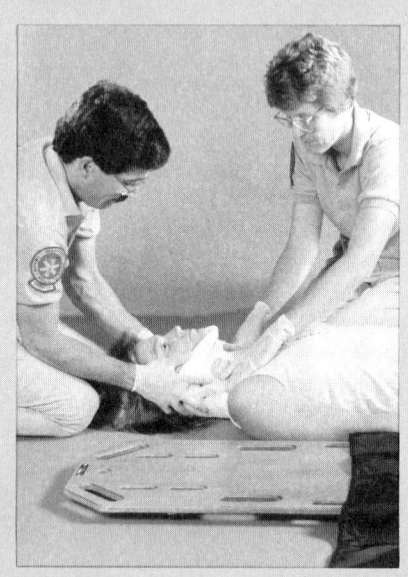

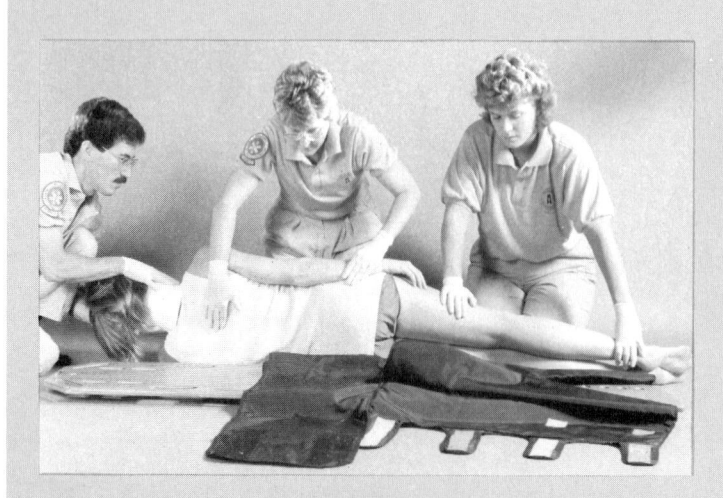

Activity 3.
Apply cervical immobilization.

Activity 4.
Log-roll patient onto backboard and PASG.

(continued)

SKILL 11-1.
PNEUMATIC ANTI-SHOCK GARMENT (continued)

ACTIVITY	HOW PERFORMED	WHY PERFORMED
5. Apply PASG to patient	Pull the abdominal section up onto the patient's abdomen, making sure the upper edge of abdominal section is at the lower border of the costal margin (Activity 5A). (In some models the abdominal section is wrapped across from each side).	Problems with respirations may develop if the thoracic area above the costal margin is covered by the PASG.
	Unroll leg sections over the patient's legs. Fasten Velcro or zipper closures (Activity 5B). Velcro should be snug and smooth.	Velcro and zipper closures secure the PASG around the patient.

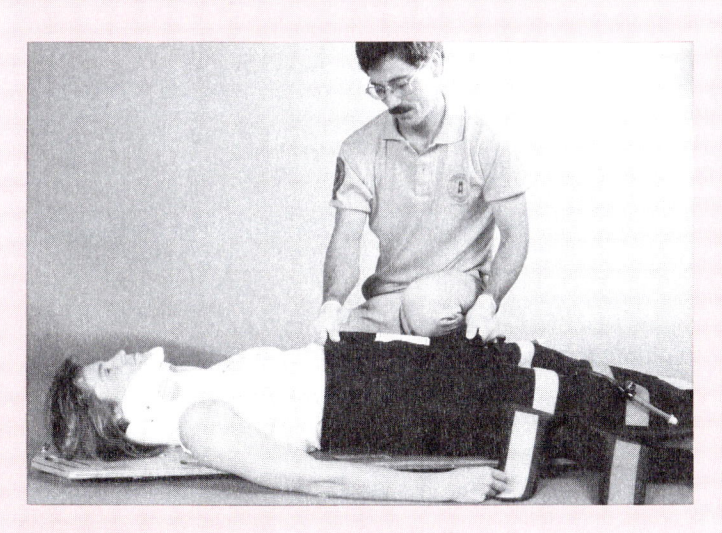

Activity 5A.
Apply abdominal section of PASG.

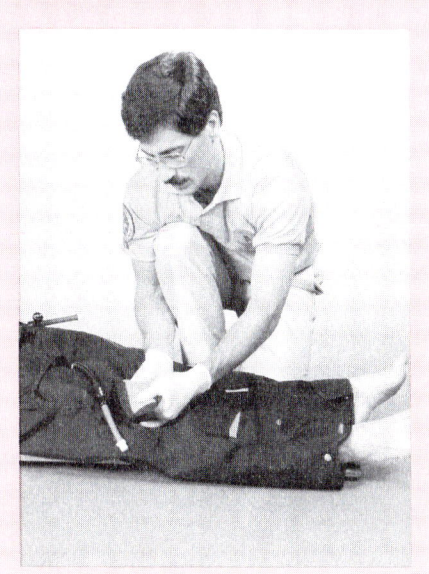

Activity 5B.
Apply PASG leg sections.

(continued)

SKILL 11–1.
PNEUMATIC ANTI-SHOCK GARMENT (continued)

ACTIVITY	HOW PERFORMED	WHY PERFORMED
6. Reassess patient	Check signs, symptoms, and vital signs to see if PASG still needs to be inflated (Activity 6).	Patient condition may change rapidly, and changes must be noted and treated. In some cases, it may be advisable to postpone the inflation of the PASG.

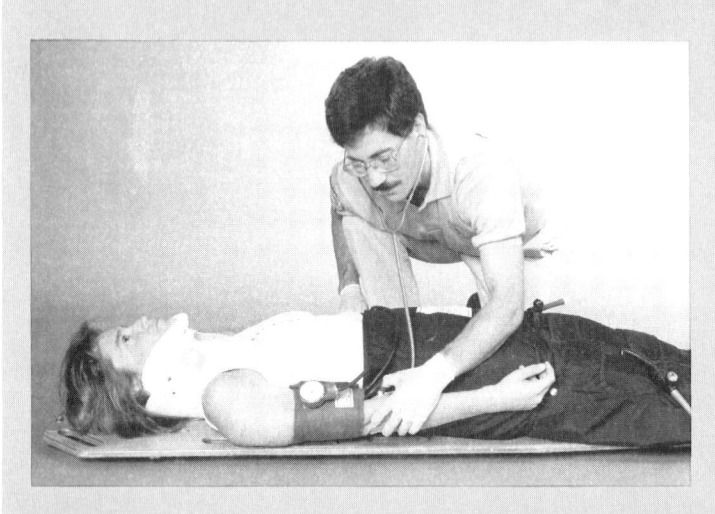

Activity 6.
Reassess patient.

7. Connect pump tubing and inflate the PASG	Connect appropriate tubing on the pants to the corresponding tubing on the inflation device (Activity 7A). Open in-line valves for sections to be inflated (Activity 7B).	These actions allow for inflation of the pants, either all at once or by sections, as indicated.

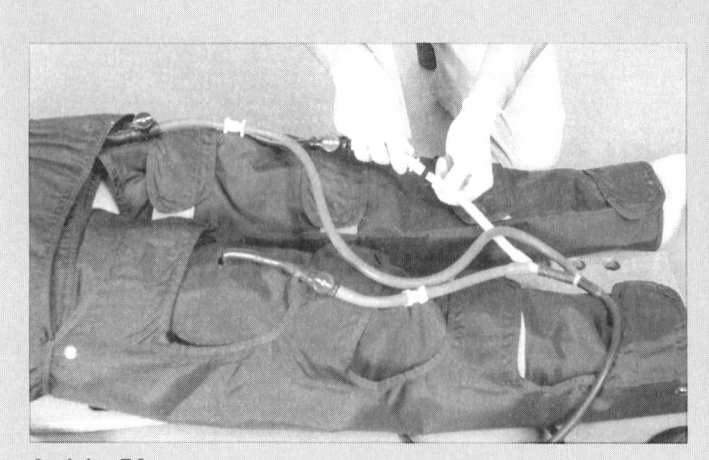

Activity 7A.
Connect pump tubing.

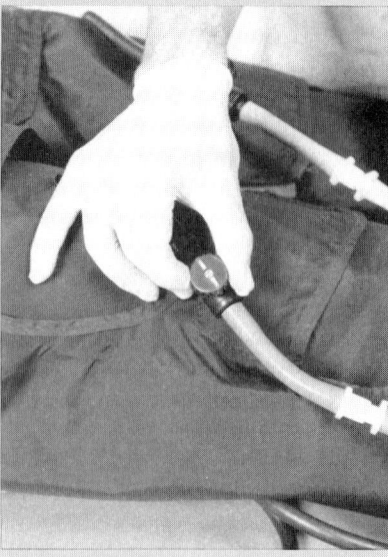

Activity 7B.
Open in-line valves.

(continued)

SKILL 11-1.
PNEUMATIC ANTI-SHOCK GARMENT (continued)

ACTIVITY	HOW PERFORMED	WHY PERFORMED
	Inflate until all sections are tight to hand pressure or until the Velcro starts to slip. Close in-line valves (Activity 7C). Reassess patient's signs, symptoms, and blood pressure (Activity 7D). If needed, inflate other sections or increase pressure in all sections.	Full inflation of all sections is the correct method unless the abdominal compartment is contraindicated.
	Inflate until clinical improvement is seen in the patient's vital signs.	Clinical improvement in vital signs is the best indicator of effective inflation.

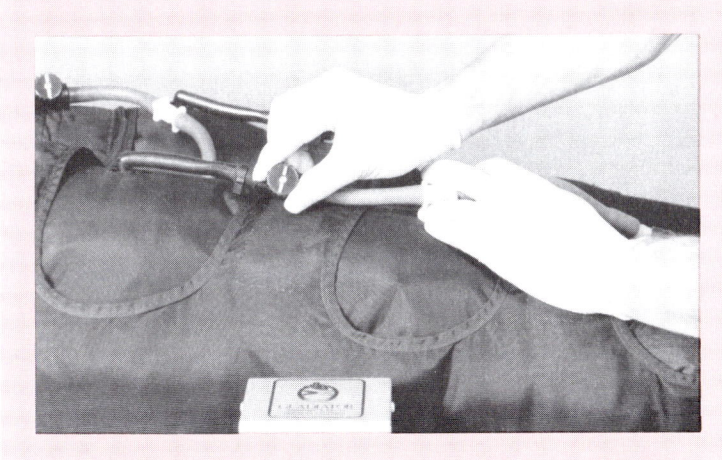

Activity 7C.
Close in-line valves.

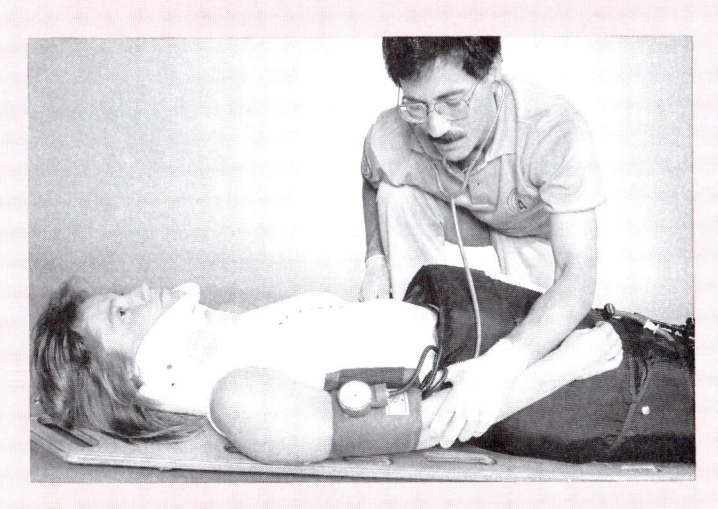

Activity 7D.
Reassess patient.

Intravenous Access. The time at which an IV line should be started depends on the situation, the personnel available, the time to the hospital, and other factors. Starting an IV line should not delay transport.

There are two reasons for starting an IV line on any patient. Each type of IV placement is done for a specific patient need. Each may require a different type of administration set up and a different technique. Before starting the IV, the paramedic must know why it is being started so that it is started correctly. Intravenous lines are started for the following reasons:

- Fluid replacement
- Medication administration

Fluid Replacement. Fluid replacement necessitates a short, large bore-needle placed in a peripheral vessel. A large vein in the forearm or the antecubital area is chosen for fluid administration or whole blood. The size of the catheter is related to the need for the fluid. In a hypovolemic patient, the fluid needs to be administered rapidly. If medication alone is needed, a "keep vein open" (KVO) or "to keep open" (TKO) rate of 25 mL per hour is acceptable. The rate at which fluids flow into the body is not related to the size of the vessel into which the catheter is placed. Veins are distensible. The limiting factor for fluid administration is that component that has the most resistance to fluid passage. Poiseuille's law of thermodynamics identifies this relationship. It states that "flow within a tube is directly proportional to its internal diameter and inversely proportional to its length." A short, large-bore tube, therefore, passes fluid at a much greater rate than does a long, narrow tube. A 14-gauge, 4-cm needle placed in a forearm vein, therefore, passes fluids approximately twice as fast as a 20-cm, 16-gauge catheter placed in the more central subclavian vein.

At least two IV sites are necessary in the hypovolemic

TABLE 11-7.
TYPES OF IV FLUIDS

IV Solution	Constituents	Osmolarity mOsm/L	Advantages	Disadvantages	Field Uses
0.9% NaCl crystalloid isotonic	154 mEq Na/L 154 mEq Cl/L	308	Fluid and sodium replacement	Pulmonary edema, congestive heart failure. Administration of large amounts may cause electrolyte depletion	Hypovolemia Dehydration Heat-related problems Freshwater drowning Diabetic ketoacidosis Fluid resuscitation for pediatrics
lactated Ringer's crystalloid isotonic	130 mEq Na/L 109 mEq Cl/L 4 mEq K/L 3 mEq Ca/L 28 mEq lactate/L	273	Approximates the electrolyte concentration of the blood	Pulmonary edema Renal failure Congestive heart failure	Hypovolemia Dehydration Burns Fluid resuscitation for pediatrics
D_5W crystalloid isotonic	50 g dextrose/L	252	Glucose nutrient solution	Used with caution in head injuries Pulmonary congestion Not appropriate for the pediatric patient	Mainly used to keep open a vein; life-line for administration of medication to adults; for dilution of IV drip drugs; IV access for emergency drugs
0.45% NaCl hypotonic	77 mEq Na/L 77 mEq Cl/L	154	Slow rehydration	Hypovolemia Administration of large amounts may cause electrolyte depletion	Patients with diminished renal or cardiovascular function where rapid rehydration is not indicated
$D_5$0.45% NaCl hypertonic	77 mEq Na/L 77 mEq Cl/L 50 g dextrose/L	406	Electrolyte and sugar replacement	Hypovolemia	Heat-related problems Diabetic TKO for patients with impaired renal or cardiovascular function
$D_5$0.9% NaCl hypertonic	154 mEq Na/L 154 mEq Cl/L 50 g dextrose/L	560	Electrolyte and sugar replacement	Impaired renal or cardiovascular function	Heat-related problems Fresh water drowning Hypovolemia Peritonitis Life-line for administration of medication to pediatrics
D_5LR hypertonic	130 mEq Na/L 109 mEq Cl/L 3 mEq Ca/L 4 mEq K/L 28 mEq lactate/L 50 g dextrose/L	525	Electrolyte and sugar replacement	Patients with renal or cardiovascular function	Hypovolemia Life-line for administration of medication to pediatrics

Note: The normal physiologic range for isotonicity is 250–310 mOsm/L

patient. As many as four sites are preferable in the patient in shock, keeping in mind that transport should not be delayed to establish IV access. For information on IV site locations and how to start an IV see Chapter 12.

An isotonic solution is usually chosen for prehospital administration. Lactated Ringer's and 0.9% sodium chloride are isotonic solutions. Although D_5W is considered an isotonic solution, it is not an acceptable choice for use in fluid resuscitation. The glucose is quickly metabolized by the liver and shortly after administration nothing but water is left. This free water is hypotonic and dilutes the blood. It then reduces the vascular oncotic pressure and is rapidly lost into the interstitial space. To stabilize the oncotic pressure, fluid travels from the cardiovascular system into the interstitial space and produces edema. This condition is particularly detrimental to the brain when ischemia is present. It is also detrimental to the heart and kidney and other organs.

Lactated Ringer's solution and 0.9% sodium chloride solution also diffuse easily into the interstitial space but do so much slower than water. However, the difference is that lactated Ringer's and 0.9% sodium chloride do not become hypotonic in the body. Patients with isolated head injuries or head injuries in the face of normotension should not be overloaded with any fluid, including lactated Ringer's or 0.9% sodium chloride, since it is the cellular edema that is particularly damaging. In the patient with significant fluid loss, capillary permeability increases. With the administration of large volumes of crystalloid solutions, extravasation of fluids into the pulmonary capillary beds can result in adult respiratory distress syndrome. Therefore, in the trauma patient, a maximum of 2 to 3 L of lactated Ringer's solution is usually administered before whole blood therapy is initiated. A summary of IV fluids is found in Table 11-7.

The rate of fluid administration in the patient who requires fluid resuscitation should be carefully monitored. In the adult, 1000 mL should be infused initially, and then vital signs reassessed. If additional fluids are required, 500 mL/hour should be administered as long as signs and symptoms of pulmonary edema are not present.

Medication. Medication administration alone is most often done through a small plastic catheter, placed in a peripheral vein and administered in association with 5% glucose and water or 0.9% sodium chloride. Medication can be administrated through a hand vein or other peripheral vein. It is a medium of transport only.

SUMMARY

Shock, in modern medical terminology, is anaerobic metabolism at the cellular level. Although an individual cell can be in shock alone, the term, by custom, applies to a generalized condition rather than a local one. The determinants of shock (anaerobic metabolism) as identified by the Fick formula are red blood cell oxygenation, red blood cell delivery, and red blood cell O_2 offloading. A failure of any of these steps can lead to anaerobic metabolism. Perfusion, the delivery of the red blood cell to the tissue, depends on the intactness of the three components of the cardiovascular system (pump, container, and fluid). Failure of any component significantly reduces perfusion. In trauma, the component most often affected is the fluid volume. This must be reestablished as rapidly as possible and the hemorrhage controlled if the patient is to survive. Adequate oxygenation, temporary hemorrhage control in the field, replenishment of lost fluid volume with lactated Ringer's solution, and delivery of the patient to the correct hospital are the hallmarks of good trauma care.

SUGGESTED READING

American Heart Association: Textbook of Advanced Life Support, 2nd ed. Dallas, American Heart Association, 1987

Campbell JE: Basic Trauma Life Support—Advanced Prehospital Care, 2nd ed. Englewood Cliffs, Prentice–Hall, 1988

Cromer AH: Physics for the Life Services. New York, McGraw-Hill, 1974

Guyton AC: Textbook of Medical Physiology, 7th ed. Philadelphia, WB Saunders, 1986

McSwain NE, Butman AM, McConnnell WK et al: Prehospital Trauma Life Support, 2nd ed. Akron, Emergency Training, 1990

McSwain NE, Kerstein MD: Evaluation and Management of Trauma. Norwalk, Appleton-Century-Crofts, 1987

Taylor C, Lillis C, LeMone P: Fundamentals of Nursing. Philadelphia, JB Lippincott, 1989

Tortora GJ, Anagnostakos NP: Principles of Anatomy and Physiology, 6th ed. New York, Harper and Row, 1990

US Department of Transportation, National Highway Traffic Safety Administration: Emergency Medical Technician-Paramedic: National Standards Curriculum. Washington, DC, US Government Printing Office, 1985

Verdile VP: Trends in IV therapy. J Emerg Serv 22(4):44, 1990

CHAPTER 12

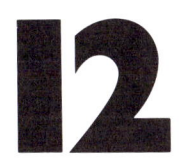

General Pharmacology

General Drug Information
Drug Sources and Legislation
Drug Names
Drug References and Resources
Forms of Drugs
Drug Pharmacokinetics
   Absorption
      Oral Administration
      Parenteral Administration
         Intradermal
         Subcutaneous
         Intramuscular
         Intravenous
         Topical
         Tracheal
   Distribution
   Biotransformation and Elimination
Drug Pharmacodynamics
   Receptors
      Autonomic Nervous System
         Sympathetic Division
            Sympathetic Receptors
            Drugs That Affect the Sympathetic Division
         Parasympathetic Division
            Vagal Stimulation

Calculating Drug Dosages
   The Metric System
      Weight Measurements
         Making Pound-to-Kilogram Conversions
      Liquid Measurements
      Common Conversions
   A Review of Decimals
      Addition and Subtraction
      Multiplication and Division
   Drug Dosage Calculations
      Intravenous Infusion Rate Calculation
Drug Administration
   Drug Packaging and Preparation
      Ampules
      Vials
      Preloaded Syringes
      Intravenous Drug Infusions
      Needles and Syringes
   Parenteral Administration
      Intradermal

Skill 12-1. Intradermal Injection
   Subcutaneous
Skill 12-2. Subcutaneous Injection
   Intramuscular
Skill 12-3. Intramuscular Injection
   Intravenous
      Peripheral
Skill 12-4. Peripheral Venipuncture
      Central
Skill 12-5. Central Line Placement (Femoral)
Skill 12-6. Central Line Placement (Internal Jugular, Anterior Approach)
Skill 12-7. Central Line Placement (Internal Jugular, Middle Approach)
Skill 12-8. Central Line Placement (Internal Jugular, Posterior Approach)
Skill 12-9. Central Line Placement (Subclavian Approach)
   Intraosseous
Skill 12-10. Intraosseous Infusion
   Sublingual
   Endotracheal
Summary

BEHAVIORAL OBJECTIVES

On successful completion of this chapter, the reader will be able to:

1. Identify four common sources of drugs
2. Differentiate between chemical, generic, and trade names of drugs
3. Explain the necessity for drug standards
4. Give a brief history of drug legislation in the United States
5. Compare and contrast local and systemic drug effects
6. Discuss advantages, disadvantages, and relative speed of absorption of the following routes of drug administration: oral, intravenous, topical, rectal, intramuscular, sublingual, subcutaneous, endotracheal, intradermal
7. Discuss factors that influence the actions of a drug on an individual patient, especially: age, body mass, physical condition, drug dosage, drug interactions

(continued)

205

BEHAVIORAL OBJECTIVES (continued)

8. Explain why the paramedic must be familiar with the following characteristics of a particular drug: actions, indications, contraindications, route and rate of administration, drug interactions
9. Describe factors that affect a drug's distribution in the body
10. Describe factors that influence the body's storage of a drug
11. Explain why impaired excretion of a drug can affect its dosage and duration of action
12. Calculate the following: the volume of drug to deliver, given the dose content and desired dose; the concentration of drug in an IV infusion; the IV drip rate of a drug infusion, given the rate in mg/min or µg/min and tubing type
13. Discuss and perform the skills for the following types of infusions: intradermal, subcutaneous, intramuscular, peripheral venipuncture, central line placement (femoral), central line placement (internal jugular, anterior approach), central line placement (internal jugular, middle approach), central line placement (internal jugular, posterior approach), central line placement (subclavian approach), and intraosseous
14. Define all of the key terms listed in this chapter

KEY TERMS

The following terms are defined in the chapter and glossary:

α-adrenergic receptors
agonists
ampules
antagonists
apothecary system
aqueous solutions
aqueous suspensions
$β_1$-adrenergic receptors
$β_2$-adrenergic receptors
blood-brain barrier
capsules
Controlled Substance Act
distribution
drug
Drug Enforcement Agency
elixirs
emulsions
extracts
Federal Trade Commission
fight or flight
fluid extracts
Food and Drug Administration
Harrison Narcotic Act of 1914
Hospital Formulary
intradermal
intramuscular(IM)
intraosseous
intravenous(IV)
liniments
lotions
magmas
metric system
ointments
parasympathetic division
parenteral drugs
pharmacodynamics
pharmacokinetics
Physicians' Desk Reference
pills
potentiation
powders
preloaded syringes
Public Health Service
pulvules
Pure Food and Drug Act of 1906
receptors
Schedule I drugs
Schedule II drugs
Schedule III drugs
Schedule IV drugs
Schedule V drugs
spirits
subcutaneous(SQ,SC)
suppositories
sympathetic division
synergistic
syrups
tablets
tachyphylaxis
tinctures
topical
United States Pharmacopeia
Valsalva's maneuver
vials

One of the primary responsibilities of a paramedic is to be able to administer medications. The basic principle of medicine is: "First, do no harm." Most experienced practitioners are reluctant to administer a medication to a patient unless it is clearly needed. The medications used in prehospital care are some of the most potent available and administration routes often leave no room for error.

To provide safe, effective care that has a positive effect on patient outcome, the paramedic must have an excellent working knowledge of both general pharmacologic principles and drugs used in the prehospital environment. The paramedic must also be familiar with common home medications. Besides anticipating possible drug interactions, knowledge about a patient's current medications can provide information about the patient's medical history and guide field management.

In learning about drug therapy, rote memorization is less effective than understanding the drug's physiologic effects. Once the drug's actions are understood, the indications, contraindications, and side effects become clear. However, rote memorization is necessary to learn information such as drug dosages.

The purpose of this chapter is to present basic pharmacologic principles that are built on in later chapters. For example, in Chapter 20, the specifics of cardiovascular drugs used by the paramedic are discussed, in addition to medications commonly taken by cardiac patients. The reader is also referred to Appendix D, for a listing of the most frequently used emergency drugs, and to Appendix E, for a listing of common home medications.

GENERAL DRUG INFORMATION

A *drug* by definition is: "Any chemical agent that affects living processes." This definition explains the wide scope of the study of pharmacology. The basic approach in the therapy of most diseases is to control or stop the disease process and allow the body to heal itself. Many of the patients encountered by the paramedic may not live long enough to heal themselves without prompt intervention; as a result, most of the drugs used in prehospital care are for stabilization of patients during resuscitation.

Risks are associated in the administration of most drugs, whether in the hospital or in the more uncontrolled prehospital environment. The *right* patient must get the *right* dose of the *right* drug, at the *right* time. Potential adverse effects also are associated with most drugs. For example, atropine is used to increase the heart rate and cardiac output in patients with unstable bradycardia. In doing so, it also increases myocardial oxygen demand and may increase the size of a myocardial infarction. While this increase may be an acceptable compromise for some patients, it may be an unreasonable risk for others.

To make risk vs. benefit decisions in the field, the paramedic must have an understanding of pathophysiology and pharmacology. This provides the background information to communicate pertinent information so that patients may be managed appropriately. Even in systems with stringent medical control, many situations occur when the paramedic must rely on a personal knowledge base to make informed, rational decisions about management options.

FEATURES OF DRUGS

Drug actions/Indications: Physiologically, how does this drug work? Why use this drug and not another? When should this drug be given?

Contraindications/Side effects: When should this drug be avoided and why? Are there any adverse symptoms the patient may experience after administration?

Dosage: What are the usual adult and pediatric dosages for this drug? Does the dosage vary if given by different routes?

Administration: By what route should this drug be given? Can it be given by other routes?

The best insurance against error is a thorough understanding of each of the drugs carried in the prehospital system. The paramedic needs to know all the features of each drug carried and must be able to answer all the questions shown in the box, "Features of Drugs," before administering any drug.

DRUG SOURCES AND LEGISLATION

At the beginning of the 20th century, most illnesses were treated by drugs manufactured solely from plant, animal, and mineral substances. Many "secret" elixirs sold to the public and allegedly effective against a wide variety of ailments were little more than alcohol or illicit drugs. As medical science began to understand the exact mechanisms of disease, researchers worked to develop more drugs to combat illnesses. Tremendous progress has been made in the development of drugs. New technologies now permit the synthetic manufacture of drugs previously unheard of. Drugs may be derived from four different sources:

1. Plants. Most parts of plants have at one time been used as drugs, including leaves, flowers, seeds, and roots. For example, digitalis, a drug used to treat heart failure, is derived from the leaves of the purple foxglove flower. Morphine and opiates are derived from the opium poppy plant.
2. Animals. Many different parts of animals have been used as drug sources, including proteins and enzymes. Substances such as epinephrine and insulin are derived from animals.
3. Minerals. Inorganic materials used as drugs are usually the refined forms of minerals, such as iodine, calcium, iron, and Epsom salts.
4. Synthetic. Most drugs used today are manufactured in a pharmaceutical laboratory, even if they were originally available in one of the previously mentioned forms.

In the early 1900s, as the number of chemical substances used to treat disease increased, it became evident that legislation was needed to protect the public. Drugs varied in strength considerably and were often impure. Since accurate dosage and predictability of response depends on uniformity of strength, it was necessary to standardize drugs. Also, the popularity of patent medicine "cure-alls" with questionable ingredients was spreading.

The first major federal drug law was known as the ***Pure Food and Drug Act of 1906***. It mandated labelling of preparations that contained certain habit-forming drugs, and it prohibited making false claims about a drug's actions. The original 1906 Act has been amended several times with relevant changes to protect the public. In 1938, a provision was added to prevent premature marketing of drugs that had not been tested for safety. It required all manufacturers to submit new drug applications to the federal government for safety review before marketing. This provision was enacted after the deaths of more than 100 people who had taken a sulfa derivative that contained a toxic solvent. In 1951, the Act was amended to restrict the refilling of prescriptions and divided drugs into two categories: those that did not require medical supervision, known as *"over-the-counter"* drugs, and those not safe for unsupervised use, requiring a prescription. In 1962, the Act was again amended in response to tragic consequences that resulted from use of a common drug. Thalidomide, a hypnotic drug widely used in Europe, caused severe birth defects in children of mothers who had taken the drug early in their pregnancy. This new amendment gave the Food and Drug Administration responsibility for the safety and efficacy of drugs. It also required that extensive testing of drugs be completed before they are made available for human use. These laws are the most protective in the world.

Another important area of drug legislation deals with control of narcotics. The first of these laws effective in the United States was known as the **Harrison Narcotic Act of 1914**. The Act regulated the manufacture, import, sale, and use of opium and cocaine and their derivatives. It also required extensive record keeping by those who prescribed, dispensed, and administered narcotics. This law has been revised many times to include new and synthetic forms of potentially addictive drugs. In 1956, the Narcotic Control Act was passed to amend the Harrison Act and increased penalties for the law's violation. This act also made possession of heroin and marijuana illegal.

In 1970, the **Controlled Substance Act** was passed, replacing the previous acts and their amendments. One component of this act classified drugs according to their usefulness and abuse potential. The following list describes the "schedules" or stratification of drugs according to this act.

Schedule I: Drugs that do not have a medical use, such as heroin, LSD, peyote, mescaline, and marijuana.

Schedule II: Drugs that have a medical use but a high abuse potential. No telephone prescriptions are allowed, prescriptions must be filled within 72 hours of when they were written and may not be refilled. Drugs in this schedule include morphine, codeine, cocaine, meperidine, and several amphetamines and barbiturates.

Schedule III: Drugs used in medical care but which have less abuse potential than Schedule II drugs. Prescriptions for these drugs must be rewritten after 6 months or 5 refills. Drugs in this schedule include combinations of codeine and other drugs, such as aspirin with codeine and Tylenol with codeine.

Schedule IV: Similar to Schedule III but the penalties for illegal possession are less severe. Drugs in this schedule include Valium, Librium, Talwin, and Darvon.

Schedule V: Drugs that have a low potential for abuse and in many states may be dispensed without a prescription, including several cough preparations that contain codeine.

Periodically, drugs may be changed from one schedule to another. The paramedic is advised to keep current with these changes to meet the reporting requirements necessary when administering these drugs. In general, drugs in Schedules II, III, and IV require meticulous record keeping by the paramedic. After the drug is administered, the paramedic must note the patient's name, the date and time the drug was given, the name of the physician who ordered the drug, and sign the drug record. In addition, the paramedic must account for the entire amount of drug dispensed, even if the whole amount is not administered to the patient. The destroyed quantity of drug must be disposed of in the presence of another person, who verifies this action on the narcotic record. Drugs in these schedules are stored in a locked compartment, and the paramedic must account for all narcotics at the end of the work shift.

Several agencies have a role in the monitoring and enforcement of drug legislation in the United States. The **Drug Enforcement Agency** is responsible for the enforcement of drug legislation. The **Federal Trade Commission** regulates drug advertising. The **Food and Drug Administration** regulates the manufacturing, research, and testing of drugs and monitors adverse effects of new drugs on the market. The United States **Public Health Service** inspects and licenses establishments that manufacture drugs.

DRUG NAMES

Each drug has an official, generic, chemical, and trade name. The *official name* of a drug is the name that is listed in the official governmental publication, the **United States Pharmacopeia**. The official name may have one or more synonymous names by which it is also listed. The *generic name* is assigned to a drug before it becomes officially listed and is often adopted by the official publication. It is usually a simple form of the chemical name of the drug. The *chemical name* is an exact description of the chemical structure. The *trade name* (also called the brand name or the proprietary name) is the name a manufacturer uses in the marketing of a drug. The trade name is a registered trademark of the company, and the first letter of the name is capitalized. The same drug may be manufactured by several different companies, each using a different trade name. Because of the confusion this practice may cause, it is necessary to be familiar with the generic and brand names of all drugs studied.

An example of the different names of a drug in common prehospital use is the following:

Chemical name: 9-fluoro-11β, 17, 21-trihydroxy-16α-methylpregna-1, 4-diene-3, 20-dione
Generic name: dexamethasone
Trade names: Decadron, Hexadrol

DRUG REFERENCES AND RESOURCES

Several easily accessible references are available to the paramedic. The **Hospital Formulary** is published by the American Society of Hospital Pharmacists. It is a loose-leaf book that may be continuously updated as new drug information is published. The **Physicians' Desk Reference** is another common resource that has advantages and disadvantages for the user. Advantages include cross indexing, which allows information to be found when only the manufacturer, generic name, or type of drug is known, and color pictures of most oral drugs, listed by manufacturer. The major disadvantage is that the product information comes directly from the manufacturer, not an objective third party, and does not include comparisons between different drugs as to efficacy or safety. Several other resources are available for reference for situations in which, for example, a patient's home medications are unfamiliar to the paramedic. It is advisable to include a drug reference as standard ambulance equipment.

FORMS OF DRUGS

Because of the paramedic's mission of acute care and resuscitation in the prehospital setting, most drugs, to be effective, must be administered quickly and show actions rapidly. Therefore, most of the medications used are injected and are usually in liquid form. Liquid drugs administered into the body by subcutaneous, intramuscular, or intravenous routes are called **parenteral drugs**. The drug forms described in the box, "Forms of Drugs," are included for a perspective on common drug preparations.

Drugs administered through the parenteral route are packaged the following ways:

Preloaded syringes: Used for administration of intravenous, intramuscular, or subcutaneous medications. They are usually packaged in tamper-proof containers, and the drug solution component and syringe must often be assembled. A variety of different systems are available; many resuscitative drugs are available with this type of packaging. They are convenient, eliminating the need to draw up the medication (Fig. 12-1).
Ampules: Breakable glass containers from which medications must be drawn up with a syringe. They are less expensive than other types of packaging and are intended for single dose use (Fig. 12-2).
Vials: Glass or plastic containers that have a self-sealing rubber stopper in the top, from which multiple doses may be drawn (Fig. 12-3).

DRUG PHARMACOKINETICS

The movement of drugs in the body as they are absorbed, distributed, metabolized, and excreted is the study of **pharmacokinetics**. Drug actions occur when the substance reaches the site of action in adequate concentration. Various factors influence the action of any drug in each individual. Some of these variables are discussed below.

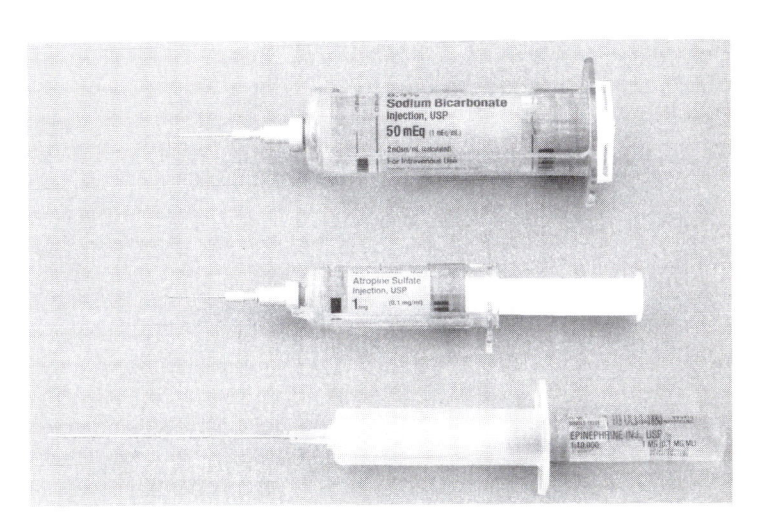

FIGURE 12-1.
Preloaded syringes.

FORMS OF DRUGS
Liquids

AQUEOUS SOLUTIONS
Drug or combination of drugs dissolved in water.

SYRUPS
Aqueous solutions of 85% sucrose. They may also be flavored to disguise an unpleasant-tasting medication.

AQUEOUS SUSPENSIONS
Preparations of finely divided solid drugs added to sterile distilled water. Heavier particles settle to the bottom of the container, requiring shaking before administration.

EMULSIONS
Suspensions of fats or oils in water with an emulsifying agent to remain in solution.

MAGMAS
Also called "milks" because of their white color. Bulky suspensions of insoluble preparations in water. They tend to settle when left standing and must be shaken before use.

SPIRITS
Concentrated alcoholic solutions of volatile substance, also called essences. The substance dissolved in the solution may be a solid, liquid, or gas and usually constitutes about 5% to 20% of the mixture.

ELIXIRS
Alcoholic preparations that have been sweetened and are used to act as a vehicle for other medications.

TINCTURES
Chemical or plant substances dissolved in an alcoholic solution. Most contain 10% to 20% drug.

FLUID EXTRACTS
The most concentrated of any fluid preparations. They are alcoholic extracts of vegetable drugs and contain 1 g of drug to 1 mL of solution. Many of them precipitate in sunlight and are usually placed in dark bottles.

EXTRACTS
Obtained by combining the active ingredients of animal or vegetable drugs with solvents and then evaporating the solvents, leaving a highly concentrated preparation. They may be liquids or powders.

LINIMENTS
Suspensions that contain oil, soap, water, or alcohol designed for external application to the skin by rubbing.

LOTIONS
Suspensions designed for external application, usually used on irritated or inflamed skin and in a form that allows application with a minimum of rubbing or friction.

OINTMENTS
Semisolid medications in a petroleum or lanolin base for prolonged contact with the skin and intended to be difficult to wash off.

Solids

CAPSULES
Made from gelatin containers designed to dissolve quickly in the stomach. They may contain powders, oils, or liquids and are a popular device used for the administration of oral medications. One disadvantage of capsules is that they may be taken apart, allowing tampering with contents.

TABLETS
Powdered drugs formed into small disks. They may be coated to enhance their visual appearance or palatability. Molded tablets usually are administered orally or sublingually. Some types of tablets are designed to be mixed with sterile water for injection.

PILLS
Mixtures of a drug with some cohesive material, which is then molded into a form convenient for swallowing. No form of pill is suitable for injection. The word "pill" is often used inappropriately by the public, as many of the medications taken by mouth are not pills but tablets or capsules.

SUPPOSITORIES
A mixture of a drug in a firm base that melts at body temperature, often cocoa butter, and is molded into a suitable shape to fit into a body orifice.

POWDERS
Finely divided or ground drug mixtures that are solid and dry.

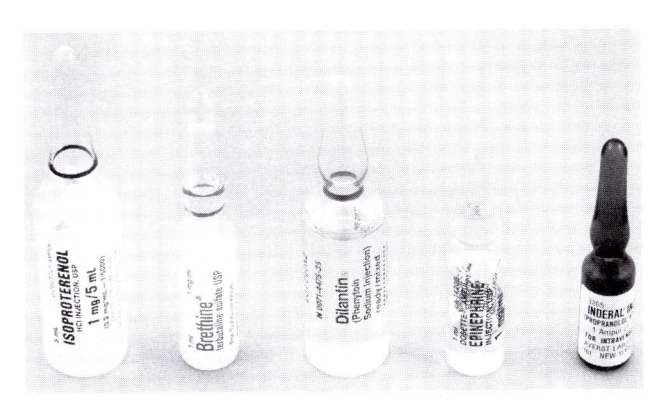

FIGURE 12–2.
Ampules.

Age: Infants have immature livers and kidneys, so it is difficult for them to metabolize and eliminate the same dosages of drugs as adults. The elderly may have impaired hepatic or renal function and slowing of elimination and excretion.

Sex: Mainly because of the percentage of body fat in males vs. females, there is a difference in body water, which may play a role in drug actions. Fat is anhydrous (without water), and muscle tissue contains substantial water. Also pregnant women must avoid certain drugs.

Body mass: The larger the body mass, the more compartment space in which the drug is diluted. For drugs to be effective, appropriate blood concentration levels must be maintained. Therefore, many medications are adjusted to body weight.

Previous exposure: Continuous previous exposure to a drug results in tolerance, and higher doses may need to be given to obtain therapeutic effects.

Disease states and drug interactions: Interactions can occur between drugs to cause altered or enhanced effects of the drugs. Patients' disease states can alter the interactions and pharmacokinetics. Several chemical interactions between drugs result in harmful or fatal effects. Therefore, the paramedic must be familiar with potential adverse effects of each drug carried and drugs that are incompatible together.

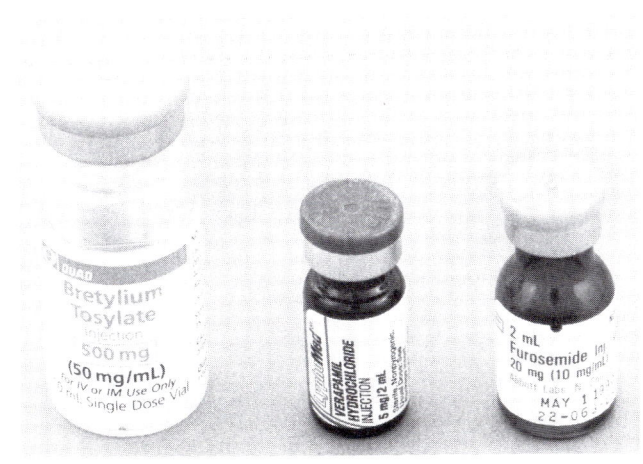

To understand how a drug produces its effects, it is important to understand what happens to that drug from the time it is administered until it leaves the patient's body (Fig. 12-4).

Absorption

Drug effects may be local, affecting only the immediate area of administration, or systemic, affecting the entire body. This effect may depend on the drug itself and the method of administration.

The administration of most drugs involves transfer to the circulatory system for distribution. With some drugs intended for local effects, such as in the gastrointestinal tract or skin, administration to the target organ may be accomplished without systemic absorption. Antacids and laxatives may be deposited directly in the intestine or stomach without absorption into the bloodstream. Most drugs, however, require absorption into the circulatory system for distribution and subsequent action. The two largest factors that affect absorption are the route of administration and the drug's ability to permeate membranes.

The "*gradient*" that forces the drug across and the surface area it is exposed to both determine the ability of a drug to move across a membrane. Since osmotic force depends on movement from higher to lower concentrations, blood flow to the area of administration affects the speed with which the drug may move across a gradient. High blood flow rapidly removes the drug, and a high pressure gradient is maintained. If the blood flow through the area is slow, tissue concentrations of the drug are high, thus slowing movement across the membrane surfaces. Vasoconstrictor drugs that must be absorbed cause local vasoconstriction at the site of deposit and are slowly absorbed. Conversely, vasodilator drugs are more rapidly absorbed because they increase local blood flow. This concept particularly important to the paramedic. Patients in shock have low perfusion to the skin and subcutaneous tissues, which act as a compensatory mechanism to preserve blood flow to vital organs. Subcutaneous epinephrine, administered to a patient with anaphylaxis and cardiovascular collapse, may stay unabsorbed at the site because of inadequate perfusion. The route of administration may deposit a drug at various sites, influencing the rate of absorption. The two basic routes of administration are oral and parenteral.

FIGURE 12–3.
Vials.

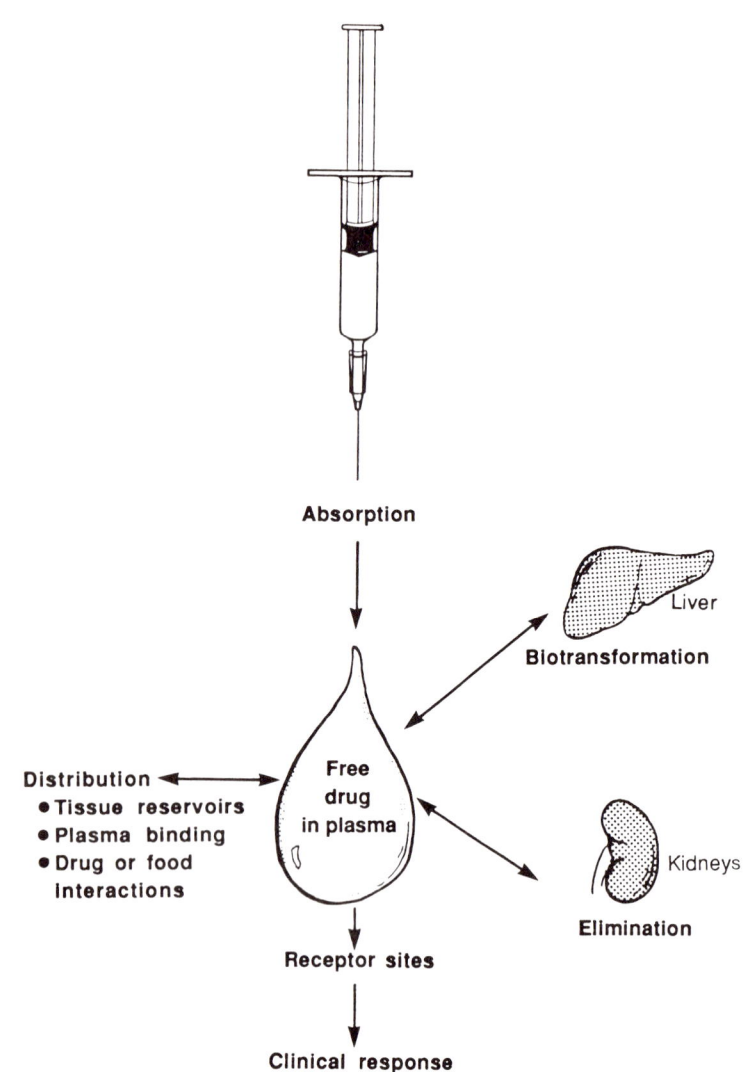

FIGURE 12-4.
What happens to a drug from the time it is administered until it leaves the body.

Oral Administration

The *oral route* (p.o. or per os) is used for absorption of drugs through the lining of the gastrointestinal tract. While some drugs, such as nitroglycerin, are placed in the mouth, under the tongue, this administration is not considered oral administration because absorption does not occur through the gastrointestinal tract. Nitroglycerin passes directly through oral mucosa into the bloodstream. The oral route is generally the most popular method of drug administration because it is a convenient, inexpensive route. Most drugs are efficiently absorbed from the gastrointestinal tract in normal circumstances. The large surface area, mixing of contents, and differences in pH enhance absorption. Some drugs, however, cannot be given orally because they are inactivated by acids and enzymes of the gastrointestinal tract before being absorbed. The presence of food in the gastrointestinal tract may retard absorption due to binding of drug molecules to food and subsequent slower movement through the gastrointestinal tract. Some drugs, however, are so irritating to the gastrointestinal tract that they should only be taken with a meal.

Since blood leaves the gut and passes through the liver before delivery to the circulatory system, doses of oral medications often must be higher than if administered by another route. Because the liver may begin to metabolize the drug before it can bind to drug receptors, greater amounts of a drug may be necessary to achieve the same effect as when given by a parenteral route. Even the form of an oral drug has an effect on absorption. A tablet, which must disintegrate and dissolve before absorption, may be much slower to act than the same drug given in liquid form. The rectal route is another form of gastrointestinal administration that may have more predictable absorption than the oral route. Few emergency drugs are manufactured in the form of suppositories; one exception is acetaminophen, which may be used for treating fevers in patients who are unable to tolerate oral medications.

Parenteral Administration

Parenteral administration is the administration of any drug by a nongastrointestinal route. Including most of the methods used by paramedics in the field, it allows bypass of the variable absorption factors involved in oral administration.

INTRADERMAL. **Intradermal** administration involves injecting a drug directly into the skin. In the field, this route generally is limited to the administration of a local anesthetic agent to numb the skin just before performing a procedure such as establishing an intravenous infusion. Drug volumes of less than 1 mL are generally sufficient for this purpose. Intradermal injections are usually performed by using a 25 to 27 gauge, ⅜ to 1 inch needle. Because capillaries in the skin absorb drugs more slowly than subcutaneous or muscle tissue, drugs delivered by this route are absorbed more slowly into the systemic circulation; however, desired drug effects are usually local rather than systemic.

SUBCUTANEOUS. **Subcutaneous (SQ or SC)** administration involves the injection of a drug into the fatty tissue beneath the skin. Volumes of drug are usually limited to quantities less than 1 mL, injected by using a 24 to 26 gauge, ½ to 1 inch needle. Subcutaneous injections are more slowly absorbed than intramuscular injections. Absorption of medications by this route is limited by the same factors that affect absorption of intramuscular drugs. One emergency medication that is routinely given by this route is 1:1,000 epinephrine, used for patients with asthma or allergic reactions. Because of the concentration of 1:1,000 epinephrine, it needs slower sustained absorption to be safe, a requirement which is met by the subcutaneous route.

INTRAMUSCULAR. **Intramuscular (IM)** administration involves the injection of small quantities of a drug into a muscle. The volume of drug administered IM is limited to quantities less than 5 mL; additional volume is unlikely to be absorbed and may cause tissue irritation. Needle length should be 1 to 1½ inches and as small a gauge as possible (limited by the viscosity of the drug solution) should be used, generally 21 to 23 gauge. Absorption is limited by the type of drug and the circulation to the muscle used for injection. Some drugs, such as phenytoin, form microcrystals in the muscle and are not absorbed. Other drugs are painful when given IM and, therefore, cannot be given this way. If a drug is injected into a poorly perfused muscle, absorption is limited. When perfusion improves, the drug sequestered in the muscle is then released to the bloodstream, often producing unpredictable effects. While it is possible to give some emergency medications by this route, it is generally avoided in favor of routes of more predictable absorption.

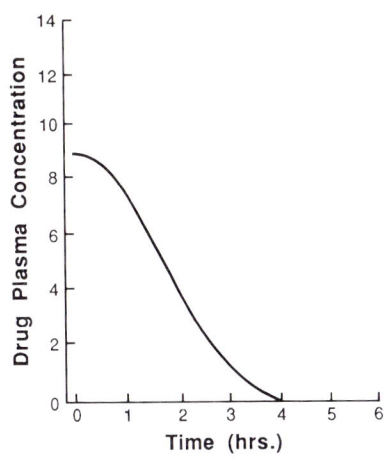

FIGURE 12–5.
Graphic demonstration of an average plasma level of an intravenous bolus injection.

INTRAVENOUS. The **intravenous (IV)** route bypasses the absorption process because the drug is injected directly into the bloodstream. While bypassing absorption barriers has many advantages, it leaves no margin for error, making IV administration a potentially dangerous technique. If circulation is adequate, drugs are delivered to target sites quickly. However, plasma drug levels peak rapidly and then drop off, a fact which may necessitate repeating the dosage or following an IV bolus with a drug infusion (Fig. 12-5). Large volumes of medications may be given quickly by this route. Because of these factors, it is the primary method of drug administration for the paramedic. Establishing IV access in unstable patients, therefore, is a routine part of care in the field. Sizes of IV catheters vary from 14 to 22 gauge to ½ to 2 inches in length.

TOPICAL. The administration of drugs through surface membranes, such as the skin and mucous membranes, is known as **topical** administration. Drugs given by these routes may have either local or systemic effects. The sublingual route is a form of topical administration for nitroglycerin, which is rapidly absorbed by the highly vascular area under the tongue. It then enters the venous system and right heart, bypassing the liver. Some drugs given by the oral route are 90% metabolized to inert chemicals by the liver before entering the circulatory system. Therefore, the sublingual route is a useful and simple route for avoiding liver circulation. Many drugs given by topical routes are used for local effects such as treatment of skin inflammation, infection, or irritation.

TRACHEAL. Because of the large surface area of the alveoli and vast blood supply of the pulmonary capillary beds that return blood to the left heart, drugs administered through the trachea are rapidly absorbed and delivered to the heart for distribution. In some cases, the bronchial tree itself is the target for drug effects. Bronchodilators, such as metaproterenol, are inhaled into the bronchial tree for relief of bronchospasm and act directly on the smooth muscle, with only a small amount entering the circulatory system. Several different drugs may be administered down the endotracheal tube, but it is important to deliver them in sufficient volume to ensure that they do not merely adhere to the inside of the tube. They may need to be diluted slightly. If peripheral IV access is impossible, several drugs can be administered through the endotracheal tube. A helpful mnemonic to remember the drugs that can be given by this route is "NAVEL":

Narcan (naloxone)
Atropine
Valium (diazepam)*
Epinephrine
Lidocaine
*Some sources disagree that diazepam can be given by the endotracheal route.

Distribution

Distribution involves the transport of an absorbed drug to its target site. Some drugs that are highly water soluble are freely distributed in the vascular system and may flow easily into other body compartments where there is body water. Other drugs become bound to serum proteins in the blood and are not immediately available to act as "free" drugs on various receptors. For example, if 5000 serum proteins were available for drug binding, the first 5000 molecules of a particular drug would become bound to the proteins. When the 5001st drug molecule enters the blood, it would be "free" to act and cause its desired effect (Fig. 12-6). These serum proteins are often called inert binding sites. Inert binding can also take place outside the vascular compartment, such as in body fat. This binding does not bring about any type of physiologic response, and bound drugs are not available for diffusion between body compartments. Bound drugs are in careful balance with free drugs. As free drugs act on receptors and are eliminated, bound drugs are released to act. This binding process limits the amount of free drug in circulation and prevents drugs from reaching their targets in a highly concentrated form. In effect, the bound drugs act as a sort of reservoir. It is important to remember that only free drugs can act at receptor sites and then be metabolized and excreted.

Some drugs have affinities for the same proteins and may compete with each other for free and bound status. For example, drug X is 98% bound, and drug Y, which has the same affinity, is administered. Drug Y may displace X and cause large percentages to become free and act on receptors. This type of action results in **synergistic** drug actions, in which their combined effects are much greater than if each were given individually. It also plays a part in **potentiation,** in which the administration of one drug enhances the effects of another. In some cases, these types of effects can result in drug toxicity.

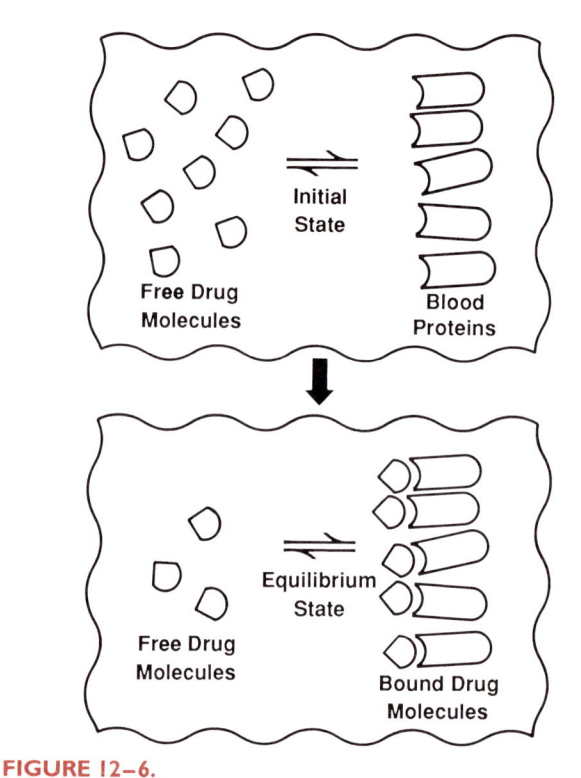

FIGURE 12-6.
The equilibrium between free and bound drug in the blood.

The body has certain protective mechanisms known as physiologic barriers. One example of this is known as the **blood-brain barrier**. It prevents many drugs from leaving the blood and crossing the cerebrospinal fluid into the brain. The blood-brain barrier is highly selective and not all drugs are allowed to cross it. In general, most drugs pass into the brain more slowly than into other tissues.

At one time, it was thought that the placenta provided a protective barrier to the fetus, but this theory is now known to be untrue. Except for some vitamins and minerals, no drugs are approved "warning free" for use in the pregnant mother. Almost all drugs are capable of crossing the placenta, except a few drugs with very large molecules. The stage of fetal development has been shown to be clearly related to risks with drug therapy. The most vulnerable time for drug-induced birth defects is the first trimester, when fetal organs are developing. During the third trimester any drugs taken may have a residual effect on the fetus. At birth, the baby must rely on its own liver and kidneys to metabolize and excrete any drugs that remain in the system while in utero. Because of the newborn's decreased ability to metabolize and excrete, toxic reactions may result. Obviously, a seriously ill mother may need medications for initial resuscitation or stabilization. This decision is clearly a difficult one that must be made in consultation with medical control.

Biotransformation and Elimination

As a drug is being distributed and starts to act, some of the free components of that drug are starting to be metabolized (*biotransformed*) into substances for elimination from the body. The primary organ used for this process is the liver. When the liver is exposed to a substance, structures in the hepatic cells called microsomes begin to react by metabolizing the drug into components capable of being excreted. As the liver is exposed to more of the drug, hepatic cells bolster production of microsomes to handle increased drug exposure and metabolism. This process may take days and reaches maximum production of microsomes after about 2 weeks. Thus, the liver is prepared to increase metabolism and elimination of a drug to which it is often exposed. When the exposure to the drug becomes less frequent or ceases altogether, the number of microsomal structures decreases.

This process of increased metabolism may eventually lead to drug tolerance. As the ability of the liver to metabolize improves, less drug is available to contact receptors and a higher dosage is needed to achieve the same physiologic response as previously experienced. A higher dose is then given, the liver develops more microsomes to metabolize the drug, and a vicious cycle begins.

Another problem that can cause decreased drug effects in an individual is **tachyphylaxis**. This occurs when the patient's tolerance for the drug is developed so rapidly that it has no pharmacologic effect on the patient.

Since the liver plays such a key role in metabolism, it is imperative to identify patients who may have impaired hepatic function. Such patients may not be able to metabolize a drug and may have prolonged effects. A normal drug dose in this type of patient could result in drug toxicity and death. The factor of liver maturity plays a major role in the determination of dosage variations in the elderly and in children. Pediatric patients have immature livers and the elderly may have impaired hepatic function.

Once biotransformed in the liver, drugs are then eliminated from the body by a variety of routes. Some volatile drugs, such as ethyl alcohol, are partially eliminated by the lungs. Many substances are eliminated by the liver through the gastrointestinal tract, but the majority are eliminated by the kidneys. Therefore, patients with impaired renal function may be unable to eliminate drugs from their systems. Some drugs, such as digoxin, are excreted by the kidney practically unchanged. Therefore, a patient with impaired renal function could develop digitalis toxicity quickly.

Any patient with an impaired ability to metabolize and excrete drugs will have sustained drug action. This reaction must be anticipated so that dosages may be adjusted accordingly or withheld.

DRUG PHARMACODYNAMICS

Pharmacodynamics is the study of the effects of drugs on the body. The major theory of drug action is called the receptor theory. It states that drugs act by associating themselves with specific molecules, often on the cell membrane, in a manner that alters the function of the cell. Receptors may be thought of as cellular "locks," and drugs are the keys. The right shape of key (*the drug*) with exactly the right code is inserted into the lock (*receptor*), and a pharmacologic response occurs.

Receptors

Receptors determine the quantity of drug necessary to effect a response. If the drug to be administered has a tremendous affinity for the receptors, the concentration necessary to produce a response may be limited. The number of receptors in an individual patient may limit the maximal effect a drug may produce. Receptors are also responsible for selective drug action. The molecular structure of a drug determines its ability or lack of ability to bind to receptor sites. A change in a drug's structure may increase or decrease a drug's affinity to bind to receptor sites. A change in structure may also alter the drug's actions.

Drugs that cause a direct change in cellular function when inserted into a receptor are called **agonists**. Receptors may also be occupied or blocked by substances called **antagonists**. An antagonist occupies a receptor site but causes no physiologic response. The chemical code (*key*) is close enough for it to fit into the receptor (*lock*) but not exact enough to cause a response. Many antagonists compete for receptors and occupy sites with greater affinity than the agonist. Naloxone is a commonly used narcotic antagonist used to treat suspected narcotic overdose and unconsciousness with unknown etiology. Naloxone binds to the receptor sites, blocking the action of the toxic drugs. Many drugs used in resuscitation and stabilization are agonists or antagonists of autonomic nervous system receptors.

Autonomic Nervous System

Prehospital advanced life support is largely involved with respiratory and cardiac emergencies. Therefore, most of the drugs carried and used in the field have some impact on one or both of these systems. To know the correct drug to use in an emergency, a good understanding of the autonomic nervous system is vital. The following material discusses the autonomic nervous system as it relates to

TABLE 12-1.
EFFECTS OF SYMPATHETIC AND PARASYMPATHETIC STIMULATION ON ORGANS

Organ	Sympathetic	Parasympathetic
Eye (pupils)	Dilated	Constricted
Sweat glands	Sweating	None
Nasal, lacrimal, parotid, submaxillary, gastric, and pancreatic glands	Vasoconstriction, slight secretion	Stimulation of copious secretion
Heart	Increased inotropic Increased chronotropic	Decreased firing of SA Decreased atrial force
Bronchial tree	Mild dilation	Mild constriction
Gut	Decreased peristalsis	Increased peristalsis
Liver	Glycogen release	Glycogen storage and production
Kidney	Decreased output	None
Blood Vessels		
Skin	Constricted	None
Abdomen	Constricted	None
Muscles	Dilated	None
Blood glucose	Increased	None
Metabolism	Increased, up to 100%	None
Adrenal Secretion	Increased	None
Mental Activity	Increased	None
Piloerector muscles (goosebumps)	Increased	None
Skeletal muscles	Increased glucose metabolism Increased strength	None None

drug therapy. A more complete discussion of the system itself can be found in Chapter 22.

The nervous system is divided into two basic components: the voluntary and the involuntary (autonomic) systems. The voluntary system is under the control of conscious thought and controls voluntary movement. It is the involuntary or autonomic nervous system that controls "*vegetative*" functions of life by affecting vital organ functions.

The autonomic system is further broken into two divisions, which tend to act in a reciprocal manner. Most organs are dominated by one component or the other. The two divisions are called sympathetic and parasympathetic; their effects on body organs are shown in Table 12-1.

SYMPATHETIC DIVISION. The **sympathetic division** (sometimes called the adrenergic division) originates in the brain. Messages are sent out to the organs by two "sympathetic chains" that leave the spinal cord at about the first thoracic vertebra and end at about the second lumbar vertebra. The term *adrenergic* stems from adrenaline, which is a synonym for epinephrine.

The primary effect of sympathetic stimulation is in-

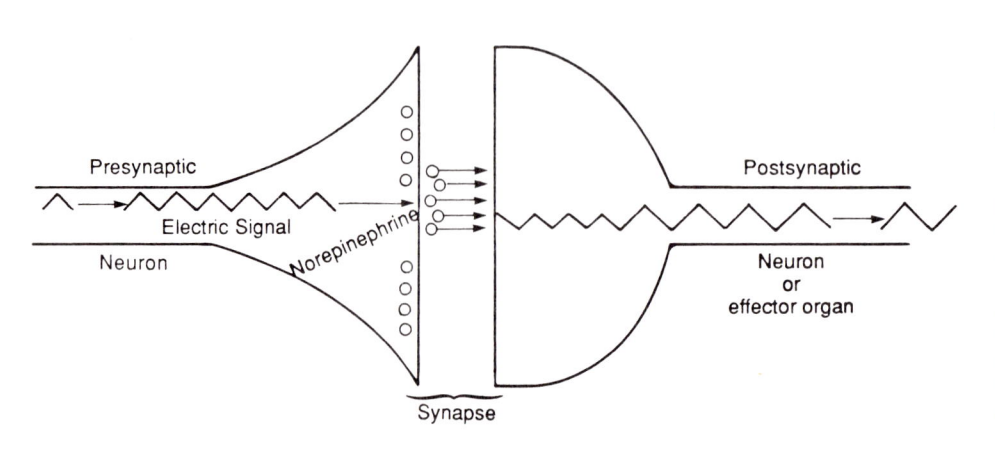

FIGURE 12-7.
A description of the synapse. An electrical signal travels down the presynaptic nerve and causes the release of norepinephrine. Norepinephrine enters the synapse and activates receptors on the postsynaptic membrane. An electrical signal is generated in the postsynaptic neuron and then travels down the postsynaptic neuron.

TABLE 12-2.
EFFECTS OF SYMPATHETIC AGONIST STIMULATION

Agonist	Heart	Bronchioles	Blood Vessels
α	No effect	Minimal constriction	Constriction
β_1	Increased heart rate, contractility, automaticity, and conduction	No effect	No effect
β_2	No effect	Slight dilatation	Dilatation in skeletal muscle

creased heart rate, bronchiole dilation, and increased metabolism and strength. These responses prepare the body for **fight or flight** from a dangerous situation. When the sympathetic division is stimulated, impulses are transmitted electrically along the nerve fibers until they reach a synapse, or nerve junction. At this point, the transfer of the impulse across the synapse is carried by a chemical neurotransmitter called norepinephrine. This transfer also occurs at the organ to be affected. Norepinephrine is stored and manufactured at the presynaptic neuron. When an impulse crosses, norepinephrine is secreted into the synapse. Then it is free to act on the organ or postsynaptic neuron. The effect of norepinephrine lasts only a few seconds. Any remaining norepinephrine is either absorbed (known as re-uptake) by the presynaptic neuron or destroyed by an enzyme known as monoamine oxidase (Fig. 12-7). In addition, whenever the sympathetic division is stimulated, epinephrine is released from the adrenal medulla, causing a more prolonged response.

Sympathetic Receptors. Two different types of receptors are in the sympathetic division. These are known as α-adrenergic and β-adrenergic receptors; β receptors are separated into β_1 and β_2.

When α-*adrenergic receptors* are stimulated, vasoconstriction results. The effect of an α agonist on any organ depends on the type and quantity of receptors. The heart is not directly affected by α agonists because it has few α-adrenergic receptors. Table 12-2 summarizes the effects of α and β agonists on selected organs.

When β_1-*adrenergic receptors* are stimulated, they cause an increase in the heart's inotropic effect (contractility and force), chronotropic effect (rate and automaticity), and dromotropic effect (conduction of impulses). They also cause slight vasodilation in skeletal muscle. Stimulation of β_2-*adrenergic receptors* results in bronchodilation.

Drugs that are sympathetic division agonists are usually described by their effect on α-adrenergic and β-adrenergic receptors. For example, a group of drugs commonly used in the treatment of asthma because of their bronchodilation effects are called β_2 agonists. Specific examples include metaproterenol and albuterol.

Drugs That Affect the Sympathetic Division. Several drugs encountered in prehospital care are sympathetic agonists or activators. While a few are pure α or β, most have both α and β effects, usually with one or another being predominant. Some drugs, such as dopamine, have dose-related effects and may act as α or β, depending on the dosages given. Some drugs are even selective in a β category, affecting β_2-adrenergic receptors only. Table 12-3 shows various adrenergic agonists and the type of receptors they affect; the box "Sympathetic Agonists" provides a more detailed discussion of various sympathetic agonists.

Another commonly encountered class of drugs is the β-blockers. They are prescribed to treat hypertension, angina, and arrhythmias because of their β antagonistic actions. They occupy β-adrenergic receptors and prevent agonists, such as some of those previously discussed, from activating receptors. One of the most common β-blockers is propranolol.

PARASYMPATHETIC DIVISION. The **parasympathetic division** of the autonomic nervous system (also called the

TABLE 12-3.
ADRENERGIC DRUGS: RECEPTOR ACTIVITY

Drug	Receptor Activity
CATECHOLAMINES	
Dobutamine	β_1
Dopamine	Dopaminergic, α (at high doses), β_1
Epinephrine	α, β_1, β_2
Isoproterenol	β_1, β_2
Norepinephrine or levarterenol	α, β_1
NONCATECHOLAMINES	
DIRECT ACTING	
Albuterol	β_1 less than β_2
Isoetharine	β_1 less than β_2
Metaproterenol	β_1 less than β_2
Phenylephrine	α, β (weak)
Terbutaline	β_1 less than β_2
DUAL ACTING	
Ephedrine	α, β, CNS
Metaraminol	α, greater than β

SYMPATHETIC AGONISTS

Epinephrine—Predominantly β with some α effects. It has potent $β_1$ effects on the heart and α effects on peripheral blood vessels. It also activates $β_2$ adrenergic receptors in some blood vessels, causing vasodilation. It is a naturally occurring substance in the body. Its effects are increased heart rate and contractility, as well as increased automaticity and irritability, and increased vascular resistance in some blood vessels. Epinephrine is a drug used in the treatment of cardiac arrest, allergic reactions, and acute bronchospasm. It is one of the most frequently used drugs in the field.

Norepinephrine—Primarily α with some $β_1$ effects. Its effects are mostly to increase vascular resistance and increase inotropic and chronotropic heart response slightly. Originally used to treat cardiogenic shock, its vasoconstrictor actions cause an increased blood pressure by increasing vascular resistance, at the expense of increased myocardial workload and oxygen demand. It is a useful drug in the treatment of low vascular resistance types of shock, such as septic and neurogenic shock.

Isoproterenol—An almost pure β agent ($β_1$ and $β_2$) and causes vasodilation, bronchodilation, and increased heart inotropic and chronotropic effects. A powerful drug used in prehospital care as a "chemical pacemaker," it is usually used in cases of symptomatic bradycardia and heart blocks that are refractory to atropine.

Dopamine—An agent that, at low doses, dilates the renal arteries. At medium doses it causes β effects, and at high doses causes β and α effects. It is used in situations of cardiogenic and low vascular resistance types of shock because of its selective, dose-related effects.

Dobutamine—A $β_1$ agent that increases heart inotropic effects without causing much increase in chronotropic activity. It is a drug primarily used in the treatment of cardiogenic shock because of its ability to increase cardiac output with a minimal increase in the heart rate, thus somewhat sparing the myocardial oxygen demand.

Metaproterenol/Terbutaline—Both of these are $β_2$ selective bronchodilator drugs, which also cause some vasodilation without much effect on the heart. They are used to treat bronchospasm in the field and are frequently encountered as home medications.

---

cholinergic division, derived from the word acetylcholine) originates in the brain and sends messages to effector organs by the cranial nerves. Pairs of cranial nerves exit directly from the brain and travel to organs without using the spinal cord as a conduit. The 10th cranial nerves, or vagus nerves, are the primary nerves of the parasympathetic division and account for about 75% of actions caused by parasympathetic stimulation, which affects the heart, stomach, and gastrointestinal tract.

Parasympathetic stimulation also causes increased activity in the gut for digestion. Its effects on the lungs are slight, causing only minimal bronchoconstriction. Blood vessels are not affected by parasympathetic stimulation.

When the parasympathetic division is stimulated, impulses travel along cranial nerves. At neuron synapses and at the junction between the nerve and effector organs, the primary neurotransmitter substance is acetylcholine. However, no indirect effect is produced in the parasympathetic division such as the adrenal glands produce in the sympathetic division.

Acetylcholine crosses the synapse to reach a postsynaptic neuron or effector organ. It then occupies receptor sites and is broken down by the enzyme cholinesterase. This action only lasts a few seconds at most. Cholinesterase breaks acetylcholine into acetic acid and choline. Choline is then transported back and used again in the manufacture of new acetylcholine (Fig. 12-8).

Atropine, a drug commonly used by the paramedic, is an acetylcholine antagonist or blocker. It occupies receptor sites and prevents a parasympathetic response. It is commonly used to increase the heart rate by increasing the discharge rate of the SA node and to increase conduction through the AV node.

It is not possible to administer acetylcholine as a drug because it is broken down by cholinesterase in the blood and at synapses before it can occupy receptors. Some drugs mimic its actions, however, and can cause parasympathetic stimulation. Muscarine, a poison found in mushrooms and pilocarpine, a drug used to treat glaucoma are examples of these drugs.

Other drugs inhibit the breakdown of acetylcholine by cholinesterase, potentiating the parasympathetic response. Poisons such as organophosphates are such inhibitors. Accidental exposure to these poisons results in severe parasympathetic overstimulation. This condition is counteracted by using atropine as an antagonist to acetylcholine. Other drugs, such as physostigmine, neostigmine, and edrophonium, are also cholinesterase inhibitors. All these drugs can be blocked by the administration of atropine.

In addition to atropine, several other drugs block acetylcholine. They are often used as antispasmodics for gastrointestinal distress. Examples include Scopolamine, Donnatal, Banthine, and Lomotil.

Vagal Stimulation. At certain times, such as in unstable patients with supraventricular tachycardia, the paramedic may attempt to cause parasympathetic or vagal stimulation in an attempt to stimulate the parasympathetic division and slow the heart rate. This state is usually accomplished by either having the patient strain and bear down as if having a bowel movement (***Valsalva's maneuver***) or by massaging the carotid sinus. Valsalva's

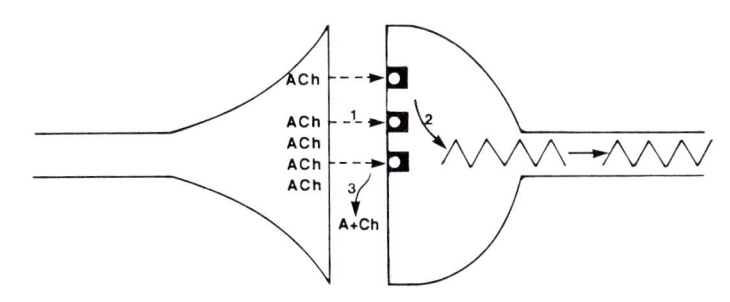

FIGURE 12–8.
The pattern of acetylcholine (ACh) release, action, and destruction at the cholinergic synapse.

1. ACh is released across the synapse and attaches to receptor
2. Receptor activation causes a pharmacologic response
3. ACh is destroyed by cholinesterase, producing acetic acid (A) and choline (Ch)

maneuver causes a bolus of blood to "hit" the carotid baroreceptors at high pressure. Massage applies direct pressure to the baroreceptors (see Chapter 20). The carotid baroreceptors sense an increased blood pressure. A high-pressure message is sent to the medulla. The parasympathetic division then sends a message via the vagus nerve to slow the heart rate.

CALCULATING DRUG DOSAGES

The paramedic needs to know not only about individual drugs but also about how to administer them in the correct amount. To master this knowledge, it is necessary to understand the units of drug measurement.

The Metric System

The two measurement systems used in the United States are the apothecary and metric systems. The *apothecary system* has a long historical background, but the scientific and medical professions have converted to the *metric system* because of its consistency, simplicity, and greater accuracy in measurement. It is rare that emergency medications are ordered in apothecary units. On occasion, however, the paramedic has to make conversions between systems.

The metric system is based on decimals, with all basic units being multiples of 10. Each unit can be multiplied by 10, 100, or 1000 to form secondary units. The metric unit of weight is the gram, fluid is measured by the liter, and distance is measured by the meter.

Weight Measurements

1 milligram (mg)	= 0.001 gram
1 gram (g)	= 10 decigrams
	= 100 centigrams
	= 1000 milligrams
	= 1,000,000 micrograms
1 milligram	= 1000 micrograms (μg)
"deci"	= tenth
"centi"	= hundredth
"milli"	= thousandth
"micro"	= millionth

MAKING POUND-TO-KILOGRAM CONVERSIONS. In apothecary terms, 1 kilogram (kg) is equal to roughly 2.2 pounds (lb). This conversion needs to be made frequently because many drugs are given according to the patient's body weight in kilograms. To make the conversion to kilograms, simply divide the weight in pounds by 2.2.

$$\text{weight in kilograms} = \frac{\text{weight in pounds}}{2.2}$$

A quick way to make pound-to-kilogram conversions is to calculate half the body weight in pounds then deduct 10%.

Example: 140 lb woman
½ of 140 lb = 70 lb
10% of 70 = 7
70 − 7 = 63 kg

Liquid Measurements

1 liter (L)	= 10 deciliters	"deci"	= tenth
	= 100 centiliters	"centi"	= hundredth
	= 1000 milliliters (mL)	"milli"	= thousandth

The liter and milliliter are commonly used in drug and IV fluid therapy. The term cubic centimeter (cc) is also used synonymously with milliliter, although the cubic centimeter is less than a milliliter by 0.000028 cc.

Common Conversions

Metric	Apothecary
1 mL	15 minims
10 mL	2.5 fluid drams
15 mL	1 tablespoon (household measurement)
100 mL	3.5 fluid ounces
1000 mL	1 quart
1 g	15 grains
10 g	2.5 drams
100 g	3.3 ounces
1000 g	2.2 pounds

Apothecary	Metric
1 minim	0.06 mL
1 fluidram	4 mL
1 fluid ounce	30 mL
1 pint	500 mL
1 quart	1000 mL (1 liter)
1 grain	60 mg
1 dram	4 g
1 ounce	30 g
1 pound	500 g

A Review of Decimals

As previously mentioned, the metric system is based on the decimal system that uses multiples of ten. Decimals consist of a whole number, which is the number before (to the left of) the decimal point, and decimal fractions, which are the numbers after (to the right of) the decimal point.

$$9.50$$
whole number . fraction

The position of a number in relationship to the decimal point gives the number its name:

hundredth / tens / units . tenth / hundredth / thousandth

For example: 0.9 = 9/10   nine-tenths
0.90 = 90/100   ninety-hundredths
0.090 = 90/1000   ninety-thousandths

Adding zeros to the right of the decimal point changes the name of the decimal fraction but not its value. To help alleviate confusion, a zero usually is placed to the left of the decimal point when the number is less than one, for example, 0.5 equals ½. Adding zeros to the left of the decimal does not change the value or name of the decimal fraction. For example, 000.5 and 0.5 both equal five-tenths.

Addition and Subtraction

To add or subtract a problem with decimals, the decimal points must be lined up, and zeros should be annexed to the right of the last numeral for clarity. For example:

Add: 7.9, 3.09, and 5.009
7.9   7.900 two zeros annexed
3.09   3.090 one zero annexed
+ 5.009 + 5.009
           15.999

The same procedure of lining the decimals up and annexing zeros must be followed when subtracting decimals. For example:

Subtract: 17.983 from 37.12
37.2   37.200
− 17.983   − 17.983
                 19.217

Multiplication and Division

To multiply decimals, use the same procedures that would be used for multiplication of whole numbers. To find the decimal point, count the total number of decimal places in the numbers to be multiplied. Then move the decimal point that same number of places to the left. For example:

7.25   There are four decimal places here (two in each
× 6.15   number), so the decimal must be moved four places
44.5875   to the left in the answer.

1.25   There are only two decimal places here (two in
× 2   1.25), so the decimal must be moved two places
2.50   to the left in the answer.

When multiplying a decimal by 10, simply move the decimal point one place to the right. When multiplying any decimal by multiples of 10, move the decimal point to the right by the number of zeros found in the multiple. For example:

7.250   There is one zero in ten; move the decimal point
× 10   one place to the right in 7.250.
72.500

12.700   There are two zeros in one hundred; move the
× 100   decimal point two places to the right in 12.700.
1270.000

1.75   There are three zeros in one thousand; move the
× 1000   decimal point three places to the right.
1750.0

Division has the following terms:

$$\begin{array}{r} 2 \text{ quotient (answer)} \\ 6\overline{)12} \end{array}$$
divisor   dividend

Change the divisor (the number you are dividing by) to a whole number by moving the decimal to the right. Then move the decimal point in the dividend (the number being divided) the same number of places to the right.

Place the decimal point in the quotient (the answer) above the decimal in the dividend, and divide as with whole numbers. For example:

3.6 divided by 0.5 $$\begin{array}{r} 7.2 \\ 0.5\overline{)3.6} \end{array}$$

Drug Dosage Calculations

Many of the drugs used in the field are premixed and premeasured, ready to deliver to the average adult patient. This convenience decreases both preparation time and likelihood of error. However, when giving certain drugs and drug infusions, calculation of volume or rate of delivery is often necessary.

Most calculations are based on the following volume calculation formula:

$$\text{Volume to Administer} = \frac{\text{Dose Desired} \times \text{Volume on Hand}}{\text{Dose on Hand}}$$

The dose desired equals the amount of drug ordered (usually expressed in mg or μg). The volume on hand equals the quantity of fluid in the drug container (usually expressed in mL). The dose on hand equals the total amount of drug present in the drug container (usually expressed in mg or μg).

For example, to give lidocaine 75 mg from a premixed syringe that contains 100 mg in 5 mL:

$$\text{Volume} = \frac{75 \text{ mg} \times 5 \text{ mL}}{100 \text{ mg}} = \frac{375}{100} = 3.75 \text{ mL}$$

A slight variation is to calculate the drug present per mL of solution:

$$\frac{100 \text{ mg}}{5 \text{ mL}} = 20 \text{ mg/mL}$$

and insert this value into the above formula:

$$\text{Volume} = \frac{75 \text{ mg} \times 1 \text{ mL}}{20 \text{ mg}} = 3.75 \text{ mL}$$

All units in the dividend must be the same as the units in the divisor, so it may sometimes be necessary to mentally convert 1 g to 1000 mg or 1 mg to 1000 μg to calculate the problem.

Intravenous Infusion Rate Calculation

The delivery rate of continuous IV drug infusions depends on the type of IV administration set used. The exact ratio of drops per mL must be known. Because this ratio varies by manufacturer, the paramedic must be familiar with the type of equipment commonly carried; if new equipment is introduced, the number of drops per mL can be found on the administration set packaging.

Two basic types of administration sets are available, each with drip chambers that allow for different rates of infusion. The standard, or *macro*, drip set infuses 1 mL for every 10 or 15 drops of solution through the chamber. Macro drops are abbreviated as "gtt" and commonly are used to describe flow rates (e.g., 30 gtt/min of lactated Ringer's solution).

The other type of set is the *micro*, or *mini*, drip set. This set allows for the infusion of 1 mL (cc) of fluid for every 60 drops. This type of set is generally standard at 60 drops/mL, but this amount also should be verified by reading the administration set container. Micro drips are abbreviated as "microgtt" to designate micro drip flow rates. The micro drip set is used when IV flow rates are to be restricted to prevent overhydration and when IV drugs are given as continuous infusions.

Intravenous infusions are often ordered to be given over a period of minutes or hours. For example, the physician may order a solution to be administered at the rate of 100 mL/hour. To calculate how many drops per minute must be infused, the number of drops per mL delivered by the administration set is a factor in the problem. The problem is set using the following rate calculation formula:

$$\frac{\text{Volume To Be Infused}}{\text{Time of Infusion in Minutes}} \times \frac{\text{Drops}}{1 \text{ mL}}$$

This formula is then used to solve the problem specified above with a micro drip:

$$\frac{100 \text{ mL}}{60 \text{ min}} \times \frac{60 \text{ drops}}{1 \text{ mL}} = \frac{6000 \text{ microgtt}}{60 \text{ min}} = \frac{100 \text{ microgtt}}{1 \text{ min}}$$

The paramedic administers several drugs by continuous IV infusion or "drip." In all cases, the solutions may be prepared in different concentrations and the infusion rate calculated to administer the correct dosage. Some common "IV drip" drugs are lidocaine, isoproterenol, dopamine, bretylium, and theophylline ethylenediamine.

Mixing and administering IV drugs require use of many of the principles of the metric system previously presented. Fortunately, most of the IV drip medications used in prehospital care are common, and most emergency medical systems have parameters for their use.

However, occasionally the paramedic may be asked to mix an infusion in a different concentration from what is standard or from one that is not available in premixed form, and this mix may change the rate of infusion. Lidocaine is probably one of the most common drip solutions used in the field. After IV bolus administration, a continuous infusion is usually started and infused at 1 to 4 mg/min. Most infusions are mixed in D_5W solution, supplied in 250-mL or 500-mL IV bags. A typical way to set up a lidocaine infusion is to inject 2 g of lidocaine in 500 mL of D_5W and infuse it at 2 mg/min.

To calculate the rate at which to run this infusion, the previous formulas are recalled, and the problem is worked in 2 steps.

1. Calculate volume by using the volume calculation formula.
2. Calculate rate by using the rate calculation formula.

For example, administer lidocaine at 2 mg/min; the premixed bag contains 2 g in 500 mL D_5W (Fig. 12-9).

1. $$\text{Volume} = \frac{2 \text{ mg} \times 500 \text{ mL}}{2000 \text{ mg}} = 0.5 \text{ mL}$$

2. (using micro drip tubing)

$$\text{gtt/min} = \frac{0.5 \text{ mL}}{1 \text{ min}} \times \frac{60 \text{ microgtt}}{1 \text{ mL}} = 30 \text{ microgtt/min}$$

For another example, administer isoproterenol at 5 μg/min; an infusion is mixed that contains 1 mg in 250 mL D_5W.

FIGURE 12-9. Preparation of lidocaine infusion.

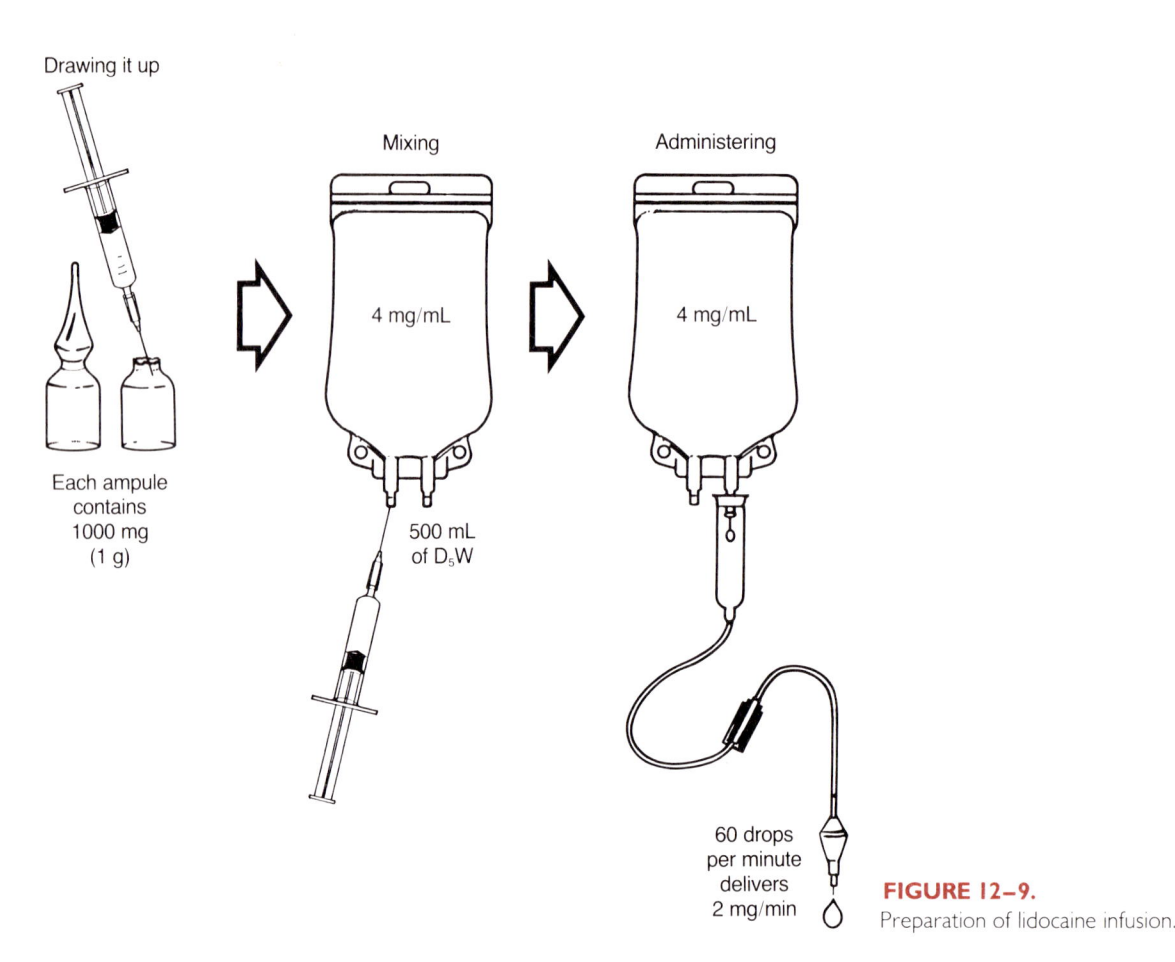

1. Volume $= \dfrac{5\ \mu g \times 250\ \text{mL}}{1000\ \mu g} = 1.25\ \text{mL}$

2. (using micro drip tubing)

   gtt/min $= \dfrac{1.25\ \text{mL}}{1\ \text{min}} \times \dfrac{60\ \text{microgtt}}{1\ \text{mL}} = 75$ microgtt/min

Because drug dosage calculations must be performed quickly and accurately in critical situations, frequent practice is necessary. Fortunately, because concentrations of drugs carried on the ambulance are generally standard and most calculations are performed routinely, the experienced paramedic is often capable of working problems mentally.

DRUG ADMINISTRATION

Drug Packaging and Preparation

Drugs may be packaged in a variety of ways, depending on the form of drug and the manufacturer. It is common in most emergency medical services systems to find any combination of the following:

- Glass ampules
- Single-dose and multi-dose vials
- Preloaded syringes
- IV solutions with premixed medications

Before using any of these, check the drug's expiration date and verify that the solution is not discolored and does not contain precipitates.

Ampules

Glass ampules are typical containers for inexpensive single-dose packaging. When using an ampule, take the following steps (Fig. 12-10):

1. Confirm the drug type, concentration, and dose.
2. Shake the ampule or tap the stem and top to shift the fluid to the bottom.
3. Place a gauze square or alcohol wipe over the neck and snap the top off.
4. Draw up the fluid with the needle and syringe selected.
5. Invert the syringe and expel any trapped air.
6. Reconfirm the drug concentration and dose.
7. Administer the drug by the desired route.

Vials

Vials are also a common form of packaging. They are supplied in either single- or muti-dose packaging. One disad-

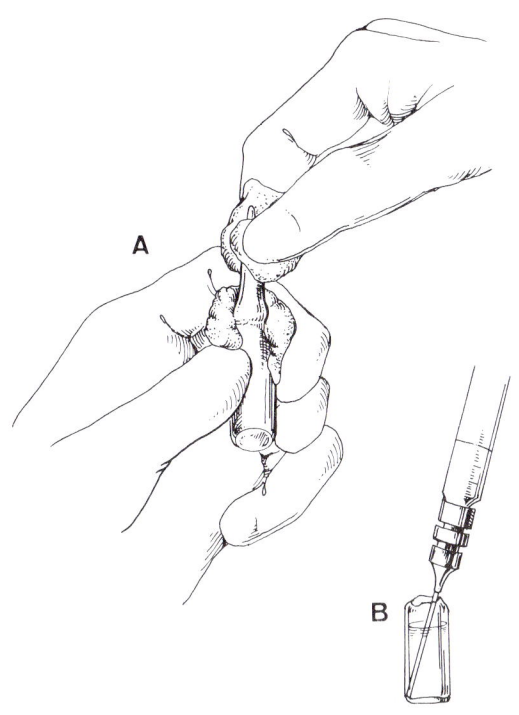

FIGURE 12-10.
A glass ampule. (**A**) The fingers are protected by a gauze square as the stem is broken off. (**B**) When the stem is removed, the drug can be easily drawn up into the syringe.

vantage is that they may be more prone to pilfering and contamination than ampules because multiple doses are often drawn from a vial before it is discarded.

When using a drug vial, take the following steps (Fig. 12-11):

1. Confirm the drug type, concentration, and dose.
2. Clean the rubber stopper with alcohol.
3. Determine the volume of drug to be withdrawn and draw that amount of air into the syringe.
4. Invert the vial, insert the needle through the rubber stopper, and inject the air into the vial.
5. Withdraw the desired amount of solution.
6. Invert the syringe and expel any trapped air.
7. Reconfirm the drug type, concentration, and dose.
8. Administer the drug by the desired route.

Preloaded Syringes

Preloaded syringes are a convenient form of packaging for emergency drugs. Some are preassembled and require no preparation, while others must be assembled before administration.

When using a preloaded syringe, take the following steps:

1. Confirm the drug type, concentration, and dose
2. If assembly is required, pop the caps off the syringe and drug cartridge and screw both together.
3. Invert the syringe and expel any excess air.
4. Reconfirm the drug type, concentration, and dose.
5. Administer the drug by the desired route.

Intravenous Drug Infusions

Common IV drug infusions, such as lidocaine and dopamine, are often available premixed in an IV solution. If the drug is not premixed, proper methods must be used to insure proper drug therapy.

To set up a continuous drug infusion that is not premixed, take the following steps:

1. Swab the bag medication port with alcohol.
2. Inject the desired amount of drug into the IV solution.
3. Invert the bag several times to mix the solution.
4. Label the bag clearly with the drug, amount added, and the calculated concentration.
5. Connect an administration set to the bag (usually microdrip).
6. Flush the drug solution through the tubing.
7. Place a 19- to 20-gauge needle on the end of the administration set and "piggy-back" the infusion into the primary IV line. Tape the needle in place. Turn off the main IV line.
8. Adjust the rate of infusion on the drug line.

Drug infusions may be placed in primary IV bags; "piggy-backing" a separate drug infusion, however, makes discontinuing the IV or changing it easier. Figure 12-12 shows an example of a piggy-back line.

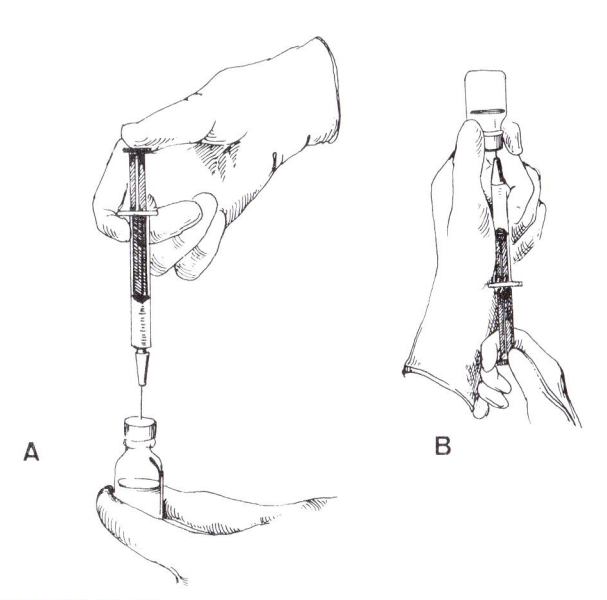

FIGURE 12-11.
A vial. (**A**) When a certain dose is being withdrawn (e.g., 1 mL), it helps to first inject an equal amount of air into the vial. (**B**) The increased pressure helps to move the solution up into the syringe when the vial is inverted.

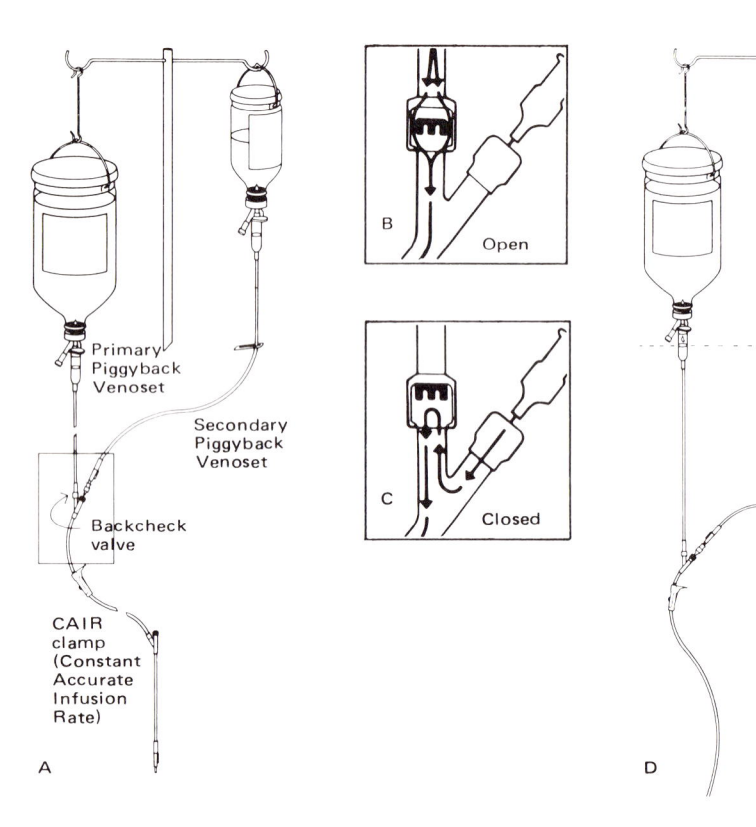

FIGURE 12-12.
(**A**) "Piggy-back" IV. On left is the primary infusion flask. Note use of extension hook (hanging from IV pole) to suspend primary flask. Backcheck valve is seen more clearly in B and C. Secondary "piggyback" source is seen on the right. (**B**) Open check-valve. Fluid from primary source flows down on either side of movable disc. Fluid from secondary source is closed off with clamp (not visible). (**C**) Closed check-valve. Note that fluid source from secondary flask (where pressure is greater because flask source is higher) is forcing movable disk upward, thereby closing off fluid from primary source. (**D**) When last of fluid from secondary source reaches the level of the fluid in the primary set drip chamber (as indicated by broken line), hydrostatic pressure between both sets will equalize. This releases check-valve; flow will shift from secondary to primary source. (Brunner LS, Suddarth DS)

Needles and Syringes

A selection of needles must be carried:

Intradermal needles: Lidocaine may be given by the intradermal to lessen the pain of IV therapy. Intradermal needles are usually 25- to 27-gauge needles, ⅜ to 1 inch long.

Subcutaneous needles: 1:1,000 epinephrine usually is given subcutaneously. Subcutaneous needles are usually 24- to 26-gauge needles, ½ to 1 inch in length.

Intramuscular needles: Many drugs can be given intramuscularly, such as diphenhydramine and meperidine. Intramuscular needles are usually 1 to 1½ inches in length and 21 to 23 gauge, although more viscous solutions, such as some antibiotics, may require larger needles, such as 19 gauge.

A selection of sterile plastic disposable syringes is needed for drawing up drugs from ampules and vials to administer parenterally. They are also used to draw blood samples. A selection of 3-mL, 5-mL, 10-mL, 20-mL, and 30-mL syringes should be on hand. Parts of a needle and syringe are shown in Figure 12-13.

Parenteral Administration

Intradermal

Intradermal injections have limited use in the field. They are most commonly used when administering local anesthesia, such as infiltrating a site before establishing IV access. A small amount of medication (usually less than 1 mL) is administered directly into the skin and is not intended to be absorbed into the circulatory system. The most commonly used local anesthetic is 1% lidocaine. The procedure for an intradermal injection is shown in Skill 12-1.

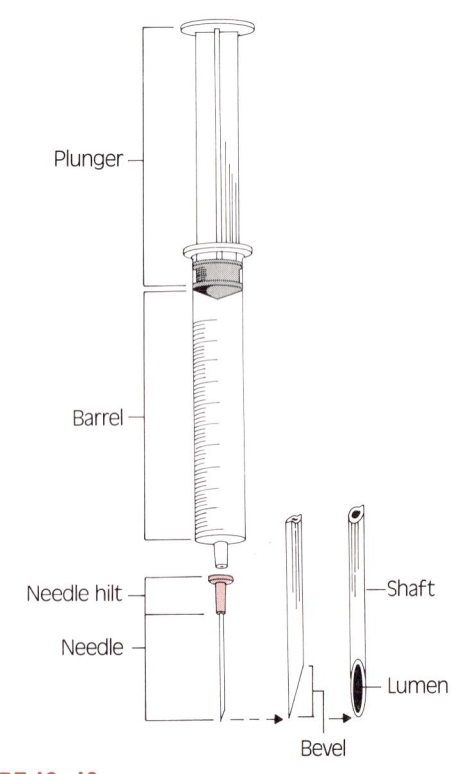

FIGURE 12-13.
Parts of a needle and syringe. (Taylor C, Lillis C, LeMone P)

SKILL 12–1.
INTRADERMAL INJECTION

ACTIVITY	HOW PERFORMED	WHY PERFORMED
1. Check: • Responsiveness • Airway • Breathing • Circulation	Establish responsiveness Stabilize neck, open the airway Assess breathing Check for a pulse Check for hemorrhage	The primary survey is a rapid evaluation, less than 45 seconds, to identify and correct any life-threatening problems.
2. Confirm and review the medication order	Repeat the order verbally if received verbally. Write the order down and consider whether the order seems appropriate and not contraindicated by any factors the physician may not be aware of. If doubt exists, ask for clarification and give reason for question.	The responsibility for accurate and appropriate administration of medication is shared by both the physician and the person giving the medication.
3. Explain procedure to patient and check for patient allergies	Explain reason for the procedure and advise of possible slight discomfort. Ask the patient about any allergies to medications.	This explanation helps calm patient and improves the patient's cooperation with the procedure. Checking for allergies to medications helps eliminate an anaphylactic reaction.
4. Assemble and check: Primary equipment (Activity 4): • Medication • 3-mL syringe • 25-gauge needle Accessory equipment and supplies: • Antiseptic swabs • Gloves	Put on gloves. Draw the proper medication into the syringe using sterile technique. Expel all but 0.1 mL of the excess air in the syringe. Turn the syringe with the needle down and flick the barrel to move the 0.1 mL of air up next to the plunger.	The 0.1 mL of air injected "behind" the medication pushes the medication fully into the subcutaneous tissue, preventing the medicine from seeping out through the injection site.

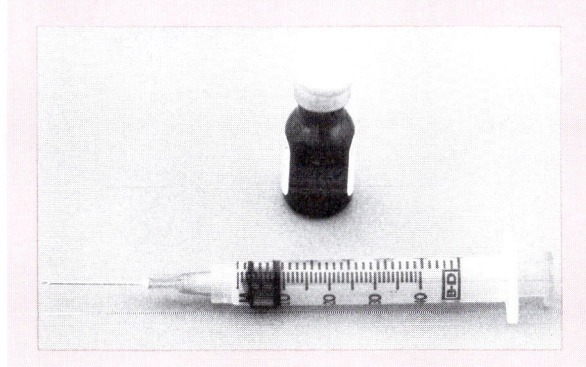

Activity 4. Primary equipment.

5. Select and prepare the injection site	Various sites may be used, depending on the purpose of the injection. In all cases, avoid an area with visible superficial blood vessels. Cleanse the site with the antiseptic swab. Allow the skin to dry before the injection (Activity 5).	Avoiding areas with superficial blood vessels reduces the risk of puncturing a blood vessel. Cleansing the site reduces the possibility of infection.

(continued)

SKILL 12-1.
INTRADERMAL INJECTION (continued)

ACTIVITY	HOW PERFORMED	WHY PERFORMED
Activity 5. Select and prepare injection site.		
6. Perform the injection	With the nondominant hand, stretch the skin over the injection site. Hold the syringe with the needle bevel up at a 10° to 15° angle to the skin (Activity 6).	The taut skin and shallow needle angle facilitate entry of the needle just under the surface of the skin.
	Insert the needle just under the skin surface and inject the medication slowly. Observe for the formation of a small wheal or bump at the injection site.	The medication must be injected slowly to keep it localized at the injection site and within the intradermal layers of the skin.
	Do not massage the site.	
Activity 6. Perform the injection.		
7. Dispose of needle	Place contaminated needle in proper container.	Eliminates the possibility of injury or infection by contact with the contaminated needle.

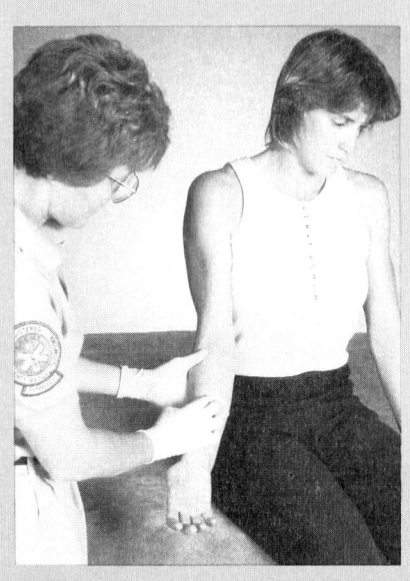

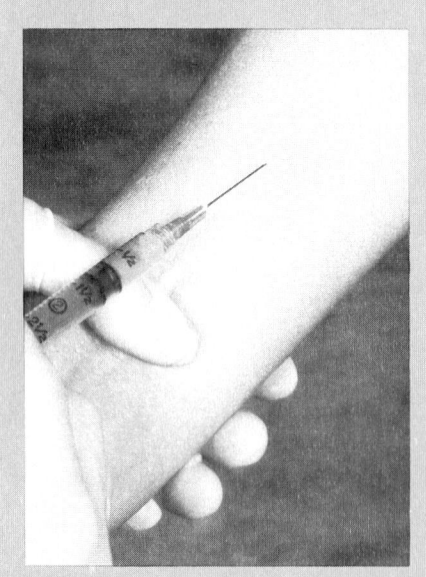

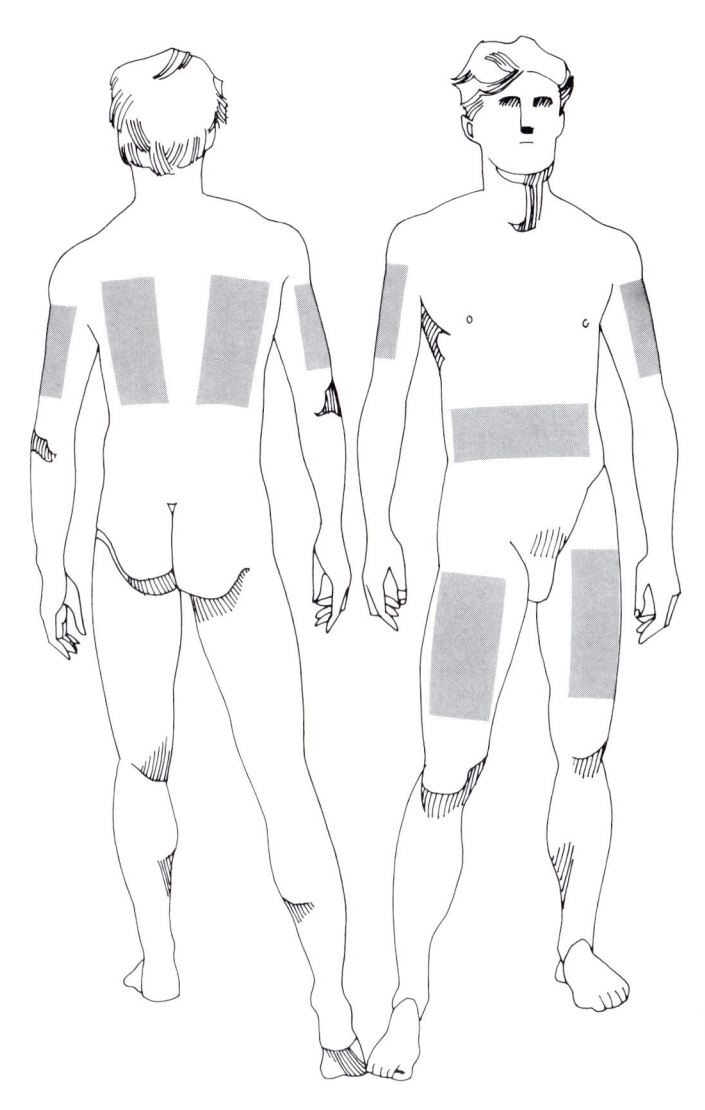

FIGURE 12–14.
The shaded areas on this diagram indicate sites where subcutaneous injections can be given. (Timby B)

Subcutaneous

Subcutaneous injections are performed when the drug to be given requires a slow but steady absorption into the blood. It places the drug under the skin but above the muscle. It also avoids tendons, nerves, and blood vessels. The best sites are areas where the skin is loose and easily pinched, such as upper arms and thighs. Figure 12-14 indicates sites for subcutaneous injections. The maximum volume that may be given subcutaneously is 2 mL. Administering larger amounts or irritating solutions could result in abscess. This route is common for 1:1,000 epinephrine or β-selective bronchodilators, such as terbutaline. The procedure for a subcutaneous injection is shown in Skill 12-2.

Intramuscular

Many drugs may be given by the IM route; however, because of the danger of decreased absorption from the muscle in low perfusion states, the IV route is often preferred. Intramuscular injection is associated with greater hazards than subcutaneous injection because of increased potential for damage to nerves. However, IM absorption is more rapid than injections into the subcutaneous fat because of the vascularity of muscle tissue. Relatively large drug volumes may be given, depending on the site: up to 2 mL may be given in the deltoid muscle (Fig. 12-15), and as much as 10 mL can be given in the buttocks (Fig. 12-16) or thigh (Fig. 12-17).

In children, the quadriceps muscle in the anterior thigh is often used for IM injection because it is large and easily palpated. Other sites in children are more likely to cause nerve damage.

The procedure for an IM injection is shown in Skill 12-3.

Intravenous

Intravenous drug administration is the route of choice for most medications used by the paramedic. While drugs

(text continues on page 230)

228 UNIT TWO: FOUNDATIONS OF EMERGENCY CARE

SKILL 12–2.
SUBCUTANEOUS INJECTION

ACTIVITY	HOW PERFORMED	WHY PERFORMED
1. Check: • Responsiveness • Airway • Breathing • Circulation	Establish responsiveness Stabilize neck, open the airway Assess breathing Check for a pulse Check for hemorrhage	The primary survey is a rapid evaluation, less than 45 seconds, to identify and correct any life-threatening problems.
2. Confirm and review the medication order	Repeat the order verbally if received verbally. Write the order down and consider whether the order seems appropriate and not contraindicated by any factors the physician may not be aware of. If doubt exists, ask for clarification and give reason for question.	The responsibility for accurate and appropriate administration of medication is shared by both the physician and the person giving the medication.
3. Explain procedure to patient and check for patient allergies.	Explain reason for the procedure and advise of possible slight discomfort. Ask the patient about any allergies to medications.	This explanation helps calm the patient and improves the patient's cooperation with the procedure. Checking for allergies to medications helps eliminate an anaphylactic reaction.
4. Assemble and check: Primary equipment (Activity 4): • Medication • 3-mL syringe • 25-gauge needle Acessory equipment and supplies: • Antiseptic swabs • Gloves	Put on gloves. Draw proper medication into the syringe using sterile technique. Expel all but 0.1 mL of the excess air in the syringe. Turn the syringe with the needle down and flick the barrel to move the 0.1 mL of air up next to the plunger.	The 0.1 mL of air injected "behind" the medication pushes the medication fully into the subcutaneous tissue, preventing the medicine from seeping out through the injection site.

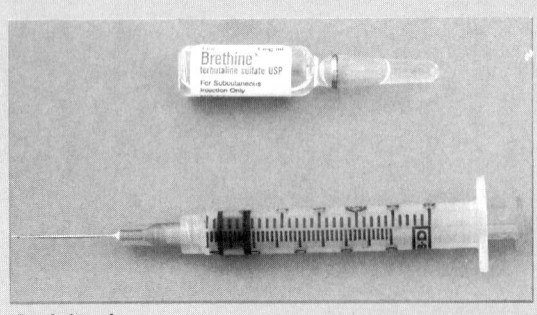

Activity 4.
Primary equipment.

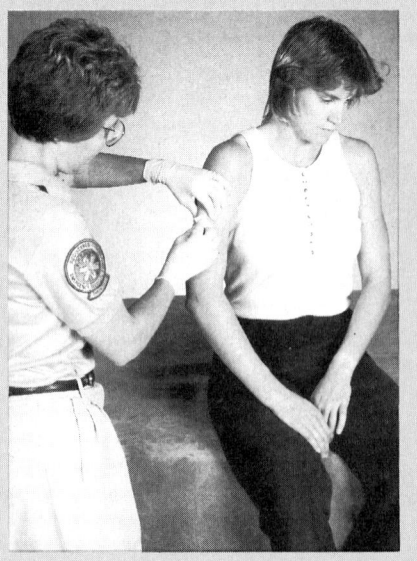

Activity 5.
Select and prepare the injection site.

| 5. Select and prepare the injection site | Usually either the lateral aspect of an upper arm or thigh is selected.

Cleanse the site with the antiseptic swab. Allow skin to dry before the injection (Activity 5). | The lateral upper arm or thigh usually has sufficient subcutaneous fat to allow proper injection and few superficial blood vessels.
Cleansing the site reduces the possibility of infection. |

(continued)

SKILL 12–2.
SUBCUTANEOUS INJECTION (continued)

ACTIVITY	HOW PERFORMED	WHY PERFORMED
6. Perform the injection	Gently pinch about a 1-inch fold of skin with the thumb and index finger of the nondominant hand. Insert the needle at about a 45° angle, until the needle tip is just below the surface (Activity 6A). Release the grasp on the skin.	Gently pinching the injection site allows the needle to enter only the subcutaneous layer of the skin.
	Pull back on the plunger slightly and observe for any appearance of blood in the syringe. If blood appears, withdraw the needle, apply pressure to stop bleeding, and start procedure over with a new needle, syringe, and new medication. If no blood appears, slowly inject the medication and quickly withdraw the needle. Apply gentle pressure to the site to prevent seepage of the medication.	Appearance of blood in the syringe indicates a blood vessel was entered, and, thus, this route is inappropriate for administration of the medication.
	Gently massage area (Activity 6B).	Massaging the area allows medication to be absorbed more readily.
7. Dispose of needle	Place contaminated needle in proper container.	Eliminates the possibility of injury or infection by contact with the contaminated needle.

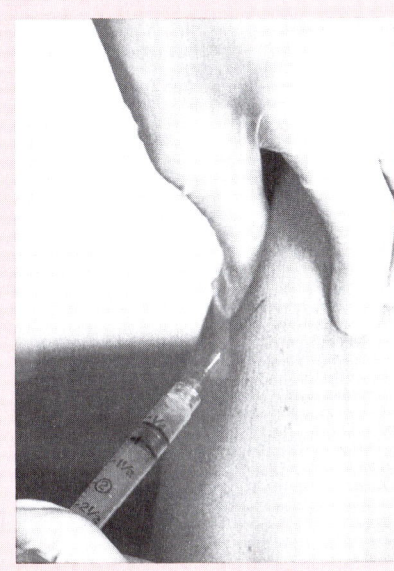

Activity 6A. Perform the injection.

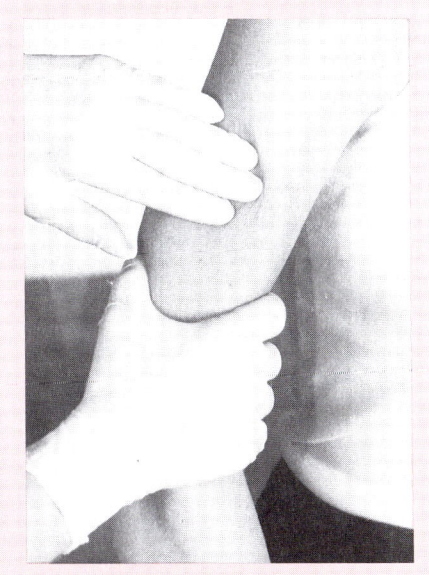

Activity 6B. Gently massage area.

may be injected directly into a vein with a syringe and needle, this action carries the risk of inadvertent injection into surrounding tissue. Therefore, IV drug administration usually is given through an existing IV lifeline. Because of this preference, IV lines are routinely placed in potentially unstable or unstable patients to facilitate the administration of drugs. Because of the osmolarity and vasoconstrictive effects of many IV drugs, it is important that infiltration into surrounding tissues does not occur, because tissue necrosis may result.

PERIPHERAL. Whenever possible, an IV lifeline should be placed in a peripheral site, such as the patient's leg or, more commonly, arm, rather than a more central portion of the body. Peripheral IV sites generally are preferred because they are easily accessible and ordinarily have a number of large superficial veins that may be reliably located (Fig. 12-18).

Many patients whose condition requires that an IV lifeline be started before they arrive at the hospital are starting a potentially long course of treatment that will require a great many venipunctures for a variety of reasons. For that reason, the paramedic should attempt to start any IV lifeline in a site that is as distal on the selected limb as possible, while still offering a viable site. This site is chosen because every venipuncture that is

(text continues on page 233)

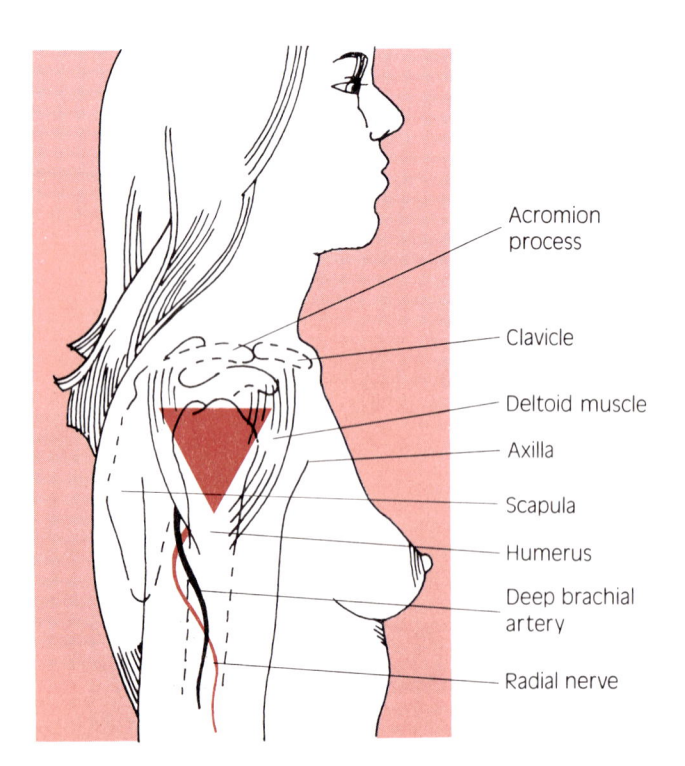

FIGURE 12-16.
The dorsogluteal site for administering an intramuscular injection is found by dividing the buttock into four quadrants. The injection is given in the upper outer quadrant. (Taylor C, Lillis C, LeMone P)

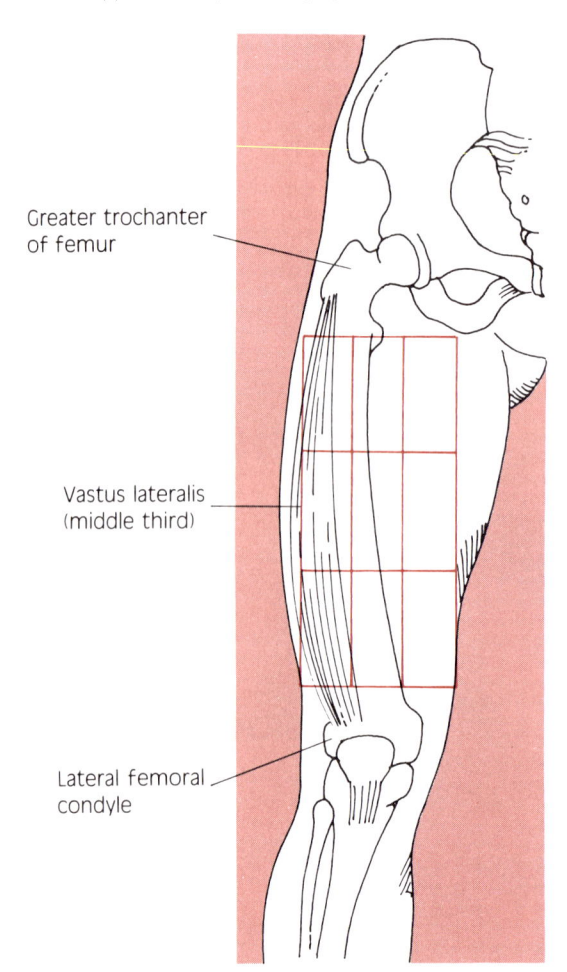

FIGURE 12-15.
The deltoid muscle site for intramuscular injection is located by palpating the lower edge of the acromion process. At the midpoint, in line with axilla on the lateral aspect of the upper arm, a triangle is formed. (Taylor C, Lillis C, LeMone P)

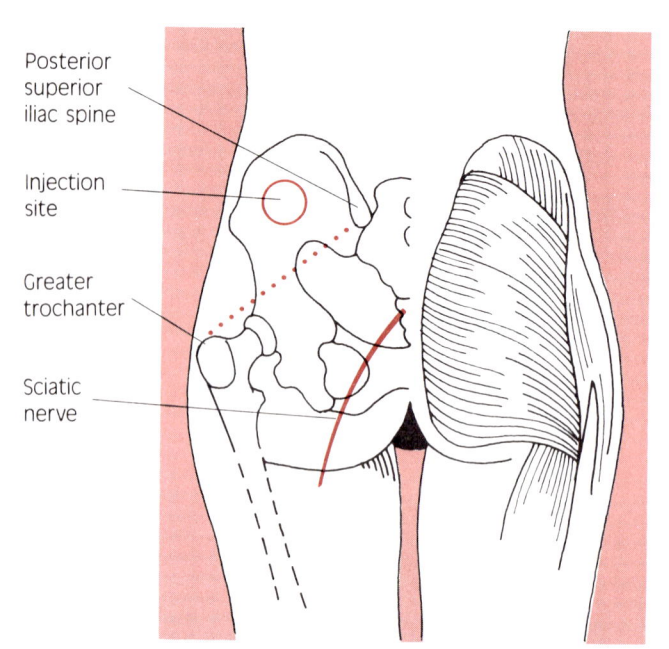

FIGURE 12-17.
The vastus lateralis site for intramuscular injections is identified by dividing the thigh into thirds horizontally and vertically. The injection is given in the outer middle third. (Taylor C, Lillis C, LeMone P)

SKILL 12-3.
INTRAMUSCULAR INJECTION

ACTIVITY	HOW PERFORMED	WHY PERFORMED
1. Check: • Responsiveness • Airway • Breathing • Circulation	Establish responsiveness Stabilize neck, open the airway Assess breathing Check for a pulse Check for hemorrhage	The primary survey is a rapid evaluation, less than 45 seconds, to identify and correct any life-threatening problems.
2. Confirm and review the medication order	Repeat the order verbally if received verbally. Write the order down and consider whether the order seems appropriate and not contraindicated by any factors the physician may not be aware of. If doubt exists, ask for clarification and give reason for question.	The responsibility for accurate and appropriate administration of medication is shared by both the physician and the person giving the medication.
3. Explain procedure to patient and check for patient allergies	Explain reason for the procedure and advise of possible slight discomfort. Ask the patient about any allergies to medications.	This explanation helps calm the patient and improves the patient's cooperation with the procedure. Checking for allergies to medications helps eliminate an anaphylactic reaction.
4. Assemble and check: Primary equipment (Activity 4): • Medication • Syringe • Needle Accessory equipment and supplies: • Antiseptic swabs • Gloves	Put on gloves. Draw the proper medication into the syringe using sterile technique. Expel all but 0.1 mL of the excess air in the syringe. Turn the syringe with the needle down and flick the barrel to move the 0.1 mL of air up next to the plunger.	The 0.1 mL of air injected "behind" the medication pushes the medication fully into the muscle, preventing the medicine from seeping out through the injection site.

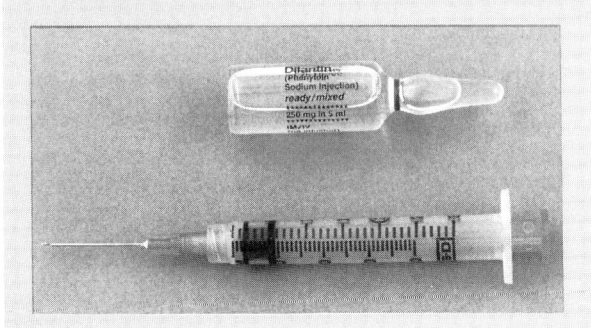

Activity 4.
Primary equipment.

5. Prepare the injection site	Usually either the deltoid muscle in the shoulder or the upper outer quadrant of the gluteal area is used. Cleanse the site with the alcohol swab. Allow skin to dry before the injection (Activity 5).	The deltoid muscle and the gluteal area have few superficial blood vessels, allowing for easier intramuscular injection. Cleansing the site reduces the possibility of infection.

(continued)

SKILL 12-3.
INTRAMUSCULAR INJECTION (continued)

ACTIVITY	HOW PERFORMED	WHY PERFORMED
	Activity 5. Prepare the injection site.	
6. Perform the injection	Use the fingers of the nondominant hand to gently stretch the skin over the injection site. Insert the needle quickly at a 90° angle to the skin and release the grasp on the skin (Activity 6A). Pull back on the plunger slightly and observe for any appearance of blood in the syringe. If blood appears, withdraw the needle, apply pressure to stop bleeding, and start procedure over with a new needle, syringe, and new medication. If no blood appears, slowly inject the medication and quickly withdraw the needle. Apply gentle pressure to the site to prevent seepage of the medication.	Gentle stretching of the skin over the injection site helps the needle enter the muscular tissue. Appearance of blood in the syringe indicates a blood vessel was entered, and, thus, this route is inappropriate for administration of the medication.
Activity 6A. Perform the injection.	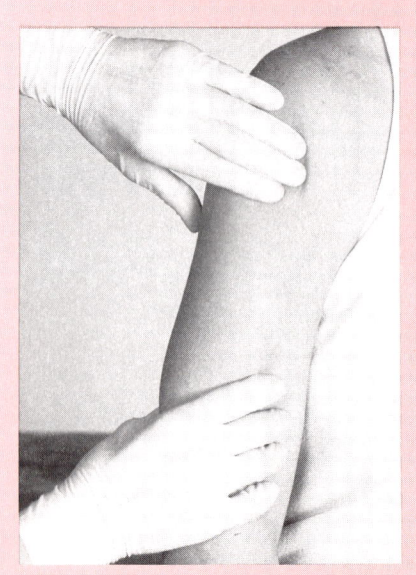	**Activity 6B.** Gently massage area.
	Gently massage area (Activity 6B).	Massaging the area allows medication to be absorbed more readily.
7. Dispose of needle	Place contaminated needle in proper container.	Eliminates the possibility of injury or infection by contact with the contaminated needle.

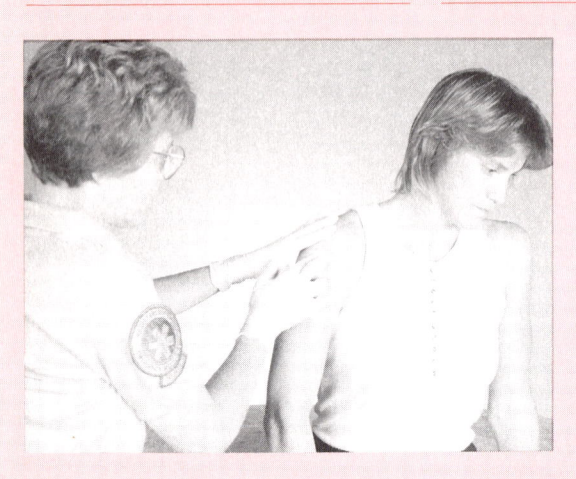

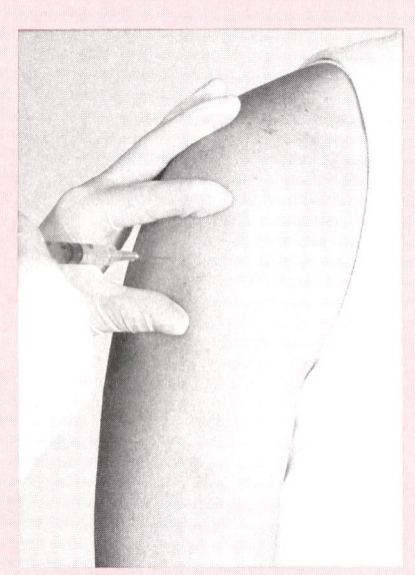

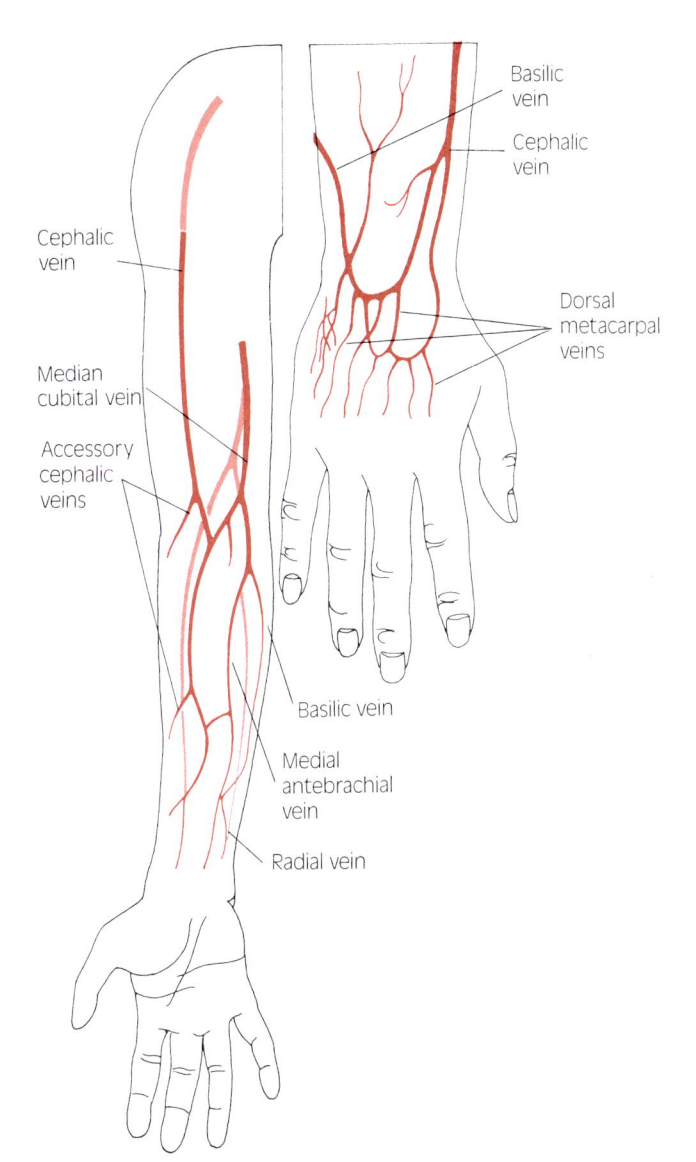

FIGURE 12–18.
Infusion sites on the ventral and dorsal aspects of the forearm and hand. (Taylor C, Lillis C, LeMone P)

required later may have to be performed at a site more proximal than the preceding one. Thus, starting the first IV in an extreme proximal location, such as in the antecubital fossa, greatly reduces the number of sites available for use in the later acute care of the patient.

A potential problem, however, is that a peripheral IV site that is too distal may be too small in diameter to offer a sufficiently large pathway for rapid infusion of fluids or medications. Similarly, the more distal the IV site, the more variable the location of veins and the more likely they are to be somewhat mobile, or able to move under the skin, which may make insertion of the IV needle more difficult.

The paramedic must make the choice of IV site based on the patient's condition, the availability of adequate veins, and the purpose for the IV lifeline. For example, a patient who needs an IV for the administration of drugs may be well served by an IV inserted in one of the small veins in the back of the hand. A patient with potentially severe trauma, however, may require a somewhat larger vein in a stable site, such as the ones on the lateral and posterior aspects of the forearm. Finally, for a patient in acute distress, the best and fastest choice may be to go directly to the large and easily found vein in the antecubital fossa.

The flow and stability of any peripheral IV are affected by the site selection and the mobility of the patient's limb. In many cases, a splint may be required, as well as communication with the patient to gain cooperation in protecting the IV site and maintaining good flow.

The procedure for a peripheral venipuncture is shown in Skill 12-4.

CENTRAL. A central IV refers to an IV lifeline placed in one of the large veins that enters directly into the trunk of the body, or central portion of the circulatory system. The most frequently used central IV routes include the femoral vein, subclavian vein, and internal and external jugular veins (Fig. 12-19).

While central IV routes provide excellent access to the circulatory system, the placement of a central IV by any of the mentioned routes is far more difficult and has many more serious complications than any of the peripheral IV routes. The difficulty of the techniques and seriousness of the complications associated with central IV insertion are the primary reasons why their use outside the hospital is limited. Rapid fluid replacement is a major reason for IV access in the field. Administration of medication is the second reason. Medication can be given as efficiently peripherally as it can be centrally. Rapid administration of fluids is better done via a peripheral vein. The rate of fluid administration is dependent directly on the internal diameter of the catheter and inversely on the length of the catheter. Generally, a peripheral catheter is larger and shorter; thus, fluids pass at a faster rate.

In some cases, however, the use of a central IV route may be warranted in the prehospital setting. In nearly every case, this use is limited to critical situations in which IV access is crucial to the survival of the patient and all efforts to establish a safer peripheral IV lifeline have failed.

Since all of the central IV routes, except the femoral, involve needle punctures near the chest and neck where extremely critical complications may occur, it is generally agreed that the safest of the central routes is the femoral vein. The procedure for a central line placement (femoral) is shown in Skill 12-5. The procedure for a central line placement (internal jugular, anterior approach) is shown in Skill 12-6. The procedure for a central line placement (internal jugular, middle approach) is shown in Skill 12-7. The procedure for a central line placement (internal

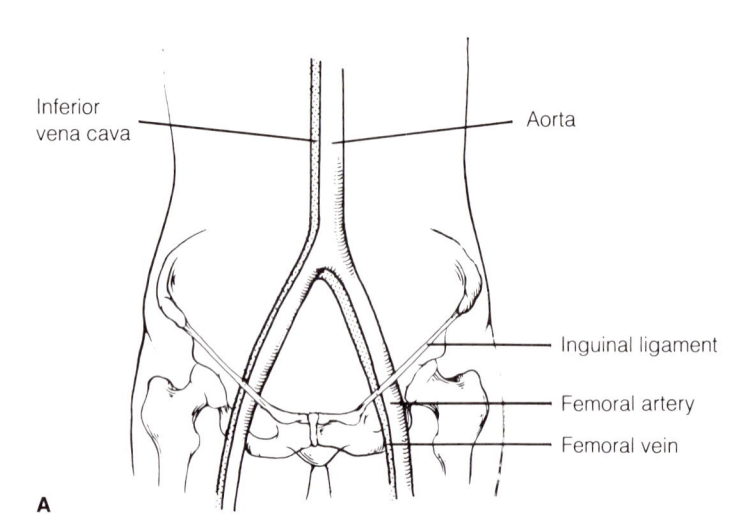

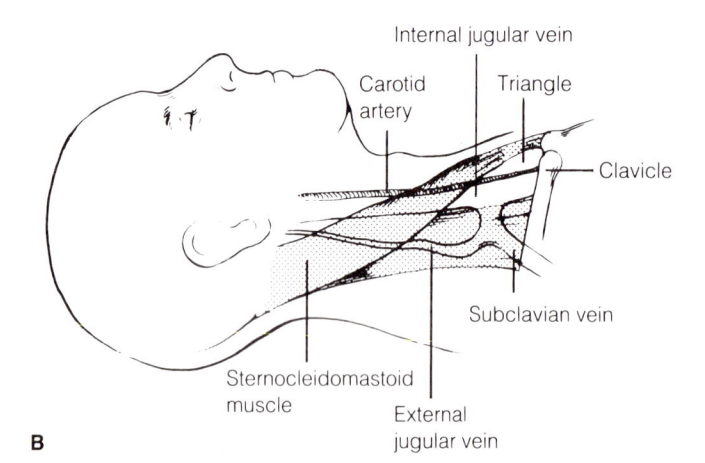

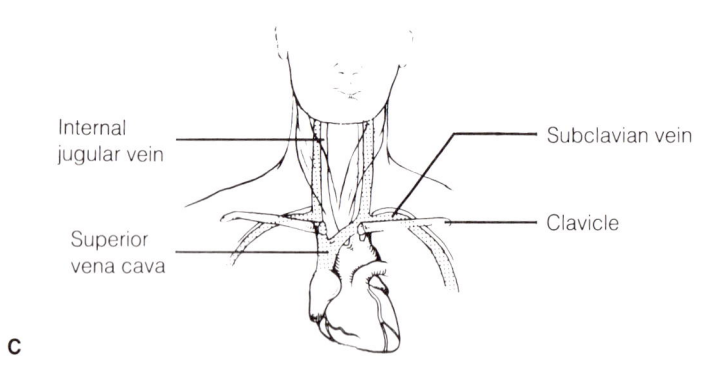

FIGURE 12-19.
Sites for central line placement. (**A**) Anatomy of femoral vein. (**B**) Anatomy of internal jugular vein. (**C**) Anatomy of subclavian vein.

jugular, posterior approach) is shown in Skill 12-8. The procedure for a central line placement (subclavian approach) is shown in Skill 12-9.

Intraosseous

Intraosseous infusion refers to the placement of a rigid needle into a bone and the infusion of fluid and medications directly into the bone marrow. Since bone marrow is highly vascular with direct communication to the peripheral circulation, both fluids and medications may be administered effectively in this way.

The technique of intraosseous infusion has been known for many years but has only recently begun to be emphasized as a relatively fast and safe means of fluid and drug administration. While it is effective in adults, the intraosseous technique is of particular value in critically ill or injured children when no other peripheral venous access

(text continues on page 247)

SKILL 12–4.
PERIPHERAL VENIPUNCTURE

ACTIVITY	HOW PERFORMED	WHY PERFORMED
1. Check: • Responsiveness • Airway • Breathing • Circulation	Establish responsiveness Stabilize neck, open the airway Assess breathing Check for a pulse Check for hemorrhage	The primary survey is a rapid evaluation, less than 45 seconds, to identify and correct any life-threatening problems.
2. Explain procedure to patient	Explain reason for the procedure and advise of possible slight discomfort.	This explanation helps calm patient and improves patient's cooperation with the procedure.
3. Assemble and check: Primary equipment (Activity 3): • Intravenous (IV) solution • IV tubing and administration set • IV catheter • Tourniquet Accessory equipment and supplies: • Antiseptic swabs • Tape • Sterile gauze squares • Syringe • Gloves	Select IV fluid and check for expiration date, contamination, cloudiness, and seal leakage. Connect infusion set to IV fluid bag. Select intravenous catheter and tear tape, and prepare dressing. Open control valve and bleed air from the line. Fill drip chamber half full. Have all items placed within easy reach. Put on gloves.	Having all equipment ready reduces time delays during the procedure and minimizes patient discomfort. To prevent blood or body fluid contact with nonintact skin.

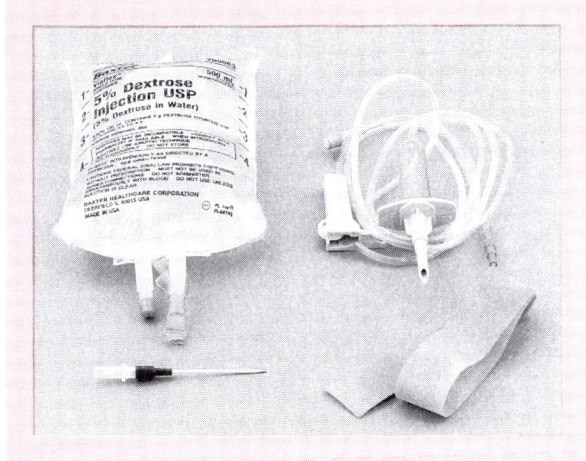

Activity 3.
Primary equipment.

4. Apply tourniquet	Place constriction band around the extremity proximal to the entry site (Activity 4). Band must be just tight enough to restrict venous, but not arterial, blood flow.	Constricting band restricts venous blood flow, causing veins to fill and distend with blood, making them easier to locate and cannulate.

(continued)

SKILL 12–4.
PERIPHERAL VENIPUNCTURE (continued)

ACTIVITY	HOW PERFORMED	WHY PERFORMED
	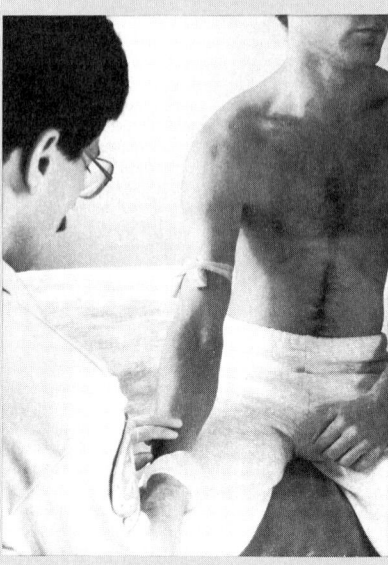 **Activity 4.** Apply tourniquet.	
5. Prepare the selected site	Cleanse the selected venipuncture site with antiseptic swabs (Activity 5).	Preparing the site reduces the possibility of infection at the venipuncture site.
	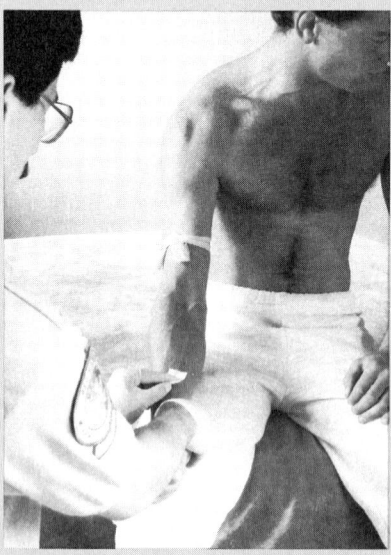 **Activity 5.** Prepare the selected site.	

(continued)

SKILL 12-4.
PERIPHERAL VENIPUNCTURE (continued)

ACTIVITY	HOW PERFORMED	WHY PERFORMED
6. Perform venipuncture	Place the fingers of the nondominant hand 1 to 2 cm distal to the selected venipuncture site and apply gentle traction distally on the skin to stabilize the vein. Hold the needle with the bevel up and directed at a 45° angle to the skin, pointing in the direction of the venous blood flow (Activity 6A). Insert the needle smoothly through the skin, and enter the vein from either the top or side (Activity 6B).	Stabilizing the vein minimizes skin and vein movement during venipuncture.
	When blood is seen in the catheter hub or "flashback" chamber, advance the needle about 1 to 2 mm further and hold the needle steady while threading the catheter off the needle (or through the needle) and into the vein (Activity 6C).	Blood return verifies the vein has been entered. Advancing the needle a tiny bit further ensures the tip of the needle and catheter are inside the vein before advancing the catheter. *Never pull the catheter back over (or through) the needle after it is even partially advanced. This action could cause the catheter to be sheared off by the sharp needle bevel, sending a foreign embolus into the patient's circulatory system.*

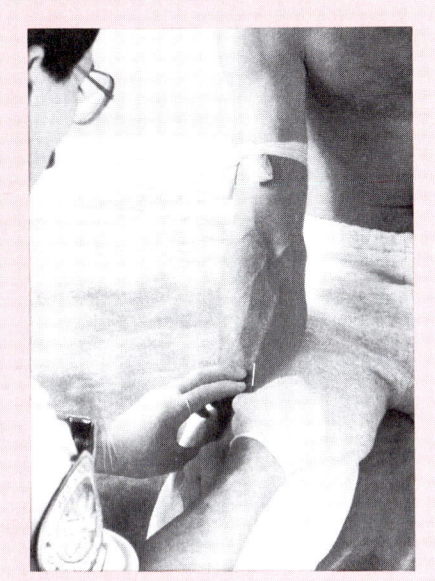

Activity 6A.
Perform venipuncture—position needle.

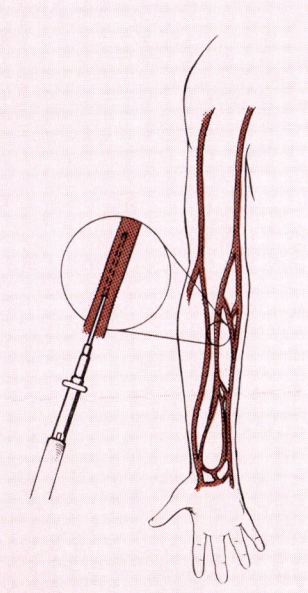

Activity 6B.
Perform venipuncture—insert needle.

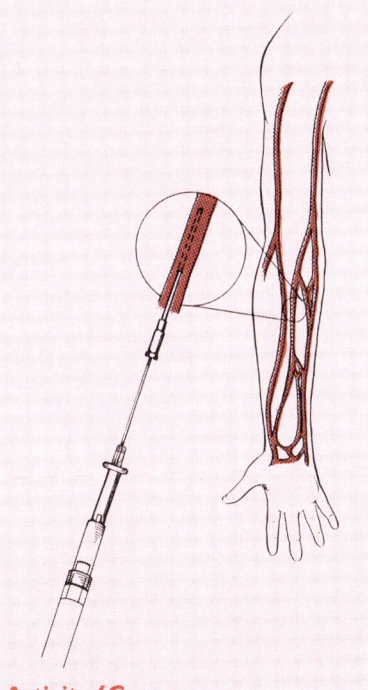

Activity 6C.
Perform venipuncture—advance needle and thread catheter into vein.

(continued)

SKILL 12-4.
PERIPHERAL VENIPUNCTURE (continued)

ACTIVITY	HOW PERFORMED	WHY PERFORMED
7. Start fluid flow	With the catheter threaded into the vein, apply pressure to the vein with fingers of the nondominant hand just proximal to the inserted catheter. Withdraw the needle, leaving the catheter in place, and attach the IV tubing to the catheter.	Proximal pressure reduces blood leakage as the needle is withdrawn and the IV tubing is attached.
	Release the tourniquet and open the IV flow clamps. Release the pressure proximal to the catheter and observe IV drip chamber for free fluid flow.	Releasing tourniquet, clamps, and proximal pressure allows free flow of IV fluid into the vein.
	Inspect the venipuncture site for any sign of fluid leakage or infiltration into the surrounding tissue.	IV fluid infiltration into tissues eliminates the effectiveness of the IV and may cause tissue damage and discomfort for the patient.
	If fluid fails to flow freely or if signs of infiltration are seen, close the IV fluid clamps, withdraw the catheter, and apply pressure over the venipuncture site to control bleeding.	
	Reattempt the venipuncture as appropriate either in another vein or at a site more proximal on the same vein.	
8. Secure the catheter	Place sterile gauze squares or commercial IV dressing over the venipuncture site and secure the tubing with tape.	Dressings protect the venipuncture site from contamination and the tape prevents accidental dislodging of the catheter during patient handling or other procedures.
9. Adjust flow rate	Adjust the clamp on the IV tubing until the number of drops per minute seen in the IV drip chamber matches the appropriate orders or protocols (Activity 9).	IV fluid flow must be carefully controlled to achieve the optimum benefit for the patient and avoid potential detrimental effects.

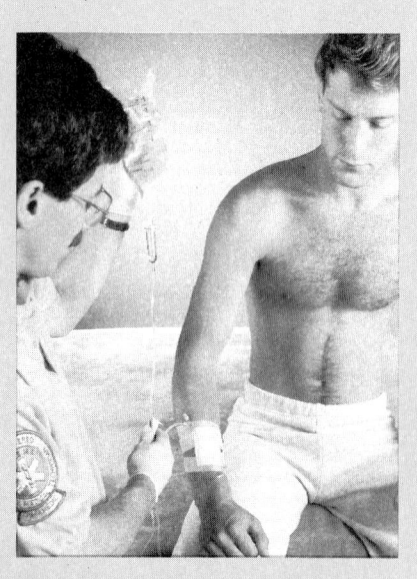

Activity 9.
Adjust flow rate.

10. Dispose of needle	Place contaminated needle in proper container.	Eliminates the possibility of injury or infection by contact with the contaminated needle.

CHAPTER 12: General Pharmacology 239

SKILL 12–5.
CENTRAL LINE PLACEMENT (FEMORAL)

ACTIVITY	HOW PERFORMED	WHY PERFORMED
1. Check: • Responsiveness • Airway • Breathing • Circulation	Establish responsiveness Stabilize neck, open the airway Assess breathing Check for a pulse Check for hemorrhage	The primary survey is a rapid evaluation, less than 45 seconds, to identify and correct any life-threatening problems.
2. Assess need for central line	Compare patient's presenting signs and symptoms with local orders or protocols to determine if procedure is indicated and appropriate.	Procedure must only be performed when indicated and appropriate according to local orders or protocols.
3. Assemble and check: Primary equipment (Activity 3): • Intravenous (IV) solution • IV tubing and administration set • 16-gauge catheter • 10-mL syringe Accessory equipment and supplies: • Antiseptic swabs • Sterile gauze squares • Tape • Protective eye wear • Mask • Gloves	Select IV fluid and check for expiration date, contamination, cloudiness, and seal leakage. Connect infusion set to IV fluid bag. Select intravenous catheter and tear tape, and prepare dressing. Open control valve and bleed air from the line. Fill drip chamber half full. Have all items placed within easy reach. Prepare 16-gauge catheter with a 10-mL syringe on the end of the catheter. Put on protective eye wear, mask, and gloves.	Having all equipment ready reduces time delays during the procedure and minimizes patient discomfort. To prevent blood or body fluid contact with nonintact skin or mucous membranes.

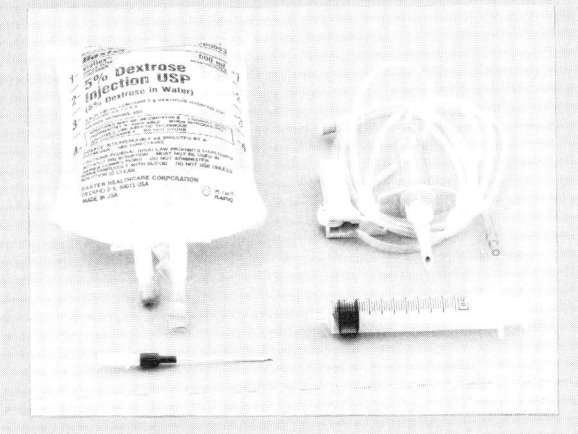

Activity 3.
Primary equipment.

4. Position the patient	Place patient supine with leg externally rotated.	External rotation of the leg brings the femoral vein closer to the surface for easier access.
5. Locate the femoral artery	Find the femoral artery by locating the femoral pulse at the midpoint of an imaginary line from the anterior superior iliac crest and the symphysis pubis (Activity 5).	The femoral vein lies just medial to the femoral artery, making the location of the artery an essential landmark.

(continued)

SKILL 12-5.
CENTRAL LINE PLACEMENT (FEMORAL) (continued)

ACTIVITY	HOW PERFORMED	WHY PERFORMED
	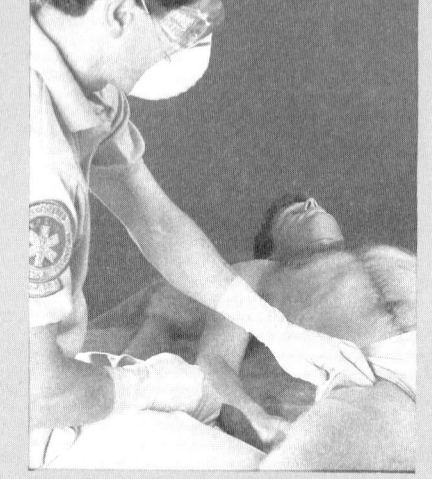 **Activity 5.** Locate the femoral artery.	
6. Prepare the selected site	Cleanse the selected venipuncture site with antiseptic swabs (Activity 6).	Preparing the site reduces the possibility of infection at the venipuncture site.
	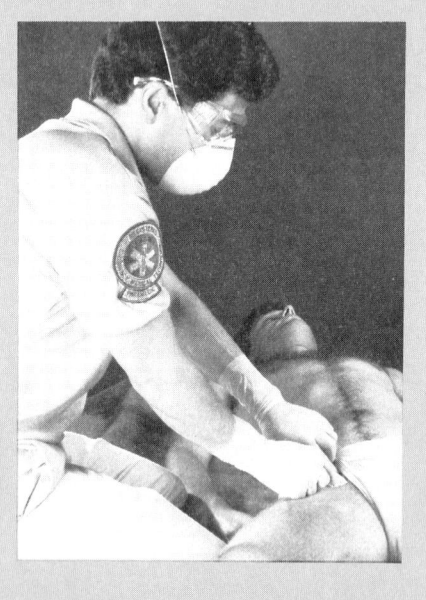 **Activity 6.** Prepare the selected site.	
7. Perform the venipuncture	Insert the needle one finger-width medial to the femoral artery, and two finger-widths inferior to the inguinal ligament. The entry angle should be 30° to 45° to the skin and directed toward the patient's head (Activity 7).	Inserting the needle medial to the artery directs it into the femoral vein.

(continued)

SKILL 12–5.
CENTRAL LINE PLACEMENT (FEMORAL) (continued)

ACTIVITY	HOW PERFORMED	WHY PERFORMED
	Aspirate the syringe as the needle is inserted. When dark red blood enters the syringe, thread the catheter into the vein.	
	If bright red blood enters the syringe, withdraw the needle and hold firm pressure on the puncture site for 10 minutes before reattempting.	*Bright red blood in the syringe indicates the femoral artery has been entered. A full 10 minutes of pressure is required to stop bleeding from the femoral artery.*
	Activity 7. Perform the venipuncture.	
8. Start fluid flow	Place firm pressure proximal to the puncture site, hold the catheter and remove the needle. Attach the IV tubing to the catheter hub and open the IV flow clamps. Observe the drip chamber for free fluid flow and inspect the venipuncture site for signs of infiltration.	Proximal pressure reduces leakage of blood as needle is withdrawn and tubing is attached.
	If fluid does not flow or if signs of infiltration are seen, withdraw the catheter and hold firm pressure on the puncture site for 10 full minutes before reattempting venipuncture.	*Absence of fluid flow or evidence of infiltration indicates misplacement of the catheter. A full 10 minutes of pressure is required to stop bleeding from the femoral vein.*
9. Adjust flow rate	Adjust the clamp on the IV tubing until the number of drops per minute seen in the IV drip chamber matches the appropriate orders or protocols.	IV fluid flow must be carefully controlled to achieve the optimum benefit for the patient and avoid potential detrimental effects.
10. Secure the catheter 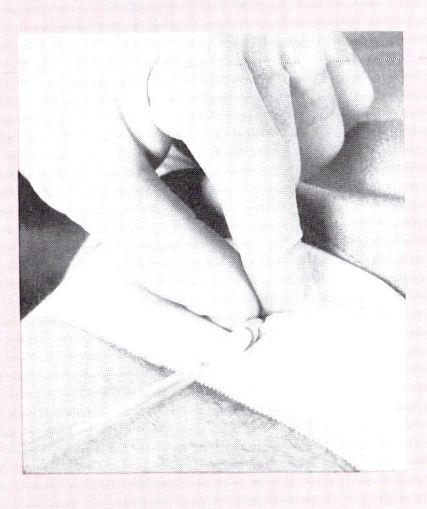	Place sterile gauze squares or commercial IV dressing over the venipuncture site and secure the tubing with tape (Activity 10).	Dressings protect the venipuncture site from contamination, and the tape prevents accidental dislodging of the catheter during patient handling or other procedures.
	Activity 10. Secure the catheter.	
11. Dispose of needle	Place contaminated needle in proper container.	Eliminates the possibility of injury or infection by contact with the contaminated needle.

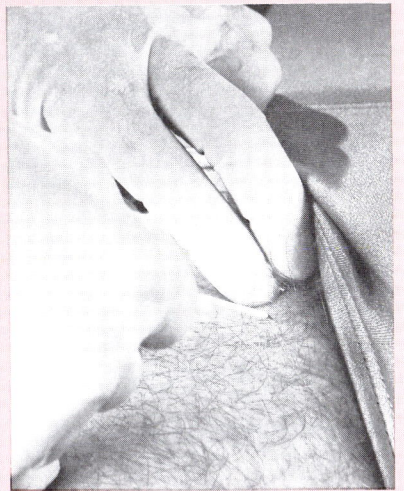

SKILL 12–6.
CENTRAL LINE PLACEMENT (INTERNAL JUGULAR, ANTERIOR APPROACH)

ACTIVITY	HOW PERFORMED	WHY PERFORMED
1. Check: • Responsiveness • Airway • Breathing • Circulation	Establish responsiveness Stabilize neck, open the airway Assess breathing Check for a pulse Check for hemorrhage	The primary survey is a rapid evaluation, less than 45 seconds, to identify and correct any life-threatening problems.
2. Assess need for central line	Compare patient's presenting signs and symptoms with local orders or protocols to determine if procedure is indicated and appropriate.	Procedure must only be performed when indicated and appropriate according to local orders or protocols.
3. Assemble and check: Primary equipment (Activity 3): • Intravenous (IV) solution • IV tubing and administration set • 16-gauge catheter • 10-mL syringe Accessory equipment and supplies: • Antiseptic swabs • Sterile gauze squares • Tape • Protective eye wear • Mask • Gloves	Select IV fluid and check for expiration date, contamination, cloudiness, and seal leakage. Connect infusion set to IV fluid bag. Select intravenous catheter and tear tape, and prepare dressing. Open control valve and bleed air from the line. Fill drip chamber half full. Have all items placed within easy reach. Prepare 16-gauge catheter with a 10-mL syringe on the end of the catheter. Put on protective eye wear, mask, and gloves.	Having all equipment ready reduces time delays during the procedure and minimizes patient discomfort. To prevent blood or body fluid contact with nonintact skin or mucous membranes.

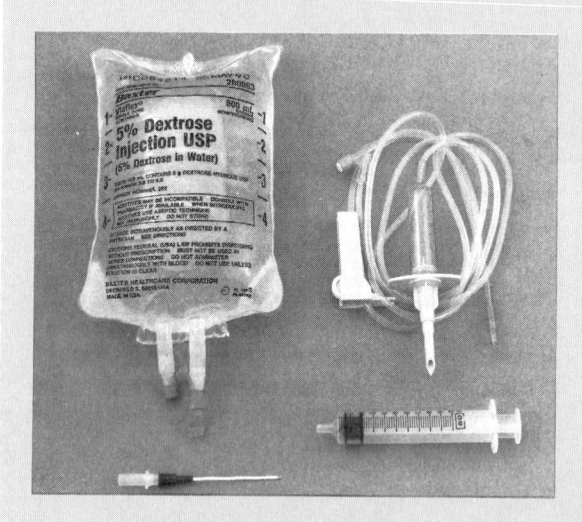

Activity 3.
Primary equipment.

4. Position the patient	Place patient in Trendelenburg's position at 15° with head turned to the opposite side of the procedure site. The right internal jugular vein is preferred.	Trendelenburg's position helps distend the internal jugular vein, and turning the head allows easier access to the area. The right internal jugular vein is usually chosen since the right lung is lower than the left, and this route does not endanger the thoracic duct.

(continued)

SKILL 12-6.
CENTRAL LINE PLACEMENT (INTERNAL JUGULAR, ANTERIOR APPROACH) (continued)

ACTIVITY	HOW PERFORMED	WHY PERFORMED
5. Find landmarks for venipuncture	Locate the point at the anterior border of the sternocleidomastoid muscle that is 5 cm above the clavicle and 5 cm below the angle of the mandible (Activity 5).	The internal jugular is located deep to this point.

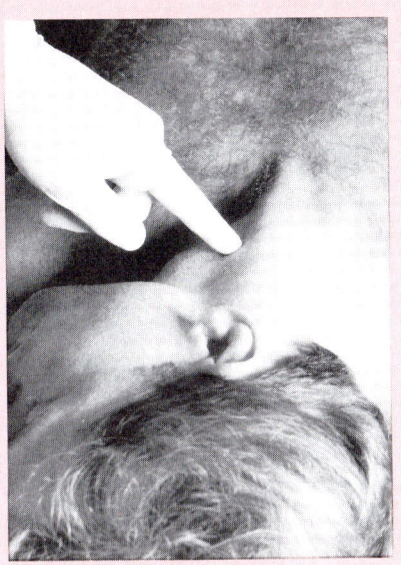

Activity 5.
Find landmarks for venipuncture.

6. Prepare the selected site	Cleanse the selected venipuncture site with antiseptic swabs (Activity 6).	Preparing the site reduces the possibility of infection at the venipuncture site.

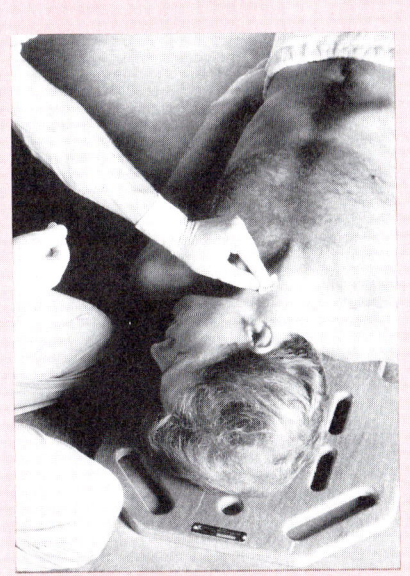

Activity 6.
Prepare the selected site.

7. Perform the venipuncture	Insert the needle toward the patient's feet at a 30° to 45°-degree angle toward the ipsilateral nipple (Activity 7).	Insertion at this angle directs the needle into the internal jugular vein.

(continued)

SKILL 12–6.
CENTRAL LINE PLACEMENT (INTERNAL JUGULAR, ANTERIOR APPROACH) (continued)

ACTIVITY	HOW PERFORMED	WHY PERFORMED
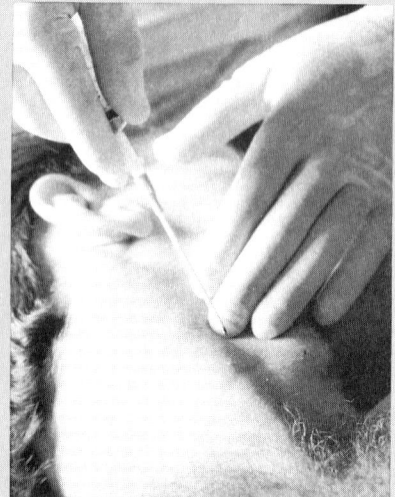 **Activity 7.** Perform the venipuncture.	While inserting the needle, aspirate the syringe until blood appears. When blood appears in the syringe, thread the catheter into the vein.	Blood in the syringe indicates the vein has been entered.
8. Start fluid flow	Holding the catheter in place, quickly withdraw the needle and attach the IV tubing to the catheter hub. Open the IV flow clamps and observe the drip chamber for free fluid flow. *If fluid does not flow or if signs of infiltration are seen, withdraw the catheter and hold firm pressure on the puncture site.*	The position of the vein does not allow pressure to reduce leaking of blood when the needle is withdrawn. *Absence of fluid flow or evidence of infiltration indicates misplacement of the catheter. Direct pressure is necessary to control any bleeding.*
9. Adjust flow rate	Adjust the clamp on the IV tubing until the number of drops per minute seen in the IV drip chamber matches the appropriate orders or protocols.	IV fluid flow must be carefully controlled to achieve the optimum benefit for the patient and avoid potential detrimental effects.
10. Secure the catheter 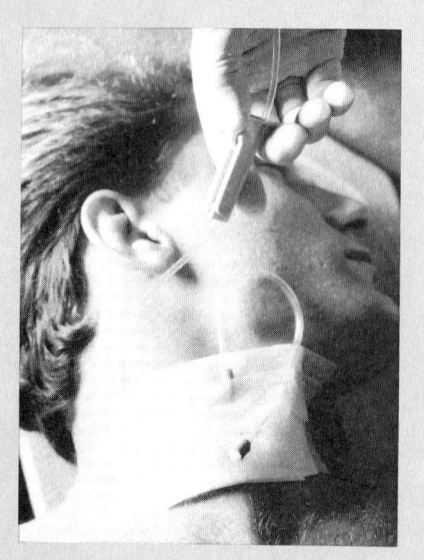	Place sterile gauze squares or commercial IV dressing over the venipuncture site and secure the tubing with tape (Activity 10).	Dressings protect the venipuncture site from contamination, and the tape prevents accidental dislodging of the catheter during patient handling or other procedures.
Activity 10. Secure the catheter.		
11. Dispose of needle	Place contaminated needle in proper container.	Eliminates the possibility of injury or infection by contact with the contaminated needle.

SKILL 12–7.
CENTRAL LINE PLACEMENT (INTERNAL JUGULAR, MIDDLE APPROACH)

ACTIVITY	HOW PERFORMED	WHY PERFORMED
1. Check: • Responsiveness • Airway • Breathing • Circulation	Establish responsiveness Stabilize neck, open the airway Assess breathing Check for a pulse Check for hemorrhage	The primary survey is a rapid evaluation, less than 45 seconds, to identify and correct any life-threatening problems.
2. Assess need for central line	Compare patient's presenting signs and symptoms with local orders or protocols to determine if procedure is indicated and appropriate.	Procedure must only be performed when indicated and appropriate according to local orders or protocols.
3. Assemble and check: Primary equipment (Activity 3): • Intravenous (IV) solution • IV tubing and administration set • 16-gauge catheter • 10-mL syringe Accessory equipment and supplies: • Antiseptic swabs • Sterile gauze squares • Tape • Protective eye wear • Mask • Gloves	Select IV fluid and check for expiration date, contamination, cloudiness, and seal leakage. Connect infusion set to IV fluid bag. Select intravenous catheter and tear tape, and prepare dressing. Open control valve and bleed air from the line. Fill drip chamber half full. Have all items placed within easy reach. Prepare 16-gauge catheter with a 10-mL syringe on the end of the catheter. Put on protective eye wear, mask, and gloves.	Having all equipment ready reduces time delays during the procedure and minimizes patient discomfort. To prevent blood or body fluid contact with nonintact skin or mucous membranes.

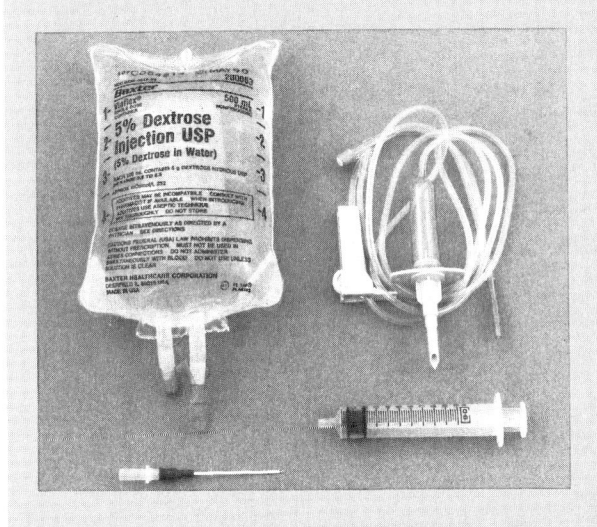

Activity 3. Primary equipment.

4. Position the patient	Place patient in Trendelenburg's position at 15° with head turned to the opposite side of the procedure site. The right internal jugular vein is preferred.	Trendelenburg's position helps distend the internal jugular vein, and turning the head allows easier access to the area. The right internal jugular vein is usually chosen since the right lung is lower than the left, and this route does not endanger the thoracic duct.
5. Find landmarks for venipuncture	Locate the triangle formed by the sternal and clavicular heads of the sternocleidomastoid muscle.	The internal jugular is located deep to the triangle.

(continued)

SKILL 12–7.
CENTRAL LINE PLACEMENT (INTERNAL JUGULAR, MIDDLE APPROACH) (continued)

ACTIVITY	HOW PERFORMED	WHY PERFORMED
6. Prepare the selected site	Cleanse the selected venipuncture site with antiseptic swabs (Activity 6).	Preparing the site reduces the possibility of infection at the venipuncture site.

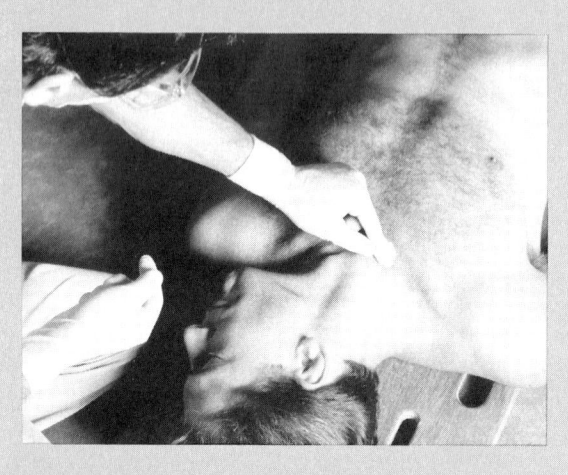

Activity 6.
Prepare the injection site.

7. Perform the venipuncture	Insert the needle in the triangle formed by the two heads of the sternocleidomastoid muscle (Activity 7). Direct the needle toward the patient's feet and somewhat lateral at a 45° to 60°-angle in the frontal plane, toward the ipsilateral nipple.	Insertion at this angle directs the needle into the internal jugular vein.
	Aspirate the syringe as the needle is inserted. When blood appears in the syringe, thread the catheter into the vein.	Blood in the syringe indicates the vein has been entered.

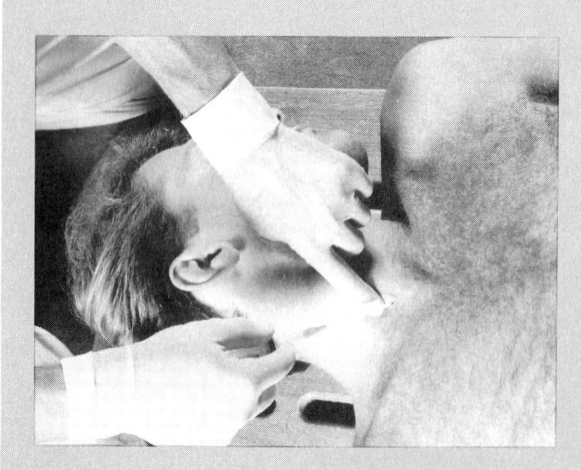

Activity 7.
Perform the venipuncture.

8. Start fluid flow	Holding the catheter in place, quickly withdraw the needle and attach the IV tubing to the catheter hub. Open the IV flow clamps and observe the drip chamber for free fluid flow.	The position of the vein does not allow pressure to reduce leaking of blood when the needle is withdrawn.

(continued)

SKILL 12–7.
CENTRAL LINE PLACEMENT (INTERNAL JUGULAR, MIDDLE APPROACH) (continued)

ACTIVITY	HOW PERFORMED	WHY PERFORMED
	If fluid does not flow or if signs of infiltration are seen, withdraw the catheter and hold firm pressure on the puncture site.	*Absence of fluid flow or evidence of infiltration indicates misplacement of the catheter. Direct pressure is necessary to control any bleeding.*
9. Adjust flow rate	Adjust the clamp on the IV tubing until the number of drops per minute seen in the IV drip chamber matches the appropriate orders or protocols.	IV fluid flow must be carefully controlled to achieve the optimum benefit for the patient and avoid potential detrimental effects.
10. Secure the catheter	Place sterile gauze squares or commercial IV dressing over the venipuncture site and secure the tubing with tape (Activity 10).	Dressings protect the venipuncture site from contamination, and the tape prevents accidental dislodging of the catheter during patient handling or other procedures.
11. Dispose of needle	Place contaminated needle in proper container.	Eliminates the possibility of injury or infection by contact with the contaminated needle.

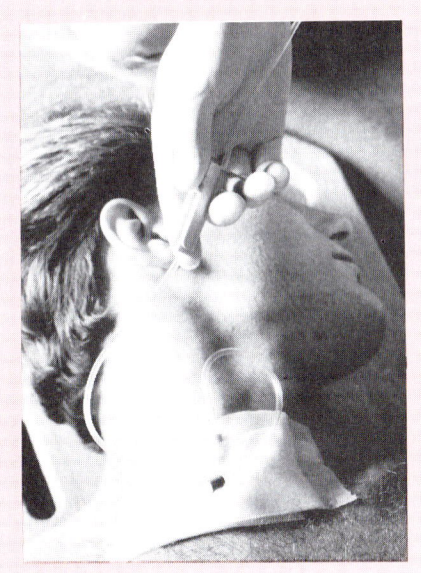

Activity 10.
Secure the catheter.

---

can be established. The marrow of virtually any bone in the body may be used for an intraosseous infusion.

The preferred site for children is the anterior proximal tibia at a point 1 or 2 finger-widths distal to the tibial tuberosity. This site is easily found, is stable, and does not interfere with other acute care of the patient. The bone marrow cavity in the child's proximal tibia is large enough to be easily entered and can accept a flow and volume of fluid comparable to a large peripheral vein. The preferred site for adults is the distal portion of the anterior tibia at a point 1 or 2 finger-widths proximal to the medial malleolus.

An additional advantage to the intraosseous route is that the bone protects the marrow cavity from outside pressure, such as the pressure from pneumatic anti-shock garments, which may restrict flow through a peripheral vein. The rigid needle, however, is left in place after insertion into the bone. The resulting portion of the needle that is sticking firmly out from the patient's leg may be an obstruction to the application of the pneumatic antishock garment.

The direct and rapid access to the peripheral circulation through an intraosseous route allows the administra-

(text continues on page 251)

SKILL 12-8.
CENTRAL LINE PLACEMENT
(INTERNAL JUGULAR, POSTERIOR APPROACH)

ACTIVITY	HOW PERFORMED	WHY PERFORMED
1. Check: • Responsiveness • Airway • Breathing • Circulation	Establish responsiveness Stabilize neck, open the airway Assess breathing Check for a pulse Check for hemorrhage	The primary survey is a rapid evaluation, less than 45 seconds, to identify and correct any life-threatening problems.
2. Assess need for central line	Compare patient's presenting signs and symptoms with local orders or protocols to determine if procedure is indicated and appropriate.	Procedure must only be performed when indicated and appropriate according to local orders or protocols.
3. Assemble and check: Primary equipment (Activity 3): • Intravenous (IV) solution • IV tubing and administration set • 16-gauge catheter • 10-mL syringe Accessory equipment and supplies: • Antiseptic swabs • Sterile gauze squares • Tape • Protective eye wear • Mask • Gloves	Select IV fluid and check for expiration date, contamination, cloudiness, and seal leakage. Connect infusion set to IV fluid bag. Select intravenous catheter and tear tape, and prepare dressing. Open control valve and bleed air from the line. Fill drip chamber half full. Have all items placed within easy reach. Prepare 16-gauge catheter with a 10-mL syringe on the end of the catheter. Put on protective eye wear, mask, and gloves.	Having all equipment ready reduces time delays during the procedure and minimizes patient discomfort. To prevent blood or body fluid contact with nonintact skin or mucous membranes.

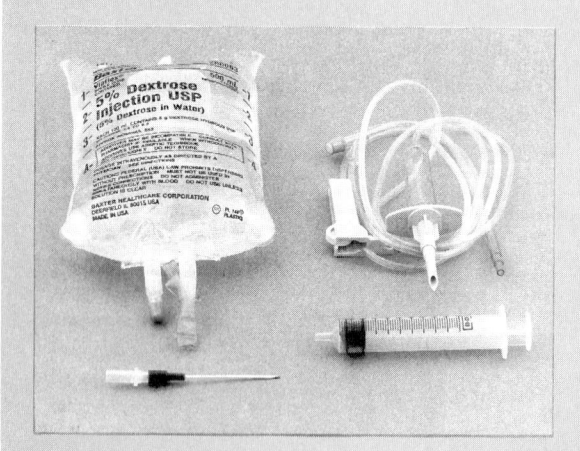

Activity 3.
Primary equipment.

4. Position the patient	Place patient in Trendelenburg's position at 15° with head turned to the opposite side of the procedure site (Activity 4). The right internal jugular vein is preferred.	Trendelenburg's position helps distend the internal jugular vein, and turning the head allows easier access to the area. The right internal jugular vein is usually chosen since the right lung is lower than the left, and this route does not endanger the thoracic duct.

(continued)

SKILL 12–8.
CENTRAL LINE PLACEMENT
(INTERNAL JUGULAR, POSTERIOR APPROACH) (continued)

ACTIVITY	HOW PERFORMED	WHY PERFORMED
	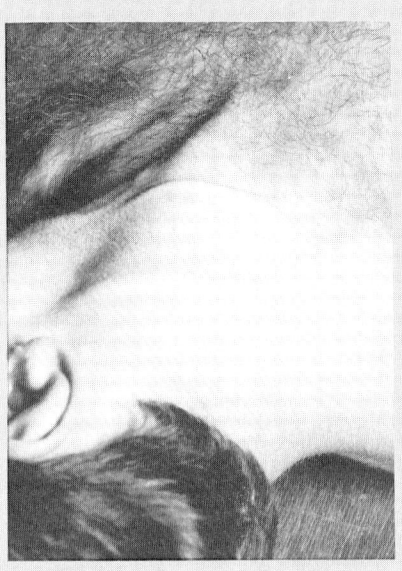 **Activity 4.** Position the patient.	
5. Find landmarks for venipuncture	Locate the midpoint of the posterior border of the sternocleidomastoid muscle. This point is just above where the external jugular vein crosses the sternocleidomastoid muscle (Activity 5).	The internal jugular vein is located deep to this point.
	Activity 5. Find landmarks for venipuncture.	

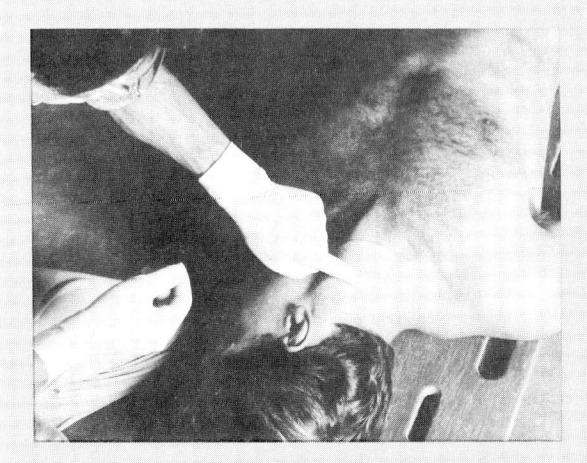

(continued)

SKILL 12-8.
CENTRAL LINE PLACEMENT
(INTERNAL JUGULAR, POSTERIOR APPROACH) (continued)

ACTIVITY	HOW PERFORMED	WHY PERFORMED
6. Prepare the selected site	Cleanse the selected venipuncture site with antiseptic swabs (Activity 6).	Preparing the site reduces the possibility of infection at the venipuncture site.

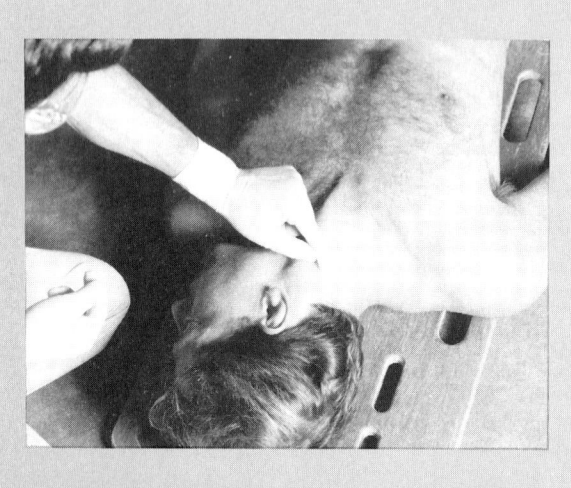

Activity 6.
Prepare the selected site.

7. Perform the venipuncture	Insert the needle under the posterior border of the sternocleidomastoid muscle, directed toward the sternal notch at an angle of 45° from horizontal (Activity 7). Aspirate the syringe as the needle is inserted.	Insertion at this angle directs the needle into the internal jugular vein.
	When blood appears in the syringe, thread the catheter into the vein.	Blood in the syringe indicates the vein has been entered.

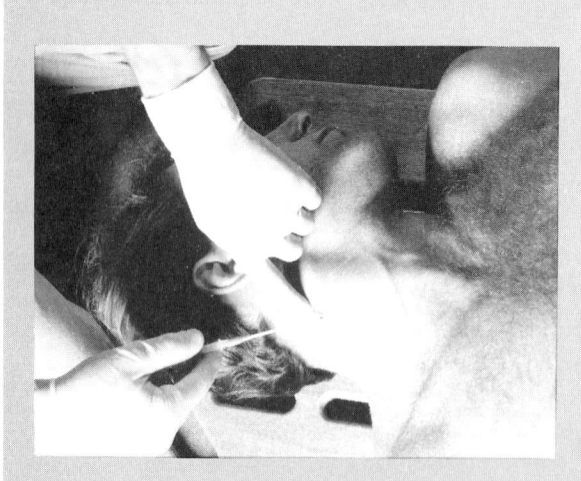

Activity 7.
Perform venipuncture.

8. Start fluid flow	Holding the catheter in place, quickly withdraw the needle and attach the IV tubing to the catheter hub. Open the IV flow clamps and observe the drip chamber for free fluid flow.	The position of the vein does not allow pressure to reduce leaking of blood when the needle is withdrawn.

(continued)

SKILL 12–8.
CENTRAL LINE PLACEMENT
(INTERNAL JUGULAR, POSTERIOR APPROACH) (continued)

ACTIVITY	HOW PERFORMED	WHY PERFORMED
	If fluid does not flow or if signs of infiltration are seen, withdraw the catheter and hold firm pressure on the puncture site.	*Absence of fluid flow or evidence of infiltration indicates misplacement of the catheter. Direct pressure is necessary to control any bleeding.*
9. Adjust flow rate	Adjust the clamp on the IV tubing until the number of drops per minute seen in the IV drip chamber matches the appropriate orders or protocols.	IV fluid flow must be carefully controlled to achieve the optimum benefit for the patient and avoid potential detrimental effects.
10. Secure catheter	Place sterile gauze squares or commercial IV dressing over the venipuncture site and secure the tubing with tape (Activity 10).	Dressings protect the venipuncture site from contamination, and the tape prevents accidental dislodging of the catheter during patient handling or other procedures.
11. Dispose of needle	Place contaminated needle in proper container.	Eliminates the possibility of injury or infection by contact with the contaminated needle.

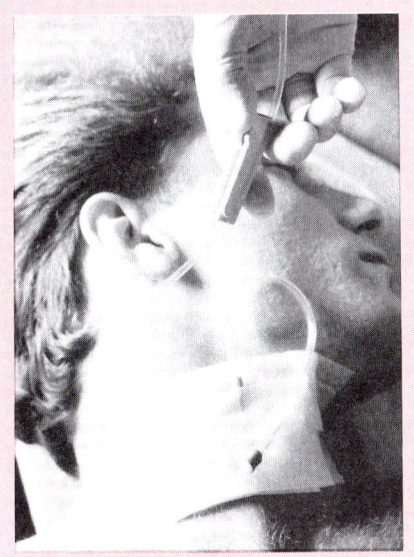

Activity 10.
Secure the catheter.

---

tion of virtually any fluid or medication that can be given through a peripheral IV site. The rate of fluid flow and rate of medication absorption through an intraosseous route is nearly identical to a peripheral IV. Blood samples for type and crossmatch may be drawn through the intraosseous route, but samples should not be used for white and red blood cell counts because of the intermixing of blood and marrow.

Indications for intraosseous infusion may include the following:

- Cardiac arrest
- Shock
- Extensive burns
- Massive trauma

Potential complications associated with intraosseous infusion may include the following:

- Leakage of blood and fluid into surrounding subcutaneous tissue
- Damage to the epiphyseal (*growth*) plate in the proximal tibia
- Misplacement of the needle, including insertion of the needle completely through the bone instead of into the marrow cavity

(text continues on page 255)

SKILL 12-9.
CENTRAL LINE PLACEMENT (SUBCLAVIAN APPROACH)

ACTIVITY	HOW PERFORMED	WHY PERFORMED
1. Check: • Responsiveness • Airway • Breathing • Circulation	Establish responsiveness Stabilize neck, open the airway Assess breathing Check for a pulse Check for hemorrhage	The primary survey is a rapid evaluation, less than 45 seconds, to identify and correct any life-threatening problems.
2. Assess need for central line	Compare patient's presenting signs and symptoms with local orders or protocols to determine if procedure is indicated and appropriate.	Procedure must only be performed when indicated and appropriate according to local orders or protocols.
3. Assemble and check: Primary equipment (Activity 3): • Intravenous (IV) solution • IV tubing and administration set • 16-gauge catheter • 10-mL syringe Accessory equipment and supplies: • Antiseptic swabs • Sterile gauze squares • Tape • Protective eye wear • Mask • Gloves	Select IV fluid and check for expiration date, contamination, cloudiness, and seal leakage. Connect infusion set to IV fluid bag. Select intravenous catheter and tear tape, and prepare dressing. Open control valve and bleed air from the line. Fill drip chamber half full. Have all items placed within easy reach. Prepare 16-gauge catheter with a 10-mL syringe on the end of the catheter. Put on protective eye wear, mask, and gloves.	Having all equipment ready reduces time delays during the procedure and minimizes patient discomfort. To prevent blood or body fluid contact with nonintact skin or mucous membranes.

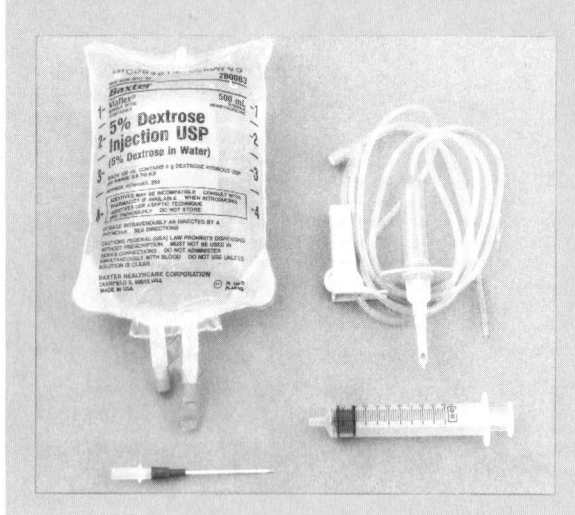

Activity 3.
Primary equipment.

4. Position the patient	Place patient in Trendelenburg's position at 15° with head turned to the opposite side of the procedure site.	Trendelenburg's position helps distend the internal jugular vein, and turning the head allows easier access to the area.

(continued)

SKILL 12-9.
CENTRAL LINE PLACEMENT (SUBCLAVIAN APPROACH) (continued)

ACTIVITY	HOW PERFORMED	WHY PERFORMED
5. Find landmarks for venipuncture	Locate the intersection of the middle and medial thirds of the clavicle (Activity 5).	The subclavian vein lies deep to this point.

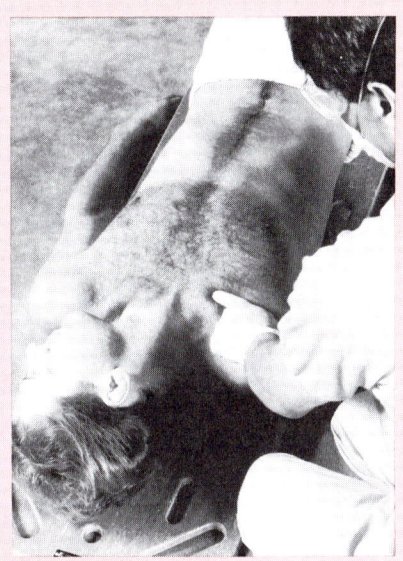

Activity 5.
Find landmarks for venipuncture.

6. Prepare the selected site	Cleanse the selected venipuncture site with antiseptic swabs (Activity 6).	Preparing the site reduces the possibility of infection at the venipuncture site.

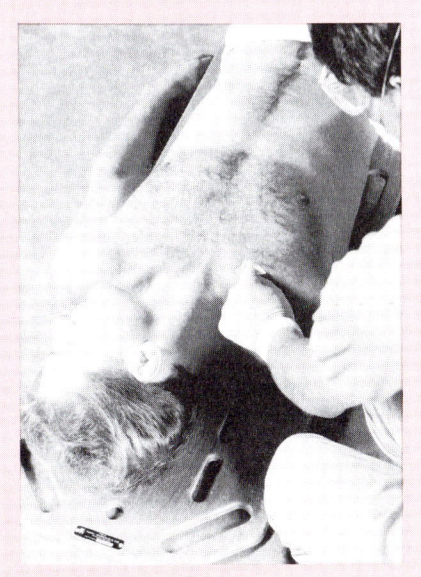

Activity 6.
Prepare the selected site.

(continued)

254 UNIT TWO: FOUNDATIONS OF EMERGENCY CARE

SKILL 12-9.
CENTRAL LINE PLACEMENT (SUBCLAVIAN APPROACH) (continued)

ACTIVITY	HOW PERFORMED	WHY PERFORMED
7. Perform the venipuncture	Insert the needle until it contacts the superior edge of the clavicle (Activity 7A). Lower the needle tip below the clavicle and direct the needle toward the sternal notch, while keeping the needle parallel to the floor (Activity 7B). Aspirate the syringe as the needle is inserted.	Insertion at this angle directs the needle into the subclavian vein.
	When blood appears in the syringe, thread the catheter into the vein.	Blood in the syringe indicates the vein has been entered.
	If no blood return is obtained or if resistance is met, redirect the needle toward the patient's opposite shoulder. *Do not, at any time, direct the needle toward the patient's feet.*	*The close proximity of the lung to the clavicle requires that the needle never be directed toward the patient's feet because a pneumothorax may be induced.*

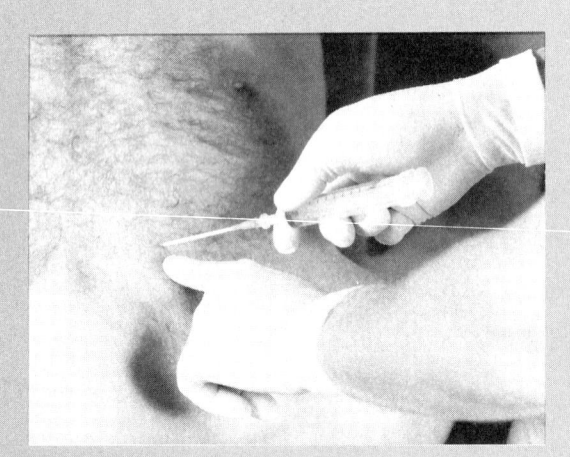

Activity 7A.
Perform venipuncture—insert needle.

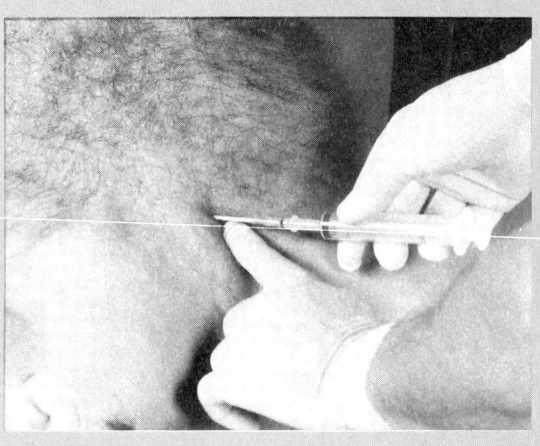

Activity 7B.
Perform venipuncture—lower needle tip.

8. Start fluid flow	Holding the catheter in place, quickly withdraw the needle and attach the IV tubing to the catheter hub.	The position of the vein does not allow pressure to reduce leaking of blood when the needle is withdrawn.
	Open the IV flow clamps and observe the drip chamber for free fluid flow.	
	If fluid does not flow or if signs of infiltration are seen, withdraw the catheter and hold firm pressure on the puncture site.	*Absence of fluid flow or evidence of infiltration indicates misplacement of the catheter. Direct pressure is necessary to control any bleeding.*
9. Adjust flow rate	Adjust the clamp on the IV tubing until the number of drops per minute seen in the IV drip chamber matches the appropriate orders or protocols.	IV fluid flow must be carefully controlled to achieve the optimum benefit for the patient and avoid potential detrimental effects.

(continued)

SKILL 12-9.
CENTRAL LINE PLACEMENT (SUBCLAVIAN APPROACH) (continued)

ACTIVITY	HOW PERFORMED	WHY PERFORMED
10. Secure catheter	Place sterile gauze squares or commercial IV dressing over the venipuncture site and secure the tubing with tape (Activity 10).	Dressings protect the venipuncture site from contamination, and the tape prevents accidental dislodging of the catheter during patient handling or other procedures.
11. Dispose of needle	Place contaminated needle in proper container.	Eliminates the possibility of injury or infection by contact with the contaminated needle.

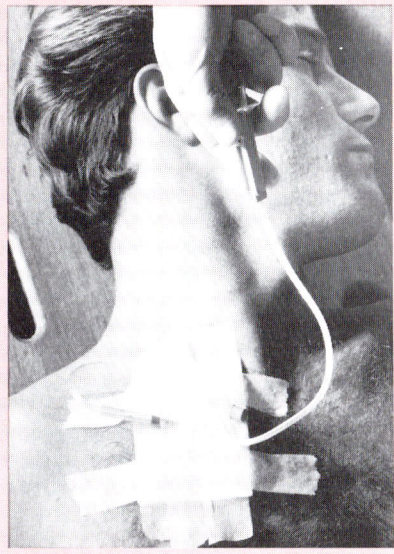

Activity 10. Secure the catheter.

- Obstruction of the application of a portion of the pneumatic anti-shock garment by the intraosseous needle
- Damage to or displacement of the intraosseous needle during patient handling and transport

Conditions may present relative contraindications to intraosseous infusion, such as the following:

- Recently fractured tibia
- *Osteogenesis imperfecta* (a congenital bone disease that makes bones fragile)
- *Osteoporosis* (loss of calcification of bones that may lead to spontaneous fractures)

Equipment for performing an intraosseous infusion must include either a rigid spinal needle with a trocar (*stylet*) strong enough to penetrate the bone or a specialized intraosseous needle, which may also include a plastic disc or other device to help secure the needle in place. An 18-gauge needle is used for children younger than 4 years of age. A 16-gauge needle is used for adults and children older than 4 years of age. Both types of needle must have a stylet of some sort to prevent clogging of the needle with bone fragments or other tissue during insertion. The procedure for intraosseous infusion is shown in Skill 12-10.

Sublingual

In rare situations when IV access is impossible, 1:1,000 epinephrine can be injected under the tongue (sublingual). The tongue is lifted and 0.5 to 1.0 mg of 1:1,000 epinephrine is injected sublingually with a subcutaneous needle. This area is highly vascular, and absorption is faster than peripheral IM or subcutaneous injection. Care must be taken to aspirate the syringe to prevent IV or intra-arterial injection of the drug.

Endotracheal

When IV access is impossible or must be delayed, some drugs can be given via the endotracheal tube. The pul-

(text continues on page 259)

SKILL 12–10.
INTRAOSSEOUS INFUSION

ACTIVITY	HOW PERFORMED	WHY PERFORMED
1. Check: • Responsiveness • Airway • Breathing • Circulation	Establish responsiveness Stabilize neck, open the airway Assess breathing Check for a pulse Check for hemorrhage	The primary survey is a rapid evaluation, less than 45 seconds, to identify and correct any life-threatening problems.
2. Assess need for intraosseous infusion	Compare patient's presenting signs and symptoms with local orders or protocols to determine if procedure is indicated and appropriate.	Procedure must only be performed when indicated and appropriate according to local orders or protocols.
3. Assemble and check: Primary equipment (Activity 3): • Intravenous (IV) solution • IV tubing and administration set • Rigid spinal needle with stylet or intraosseous needle • 10-mL syringe filled with sterile saline Accessory equipment and supplies: • Antiseptic swabs • Tape • Sterile gauze squares • Protective eye wear • Mask • Gloves	Select IV fluid and check for expiration date, contamination, cloudiness, and seal leakage. Connect infusion set to IV fluid bag. Select intravenous catheter and tear tape, and prepare dressing. Open control valve and bleed air from the line. Fill drip chamber half full. Have all items placed within easy reach. Put on protective eye wear, mask, and gloves.	Having all equipment ready reduces time delays during the procedure and minimizes patient discomfort. To prevent blood or body fluid contact with nonintact skin or mucous membranes.

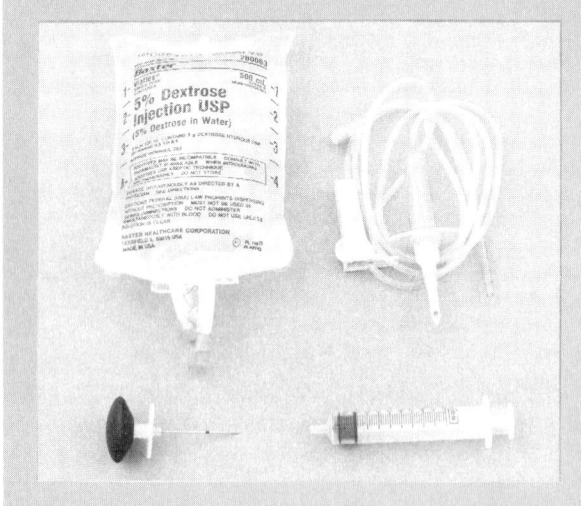

Activity 3.
Primary equipment.

4. Position the patient	Externally rotate the leg to expose the medial aspect of the leg.	Externally rotating the patient's leg allows better access to the puncture site.
5. Find landmarks for needle insertion and prepare the site	For a child, palpate the proximal tibia to find the tibial tuberosity. Locate a point on the flat aspect of the tibia 1 to 2 finger-widths distal to the tibial tuberosity (Activity 5A).	The child's proximal tibia has a larger marrow cavity, which allows easier placement.

(continued)

SKILL 12–10.
INTRAOSSEOUS INFUSION (continued)

ACTIVITY	HOW PERFORMED	WHY PERFORMED
	For an adult, palpate the distal tibia to find the medial malleolus. Locate a point on the tibia 1 to 2 finger-widths proximal to the medial malleolus (Activity 5B).	The adult's distal tibia offers an easily found and relatively complication-free puncture site.
	Cleanse the site with antiseptic swabs.	Cleansing the site reduces the possibility of infection.

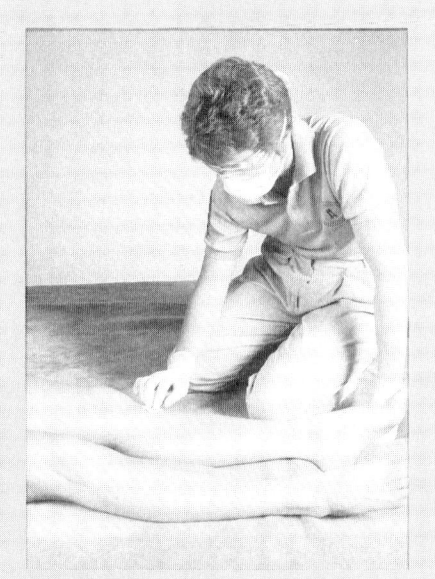

Activity 5A.
Child: Find landmarks for needle insertion; prepare site.

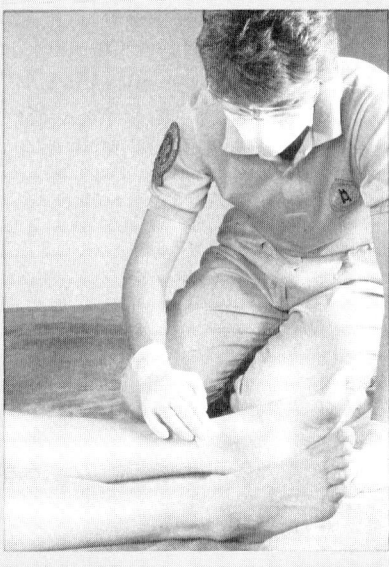

Activity 5B.
Adult: Find landmarks for needle insertion; prepare site.

6. Perform procedure

For a child, hold the needle at a right angle to the tibial plate and angle it toward the foot and away from the knee (Activity 6A).

Angling downward avoids damage to the epiphyseal growth plate.

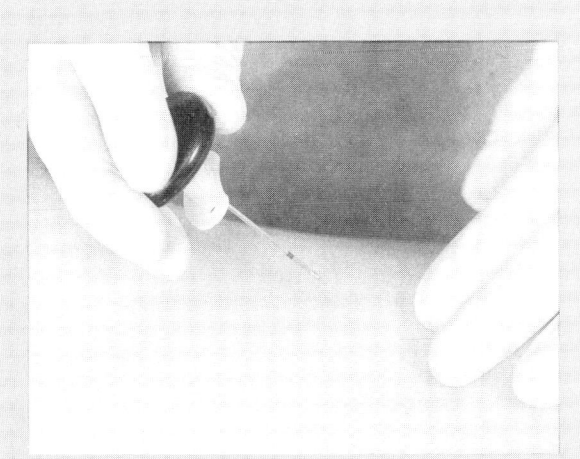

Activity 6A.
Child: Perform procedure.

(continued)

SKILL 12–10.
INTRAOSSEOUS INFUSION (continued)

ACTIVITY	HOW PERFORMED	WHY PERFORMED
	For an adult, hold the needle at a right angle to the tibial plate and angle it slightly toward the patient's head (Activity 6B). Insert the needle firmly through the skin and subcutaneous tissue first, then through the periosteum of the bone using a twisting motion, until a "pop" or "give" is felt. Do not advance the needle further.	Directing the needle slightly toward the adult patient's head avoids the ankle joint and places the needle in the largest portion of the marrow cavity. The sudden loss of resistance indicates entry into the marrow cavity. Only 2 mm to 4 mm insertion depth is needed in the child.
	Withdraw the stylet, attach the saline-filled syringe and aspirate a small amount of blood and marrow (Activity 6C).	Ability to aspirate a blood-marrow mixture verifies placement in the marrow cavity.

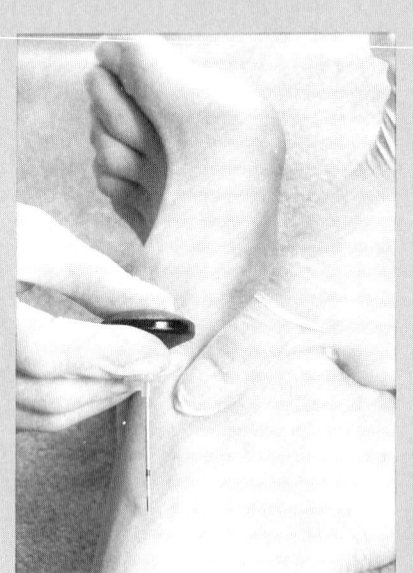

Activity 6B. Adult: Perform procedure.

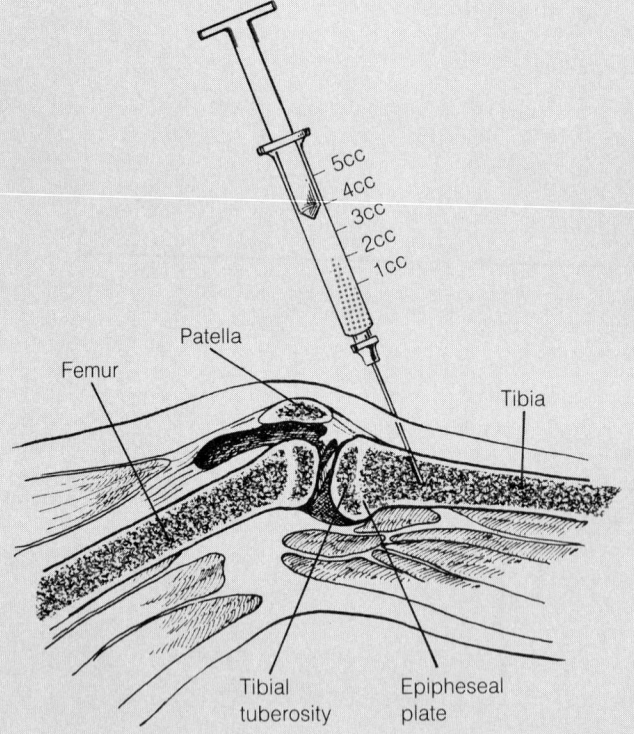

Activity 6C. Aspirate small amount of blood and marrow.

7. Start fluid flow	Remove the syringe and attach IV tubing. Open the IV flow clamps and observe the drip chamber for free fluid flow.	Free flow of fluid indicates an open line into the bone marrow.
8. Adjust flow rate	Adjust the clamp on the IV tubing until the number of drops per minute matches the appropriate orders or protocols.	IV fluid flow must be carefully controlled to achieve the optimum benefit for the patient and avoid potential detrimental effects.

(continued)

SKILL 12–10.
INTRAOSSEOUS INFUSION (continued)

ACTIVITY	HOW PERFORMED	WHY PERFORMED
9. Secure the needle	Secure the needle in place with a protective disc or other commercial device if present. Place sterile gauze squares around the needle and secure with tape (Activity 9A, Activity 9B).	Protective discs and dressings help hold the needle in place during patient handling and other procedures, as well as protect the site from contamination.

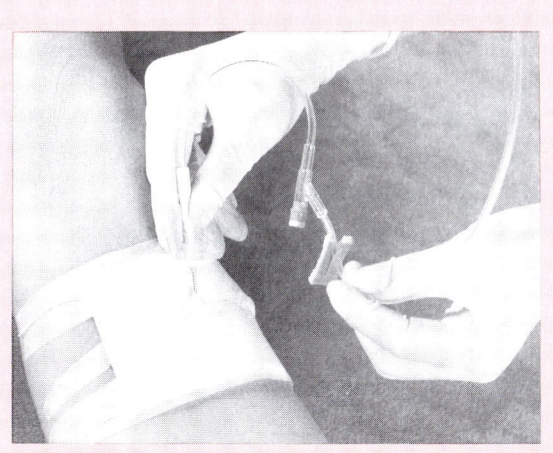

Activity 9A.
Child: Secure needle.

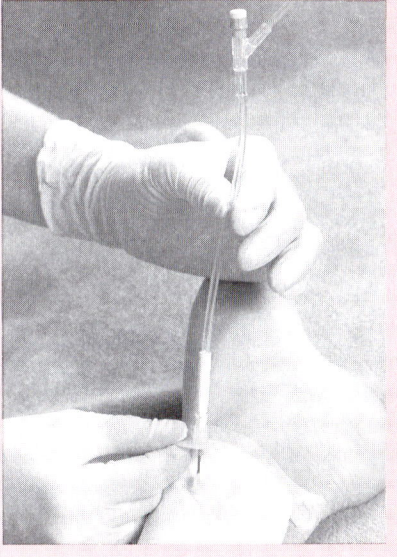

Activity 9B.
Adult: Secure needle.

10. Dispose of needle	Place contaminated needle in proper container.	Eliminates the possibility of injury or infection by contact with the contaminated needle.

---

monary tree is highly vascular and absorbs certain drugs well. To remember the drugs that can be given endotracheally, recall the helpful mnemonic "*NAVEL*," which stands for *N*arcan, *A*tropine, *V*alium, *E*pinephrine, and *L*idocaine.

Other drugs are poorly absorbed by the pulmonary tree or severely irritate the tissue and may not be given by this route.

To administer a drug by the endotracheal route, take the following steps:

1. Draw up the drug in the correct dose and concentration.
2. Remove the needle from the syringe if the needle is separate from the syringe. Needles may be inadvertently squirted into the bronchial tree.
3. Stop cardiopulmonary resuscitation if it is in progress, remove the ventilation device from the tube, and inject the desired dosage of drug down the endotracheal tube.
4. Ventilate the patient several times before starting compressions. This action pushes the drug into the bronchial tree and prevents reflux back to the tube and ventilation device.
5. Resume cardiopulmonary resuscitation.

SUMMARY

The knowledge of pharmacology is not limited to knowing *how* to administer drugs but includes understanding *why* a drug is given for a particular problem. Therefore, basic concepts of physiology and pathophysiology are critical. These concepts have been presented in this chapter and are built on throughout the text.

With the ability to administer medications, the paramedic acquires tremendous potential for positively affecting a patient's outcome. An accurate dosage of the appropriate drug, administered at a precise rate by the correct route, can relieve pain, terminate lethal arrhythmia, or ease dyspnea. However, if the paramedic's knowledge of that drug is incomplete, the patient may suffer disastrous consequences. Death may result from administering the wrong drug, from giving it too rapidly or too slowly or by the wrong route, by giving too much or too little drug, or from not anticipating adverse drug reactions.

In addition to the drugs carried in the ambulance, the paramedic must be familiar with common home medications to recognize possible adverse reactions, prevent potential drug interactions, and deduce information regarding a patient's medical history. Because new drugs are constantly placed on the market, maintaining current knowledge is an ongoing challenge for the paramedic. Appendix D describes individual drugs most commonly encountered in the field. Appendix E lists common home medications.

SUGGESTED READING

American Hospital Formulary Service: Drug Information 1991. Bethesda, American Society of Hospital Pharmacy, 1991

Baer CL, Williams BR: Clinical Pharmacology and Nursing. Springhouse, PA, Springhouse Publishing Co, 1988

Bledsoe BE, Bosker G, Papa FJ: Prehospital Emergency Pharmacology, 2nd ed. Englewood Cliffs, Prentice-Hall, 1988

Edmunds MW: Introduction to Clinical Pharmacology. St. Louis, Mosby Year Book, 1991

Gahart BL: Intravenous Medications, 7th ed. St. Louis, Mosby Year Book, 1990

Gilman AG, Goodman LS, Rall TW et al: The Pharmacological Basis of Therapeutics, 7th ed. New York, Macmillan, 1985

Krieger JN, Sherrard DJ: Practical Fluids and Electrolytes. Norwalk, Connecticut, Appleton and Lange, 1991

Physicians' Desk Reference, 45th ed. Oradell, Medical Economics, 1991

Scherer JC: Introductory Clinical Pharmacology, 3rd ed. Philadelphia, JB Lippincott, 1987

Scherer JC: Lippincott's Nurses' Drug Manual. Philadelphia, JB Lippincott, 1987

US Department of Transportation, National Highway Traffic Safety Administration: Emergency Medical Technician-Paramedic: National Standards Curriculum. Washington, DC, US Government Printing Office, 1985

UNIT THREE

Trauma

CHAPTER 13

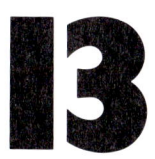

Kinematics of Trauma

Physics
    Conservation of Energy Law
    Newton's First Law of Motion
    Newton's Second Law of Motion
    Kinetic Energy
    Energy Exchange
        Density of Body Tissue
        Particle Motion
Penetrating Trauma
    Profile
    Tumble or Rotation
    Fragmentation
    Cavitation
    Energy
    Mechanism of Injury

Anatomical Considerations
    Head
    Neck
    Thorax
    Abdomen
    Extremities
Blunt Trauma
    Automotive Injuries
        Frontal Collisions
            Down and Under
            Up and Over
        Rear-end Collisions
        Lateral Collisions
        Rotational Collisions
        Rollover Collisions
    Pedestrian Injuries

Motorcycle Injuries
    Motorcycle Injury Patterns
        Head-on
        Angular
        Ejection
        Laying the Bike Down
Sports Injuries
Anatomical Considerations
    Head
    Neck
    Thorax
    Abdomen
    Extremities
Blast Injuries
    Light
    Heat
    Pressure
Summary

BEHAVIORAL OBJECTIVES

On successful completion of this chapter, the reader will be able to:

1. Explain the conservation of energy law, Newton's first law of motion, Newton's second law of motion, and kinetic energy
2. Explain the amount of energy exchange relative to density of body tissue and particle motion
3. Discuss mechanism of injury in an accident situation
4. Discuss the three factors that affect the frontal area of a penetrating object
5. Describe the anatomical considerations in penetrating trauma
6. List and describe five patterns of automobile collisions
7. Discuss energy exchange and injuries in pedestrian accidents
8. Discuss energy exchange and injuries in motorcycle collisions
9. Discuss energy exchange and injuries in sports injuries
10. Describe the anatomical considerations in blunt trauma
11. List and discuss the three forces of blast injuries
12. Define all of the key terms listed in this chapter

KEY TERMS

The following terms are defined in the chapter and glossary:

acceleration
blast
blunt trauma
braking distance
cavitation
Conservation of Energy law
deceleration
density
drag
elasticity
energy exchange
force
fragmentation
frontal collisions— down and under, up and over
kinematics
kinetic energy
lateral collisions
malleability
mass
mechanism of injury
momentum
Newton's first law of motion
Newton's second law of motion
O'Donohue's triad
penetrating trauma
permanent cavity
physics
pressure waves
profile
pseudoaneurysm
reaction distance
rear-end collisions
rollover collisions
rotational collision
stopping distance
stretch
temporary cavity
velocity
whiplash

The accuracy of scene assessment and management of a trauma victim is enhanced when the paramedic combines the knowledge of anatomy and physiology with kinematics of trauma. **Kinematics** of trauma is the science of motion that involves the transfer of energy from an external source to the victim's body.

On arrival at the accident scene, the astute paramedic surveys the scene, asks pertinent questions to reconstruct the events that caused the trauma, and uses this information in the physical assessment of the trauma victim. For example, in an automobile collision, the paramedic should quickly look at the damage to the car. If it is damaged extensively, the occupants are most likely injured. What type of collision was it, rear end or frontal? Can approximate speed be estimated? Were the occupants wearing seat belts or were they ejected from the car? The paramedic should mentally picture the occupants of the car during the crash phase. What did the occupants impact to slow and stop their motion? What stopped their motion? What body parts were likely crushed, stretched, or lacerated during the collision? Asking the victims or bystanders "what happened?" provides additional information as to the kinematics of trauma involved in the crash.

The paramedic's sensitivity to the significance of the mechanism of injury increases the accuracy and completeness of the physical examination that is used to confirm suspicions derived from the accident history. The mechanism of injury may not totally identify all injuries. Such injuries should not be discounted simply because the mechanism does not seem correct. To obtain an accurate accident history, an understanding of the physical principles and pathologic conditions that occur during trauma is essential. Understanding the mechanism of injury reduces the potential for overlooked injuries and ensures that potentially devastating injuries will be identified early. In this chapter, selected principles of physics are explained and applied to the mechanism of injury and three types of trauma: penetrating, blunt, and blast.

PHYSICS

Physics is the study of space, time, and matter and their interaction with one another. When caring for the trauma victim, the paramedic must understand several laws of physics to obtain a precise history and correctly interpret the conditions of the incident. With this historical data, the patient's potential injuries can be predicted with moderate accuracy.

Conservation of Energy Law

The **Conservation of Energy law** states that energy can neither be created nor destroyed, but the form can be changed. Two examples explain this concept. One example is the braking of a rapidly moving vehicle. The energy of speed is converted to heat in the brake system. The vehicle comes to a halt over a distance of perhaps several hundred feet. A trail of rubber left behind as energy is dissipated by the friction between the tires and the asphalt. In this case, the energy of movement is exchanged for energy of

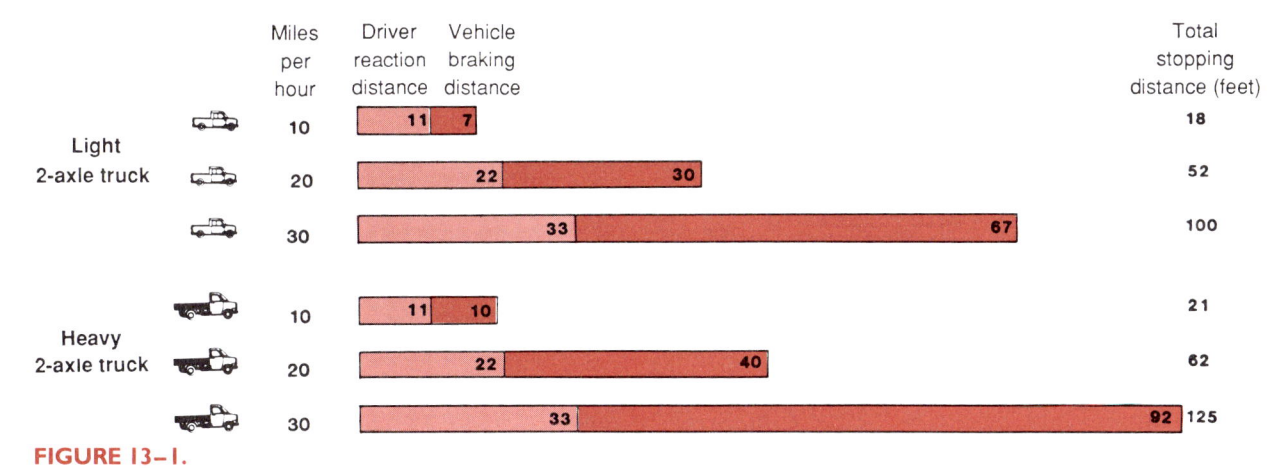

FIGURE 13-1.
Total stopping distances for light and heavy two-axle trucks traveling at various speeds. Total stopping distance is equal to driver reaction distance plus vehicle braking distance.

	Miles per hour	Driver reaction distance	Vehicle braking distance	Total stopping distance (feet)
Light 2-axle truck	10	11	7	18
	20	22	30	52
	30	33	67	100
Heavy 2-axle truck	10	11	10	21
	20	22	40	62
	30	33	92	125

heat and tire destruction. Figure 13-1 illustrates total stopping distances at various speeds for light and heavy two-axle trucks. Total **stopping distance** is equal to reaction distance plus braking distance. **Reaction distance** is the distance the vehicle travels from the time the driver recognizes the need to stop until brake pedal movement begins. **Braking distance** is where energy is exchanged and is the distance from the first brake pedal movement until the vehicle comes to a full stop. Both the speed of the vehicle and its mass affect the amount of energy to be exchanged.

Another example is a speeding car that suddenly strikes a brick wall. Because energy can neither be created nor destroyed, the energy of this forward motion must be absorbed. When the collision occurs, the front portion of the car stops its forward motion, but the rear of the car remains in motion. It is only after the front frame is bent and the body twisted that the rear portion of the car is halted. The amount of force is determined by the weight of the vehicle and the rate at which it slows.

Newton's First Law of Motion

Newton's first law of motion states that a body, whether in motion or at rest, remains in that state until acted on by an outside force. Newton's first law of motion applies in automobile collisions. A car remains in forward motion on the road surface until an outside force, such as the application of the brakes or collision with another car, halts its forward **momentum** (motion).

The same law of motion affects the occupants of the car. In car collisions, unrestrained drivers and passengers continue to move forward, backward, or sideward, depending on the motion of the vehicle. They remain in motion until their bodies collide with the dashboard, steering wheel, rear window, or other occupant. Colliding with any of these objects or persons stops their forward motion. Therefore, the outside force that restricts the forward motion of the occupants of colliding cars is the interior of the car or the other occupant.

Newton's Second Law of Motion

Newton's second law of motion states that the **force** of an object is equal to its **mass** (weight) multiplied by its **acceleration** (change in velocity), or:

F (force) = m (mass) × a (acceleration or deceleration)

Stated differently, an object m acted on by a total force F has an acceleration a in the direction of F. Examples are shown in Figure 13-2.

Obviously, a speeding semi-truck has more force than a car traveling 10 mph. Because the mass or weight and the acceleration or speed of the truck are greater, if the truck hits a telephone pole, the damage to the telephone pole, the truck, and the driver is more extensive than that of a car that is traveling at 10 mph. The force applied to a moving body to stop or reduce its motion is called **drag** or **deceleration**. Recall that acceleration is in the direction of F. Therefore, once the moving body stops or slows its motion, the degree of F is not as great. If, however, the truck suddenly is halted by a collision with a telephone pole, rapid deceleration or drag results in damage to the moving bodies, both the truck and the driver, and anything in the truck's path, in this case the telephone pole. The energy that results from the crash causes deformity of all the objects and persons involved.

Kinetic Energy

Kinetic energy is the energy of motion. The kinetic energy of a moving body is equal to one half of the mass

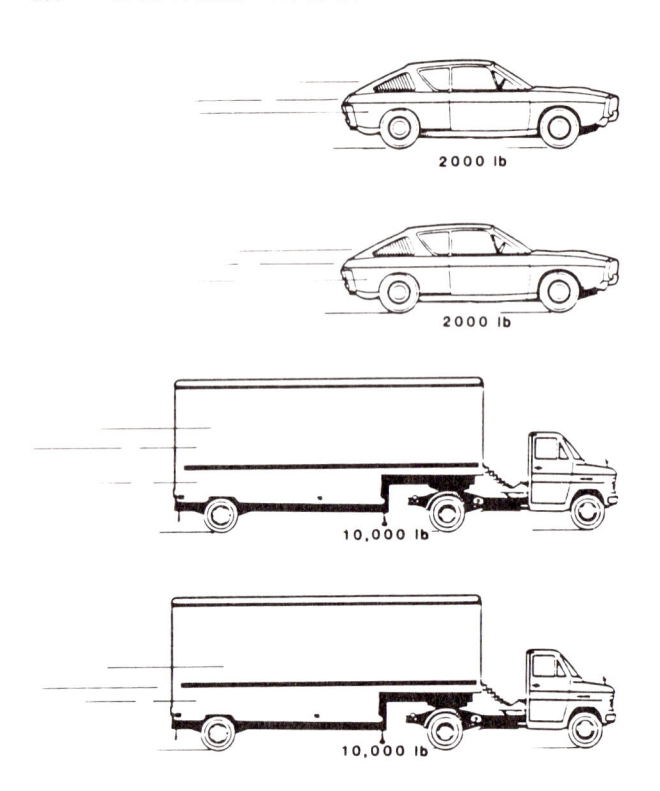

x 10mph = 20,000 units
2000 lb

x 30 mph = 60,000 units
2000 lb

x 10 mph = 100,000 units
10,000 lb

x 30 mph = 300,000 units
10,000 lb

FIGURE 13–2.
A 2000-lb car and 10,000-lb semi-truck are shown traveling at 10 mph and 30 mph. The total force of the vehicles is shown by mass times velocity and is given in units.

(weight) multiplied by the **velocity** (speed) squared. The formula is given as the following:

$$\text{kinetic energy} = \frac{m\ (\text{mass})}{2} \times v^2\ (\text{velocity})$$

For example, an 8000 lb parked truck has no kinetic energy.

$$\text{kinetic energy} = \frac{\text{mass (8000 lbs)}}{2} \times \text{velocity}^2\ (0\ \text{mph})$$

kinetic energy = 0 units of energy

For the purpose of this discussion, no specific physical unit is implied for kinetic energy. This method simply illustrates the change in force. While the parked truck has a potential force, the 8000-lb mass, only moving bodies have kinetic energy. In the determination of the amount of kinetic energy of a moving body, velocity is more significant than mass. While doubling the mass doubles the kinetic energy, doubling the velocity increases the kinetic energy fourfold. Therefore, when the mass is the same, a rapidly moving object has much more kinetic energy than a slowly moving object. To illustrate, compare the kinetic energy in a crash of an 8000-lb truck traveling 50 mph with that of the same weight truck traveling 25 mph.

50 mph crash	25 mph crash
$\dfrac{8000\ \text{lb}}{2} \times 50\ \text{mph}^2$	$\dfrac{8000\ \text{lb}}{2} \times 25\ \text{mph}^2$
kinetic energy =	
10,000,000 units of energy	2,500,000 units of energy

The truck traveling at 50 mph has 10,000,000 units of kinetic energy, while the same truck traveling at 25 mph has 2,500,000 units of kinetic energy. Recall that the total amount of kinetic energy must be absorbed in the crash. Obviously, the 50-mph crash results in four times the damage to the persons and objects involved as does a collision at 25 mph. This example illustrates, dramatically, the importance of estimating the speed of vehicles involved in a crash to more accurately estimate the potential injury to the patients.

Energy Exchange

In the interaction between two bodies moving at different rates of speed, the two speeds attempt to equalize. The loss of velocity or energy by one body to the other is known as **energy exchange**. How fast this exchange occurs and the amount of damage produced to either of the bodies is dependent on the **density** (number of particles per volume) of the tissues involved and the area of contact between the two. Contrast holding one's hand out of the window of a moving car. With the hand turned with the thumb and index finger only into the flow of air, there is not much pressure forcing the hand backward. Change the position of the hand so that the flat of the hand is into the flow of air, and the force on the hand becomes much greater. This change is due to the increase in the frontal area facing the wind and an increase in the number of air molecules that strike the hand. This analogy demonstrates the two major factors of energy exchange: Density and frontal projection. The energy exchange that occurs is directly related to the collision between the particles of the two bodies.

CHAPTER 13: Kinematics of Trauma   267

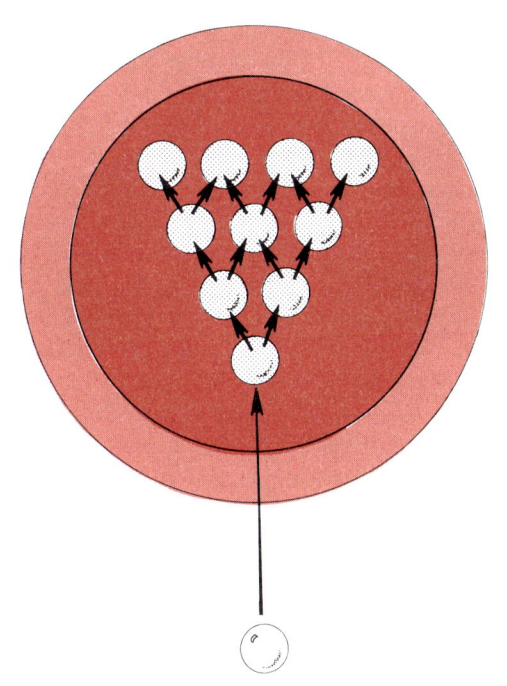

FIGURE 13–3.
Energy is dissipated by the cue ball when it hits a rack of balls.

FIGURE 13–5.
If hit directly, the pool ball travels in the same direction as the force exerted by the cue ball.

Density of Body Tissue

The density of the body tissue involved influences the amount of damage that results from a collision with a moving body. The game of pool provides a visible example of this concept. A cue ball that is rolling down a pool table loses no energy until it hits another ball. However, if the cue ball is directed into and hits a rack of balls, its energy is rapidly dissipated, causing the pool balls, previously motionless, to roll around the table (Fig. 13-3). In contrast, if the cue ball hits only one or two balls, it loses less of its energy (Fig. 13-4). The situation in the human body is similar: organs and tissues in close proximity stand a greater chance of being damaged in any type of trauma. Also, a moving object meets little resistance moving through hollow organs, such as the intestines, or through gaseous organs, such as the lungs. However, when the moving body encounters denser tissue, such as skin, muscle, or bone, an increased energy exchange occurs. If tissue as dense as bone is hit, extensive energy exchange causes the bone to fracture or shatter. The bone fragments become missiles themselves, increasing the potential for more extensive tissue damage to adjacent blood vessels, peripheral nerves, muscles, and ligaments.

Particle Motion

As the moving object hits body tissue, the tissues move away at an angle equal to the one by which they were hit. Tissue involved in **blunt trauma** moves in an anterior—posterior direction consistent with the angle of impact. In contrast, the tissue involved in **penetrating trauma** moves in a lateral direction away from the penetrating instrument. This motion away from the impacting object creates a cavity in the tissue.

Consider, again, the pool ball analogy. The pool ball hit directly by the cue ball moves in the direction that the cue ball was traveling (Fig. 13-5). The pool ball hit at an angle moves away from the cue ball at an opposite angle (Fig. 13-6). These motions are similar to the impact of a moving body on human tissue. This reaction is similar in human accident victims, in which each body tissue hit absorbs some of the energy from the original source until no more energy exists. When body tissues are displaced, a hole or cavity is created. The human body, when hit by objects with high energy, whether due to extensive mass or high velocity, sustains trauma at a distance from the impact point as the cavity expands. The cavity is at least

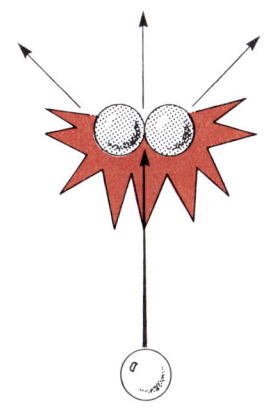

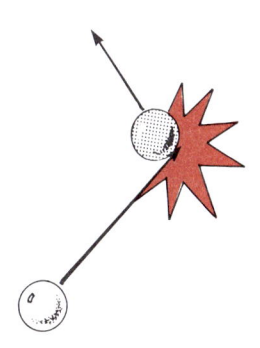

FIGURE 13–4.
Less energy is lost by the cue ball if it hits fewer pool balls.

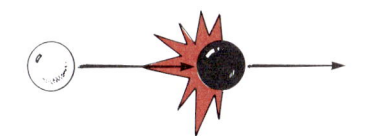

FIGURE 13–6.
When the pool ball is hit at an angle, it moves away in an opposite angle.

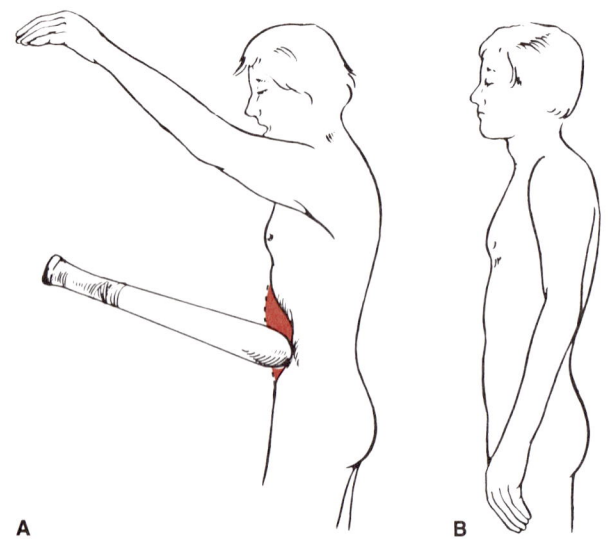

FIGURE 13-7.
(**A**) A temporary cavity is formed when the abdomen is struck by a baseball bat. (**B**) The abdominal wall returns to its original position because of the elasticity of the tissues. No permanent cavity is formed.

temporary and is possibly permanent. The size of the **permanent cavity** depends on the resiliency of the tissues or organs involved. For example, when the abdominal wall is hit with a baseball bat, the abdominal wall tissues are displaced posteriorly, away from the point of impact, producing a **temporary cavity** (Fig. 13-7). However, the resiliency of the muscular abdominal wall is such that shortly after impact it returns to its original position. In contrast, when the cranium is hit, it is likely to produce a depressed skull fracture. After a forceful blow to the head, cavitation that results from the fractured bones is visible. The cavity remains until definitive management is initiated (Fig. 13-8). Therefore, the extent of permanent damage depends on the **elasticity** of the damaged tissue. Consider the difference between hitting a hollow metal drum and a roll of foam rubber with the same baseball bat and the same energy. Although the energy exchange and the temporary cavity were the same, the permanent cavity is very different.

All penetrating objects leave a temporary cavity in their wake, as the body tissues move laterally away from the penetrating object (Fig. 13-9). The greater the size and velocity of the penetrating object, the greater the size of the temporary cavity or hole. For example, the bullet sizes of the .22 caliber and M 16 firearms are similar, yet the internal cavity and damage that result from them are considerably different. The wound caused by the M 16 is much more extensive. In this case, the velocity of the firearm makes the difference. As one would suspect, given the same type of tissue hit, a larger temporary cavity results in greater damage.

As with blunt trauma, the extent of trauma to the individual from penetrating injuries depends on the type and elasticity of the body tissue that is hit. For example, the tissue density of liver and muscle are similar. While the temporary cavity that results from a penetrating injury is similar, the permanent cavity in liver trauma is much more extensive and longer lasting. This difference lies in the fact that the physiologic elastic properties of muscles cause them to **stretch** and contract to their original at-rest position. In contrast, the liver contains little elastic tissue and tends to rupture. The result is that the extent of permanent liver damage approaches the size of the temporary cavity produced by the original injury.

PENETRATING TRAUMA

Several principles of physics learned in the beginning of this chapter deal with penetrating injuries. Kinetic energy is the energy that a striking object has based on

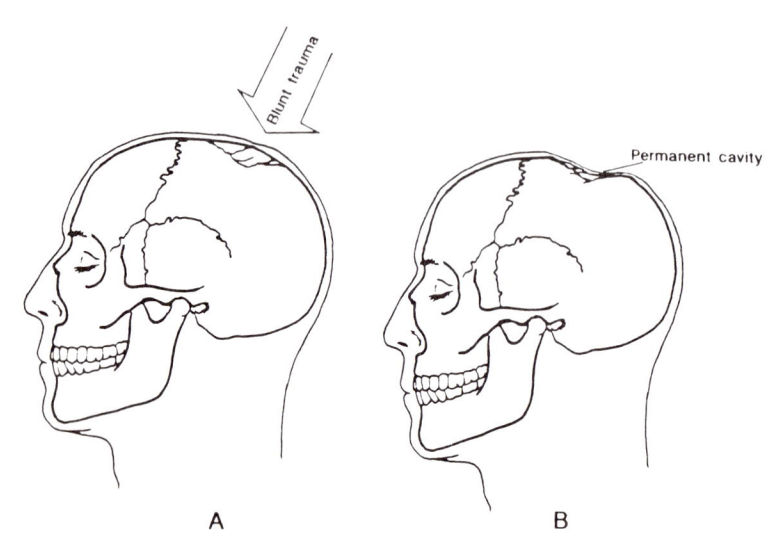

FIGURE 13-8.
(**A**) Blunt trauma to the head causes a depressed skull fracture. (**B**) A permanent cavity is formed.

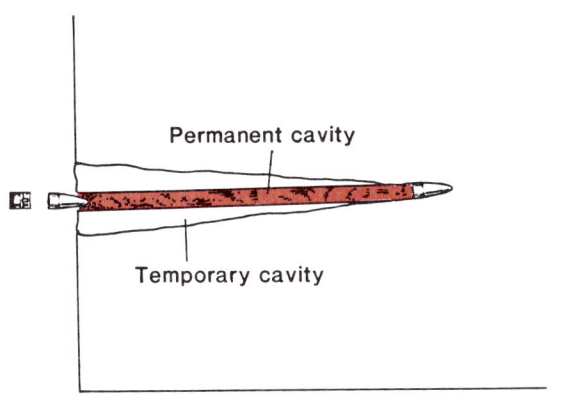

FIGURE 13-9.
Diagram of a bullet that is passing through human tissue shows how a temporary and permanent cavity are formed.

weight and velocity. It is important to remember that energy cannot be created or destroyed but can be changed in form. For example, a bullet has no force until the hammer of the gun hits the brass casing of the bullet. The powder contained in the brass casing explodes, forcing the nose of the bullet to move out of the gun. According to Newton's first law of motion, once the force has been applied to the bullet, the bullet remains at that energy level (speed) until it is acted on by an outside force. When, for instance, the bullet hits the human body, it impacts tissue. The speed and energy of the bullet are exchanged for the force that moves tissue away from the path of the bullet.

Three factors that affect the frontal area of the penetrating object are the following:

- The profile or size of the penetrating object
- The tumble or rotation of the missile
- Fragmentation of the missile

Profile

A narrow object, such as an ice pick, has a much smaller *profile*, or frontal area, than a wider object (baseball bat). One property of some projectiles that changes the profile is the **malleability** (the ability of the projectile object to change shape.) The hollow-point rifle bullet is an example of a projectile with such changeable frontal profile (Fig. 13-10). As the hollow-point bullet speeds through the air, impacting only a few particles, its frontal profile is altered little. As it impacts denser tissue, such as skin or bone, the frontal profile widens rapidly. The missile slows rapidly as its energy is exchanged with the tissue in its path.

Tumble or Rotation

A sharply pointed bullet contacts less body tissue than if the same bullet is rotated 90° after the initial thrust into the body. This rotation increases the amount of energy exchange dramatically, as more tissues are encountered, resulting in more extensive tissue damage. The cavity profile of a .22 long rifle shows this rotational effect (Fig. 13-11).

Fragmentation

A bullet that breaks into many small fragments on impact or one that fragments as it leaves the gun, such as a shotgun bullet, increases the frontal area significantly. Because the multiple fragments hit more body tissue, the energy exchange and resulting tissue damage extend to all tissues hit. While the energy exchange slows down the shotgun pellets, thereby diminishing their energy, the tissue damage occurs over a wider area of the body. When this **fragmentation** has resulted in total energy exchange, the pellets lack sufficient energy to exit the patient's body (Fig. 13-12). The effect is the same when a rifle or pistol bullet breaks into several parts.

Cavitation

The acceleration of tissue particles away from the pathway of the missile creates a cavity, or **cavitation,** away from the point of impact. The pool ball analogy demonstrates this situation well. The impacting object crushes the tissue ahead of it, and the surrounding tissue is stretched as the cavity expands. This cavitation produces tissue injury throughout the area.

Energy

As stated earlier, the kinetic energy of any moving object is determined to a large extent by its velocity. In a stab wound, the velocity of the instrument depends on the size and strength of the person thrusting it, but, nonethe-

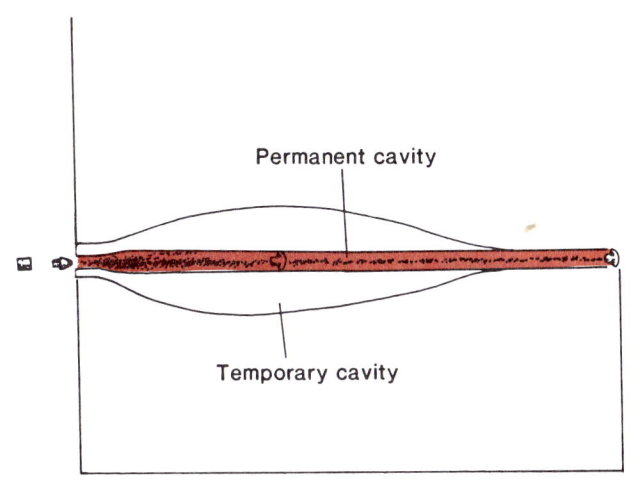

FIGURE 13-10.
Wound profile of a .22 long rifle rimfire bullet (lead hollow-point). This bullet deforms to the typical "mushroom" form of the expanding-type bullet.

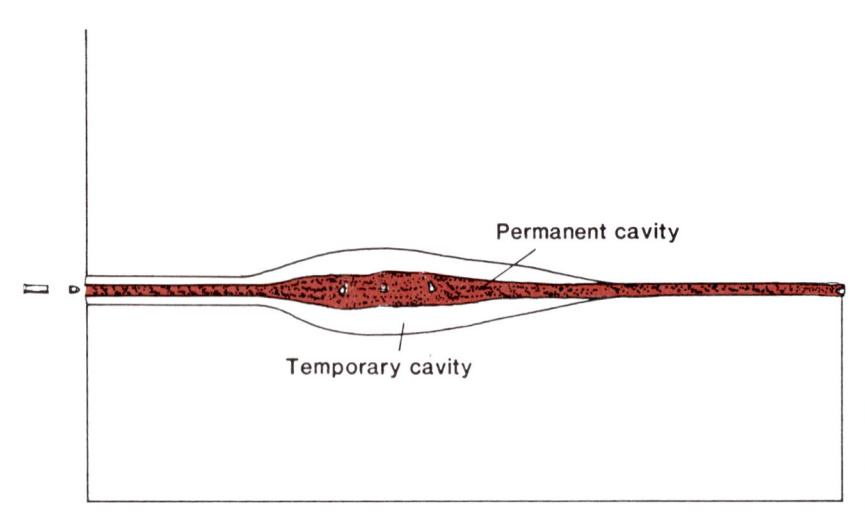

FIGURE 13–11.
Wound profile of a .22 long rifle rimfire solid-lead bullet. This bullet shows no deformity from passing through animal soft tissue.

less, it is low. Therefore, it is a low-energy penetration. Only a small temporary cavity is created. The injury produced is mainly from the sharp edges of the knife. However, in gunshot wounds, multiple variables affect the kinetic energy of the penetrating missile, including the type of gun, the length of the gun barrel, the distance between the perpetrator and the victim, and the muzzle velocity of the bullet. Penetrating injuries are divided into three energy categories: low, medium, and high. Table 13-1 differentiates these categories.

Some weapons, such as the .44 magnum with a 10-inch barrel and the .22 Hornet, are borderline between medium- and high-energy weapons. In general, low-energy missiles create a minimal temporary cavity and lacerate the body tissues that come in direct contact with the cutting surface of the instrument. Medium energy missiles create a temporary cavity that may be three to four times the size of the missile. In most instances, the permanent cavity that results from body penetration by a medium-energy missile is smaller than the diameter of the missile. In contrast, high-energy missiles create a cavity many times the diameter of the missile (Fig. 13-13). The size of the permanent cavity is proportional to the elasticity of the tissue hit. Recall that nonencapsulated tissue, such as striated muscle, is much more elastic than encapsulated organ tissue. Also, because the eye, brain, and spinal cord are more fragile than other body organs, penetrating trauma to these organs tends to result in larger permanent cavities.

Mechanism of Injury

The paramedic who arrives at the accident scene reconstructs the incident. The laws of physics previously discussed are applied to determine the **mechanism of injury**. This is prerequisite to accurate physical assessment

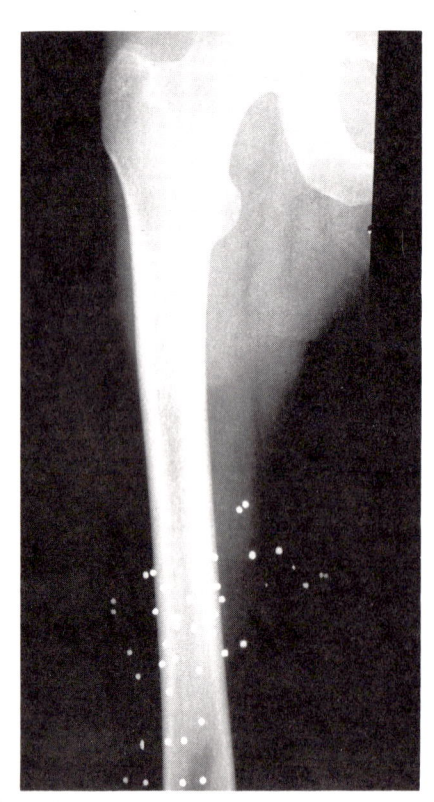

FIGURE 13–12.
Shotgun pellets are shown in the muscle that surrounds the femur.

TABLE 13–1.
ENERGY CATEGORIES FOR PENETRATING INJURIES

Energy Category	Examples
Low	Needle, ice pick, knife
Medium	Handgun, .22 rifle
High	Military and hunting rifles

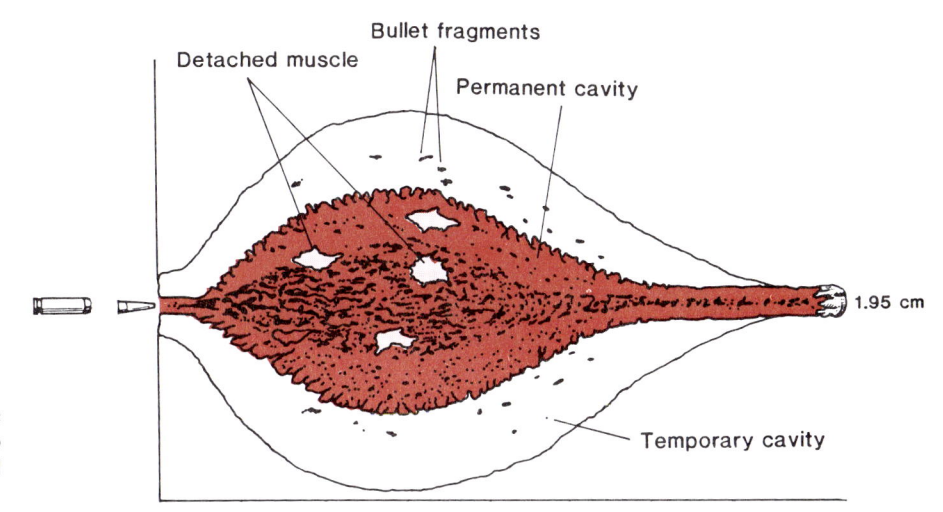

FIGURE 13-13.
Wound profile of a high-energy weapon. Note the difference in cavity size when compared to lower energy weapons in Figures 13-10 and 13-11.

of the patient. For example, recall that the occupants and the car involved in a collision are alike in their response. Recognizing the potential internal trauma to the occupants resulting from acceleration-deceleration motions at the time of the car collision, the paramedic considers the three crashes that have occurred: the car, the occupants, and the persons' internal tissues and organs.

After a quick survey of the damage to the car, it is essential to obtain a precise history of the incident (Fig. 13-14). Accurate estimation of the forces that caused the accident and the amount of energy that has been absorbed by the patient's body during a collision, combined with knowledge of anatomy, focuses the paramedic's initial physical examination of the patient. Valuable time is saved when the initial consideration of the paramedic is to determine the mechanism of injury. In addition, this determination provides essential information for subsequent care providers. Astute observation of the environment and focused questioning to reconstruct the accident can ensure accurate assessment, stabilization, and definitive care of the trauma patient.

Anatomical Considerations
Head

Penetration of the skull requires significant energy, which significantly reduces the speed and energy of the missile. However, if the missile lacks sufficient force to exit the skull opposite the entry site, it ricochets around the interior of the skull and rebounds into brain tissue until all of its energy is dissipated. Because of the closed structure of the skull, the missile's exchanged energy is absorbed by the brain. This *absorption* results in far more tissue destruction than if the missile had penetrated the more elastic tissue of the extremities or abdomen. Despite what appears to be a fatal injury, some patients incur penetrating skull injuries to areas of the brain that are not critical

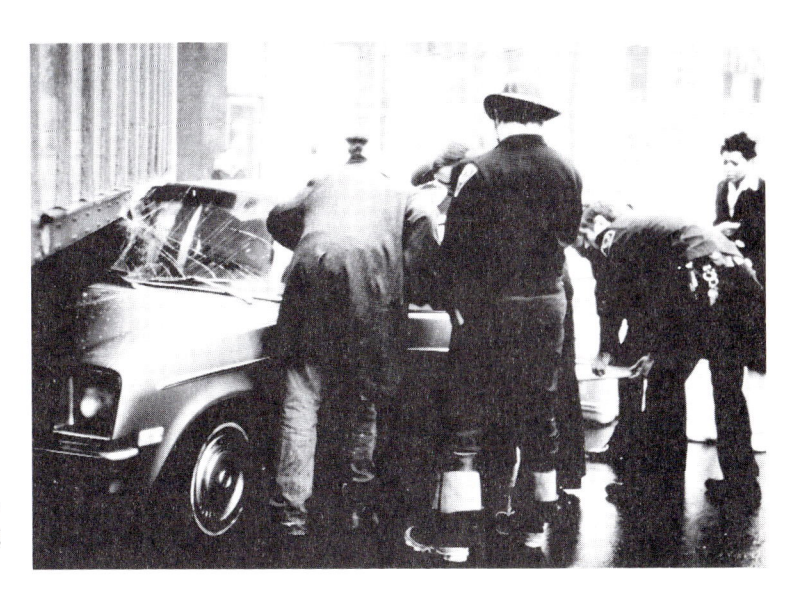

FIGURE 13-14.
Determining the mechanism of injury and the history of the accident are important factors in gathering information.

to the function of the brain and body. Therefore, patients with penetrating skull injuries should be carefully assessed and resuscitation measures initiated, in spite of the apparently fatal injury. As indicated previously both energy and anatomy are important factors in determining injury. Some portions of the brain are more critical to survival than others.

Neck

From an energy absorption standpoint, the neck contains six types of structures: muscle, esophagus, trachea, blood vessels, spinal cord, and vertebrae. Because of the proximity of these structures within a relatively small area, penetrating neck injuries can be devastating. Neck muscles respond to penetrating injuries in the same manner as muscles in the extremities, with initial cavitation and almost immediate return to their normal position. Esophageal injury is difficult to assess on site, as gastrointestinal leakage may not produce symptoms for 48 to 96 hours after injury. Tracheal trauma is substantiated by the presence of subcutaneous emphysema and the dyspneic condition of the patient. When blood vessels are penetrated, external or internal bleeding can be significant. A hematoma near the trachea may compress it to the point of airway compromise. Hematoma formation and vascular compression may be evidenced by weakening or loss of pulses distal to the injuries. However, some blood vessel injuries do not result in loss of pulses. These include compression of the intima of the vessel without complete disruption of blood flow, delayed thrombus formation at the site of injury, and formation of an arteriovenous fistula when both artery and vein are penetrated.

When the spinal cord is damaged by a penetrating injury, the result is an alteration in motor and sensory function below the level of the lesion.

Thorax

The thorax contains five types of tissue: muscle, bone, blood vessels, lungs, and heart. Initially, the intercostal muscles deviate laterally from the penetrating object and rebound to near their normal position. Bone fractures into smaller particles, which become penetrating missiles themselves. Because of the air content of the lungs, penetrating missiles travel through the lungs with minimal exchange of energy. A relatively small temporary and permanent cavity is created in the lung. The resultant hemorrhage and tissue damage (known as contusion) reduces the ventilatory capacity of the lung. When the heart is pierced, the bleeding may be contained in the pericardial sac. This condition, cardiac tamponade, requires immediate decompression. Penetration of the blood vessels produces hemorrhage. Because less protective tissue surrounds the blood vessels in the thorax, blood volume loss is generally great. Thus, hemothorax requires volume replacement. As described previously in neck trauma, penetration of blood vessels can also produce arteriovenous fistulas or alveolar-vascular fistulas. The alveolar-vascular fistula can produce an air embolus.

Abdomen

More than one half of the abdominal cavity is encased by or proximate to bony structures. The upper third of the abdomen is protected by the rib cage. The lower fourth of the abdomen is inside the pelvis. A small posterior portion is near the vertebral column. As in other parts of the body, bone fragments become missiles themselves. When the solid tissues of the abdomen, such as the liver and spleen, are penetrated, the temporary cavity created by the missile expands rapidly. Hemorrhage from these vascular organs can be extensive.

In contrast to the response of solid organs, the air- and fluid-filled organs of the abdomen respond to penetration much like the skin. A significant amount of the energy from the missile is absorbed at the entrance and exit sites but little energy exchange occurs in the air-filled center. The air-filled hollow structures of the abdomen include the colon, small bowel, and stomach. The fluid-filled hollow structures of the abdomen are the bladder, gallbladder, aorta, and other blood vessels. The potential expansion of the hollow abdominal structures depends on the density of the material within the cavity. Those with greater density, such as the gallbladder and blood vessels, absorb more energy from a penetrating object than the air-filled structures, such as the stomach or intestines. However, if the stomach is filled with food or the colon with feces, the energy exchange is greater, producing a larger cavity. All of the abdominal organs and vessels are surrounded by elastic muscle tissue.

The extent of abdominal trauma from penetrating injuries depends on the thickness, strength, and elasticity of the muscle surrounding the abdominal structures and on the amount of energy exchange and resulting temporary cavity produced by the penetrating object. Penetration by medium- and high-velocity missiles frequently results in peritonitis, as the contents of the penetrated organs leak into the peritoneum. The signs and symptoms of such a condition are increased abdominal girth and complaint of severe abdominal pain and tenderness. However, these signs and symptoms may not develop for several hours. The paramedic must respond based on the potential of injury. Assessment of potential injury is based on the understanding of the kinematics involved.

Extremities

The major structural difference in extremities versus other parts of the body is the presence of more bone. Muscles in the extremities react to penetrating injuries with the same rebound effect as they do in other parts of the body. Because of the proximity of blood vessels and peripheral nerves to the bones in the extremities, bone fragmentation frequently results in laceration of these structures. As a rule of thumb with bone trauma, assume associated injuries to adjacent blood vessels and nerves. The astute paramedic assesses pulses and neurologic sensory and motor function distal to the injury and observes for signs of an expanding hematoma.

BLUNT TRAUMA

Blunt trauma differs only from penetrating trauma in that the impact of energy is spread out over an area so large that the skin cannot be broken. It can be caused by a direct blow with a moving object, such as a baseball bat, or, more commonly, by acceleration-deceleration vehicular collisions. When an individual is struck by a baseball bat, the energy from the weight and velocity of the moving bat is transferred to the skin and underlying tissue in the body area of the impact. The impact compresses the tissues. As the surrounding tissue is compressed and stretched, the cavity expands in an anterior–posterior direction.

In auto collisions, the extent of trauma to the individual depends on whether safety equipment, such as seat belts, supplemental inflatable restraints (air bags), and properly positioned head rests, are used. In rear-end collisions, if the head rest is in the down position, the part of the occupant's body that touches the seat is accelerated forward, but the head is not. The neck is then hyperextended backward over the top of the seat. This movement opens up the anterior portion of the intervertebral space and compresses the posterior elements (see later discussion of whiplash under "Rear-End Collision"). In contrast, if the occupant's head rest is elevated and the seat belt properly applied, the occupant's head and neck are propelled forward by the seat and head rest as a unit. The neck is protected. The occupant may move forward into the steering wheel or dashboard if the auto impacts another car in front of it. Compression and deceleration injuries occur as the forward motion of the person's body is suddenly halted, as in head-on collisions. This impact results in stretching and compression of body tissue, laceration or rupture of blood vessels and organs, and tearing of the organ attachments from the aorta. Most high speed auto collisions cause both acceleration and deceleration injuries. Regardless of the type of collision, the resulting energy is directed to the occupant.

In order of occurrence, the most common sites of injury in automotive trauma without restraints are the head, thorax, abdomen, and long bones. To decrease the mortality and morbidity that results from car collisions, the most common cause of blunt trauma, automobile safety devices have been invented. Examples include seat and shoulder belts, supplemental inflatable restraints (air bags), padded dashboard and steering wheels, and adjustable head rests. The single most effective device, ac-

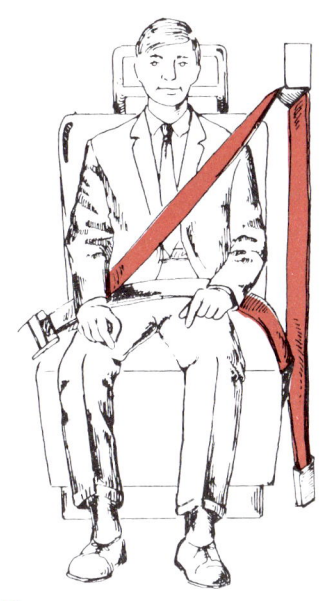

FIGURE 13–15.
Correct application of a safety belt.

cording to the National Association of Stock Car Auto Racing (NASCAR), the authority on race car safety, is the safety belt. It is considered the most effective system available to prevent crushing injuries. Properly applied safety belts restrict the movement of the occupant in all types of car collisions. Correct application is illustrated in Figure 13-15. The lap portion of the belt restrains the lower torso while the shoulder portion restrains the chest.

While safety belts may cause some compression of underlying organs and tissues in high-velocity collisions, they prevent the body from colliding with the solid dashboard or windshield. Many states have enacted laws that require the use of safety belts. Air bags provide no protection for the occupants in side, rollover, or second collisions. However, they significantly reduce the deceleration and compression forces that result from head-on collisions, the most common type. The paramedic must be alert to the use or nonuse of these safety devices in determining the mechanism of injury and potential trauma in car collisions. For the sake of clarity, blunt trauma is categorized according to the following causes of this type of injury: automotive, pedestrian, motorcycle, sporting, and blast.

Automotive Injuries

Automotive injuries are subdivided into patterns of collisions: frontal, rear end, lateral, rotational, and rollover. The five patterns of collisions are summarized in Figure 13-16. The structural damage to the car is similar to the damage sustained by the patient, in both location and amount of energy exchange. Therefore, by assessing the location and extent of car damage, the paramedic can anticipate the injuries the patient may have sustained. As

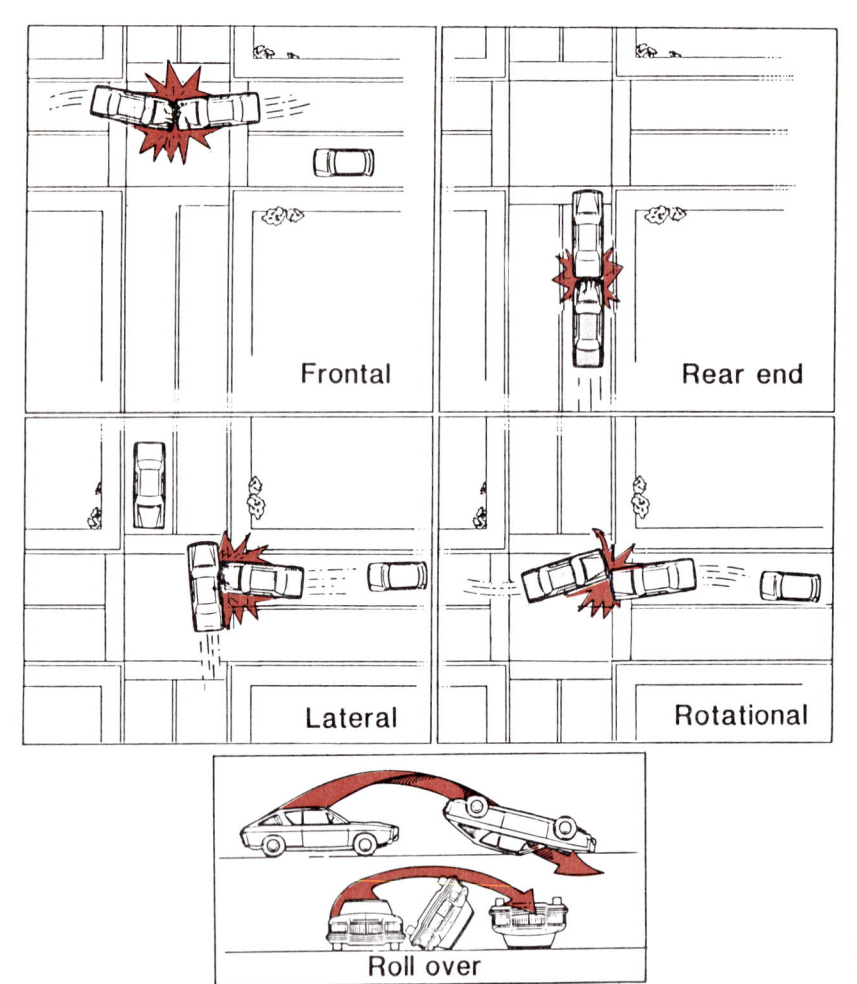

FIGURE 13-16.
Five patterns of automobile collisions.

stated, the force of an object is equal to its weight multiplied by its change in velocity; therefore, the force of impact in car collisions is absorbed by deformation of the patient's body before the person's momentum is halted. The greater the force, the greater the deformity. Because of this fact, noting the type and force of collision is essential to the accuracy of on-site and subsequent patient care.

Frontal Collisions

According to Newton's first law of motion, when a car moves through time and space, its occupants move at the same speed. There is minimal energy exchange between the car and the occupants. However, in ***frontal collisions,*** if the car suddenly stops or hits an object in its way, the occupants continue in forward motion until something restrains or stops them. Unless a safety belt is worn, absorbing some of the energy that results from a sudden stop, the occupants hit the dashboard, steering wheel, or windshield. In frontal collisions, the unrestrained occupant's body can follow one of two pathways: down and under or up and over.

DOWN AND UNDER. In a ***down-and-under frontal collision*** pattern, the unrestrained occupant's body travels down into and slides over the edge of the car seat. In this case, the knees or feet are the lead points. However, if the feet are firmly planted on the car floor, much of the energy is dissipated at the ankle joint, resulting in ankle dislocation or open fracture. If the knee is the lead point, it collides with the dashboard on the tibia or patella and femur (Fig. 13-17). If the tibia is the point of impact, damage to the supporting structures of the knee results. The popliteal artery, which is tightly bound by collateral vessels to the femur and tibia, is stretched. In this case, popliteal artery disruption or thrombosis should be suspected. In other cases, the popliteal vessel is not severed, but stretching of the popliteal artery damages the inner layer of the vessel. The resulting decreased blood flow may not be apparent for several days. When damage to the popliteal artery is suspected, an arteriogram should be obtained shortly after arrival at the emergency department.

When the patella or the femur is the point of impact, either the energy is absorbed by fracturing the midshaft of the femur or the pelvis overrides the head of the femur (see Fig. 13-17). If the pelvis overrides the femur, the head of the femur is positioned posterior to the acetabulum and is frequently associated with a fracture of the socket. In this situation, if the patient has the leg flexed at the hip when the paramedic arrives on scene, the hip

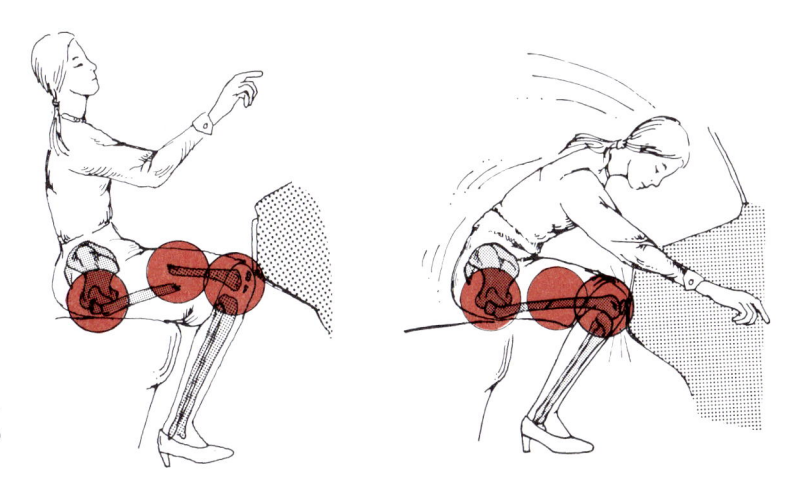

FIGURE 13-17.
In the down-and-under pathway, the unrestrained occupant's knees are the lead points. Damage can result to the knee, femur, or hip.

joint should not be forcibly extended. Extension of the hip joint may increase the extent of damage to the joint, femur, and the surrounding tissues.

In down-and-under collisions, after the femur and pelvis have stopped their forward motion, the upper torso continues toward the steering wheel on the driver's side and the dashboard on the passenger's side. When the person's chest hits one of these structures, the sternum and anterior chest wall are pushed into the thoracic cavity. This push causes compression of the lungs and heart in the chest, and the temporary cavity results in a forceful compression of the liver and pancreas in the abdomen.

The internal organs of both the thoracic and abdominal cavities continue their forward motion even after the torso has stopped. The most vulnerable structures in the thoracic cavity are the heart and the aortic complex. In the abdomen, the most vulnerable organs are the spleen, liver, kidneys, and intestines that are attached by a pedicle to the posterior abdominal wall.

After the torso stops, the forward motion of the head propels it into the windshield, which suddenly stops its forward motion. Unfortunately, the brain continues its forward motion until stopped by the person's skull. If the energy from the impact has not been totally absorbed at this point, the cervical spine is compressed or either flexed forward or backward. Trauma to the cervical area produces neurologic damage because of the compression and stretching of the fragile cervical spinal cord.

UP AND OVER. In the *up-and-over frontal collision* pattern, the head of the unrestrained occupant is the lead point of the human missile. It hits the windshield without any previous dissipation of energy. Even after the head has stopped, the brain continues its forward motion, followed by the neck, and, lastly, the torso. Compression, extension, or flexion of the cervical spine occurs. Unstable vertebral fractures should be suspected with bull's-eye fractures of the windshield or any head and neck injuries above the spine.

The thorax and abdomen then impact the dashboard or steering wheel, producing compression and decelera-

tion injuries similar to those described with the down-and-under pathway. In up-and-over collisions, the initial and greater energy is absorbed by the head and neck. Such patients are always immobilized with a backboard and cervical collar.

Rear-End Collisions

The unrestrained occupants of a slow-moving or stopped car are extremely vulnerable when hit from behind by another vehicle. In a *rear-end collision* the energy from the car behind is transferred to the car in front, suddenly increasing the front car's speed. This action also rapidly accelerates the bodies of the occupants. If the head rest is improperly positioned, the cervical spine is the recipient of the initial energy exchange, with backward extension over the top of the seat (Fig. 13-18). The initial backward

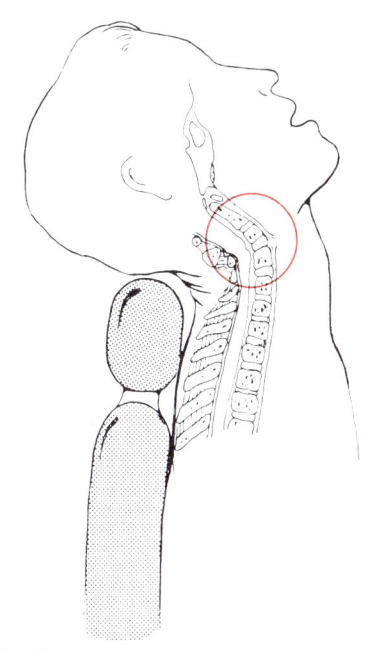

FIGURE 13-18.
"Whiplash" is caused by the rapid backward extension of the cervical spine. If the head rest is improperly positioned, tearing and stretching of the cervical ligaments and tendons may occur.

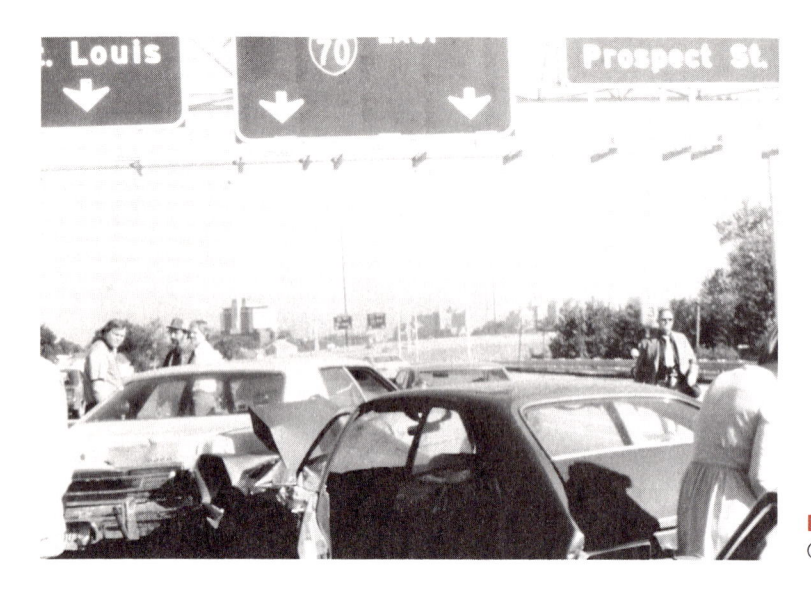

FIGURE 13-19.
Chain reactions can easily occur in rear-end collisions.

extension of the neck causes stretching and, frequently, tearing of the neck ligaments and tendons, which may even be torn away from the vertebrae. Severe cervical strains, commonly called **whiplash**, can result. If, however, the head rest is adjusted to touch the occipital area of the skull, the backward extension motion is prevented.

Frequently, in rear-end collisions, another car is in the line of traffic. In rear-end collisions, the occupants of the second car (the car that struck the rear end of the first car) sustain the same injuries previously described in the frontal collision, but with less force. If other cars are involved, as in a chain reaction, similar acceleration-deceleration injuries occur (Fig. 13-19).

Lateral Collisions

Lateral collisions occur most often at intersections (called *T-bone collisions*) or when an out-of-control car skids sideways into a fixed object, such as a telephone pole. Although the intersection collision produces an acceleration force and the telephone pole collision produces a deceleration force, the amount and direction of energy exchange is similar.

When lateral collisions occur, the car door hits the person's body. Initially, bony areas are affected: the thorax, pelvis, and possibly the arm. If the occupant's arm does not rotate out of the way, in other words, if it is located between the person's chest and the car door, the energy is transferred to the head of the humerus and the clavicle. Because the clavicle is a long, thin bone with minimal support tissue, it is extremely vulnerable to fracture. If the arm rotates out of the way, the ribs, in contact with the car door, form a cavity inward, producing multiple rib fractures with a lateral flail chest. Energy is dissipated into the thoracic cavity, causing compression and possibly contusion of the lung. The energy exchange between the thoracic aorta, which is tightly attached to the vertebral column, and the relatively mobile heart causes the arch of the aorta to shear at the distal end of the arch, where the arch ends and the descending aorta (tightly attached portion) begins.

In some cases, the shearing forces tear the inner layer, muscularis, and adventitia of the aorta. This tear results in immediate exsanguination. Approximately 80% of shear injuries are full thickness. In other instances, 20% of the patients sustain a partial disruption of the aortic wall, with the adventitia containing the hemorrhage. This condition is called **pseudoaneurysm**. While a pseudoaneurysm prevents immediate death, one third of pseudoaneurysms rupture within 6 hours of the injury. Another one third rupture within 24 hours, and the final one third within the next 72 hours unless surgical repair is initiated. Suspicion of such injuries is based on the pattern of the collision. The paramedic is responsible for communicating this information so that appropriate diagnostic tests and definitive surgical treatment can be initiated on arrival at the trauma center.

As stated earlier, one third of the abdominal contents are encased in the thoracic cage. During maximal expiration, the diaphragm reaches as high as the fourth intercostal space anteriorly and the sixth intercostal space laterally. Because of this fact, the risk of abdominal organ injury with thoracic wall compression is increased.

Abdominal organs at greatest risk in lateral collisions are the spleen of the driver and the liver of the passenger in the right front seat. Kidney trauma should be suspect in all deceleration accidents. In the lower torso, the greater trochanter of the femur is the point first impacted in lateral collisions. The head of the femur penetrates the acetabulum, frequently resulting in fragmentation of the joint and possible fracture of the head of the femur. If the car door reaches the wing of the ilium, the entire pelvis can be fractured. When pelvic bones are fractured, major blood loss should be anticipated. Another area likely to be injured in lateral collisions is the cervical spine. The person's torso is suddenly moved from under the head. The lateral momentum of the torso results in lateral flexion of the neck and rotation of the head in the direction opposite the torso. Because the head of the average adult weighs 13 lb, lateral flexion to the cervical spine can be severe.

Clinically significant cervical spine injuries are more common in lateral collisions than in rear-end collisions. The damage sustained by the brain is also lateral in direction, resulting in compression of the lateral aspects of the frontal, parietal, and temporal lobes against the skull.

Rotational Collisions

Not all collisions occur at the center point of the front, rear, or side of a car. When a car is hit at the front or rear quarter, the portion hit comes to an immediate stop (Fig. 13-20). However, the opposite portion does not. The resulting force causes the car to rotate. In **rotational collisions,** the occupant sustains a combination of the injuries caused by lateral and front-end collisions. Because the injuries are related to the directional force during the collision, the paramedic should attempt to discover the direction in which the car rotated.

Rollover Collisions

In **rollover collisions,** it is extremely difficult to predict the injury pattern. As the car flips, the unrestrained occupant is thrown around the interior of the car and propelled into various structures: the windshield, roof, seats, a and b pillars, and, possibly, the floor. Each directional change causes an energy exchange with the person's body. Although these exchanges are multiple and varied, the same compression and stretch injuries occur as in other patterns of collision.

The paramedic should inquire about the direction of the rollover, whether front-over-rear, lateral, or mixed. Using the information previously presented and knowing the directional pattern of the rollover, the paramedic can evaluate the most probable injuries the patient has sustained (Fig. 13-21).

Pedestrian Injuries

The energy exchange in pedestrian trauma is similar to the exchange that occurs in other kinds of blunt trauma, with one exception. The pedestrian has less protection. In car collisions, the car occupants are protected by the car frame, which absorbs a substantial amount of collision energy. If the occupants are wearing safety belts, they have additional protection. This protection is not available in pedestrian injuries.

Pedestrian-car collisions occur in three stages: the car-body impact, the body-to-car hood thrust, and the body-to-ground fall. Each of these changes in momentum causes injury to another part of the person's body. In the adult victim, the initial body contact with the car bumper is at or just below the knee. Because the person's foot is firmly planted on the ground surface, the knee is pushed rapidly in the same direction in which the car is traveling. If the knee is hit from the lateral side, the knee is pushed inward or medially (Fig. 13-22A). This type of injury causes stretching or tearing of the cruciate ligaments and, frequently, the cartilage. This condition results in an injury characterized by severe localized pain, joint deformity and dysfunction, and ecchymosis. This complex (called **O'Donohue's triad**) results is cartilage injury with a tear in the lateral collateral and cruciate ligaments. This injury was first described in football players. When the pedestrian is hit from the front, the knee is pushed backward or posteriorly.

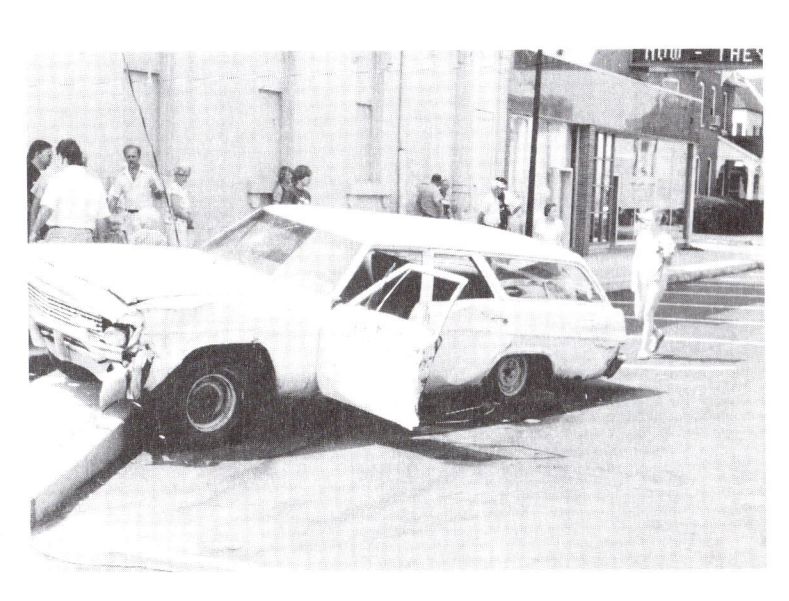

FIGURE 13-20.
Rotational collisions occur when a force causes the car to spin at an angle.

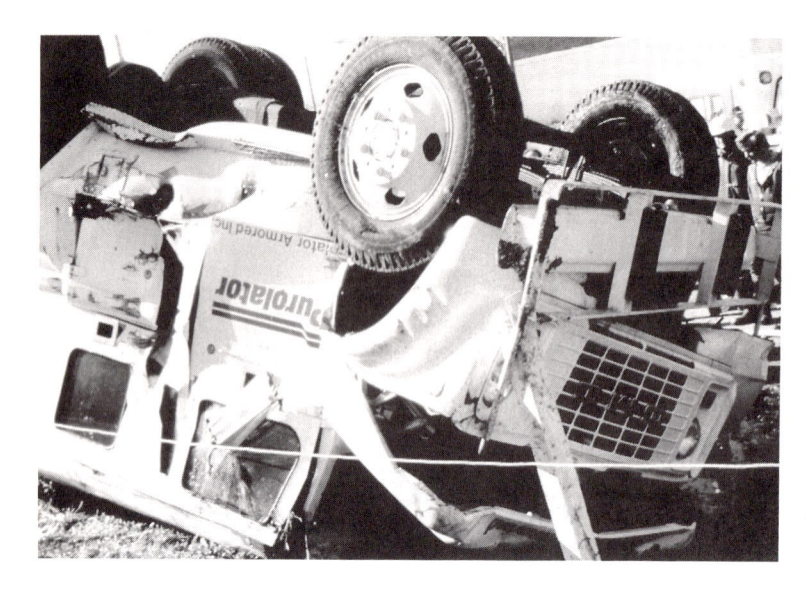

FIGURE 13-21.
The mechanism of injury is important to establish in a rollover collision.

Frontal injuries cause posterior dislocation of the tibia and fibula with destruction of all of the cruciate ligaments. Because of the hyperextension and dislocation of the knee, damage to the popliteal artery and vein is probable. Only in rear-end collisions does the knee bend naturally. While this type of injury produces less damage to the lateral ligaments and tendons, the posterior popliteal vessels are extremely vulnerable to injury. In assessing the extent of knee injury, the paramedic should always palpate the distal pulses. Generally, knee injuries are splinted from pelvis to foot. A long backboard can be used to protect the legs as well as the entire spine. However, if knee extension causes severe pain, the paramedic should splint the patient's knee in the flexed position.

The second stage of the car-pedestrian accident occurs as the pedestrian's body is impacted by the car hood. The type of injury sustained depends on the position of the person before the accident. If the hit was front-on or lateral, the result may be a lateral or anterior flail chest. If the person was hit from behind, hyperextension of the lumbar and thoracic spine can open and tear the anterior ligaments. This type of motion may also shear the posterior supporting vertebral structures, resulting in dislocation and possible spinal cord damage with neurologic loss.

The third stage occurs as the pedestrian hits the ground. If the person falls head-first off the car hood, the potential for cervical spine fractures is as great as the potential for brain trauma. Proper immobilization is required.

Several differences must be considered with the pediatric pedestrian accident victim. First, the point of car-body impact depends on the child's height (Fig. 13-22B). In the case of a 2-year-old child, the car bumper may hit the child's head. Another difference is the natural curi-

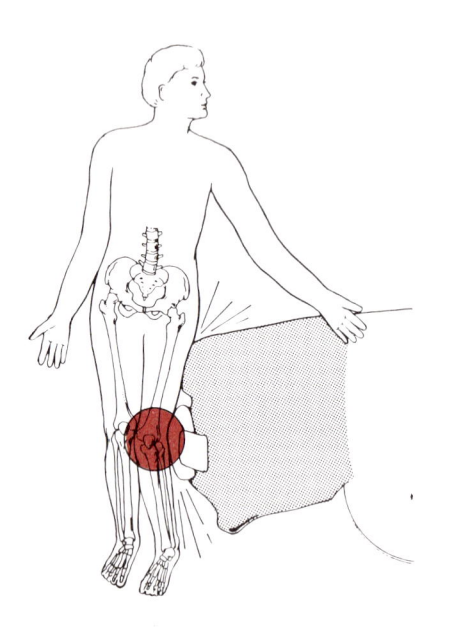

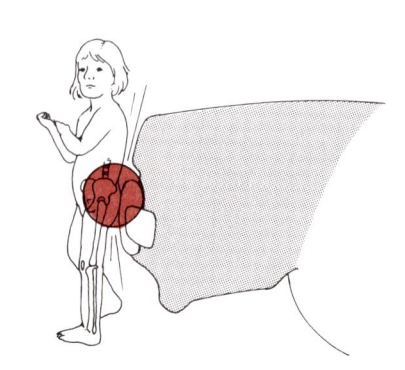

FIGURE 13-22.
(**A**) Stretching or tearing injuries occur when the adult pedestrian's knee is hit from the side. (**B**) A child's height determines the injuries likely sustained when hit by the bumper of a car.

osity of the child. While the adult attempts to escape from the impact, a young child looks to see what is happening. This action may result in frontal injury rather than lateral or posterior (more common in the adult).

Significant kinematic information that the paramedic should note in car–pedestrian accidents includes the speed of the car, initial and subsequent positions of the pedestrian, age and height of the victim, and reconstruction of the stages of the accident.

Motorcycle Injuries

Although the same energy forces are involved in motorcycle collisions as in car collisions, there are two major differences. The cyclist lacks the structural protection of the steel car frame, and some cyclists neglect to wear protective helmets and clothing. These factors increase the risk of significant trauma in cycle collisions. While professional motorcycle riders are required by the American Motorcyclist Association to wear protective clothing during competitive events, most recreational cyclists do not do so. Cyclists should realize that, without head protection, the increased risk of head injury is 300%. As substantiated by comparison research studies conducted in Kansas, Louisiana, and Texas of more than 25,000 collisions, the long-term disability and higher medical costs and money lost by society that result from nonfatal head injuries are far greater when helmets are not worn by cyclists.

Many states have enacted laws that require cyclists to wear protective helmets. In Louisiana, the law was based on the premise that citizens should not have to pay increased taxes or hospitalization insurance rates to provide care for cyclists who refused to use available helmet protection.

Motorcycle Injury Patterns

Motorcycle injuries result from four types of collisions: head-on, angular, ejection, and laying the bike down. To make accurate assessments and provide information to emergency department personnel, the paramedic must be familiar with the pattern of injury and the kinematics of cycle trauma (Fig. 13-23).

HEAD-ON. The center of gravity of the motorcycle engine is above the pivot point at the front axle. However, the rider's center of gravity is higher, at hip level. In a head-on collision, the rider is ejected up and over the front of the cycle. The rider's face, chest, or abdomen can hit the handle bars, producing significant cavitation of the body part hit. If the cyclist's feet are on the pegs, the femurs hit the handle bars, resulting in bilateral femoral fractures.

ANGULAR. When the motorcycle hits an object other than head-on, the cycle and the object come together, with the cyclist's legs trapped in between. In this situation, open fractures of the tibia and fibula are the result, primarily near the ankle.

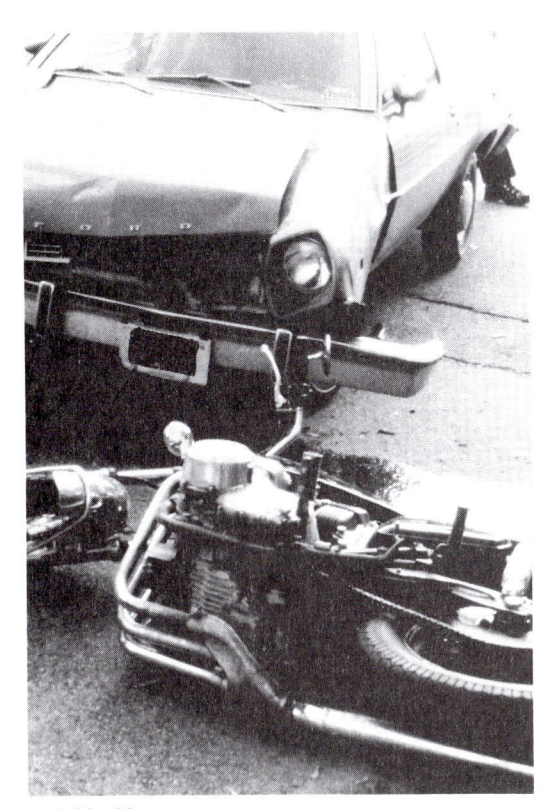

EJECTION. An ejected rider becomes a human missile. The cyclist hits the same objects the cycle has hit, the road surface and objects on the other side of the road. When the cyclist's body hits the ground, body tissues are compressed, and unattached or loosely attached body organs are subject to all the acceleration-declaration injuries described previously in head-on collisions.

LAYING THE BIKE DOWN. Laying the bike down is a maneuver that professional and some recreational riders use to separate themselves from the bike before a crash. The purpose of this protective mechanism is to prevent ejection and crash. The process of laying the bike down involves turning the cycle sideways, at a 90° angle to the potential crash site, dropping the inside leg to the ground, and stepping or jumping away from the cycle. Protected against the crash, the rider slides along the ground surface. If protective leather clothing and boots are not worn, severe abrasions, degloving injuries, and fractures of the extremities or torso can occur.

FIGURE 13-23.
The kinematics of trauma is an important concept in the determination of motorcycle injury patterns.

Sports Injuries

Injuries sustained in athletic events are unique to the specific sport being played. Most sports injuries can by predicted by the activity involved in the game. For example, in football, head-on tackles can cause cervical spine injuries, while lateral knee hits result in trauma to the knee ligaments. In baseball, if the base runner's foot is caught on the base pad, the torso overrides the leg, possibly dislocating or fracturing the ankle. While the marathon runner is subject to shin splints, the rebounder on a basketball team may sustain ankle trauma. Organized amateur and professional athletes are required to participate in training programs and wear protective padding and helmets. Examples are the knee pads worn by volleyball, football, and soccer players and the helmets worn by bike racers, football, hockey, and baseball players.

Athletic training programs focus on increasing muscle strength and mass. Unfortunately, participants in "street" or "pick-up" games frequently do not wear protective clothing and most are not in peak physical condition. These factors place them at additional risk for injury. The majority of sports injuries are caused by blunt trauma. Just as the occupants in car collisions absorb the energy from a collision, the athlete's body must absorb the energy generated by colliding with another person or the ground.

Anatomical Considerations

Head

When an athlete, such as a boxer or football player, sustains a forceful blow to the head, the skull may be fractured or a contusion of brain tissue may result. Similar injuries result from the driver's head hitting the windshield in a car collision. In skull fractures, the skull fragments lacerate brain tissue; however, contusion of the brain with cerebral hemorrhage more commonly is caused by contact with the irregular configuration of the skull bone interior. Deceleration injuries to the brain result in a tearing away of the brain tissue from its supporting structures, resulting in either venous subdural or arterial epidural hemorrhage. Epidural hemorrhage frequently is associated with temporal skull fractures. When the artery is disrupted, hemorrhage into the closed skull compresses the brain, producing ischemia and necrosis. Prompt medical attention is essential. In extremely forceful injuries, the brain can be separated from the spinal cord at the brain stem; the outcome of this condition is fatal.

Neck

Neck injuries associated with sports are more common with diving and football. Victims of car collisions may sustain acceleration or deceleration injuries. The types of neck injuries include cervical compression and vertebral fractures due to hyperextension, hyperflexion, or lateral flexion. The most common site of vertebral fractures are at C-1, C-2, C-5, and C-6. Dislocation of the vertebrae reduces the lumen of the spinal canal, thereby impinging on the spinal cord. This condition can cause spinal cord edema, ischemia, or cord separation. At the C-3 level, the spinal canal is smallest in diameter and the cervical spinal cord is largest, with less than 1 mm of clearance between the cord and canal. Because of this fact, trauma at C-3 results in severe injury with a high probability for permanent neurologic damage for survivors.

Thorax

A forceful thoracic blow, such as that which occurs when the driver's chest impacts the steering wheel, can produce a flail chest and compression injuries to the heart and lung. Contusion of the lung results in compromised oxygenation. With lung contusions, there is an increase in the amount of interstitial fluid between the alveoli and the capillaries and in the potential for blood accumulation in the alveolar spaces. Oxygen transport across the alveolar-capillary membrane is reduced. Severe compression or lacerations may cause air to accumulate in the pleural space (*pneumothorax*). The lung, therefore, is compressed and cannot properly expand. Compression of the inflated alveolar sac may cause the sac to rupture, and air again leaks into the pleural space. In an accident situation, when faced with the impending disaster, the victim instinctively takes a deep breath and closes the glottis. When external compression occurs as the chest impacts the steering wheel (or some other object), internal pressures build up within the lung. The resulting "*paper bag*" effect is illustrated in Figure 13-24. A paper bag expanded with air and held tightly at the neck pops when rapidly compressed with the other hand. Actually, this cause of pneumothorax is more common than rib penetration of the lung.

Compression of the heart injures the conduction system, evidenced by arrhythmias or a bundle-branch block. Damage to the muscle wall (cardiac contusion) can be a mild injury with no clinical significance, or rupture of the myocardium (cardiac concussion), which results in cardiac tamponade, can occur.

In deceleration injuries, the aortic complex is the structure most affected. The descending aorta is bound by strong attachments to the thoracic vertebral column. The arch of the aorta and the heart are more freely movable. When rapid deceleration occurs, whether from lateral or frontal impact, the stationary thoracic aorta remains with the chest wall, and the heart and aortic arch swing like a pendulum. The intensity of the shearing and stretch forces are greatest at the point where the descending aorta is attached to the vertebral column. Obviously, these forces result in tremendous blood loss. Eighty percent of patients exsanguinate in the first hour. Twenty percent survive to allow efficient transportation to the hospital.

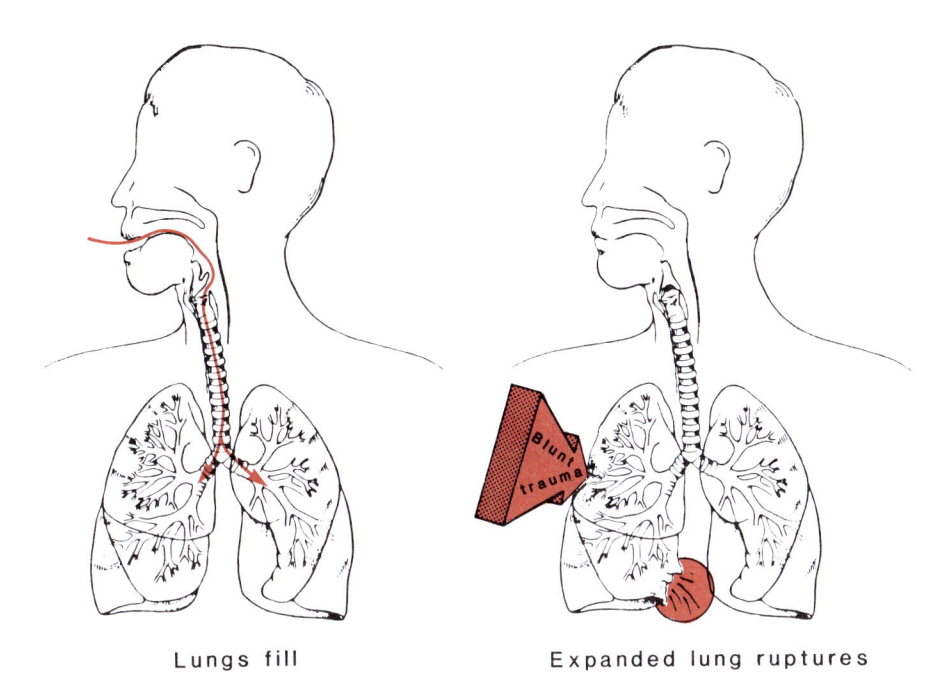

FIGURE 13-24.
If blunt trauma to the lungs occurs when they are full of air, the resulting "paper bag" effect causes rupture of the lungs.

Lungs fill   Expanded lung ruptures

Abdomen

Compression of the abdominal cavity produces cavitation toward the posterior of the body. Recall, however, that one third of the abdominal cavity is encased in the rib cage. If the lower ribs are fractured, the victim is likely to sustain liver or spleen injuries. Severe compression of the abdominal organs results, first, in displacement and, then, in possible rupture, causing peritonitis. In addition, when abdominal blood vessels are injured, rapid blood loss can occur. Massive hemorrhage causes outward expansion of the abdomen.

A marked increase in intra-abdominal pressure produced by impact with the steering wheel or the dashboard can rupture the diaphragm. The abdominal contents migrate into the thoracic cavity. Definitive diagnosis of this condition requires radiographic examination.

Rapid deceleration injuries frequently affect the pedicle organs, such as the spleen, kidneys, and small intestine, resulting in either stretch, tears, or rupture. Deceleration liver injuries are unique. These types of injuries are caused by frontal automobile collisions when the occupant follows the down-and-under pathway, falls from heights, or skiing accidents. Attached only to the diaphragm, the liver descends into the abdominal cavity and is stopped by the ligamentum teres in the perineal area. The capsule can split like cutting cheese. The result is a midpoint laceration of the liver.

Extremities

In most sports, the extremities are not protected by padding. The most common extremity injury is joint sprain and muscle stretch, both of which are extremely painful. In addition, joint dislocation and bone fractures are a likely potential when the force of collision is great. These conditions can occur with any sport but should be suspect in football, soccer, and skiing. Either open or closed fractures can occur.

Car and motorcycle accident victims sustain various types of fractures and dislocations depending on the type of impact.

Blast Injuries

A ***blast*** is an explosive force. Blast injuries are not necessarily associated with wars or terrorist attacks. An explosion can result from civilian-type actions, such as dynamite explosions on construction sites. In explosions, the energy contained in the burning substance is converted into light, heat, and pressure. The extent of damage to the individual from each of these forces depends on the force of the blast and the distance between the blast and the individual (Fig. 13-25).

Light

Light, traveling at 186,000 mph, is the first force to reach the victim. If the person is looking directly at the blast, damage to the eyes can occur. This damage is usually temporary.

Heat

Two factors influence the extent of body burns sustained by the victim: distance from the blast and the protection available to the person. Burns produced by the heat wave are inversely proportional to the distance between the blast site and the victim. As the distance is increased, the more heat is dissipated, leaving lesser amounts for

FIGURE 13-25.
Blast injuries can occur several feet or many yards away from the incident.

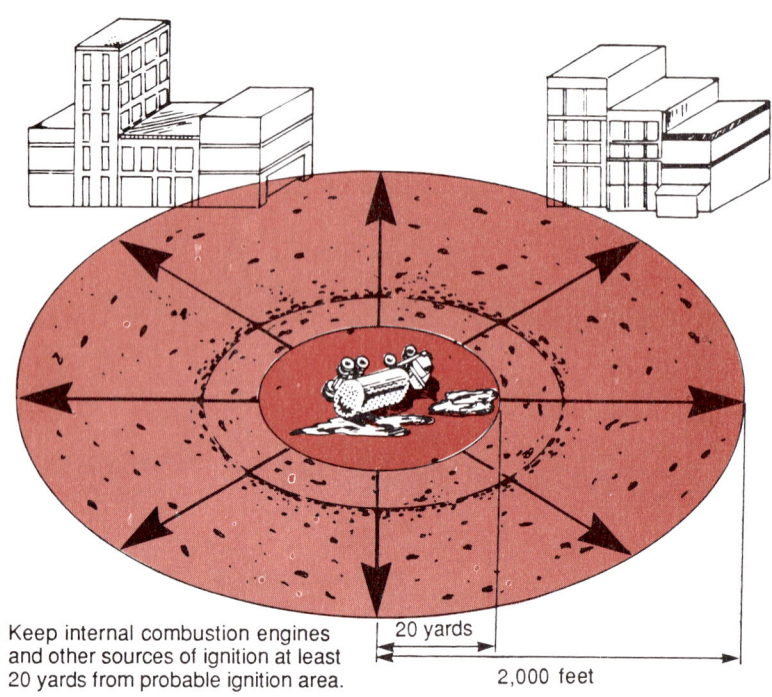

Keep internal combustion engines and other sources of ignition at least 20 yards from probable ignition area.

20 yards

2,000 feet

In case of explosion, the minimum safe distance from flying fragments is 2000 feet in all directions.

absorption by the victim's skin. The second factor that influences the amount and degree of skin heat absorption is protection, which may be a wall, building, or clothing. The burn patterns on the victim indicate the protection used.

Definitive management of major burns requires prompt transport to the hospital after extinguishing any smoldering material and applying wet compresses to burned skin areas. The problem of smoke inhalation should be considered in the initial assessment and management, especially for explosions in closed areas.

Pressure

Pressure waves that radiate outward from the blast are known as *"over-pressure."* Three major components of waves result from explosions. The first component is the explosive force that transfers energy to any object in the immediate vicinity. These objects, whether pieces of wood, rocks, or metal are hurled away from the site with extensive force. If these missile objects hit an individual, they can cause either blunt or penetrating trauma.

The second component exerts pressure on the victim's body, which is forcefully moved from its original position. The victim actually becomes a missile, traveling a distance proportional to the force of the blast. The person can be hurled into other objects or the ground. The injuries sustained are similar to those of the cyclist who is ejected from the motorcycle or the pedestrian hit by a car. When hurled to the ground, the victim tries to break the fall and frequently sustains extremity fractures or severe compression injuries.

The third component of pressure waves produces a sudden difference between the external and internal body pressures. Two organs most susceptible to pressure changes are the ears and the lungs. The ear's tympanic membrane separates the middle ear from the external environment. The middle ear is connected via the eustachian tube to the oropharynx. A sudden increase in external pressure forces the tympanic membrane inward. If this inward stretching exceeds the tensile strength of the membrane, a tympanic rupture occurs. The lungs experience a similar sudden differential in the internal-external pressure gradient. This sudden compression of the thoracic cavity produces rupture of the alveoli (pneumothorax), contusion and hemorrhage of the alveolar-capillary membrane (decreased gas exchange), and hemorrhage into the alveolar sac (decreased ventilation).

The astute paramedic at the scene of a blast accident is alert to the three blast forces that cause injury and assesses the victim for eye, lung, ear, extremity, and thermal injuries.

SUMMARY

The paramedic at the accident scene is the most reliable source of information about the kinematics of the traumatic event and the injuries sustained. The accuracy and completeness of the accident scene information regarding the mechanism of injury is vital to accurate assessments and appropriate interventions. Laws of physics are applied to determine the mechanism of injury. The energy caused by a traumatic event is absorbed by the body of the victim. The physical damage to the tissues results in major or minor dysfunction of the organs involved. The extent of damage and deformity is directly related to the force of the blow or impact. Familiarity with these laws of physics, combined with knowledge of anatomy and physiology, increases paramedics' accuracy and thoroughness of accident scene assessment and their ability to identify possible injuries and, thereby, to institute correct management immediately.

Reconstruction of the accident includes noting the protective devices, equipment, and clothing that prevented more extensive trauma to the person involved, whether it was a vehicular, sporting, or blast accident. This vital information must be communicated to emergency department personnel to ensure effective patient care.

SUGGESTED READING

Campbell JE: Basic Trauma Life Support, 2nd ed. Englewood Cliffs, Brady, 1988

Carter WA: Arming yourself to treat gunshot wounds. J Emerg Med Serv 15(9):34, 1990

Gandy PS: Trauma course: Take your pick. J Emerg Med Serv 22(4):57, 1990

Garza MA: Who cares about trauma. J Emerg Med Serv 15(3):32, 1990

McSwain NE, Belleo A: Medical and financial impact of motorcycle helmet laws. J Trauma, Oct, 1990

McSwain NE, Butman AM, McConnel WK et al: Pre-hospital Trauma Life Support. Akron, Emergency Training, 1990

McSwain NE, Kerstein MD: Evaluation and Management of Trauma. Norwalk, Appleton—Century—Crofts, 1987

Stewart C:. Mechanisms of injury. Journal of Emergency Care and Transportation 18(1): 21, 1989

Turnkey D, Lewis F: Current Therapy of Trauma—2. Philadelphia, BC Decker, 1986

US Department of Transportation, National Highway Traffic Safety Administration: Emergency Medical Technician—Paramedic: National Standards Curriculum. Washington, DC, US Government Printing Office, 1985

CHAPTER 14

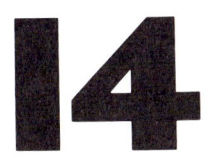

Soft-Tissue and Burn Injuries

Anatomy and Physiology of the Skin
- Structure
- Function

Soft-tissue Injuries
- Closed Wounds
- Open Wounds
  - Abrasion
  - Laceration
  - Major Arterial Laceration
  - Puncture Wound
  - Avulsion
  - Amputation
  - Impaled Object
- Assessment
- Management
  - Closed and Open Wounds
  - Amputations
  - Impaled Objects

Burn Injuries
- Major Sources of Burn Injury
- Pathophysiology of Burn Injury
  - Local
  - Systemic

Classifications of Burn Injury
- Superficial
- Partial-thickness
  - Superficial Partial-thickness
  - Deep Partial-thickness
- Full-thickness

Calculation of Body Surface Area
- Rule of Palms
- Rule of Nines
- Lund—Brower Chart

Severity of Injury
- Factors That Affect Severity of Injury
  - Depth of the Burn
  - Extent of the Burn
  - Location
  - Age
  - General Health
  - Associated Injuries
- Categories of Burn Injury Severity

Categories of Injuries
- Inhalation Injuries
  - Carbon Monoxide
  - Smoke Inhalation
- Thermal Injuries
- Eye Injuries

Patient Assessment
- Scene Survey
- Primary Survey
  - Responsiveness
  - Airway
  - Breathing
  - Circulation
- Secondary Survey

Management
- Thermal Burns
- Electrical Burns
- Chemical Burns
- Radiation Burns
- Inhalation Injuries
- Eye Injuries

Fluid Resuscitation

Prevention and Patient Education

Summary

BEHAVIORAL OBJECTIVES

On successful completion of this chapter, the reader will be able to:

1. Describe the structure of the skin
2. Describe a closed wound
3. Describe the seven open wounds and include assessment and management
4. State the four major sources of burn injuries
5. Describe the local and systemic pathophysiology of burn injury
6. Describe the three classifications of burn injury
7. Given a diagram, calculate the percentage of body surface area burned by the rule of palms, rule of nines, and Lund—Brower
8. List the six factors that affect severity of burn injury
9. Describe a minor, moderate, and major burn using the American Burn Association Burn Severity Index
10. Explain a primary and secondary survey that deals with the burn patient
11. Describe the management of thermal, electrical, chemical, and radiation burns
12. Describe the management of inhalation injuries
13. Describe the five formulas for fluid resuscitation
14. List ten safety measures for the prevention of burns
15. Define all of the key terms listed in this chapter

KEY TERMS

The following terms are defined in the chapter and glossary:

abrasion
amputation—
   complete, partial,
   degloving
avulsion
body surface area
   (BSA)
burns—superficial
   (first-degree),
   partial-thickness
   (second-degree),
   full-thickness
   (third-degree)
carbon monoxide
chemical burns
closed wound
contusion
cutaneous membrane
dermis

ecchymosis
electrical burns
epidermis
hematoma
impaled object
laceration
Lund—Brower chart
melanocytes
melanin
open wound
puncture wound
radiation burns
rule of nines
rule of palms
subcutaneous connec-
   tive tissue
tetanus
thermal burns

The skin is the organ most affected by soft-tissue and burn injuries. Soft-tissue injuries are usually easily managed in the field unless a vital organ is affected, such as a puncture wound that creates a pneumothorax, or if amputation occurs.

Millions of people around the world are hospitalized for treatment of burns every year, and thousands of these people die. Smoke inhalation accounts for more than half of the deaths. Thousands are disfigured or disabled for life. A recognition of the severity and necessary treatment of caring for the burn patient is crucial for the paramedic. This chapter presents information on the four major sources of burn injuries and the pathophysiologic response of the body to these injuries. Severity of burn injury is shown to depend on several factors. Treatment and management of the burn-injured patient depend on these factors.

ANATOMY AND PHYSIOLOGY OF THE SKIN

The severity of the consequences of soft-tissue and burn injuries emphasizes the importance of the human body's largest organ system, the integument, more commonly known as the skin.

Structure

The skin is a relatively thin, flat organ. It is composed primarily of two layers; an outer, thinner layer, known as the epidermis, and an inner, thicker layer, known as the dermis. The **epidermis** is the body's first line of defense against the external environment. Four distinct layers of cells comprise the epidermis. The outer two layers of the epidermis are composed of dying or dead cells that are continuously replaced by new cells from the deeper layers of the epidermis. The deeper two layers of the epidermis are composed of living cells. These cells perpetually divide and, thus, give rise to the cells of the outer layers. Certain cells, known as **melanocytes,** can be found in the deeper aspects of the epidermis. Melanocytes synthesize **melanin,** which is responsible for skin pigmentation. The darkness of a person's skin is directly proportional to the amount of melanin present. Melanin serves in a protective capacity by hindering the penetration of ultraviolet rays, which could harm or injure the dermis and underlying tissues.

Beneath the epidermis lies a thicker layer of tissue known as the **dermis**. Also called the *corium* (true skin), the dermis can be described as a thick layer of dense fibrous connective tissue. Like the epidermis, it, too, is composed of layers of tissue; yet the tissue of the dermis is thicker, tougher, and much more elastic than the epidermis. The dermis has two principal layers. The outer layer of the dermis, which is relatively thinner than the deeper layers, contains specialized structures that enable the skin to perform many of its vital functions. Therefore, a vast array of sensory nerve endings, blood vessels, *sudoriferous* (sweat) *glands, sebaceous* (oil) *glands,* and hair follicles are found in this part of the dermis. The deeper structures of the dermis consist of a dense network of both connective and elastic fibers. These provide for important qualities of the skin, such as toughness and the ability to stretch.

The skin, both the epidermis and dermis collectively, is often referred to as the **cutaneous membrane**. Just below the dermal layer of the skin is an adherent layer of *adipose* (fatty) tissue called **subcutaneous connective tissue**. This layer of fatty tissue is beneath the layers of the skin and above the fascia, which covers the muscles. Bundles of fibers extend from the dermis into the subcutaneous tissue, attaching the two structures firmly to each other. The thickness of the subcutaneous layer varies among individuals. In lean people, for example, the subcutaneous layer is deficient in various areas; whereas, obese people have an excess of this tissue. Furthermore, its degree of thickness varies according to the area or part of the body that it covers. For instance, subcutaneous tissue of the eyelids is extremely thin, while it is thick over the abdomen and buttocks.

Though the subcutaneous tissue is not considered actually to be part of the skin, it is often injured in soft-tissue injuries and in full-thickness (third-degree) burn injuries. Injuries to the subcutaneous tissue layer can be life threatening, since it serves as the body's insulator, thus helping to maintain homeostatic temperature levels in the body.

Figure 14-1 shows the structure of the skin.

Function

The skin acts as a barrier between the body's more delicate tissues and organs and the outside world. Covering the entire body and its various orifices, the skin protects the deeper tissues from injury. These injuries can range from those caused by temperature extremes, traumatic events, and invasion by foreign intruders, such as bacteria.

The skin serves multiple functions. It helps to regulate body temperature by preventing heat loss when the core temperature falls and facilitating heat loss when the core temperature rises. Other functional capacities of the skin include preventing excessive water loss and drying of tissues, thus helping to maintain a homeostatic environment, and functioning as a receptor (sense) organ for touch, pain, heat, and cold. Therefore, substantial damage to the skin can result in serious complications. The body becomes defenseless against harmful bacterial agents, marked temperature changes, and costly disturbances in fluid balance.

SOFT-TISSUE INJURIES

In the injured patient, the skin may itself be the site of damage. The entire surface of the body, therefore, must be examined for soft-tissue injuries. Although this type of injury may be the most obvious and dramatic, it is seldom the most serious, unless it compromises the airway or is associated with massive hemorrhage. The paramedic, therefore, must survey the patient in a systematic and thorough way to detect other injuries or life-threatening conditions that may exist, before treating the trauma to the soft tissues.

Soft-tissue injuries involve the skin and underlying musculature. An injury to these tissues is commonly referred to as a wound. More specifically, a wound is a trau-

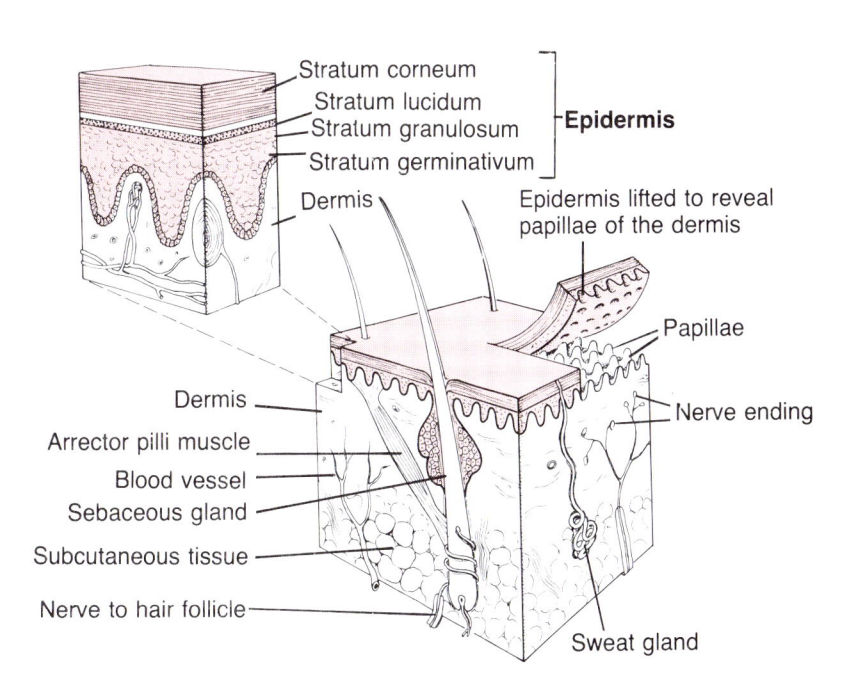

FIGURE 14-1.
Structure of the skin. (Rosdahl CB)

matically induced injury to the body that disrupts the normal continuity of the tissue, organ, or bone affected.

Closed Wounds

When a blunt object strikes the body, it may crush the tissue beneath the skin. Although the skin does not break, severe damage to tissue and blood vessels may cause bleeding within a confined area. This is called a **closed wound**. Types of closed wounds include contusions, hematomas, and crush injuries. A **contusion** is a bruise. Blood collects under the skin or in damaged tissues. Swelling at the site may occur immediately or 24 to 48 hours later. As blood accumulates in the area, a characteristic black and blue mark, called **ecchymosis**, is seen. A blood clot that forms at the injury site is called a **hematoma**. Hematomas are generally caused when large areas of tissue are damaged. When a large bone such as the femur or pelvis is fractured, as much as 1 L of blood can be lost in a confined space within the soft tissue.

Crush injuries are usually caused by extreme external forces that crush both tissue and bone. Even though the skin remains intact, severe damage may occur to underlying organs.

Open Wounds

In an **open wound**, the skin is broken and the patient is susceptible to external hemorrhage and wound contamination. An open wound may be the only surface evidence of a more serious injury, such as a fracture. Open wounds include abrasions, lacerations, major arterial lacerations, puncture wounds, avulsions, amputations, and impaled objects.

Before managing any patient with open wounds, the paramedic should put on a pair of latex gloves for personal protection against the transmission of blood-borne diseases, such as AIDS or hepatitis, and for the patient's protection from further contamination. In general, the patient with open wounds should be transported if affected by the following conditions:

- The wound has spurted blood (even if bleeding has been effectively controlled)
- The wound is deeper than the outer skin layer
- Hemorrhage is uncontrolled
- There is embedded debris, an impaled object, or extensive contamination
- The wound involves nerves, muscles, or tendons
- The wound involves the mouth, tongue, face, genitals, or a place where a scar would be noticeable or disfiguring
- The wound is from a human or animal bite

Abrasion

An **abrasion**, the least serious type of open wound, is little more than a scratching of the skin surface without penetration of all layers of the skin (Fig. 14-2). Usually, only the epidermis and part of the dermis is lost. A little bleeding may result, but rarely do more than a few drops ooze from injured capillaries. All abrasions, regardless of size, are extremely painful because of the nerve endings involved. A large amount of dirt may be ground into the wound, so contamination should be expected, even though the extent of injury may appear to be minor. Abrasions can pose a threat if large areas of skin are involved as, for example, is often associated with motorcycle accidents when the rider is thrown against the road.

Laceration

A **laceration** results from the snagging or tearing of tissues that leaves a jagged wound that bleeds freely (see Fig. 14-2). However, a laceration can also result from a severe blow or impact from a blunt force. It is usually difficult, by surveying the outside of a laceration, to see what important structures have been damaged, since the jagged edges of the wound tend to fall together and obscure depth. Because the edges of the wound are jagged, healing is not as good as in *incisions* (sharp, even cuts with smooth edges). Skin tissue may be partly or completely torn away, and the laceration may contain foreign matter that can lead to infection. An example of a laceration would be a wound caused by a broken bottle or a jagged piece of metal. Figure 14-3 shows a large laceration caused by a bike-car accident.

Major Arterial Laceration

Lacerations can cause significant bleeding if the sharp or jagged instrument also cuts the wall of a blood vessel, especially an artery (see Fig. 14-2). Bleeding is especially a problem in areas where major arteries lie close to the skin surface, such as in the wrist. Blood loss of 1500 to 2000 mL can be severe in an adult. Children do not tolerate blood loss as well as adults, although initially their compensatory mechanisms may mask signs and symptoms of shock. Though the body has natural mechanisms of defense against bleeding, namely vasoconstriction and clotting mechanisms, if damage is severe enough, clots physically cannot occlude the damaged arteries. If uncontrolled, major arterial bleeding can result in shock and death.

Puncture Wound

A **puncture wound** can result from a number of causes, such as from sharp, narrow objects like knives, nails, and ice picks (see Fig. 14-2). Punctures also can be caused by high-velocity penetrating objects, such as bullets. The apparent damage caused by a puncture is often deceptive; the entrance wound may be small with little or no bleeding, giving no clue to the extent of damage to organs and blood vessels below. A puncture usually does not cause a bleeding problem unless it is located in the chest or ab-

A. Abrasion **B. Laceration**

C. Major arterial laceration
Blood vessel

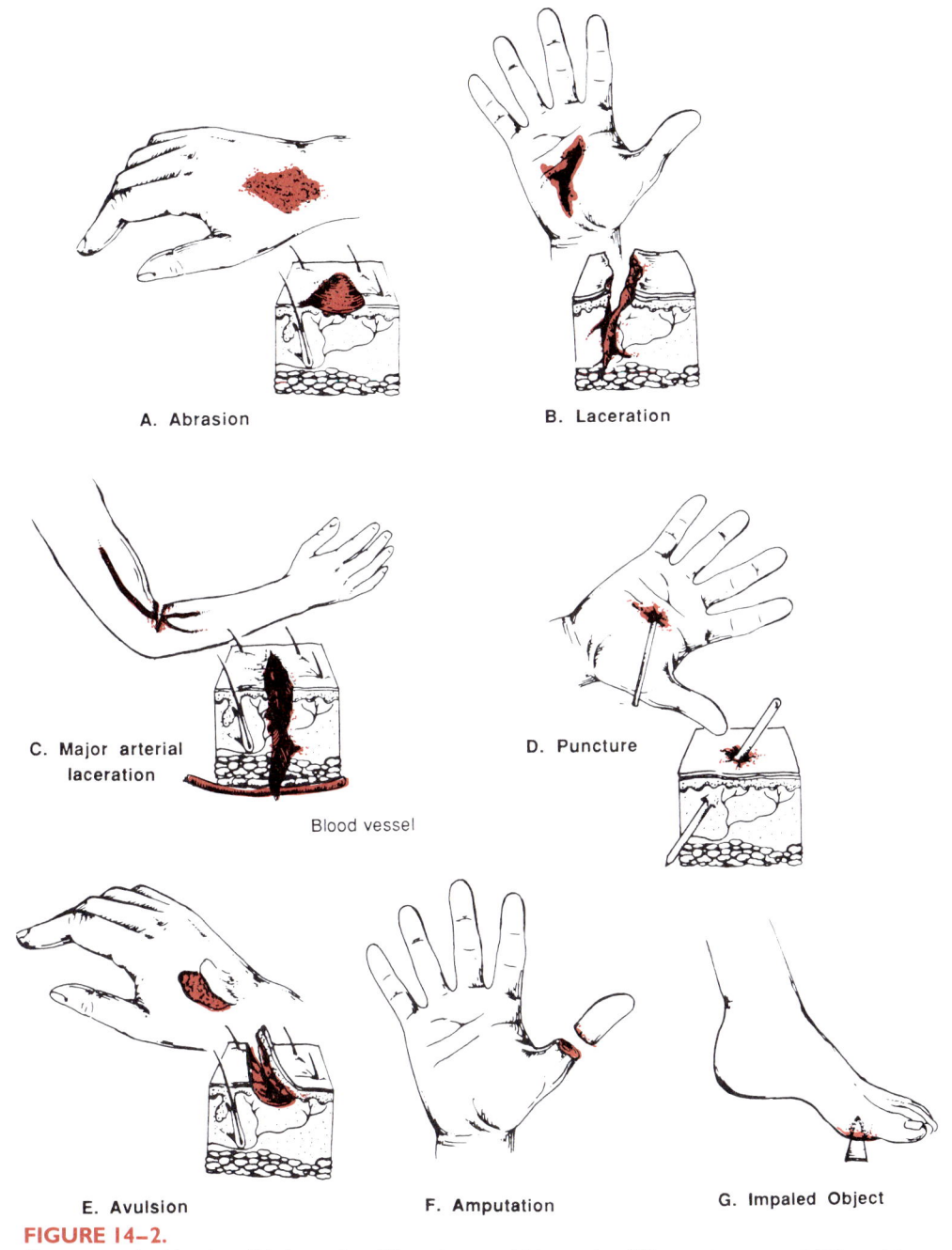

D. Puncture

E. Avulsion **F. Amputation** **G. Impaled Object**

FIGURE 14-2.
Open wounds. Abrasion (**A**), laceration (**B**), major arterial laceration (**C**), puncture wound (**D**), avulsion (**E**), amputation (**F**), and impaled object (**G**).

domen. Bleeding from these areas can be rapidly fatal. Bullets and long, sharp objects can penetrate completely through a body part; thus, a search should be made for exit wounds.

Tetanus can be a serious complication of any open soft-tissue injury. This disease is caused by a soil bacterium introduced into open wounds. As the bacteria grow, they produce a toxin that provokes serious muscle spasms and interferes with breathing. Puncture wounds are fertile ground for the tetanus organism, which flourishes in an oxygen-poor environment. Wounds that are deep and small in diameter are more likely to be oxygen-free. All open wounds are susceptible, however, especially those contaminated by soil. To prevent tetanus, people should be fully immunized in infancy and have a booster immunization of toxoid every 10 years. A booster immunization should be given after an open wound if the patient has not had such an immunization within 5 years.

Avulsion

An ***avulsion*** is the tearing loose of a flap of skin, which may either remain hanging or tear off altogether (see

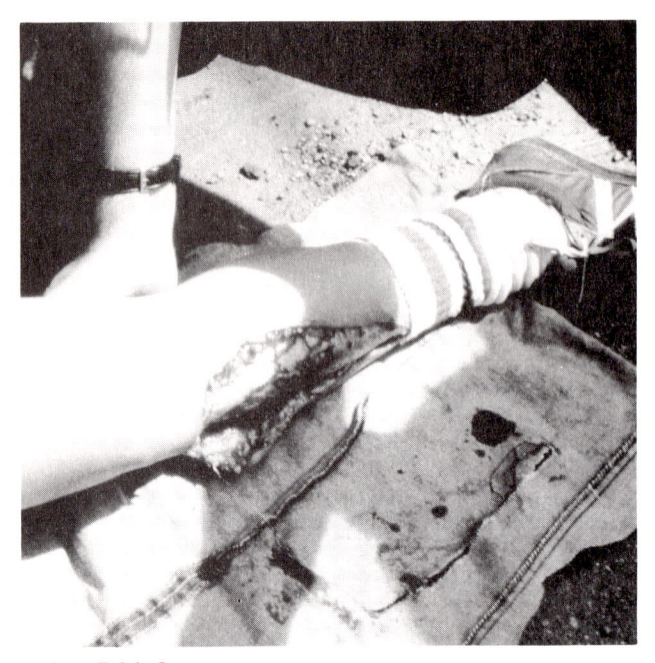

FIGURE 14-3.
Long, jagged laceration caused by a car that hit a child on a bike. Note that the tibia is exposed.

Fig. 14-2). Scarring is often extensive, and avulsions usually bleed profusely. If the avulsed skin is still attached by a flap of skin and the skin is folded back, circulation to the flap can be severely compromised. The paramedic should take care to ensure that the flap is lying flat and that it is aligned in its normal position.

The most commonly avulsed skin on the body is that on the fingers and toes, hands, forearms, legs, feet, ears, nose, and penis. Most often, the patient who presents with an avulsion works with machinery. Home accidents that involve lawn mowers and power tools are common. Avulsions also occur in automobile and motorcycle accidents.

Amputation

The ripping, tearing force of industrial and automobile accidents is often great enough to tear away or crush limbs from the body and cause an ***amputation***. Jagged skin and bone edges characterize the wound, and bleeding may be massive. The initial emergency management of the patient and of the dismembered limb, therefore, is critical.

There are three general types of amputation (Fig. 14-4):

Total or ***complete amputation:*** The body part is completely severed.
Partial amputation: More than 50% of the body part is severed.
Degloving amputation: Skin and adipose (fatty) tissue are torn away, but underlying tissue is left intact.

Because blood vessels are elastic, they tend to have spasms and retract into surrounding tissue in cases of complete amputation; therefore, complete amputations usually cause less bleeding than partial or degloving amputations, in which lacerated arteries continue to bleed profusely.

The most common sites of amputation include: fingers, hands, forearms, ears, toes, below the knee, through the knee, above the knee, penis, and the nose. Figure 14-5 shows a complete amputation.

Impaled Object

A special case of the puncture wound is the ***impaled object*** wound, in which the instrument that causes the injury remains impacted in the wound (see Fig. 14-2). The object could be anything—a stick, a piece of glass, an arrow, a knife, a steel rod—that penetrates any part of the body. This type of injury requires careful immobilization of the patient and the injured part. Any motion of the impaled object can cause additional damage to the surface wound and, particularly, the underlying tissues.

Assessment

The assessment should always begin with an evaluation that notes the patient's responsiveness, airway, breathing, and circulation. As stated earlier, although soft-tissue injuries at times may be visually overwhelming, they are seldom the most serious injury, unless they compromise

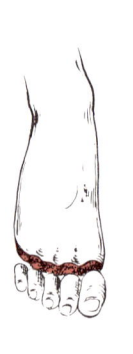

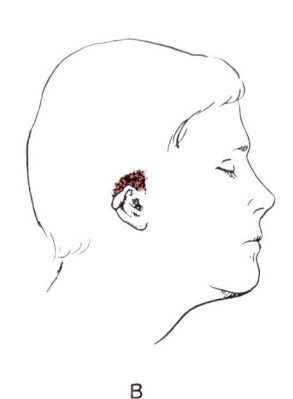

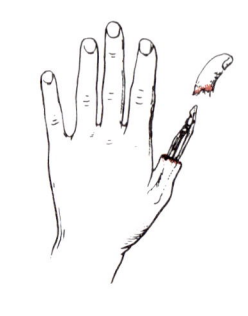

FIGURE 14-4.
Types of amputations. Complete (**A**), partial (**B**), and degloving (**C**).

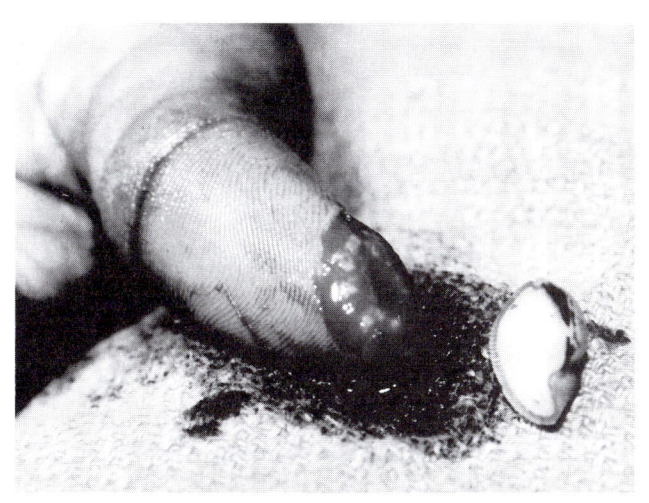

FIGURE 14–5.
Complete amputation of the tip of the thumb.

the patient's airway or circulation (when associated with massive hemorrhage).

The nature of the wound needs to be thoroughly examined when all life-threatening injuries have been ruled out. Once this examination is complete, the wound should be inspected as thoroughly as is possible in the field to gather necessary information about the extent of the wound and involvement of underlying tissues.

Management

Closed and Open Wounds

Management of closed soft-tissue wounds is usually handled by using cold packs or ice. If a closed wound has caused underlying damage, the wound should be handled appropriately, for example, as a fracture would be handled. Management of open soft-tissue wounds is similar in all cases, except with amputation injuries and impaled objects. Bleeding needs to be controlled initially with direct pressure and elevation. Sterile gauze should be used to cover the wound. Once bleeding is controlled, surface dirt and loose debris should be removed. Wound cleaning should be left to hospital personnel. Next, the wound should be covered with a sterile dressing. A roller bandage and 4 × 4 gauze are usually effective as a pressure dressing, which helps to control bleeding. Elevation of the affected part above the level of the heart is effective in the control of both pain and bleeding. At times, it may be necessary to splint and immobilize the injured part. These actions also help to control profuse bleeding and reduce pain. The paramedic should be able to recognize potential injuries that are likely to cause shock and, thus, treat them aggressively. Anytime shock is present, the patient should be properly immobilized and packaged and then transported immediately to the hospital.

Amputations

Management of amputations includes maintaining the patient's vital functions. Remember that trauma great enough to cause an amputation may also cause other bodily injury.

The limb, if crushed, may not bleed a great deal. Any hemorrhage should be controlled by direct pressure and elevation. The use of a tourniquet should be reserved as a last resort and only as a lifesaving means. Care should be taken so that blood vessels are never clamped in an attempt to control bleeding. Rather, the injured blood vessels should be preserved in case the amputated part can be reconstructed. If necessary, a blood pressure cuff or pneumatic anti-shock garment can be used to help control bleeding.

After bleeding has been controlled, apply a dressing to the amputated stump and wrap the end of the stump with an elastic bandage to replace hand pressure. Monitor the wound for a recurrence of bleeding. If the amputation was a degloving injury, apply a saline-soaked dressing held in place with a bandage. Never apply ice.

Do not waste time in the field searching for amputated parts, and do not neglect patient care to search for amputated parts. If they cannot be found easily, assign someone to the task. Amputated parts should be handled in the following manner:

1. Put on latex gloves.
2. Separate the severed part from dirt and other foreign matter; rinse with a saline solution, but do not immerse in liquid. Dry the part with sterile gauze or other absorbent material.
3. Wrap the part in dry, sterile gauze, a clean towel, or a clean sheet. Cover the open end with a surgical sponge that has been moistened with saline; hold the sponge in place with sterile gauze.
4. Place the severed part in a plastic bag and seal it shut; place the first bag in a second plastic bag, and seal it shut. The second bag provides added protection against moisture loss.
5. Place the sealed bags in a container of ice or ice water. Never use dry ice.
6. When possible, transport the part with the patient.

Proper handling of a severed part may allow it to be reattached as long as 24 hours after the injury, although reattachment is best within 6 hours.

Impaled Objects

Proper emergency care of impaled objects involves stabilizing the object with a bulky dressing; the technique is best accomplished with the help of a partner. The only time an impaled object should be removed in the field is when it is causing an airway obstruction. For example, if the object is impaled in the cheek, bleeding into the mouth and throat can impair breathing.

If it becomes necessary to remove an object, such as in the above example, a few key points should be kept in mind. Before removing the object, inspect and palpate the inside of the patient's mouth to ascertain if the object has penetrated completely. It is extremely important when removing the object to pull it in the direction in which it entered. This action helps to minimize further damage to the tissues and helps to reduce bleeding at the site. After removal, aggressively control any active bleeding and dress the wound properly. It may be necessary to pack the inside of the cheek, between the cheek wall and the teeth, with sterile gauze to help control bleeding and, thus, decrease the risk of aspiration.

In cases of other impaled objects, clothing should be removed from around the wound, taking painstaking measures to ensure the object is not moved or disturbed. Though bleeding is best controlled by direct pressure, do not exert any pressure on the impaled object itself or on the tissue margins around the cutting edge of the object. The object is best stabilized with bulky dressings and bandage. The impaled object itself must be completely surrounded by bulky dressings. The goal is to pack dressings around the object and tape them securely in place so that motion is reduced to a minimum. If possible, at least three fourths of the object must be covered by dressings. The use of a doughnut-type ring pad may also help in stabilization.

Never attempt to cut off, break off, or shorten an impaled object unless transportation is impossible with it in place. If it must be reduced, stabilize it securely before cutting. Remember that any motion is transmitted to the patient and can cause additional tissue damage and shock.

BURN INJURIES

Major Sources of Burn Injury

There are four major sources of burn injury: thermal, electrical, chemical, and radiation (Table 14-1). **Thermal burns,** also called *heat burns*, are a result of heat conducted by hot liquids, solids, and super-heated gases, as well as flame burns that result from fire. **Electrical burns** are caused from contact with low- or high-voltage electricity. Lightening injuries are also considered to be electrical burns. The amount of damage caused by electrical injuries is determined by the type of current, duration of current, voltage and amperage of the current, resistance of the tissue, and path of the current through the body. The damage is actually created by the generation of heat. As the current of electricity flows through the tissue, heat is generated by the resistance of this tissue. Effects from an electrical injury are special and differ from other types of burn injury. Fractures may occur from severe muscular contractions. Special consideration should be given to the spine, since this is a common area injured when electrical current causes violent contractions. Passage of high-voltage electrical current through the heart can disrupt normal electrical activity and result in cardiac standstill, ventricular fibrillation, and, possibly, death. Asphyxiation may also be present. Respiratory arrest may occur if the passage of current includes the brain.

Electrical burns can present with four types of injuries:

Contact burns: These result from the passage of electrical current through tissue. On observation, only a charred entrance and exit wound may be seen, but the greatest amount of damage is internal, with coagulation of blood vessels and tissue necrosis all along the path of the current. Most of the tissue that is injured or destroyed lies deep within the body.

Arc injuries: These occur by an arcing of electricity between two contact points on the skin. Injuries are localized at the termination of current flow. Joints that are flexed are commonly involved; the electrical current exits and reenters skin in an attempt to find the shortest pathway.

Flame or flash burns: These occur when the patient is too close to the electrical source and clothes ignite. The result is a thermal burn.

Lightning injuries: These are caused by a natural phenomenon. Lightning strikes with many thousands of volts and takes only a fraction of a second to strike the ground. The pathophysiology of lightning injuries follows the same laws of physics that high-voltage electricity does. Figure 14-6 shows the exit wound of a lightning burn.

Chemical burns result when wet or dry corrosive substances come in contact with the skin. The amount of injury with a chemical burn depends on the concentration and quantity of the chemical agent. Mechanism of cell death is from coagulation of proteins. Exposure is caused by contact, ingestion, inhalation, or injection.

Radiation burns are similar to thermal burns and can occur from overexposure to ultraviolet light (*sunburn*) or from the heat of an atomic explosion. Nuclear radiation burns can vary in severity, depending on the distance between the patient and the heat of the atomic explosion.

TABLE 14-1.
MAJOR SOURCES OF BURN INJURY

Type	Source
Thermal	Hot liquids, solids, super-heated gases, flames
Electrical	Low- or high-voltage current, lightning
Chemical	Wet or dry corrosive substances
Radiation	Ultraviolet light (sunburn), atomic explosion

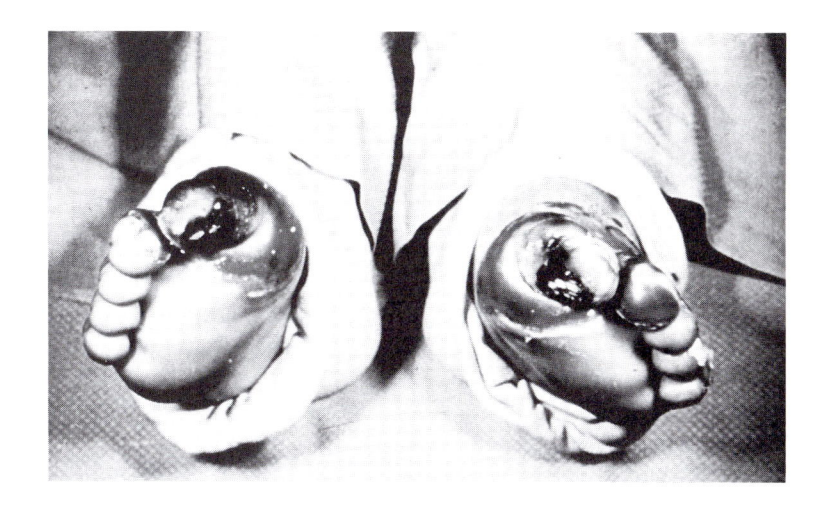

FIGURE 14-6.
Exit wound in the feet caused by a lightning burn.

Pathophysiology of Burn Injury

Loss or damage of the skin from any source results in tremendous local and systemic changes in the physiology of the burn patient. Although the body can sustain burn injury by various means, the local and systemic effects may be common to all. Successful management and treatment of the patient requires understanding the pathophysiology of the burn injury.

Local

Immediately after a burn, venules have spasms, arterioles undergo vasoconstriction, and capillaries dilate. Increased capillary permeability allows fluid to leak into the interstitial space for several hours and is accompanied by inflammation. Fifty percent of extracellular fluid volume may be lost in a major burn through capillary permeability, intracellular shifting into injured cells, and evaporation through destroyed skin. These fluid shifts result in hemodynamic instability, the classic burn shock, if not corrected with adequate fluid resuscitation. The resulting hypovolemia must be treated with large amounts of fluid to maintain cardiovascular homeostasis. Capillary permeability gradually returns to normal in 48 hours, and the resorption of edema fluid begins.

Systemic

Systemic changes are taking place in the body at the same time that local events are occurring. Among the most immediate and severe changes are those in the heart and blood vessels. A drop in cardiac output of as high as 50%, due to intravascular fluid loss, occurs within 3 hours after a major burn. As the intravascular volume falls, the cardiac output decreases further until levels as low as 20% of normal are reached. Myocardial failure can ensue.

The physiologic response presented with inhalation injuries starts with laryngeal spasm and bronchospasm due to steam or toxic fumes that cause smooth muscle reflexes. Marked edema can lead to upper airway obstruction. Eventually alveolar collapse occurs, resulting in atelectasis and unoxygenated blood flows from the right to the left side of the heart, and, finally, pulmonary edema develops. Most patients with inhalation injuries have damage to the tracheobronchial mucosa as a result of inhalation of the noxious products of combustion.

The immune system is depressed by burn injury. Burn patients are more susceptible to infection. Necrotic, moist tissue from a burn provides a perfect medium for pathogen growth, allowing for rapid bacterial proliferation.

Classifications of Burn Injuries

Classification of burn injuries depends on the depth or tissue layers of the skin that are involved. Factors that determine the depth of the burn include the agent of burn, temperature, and length of time exposed. The agent of burn varies according to the source: thermal, electrical, chemical, or radiation. Human skin tolerates temperatures as high as 137°F (44°C) for brief periods of time given certain variations in biologic structure. Above this temperature, tissue destruction occurs. Length of time exposed is determined by how long the agent of burn has been active. Burns can also convert to a deeper degree injury from infection and mishandling.

Once the factors that affect the depth of the burn are understood, burns can be separated into three classifications of injury: superficial (first-degree); partial-thickness (second-degree), either superficial or deep; and full-thickness (third-degree). It should be noted, however, that the depth of tissue burned is not uniform throughout the injury. Full-thickness burns, for example, can have superficial or partial-thickness injuries located around the full-thickness wound. Table 14-2 describes these wounds in detail.

Superficial

Superficial (first-degree) burns are confined to the epidermal layers of the skin. Wounds are characterized by

TABLE 14-2. EVALUATION OF DEPTH OF A BURN

Cause of Burn	Skin Involvement	Symptoms	Appearance	Course
SUPERFICIAL (FIRST-DEGREE)				
Sunburn Low-intensity flash	Epidermis	Tingling Hyperesthesia Painful Soothed by cooling	Reddened; blanches with pressure Minimal or no edema	Complete recovery within a week Peeling
PARTIAL-THICKNESS (SECOND-DEGREE)				
Scalds Flash flame	Epidermis and part of dermis	Painful Hyperesthesia Sensitive to cold air	Blistered, mottled red base; broken epidermis; weeping surface Edema	Recovery in 2–3 weeks Some scarring and depigmentation Infection may convert to third-degree
FULL-THICKNESS (THIRD-DEGREE)				
Fire Prolonged exposure to hot liquids	Epidermis, entire dermis, and sometimes subcutaneous tissue	Painless Symptoms of shock Hematuria and hemolysis of blood likely	Dry; pale white or charred Broken skin with fat exposed Edema	Eschar sloughs Grafting necessary Scarring and loss of contour and function

(Brunner LS, Suddarth DS)

---

erythema (redness), which blanches on pressure. Discomfort occurs from tenderness and edema of the skin. Skin appears dry with no blistering. Most superficial burns are a result of prolonged exposure to the sun or minor scalding injuries. Pain normally subsides after 48 to 72 hours. There is no scarring, and healing time is generally 3 to 7 days with peeling of the outer epidermal layers. Figure 14-7 illustrates a superficial burn.

Partial-Thickness

Partial-thickness (second-degree) burns are further classified into superficial partial-thickness and deep partial-thickness (see Fig. 14-7).

SUPERFICIAL PARTIAL-THICKNESS. *Superficial partial-thickness burns* involve the deep epidermal layers of the skin

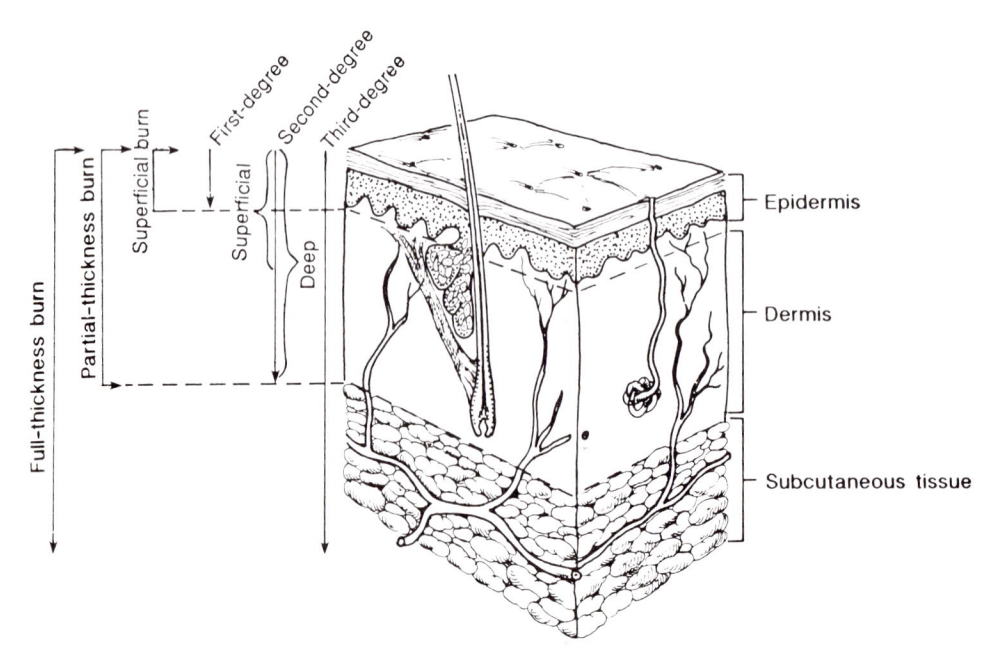

FIGURE 14-7.
Classification of burn injury.

and always cause injury to the upper layers of the dermis. Blisters are formed due to the detachment of the epidermis from the underlying dermis. The burn surface is erythematous, moist, weeping, and very painful. In absence of infection, these burns heal in about 6 to 14 days.

DEEP PARTIAL-THICKNESS. *Deep partial-thickness burns* involve the entire epidermis and extend deep into the dermis. Damage to sweat glands, hair follicles, and sebaceous glands may occur, but tissue death is not complete. Blisters, severe pain, generalized swelling, and edema characterize this type of burn. The skin may appear pink, white, or tan. Scarring is common. Healing time is 14 to 21 days and some grafting may be required.

Full-Thickness

Full-thickness (third-degree) burns are characterized by destruction of both the epidermis and dermis (see Fig. 14-7). Tissue death extends below the hair follicles and sweat glands. The skin appears dry, hard, white, charred, or tan. The area becomes leathery, and clotted vessels may be visible under the burned skin. Full-thickness burns are insensitive to pain immediately after injury because of the destruction of nerve endings. The skin cannot heal itself, and grafting is required. Severe full-thickness burns may even involve damage to the subcutaneous tissue, muscle, and bone. Healing time may take several weeks or months. Scarring is a serious problem. Figure 14-8 shows a full-thickness burn.

Calculation of Body Surface Area

The extent of ***body surface area (BSA)*** burned can be estimated several different ways. Each method calculates the percentage of body surface occupied by individual sections of the body. To determine the extent of BSA burned, the percentage of superficial, partial-thickness, and full-thickness burns should be recorded. This process may seem easy; however, initial evaluation of the extent of injury is often poorly estimated.

Rule of Palms

One method, called the **rule of palms,** is based on the assumption that the palm size of the burn patient is about 1% of the patient's total BSA. Therefore, estimating the number of "palms" that are burned approximates the percentage of BSA involved. This method gives a rough estimate and only should be used to calculate surface area that is minimally burned.

Rule of Nines

The **rule of nines** is another and more accurate method of determining the extent of burn injury (Fig. 14-9). With this technique, in the adult, 9% of the skin is estimated to cover the head and each upper extremity, including front and back surfaces. Twice as much, or 18%, of the total skin area covers the front and back of the trunk and each lower extremity, including front and back surfaces. The area around the genitals, called the perineum, represents the additional 1% of BSA. In the infant or child, the percentages remain the same with the exception of the head, which is 18%, and each lower ex-

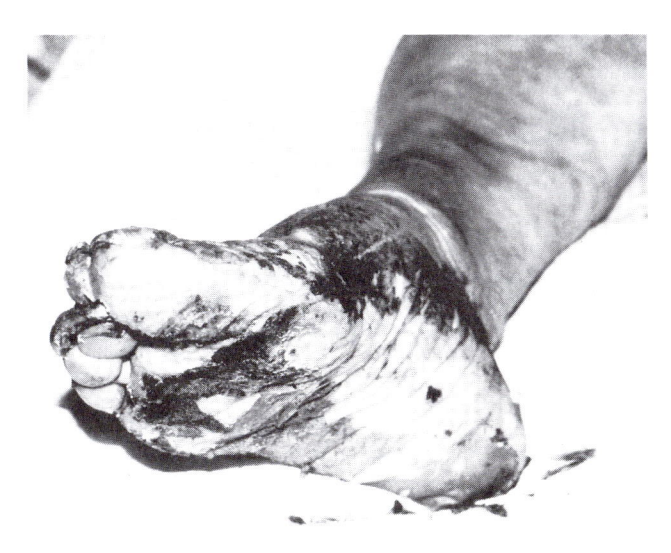

FIGURE 14–8.
Full-thickness burn to the foot. Some partial-thickness burns are also noted.

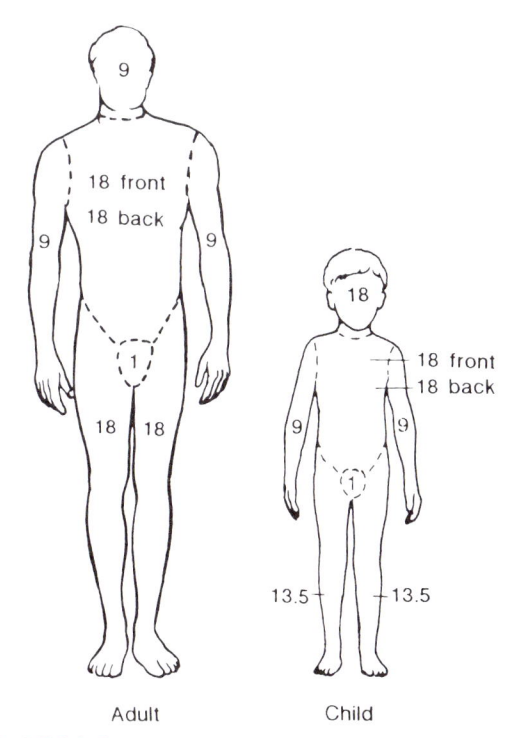

FIGURE 14–9.
Rule of nines.

tremity, which is 13.5% of total BSA. The rule of nines works well in adults but does not reflect the various anatomical growth differences seen in children.

Lund—Brower Chart

A special table, called the **Lund—Brower chart,** is the most accurate method of assessing the extent of the burn (Fig. 14-10). Consideration is given to both the growing child's head-to-chest ratio, which is greater than in adults, and the extremities, which are of a different proportion. Figure 14-11 is an example of an actual burn chart.

Severity of Injury

Factors That Affect Severity of Injury

When burns involve large areas of the skin, treatment and prognosis for recovery depend in a large part on the severity of the burn. The severity of injury is determined by the depth of the wound as well as the extent (percent of BSA burned) of the wound. Additional factors include location, age and general health of the patient, and associated injuries, as shown in the box, "Factors That Affect Severity of Injury."

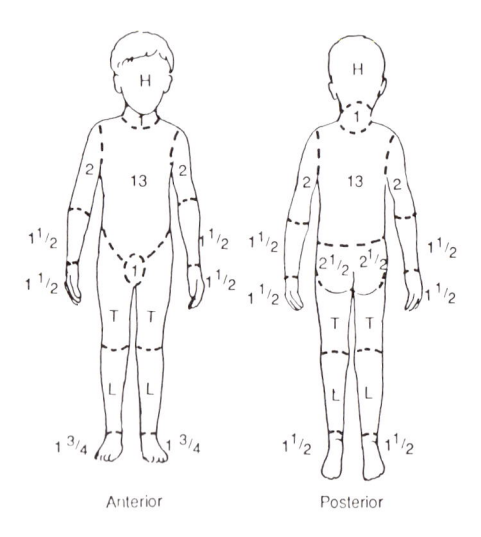

FACTORS THAT AFFECT SEVERITY OF INJURY

Depth of the burn
Extent of the burn
Location
Age
General health
Associated injuries

DEPTH OF THE BURN. It has already been shown that the depth of the wound is determined by the tissue layer of the skin involved. The greater the depth, the more severe the wound.

EXTENT OF THE BURN. Extent of the burn can be determined from one of three methods previously discussed: rule of palms, rule of nines, and the Lund—Brower chart.

LOCATION. The location of the burn injury is another factor in severity. Burns of the face, neck, hands, perineum, and feet even if small can become debilitating, requiring hospitalization and special care. Each of these areas present specific consideration regarding treatment, reconstruction, and eventual rehabilitation.

AGE. The age of the patient is an important factor in determining the outcome; the infant, child, and elderly are seriously affected by burn injuries. These age groups are not able to handle severe stress well, and the thickness of the dermal layer of the skin is thinner in the very young and old. The same injuries that cause a partial-thickness burn in a young adult could result in a full-thickness burn in the thinner skin of a very young or old person. The people who respond best to therapy are those between 5 and 34 years of age. The mortality rate can be estimated by subtracting from the patient's age the percentage of full-thickness burn involved. Therefore, a patient who is 50 years old with 30% full-thickness burns would have a 20% chance for survival.

GENERAL HEALTH. Along with age, the underlying health of the patient before the burn injury plays a major role. Prior existing disease states, such as diabetes, hypertension, and cardiac or pulmonary diseases, often complicate the treatment and increase mortality. Medications taken because of preexisting disease are also considered a factor.

ASSOCIATED INJURIES. Associated injuries can complicate the care of the burn-injured patient. Fractures or internal injuries that may be suffered from explosions, motor vehicle accidents associated with fire, or falls when jumping from burning buildings can alter the eventual outcome of the burn-injured patient.

Lund-Brower Method for % Burn Injury

Age (years)	0	1	5	10	15	Adult
H - 1/2 of head	9 1/2	8 1/2	6 1/2	5 1/2	4 1/2	3 1/2
T - 1/2 of thigh	2 3/4	3 1/4	4	4 1/4	4 1/2	4 3/4
L - 1/2 of leg	2 1/2	2	2 3/4	3 1/4	3 1/4	3 1/2

% Second-Degree + % Third-Degree = Total % Burned

FIGURE 14–10.
Lund–Brower chart. This method takes into consideration changing BSA due to growth.

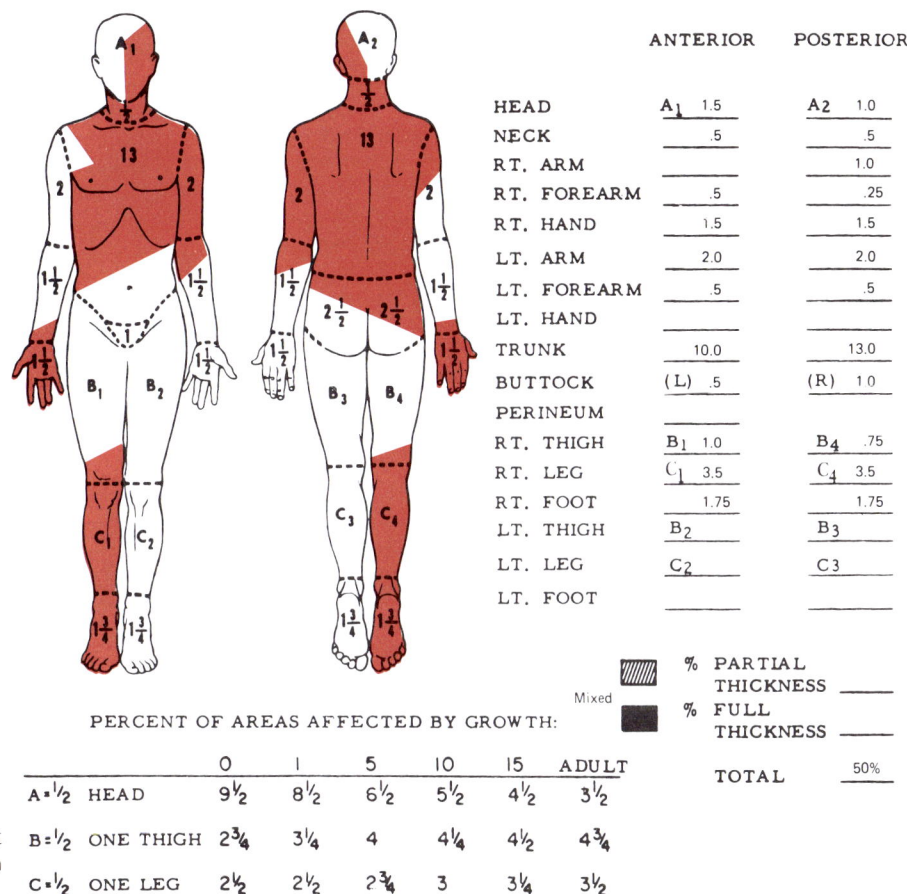

FIGURE 14-11.
Burn evaluation chart estimates percent of body burns. (Brunner LS, Suddarth DS)

Categories of Burn Injury Severity

A careful calculation of the percent BSA injured and associated factors forms the basis of the American Burn Association Burn Severity Index (Table 14-3).

Categories of Injuries

Inhalation Injuries

Suspicion of an inhalation injury should never be ruled out. This type of injury demands immediate and intense therapy. Inhalation injuries most commonly result from steam or toxic fumes. Fire victims surrounded by smoke and fire in a closed space are likely candidates for this type of injury. Inhalation injuries account for more than half of the burn deaths every year.

CARBON MONOXIDE. Carbon monoxide poisoning presents itself in a patient trapped in a closed, poorly ventilated space. A house fire produces vast amounts of carbon monoxide. The fire consumes all the available oxygen, and carbon monoxide is a product of incomplete combustion. Exhaust fumes from a motor vehicle running in a closed garage or furnaces with poor ventilation create harmful levels of this toxic gas. **Carbon monoxide** is a colorless, odorless, and tasteless gas. It passes through the lungs and combines with hemoglobin to produce *carboxyhemoglobin*. Oxygen is displaced, since carbon monoxide has an affinity for hemoglobin 200 times greater than oxygen. The greatest component of damage, however, is at the cellular level in the mitochondria. Early signs and symptoms are headache, nausea, and vomiting with loss of manual dexterity. The skin has a pink color, and mucous membranes are cherry red, unless associated hypoxia is present. Moderate levels in the blood produce confusion, lethargy, depressed ST segments as well as all the early signs. Eventually, coma and death ensue if intervention does not occur. The hypoxia that results from carbon monoxide poisoning is caused by a decrease in circulating oxygen and may result in permanent or recurring central nervous system damage.

SMOKE INHALATION. Smoke inhalation damages the lungs and is caused by products of incomplete combustion. More than 200 toxic fumes are produced from wood and too many to determine from burning synthetics. Burning synthetics, such as polyvinyl chlorides, produce hydrochloric acid (HCL) gas. Burning Freon produces phosgene (mustard) gas. Others have cyanide gas as a by-product. Many of these products are toxic to airway

TABLE 14-3. AMERICAN BURN ASSOCIATION BURN SEVERITY CLASSIFICATION

Burn Classification	Characteristics	Implications for Treatment
Minor burn injury	1° burns 2° burn <15% BSA in adults 2° burn < 5% in children/aged 3° burn < 2% BSA	These patients may qualify for outpatient therapy.
Moderate burn injury	2° 15%–25% BSA in adults 2° burn 10%–20% BSA in children/aged 3° burn <10% BSA	Hospitalization is required. Given adequate staff and facilities, a community hospital may suffice.
Major burn injury	2° burn >25% BSA in adults 2° burn >20% BSA in children/aged 3° burn >10% BSA Burns that involve hands, face, eyes, ears, feet, or perineum Most patients with inhalation injury, electrical injury, concomitant major trauma, or significant preexisting diseases	Care in a specialized burn center is indicated.

mucosa because of their acidity. They may cause severe inflammation, congestion, and marked pulmonary edema. Signs and symptoms may be delayed as long as 12 to 36 hours. It is a general rule that, the earlier the signs and symptoms appear, the more severe the damage.

Signs and symptoms of smoke inhalation include hoarseness, cough, either nonproductive or with production of carbonaceous sputum, singed nasal hair, blisters around the mouth, labored or rapid breathing, facial burns, and restlessness or confusion. Breath sounds may be normal for the first hour or two, with the onset of rales an ominous sign.

Thermal Injuries

Thermal injury to the upper or lower airway is caused by super-heated gases. Dry heat is usually limited to upper airway damage, but steam can penetrate the lower airway. Suspect a thermal injury if facial burns are present. Be alert to the signs and symptoms of any inhalation injury, especially with the onset of rales, which can indicate pulmonary edema.

Eye Injuries

Damage to the eye or eyelid should always be suspected if head or facial burns are present. As a rule, in chemical burns, alkalis are more dangerous than acids since they penetrate the skin faster.

Patient Assessment

A careful history and physical assessment modified to accommodate special considerations for the burn patient should be performed. Since safety is always the main objective, the discussion begins with scene survey.

Scene Survey

The scene survey is the quick, yet observant, evaluation of potential hazards, mechanism of injury, and clues to medical illness that are provided by the patient's environment. An important aspect of scene survey is the assessment of potential hazards to the paramedic and patient. The presence of power lines down, toxic substances, or flames should all be quickly evaluated. In burn emergencies, the number one priority is the safety of the rescuers. Once trained rescue personnel are on the scene, the patient needs to be removed from the source, or in some cases, such as chemical spills, the source needs to be removed from the patient.

Primary Survey

The primary survey is always the first step once the paramedic is at the patient's side. The primary survey includes responsiveness, airway, breathing, and circulation.

RESPONSIVENESS. Checking the patient's responsiveness is the initial determination of the patient's overall level of cerebral function. The cerebrum is the seat of conscious mental processes, and deterioration in this status is one of the earliest signs of hypoxia.

AIRWAY. Evaluate for respiratory distress: look for singed nasal or facial hair, any facial burns, carbonaceous sputum, and carbon or blisters around or in the mouth. Listen for air movement: is it stridulous, labored? Feel for the movement of air.

BREATHING. Continue evaluation for respiratory distress. Be sure to include the trachea as well as the chest wall in the evaluation of breathing. Observe the rate of breathing. Look for any open wounds, watch the rise and fall of the chest, and look for circumferential chest burns that may limit respiratory effort. Listen to the lungs for presence or absence of lung sounds or developing pulmonary edema. Feel for the integrity of the chest wall and the presence of any subcutaneous emphysema.

CIRCULATION. Feel for radial and carotid pulses, and evaluate their strength and rate. Observe for any serious bleeding. Be suspicious of internal bleeding into the chest or abdomen if unexplained signs of shock persist. Check the capillary refill.

Secondary Survey

Perform a head-to-toe survey. Evaluate the extent and depth of the burn and its location, and observe for smoke inhalation or associated injuries. A burn history and medical history should also be conducted, as shown in the boxes, "Burn History" and "Medical History."

BURN HISTORY

How long ago did the burn occur?

Has any treatment been rendered?

Was the patient in an enclosed space?

Did the burn involve steam, smoke, or combustive products?

For what period of time was the patient exposed to the source of the burn?

Did loss of consciousness occur?

What was the specific source of the burn?

Did an explosion occur?

MEDICAL HISTORY

A—Allergies

M—Medications

P—Past medical history

L—Last oral intake

E—Events leading up to this incident

Management

Thermal Burns

Stop the burning process; secure airway and breathing; administer 100% oxygen by mask (humidified is preferred) if breathing is adequate and unlabored. If the patient is unconscious or unresponsive, intubate with an endotracheal tube immediately after hyperventilating with a bag-valve-mask device. Assist breathing with the bag-valve-mask device in the patient who may be awake but breathing inadequately.

Restore circulation and treat for shock. If the patient is in hemorrhagic shock due to associated injuries, apply the pneumatic anti-shock garment if the blood pressure is less than 90 systolic accompanied by a heart rate greater than 120. If the legs or abdomen are burned, place a sterile or clean sheet between the pneumatic anti-shock garment and the patient's skin. If the patient is in shock due to loss of fluid from the burn, start one or two large-bore intravenous cannulas in either burned or unburned areas. Follow one of the burn formulas presented in Table 14-4 for type of fluid and infusion rate. These formulas are calculated based on the patient's body weight and percent BSA burned. In the field, rough estimates of the percent BSA burned can be calculated by using one of the methods described earlier in this chapter. If the situation is extremely urgent, it may be more practical in the field to monitor the blood pressure and heart rate closely, increasing the rate of fluids accordingly.

Remove all jewelry and clothing. Cut around clothes that are burned to the skin; do not pull them off. Maintain integrity of blisters if possible. Bring burned clothing with the patient. Protocol of wet versus dry dressings is still controversial and varies from area to area. The general consensus of many physicians is that, if the BSA involved is less than 15%, high risk problems will not be presented relative to a wet dressing. If BSA is more than 15%, cover burns with dry, sterile dressings. Allowing wet dressings to remain even on small burn injuries invites hypothermia and infection. The paramedic has to evaluate the external environment to avoid overcooling the patient. In any case, follow local protocol established by medical control. Never allow anything, such as creams, ointments, aloe, salves, and butter, to be rubbed onto any burn injury. Separate fingers and toes with moist sterile pads.

If given in the prehospital setting, analgesics should be cautiously prescribed. Always give morphine or meperidine intravenously and in small amounts until the desired effect is achieved. If nitrous oxide is used, be sure it is administered by the patient. Always give patients reassurance. They will have great concern over disfiguration and the extent of care that will need to be provided.

Electrical Burns

Management of an electrical burn includes ensuring that the patient is no longer in contact with the source of current. Defer to rescue, fire, or power company personnel to remove the patient from the electrical current. Treatment of a patient who is suffering an electrical injury often begins with cardiopulmonary resuscitation because of cardiac standstill or ventricular fibrillation. Airway and

TABLE 14-4.
GUIDELINES AND FORMULAS FOR FLUID REPLACEMENT IN BURN PATIENTS

Burn Formula	Colloid	Electrolyte	Water	Rate of Administration
Baxter		4 mL × kg × % BSA burn (no upper limit)		1/2 first 8 hr 1/4 second 8 hr 1/4 third 8 hr
Brooke	0.5 mL × kg × % BSA burn	1.5 mL × kg × % BSA burn (up to 50% max.)		1/2 first 8 hr 1/4 second 8 hr 1/4 third 8 hr
Evans	1 mL × kg × % BSA burn	1 mL × kg × % BSA burn (up to 50% max.)	2000 mL	1/2 first 8 hr 1/4 second 8 hr 1/4 third 8 hr
Parkland		4 mL × kg × % BSA burn (up to 50% max.)		1/2 first 8 hr 1/4 second 8 hr 1/4 third 8 hr
Hypertonic saline	NaCl and lactate with concentration of 300 mEq of sodium may be administered to manage the burn patient without overloading the patient with water. The goal is to increase serum sodium levels and osmolality to reduce edema and lung complications. Several formulas are based on close monitoring of serum sodium and potassium levels or on giving specific volumes based on patient weight. Burn centers that use this technique have specific methods. These methods should be followed.			

breathing control is instituted just as for any burn injury, along with fluid resuscitation. Large amounts of intravenous fluids are used to flush the kidneys of *myoglobin,* a by-product of the breakdown of muscle tissue. Cardiac monitoring is essential if cardiac arrest or arrhythmias occur. Rhythm problems should be treated as any other cardiac problem would be. Dress the injuries with dry, sterile bandages. Be sure to look for any associated injuries, especially fractures of the spine.

Chemical Burns

Chemical burns differ from thermal burns because the topical agent adheres to the skin. Begin flushing immediately with copious amounts of water. Do not use neutralizing agents since these may cause an additional reaction. Flushing should be continued for at least 20 to 30 minutes. It is wise to begin flushing and continue through the transport time. The ideal irrigation fluid is normal saline or sterile water. If a shower or running water is available, take advantage of either for the initial flush of the chemical. Contact lenses should be removed in the case of eye injuries. Flush under eyelids for a minimum of 15 to 20 minutes. Close and cover eyes with a loose sterile dressing after flushing.

Special considerations include chemical irritants such as dry lime. Brush off as much of the chemical as possible, remove clothing, and proceed with flushing. Carbolic

SPECIAL CASES OF CHEMICAL BURNS
Carbolic Acid (Phenol)

Rinse with alcohol if possible before flushing with water. Keep alcohol out of eyes.

Dry Lime

Brush away as much as possible before flushing with water.

Remove all contaminated articles of clothing.

Flush with copious amounts of water.

Hydrofluoric Acid

Flush with copious amounts of water for a minimum of 15 minutes.

Remove all contaminated articles of clothing.

Administer 100% oxygen.

Lye

Do not induce vomiting if ingested.

Flush with copious amounts of water if external.

Sulfuric Acid

Rinse with soapy solution, if possible, before flushing with water.

acid (Phenol) is widely used as a cleaning solvent. Since it is not water soluble, alcohol should be used for flushing. Do not put alcohol in the patient's eyes. If alcohol is unavailable, large amounts of water will suffice. Lithium and sodium metals react with water, releasing toxic fumes as well as heat. Large chunks should be placed in oil. Copious amounts of water should be used to irrigate.

The box "Special Cases of Chemical Burns" discusses management of some of these burns.

Radiation Burns

Radiation injuries should be handled the same as thermal injuries, making sure the patient is away from the source. Associated injuries from possible explosions should be handled appropriately.

Inhalation Injuries

Close observation of the upper airway is required in inhalation injuries to avoid serious complications. Management may require endotracheal intubation in unconscious patients. If patients are awake, place them in a comfortable position, usually high Fowler's. Administer 100% (humidified preferred) oxygen. A demand valve or a bag-valve-mask device should be used if respirations are inadequate. Significant laryngeal edema demands early endotracheal intubation to avoid upper airway occlusion.

Eye Injuries

Chemical burns to the eyes are extremely serious. The body's response to foreign material is to tightly close the eyes. The eyes must be open for irrigation. Remove contact lenses immediately and begin flushing with water or saline. Never use anything that may cause further injury to the eye. Alkali burns are always more severe, as they penetrate the tissue deeper than acid burns. Minimum flushing time in any case is 15 to 20 minutes. If transport time is not complete after flushing for 20 minutes, skin and eyes can be bandaged with dry, sterile dressings.

Fluid Resuscitation

Several formulas have been developed for fluid resuscitation. Each serves only as a guideline, since appropriate fluid resuscitation is determined by the observation of the patient and vital signs. The greatest loss of intravascular fluid occurs in the first 8 to 12 hours, followed by a continued, more moderate loss over the next 12 to 16 hours. The goals of fluid resuscitation are to replace and maintain effective plasma volume during the period of increased capillary permeability and evaporated surface losses. A large-bore intravenous cannula must be inserted to allow administration of the large quantities of fluid required for resuscitation. Frequently, finding adequate intravenous sites is difficult, especially with burns that involve all four extremities. During the resuscitative phase, access for an intravenous cannula is more important than violation of the burn wound.

Massive fluid resuscitation in the absence of underlying cardiac disease is tolerated well in most burn patients. The burn-injured patient needs a sufficient amount of fluid in the first 24 hours after the burn. Most burn formulas used to calculate fluid resuscitation are based on the patient's body weight and the percent BSA burned (see Table 14-4).

An example of fluid replacement can be illustrated using the Baxter formula as follows: A 132-lb (60 kg) 52-year-old female has suffered 15% partial-thickness and 5% full-thickness burns to her lower extremities.

Fluid: lactated Ringer's or 0.9% NaCl solution
Rate of infusion:

$$\text{Baxter formula: } 4 \text{ mL} \times 60 \text{ kg} \times 20\% \text{ BSA}$$

$$\text{Calculate } 4 \times 60 \times 20 = 4800 \text{ mL/24 hours}$$

Plan to administer: First 8 hours infuse one half of 4800 mL, or 2400 mL = 300 mL/hour; next 16 hours = 2400 mL = 150 mL/hour

The primary goal of fluid resuscitation is to keep the heart rate below 110, the level of normal consciousness, and to keep urine output at least 30 mL/hr. Monitoring and maintaining these vital functions ensure adequate perfusion to the heart, brain, and kidneys.

Prevention and Patient Education

It has been estimated that 75% of all burn injuries can be prevented. Burns usually result from accidents in the home caused by carelessness and ignorance. Clothing is almost always involved in fatal burns. The public must be encouraged to read labels. Flame-resistant clothing is essential, especially for children.

Safety measures that can be employed in the home include the following:

- Avoid oily mops, which can ignite spontaneously
- Do not store paint near sources of heat
- Avoid accumulation of grease on burners and broilers
- Avoid overloading circuits
- Use fuses that are the correct size
- Do not use frayed wires or cords
- Never use electric lights on an artificial Christmas tree
- Screens should be in place in front of fireplaces
- Keep towels, curtains, and clothing away from flames
- Do not smoke in bed
- Use a flashlight instead of matches
- Keep flammable liquids out of the reach of children
- Don't leave children alone with open flames or any other electrical instrument
- Check temperature of bath water before immersing children
- Do not allow children to put fingers in electrical sockets

SUMMARY

Soft-tissue injuries are classified as closed or open. Care should be taken not to cause further contamination of the area injured. Underlying problems, such as shock, should be handled appropriately.

Burn injuries can be devastating to victims. Prehospital care makes a difference in the eventual outcome of these patients. Remember the important points. Put out the fire. Aggressively manage the airway and breathing with necessary oxygen and ventilation. Treat fluid loss with fluid. Treat hemorrhagic shock with the pneumatic anti-shock garment and intravenous fluids, and transport as rapidly as possible to the closest, appropriate facility. The stress of a major burn is often prolonged and unrelenting. The psychological aspect of care is important. Patients need reassurance about their own survival and that of other family members that may have been involved. Recognition of the complexity and severity of the burn is the key to management and treatment of the patient.

SUGGESTED READING

American Academy of Orthopedic Surgeons: Emergency Care and Transportation of the Sick and Injured, 4th ed. Park Ridge, Illinois, ORCO, 1987

Bourn MK: Fire and smoke: Managing skin and inhalation burns. J Emerg Med Serv (14)9:62, 1989

McSwain NE, Kerstein MD: Evaluation and Management of Trauma. New York, Appleton—Century—Crofts, 1987

Rosdahl CB: Textbook of Basic Nursing, 5th ed. Philadelphia, JB Lippincott, 1990

Taylor C, Lillis C, LeMone P: Fundamentals of Nursing. Philadelphia, JB Lippincott, 1989

Tortora GJ, Anagnostakos NP:Principles of Anatomy and Physiology, 6th ed. New York, Harper and Row, 1990

Turnkey D, Lewis F: Current Therapy of Trauma—2. Philadelphia, BC Decker, 1986

US Department of Transportation, National Highway Traffic Safety Administration: Emergency Medical Technician—Paramedic: National Standards Curriculum. Washington, DC, US Government Printing Office, 1985

CHAPTER 15

Injuries to the Head, Neck, and Spine

Injuries to the Head
  Ear Injuries
    Anatomy and Physiology
    Pathophysiology
    Assessment
    Management
  Eye Injuries
    Anatomy and Physiology
    Pathophysiology
    Assessment
    Management
  Nose Injuries
    Anatomy and Physiology
    Pathophysiology
    Assessment
    Management

Skull and Brain Injuries
  Blood Flow to the Brain
  Pathophysiology
  Cerebral Herniation
    Level One
    Level Two
    Level Three
  Cerebral Concussion
  Cerebral Contusion
  Skull Fracture
    Depressed
    Basilar
  Intracranial Hematomas and Hemorrhage
    Epidural Hematoma
    Subdural Hematoma
    Subarachnoid Hemorrhage
    Intracerebral Hemorrhage
  Assessment
  Management

Soft Tissue Injuries to the Neck
  Pathophysiology
  Assessment
  Management
Injuries to the Spine
  Mechanism of Injury
  Pathophysiology
  Assessment
  Management
Summary

BEHAVIORAL OBJECTIVES
On successful completion of this chapter, the reader will be able to:

1. Describe the anatomy and physiology of the ear
2. Explain how infections can spread by way of the eustachian tube
3. Describe how to assess the ear for external and internal damage
4. Describe the management techniques for soft tissue injuries to the ear and for foreign objects in the ear
5. Describe the anatomy and physiology of the eye
6. List common injuries to the eye, giving the assessment and management techniques for each
7. Describe the anatomy and physiology of the nose
8. List the common causes of bleeding from the nose, giving the assessment and management for each
9. Describe the blood flow to the brain and explain the various pressures involved in cerebral blood flow
10. Explain cerebral herniation, including the signs and symptoms found as each part of the brain stem is involved
11. Describe cerebral concussion, cerebral contusion, skull fractures, epidural hematoma, subdural hematoma, subarachnoid hemorrhage, and intracerebral hemorrhage

(continued)

BEHAVIORAL OBJECTIVES (continued)

12. Explain the assessment and management techniques for a head-injured patient
13. Describe pathophysiology, assessment, and management of soft tissue injuries to the neck
14. Describe how mechanism of injury relates clues to types of injury to the spine
15. Describe the pathophysiology, assessment, and management for injuries to the spine
16. Define all of the key terms listed in this chapter

KEY TERMS

The following terms are defined in the chapter and glossary:

amnesia
antegrade amnesia
anterior chamber
aqueous humor
arousal
auricle
basilar skull fractures
Battle's sign
cataract
cerebral concussion
cerebral contusion
cerebral herniation
cerebral perfusion pressure
cerebrospinal fluid (CSF)
cerumen
consciousness
conjunctiva
conjunctivitis
cornea
cribriform plate
Cushing's triad
decerebrate
decorticate
depressed skull fracture
epidural hematoma
epistaxis
eustachian tube
exsanguinate

foramen magnum
hemiparesis
intracerebral hemorrhage
intracranial pressure
iris
kyphosis
lacrimal gland
lens
mastoiditis
mean arterial pressure
ossicles
paresis
priapism
raccoon's eyes
reticular activating system
retina
retrograde amnesia
sclera
sebaceous glands
spinal shock
subarachnoid hemorrhage
subdural hematoma
transtentorial herniation
tympanic membrane
vitreous body
vitreous humor

Each year, thousands of people die from injuries that involve the head, neck, and spine. A majority of victims of motor vehicle accidents have some degree of head injury in addition to neck and spine injuries. Falls, gunshot wounds, assaults, and sports injuries account for most of the remaining incidence of nervous system trauma.

Head trauma is the leading cause of trauma deaths. Typically, these victims are young adults who have been involved in a motor vehicle accident and who have a history of drug or alcohol abuse. Often times, these patients become combative, making patient care difficult to perform. The paramedic should exercise particular caution in approaching and dealing with these patients, since the effects of drug or alcohol consumption may mask the seriousness of the head injury. Skilled care and prudent thinking by the paramedic can often make the difference between recovery and serious neurologic deficits or death. In any significant head injury, cervical spine injury must always be assumed until proven otherwise.

INJURIES TO THE HEAD

Ear Injuries

Cuts and lacerations of the ear can occur frequently; occasionally, a section of the ear may be severed. Treatment for ear injuries should be the same as for other soft tissue injuries. Any avulsed parts should be saved and transported with the patient. To dress an injured ear, part of the dressing should be placed between the ear and the side of the head.

Anatomy and Physiology

The ear functions in hearing and equilibrium. The ear has three divisions: the outer, middle, and inner ear (Fig. 15-1).

The outer ear is comprised of the **auricle** (pinna), a skin-covered cartilaginous framework that projects from the head, and the external auditory canal. This canal, lined with hairs and glands that secrete earwax (**cerumen**), is S-shaped and about 1 inch long and extends to the middle ear.

The eardrum (**tympanic membrane**) separates the external auditory canal from the middle ear. In the middle ear, three tiny movable bones (the **ossicles**) modify and conduct sound vibrations from the eardrum to the inner ear. The eardrum and the ossicles are so delicate that violent vibrations of the air, like those caused by the explosion of a bomb or the firing of a heavy gun, may injure them. The three ossicles of each ear, called the *malleus, incus,* and *stapes,* resemble a miniature hammer, anvil, and stirrup, respectively.

304

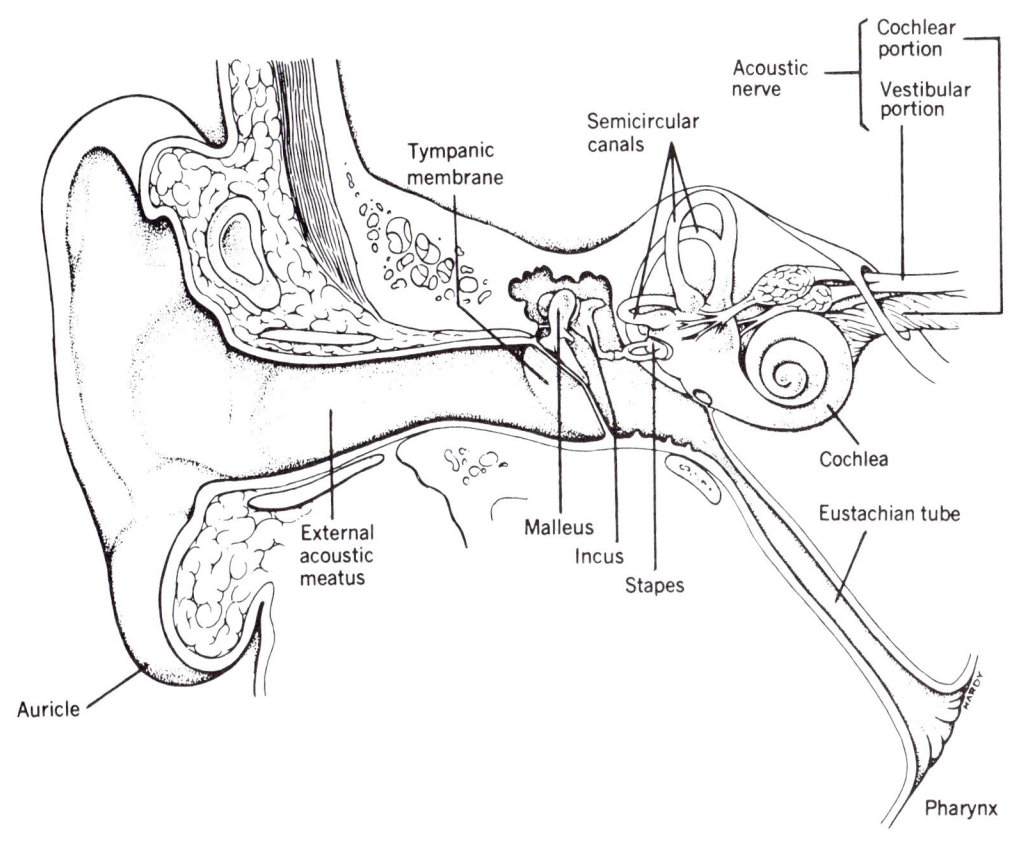

FIGURE 15-1.
Diagram of the ear, showing the external, middle, and internal subdivisions. (Rosdahl CB)

Pathophysiology

Air passes into or out of the middle ear through the *eustachian tube,* which leads to the upper part of the throat. The eustachian tube allows air pressure in the middle ear to equal that of the air that enters the external ear canal. A nose or throat infection can spread to the middle ear by way of the eustachian tube. Blowing the nose may force the infected material into the middle ear. An infection of the middle ear may abscess (form pus), resulting in a discharge from the ear. Sometimes infection may extend from the middle ear to the mastoid cells in the temporal bone and cause *mastoiditis* (inflammation of the mastoid process). When this condition occurs, a brain abscess or permanent deafness may result.

Vibrations of the eardrum caused by sound waves are carried by the ossicles to the inner ear, which is a series of fluid-filled chambers hollowed out of bone. The fluids in the inner ear then vibrate, stimulating various nerve endings, which send impulses to the auditory center in the brain; these are interpreted as sound. When the head and body change positions, the fluid moves; the inner ear has receptors that react to the motion and indicate to the brain which position the head is in and its motion. The brain can then make adjustments to maintain balance. Infections of the inner ear can interfere with these receptors, causing dizziness and imbalance.

In addition to various types of infections that affect the ear, foreign objects can also cause serious damage. Foreign objects in the external ear are a common problem, especially among children. Some children have an irresistible compulsion to stuff their ears with small objects, such as beans and peanuts.

Assessment

Assessing a patient for injury to the ear takes place in the secondary survey or exam. The ear should be assessed for any external damage or bleeding. Blood alone coming from the ear may be the result of damage to the soft tissue of the ear itself. Sometimes this determination is difficult to assess in the field. Both ears should be inspected for blood and clear fluid. A pen light may help perform this assessment. The brain and spinal cord are cushioned and nourished by a clear waterlike fluid called *cerebrospinal fluid (CSF).* A break in the skull can result in the loss of this fluid into the nearby cavities and eventually out through the ears or nose or both. Loss of fluid is an important sign both of basilar skull or cribriform plate fracture. Blood mixed with this fluid is an indication of a fracture to the base of the skull.

Management

Cuts and lacerations about the ear should be treated like other soft tissue injuries. Bleeding is often stopped by direct pressure. It may be necessary to wrap the wound in dry sterile dressings. If CSF is observed leaking from the ear, the ear should be gently packed with sterile dressings. Although blood and CSF leaking from the ear is not a good sign, release of this fluid inadvertently decreases the pressure within the skull. Thus, direct pressure to stop this blood and fluid from leaking should be avoided since this action can, in turn, increase the intracranial pressure.

If a foreign object is lodged within the ear canal, the ear should be left alone, and the patient should be transported to the hospital. An attempt to remove the object in the prehospital setting may cause further damage to the ear and may also create a greater obstruction. The best care for this patient is at the hospital, where good lighting and appropriate equipment are available.

The one possible exception to this rule is when the object, such as corn, beans, or peas, absorbs water and, thus, will swell rapidly within the ear canal. If the distance to the hospital is great, the paramedic may wish to try to flush out the foreign object before transport.

If it is certain that the eardrum has not been perforated, the following measures can be taken:

1. Fill a bulb syringe with alcohol. The alcohol should be close to body temperature.
2. Lie the patient down with the affected ear over a basin. In the case of a small child, the paramedic needs assistance to keep the child still.
3. Place the tip of the syringe near the top part of the entrance to the ear canal, and rapidly flush in the alcohol.
4. Use gentle pressure because forceful flushing can drive the object deeper into the ear canal.
5. If the object cannot be flushed out easily, transport the patient without further attempts.
6. All patients with foreign bodies in the ear should go to the hospital to have the tympanic membrane and the deep portions of the ear canal examined for injury and checked for other foreign bodies.

Eye Injuries

Few true eye emergencies occur; when they do, however, they tend to be urgent. It is important that the paramedic be well enough informed to suspect an eye emergency in the appropriate settings.

Anatomy and Physiology

The eye is a sphere, about 1 inch in diameter, formed by a tough outer coat called the *sclera* and a clear front portion known as the *cornea.* Six muscles are attached to the sclera, and they work in various combinations to move the eye.

The cornea is the window through which light enters the eye. There are no blood vessels in the normal cornea, and it is extremely sensitive and especially susceptible to injury or infection. If scarring occurs from injury, the cornea loses its transparency at the site of the scar, a loss which may markedly impair vision. The cornea has an extremely high concentration of nerve fibers that make it sensitive. A superficial scratch, abrasion, or the smallest foreign object can cause extreme pain with reflex tearing and redness (inflammation) of the eye.

The exposed portion of the white part of the eye (sclera) is lined with a paper-thin covering called the **conjunctiva**; it does not cover the cornea. The conjunctiva may become infected and produce a red eye with a variable amount of pus, mucus, or watery discharge. This infection is called **conjunctivitis.**

The internal portions of the eye are the anterior chamber, iris, lens, vitreous body, and retina. The **anterior chamber,** a space filled with watery fluid called **aqueous humor,** lies between the cornea and the colored portion of the eye (**iris**). The iris is a pigmented muscular structure that opens and closes the pupil to allow more or less light to enter the eye, depending on the level of illumination. This process works much the same as the iris diaphragm on a camera, which controls the amount of light that enters the camera.

Just behind the iris is a structure known as the **lens,** which can change shape to focus light rays on the back of the eye. When the lens becomes cloudy, the condition is called a **cataract.** In middle age, the lens usually becomes less flexible, making it necessary to get glasses for close vision or even for both distant and close vision. Behind the lens is the *vitreous body,* a cavity filled with a clear jelly known as the *vitreous humor.*

The innermost layer of the eye is the *retina,* which has specialized nerve cells that are sensitive to light and color. The retina acts much the same as the film in a camera, except that the retina receives the light rays and converts them into nerve impulses that are transmitted to the brain by the optic nerve. In the brain, the nerve impulses are interpreted as sight.

A *lacrimal gland* (tear gland), located under the outer part of the upper lid, constantly produces tears to keep the eye moist and lubricated so that the eyeball can glide smoothly under the eyelid. When the eye is irritated, tear production is increased to help wash away the irritant.

The eye is protected and cleansed by the eyelids. They spread tears over the front of the eye and tend to wipe away dust and other foreign particles. Along the edges of the eyelids are openings of many small oil glands that help prevent the tears from evaporating too rapidly. The lashes and eyebrows help to prevent foreign material from entering the eye. Figure 15-2 illustrates the anatomy of the eye.

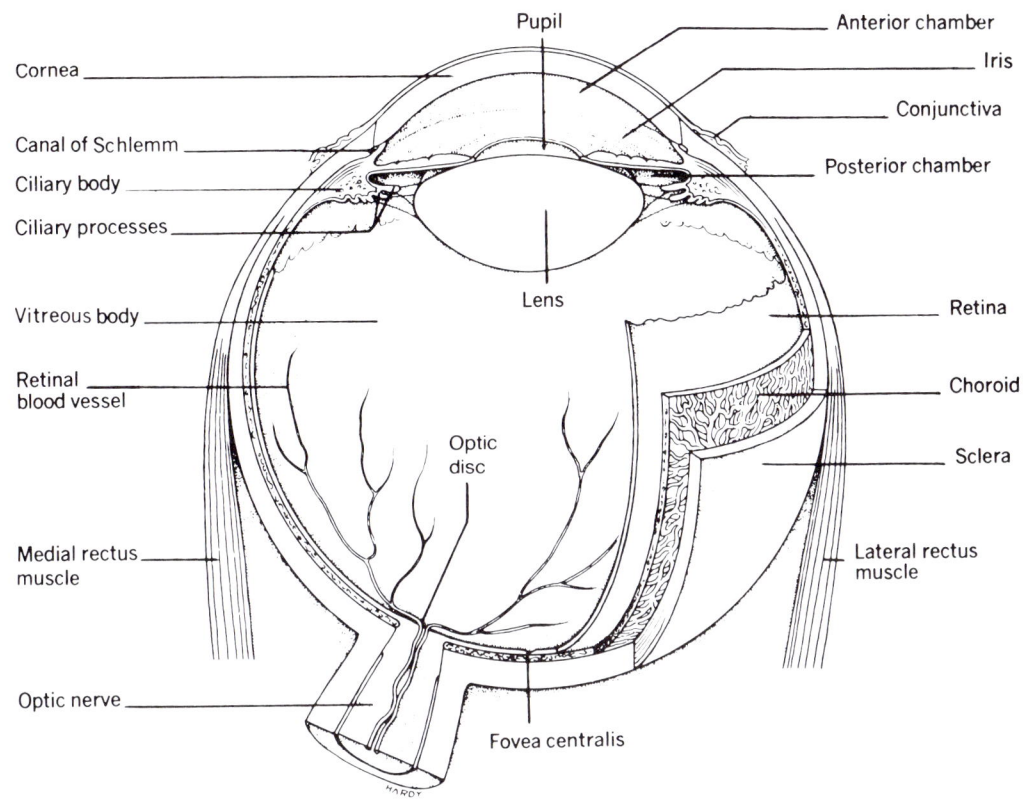

FIGURE 15–2.
Transverse section of the eye. (Brunner LS, Suddarth DS)

Pathophysiology

Eye injuries can be grouped into those caused by foreign objects, those caused by lacerations and contusions, and those caused by chemical, heat, and light burns. The general signs and symptoms of injuries to the eyes include an obvious foreign object protruding from the globe, a swollen or lacerated globe, a bloodshot sclera, a scratched cornea, or a distorted pupil.

The most common eye injuries are caused by flying particles that lodge in the outer surface of the eyeball or under the lid. This type of injury, although relatively minor, is remarkably disabling while the object is present. Most foreign particles are washed away by tears caused by irritation of the globe. The tears are one of the body's defense mechanisms.

Injuries to the soft tissues around the eyes take the form of lacerations and contusions. As in many soft tissue injuries about the face, the outward appearance may not be an accurate indication of the seriousness of the injury. A laceration of the eyelid may appear to be serious, but, as long as the globe itself is not damaged, the person's sight will probably not be lost. On the other hand, a laceration of the cornea or of the sclera, even with no injury to the eyelid, may cause the loss of vision. Lacerated eyelids usually bleed profusely because of the rich blood supply. Direct pressure or a pressure dressing usually is sufficient to stop the bleeding.

Immediate emergency care is absolute when a person's eyes are burned by a chemical. If acid or alkali burns are not treated immediately, irreparable damage may result. In addition, when a person suffers burns of the face from a fire or explosion, the person's eyes usually close instantly in response to the heat; thus, the eyes are protected. The eyelids remain exposed, however, and they may be burned along with the face.

Assessment

Patients with injuries or medical problems that involve the eye should be thoroughly questioned. When did the accident or pain occur? What did the patient first notice? Were both eyes affected? If so, in what way?

Physical assessment of the eyes involves evaluation of the following:

- The *orbits* (eye sockets), for *ecchymosis* (bruising), swelling, laceration, and tenderness
- The lids, for ecchymosis, swelling, and laceration
- The conjunctivae, for redness, pus, and foreign bodies
- The *globe* (eyeball), for redness, abnormal coloring, and laceration
- The pupils, for size, shape, equality, and reaction to light
- Eye movements in all directions, for abnormal gaze, paralysis of gaze, or pain on movement

- A rough assessment of visual sharpness should be made; the paramedic should ask the patient to read newsprint or should employ another simple test; this test is important because it provides aid to the emergency physician in subsequent assessment of the patient

Management

Proper emergency care of the injured eye first requires a thorough examination to determine the extent and nature of any damage. The examination should be performed with great care so as not to aggravate existing injury. Correct initial emergency management minimizes pain and may help prevent permanent loss of vision.

Though most foreign objects are flushed away by the body's natural defense of increased lacrimation, in some cases it is necessary to flush the eye with a sterile solution. Objects that cannot be washed away are usually lodged in the underside of the upper lid. The space under this lid is so extensive that the person is rarely able to extract the foreign body. The paramedic may be able to remove a foreign object by the following technique:

1. Flush the eye with 500 to 1000 mL of warm 0.9% NaCl, holding the eyelids apart.
2. Often, a foreign object lodged under the upper eyelid can be removed by drawing the upper lid down over the lower lid; as the upper lid returns to its normal position, the undersurface is drawn over the lashes of the lower lid, and the foreign body is removed by the wiping action of the eyelashes.
3. A foreign object in the eye may also be removed by grasping the eyelashes of the upper lid and turning the lid over a cotton swab or similar object. The particle may then be carefully removed from the eyelid with the corner of a piece of sterile gauze.
4. Particles lodged under the lower lid may be removed by pulling down the lower lid, exposing the inner surface. The corner of a piece of sterile gauze can be used to remove the foreign object.

If a foreign object becomes lodged in the eyeball, no attempt should be made to disturb it, as it may be forced deeper into the eye and result in further damage. Carefully place a bandage compress over both eyes. Gentleness is essential in handling eye injuries. If difficulty is experienced in removing a foreign object from the eye, the paramedic should transport the patient to the hospital at once.

As previously stated, lacerated eyelids tend to bleed profusely since they are highly vascular. In management of this type of injury, direct pressure to the wound or use of a pressure dressing is usually adequate. Before applying pressure or a pressure dressing to the injured eyelid, make sure that the globe is not injured. If the globe is lacerated, do not use pressure even to stop profuse bleeding from the lid. Instead, cover the bleeding lid with a loose dressing; the dressing absorbs blood, aids in the clotting process, and discourages contamination.

If the jellylike vitreous humor is squeezed from the globe, it cannot be replaced, nor can the body replace the fluid by the natural regenerative processes. Loss of the globe results in blindness.

Torn eyelids should be handled carefully to prevent further injury. They may be covered with a loose dressing, if necessary. Any fragment of eyelid skin that is torn loose should be recovered, wrapped in a wet dressing, and taken to the medical facility with the patient. The physician may be able to use the fragment to repair the damaged eyelid.

An avulsed eye, one that is torn from the socket, should be treated in the same manner as an eye impaled by an object. A dressing should be prepared composed of several layers of a bulky dressing material. A hole should be cut in the center of this pad, and the pad should be placed over the eye so that the injured globe protrudes through the hole. The pad should be moistened so that the globe does not become dry. A protective cup should be secured over the pad with a soft, self-adherent roller bandage. The uninjured eye should also be bandaged to prevent sympathetic eye movement.

Blunt injuries to the eye can be identified by blood that covers the iris or the pupil. In this situation, little can be done except to cover the injured eye and transport the person to a medical facility. A commercially available rigid eye shield is excellent for cases of blunt trauma to the eye.

If injury to the eye occurs as a result of burns—chemical, heat, or light—the only emergency care measure practical is to dilute the chemical by flushing the injured eye with copious amounts of warm sterile water or 0.9% NaCl. Either solution usually is readily available. In any event, never delay treatment. In this technique, the patient's face should be held up under the running water or saline solution. The patient's eyes should be held open so that the globes and underside of the lids may be thoroughly irrigated. Because closing the eyes when they are irrigated is a natural reaction, the patient may find it difficult to keep the eyes open. The paramedic may have to assist the patient by applying traction to the lids while the eyes are being flushed.

If injury is the result of heat, as from an explosion or fire, special treatment is required. Unfortunately, these procedures are not practical in the prehospital setting. Therefore, it is best to transport the patient immediately, without further examination of the eyes. The burned lids should be covered with loose, moist, sterile dressings during transport to the medical facility.

Light injuries can be caused by the flash from an arc welder or by the extreme brightness of the sun as reflected by sand or snow; these burns are generally painful. The patient can be made more comfortable and some of the pain can be relieved if the eyes are covered with dark patches.

Nose Injuries

A specialized structure of the face, the nose is prone to injury primarily because of its location. While injuries to the nose are often minor, they can be life-threatening because they compromise the upper airway, thus impairing the patient's ability to breathe.

Anatomy and Physiology

The nose consists of an external and internal portion. The external portion, that is, the part that protrudes from the face, consists of a bony and cartilaginous framework overlaid by skin that contains many **sebaceous** (oil) **glands.** The internal nose or nasal cavity lies over the roof of the mouth where the *palatine bones*, which form both the floor of the nose and the roof of the mouth, separate the nasal cavities from the mouth cavity. The roof of the nose is separated from the cranial cavity by a portion of the *ethmoid bone* called the **cribriform plate.** The cribriform plate is perforated by many small openings that permit branches of the *olfactory nerve* responsible for the special sense of smell to enter the cranial cavity and reach the brain.

Separation of the nasal and cranial cavities by a thin perforated plate of bone presents real hazards. If the cribriform plate is damaged as a result of trauma to the nose, it is possible for potentially infectious material to pass directly from the nasal cavity into the cranial fossa and surround the brain.

The hollow nasal cavity is separated by a midline partition, the *septum*, into a right and left cavity. In the adult, the nasal septum frequently is deviated to one side or the other, interfering both with respiration and with drainage of the nose and sinuses. The nasal septum has a rich blood supply. Nosebleeds (**epistaxis**) often occur as a result of septal contusions caused by a direct blow to the nose.

The external openings into the nasal cavities (*nostrils*) have the technical name of *anterior nares*. They open into an area covered by skin that is reflected from the wings (*ala*) of the nose. This area called the *vestibule* is located just inside the nasal cavity. Coarse hairs called *vibrissae*, sebaceous glands, and numerous sweat glands are found in the skin of the vestibule. Once air has passed over the skin of the vestibule, it enters the respiratory portion of each nasal passage. The anatomy of the nose is depicted in Figure 15-3.

The nose serves as a passageway for air that goes to and from the lungs. Air that enters the respiratory system through the nasal cavity is filtered of impurities, warmed, moistened, and chemically examined for substances that might prove irritating to the delicate lining of the respiratory tract. In addition, the hollow sinuses act to lighten the bones of the skull and serve as resonating chambers for speech. Finally, the highly sophisticated network of the olfactory system makes the special sense of smell possible.

Pathophysiology

Blood that flows from the nostrils is the most obvious sign of nasal injury. Bleeding may be slight or severe, depending on the location and the severity of the injury. When bleeding from the nose is caused by an injury, look closely for bleeding from the ears and for clear, waterlike CSF; both signs are reliable indicators of a basilar skull fracture or fracture of the cribriform plate. Cerebrospinal fluid

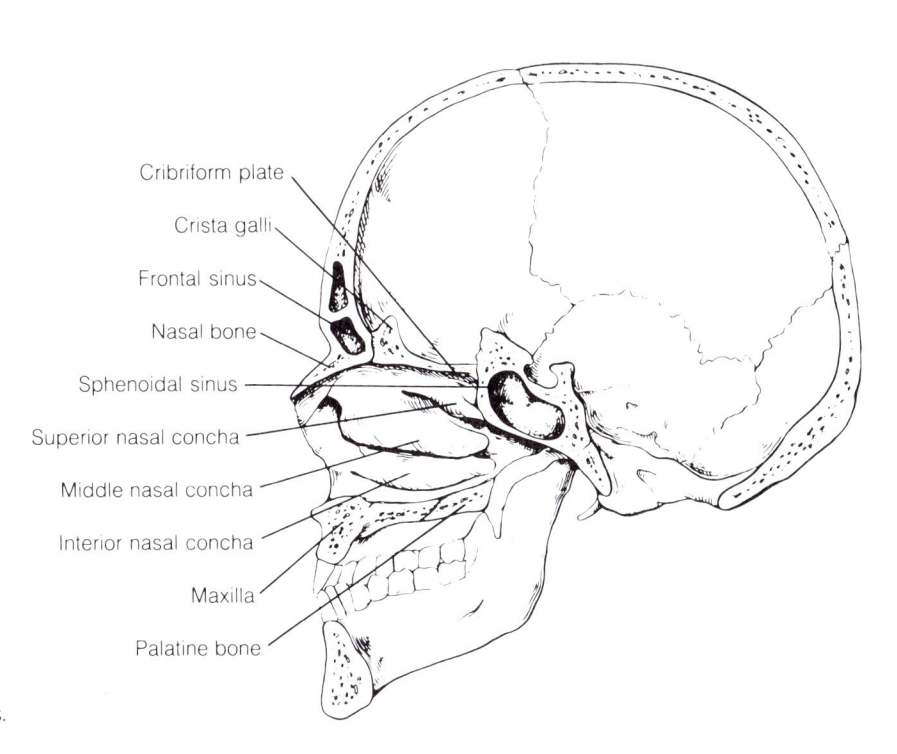

FIGURE 15-3.
Transverse section of the nasal passages.

mixed with blood looks like blood. The CSF can be found by placing a drop of the discharge onto an absorbent piece of paper, such as a paper towel or filter paper. A clear ring "halo" on the outside of the blood is CSF. When bleeding from the nose is attended by pain, swelling, and deformity, fracture of the nasal bones is probable. The nose is not composed entirely of bone. The outermost portion is cartilage; only the rearward third is actual bone.

Bleeding from the nose can result from a number of causes:

1. A fracture of the skull allows blood to seep from the cranium into the sinus cavities and then out the nostrils.
2. Facial injuries that result from blunt trauma usually cause a nosebleed as the delicate blood vessels in the nose are ruptured.
3. Infections within the nose, bleeding diseases, sinusitis, and high blood pressure can all cause a nosebleed.

Beside the bleeding, a problem associated with a nasal fracture is the blockage of the airway. Every effort must be made to assure that the injured person has an open airway. Careful application of cold helps to reduce swelling, bleeding, and pain.

Assessment

Though injuries to the nose may not appear severe, they should never be underestimated. While a nosebleed is usually of little consequence, at times it may be a sign of serious injury. Prolonged uncontrolled bleeding of any type can cause shock.

Management

Caring for nasal injuries usually is conservative, directed toward stopping the flow of blood and positioning the injured person so that blood does not drain into the throat and, thus, into the stomach. Since blood is an irritant to the lining of the stomach, nausea and vomiting are likely to ensue, potentially resulting in aspiration of the vomitus into the lungs.

When a skull injury is indicated by blood, clear fluid, or a mixture of the two flowing from the nose and ears, no attempt should be made to stop the flow. This charge may seem contrary to the principle of controlling hemorrhage; allowing the fluids to flow, however, actually vents dangerous pressures that may result from the build-up of fluid within the cranium, pressures that can injure vital brain centers.

Bleeding from causes other than a skull fracture can be controlled by a simple technique. Keep the person in a sitting position, if possible; this position prevents blood that is flowing into the back of the throat from being automatically aspirated into the lungs. If no complicating nasal fractures exist, the nostrils should be pinched closed. This action applies direct pressure to the bleeding vessels, most commonly located in the venous plexus on the anterior nasal septum. Simple bleeding usually stops within a few minutes after pressure is applied in this manner. It is important to keep the person quiet. Anxiety tends to increase blood pressure, and increased pressure causes increased blood flow at an injury site. Associated conditions that produce hemorrhage, such as hypertension, must be ruled out.

Having to stand and hold a person's nostrils pinched shut may not be practical, especially if there are other people to care for in a multiple casualty situation. Several alternatives are available. The injured person may be able to pinch the nostrils together, or a rolled bandage can be placed between the person's upper lip and gum and held in place. These techniques should control the bleeding. Application of cold also helps to stop a nosebleed since cold constricts blood vessels. An ice pack or a chemical cold pack can be used. Lacking these, even a cold, wet cloth can be applied to the injured person's nose, making sure the head is tilted forward.

If bleeding cannot be controlled by any of the techniques described, it may be necessary to pack the patient's nostrils with gauze and then apply pressure with the fingers. A short tail of gauze is left protruding from the nostrils so that the pack can be easily removed.

Nasal fractures rarely need to be immobilized in the field. However, one technique can be applied if unusual situations arise and immobilization is indicated. A roll of narrow bandage can be placed along each side of the nose and held in place with tape.

Like the ears, a variety of foreign objects find their way into nostrils, especially in those of children. Flying insects can be inhaled as well. If the object protrudes, do not pull it out. If it is sharp, it may have penetrated the septum or the tissues high in the nose; carefully transport the person without disturbing the object.

If the object cannot be seen, do not probe for it. Probing may only force the object higher into the nose, thus complicating its removal by a physician. Have the person gently blow through the nose but not while holding one nostril closed, as seems the natural thing to do. Do not allow the person to blow forcefully. If the object cannot be dislodged in this manner, transport the person to a medical facility.

Injuries with sharp objects may result in avulsion of the tip of the nose. A pressure dressing should be placed on the injury site, and the avulsed part should be recovered, if possible. Pack the part in a cool, wet, sterile dressing and transport it with the patient to a medical facility.

Skull and Brain Injuries

Collision of the head with a fixed object can cause multiple skull and brain injuries. Damage depends on the speed at which the head was traveling and its position just before contact. It is essential to report this information to the base physician at the hospital, because concerns about patient care are based, in part, on mechanisms of injury.

The incidence of head injuries is high because the head has relatively little support. The bony cranium, or skull, forms a tightly closed box around the brain with an opening for the spinal cord called the **foramen magnum.** It is especially thin in the temporal region. The base of the skull is rough and irregular, and these irregularities can bruise and lacerate the brain when the head is jarred suddenly or when rapid deceleration occurs. Anatomy and physiology of the skull and brain is found in Chapter 22.

Blood Flow to the Brain

Blood flow to the brain is remarkably constant despite changes in blood pressure, temperature, and internal activity. Cerebral blood flow begins to decrease when the **mean arterial pressure** drops to 60 mm Hg.

$$\text{Mean arterial pressure} = \frac{\text{pulse pressure}}{3} + \text{diastolic pressure}$$

(Pulse pressure is equal to the systolic pressure minus the diastolic pressure)

Arterial $PaCO_2$ concentration has a profound effect on cerebral blood flow. When $PaCO_2$ rises above normal (35–45 mm Hg), cerebral blood vessels dilate. When $PaCO_2$ drops below 30 mm Hg, the vessels constrict, therefore taking up less space. This response results in temporary lowering of the intracranial pressure.

The **cerebral perfusion pressure** depends on the mean arterial pressure and the **intracranial pressure.**

Cerebral perfusion pressure
= mean arterial pressure − intracranial pressure

The difference between these pressures (the mean arterial pressure and the intracranial pressure) is normally sufficient to maintain adequate cerebral perfusion. However, if the intracranial pressure is increased through cerebral edema or hemorrhage, cerebral perfusion pressure is decreased and blood flow to the brain is decreased. The change in cerebral perfusion pressure is the same with rising intracranial pressure or a falling mean arterial pressure. If the intracranial pressure becomes equal to or exceeds the mean arterial pressure, blood flow to the brain effectively ceases. Therefore, it is necessary to maintain an adequate mean arterial pressure as well as reduce an elevated intracranial pressure in the head-injured patient.

Pathophysiology

Unconsciousness stems from injury either to the cerebral cortex or the brain stem's reticular activating system. The **reticular activating system** functions in general wakefulness (**consciousness**) and causes **arousal**, that is, awakening from deep sleep. Nerve impulses pass upward from the brain stem and disperse to widespread areas of the cerebral cortex (Fig. 15-4). An increase in intracranial pressure and a decrease in cerebral blood flow, no matter what the cause, can depress the level of consciousness. Rising intracranial pressure produces complications because the brain is enclosed in a rigid box. An increase in one area occurs at the expense of another compartment. If the brain tissue itself swells, or if a rapidly growing hematoma is present, all possible CSF is eliminated and blood volume is reduced to as low a level as is compatible with life.

The pressure in the arteries of the skull normally exceeds the intracranial pressure by a considerable margin. When the intracranial pressure increases and approaches the mean arterial pressure, the blood vessels are squeezed from the outside. Blood flow throughout the arteries becomes more and more restricted. The baroreceptors, sensing the resulting drop in blood pressure, stimulate the sympathetic defenses, and the blood pressure increases.

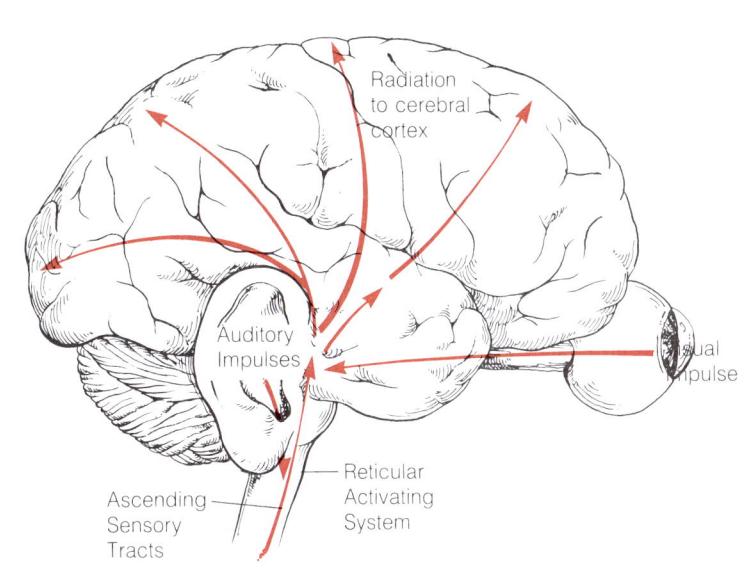

FIGURE 15–4.
Reticular activating system.

The respiratory defenses and various changing respiratory patterns occur based on the chemoreceptors' sense of changes in the blood chemistry. The increasing intracranial pressure also applies pressure on the vagus nerve, resulting in a slowing pulse. This threefold phenomenon associated with increasing intracranial pressure—rising blood pressure, slowing pulse rate, and changes in respiratory pattern—is known as **Cushing's triad** (or response) and when seen should be recognized as a clear but late sign of increasing intracranial pressure.

Increases in intracranial pressure cause alterations in the level of consciousness, leading to unconsciousness, deficits in vital function, and, ultimately, brain death due to loss of adequate cerebral perfusion pressure. Cerebral perfusion must be maintained to keep the brain alive. If edema continues, or if a hematoma continues to enlarge, the brain has nowhere to go except to herniate through the tentorium and eventually through the foramen magnum.

Cerebral Herniation

Cerebral herniation is the protrusion of a portion of the brain through an opening in the wall of the cranial cavity. The tentorium, a portion of the dura, forms a covering over the cerebellum. There is an opening called the incisura in the tentorium at the junction of the midbrain and the cerebrum. The brain stem lies almost directly below this opening. The incisura is the weakest point in an otherwise closed cranial vault. Therefore, increasing intracranial pressure can force a portion of the temporal lobe to herniate through this opening. **Transtentorial herniation** occurs when the falx cerebri is displaced. The *falx cerebri* is a sickle-shaped fold of the dura mater that is found in the longitudinal fissure (the structure that separates the two cerebral hemispheres). Progressing in a head-to-toe direction, the expanding brain herniates through the falx, tentorium, and then through the foramen magnum.

One of two clinical pictures may be observed once the brain begins to herniate. If the brain stem is compressed directly from above, the condition is called *central syndrome* (Fig. 15-5). In this type of herniation, the downward movement of the brain displaces the ventricular system. This condition occurs from masses such as large cerebral contusions, frontal lobe tumors, and subdural hematomas. The other type of herniation is referred to as the *lateral* or *uncal syndrome* (see Fig. 15-5). This condition involves the compression of the midbrain and brain stem by the herniating tip of the temporal lobe (the uncus) through the tentorial notch. Uncal herniation may result from an epidural hematoma (middle meningeal artery bleed) or linear skull fractures of the temporal bone, which also carry a high risk of lacerating the middle meningeal artery.

Differing signs and symptoms occur as pressure intensifies and lower areas of the brain stem are affected. They can be categorized or grouped into three levels that correspond to the amount of brain involvement. All three levels measure or involve vital signs, pupil reaction, and response to stimuli.

LEVEL ONE. As the cerebral cortex and upper brain stem become involved, blood pressure rises and the pulse rate slows. Pupils may be constricted but remain reactive. The patient may go from slow shallow breaths to rapid deep breaths, returning to slow shallow breaths again, followed by a period of apnea. Then the pattern is repeated. This type of breathing is called Cheyne-Stokes respiration and is a response to lowering PaO_2 and rising $PaCO_2$.

Patients initially try to localize and remove painful stimuli. Later they withdraw from pain, and, still later, pain evokes **decorticate** posturing (flexion of the upper extremities with the lower extremities rigid and extended). This stage of compression usually is reversible with prompt surgical intervention to remove the compressing force. The need for rapid transportation and hyperventilation to reduce intracranial pressure is clearly evident in this case.

LEVEL TWO. As the middle portion of the brain stem becomes involved, the blood pressure continues to rise. The pulse rate becomes slower. The pupils become fixed at 3 to 5 mm and become nonreactive or only sluggishly reactive to light. The abnormal respiratory pattern continues (Cheyne–Stokes respiration) and often becomes that of central neurogenic hyperventilation, that is, a fast shallow panting. When a painful stimulus is applied, the patient may exhibit **decerebrate** posturing (upper extremities extended and rotated inward with palms facing lateral; lower extremities extended and rigid). Few patients who reach this stage ever function normally again.

LEVEL THREE. As the lower portion of the brain stem is compressed, one or both pupils may become fixed and dilated. A "blown" pupil is on the same side as the hematoma or swelling that is causing herniation. The crossover of the nervous system, which creates the effect that the right side of the brain controls the left side of the body, basically occurs at the level of the spinal cord (just below the eyes). Hence, the right pupil is controlled by the right side of the brain and the left pupil by the left side. It is important to remember which pupil dilated first. This information is a clue to which side of the brain has the hematoma. Structures innervated by cranial nerves produce signs on the same side as the lesion.

Ventilation may become *ataxic* (erratic breathing with no rhythm) or absent. No response to painful stimuli is found, and the patient becomes flaccid. At this stage, the medulla oblongata becomes involved. The pulse becomes rapid and irregular, and the blood pressure drops. It is important to recognize these developing signs and react to them rapidly.

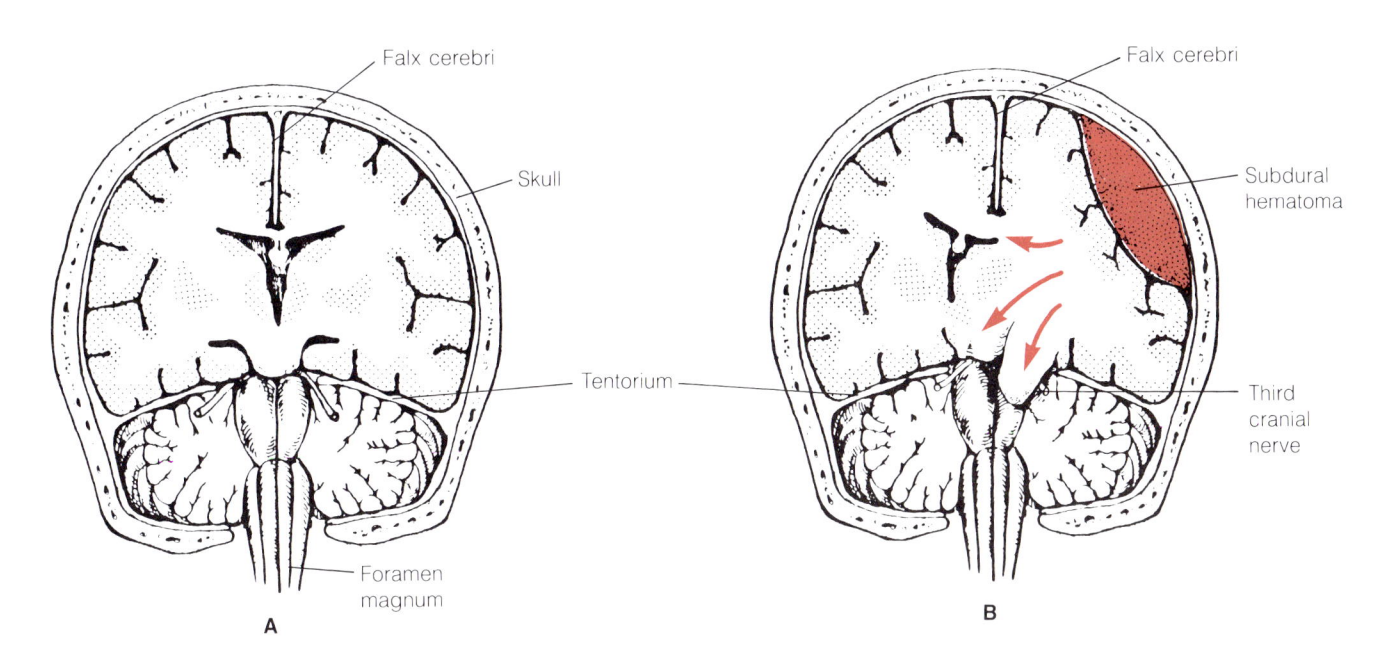

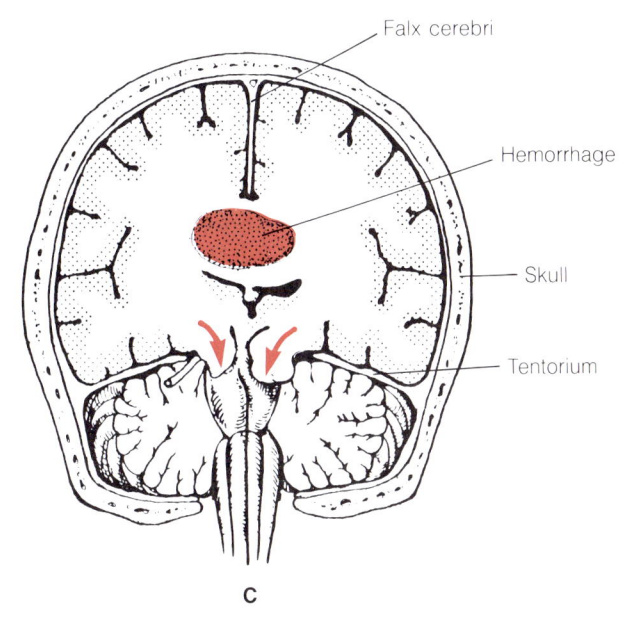

FIGURE 15–5.
(**A**) Normal relationship of intracranial structures. (**B**) Uncal herniation syndrome. (**C**) Central herniation syndrome.

Combinations of these three levels may be seen. Although central and uncal syndromes are two distinct and well-recognized syndromes, it should be realized that, in the seriously head-traumatized patient, the two often overlap. Symptoms may not occur with precise definition as compression moves down the brain stem.

Cerebral Concussion

A **cerebral concussion** has classically been defined as a transient episode of neuronal dysfunction (change in brain function) after a violent jar or shock to the brain with a rapid return to normal neurologic activity. Although most physicians consider a history of loss of consciousness necessary for this diagnosis, others suggest that a wide variety of disturbances in neurologic function, including confusion, dizziness, amnesia, nausea, and vomiting, are sufficient to make the diagnosis even with no loss of consciousness. Anatomically, no gross brain damage is noticeable. A traumatic temporary loss of consciousness, along with the associated memory deficit without underlying brain injury, generally is considered a hallmark of cerebral concussion. Memory deficits (**amnesia**) include inability to remember events before (**retrograde amnesia**) or after (**antegrade amnesia**) the event. Short-term memory loss produces repetition of questions.

A major cause of this type of behavior is frontal lobe injury, and some of these patients may be combative. A simple way to determine this condition is to ask the patient to describe the details of the incident. Although some patients may say they know what happened, when asked to describe it, they cannot.

The period of unconsciousness typically is short lived, lasting from several seconds or minutes to several hours. Loss of consciousness is thought to be caused by a disturbance in the functioning of the reticular activating system in the brain stem. The most common knockout blow is one that makes contact with the mandible or the side of the face. The reticular activating system is overwhelmed by the brain stem being twisted as well as violent brain movement against the side of the skull and sends an immediate surge of nerve impulses to the brain, resulting in unconsciousness.

Patients unconscious for longer that 5 minutes or those who have persistent symptoms such as vomiting should generally be admitted to the hospital for 24 hours of observation. The duration rather than the severity of a memory deficit determines the prognosis. When posttraumatic amnesia persists for more than 24 hours, the concussion is regarded as severe. It is extremely important to document at the scene the patient's historical loss of consciousness, present neurologic status, and memory deficits. This baseline evaluation helps to determine if the patient's condition is deteriorating or improving.

Cerebral Contusion

Contusions and lacerations occur characteristically in the frontal and temporal poles of the brain and on the inferior surfaces of the frontal and temporal lobes, where brain tissue comes in contact with bony protuberances at the base of the skull. Simply stated, a **cerebral contusion** is the bruising and bleeding of the brain (Fig. 15-6).

Depending on the area of brain involved, a neurologic deficit may or may not be evident. *Coup* contusions occur at the site of the injury. *Contrecoup* contusions occur in the brain opposite to the point of injury. Frontal and temporal lobes are common sites of contrecoup contusions, as the occipital lobe is frequently a site of injury. When a large area of brain is contused, intracranial pressure can increase significantly.

Skull Fracture

Skull fractures may be of two types: a closed break in the bone that does not break the skin or bone covering (*periosteum*), or an open one that does break the skin and periosteum. If the impact is powerful enough, the impact site may be depressed, and bony fragments are driven into the brain tissue. Contact sports, especially if the head is not protected properly, can result in skull fractures. The seriousness of a skull fracture is not the fracture itself but the associated cerebral injury or subsequent hematoma formation that might result. A high velocity gunshot wound may only minimally deform the skull but cause damage by the tremendous shock waves, the missile itself, and the bony fragments.

DEPRESSED. While any type of skull fracture can be associated with a brain injury, more extensive damage can be seen in a **depressed skull fracture** (Fig. 15-7). Bone fragments are driven into the brain. Because of the brain's exposure to the open air, open fractures also carry a risk of severe secondary injury due to infection.

BASILAR. **Basilar skull fractures** are usually the result of the extension of linear fractures onto the floor of the skull (Fig. 15-8). They are more often diagnosed by physical examination (*i.e.*, mechanism of injury) rather than by radiographic examination. A basilar skull fracture may be

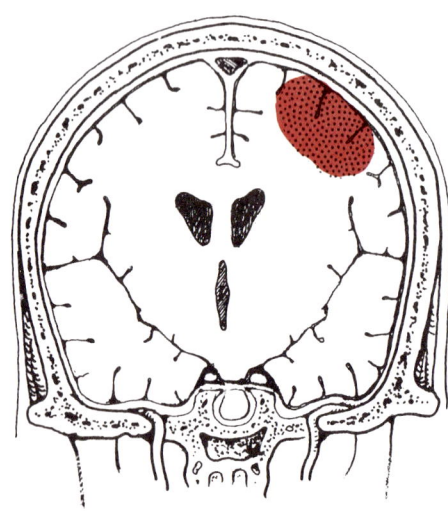

FIGURE 15-6.
Cerebral contusion.

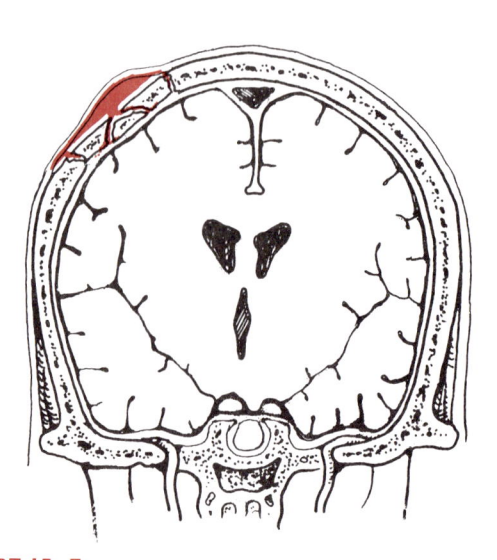

FIGURE 15-7.
Depressed skull fracture.

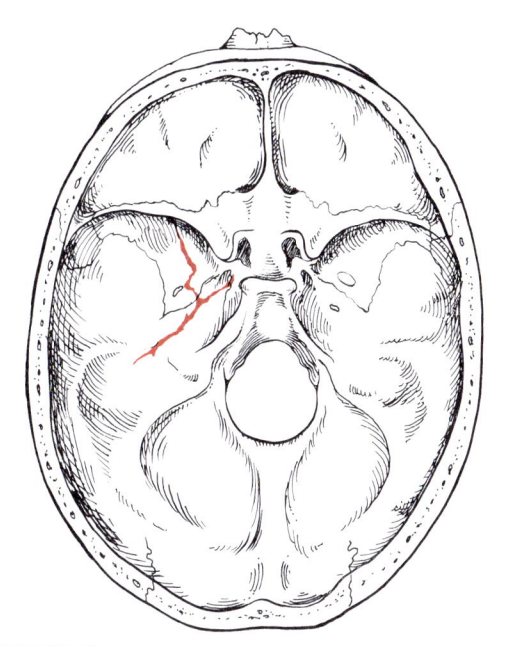

CHAPTER 15: Injuries to the Head, Neck, and Spine   315

FIGURE 15-8.
Basilar skull fracture.

associated with a tear of the middle meningeal artery, and an epidural hematoma may develop (Fig. 15-9). Note that skull fractures may be small and difficult to diagnose even with radiography. A basilar skull fracture should be suspected if blood or CSF is seen coming from the ears or nose.

Bleeding caused by basilar skull fractures often presents a dramatic appearance within hours of injury. Blood can travel into the periorbital subcutaneous tissue, producing the typical **raccoon's eyes** (periorbital ecchymosis) appearance. This sign may also be seen with direct orbital (eye) trauma. Occipital basilar skull fractures bleed into the subcutaneous tissue behind the ear, producing **Battle's sign** (discoloration behind the ears). Keep in mind that, though raccoon's eyes may be seen relatively soon after the injury (usually 6–12 hours, not immediately), Battle's sign does not develop for 24 to 36 hours. A person who has this physical finding immediately after an accident has sustained trauma to the mastoid area but has not necessarily sustained a basilar skull fracture.

If no associated brain injury, hematoma, subsequent infection, or CSF leak is present, skull fractures usually present no danger to the patient. In general, patients who have sustained a skull fracture are admitted to the hospital for observation for 24 hours.

Intracranial Hematomas and Hemorrhage

Traumatic intracranial hematomas and hemorrhage can produce devastating neurologic consequences in the head-injured patient. Hemorrhage can occur in several places: between the skull and dura mater, the dura mater and arachnoid, and the arachnoid and brain, and within the brain tissue itself.

EPIDURAL HEMATOMA. Epidural bleeds represent 2% of head injuries that result in hospitalization. They almost always occur from a tear in the middle meningeal artery. About 15% to 20% of these patients die. This percentage remains nearly the same when the problem is recognized and treated and is even greater when the condition goes unrecognized.

In an **epidural hematoma** (see Fig. 15-9), bleeding occurs when the meningeal arteries, which are located be-

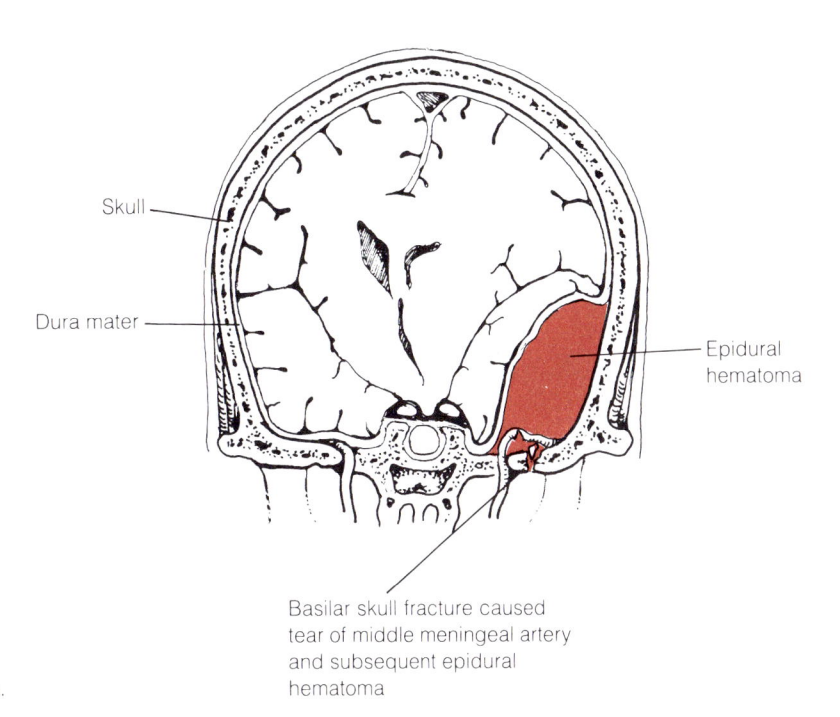

FIGURE 15-9.
Epidural hematoma.

tween the internal surface of the skull and dura mater (epidural space), are torn. These hematomas usually are produced by low velocity blows to the head, such as those that occur in fist fights or when hit by a baseball, by contrecoup arterial tears, or by lacerations that occur as the dura is pulled away from the skull by deceleration. Such injuries usually are associated with skull fractures.

An epidural hematoma creates an increase in intracranial pressure over several hours. Signs and symptoms include the following:

- Loss of consciousness, followed by a lucid interval
- Secondary depression of consciousness
- Developing **hemiparesis** (muscular weakness or partial paralysis that affects one side of the body) on the opposite side of impact
- A dilated and fixed pupil on the side of impact (commonly)
- During the lucid period, the patient's complaint of headache and sleepiness (possibly)

SUBDURAL HEMATOMA. A **subdural hematoma** occurs when bleeding is present between the dura mater and arachnoid membrane usually as a result of injury (Fig. 15-10). Surrounding brain tissue can be damaged. Although similar to an epidural hematoma, a subdural hematoma results from bleeding that is venous in nature, allowing pressure to build up more slowly. Because of this fact, the injury may not be noticed for several hours or days from onset.

SUBARACHNOID HEMORRHAGE. A **subarachnoid hemorrhage** occurs when bleeding is present between the arachnoid membrane and the pia mater. In a healthy person, CSF is found in this space. Typically, the hemorrhage is caused by a congenital arterial aneurysm (located in the subarachnoid space) that ruptures spontaneously, often during exertion. A subarachnoid hemorrhage is characterized by the severity and abrupt onset of a headache. Nausea and vomiting frequently accompany this condition, and a low-grade fever may be present.

INTRACEREBRAL HEMORRHAGE. **Intracerebral hemorrhage** occurs from bleeding within the brain itself. This condition typically is associated with penetrating head injuries, such as bullet wounds. The uninjured brain tissue is forced against the sides of the skull as the hemorrhage increases. Signs and symptoms may mimic a stroke. Prognosis and signs and symptoms are based on degree of injury and location of the hemorrhage.

Assessment

The first step in assessment of the head-injured patient is evaluation of responsiveness, airway, breathing, and circulation. Historical data obtained from even the most lucid head-injured patient is often of limited value. The patient's own judgment of the occurrence or duration of unconsciousness may not agree with the reports of witnesses. A patient who was alert and conversant immediately after the accident and later can only open the eyes, flex the arms, and vocalize in response to noxious stimuli has sustained a serious injury. A change in the level of consciousness is the earliest sign of neurologic deterioration after a brain injury.

Several abnormal ventilatory patterns are associated with a head-injured patient. An acute rise in intracranial pressure causes a slowing of the breathing rate. As the rise in intracranial pressure continues, the rate becomes rapid. Trauma to the cervical spine, which must always be assumed, may produce respiratory distress or arrest.

An elevated blood pressure without a therapeutic explanation reflects a rise in intracranial pressure. As intracranial pressure increases, the systolic pressure rises with a widening pulse pressure. Hypotension is a rare and terminal event in closed head trauma, and bleeding should be looked for elsewhere. Changes in the pulse rate may also be related to increasing intracranial pressure. Eleva-

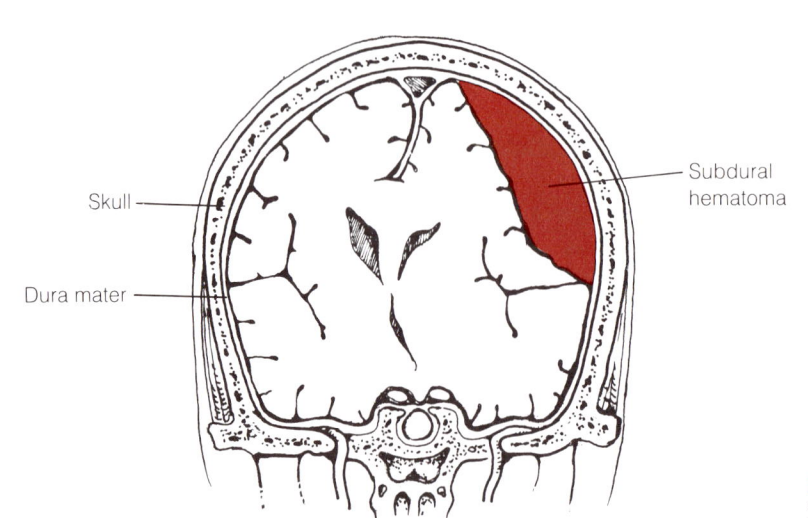

FIGURE 15-10.
Subdural hematoma.

tion of intracranial pressure may produce bradycardia. Bradycardia with hypertension suggests a rapidly expanding hematoma (Cushing's triad). A rapid pulse is a grave sign, unless another cause is found. Continued rise of intracranial pressure can produce tachycardia, which is a preterminal event.

The Glasgow Coma Scale (see Appendix C) relates consciousness to the parameters of motor response, verbal response, and eye opening. In each of these categories, the paramedic determines the best response the patient can make to a set of standardized stimuli. The point score increases as the patient's response approaches that of a person with a normal level of consciousness. This is one of the best evaluation techniques for brain injury that the paramedic has. It should be measured and recorded on every patient (medical or trauma) with an altered level of consciousness.

Although much attention is given to pupillary asymmetry after trauma, almost 20% of the population has a nonmeasurable pupillary asymmetry, and almost 5% have a measurable (greater than 1 mm) difference in pupil size. However, the more depressed the level of consciousness, the more likely it is that a one-sided fixed and dilated pupil represents herniation of brain structures secondary to increased intracranial pressure. This sign generally indicates compression of the third cranial (oculomotor) nerve.

Any scalp wound draws attention to the fact that the patient has sustained a head-injury. Not all external signs of recent head trauma, however, indicate traumatic brain injury. Such injuries can occur, for example, with the onset of a cerebral vascular accident, during which patients fall and strike their heads during the course of unconsciousness. Fluid from the ears or nose, however, should be checked to see if it contains CSF.

Any trauma above the clavicle suggests cervical spine injury. The patient should be properly immobilized if any of the following are present:

- A mechanism of injury that suggests violent action to the spine
- Any severe head injury
- Any head injury that results in a loss of consciousness or a markedly altered level of consciousness
- Specific signs of neurologic deficit, either motor or sensory

Management

Prehospital treatment of any patient with head injury focuses on maintaining adequate oxygenation and cerebral blood flow. Hyperoxygenation is effective in providing oxygen to hypoperfused cells. Carbon dioxide should be blown off by hyperventilating the patient at the rate of 24 to 30 breaths per minute. Rapid ventilations alone are not the factor. It is important to deliver 800 ml per breath for the adult. The patient's spine must be protected, and the patient must be rapidly transported to the hospital for definitive treatment.

As with any patient, the airway has first priority. The patient may require insertion of an endotracheal tube to maintain and protect the airway. Since it must be assumed that the patient has a cervical spine injury, in-line support must be maintained while establishing and managing the airway.

Head-injured patients are likely to vomit. Unconscious patients must be protected against aspiration. Suction equipment and a tonsil-tip or large-bore suction catheter must be available. Patients must be well immobilized to the backboard in case they have to be turned quickly. Once the neck is manually stabilized, the airway controlled, and ventilation is adequate, bleeding can be controlled and circulation reestablished. Bleeding scalp vessels are easily compressed by gentle and continuous direct pressure. If obvious deformity or a palpable bony defect or instability is seen, the bleeding can be controlled by compressing the area of the scalp around the wound, taking care to press against a stable area of the skull. Shock may occur as a result of gross bleeding, as the face and scalp are vascular. Be especially alert to this possibility in children.

Look for other internal injuries. Shock in an adult trauma victim who has not had excessive bleeding from the face or scalp or other injuries cannot be due to brain injury, unless it is the terminal event. The multiply injured patient with head trauma who is in shock should be managed like any other trauma patient in shock: with Trendelenburg positioning, thermal control, and control of major hemorrhage.

In addition, immediate rapid transportation to the closest appropriate hospital must be done and the use of advanced life support to provide the patient with fluid resuscitation (intravenous [IV] electrolyte solution and pneumatic anti-shock garment) as needed. Even the injured brain must be perfused with blood under adequate pressure to survive. The patient with an isolated head injury should be fluid restricted to help minimize cerebral edema. An IV line of Ringer's lactate or normal saline at a to-keep-open (TKO) rate should be started in case signs of shock appear. If the vital signs are adequate, the flow of the IV should be kept to 50 mL/hour. The flow rate must be monitored closely to prevent overhydration en route to the hospital.

Obviously, surgery cannot be done in the field to relieve increasing intracranial pressure. The method that can be used to decrease intracranial pressure and prevent brain stem herniation is hyperventilation with 100% oxygen, which causes cerebral vasoconstriction and subsequently decreases intracranial pressure, as described earlier. It is well known that hypoxia and hypercarbia aggravate brain swelling. In the deteriorating patient, a $PaCO_2$ of 30 mm Hg or lower is desirable and can be achieved by increasing the ventilatory rate from the usual

12 to 16 breaths per minute to 24 to 30 breaths per minute. It is essential that enough time for exhalation be allowed between positive-pressure inhalations, or the patient retains CO_2, being unable to blow it off.

A variety of medications (*e.g.*, Mannitol, Lasix, and other diuretics) are used to draw fluid from the interstitial and intracellular spaces, thereby reducing cerebral edema and decreasing intracranial pressure. These drugs work well but, like hyperventilation, are only temporary agents. While causing a decrease in cerebral edema or circulating blood volume and lowering intracranial pressure, they may also allow for a more rapid expansion of the intracranial hematoma. Because of this danger, diuretics and a wide range of other medications should be used only in the hospital and not in the prehospital setting.

SOFT TISSUE INJURIES TO THE NECK

Pathophysiology

The neck contains several vital structures but lacks the protection of a surrounding skeleton. Partial protection is offered by the thick musculature and surrounding skeleton of the cervical spine and shoulders. Blunt injuries to the neck can occur in a variety of accident situations. In a head-on vehicle accident, the unrestrained driver may pitch forward on impact and strike the anterior neck against the steering wheel, and the unrestrained passenger may strike the anterior neck on the projection of the dashboard. In these circumstances, the larynx is compressed against the cervical spine. A person may be seriously injured in nothing more than a simple fall if the neck strikes some object, or a person may suffer life-threatening blunt trauma to the neck if the throat is struck forcefully.

Regardless of the cause, the danger of a blunt injury to the neck in the adult is fracture of the larynx. A child, however, can sustain a fractured larynx because the larynx is better protected by the mandible and hyoid bone. A child's trachea also has more elasticity and mobility, and the laryngeal cartilages are more resistant to crush injuries and fractures.

The trachea can also be damaged in both the adult and child. The trachea is a semirigid tube that, once collapsed, cannot spring back to its original shape.

It is important to remember that if the accident was serious enough to produce blunt injury to the neck, it may have also produced an injury to the cervical spine. If life-saving measures must be taken for a neck injury before the condition of the spine can be determined by a field examination, extreme care must be taken not to move the person's head any more than is absolutely necessary. Aggravation of a cervical spine injury can cause permanent paralysis and lead to death.

The large blood vessels in the neck carry blood to and from the brain, and they are located close to the surface of the neck. Sharp injuries to these vessels may produce catastrophic bleeding. As in all wounds, arterial bleeding is characterized by bright red blood spurting from the wound, while venous bleeding produces a steady flow of dark red or even maroon-colored blood. A potential complication of vascular injury in the neck is air embolism. This condition may present as the sudden development of tachypnea, tachycardia, and hypotension in a patient who was previously stable.

Assessment

The principal signs for injury to the soft tissues of the neck include the loss of voice, hoarseness, a noticeable depression or palpable fracture over the anterior neck, and an obvious airway obstruction with respiratory distress. Evidence may also be seen of a condition known as subcutaneous emphysema, which is the result of air leaking into the soft tissues of the neck. Swelling and a crackling sensation under the skin are characteristic signs of subcutaneous emphysema. The integrity of the larynx, mandible, and other bony structures of the face and neck should be carefully evaluated.

Management

In blunt neck injuries, the patient's mouth should be cleared of blood, vomitus, broken teeth, dentures, or other foreign bodies to ensure a patent airway. High concentrations of oxygen should be administered. If the collapse of the larynx or trachea is severe, the patient should be ventilated with oxygen from a bag-valve-mask device. This process may be the only way to force air past the obstruction. If any question of airway compromise arises, active airway management should be instituted as early as possible. If endotracheal intubation is not possible, cricothyroidotomy (see Chapter 10) becomes the procedure of choice. If injury to the cervical spine is suspected, immobilization of the cervical vertebra is imperative.

If the neck injury is the result of a sharp object, bleeding may be so severe as to cause a person to **exsanguinate** (bleed to death). An ordinary pressure dressing may not stop the flow of blood from an artery in the neck because of the open weave of the dressing and the force of the blood. If it seems that an ordinary pressure dressing will not be sufficient to control blood flow, a gloved finger can be placed firmly in the wound against the open vessel. While this measure is extreme, it may be the only means by which bleeding from an open artery in the neck can be controlled.

An especially dangerous situation is created when a large vein in the neck is severed. Since blood is being returned to the heart through the vessel, it is possible for air to be sucked in through the wound and travel to the heart in the form of a bubble. This condition is known as air embolism and usually is fatal. An ordinary pressure dressing is not suitable for this type of injury because of the open weave. An occlusive dressing should be applied to the wound. Plastic wrap is well suited for this purpose. The wrap should be sealed on all sides to make the seal airtight. Direct pressure should be applied over the occlusive dressing to control bleeding.

Transportation to a medical facility should be taken without delay. Oxygen concentrations approaching 100% should be administered. The patient should be positioned in a way that facilitates the removal of any blood or vomitus (unless other known or suspected injuries prevent this positioning).

INJURIES TO THE SPINE

Spine trauma, if not recognized and properly managed in the field, can result in irreparable damage and leave the patient paralyzed for life. Some patients suffer immediate spinal cord damage as a result of an accident. Others suffer an injury to the spinal column that does not initially damage the cord, but cord damage may result later with movement of the spine. The central nervous system does not regenerate; a severed cord cannot be repaired. The consequences of moving patients with missed spinal injuries or allowing them to move can be devastating. Failure to properly immobilize a fractured spine, for example, can produce a much worse outcome than failing to properly immobilize a fractured femur.

Spinal injury can occur at any age; however, it is commonly found in patients 16 to 35 years old, since this age group is involved in the most violent activities. The largest number of spine trauma patients fall into the group between 16 and 20 years of age. The second largest group is patients between 21 and 25, and the third largest group is between 26 and 35.

Sudden violent forces that act on the body can move the spine beyond its normal range of motion, by either impacting on the head or neck or by driving the torso out from under the head. Three concepts help make the possible effect on the spine clearer when evaluating the potential of injury:

1. The head is like a bowling ball perched on the neck; its mass often moves in different directions from the torso, resulting in strong forces being applied to the neck.
2. Objects in motion attempt to stay in motion and objects at rest attempt to stay at rest.
3. Sudden or violent movement of the upper legs displaces the pelvis, resulting in forceful movement of the lower spine. Because of the weight and inertia of the head and torso, force in a contrary direction is applied to the upper spine.

The spine is composed of bony vertebrae, ligaments, the spinal cord, and branches of the spinal cord called nerves (see Chapter 22). Any of these structures can be damaged in many ways.

Mechanism of Injury

The bony spine can normally withstand forces of up to 1000 ft-lb of energy. High-speed travel and contact sports routinely cause forces well in excess of this amount to be exerted on the spine. Even in a low-speed automobile collision, the body of an unrestrained 150-lb person can easily place 3000 to 4000 ft-lb of force against the spine, as the head is suddenly stopped by the windshield or roof. Similar force can occur when a motorcyclist is thrown over the front of the cycle or when a high-speed skier collides with a tree.

The specific mechanisms of injury that cause spine trauma are axial loading, excessive flexion or hyperextension, hyper-rotation, sudden or excessive lateral bending, and distraction.

Axial loading can occur in several ways. Most commonly, this compression of the spine occurs when the head strikes an object and the weight of the still-moving body bears against the stopped head, such as when the head of an unrestrained occupant strikes the windshield or when the head strikes an object in a shallow water diving accident.

Compression and axial loading also occur when the patient sustains a fall from a substantial height and lands standing. This landing drives the weight of the head and thorax down against the lumbar spine, while the sacral spine remains stationary. Twenty percent of falls greater than 15 ft involve an associated lumbar spine fracture.

During such an extreme energy exchange, the spinal column tends to exaggerate its normal curves, and fractures and compressions occur at such areas. The spine is S-shaped, hence it can be said that the compressive forces tend to break the patient's "S."

Excessive flexion, excessive extension, and excessive rotation can cause bone damage, tearing of muscles and ligaments, and tearing of the spinal cord.

Lateral bending requires much less movement before injury occurs than does flexion or extension. A sudden lateral thrust can more easily cause significant injury or fractures to the cervical spine than an impact from the rear. During lateral impact the torso and the thoracic spine are moved laterally. The head tends to remain in place until pulled along by the cervical attachments. The center of gravity of the head is above and anterior to the cervical spine; therefore, the head tends to roll sideways and rotate. This movement often results in dislocations.

Distraction, which is overelongation of the spine, usually occurs when the head suddenly is stopped while the weight and momentum of the torso pull away from it. This "pulling apart" of the spine can easily cause stretching and tearing of the cord. This mechanism of injury is common in children's playground accidents and in hangings.

Although any one of these types of violent movement can be the dominant cause of spinal injury in a given patient, such injuries are seldom isolated; one or more of the others usually is also involved. As a guideline, the presence of spine injury and an unstable spine must be assumed with the following:

- Any mechanism that impacts violently on the head, neck, torso, or pelvis, since these impacts must be assumed to have caused violent sudden movement of the spine
- Accidents that produce sudden acceleration, sudden deceleration, or sudden lateral bending
- Falls from a significant height, regardless of whether the patient landed on the head or feet, since these must be considered to have resulted in axial loading and compression
- Any falls in which one part of the body was suddenly stopped while the rest continued to fall
- Any unrestrained victims in a vehicular roll-over, victims ejected from a moving vehicle, or victims of an explosion
- Any victim of a shallow water diving accident

Other injuries that commonly have spine damage associated with them include head injuries with any alteration in level of consciousness, the presence of any significant helmet damage, significant blunt injury above the clavicles, impacted or other deceleration fractures of the legs or hips, and significant localized injuries to the area of the spinal column.

Wearing proper seat belt restraints has been proven to save lives and reduce head, face, and thoracic injuries, but it is not valid grounds for ruling out the possibility of spine injury. In frontal impact accidents when sudden deceleration occurs, the restrained torso stops suddenly, but the unrestrained head attempts to continue its forward movement. Held by the diagonal shoulder strap, the chest can only move forward slightly, and then, the head rotates down and around the strap. Such rapid forceful hyperflexion and rotation of the neck can result in rotation of the cervical vertebrae and stretching of the spinal cord. Different mechanisms can also cause spine trauma in restrained victims of rear or lateral collisions. The amount of damage to the car and the patient's other injuries are the key factors in determining if the patient needs to be immobilized.

The patient's ability to walk should also not be a factor in determining whether or not a patient needs to be treated for spine injury. In a recent study of trauma patients who required surgical repair of unstable spine injuries, 17% were found "walking around" at the scene by the arriving paramedics, or they walked into the emergency department at the hospital. An unstable spine can only be ruled out by radiography.

Pathophysiology

The types of injuries that may occur to the spine are varied. Most common are the following:

- Compression fractures of a vertebra, which often result in the vertebra having a wedgelike shape
- Fractures that produce small extremely sharp teardrop fragments of bone, which may lie in the canal near the cord
- *Subluxation* (partial or complete dislocation of a vertebra from its normal alignment in the spinal column)
- Overstretching or tearing the ligaments and muscles, which often results in the loss of their ability to keep the vertebra in proper alignment if the patient moves about (or is moved)

Any of these skeletal or ligamentus injuries may, at the time of insult, immediately result in the irreversible cutting of the cords or may pinch, stretch, or bruise the cord. In many patients, however, damage to the vertebrae results in an unstable spinal column but does not result in a cord injury at the time of insult.

A lack of neurologic deficit does not rule out an unstable spine. Although the presence of good motor and sensory responses in the extremities indicates that at that point in time the cord is intact, it does not indicate an absence of injured vertebrae or damage to the muscles and ligaments that support the spinal column. Some patients with an unstable bony spine have no neurologic deficit.

Shock secondary to spinal cord injury represents a significant additional finding. Neurogenic **spinal shock** is due to two mechanisms that result from the neurologic deficits caused by injury to the spinal cord. As well as the classical signs of shock, spinal shock provides a unique presentation of the skin. When the cord is disrupted, the body's sympathetic compensatory mechanism cannot maintain control of the muscles in the walls of the blood vessels below the point of disruption. These arteries, arterioles, and veins dilate, enlarging the size of the vascular container and producing relative hypovolemia. Above the point of injury, the sympathetic defenses may produce vasoconstriction, and the skin is pale or white, cool or cold, and clammy or with marked diaphoresis. However, since no vasoconstriction occurs below the point of injury, the skin there remains pink, warm, and dry.

Instead of the tachycardia commonly associated with hypovolemic shock, this type of injury produces a normal heart rate or a slight bradycardia, since the unchecked vagal stimulus may override the normal sympathetic shock response and cause a drop in the pulse rate.

Assessment

The assessment for spinal injury, as with other conditions, must be done in perspective with the priorities for assessing and treating other injuries and conditions. This assessment includes checking the patient's responsiveness, airway, breathing, and circulation; however, these often cannot be assessed or treated without some movement of the patient. Therefore, a rapid survey of the scene, the situation, and the history of the event helps determine if a spinal injury is likely to exist.

If a cervical spine injury might exist, the paramedic must assume it does exist, and the patient's spine must be manually protected. The head, unless contraindicated, should be brought into a neutral in-line position. It must be maintained in that position until the manual immobilization is replaced with a spine immobilization device, such as a half backboard, long board, or vest-type device. Any necessary movement involved in assessing and treating the airway, breathing, or circulation must include continuous manual protection of the spine.

The patient's other injuries must also be considered when evaluating the mechanism of injury and the forces involved. Any significant blunt trauma to the head, neck, or torso can result in compression or sudden movement of the spine beyond its normal range. For example, any injury to the head that involved enough force to result in unconsciousness (or helmet damage) must be assumed to have violently and suddenly moved the head and neck and produced a spinal injury.

Physical indications of spinal trauma are pain or pain on movement, point tenderness, deformity, and guarding of the spine area. Neurologic signs include bilateral paralysis, partial paralysis, **paresis** (weakness), numbness, prickling or tingling, and neurogenic spine shock below the level of injury. In males, a continuing erection of the penis, called **priapism,** may be an additional indication of spinal cord injury. Note, however, that the absence of these signs does not rule out bony spine injury.

Indicators of spine trauma that requires treatment are the following:

- The mechanism of injury, regardless of the absence of any other signs or symptoms
- Other injuries that indicate violent forces acted on the spine
- Pain to the neck or back
- Pain on movement of the neck or back
- Pain on palpation of the posterior neck or midline of the back
- Any deformity of the spinal column
- Guarding or splinting of the neck or back
- Paralysis, paresis, numbness, or tingling in the legs or arms at any time after the insult
- Signs and symptoms of neurogenic shock
- In males, priapism

Management

The management of a patient with a suspected unstable spine is immobilization of the patient supine on a rigid spine board in a neutral in-line position. To avoid any further movement of the unstable spine that could result in damage to the cord, the head, neck, torso, and pelvis must each be immobilized in a neutral in-line position. This positioning follows the common principle of fracture management of immobilizing the joint above and the joint below an injury. Because of the anatomy of the spinal column and the interaction caused by forces that affect any part of the spine, this principle simply needs to be extended. Effectively, the *joint above* the spine means that the head must be immobilized, and the *joint below* means that the chest and pelvis must be immobilized.

Moderate anterior flexion or extension of the arms does not cause significant movement of the shoulder girdle. However, extending the arm to the side or elevating it above the head causes angulation of the shoulder girdle and substantial movement of the cervical spine.

Any movement or angulation of the pelvis results in movement of the sacrum and the vertebrae above it. For example, lateral movement of both legs together can result in angulation of the pelvis and lateral bending of the spine.

The body is considerably wider at the hips than at the ankles. When people are rolled to the side and the lower legs are allowed to remain on the ground, they move out of lateral alignment, possibly causing angulation of the pelvis and resulting in movement of the lower spine and mid-spine. Therefore, in patients with suspected spine injury, the legs need to be maintained in a mid-line neutral position in line with the rest of the body. Log-rolling methods that call for elevating an arm over the head or that do not include keeping the ankles elevated off the ground when the patient is rolled on the side are not recommended, since they can cause movement of both the cervical and lower spine.

Fractures of one area of the spine are commonly associated with fractures of other areas of the spine. Therefore, the entire weight-bearing spine (cervical, thoracic, lumbar, and sacral) must be considered as one entity, and all of the spine must be immobilized and supported (splinted) for proper immobilization to be achieved. The supine position is the most stable position to assure continued support during handling, carrying, and transporting the patient. It also provided the paramedic with the best access for further examination, monitoring of the airway, breathing, and circulation, and additional resuscitation and treatment of the patient. Only when the patient is supine is easy simultaneous access to the airway, mouth and nose, eyes, chest, and abdomen possible.

Patients with a suspected unstable spine usually present in one of four general postures: sitting, semiprone, supine, or standing. The patient's spine must be protected and immobilized immediately and continuously from the time the patient is discovered until mechanically secured to the long backboard. Techniques and equipment, such as manual immobilization, half backboards, immobilization vests, scoop litters, log rolls, or rapid extrication with full manual immobilization, are all necessary interim techniques used to protect the spine and allow safe movement

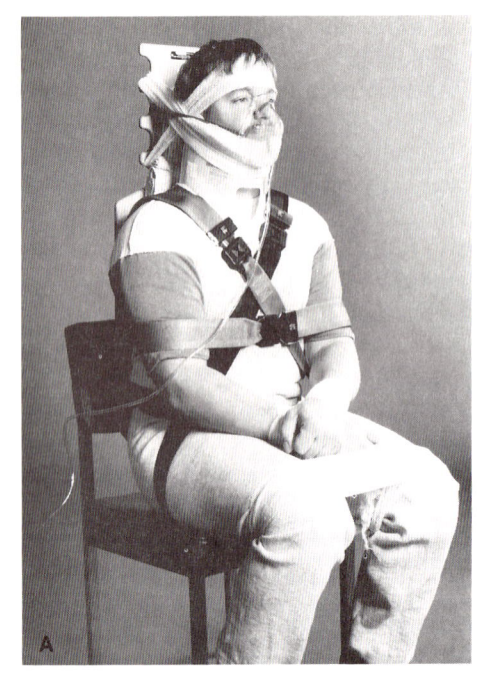

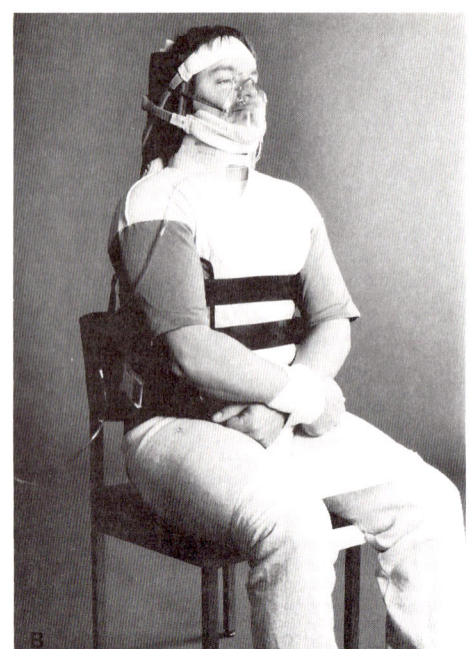

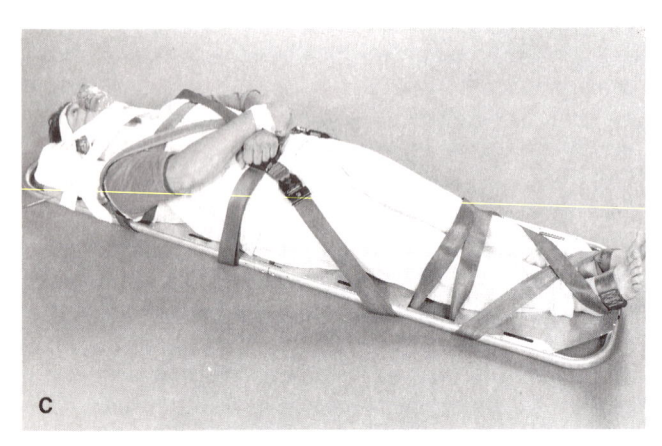

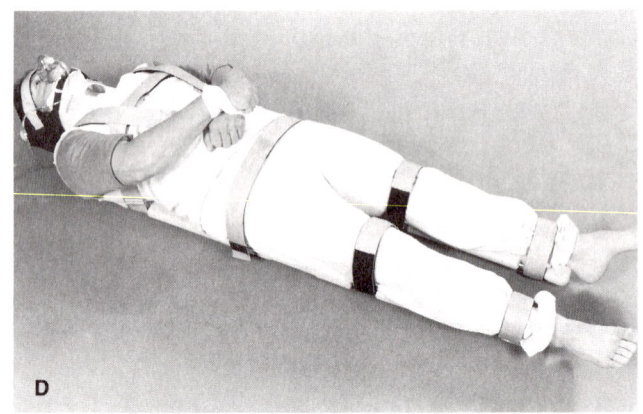

FIGURE 15–11.
Spinal immobilization devices. (**A**) Short backboard. (**B**) Kendrick extrication device. (**C**) Long backboard. (**D**) Miller board.

of patients from the position in which they were found until full immobilization supine on the rigid long board can be achieved. Several immobilization devices are shown in Figure 15-11.

The paramedic must practice and be familiar with a variety of particular devices and techniques. However, in the past, too much focus has been placed on the particular devices without an understanding of the principles of immobilization and how to modify these principles to meet each individual patient's needs.

Specific devices and immobilization methods can only be safely used with an understanding of the anatomical principles that are "generic" to all methods and equipment. Any inflexible detailed method for using a device does not meet the varying problems found in the field.

Regardless of the specific equipment or method used, the treatment of any patient with an unstable spine should follow these general steps:

- Provide manual in-line immobilization
- Evaluate responsiveness, airway, breathing, circulation, need for immediate resuscitation and check motor, sensory, and circulation in all four extremities
- Examine the neck and apply a cervical collar
- Immobilize the torso to the device so that the torso cannot move up or down or left or right
- Evaluate the torso straps and adjust as needed
- Pad behind the head as needed for adult patients and under the thorax as needed for pediatric patients (7 years or under)

- Immobilize the head
- Once on the long board, immobilize the legs and arms to the board
- Recheck responsiveness, airway, breathing, and circulation and recheck motor, sensory, and circulation in all four extremities

It is important to note that, as a person grows to adulthood, the spinal changes (**kyphosis**) that occur place the posterior part of the head more anterior than the posterior aspect of the thorax. In most adults, neutral in-line positioning produces a space between the back of the head and the ground or device. When such a space exits, padding must be placed behind the head to maintain neutral alignment. Children are the opposite: the head is large, and the posterior musculature is not well developed. If placed on the ground or on a rigid board, a child's head is typically moved to severe flexion. When immobilizing children, padding under the torso usually is necessary to offset the problem.

Cervical collars alone do not immobilize, they simply help support the neck and promote a lack of movement. A cervical collar must always be used in conjunction with manual in-line immobilization or with a mechanical immobilization device, such as a half backboard, vest, or long board. It is important to note that, regardless of the method or device used and whether support and immobilization are achieved manually or mechanically, they are either properly achieved or they are not. If they are properly achieved, the spine is protected; if they are not properly achieved, regardless of the method or amount of equipment, the spine is not protected.

SUMMARY

Injuries to the ear, eyes, and nose are usually soft tissue injuries. Foreign objects are sometimes found in the young child's ear and may be removed or left in place until arrival at the hospital. Chemical and burn injuries to the eyes can be serious and should be treated with care. Head injuries can result in a number of clinical syndromes. Each must be assessed and managed appropriately. The presence of spine trauma and the need to immobilize the patient can be indicated by the mechanism of injury, by the presence of other injuries that could occur with the sudden violent forces that act on the body, or by specific signs and symptoms of bone or cord injury. Immobilization of spinal fractures, as with other fractures, requires immobilization of the joint above and the joint below the injury.

SUGGESTED READING

Campbell JE: Basic Trauma Life Support Advanced Prehospital Care, 2nd ed. Englewood Cliffs, NJ, Prentice-Hall, 1988

Caroline NL: Emergency Care in the Streets, 3rd ed. Boston, Little, Brown & Co, 1987

Grant HD, Murry RH, Bergeron JD: Emergency Care, 5th ed. Englewood Cliffs, NJ, Prentice-Hall, 1990

McSwain NE, Butman AM, McConnell WK, Vomacka RW: Pre-hospital Trauma Life Support, 2nd ed. Akron, Emergency Training, 1990

McSwain NE, Kerstein MD: Evaluation and Management of Trauma. Norwalk, CT, Appleton-Century-Crofts, 1987

O'Brien J: Vasogenic Shock: Lost connections and overwhelming infection. Journal of Emergency Medical Services 14(3):32, 1989

Smith M, Bourn S, Larmon B: The ties that bind: Immobilizing the injured spine. Journal of Emergency Medical Services 14(4):28, 1989

Trunkey DD, Lewis FR: Current Therapy of Trauma, 2. Philadelphia, BC Decker, 1986

US Department of Transportation, National Highway Traffic Safety Administration: Emergency Medical Technician–Paramedic: National Standards Curriculum. Washington, DC, US Government Printing Office, 1985

CHAPTER 16

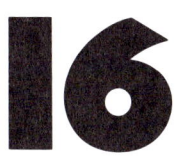

Thoracic Injuries

Assessment of Thoracic Injuries
  Primary Survey
  Secondary Survey
    Auscultation
Pathophysiology of Thoracic Injuries

Injuries That Cause Inadequate Ventilation
  Rib Fractures
  Flail Chest
  Pulmonary Contusion
  Ruptured Diaphragm
  Simple Pneumothorax
  Tension Pneumothorax
Skill 16-1. Thoracentesis
  Open Pneumothorax
  Hemothorax

Injuries That Cause Inadequate Cardiac Output
  Cardiac Contusion
  Cardiac Tamponade
Skill 16-2. Pericardiocentesis
Injuries That Cause Inadequate Circulating Blood Volume
Summary

BEHAVIORAL OBJECTIVES
On successful completion of this chapter, the reader will be able to:

1. Describe how to conduct a primary and secondary survey on a patient with thoracic injuries
2. Explain the mechanism for blunt and penetrating thoracic injuries
3. Describe the assessment and management of the eight injuries that cause inadequate ventilation
4. Describe the assessment and management of injuries that cause inadequate cardiac output
5. Describe the assessment and management of injuries that cause inadequate circulating blood volume
6. Given the proper equipment, demonstrate the procedure for pericardiocentesis and thoracentesis
7. Define all of the key terms listed in this chapter

KEY TERMS

The following terms are defined in the chapter and glossary:

cardiac contusion
cardiac tamponade
flail chest
hemothorax
mediastinal shift
needle chest decompression
paradoxical motion
pericardial sac
pericardiocentesis
pneumothorax—simple, tension, open
pulmonary contusion
thoracentesis

Thoracic injuries include injuries to structures within the thorax, such as lungs, tracheobronchial tree, heart, great vessels including the aorta, vena cavae, and pulmonary circulatory system. Injuries to the structures that form the thoracic cavity itself, such as the ribs and diaphragm, are also included.

Because of the vital life-sustaining functions performed by and within the thorax, any injury that causes an interruption or compromise of those functions may be critical. In many cases, the patient may rapidly deteriorate without aggressive treatment and expeditious transport to a qualified trauma center.

Unfortunately, many serious thoracic injuries outwardly appear to be relatively minor, especially in the young, otherwise healthy patient, whose cardiovascular and respiratory systems are capable of compensating for profound injuries for an extended but limited time. It is the responsibility of the paramedic to rapidly examine the patient, assess the scene, and evaluate the history and mechanisms of injury to detect clues that may lead to the discovery or suspicion of potentially life-threatening injuries.

ASSESSMENT OF THORACIC INJURIES

Assessment for thoracic trauma begins with the primary survey by looking at the skin to determine if cyanosis is present, observing the chest for thoracic movement, listening to the lungs to identify absent or decreased breath sounds, feeling the pulse to identify its rate, strength, and character, and listening to the heart to identify muffled heart sounds. The secondary survey proceeds by reassessing the lungs with the stethoscope for breath sound changes, evaluating the external jugular veins for distension, and feeling the chest wall for crepitus, abnormal rib motion, palpable paradoxical segments, or pain.

Primary Survey

Initial assessment in the primary survey is a simultaneous evaluation of the patient's responsiveness, airway, breathing, and circulation. If the patient is unconscious, the appropriate measures to open the airway and check breathing and circulation should be used. In the conscious patient, the paramedic takes hold of the patient's wrist, feels for a pulse, and begins a silent assessment of the pulse rate and character while asking the patient what happened. The patient's description of the accident identifies the airway status, ability to move air, and level of consciousness while the skin temperature, skin color, and capillary refill are being evaluated.

Secondary Survey

Recall from Chapter 9 that a complete secondary survey should always be performed if time and the patient's condition permit. Since the focus of this chapter is on the thoracic area, discussion begins by inspection of the patient's chest. The anterior and lateral chest wall is evaluated first. The posterior thoracic visual evaluation along with that of the posterior part of the abdomen is accomplished as the patient is log-rolled (to protect the cervical spine) into the right or left lateral position. The chest wall is inspected for perforations (indicating an entrance or exit wound), bruises, and abrasions, all of which could indicate fractured ribs or flail chest. A possible cardiac contusion would be associated with a bruise of the sternum from the steering column. Thoracic compression associated with this type of bruise could produce a pneumothorax.

If the damage to the vehicle is lateral, the lateral chest wall, which covers the lung, liver, and spleen, should be checked. Acceleration injuries to the thoracic aorta and cervical spine fractures must not be forgotten.

The patient's entire rib cage should be palpated anteriorly, posteriorly, and laterally, including the sternum and clavicle. Each rib should be examined individually, feeling for pain, areas of instability, crepitus, paradoxical movement, and subcutaneous emphysema. Percussion for the hyper-resonance associated with pneumothorax can be done when the environment is quiet enough to permit. The cardiac tones are checked while evaluating the neck veins for distension.

Auscultation

Identifying disorders with the stethoscope requires understanding of the variations in the sounds heard and a paramedic experienced enough to differentiate normal from abnormal sounds. This expertise cannot be gained with only one or two experiences with the stethoscope, but must be obtained during the initial training program with continued exposure to the possible variations of breath sounds. It is a skill that, if not pursued with diligence, can be lost. Once obtained, the skill must be practiced daily to be maintained.

Auscultation of the chest wall is initially done over both of the anterior lung fields and over the epigastrium. This quick listen identifies only the presence of breath sounds in each of the lung fields and their absence in the stomach. This identification helps to ensure that whichever method of airway management has been chosen is effective or that controlled ventilation is adequately ventilating both lungs. Auscultation is next done in the anterior lung fields at the apex by placing the stethoscope in the second or third intercostal space, midclavicular line, just inferior to the clavicle. Placement at this point is for comparison of breath sounds in each lung field to identify the presence of a pneumothorax.

A pneumothorax is identified by *unilateral* (one-sided) "absence of breath sounds." In reality, though, breath sounds are not absent but are merely diminished. These diminished breath sounds can be extremely difficult to distinguish from the breath sounds on the other side or from tracheal sounds. Frequently, several comparative listening maneuvers must be done to make this distinction. Several comparisons must be made. With a pneumothorax, the lungs tend to be compressed toward the mediastinum, and the air tends to rise.

The high anterior chest wall, near the apex of the lung, is the preferred area for identification of decreased or absent sounds. There are several reasons for choosing this point in the acutely injured patient. It is convenient for the paramedic who has just established the airway. The lung falls toward the mediastinum, and air rises to the anterior superior part of the thoracic cavity. Finally, the patient can be examined without log-rolling to the side, thus protecting the cervical and thoracic spine.

PATHOPHYSIOLOGY OF THORACIC INJURIES

Traumatic thoracic injuries may be caused by either blunt or penetrating forces. Penetrating forces include gunshot wounds, stab wounds, and lacerations that pierce the thoracic cavity and, frequently, structures and organs within the thorax. Blunt forces include striking steering wheels, body blows, falls, and other insults that do not directly pierce the thoracic wall or any thoracic structure.

In many cases, both blunt and penetrating injuries occur from the same mechanism of injury. Blunt forces may frequently cause related penetrating injuries as in the example of a blunt force that causes a rib fracture and further forces the sharp end of the fractured bone into the thorax where it penetrates a lung. Similarly, a gunshot wound from a high-caliber weapon not only creates a penetrating injury, but the tremendous ballistic force of the bullet as it enters the body also causes blunt injuries to tissues and structures near its path.

The variety of injuries that may occur within the thorax as a result of blunt and penetrating traumatic forces may be generally divided and described by the effects that they have on the function of the respiratory and cardiovascular systems. The effects of these injuries fall into three basic groups:

- Injuries to the chest wall, diaphragm, or lungs that disrupt the respiratory mechanisms and cause inadequate ventilation
- Injuries to the heart that compromise the circulatory system, resulting in inadequate cardiac output
- Injuries to the thoracic vascular system that cause blood loss, leading to inadequate circulating blood volume

INJURIES THAT CAUSE INADEQUATE VENTILATION

Rib Fractures

Even the simple fracture of a single rib may have an adverse effect on the patient's ability to breathe. Frequently caused by blunt trauma, a rib fracture may compromise ventilation as a result of the substantial pain caused when the chest wall moves in the process of normal breathing. The patient's natural reaction is to minimize the movement of the chest wall to reduce the pain. By voluntarily reducing the movement of the chest wall, the patient also reduces the volume and depth of ventilation. Prolonged reduced ventilation in a small component of the lung leads to atelectasis and pneumonia. If other injuries are present, the reduced ventilation may be an additive factor to worsen the overall response to the other injuries (*synergistic effect*).

Isolated, uncomplicated rib fractures require little in the way of specialized treatment. The best care, generally, is to allow the patient to sit or lie in the most comfortable position and provide supplemental oxygen to overcome the effect of reduced ventilation. Taping, binding, or otherwise attempting to immobilize rib fractures serves only to reduce further the volume and depth of ventilation and does little to help heal the fractures.

The most important consideration in treating a rib fracture is to recognize the potential for associated injuries, such as pneumothorax or pulmonary contusion, and to observe aggressively for signs or symptoms of more serious problems.

Flail Chest

A ***flail chest*** usually is defined as two or more adjacent ribs that are each fractured in at least two places (Fig. 16-1). This combination of fractures creates a "*flail*" segment of the chest wall, which is made up of the segments of the fractured ribs between the fractures that no longer have a firm bony attachment to the rest of the rib cage. In some cases, a series of rib fractures around the sternum may cause the sternum itself to be the flail segment.

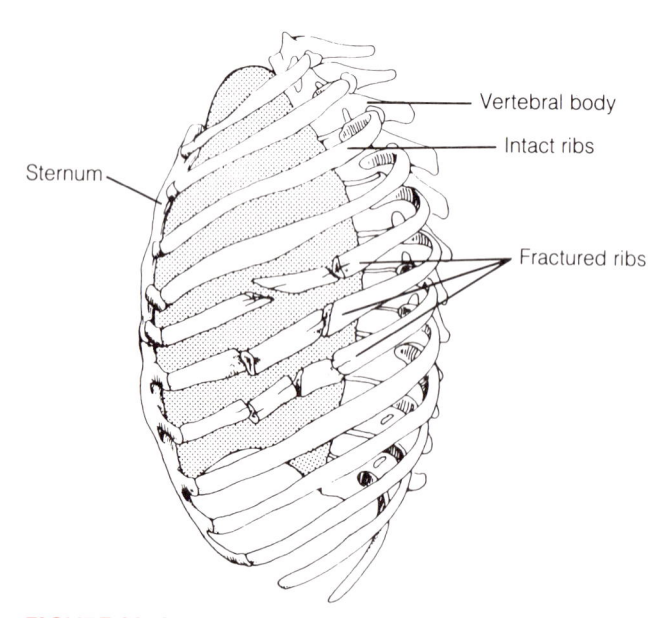

The major pathologic process of a flail chest is the damage (pulmonary contusion) to the lung beneath. The decreased oxygenation associated with a pulmonary contusion requires the primary focus to be patient care. ***Paradoxical motion*** occurs when the flail segment of the chest moves in a direction opposite to that of the rest of the chest wall during respiration. In the normal chest, the inspiratory phase of respiration consists of the diaphragm's contracting and moving downward as the intercostal muscles contract and raise the ribs slightly to expand the chest cavity. These two motions enlarge the chest cavity, reducing the atmospheric pressure in the chest and allowing air to move into the lungs. On expiration, the relaxing of the diaphragm and intercostal muscles causes a reduction in the size of the chest cavity, which creates a somewhat higher pressure in the chest and allows passive exhalation of air.

When a flail segment is present, however, the negative pressure in the chest during inspiration causes the flail segment of the chest to be pulled inward instead of expanding outward with the rest of the chest wall. Similarly, during expiration, the higher pressure in the chest causes the flail segment to move outward instead of relaxing inward with the rest of the chest wall (Fig. 16-2).

If the flail segment is relatively small, the effect of the flail chest is little worse than a simple rib fracture. A larger flail segment, however, such as one that involves three or more ribs or the sternum itself, may significantly reduce the volume and depth of respiration possible because of the paradoxical motion of the flail segment.

In the examination of a patient with a flail chest in the first few hours after the injury, the paradoxical motion of the flail segment is not be easily visible. It may only be detectable by placing the palm of the hand on the chest wall and feeling the subtle paradoxical motion. Muscle spasm and voluntary reduction of thoracic movement because of pain make paradoxical movement of the chest wall a late sign. Its absence should not indicate that the lung beneath is not injured. Obviously, it is imperative that a patient with thoracic injuries have all clothing removed and all areas of the thorax carefully palpated and examined to detect such subtle but significant signs.

Treatment of a patient with a flail chest should be focused on providing supplemental oxygen to overcome the hypoxemia that may accompany the reduced ventilatory capacity and aggressive treatment of any associated injuries. If a large flail segment is present, endotracheal intubation and positive pressure ventilation may be necessary to provide adequate ventilation.

Pulmonary Contusion

A common result of blunt trauma to the chest is a ***pulmonary contusion,*** or bruise, that frequently accompa-

FIGURE 16-1.
Ribs that are fractured in one or more places, because they have no attachment to either the sternum or vertebral bodies, have no stability and are free floating. This condition is known as a flail chest.

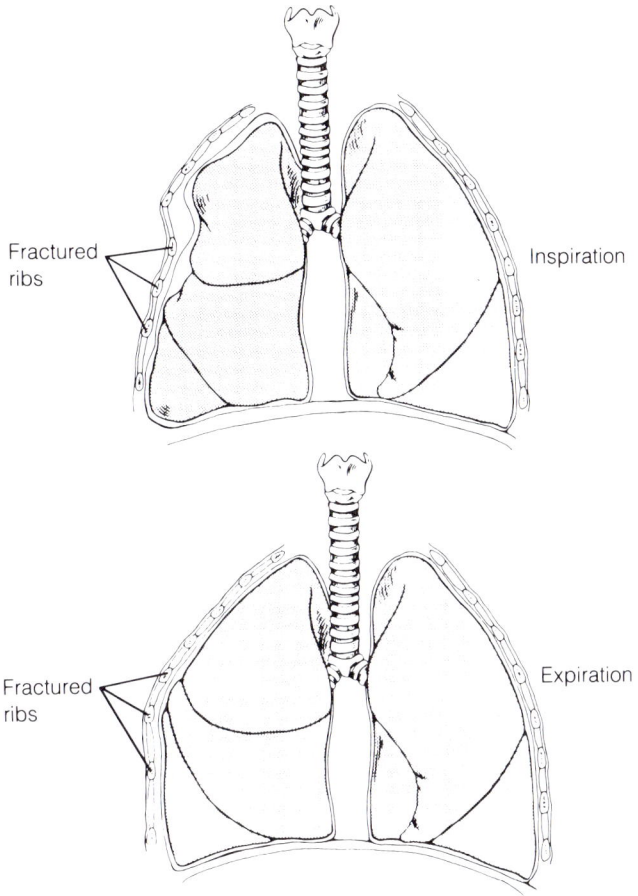

nies rib fractures and flail chest. While a contusion to other body tissues is a relatively minor problem, the contusion of lung tissue causes disruption of the alveoli and their surrounding capillaries. The resultant filling of the alveoli and interstitial spaces with fluid and blood reduces or eliminates that portion of the lung tissue from providing effective gas exchange (Fig. 16-3). Although blood is still perfusing most of the capillaries, the hemorrhage into the alveolar capillary membrane reduces transfer of oxygen into the capillary. As the alveoli fill with blood or fluid and are no longer ventilated, these portions are eliminated completely from the oxygenation process.

The detrimental effect of a pulmonary contusion is directly related to the size of the contused area and the amount of lung tissue that cannot function effectively. Since pulmonary contusion frequently is accompanied by other ventilation-compromising injuries, the cumulative effect of all the injuries on the patient's ability to breathe may be profound. The pulmonary contusion is the major pathologic process that effects the morbidity and mortality associated with a flail chest.

Ruptured Diaphragm

In cases of extreme blunt force to the abdomen, such as may occur from a steering wheel but may infrequently be due to the seat belt, the force on the abdomen may be so great as to cause the diaphragm to rupture (like the paper bag effect) and allow contents of the abdominal cavity, such as the spleen, liver, or bowel, to protrude into the thoracic cavity (Fig. 16-4).

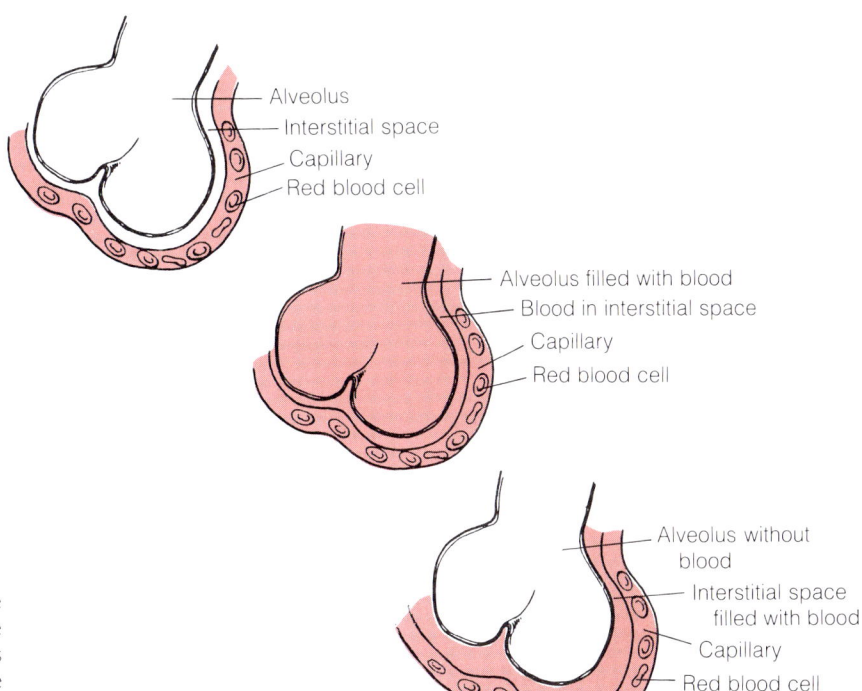

FIGURE 16–2.
A flail segment moves inwardly on inspiration and outwardly on expiration, as the segment cannot resist changes in intrathoracic pressure. This condition is called paradoxical movement or paradoxical respiration.

FIGURE 16–3.
Hemorrhage into the alveolus reduces the amount of air for exchange. Increasing the fluid (blood or edema) in the interstitial spaces reduces the rate of oxygen diffusion into the red blood cells and the exchange of carbon dioxide from the plasma.

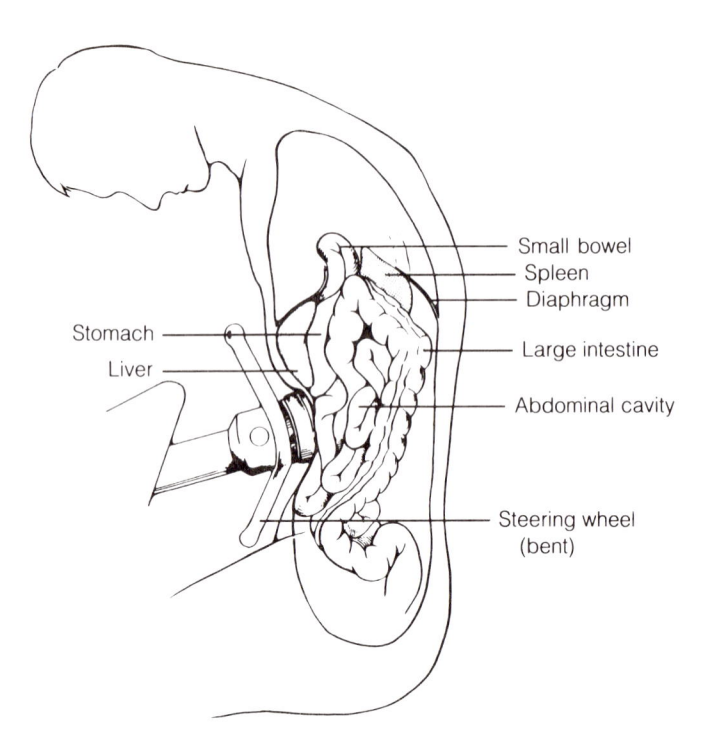

FIGURE 16-4.
Compression of the abdominal cavity by the steering wheel increases intra-abdominal pressure. The weakest wall is the diaphragm, which is only 0.5 cm in thickness without strong supporting fascia. Small bowel, stomach, spleen, and colon can be forced through the defect on the left and the liver can be forced through a defect on the right.

When such a rupture of the diaphragm occurs, not only is the diaphragm significantly impaired from contracting as usual with respiration, but the volume of the chest cavity is also reduced by the presence of the abdominal contents, which further reduces the capacity of the chest for respiration.

Though difficult to detect in the field, a telltale finding that indicates a ruptured diaphragm is the presence of bowel sounds in the chest. A significant consideration with a ruptured diaphragm is that further abdominal pressure, such as that provided by the pneumatic anti-shock garment, may worsen the respiratory compromise. This condition is one of the few that require the pneumatic anti-shock garment to be deflated in the field.

Blunt trauma to the abdomen can also affect the heart by producing a pulse of retrograde blood flow up the aorta and against the aortic valve (Fig. 16-5).

Simple Pneumothorax

A *pneumothorax* is the presence of air in the pleural space between the visceral pleura, which covers the lungs, and the parietal pleura, which covers the inner chest wall. Normally only a "*potential space*" of negative pressure, the pleural space serves to keep the lungs expanded fully to the chest wall, while allowing lubricated movement of the lungs along the chest wall. When the pleural space is occupied with air, the lung does not expand completely. This reduced pulmonary volume disrupts its ability to respond normally to respiratory efforts. The greater the amount of unexpanded lung, the greater the reduced oxygenation that occurs.

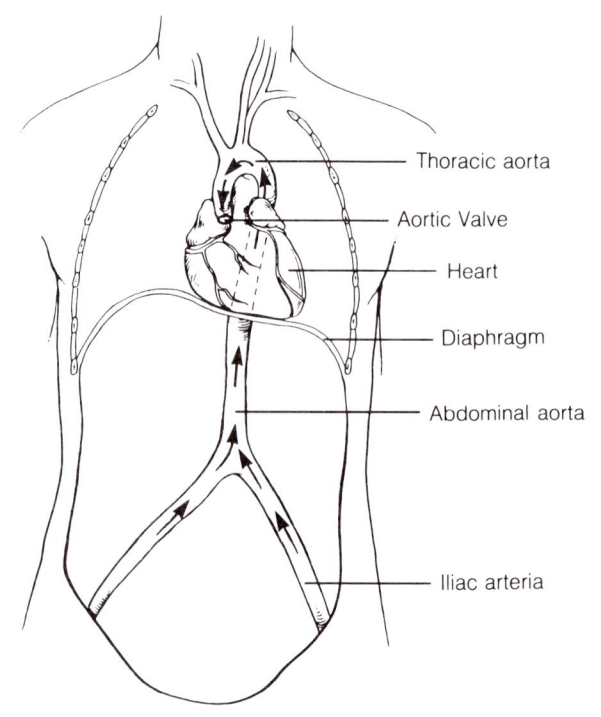

FIGURE 16-5.
Increased intra-abdominal pressure from the steering wheel or dashboard forces blood retrograde out of the abdomen, up the thoracic aorta, and against the aortic valve. Such pressure can rupture the leaflets of the valve and produce sudden severe aortic insufficiency.

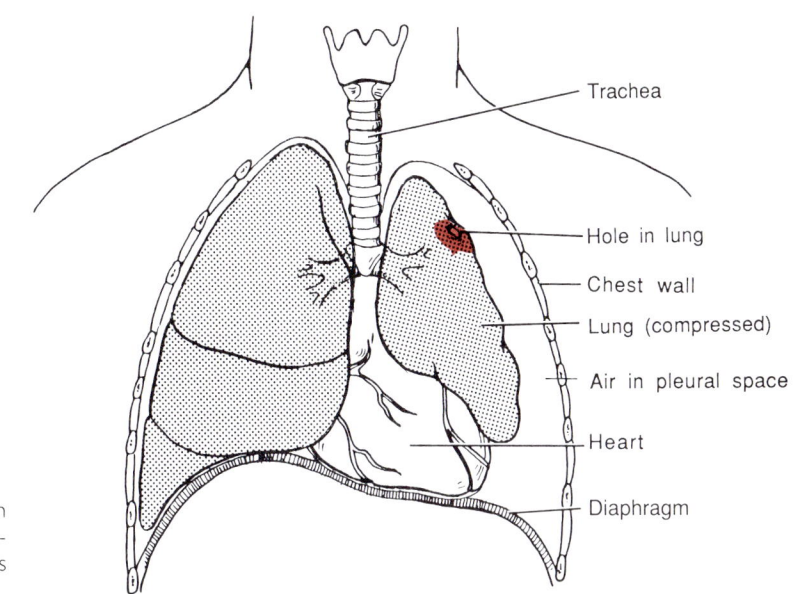

FIGURE 16-6.
Air that is leaking into the pleural space from a hole in the lung becomes a space-occupying lesion that prevents expansion of the lung during inspiration. This condition is known as a simple pneumothorax.

A **simple pneumothorax** may result from a fractured rib that punctures lung tissue, allowing air into the pleural space, or from a blunt force to the chest that simply ruptures a weak portion of the lung tissue, allowing air leakage into the pleural space (Fig. 16-6). It is also possible for a simple pneumothorax to occur spontaneously in an otherwise normal patient for no apparent reason. In these cases, a weak portion of the lung tissue apparently ruptures spontaneously, creating a small pneumothorax.

In a normal, otherwise healthy patient, a small simple pneumothorax may be tolerated rather well, since the normal lung usually has a good deal of reserve capacity. In a patient with multiple injuries, respiratory compromise may be serious, since positive pressure ventilation increases the size of a pneumothorax or even converts it to a tension pneumothorax.

The patient with a simple pneumothorax normally does not complain of shortness of breath unless the pneumothorax is large. Reduced breath sounds may be noted over a portion of the affected lung. Provided that the shortness of breath does not worsen or that the area of decreased breath sounds does not enlarge, the provision of supplemental oxygen and transport to a hospital probably is sufficient field treatment. However, if the shortness of breath worsens or if the area of decreased breath sounds enlarges, a much more serious tension pneumothorax may be developing.

Tension Pneumothorax

A **tension pneumothorax** may result from the same mechanisms that cause a simple pneumothorax. The major difference, however, is that, in a tension pneumothorax, the leakage of air into the pleural space continues to occur, with no avenue of escape from the pleural space for the accumulating air and pressure (Fig. 16-7).

The result of the continued accumulation of air in the pleural space is a progressively increasing pressure, which further collapses the affected lung and, therefore, increasingly compromises ventilation. The principal danger of a tension pneumothorax occurs when the pressure accumulated in the affected side gets so great that, not only is the one lung collapsed, but the excessive pressure begins to push the mediastinal structures over into the opposite hemothorax to put pressure on the other lung. This shift of pressure, known as **mediastinal shift,** creates a profound compromise of ventilation and reduces cardiac output because it reduces blood flow into the left atrium by kinking the vena cava and increasing pulmonary vascular resistance.

The classic signs of a tension pneumothorax are progressive shortness of breath and absence of breath sounds on the affected side, distended neck veins, cyanosis, hypotension, and deviation of the trachea away from the affected side.

Depending on several other circumstances, however, some of the signs of a tension pneumothorax may not be present or easily detectable. For example, a hypovolemic patient may not show distended neck veins, and it may be difficult to determine if hypotension is due to hypovolemia or a tension pneumothorax. The shift of the trachea often is only clear on a radiograph, since the most mobile portion is low on the trachea and not in the neck. Cyanosis is often difficult to detect in the field.

Worsening of a tension pneumothorax may be rapidly fatal without aggressive intervention to reduce or eliminate the increasing pressure. In the field, the fastest and easiest treatment is to perform a **thoracentesis** by insert-

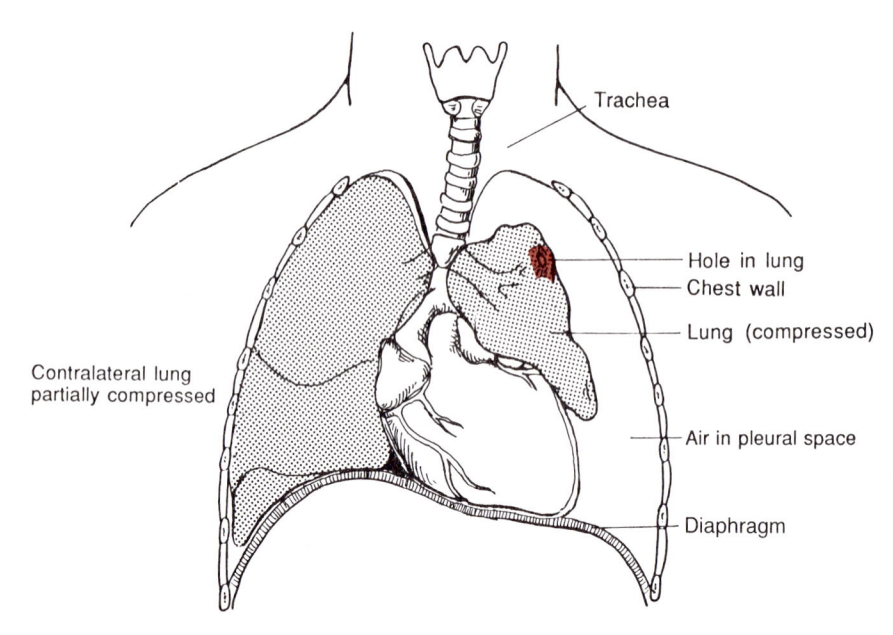

FIGURE 16-7.
Continued increase of pressure in the pleural space compresses the lung and pushes the mediastinum into the opposite side of the thorax. This action compresses the opposite lung and decreases the ventilation capacity of it. The increased intrathoracic pressure and kinking of the vena cava reduce blood return to the heart. This condition is known as a tension pneumothorax.

ing a needle into the wall of the affected chest to relieve the accumulating pressure. In a severely compromised patient, this field thoracentesis can quickly produce dramatic improvement.

The purpose of the field thoracentesis is to convert the tension pneumothorax into an open pneumothorax by allowing an escape for the air that is accumulating in the pleural space. While still serious, the open pneumothorax is far less life-threatening and is easier to treat with supplemental oxygen and positive pressure ventilation.

Thoracentesis is indicated in the field only in the face of a life-threatening tension pneumothorax. In that situation, there are essentially no contraindications since the only alternative is almost certain death.

The potential complications of thoracentesis include the following:

- Puncture or laceration of lung tissue
- Bleeding from laceration of intercostal vessels
- Inducing a pneumothorax unnecessarily if performed when a tension pneumothorax is not actually present.

The technique of thoracentesis, also known as **needle chest decompression,** is usually performed with a large-bore over-the-needle catheter inserted in the second intercostal space in the midclavicular line on the affected side of the chest.

An improvised or commercial valve may be attached to the needle to only allow air to escape from the pleural space and not allow any air to enter through the needle. In many cases, however, it is felt that the escape of the air under pressure in the pleural space is the primary con-

(text continues on page 335)

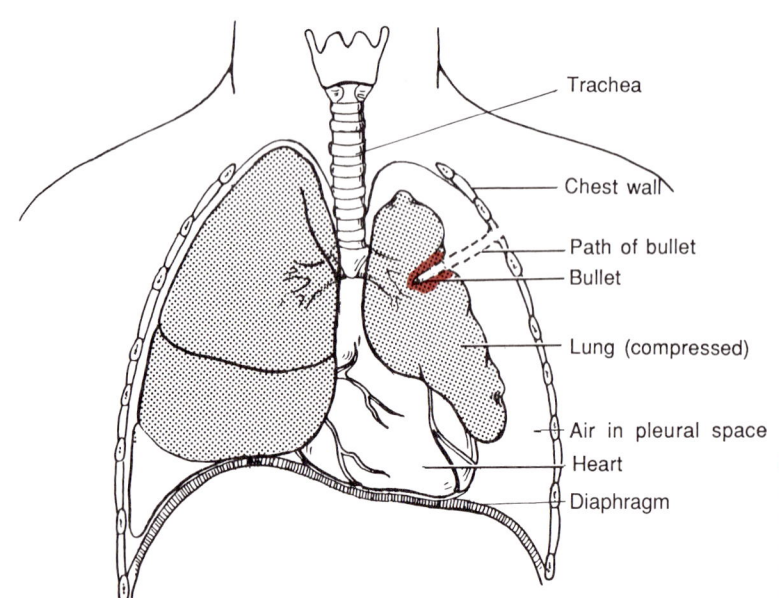

FIGURE 16-8.
A hole in the chest wall allows air passage into the pleural space when intrathoracic pressure is negative. The lung falls inward toward the mediastinum, expansion is reduced, and ventilation is not complete. This condition is known as an open pneumothorax.

SKILL 16–1.
THORACENTESIS

ACTIVITY	HOW PERFORMED	WHY PERFORMED
1. Check: • Responsiveness • Airway • Breathing • Circulation	Establish responsiveness Stabilize neck, open the airway Assess breathing Check for a pulse Check for hemorrhage	The primary survey is a rapid evaluation, less than 45 seconds, to identify and correct any life-threatening problems.
2. Assess the need for thoracentesis	Evaluate patient's presenting signs and symptoms to determine if procedure is indicated and appropriate.	Procedure must only be performed when indicated and appropriate, usually on orders from medical control.
3. Assemble equipment: Primary equipment (Activity 3): • 14-gauge over-the-needle catheter Accessory equipment and supplies: • Flutter valve (if available) • Antiseptic swabs • Protective eye wear • Mask • Gloves	Attach the needle to an improvised or commercial flutter valve. This procedure may also be performed without a flutter valve if one is unavailable. Place all equipment within easy reach. Put on protective eye wear, mask, and gloves.	Flutter valves allow air to escape from the chest but do not allow air to enter the chest. Having all equipment ready reduces time delays during the procedure. To prevent blood or body fluid contact with non-intact skin or mucous membranes.

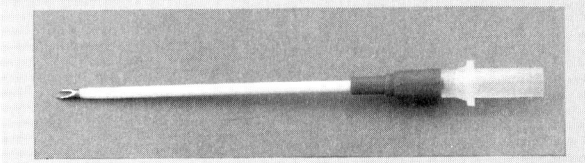

Activity 3.
Primary equipment.

4. Position the patient	Place the patient supine (Activity 4.)	This is the best position to perform the procedure.

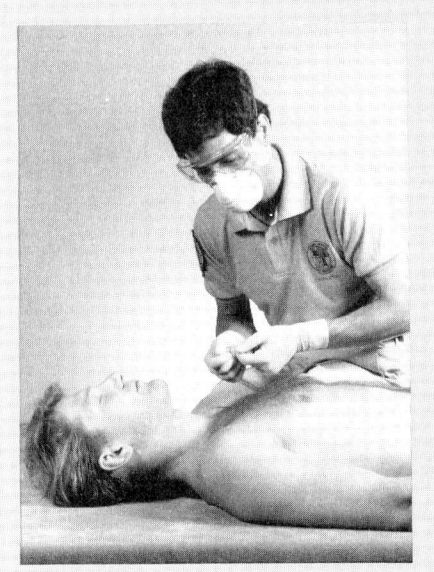

Activity 4.
Position the patient.

(continued)

SKILL 16–1.
THORACENTESIS (continued)

ACTIVITY	HOW PERFORMED	WHY PERFORMED
5. Find landmarks for thoracentesis and prepare the site	On the affected side of the chest, locate the point in the second intercostal space at the midclavicular line (Activity 5A). Cleanse the area with antiseptic swabs (Activity 5B).	This location is in the upper lobe of the lung cavity, providing access to relieve the accumulating air pressure with the least possibility of damage to the lung. Cleansing the area reduces the possibility of infection.

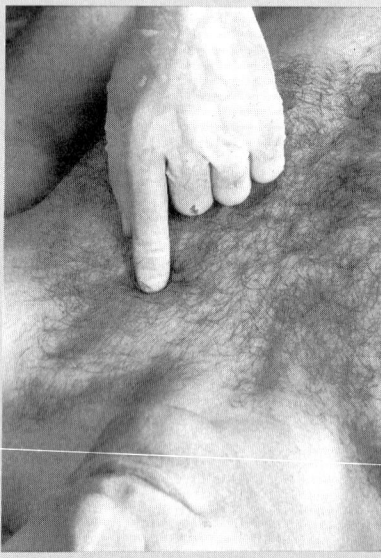

Activity 5A. Find landmarks for thoracentesis.

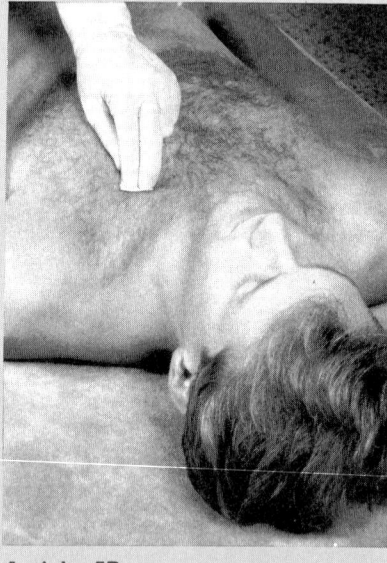

Activity 5B. Prepare the site.

6. Perform the thoracentesis	Insert the needle at the second intercostal space at the midclavicular line, directing the needle just over the top of the third rib. (Activity 6A shows the procedure without a flutter valve; Activity 6B shows a flutter valve.)	Following the top of the third rib avoids the intercostal nerve and blood vessels that lie along the bottom of each rib.

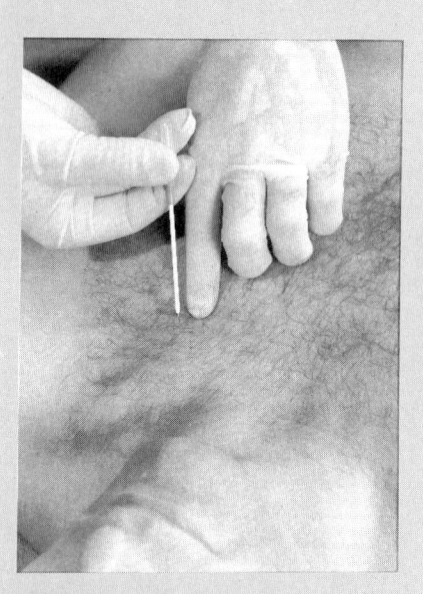

Activity 6A. Perform the thoracentesis. Insert needle *without* the flutter valve.

(continued)

CHAPTER 16: Thoracic Injuries   335

SKILL 16–1.
THORACENTESIS (continued)

ACTIVITY	HOW PERFORMED	WHY PERFORMED
	With the needle fully inserted into the chest, hold the catheter in place and withdraw the needle (Activity 6C).	Leaving the flexible catheter in place allows continued escape of air that might otherwise be trapped in the pleural space.
Activity 6B. Insert the needle *with* flutter valve.	**Activity 6C.** Hold catheter in place and withdraw needle.	
7. Dispose of needle	Place contaminated needle in proper container.	Eliminates the possibility of injury or infection by contact with the contaminated needle.

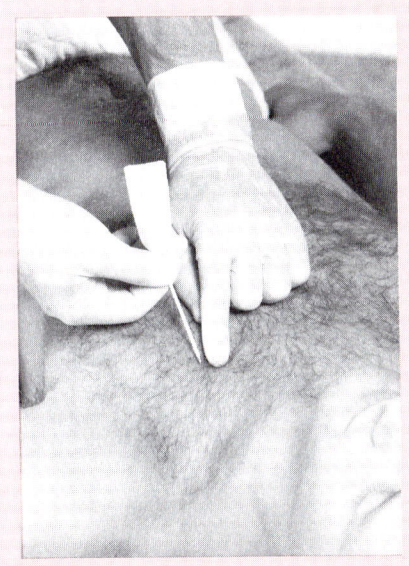

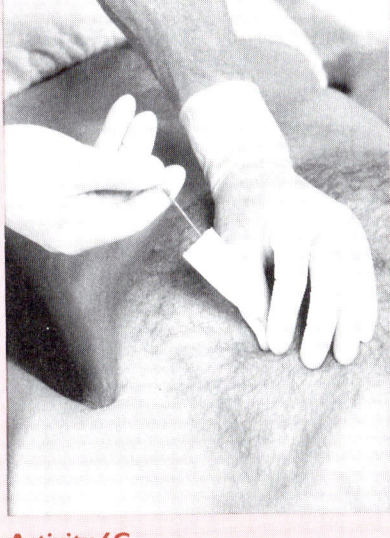

cern, and allowing some air to enter through the needle is of minor importance, provided the needle remains in place to keep pressure from accumulating again. A gloved finger can be placed over the needle during inspiration and removed during expiration to achieve the same effect. Another method is to attach an intravenous administration set to the needle, cut off any valves in the set, then place the cut end under water. Any method to achieve one-way flow of air out of the chest but not into it is acceptable.

The procedure for thoracentesis is shown in Skill 16-1.

Open Pneumothorax

An **open pneumothorax** is similar to a simple pneumothorax except that an open wound connects the pleural space to the outside (Fig. 16-8). Such an open wound may be the result of a variety of penetrating trauma forces such as gunshot or stab wounds.

In many cases, the wound of an open pneumothorax may remain at least partially open, resulting in a rush of air into the pleural space with each inspiratory effort by the patient. This rush of air gives rise to the expression "*sucking chest wound*" frequently applied to such injuries. Because of the elastic nature of the skin, however, it is common for a penetrating wound to the chest to become sealed over by the elastic skin and tissue of the chest wall. It is, unfortunately, a common error for such a wound to be assumed to be superficial when it is not carefully examined for evidence that the thoracic cavity was penetrated.

In addition to the external wound, the patient with an open pneumothorax displays many of the same signs and symptoms of a simple pneumothorax, such as shortness of breath and reduced breath sounds.

The common treatment for all open chest wounds is to seal the external wound with an airtight dressing and provide supplemental oxygen. It is important to appreciate, however, that the patient with an open pneumothorax may easily develop a tension pneumothorax either because of the nature of the external wound or the treatment applied in the field.

In the case of the chest wound that is naturally sealed over by the mobile skin of the chest wall, if damage to the lung tissue continues to allow leakage of air into the pleural space, that air may become trapped and may begin to build in pressure to form a tension pneumothorax.

Similarly, if the wound is sealed with an airtight dressing and sufficient damage to the lung tissue allows continued leaking and trapping of air in the pleural space, a tension pneumothorax may quickly develop. In this instance, however, if the signs of a tension pneumothorax are seen, the pressure may be easily relieved by simply briefly removing the airtight dressing over the wound and releasing the building pressure.

It should be clear that any patient with a blunt or penetrating chest injury must be carefully evaluated and continuously monitored for any indications that a simple or open pneumothorax exists and, if so, whether or not it is progressing to a tension pneumothorax, which requires rapid decompression.

Hemothorax

A **hemothorax** is a condition in which blood has accumulated in the pleural space because of blunt or penetrating trauma or other insult in much the same way as air accumulates in a pneumothorax (Fig. 16-9).

Frequently occurring along with a pneumothorax, a hemothorax produces many of the same signs and symptoms as a pneumothorax. Notably, however, the blood accumulation in a hemothorax most often moves to the lower lung fields, producing reduced breath sounds much lower than those found in a pneumothorax. The patient with a hemothorax may also become hypovolemic, since the chest cavity has room for a substantial accumulation of blood.

INJURIES THAT CAUSE INADEQUATE CARDIAC OUTPUT

Cardiac Contusion

Like any muscle, the heart can be bruised by blunt trauma from a variety of sources. A bruise or contusion to the heart (**cardiac contusion**) may have a number of different effects, including disturbances in the electrical conduction system, producing arrhythmias, reduced cardiac output due to muscle weakening, and even rupture of the heart muscle or valves. Rupture of the myocardium may lead to cardiac tamponade.

In any patient with potential for cardiac contusion as evidenced by apparent mechanisms of injury, such as a bent steering wheel, an electrocardiogram should be done. When cardiac contusion affects the electrical system of the heart, it may cause a tachycardia due to the amount of blood loss, multiple premature ventricular contractions, or atrial fibrillation. A bundle-branch block, usually caused by a right muscular contusion, produces ST-segment elevation and enzyme changes.

Cardiac Tamponade

Either blunt or penetrating trauma, as well as some disease conditions, can produce bleeding from the heart into

(text continues on page 339)

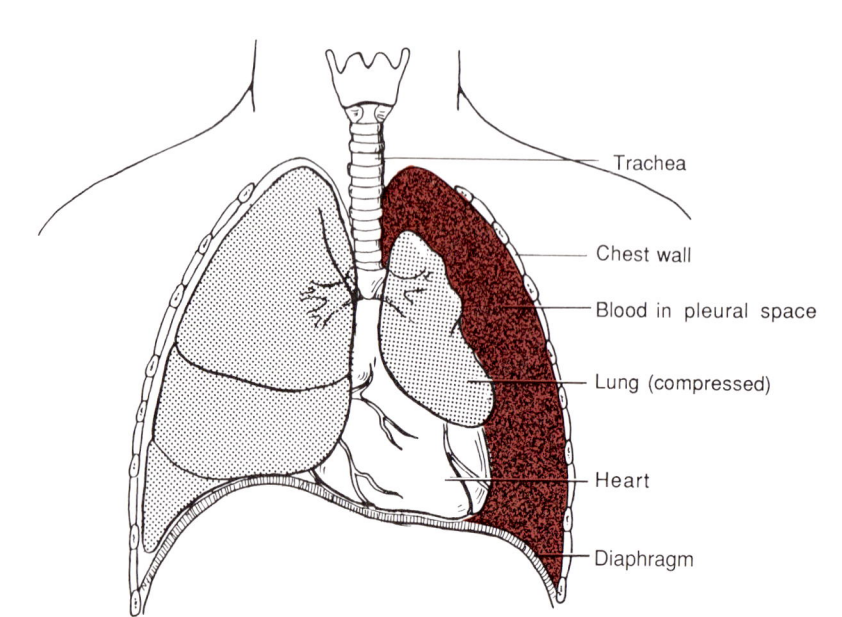

FIGURE 16-9.
Blood in the pleural space produces the same type of problems a pneumothorax does by reducing expansion of the lung. It can also progress to a tension hemothorax. A further complicating factor is the volume of blood lost in the chest cavity.

SKILL 16–2.
PERICARDIOCENTESIS

ACTIVITY	HOW PERFORMED	WHY PERFORMED
1. Check: • Responsiveness • Airway • Breathing • Circulation	Establish responsiveness Stabilize neck, open the airway Assess breathing Check for a pulse Check for hemorrhage	The primary survey is a rapid evaluation, less than 45 seconds, to identify and correct any life-threatening problems.
2. Assess the need for pericardiocentesis	Evaluate patient's presenting signs and symptoms to determine if procedure is indicated and appropriate.	Procedure must only be performed when indicated and appropriate, usually on orders from medical control.
3. Assemble equipment: Primary equipment (Activity 3): • 18-gauge spinal or cardiac needle • Syringe Accessory equipment and supplies: • Antiseptic swabs • Protective eye wear • Mask • Gloves	Assemble the needle and syringe. Place all equipment within easy reach. Put on protective eye wear, mask, and gloves.	Having all equipment ready reduces time delays during the procedure. Prevents blood or body fluid contact with non-intact skin or mucous membranes.

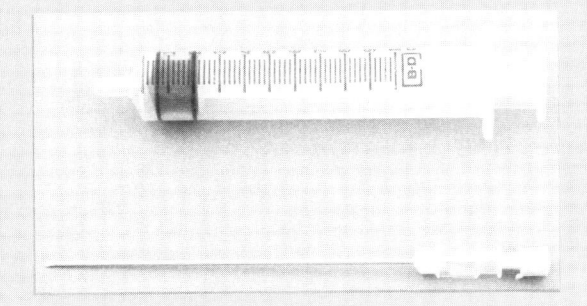

Activity 3.
Primary equipment.

4. Position the patient	Place the patient supine.	Positioning the patient supine allows for better access to the infraxiphoid area.
5. Find landmarks for pericardiocentesis and prepare the site	Locate a point just below and to the left of the xiphoid process. Cleanse the site with antiseptic swabs (Activity 5).	This point allows insertion of the needle just under the lower sternal border, from which it can be directed to the pericardial sac. Cleansing reduces the possibility of infection.

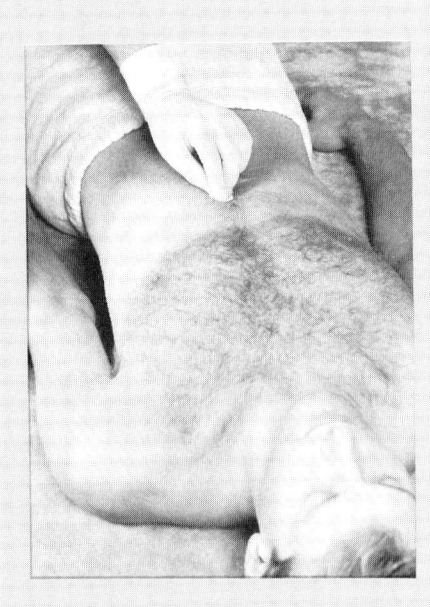

Activity 5.
Prepare the site.

(continued)

CHAPTER 16: Thoracic Injuries 337

SKILL 16–2.
PERICARDIOCENTESIS (continued)

ACTIVITY	HOW PERFORMED	WHY PERFORMED
6. Perform the pericardiocentesis	Insert the needle through the skin at a 90° angle to the skin (Activity 6A). Advance the needle about 1 cm, then direct the needle at a 45° angle toward the inferior tip of the patient's left scapula (Activity 6B). As the needle is advanced, pull gently on the plunger of the syringe attached to the needle (Activity 6C). Stop advancing the needle when blood appears in the syringe, but continue to aspirate all the blood that can easily be withdrawn. Withdraw the needle from the chest.	The perpendicular insertion directs the needle tip under the sternum. The described angle directs the needle toward the pericardial sac. When the pericardial sac is entered, blood is aspirated into the syringe. Removal of the accumulated blood should produce a rapid and dramatic improvement in the patient's condition.

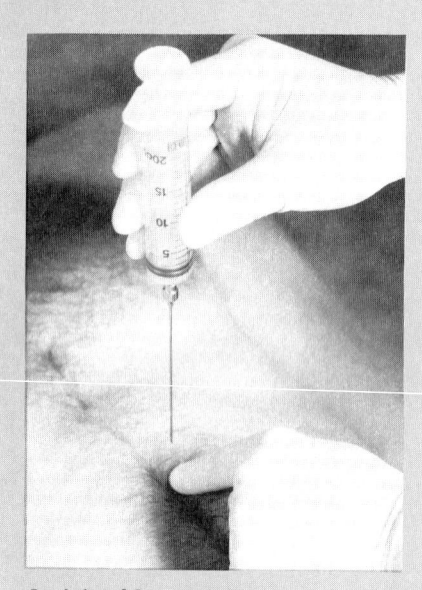

Activity 6A.
Perform the pericardiocentesis. Insert the needle.

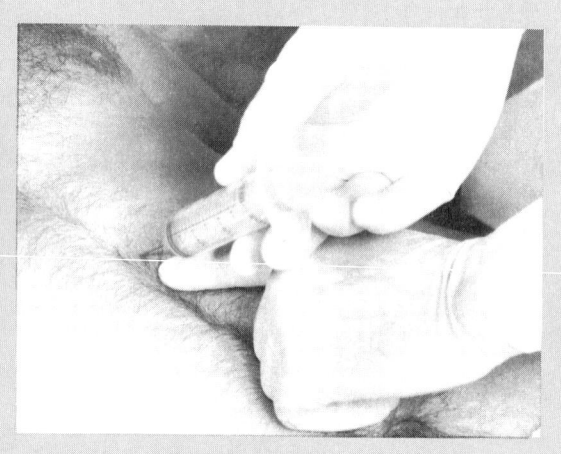

Activity 6B.
Advance and direct needle.

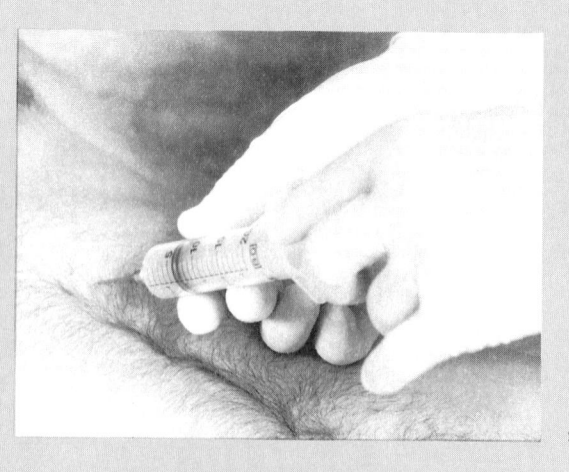

Activity 6C.
Pull gently on plunger of syringe.

7. Dispose of needle	Place contaminated needle in proper container.	Eliminates the possibility of injury or infection by contact with the contaminated needle.

CHAPTER 16: Thoracic Injuries 339

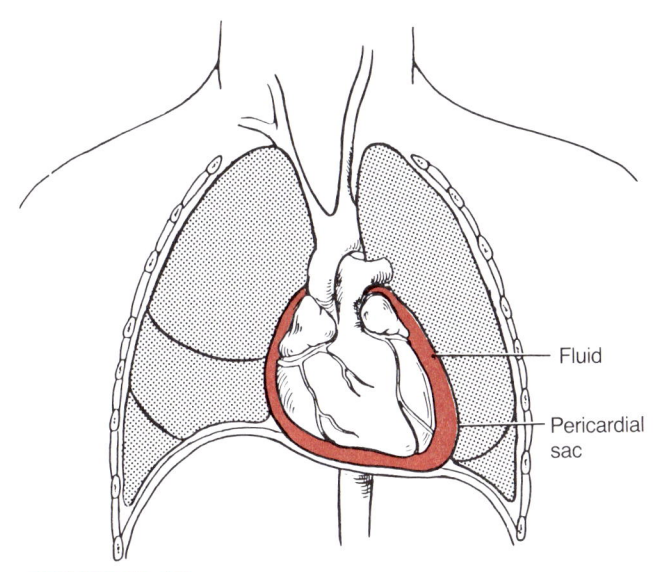

FIGURE 16-10.
Hemorrhage into the pericardial space compresses the heart and restricts the volume of blood that returns to the heart. Less blood is available for cardiac output during each contraction. This condition is known as cardiac tamponade.

the *pericardial sac* that surrounds the heart (Fig. 16-10). This condition is known as a *cardiac tamponade*. The pericardial sac, however, is an extremely tough and inelastic membrane that does not stretch or give as blood accumulates.

The result of this bleeding into the pericardial sac is similar to that of a tension pneumothorax; the heart muscle is compressed with the increasing pressure of the accumulating blood. This rising pressure restricts the amount of blood that can flow into the heart chambers during diastole. This restriction reduces the volume of blood pumped out of the heart during systole. This rapid and profound decrease in cardiac output and increase in preload gives rise to the signs and symptoms of cardiac tamponade, which include hypotension out of proportion to apparent blood loss, distended neck veins, narrowing pulse pressure, muffled heart sounds, and paradoxical pressure and pulse.

Without aggressive treatment, cardiac tamponade can be rapidly fatal. The only effective emergency treatment for life-threatening cardiac tamponade is ***pericardiocentesis***, a procedure that involves the insertion of a needle into the pericardial sac and aspiration of the accumulating blood.

The only indication for pericardiocentesis in the field is life-threatening cardiac tamponade. Given the relative certainty of death if the cardiac tamponade is not relieved, no real contraindications to the procedure exist.

The complications of pericardiocentesis, however, are so substantial that the diagnosis of cardiac tamponade must be carefully established. Complications of the technique include pneumothorax, puncture or laceration of the heart or coronary arteries, and cardiac arrhythmias.

A large-bore spinal or intracardiac needle, with or without an over-the-needle catheter, is inserted just below the xiphoid process and directed toward the inferior tip of the left scapula. As the needle is advanced into the pericardial sac, a syringe is used to aspirate the accumulated blood.

The procedure for pericardiocentesis is shown in Skill 16-2.

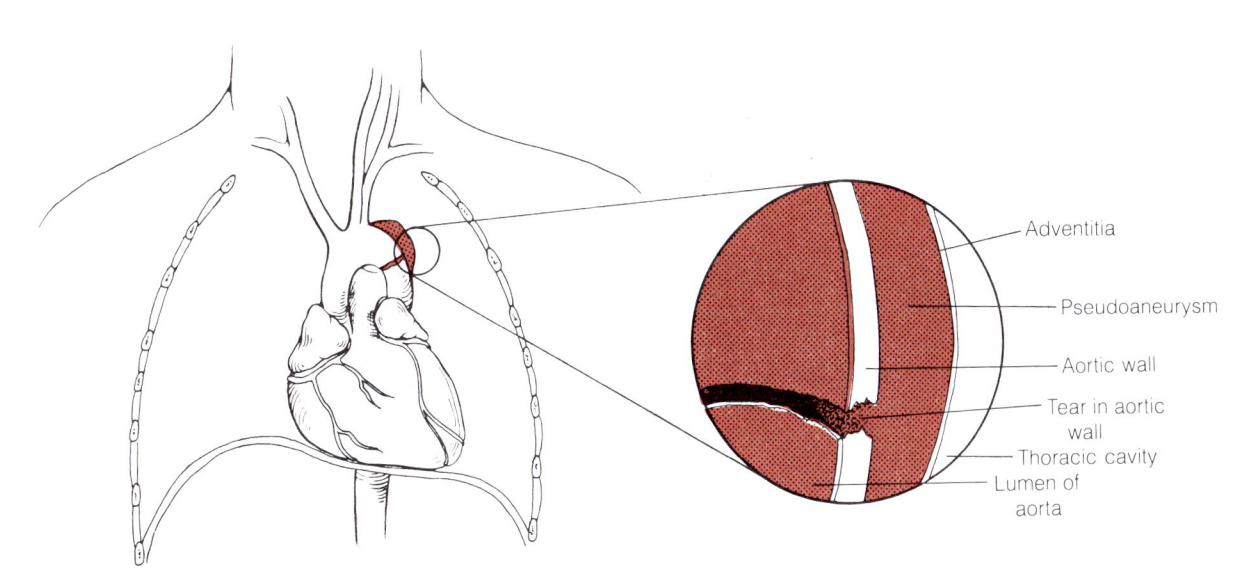

FIGURE 16-11.
Eighty percent of the decelerating tears of the aorta rupture into the free thoracic cavity within 1 hour after the tear occurs. Twenty percent are contained by the adventitia. This pseudoaneurysm may remain intact for only a few hours. Transportation of the patient to a trauma center is critical if the patient is to survive.

INJURIES THAT CAUSE INADEQUATE CIRCULATING BLOOD VOLUME

The thoracic cavity and the organs that lie within it are richly supplied with blood vessels that range from the smallest to the largest in the body. Virtually any of the injuries discussed previously may include bleeding within the thorax, and isolated injuries to vessels in the thorax may occur as well. The severity of bleeding may range from slight to substantial to exsanguinating life-threatening hemorrhage from major vessel damage.

A significant difficulty with any intrathoracic bleeding is that the presence of even major hemorrhage may not be evident on the exterior of the body. In virtually all cases, the presence of internal thoracic bleeding must be suspected from such clues as vital sign changes, mechanisms of injury, and patterns of other injuries.

Where major vascular damage has occurred, such as in a deceleration injury that causes a tearing of the aorta (Fig. 16-11), the only possibility of saving the patient is early suspicion of the injury and expedient transport to a qualified trauma center. Other less ominous vascular injuries are similar in that little other than general supportive care and expeditious transport can be provided in the field.

In these cases, the primary responsibility of the paramedic is to assess and examine the patient and the surroundings, rapidly appreciate the possibility of the presence of such injuries, and transport the patient without delay, performing most all treatment and detailed examination en route to the hospital.

SUMMARY

The most important component of management of thoracic trauma is prevention of hypoxia and anaerobic metabolism. As recalled from Chapter 11, the first step in this process is red blood cell oxygenation in the lungs. To achieve this step, oxygen must reach the alveoli. If some are compromised, extra oxygen must be given to the rest of them. Therefore, the first step is to administer a FiO_2 of 0.85 or greater. The second step is to provide adequate ventilation, which is assisted as necessary to achieve 800 to 1200 mL/ventilation. The third step is to treat the specific pathophysiologic process if prehospital management is indicated.

SUGGESTED READING

Ferko JG, Singer EM: Injuries to the thorax. J Emerg Med Serv 22(4):20, 1990

Howard CA, Easterday UJ: Respiratory Dysfunctions: Manual of Critical Care. St. Louis, CV Mosby, 1988

US Department of Transportation, National Highway Traffic Safety Administration: Emergency Medical Technician—Paramedic: National Standards Curriculum. Washington, DC, US Government Printing Office, 1985

CHAPTER 17

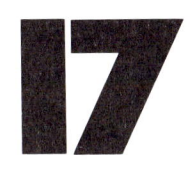

Abdominal Trauma

Mechanisms of Abdominal Trauma
Complications of Abdominal Trauma
Specific Intra-abdominal Injuries
    Splenic Injury
    Injury to the Liver
    Injury to the Large Intestine
    Injury to the Small Intestine
    Injury to the Stomach
    Assessment
    Management
Summary

BEHAVIORAL OBJECTIVES
On successful completion of this chapter, the reader will be able to:

1. Describe the mechanisms of blunt and penetrating abdominal trauma
2. List the solid and hollow organs of the abdomen
3. Describe the clinical manifestations of splenic injury and injury to the liver, large intestine, small intestine, and stomach
4. Explain how to assess a patient who is suspected of having an injury to the abdomen
5. Describe tenderness, rebound, and guarding in relation to palpation of the abdomen
6. Explain the management of a patient who has sustained an abdominal injury
7. Define all of the key terms listed in this chapter

KEY TERMS

The following terms are defined in the chapter and glossary:

Kehr's sign
rebound
guarding
peritonitis
tenderness

Major abdominal trauma represents a serious and potentially life-threatening form of injury. While abdominal trauma formerly carried with it a high mortality, recent recognition that the management of the trauma patient is improved by rapid surgical intervention has substantially reduced the incidence of poor outcome. Because definitive surgical treatment can be provided for many victims of abdominal trauma, the paramedic's role in the management of such patients has become increasingly important. The paramedic's skill in assessing, managing, and transporting the victim with major abdominal trauma to a trauma center that has surgeons and an operating room immediately available is of key importance to the patient's outcome.

MECHANISMS OF ABDOMINAL TRAUMA

Knowledge of the location of various abdominal organs in reference to the *four-quadrant system* allows the paramedic to assess the location of an injury (see Chapter 23) and greatly facilitates communication between health care workers. The importance of this knowledge is illustrated in the following scenario: The patient is a 23-year-old male who sustained blunt trauma to the abdomen. He is hypotensive with a blood pressure of 80/60 and has marked pain and guarding in the left upper abdominal quadrant. Since the spleen is the major abdominal organ subject to blunt injury in the left upper abdominal quadrant, such a description clearly conveys both the external location of the patient's injury as well as the possible internal injuries that may have resulted.

For descriptive purposes, traumatic abdominal injuries are classified as either *closed* or *open*, depending on the intactness of the abdominal wall. Closed (*i.e.*, blunt) abdominal injury defines those cases in which external trauma to the abdomen produces damage without penetrating the abdominal wall. The mechanism of injury in such cases can involve several types of physical forces; the common denominator is blunt trauma to the abdominal region. A direct blow, a fall, and a motor vehicle accident are all examples of cases in which significant closed abdominal trauma may result. Open (*i.e.*, penetrating) abdominal injuries occur when the continuity of the abdominal wall has been broken. Frequently, this type of trauma results in penetration of a foreign body into the abdominal cavity. Examples include gunshot wounds, stab wounds, and impaled objects.

COMPLICATIONS OF ABDOMINAL TRAUMA

Traumatic abdominal injury may result in hemorrhage, inflammation, infection, or loss of organ function. The particular complication that predominates often depends on the type of abdominal structure that has been injured (Table 17-1). For this reason, it is convenient to classify the abdominal structures into the following groups:

- Solid organs
- Hollow organs
- Vascular structures

TABLE 17–1.
ANATOMICAL CLASSIFICATION OF ABDOMINAL STRUCTURES AS RELATED TO MAJOR TYPE OF COMPLICATION AFTER INJURY

Category	Structures	Complication
Solid organs	Liver	Hemorrhage
	Spleen	
	Pancreas	
	Kidney	
Vascular structures	Aorta	Hemorrhage
	Inferior vena cava	
Hollow organs	Stomach	Peritonitis
	Gallbladder	
	Bladder	
	Small intestine	
	Large intestine	

The *solid organs* include the liver, spleen, pancreas, and kidneys. Each of these structures is characterized by possession of an extensive blood supply. As a result, injury to any of the solid organs is often complicated by major internal hemorrhage and hypovolemic shock.

The *hollow organs* include the stomach, bladder, large intestine, small intestine, and gallbladder. These structures all possess a hollow lumen, inside of which are a variety of liquid or solid materials. Injury to the hollow abdominal organs, especially in cases of penetrating trauma, is frequently complicated by spillage of the contained materials into the abdominal cavity. This spillage frequently results in severe irritation and inflammation (e.g., peritonitis) and may produce life-threatening infection.

The intra-abdominal *vascular structures* of prime importance are the aorta and the inferior vena cavae. Both of these structures carry large volumes of blood between the heart and body tissues. As a result, injury to either of these structures may produce major bleeding and hypovolemic shock.

SPECIFIC INTRA-ABDOMINAL INJURIES

Splenic Injury

The *spleen* is a flat oblong organ, about one-half foot in length, situated in the left upper abdominal quadrant. In the adult, it participates in a variety of important, though not life-essential, immunologic functions. Two characteristics of practical importance are the extensive vascularity of the spleen and its close anatomical relation to the lower left thorax. Because the spleen lies directly beneath the lower ribs of the left side of the thorax, any injury or fracture of the eighth, ninth, or tenth ribs on this side carries with it a high risk of splenic injury. For this reason, patients who have sustained trauma to the chest wall should be carefully evaluated for rib fractures. Localized tenderness, deformity, and pleuritic chest pain referred to the lower left rib cage all suggest rib fracture; the possibility of associated splenic injury should be considered. The large blood supply and soft consistency of the spleen make it particularly vulnerable to hemorrhage. In fact, major hemorrhage that results in hypovolemic shock is a serious and frequent complication of splenic fracture. Therefore, splenic rupture should always be considered in cases of trauma that involve the lower left rib cage and in all patients with abdominothoracic trauma complicated by unexplained hypovolemia.

Assessment of the patient with presumed splenic rupture often reveals some combination of the following:

- Blunt trauma to the left upper quadrant
- Trauma to the lower left rib cage
- Abdominal tenderness
- Involuntary guarding
- **Kehr's sign:** pain radiating to the left shoulder
- Hypotension
- Pallor
- Diaphoresis
- Tachycardia

Because definitive treatment requires surgical intervention, patient transport should be undertaken as rapidly as possible. Close monitoring and support of vital body functions with special attention to the patient's hemodynamic status are essential.

Injury to the Liver

The *liver* is a large, wedge-shaped, solid organ, the bulk of which occupies the right upper abdominal quadrant. Its superior surface lies directly beneath the right half of the diaphragm, and the major portion of the organ is protected by the overlying rib cage. Because of its large size, it is frequently subject to injury; in fact, in cases of both blunt and penetrating abdominal trauma, it ranks as one of the most frequently injured abdominal structures. The close association between the liver and the overlying rib cage should cause suspicion of the possibility of hepatic injury whenever fractures of the right rib cage are encountered. Clinical manifestations of injury to the liver may include the following:

- Right upper quadrant tenderness
- Rebound
- Involuntary guarding
- Referred pain to the right shoulder
- Hypotension
- Right hemothorax (in cases of associated diaphragmatic injury)

Since uncontrollable hemorrhage is the major cause of early death in patients with hepatic (liver) injury, rapid transport to a trauma facility for definitive surgical intervention and careful monitoring of the patient's hemodynamic status is crucial.

Injury to the Large Intestine

The *large intestine* is a hollow organ that measures about 1.5 m in length. Beginning in the right lower abdominal quadrant where it joins the terminal portion of the small intestine, it skirts the periphery of the abdominal cavity in the form of an arch. It ascends on the right side (*the ascending colon*) until it reaches the liver, then it makes a 90° bend and travels transversely across the abdomen (*the transverse colon*) until it reaches the spleen, where it again makes a 90° turn and descends along the left side (*the descending colon*) to the left iliac fossa, where it becomes more convolute (*the sigmoid flexure*) and enters into the pelvis to form its most terminal portion (*the rectum*).

Although subject to both blunt and penetrating trauma, injuries to the large intestine commonly involve a firearm of some sort, less commonly a knife. The close proximity of the colon to the small intestine and other structures accounts for the infrequency of isolated colonic injury; in the great majority of cases, other abdominal structures, most frequently the small intestine, are involved.

Assessment of the patient with colonic injury may reveal general signs of **peritonitis**; perforation allows the escape and spread of bacteria-laden intestinal contents throughout the abdomen. Tenderness, rebound, and involuntary guarding may all be present. However, peritonitis from infection usually takes several hours to develop, and these signs are not usually found in the prehospital patient. If, as is commonly the case, injury to other organs is found, then uncontrolled hemorrhage and its associate clinical signs may be present. Treatment should be supportive with rapid transport to a trauma facility where surgical exploration can be undertaken.

Injury to the Small Intestine

The *small intestine* is a long, tubular, hollow organ that begins at the pylorus and continues to the ileocecal valve, at which it ends by joining the large intestine. It is subdivided into three segments, the *duodenum, jejunum,* and *ileum.* Its combined length measures about 7 m and is bounded superiorly and laterally by the large bowel. The small intestine occupies a generous portion of the abdomen. Its presence in all four abdominal quadrants makes the small bowel particularly vulnerable to injury by penetrating trauma. Blunt trauma, though less common, may produce damage by crushing the small bowel against the vertebral column or by tearing it at any one of its several fixed locations. As with injury to the other hollow abdominal viscera, perforation of the small intestine results in general signs of peritonitis; tenderness, guarding, and rebound may all be found, but not early. Since infection is a major complication of small bowel injury, all patients must be rapidly transported to a trauma facility where surgical repair can be effected.

Injury to the Stomach

The *stomach* is a hollow muscular organ situated predominantly in the left upper abdominal quadrant. Possessing a *crescent shape*, it is subdivided into the cardiac portion, fundus, body, and pyloric portion. Gastric injury is significantly more frequent with penetrating trauma than with blunt trauma. The clinical manifestations, for the most part, are nonspecific; they are the result of the release of highly acidic and irritative contents from the stomach, which invariably occurs after perforation. Tenderness, rebound, and involuntary guarding may all be seen. Once again, transport to a medical facility with support of vital body functions is the prescribed mode of treatment in the prehospital setting.

Assessment

The initial evaluation of abdominal trauma is vital to both the immediate provision of prehospital care and to the establishment of a baseline by which physicians and nurses can monitor the patient's progress. The assessment should encompass the history, primary survey, and secondary survey (see the box "Approach to the Patient With Abdominal Trauma").

Obtaining a history in cases of major abdominal trauma may be complicated by the patient's condition. The paramedic should obtain as much pertinent information as possible without unduly delaying subsequent treatment and transport. The primary survey should, as always, be aimed at detecting and correcting any life-threatening conditions. Once the patient's responsiveness, airway, breathing, circulation, and cervical spine have been attended to, the paramedic can proceed with the secondary survey.

The secondary survey should start with the head and progress to the abdomen. Since internal hemorrhage is a major complication of abdominal trauma, its presence should be actively sought. Serial measurements of blood pressure and pulse should be recorded and interpreted in association with the patient's clinical condition. The finding of either hypotension or a pattern of decreasing blood pressure and increasing pulse rate in the patient with suspected abdominal injury and no evident source of blood loss should immediately suggest significant intra-abdominal injury with hemorrhage until proven otherwise. This possibility is a major reason for rapid assessment, resuscitation, packaging, and transport to the hospital.

The patient's abdomen should be inspected for any evidence of blunt or penetrating trauma. Gross signs of major penetrating trauma, such as abdominal eviscerations, impaled objects, or large entrance wounds, should

APPROACH TO THE PATIENT WITH ABDOMINAL TRAUMA

History
- Description of pain
- Mechanism of injury
- Prior alcohol or drug ingestion
- Time of most recent meal
- Preexisting medical conditions
- Medication and allergies

Primary Survey
- Responsiveness
- Airway and cervical spine
- Breathing
- Circulation and bleeding

Secondary Survey
- Vital signs
- Head and neck examination
- Pulmonary examination
- Cardiac examination
- Abdominal examination
    - Inspection
    - Auscultation (optional)
    - Palpation
- Musculoskeletal examination
- Neurologic examination

Management
- Monitor vital signs
- Ensure adequate ventilation and oxygenation
- Maintain adequate hemodynamic status (establish an intravenous line as needed)
- Monitor for cardiac arrhythmias
- Bandage abdominal wounds
- Apply pneumatic anti-shock garment for hemorrhage control
- Manage other injuries

Transport
- Undertake as soon as possible
- Notify receiving medical facility
- If appropriate, transport to a trauma center

---

be noted. More subtle yet equally dangerous small puncture wounds should be searched for, as these may be easily overlooked. If penetrating trauma is evident on inspection, an attempt to ascertain an entrance wound, exit wound, and probable path of the penetrating object should be made. With knowledge of the anatomical make-up of the abdomen, a reasonable guess may be made as to which organs are likely to have been injured. If no signs of penetrating trauma are evident, then indications of blunt abdominal trauma should be looked for. Are there areas of discoloration (ecchymosis) to suggest bleeding? Does the abdomen appear abnormally distended? The internal hemorrhage of blunt trauma may produce a distended abdomen.

After inspection, the next phase in assessing the abdomen is *auscultation*. The use of auscultation in cases of abdominal trauma must be guided by the clinical status of the patient and the particular situation at hand. The bell of the stethoscope is placed below the umbilicus in an effort to detect the normal pattern of bowel sounds. Diminished or absent bowel sounds may be a clue to intra-abdominal trauma with its resultant peritonitis and decreased gut motility (*ileus*). This component of the abdominal examination does not provide much useful information for the prehospital care provider, and it usually is eliminated. Percussion of the abdomen is frequently difficult in the prehospital setting and, for the most part, may be omitted also.

The last step in the physical examination of the abdomen, after inspection and auscultation, is *palpation*. Palpation of the victim of abdominal trauma is aimed at determining the presence or absence of tenderness and guarding and searching for the clinical manifestations of the irritant and inflammatory processes that result from intra-abdominal hemorrhage or leakage of normally contained fluids (e.g., intestinal contents, gastric fluid, bile). The following terms should be understood in relation to abdominal palpation:

Tenderness: An area that demonstrates an increased sensitivity to touch. Clinically, light palpation of the abdomen elicits a painful response.

Rebound: Pain that occurs when the peritoneal surfaces are rubbed together. Clinically, pressure is exerted over the abdominal wall with the gloved hand and then quickly released. The result is pain, either at or remote from the site. However, this method should not be used to elicit rebound tenderness because it produces confusing and falsely positive signs of guarding. The patient is instinctively taught that a hand on the abdomen produces pain. The patient then protects the abdomen by voluntarily tensing the abdominal musculature in a way similar to guarding. Such a technique should not be used to evaluate the abdomen. Rebound is best detected by having the patient cough or by gently shaking the cot or bed to see if pain is produced.

Guarding: Contraction of the abdominal wall musculature, either reflexively (*involuntary guarding*) or consciously (*voluntary guarding*). Clinically, in attempting to palpate the abdomen, the examiner's gloved hand meets with resistance or possibly rigidity.

Palpation is carried out by placing the outstretched gloved hand onto the abdomen with the fingers together and gently pressing inward about one-half inch. The entire abdomen should be quickly palpated in this fashion, leaving for last any localized areas of pain reported by the patient. A rough idea of the status of the patient's abdominal wall is desired. Is there tenderness? If so, is it localized or generalized? Does the abdomen feel soft or is it rigid and boardlike, or something in between? These are the questions that should be answered. The entire examination should be quick and take no more than 30 seconds. Deep and detailed palpation of the abdomen and its viscera is not indicated in the prehospital setting in cases of abdominal trauma. After the assessment of the abdomen is complete, the secondary survey should be continued with examination of the other body areas as described in Chapter 9.

Trauma of a magnitude sufficient to produce major abdominal injury may also result in significant injury to other body systems; conversely, major injury to other body areas can be associated with significant abdominal injury. The importance of a good secondary survey is well illustrated in the following scenario: An ambulance is dispatched for a 28-year-old male who has sustained a small-caliber gunshot wound to the left upper abdominal quadrant. The patient is conscious, breathing spontaneously, and without evidence of external hemorrhage or cervical spine injury. He is cool, pale, and diaphoretic with the following vital signs: blood pressure 90/60, pulse 110 weak and regular, respirations 28 and regular.

Without a good secondary survey, this patient might be rapidly transported with a diagnosis of penetrating abdominal trauma complicated by intra-abdominal hemorrhage. Only through a quick but complete secondary survey would the paramedic realize that the bullet had struck the spinal column, deflected upward, penetrated the left part of the diaphragm, and left the body through a small exit wound in the upper posterior thorax. The patient, in addition to penetrating abdominal trauma, also had sustained left pneumothorax and hemothorax with injury to the spinal cord. The key lesson is that one must always conduct a good, although at times abbreviated, secondary survey, keeping in mind the possibility of injury to multiple systems.

Management

Management of major abdominal trauma is highly patient specific; that is, the particular treatment modalities employed must be tailored to the particular needs of the patient. However, certain basic principles of trauma care apply more or less across the board. The airway must be maintained and kept free of foreign debris, blood, or vomitus. Breathing should be carefully monitored: patients with abdominal injury or associated thoracic injuries may have difficulty maintaining adequate ventilation and oxygenation. Supplemental oxygen administration is advisable in most cases of major abdominal injury to ensure adequate oxygenation. The circulatory status should

---

TREATMENT OF MAJOR ABDOMINAL TRAUMA

Administer supplemental oxygen

Monitor vital signs

Start an intravenous line
    Use large-bore administration set (macro drip)
    Use large-bore catheter (*i.e.*, 14 or 16 gauge)
    If hypovolemia exists and if it is feasible, two separate intravenous lines should be placed

Apply pneumatic anti-shock garment
    If clinical indications of marked hypovolemia are present, inflate pneumatic anti-shock garment

Initiate cardiac monitoring

Bandage any abdominal wounds
    Impaled objects should be stabilized with bulky dressings
    Abdominal eviscerations should be sealed with a sterile dressing to prevent loss of moisture

Initiate transport as soon as feasible

---

be closely monitored with frequent measurements of blood pressure and pulse rate. Cardiac monitoring is advisable to detect any arrhythmia that may develop. In cases of penetrating trauma, abdominal wounds should be bandaged and impaled objects should be stabilized with bulky dressings. In cases of abdominal evisceration, the protruding organ should be sealed with an occlusive dressing to preserve sterility and prevent excessive loss of moisture.

Because intra-abdominal hemorrhage is a major complication of abdominal trauma, its presence should be actively sought and treated. If clinical signs of hypovolemia are present, the measures of establishing intravenous access with volume replacement and applying the pneumatic anti-shock garment should be considered.

Intravenous access should be established with a 14- or 16-gauge catheter. At least one, and if possible two, intravenous lines should be placed to facilitate rapid fluid replacement. Volume replacement should be with normal saline or lactated Ringer's solution. If hypovolemia is significant, the pneumatic anti-shock garment should be applied and inflated. While these measures are helpful, definitive treatment usually requires rapid transport to a designated trauma facility for surgical intervention. The box "Treatment of Major Abdominal Trauma" outlines management procedures.

SUMMARY

Abdominal trauma can be extensive and difficult to assess in the prehospital setting. Traumatic abdominal injury can affect the solid or hollow organs in the abdominal compartment. Vascular structures can also be damaged. Large amounts of blood can be lost in the abdomen and not be noticed until extensive hemorrhage has occurred. Definitive treatment of abdominal injuries usually requires rapid transport to a designated trauma center for surgical intervention.

SUGGESTED READING

Campbell JE:Basic Trauma Life Support, 2nd ed. Englewood Cliffs, Prentice–Hall, 1988

Edwards FJ: Liver trauma. The Journal of Emergency Care and Transportation 19(3):28, 1990

Grant HD, Murray RH, Begeron JD:Emergency Care, 5th ed. Englewood Cliffs, Prentice–Hall, 1990

McSwain NE, Butman AM, McConnell WK, Vomacka RW: Pre-hospital Trauma Life Support, 2nd ed. Akron, Emergency Training, 1990

US Department of Transportation, National Traffic Highway Administration: Emergency Medical Technician–Paramedic: National Standards Curriculum. Washington, DC, US Government Printing Office, 1985

Walters DT et al:Abdominal Pain. Prim Care 13:3, 1986

CHAPTER 18

Musculoskeletal Injuries

Anatomy and Physiology of the Muscular System
  Skeletal Muscle
  Smooth Muscle
  Cardiac Muscle
  Energy Production
Anatomy and Physiology of the Skeletal System
  Functions
  Skeletal System
    Axial Skeleton
      Skull
      Spinal Column
      Sternum and Ribs
    Appendicular Skeleton
      Upper Extremity
      Lower Extremity
      Joints

Injuries to Muscle
  Strain
  Sprain
  Assessment
  Management
Injuries to Bone
  Fracture
    Assessment
    Management
  Dislocation
    Assessment
    Management
Summary

BEHAVIORAL OBJECTIVES
On successful completion of this chapter, the reader will be able to:

1. Locate on a diagram 20 of the principal superficial muscles of the body and give the action of each
2. Describe the anatomy and physiology of the three types of muscle tissue
3. Describe the principal structures of bone
4. Explain the five functions of bone
5. Locate and identify on a diagram all of the bones of the axial and appendicular skeleton
6. Describe six different types of joint movement, giving examples of each
7. Distinguish between a strain and sprain and discuss the management of each
8. List and describe the eight types of fractures
9. Describe how to properly perform an assessment on a patient with a fracture
10. Discuss the various management techniques for fractures, listing required equipment
11. Describe the assessment and management of dislocations
12. Define all of the key terms listed in this chapter

KEY TERMS

The following terms are defined in the chapter and glossary:

appendicular skeleton
articular cartilage
articulation
avulsion fracture
axial skeleton
bone
cardiac muscle
cartilaginous joint
comminuted fracture
compression fracture
crepitus
depressed fracture
diaphysis
dislocation
epiphyses
fascia
fibrous joint
fracture
greenstick fracture
hemopoiesis
impacted fracture
intervertebral disc
Le Fort's fractures

ligaments
manubrium
medullary cavity
oblique fracture
orthopaedic
osteoblasts
patella
periosteum
skeletal muscle
smooth muscle
spiral fracture
sprain
sternum
strain
synovial joint
tendons
transverse fracture
vertebrae
vertebral foramen
xiphoid process

Injuries to muscles, bones, and joints are some of the most common problems encountered by prehospital care providers. The seriousness of these injuries varies widely from simple injuries, such as a fractured finger, to major life-threatening conditions, like an open femur fracture or compromising spinal damages. Early intervention is crucial for preventing permanent impediments. A thorough, systematic survey of the patient and the mechanisms of injury involved is essential so that concealed injuries are not overlooked.

There is little difference in the management of a musculoskeletal injury between the basic or advanced life support level. Management consists of identification of the injury, control of hemorrhage, stabilization of the fracture or dislocation, and transportation to the hospital. The paramedic is expected to have a good understanding of the kinematics of such an injury and to be able to anticipate the injuries that will be present, as well as to have an in-depth knowledge of the anatomy of the muscles, bones, joints, and blood vessels.

ANATOMY AND PHYSIOLOGY OF THE MUSCULAR SYSTEM

Muscle tissue is made up of specialized cells, which, because of their distinctive properties, such as irritability, contractility, extensibility, and elasticity, are responsible for movement either of the body as a whole (locomotion) or of its parts (Table 18-1). The size of the body's framework is determined by the skeleton, but the muscles and fat determine body shape (Figs. 18-1 and 18-2). Though movement is the most familiar function of muscles, they also play a significant role in the production of body heat, and they aid in the maintenance of posture.

Muscle tissue is augmented by connective and nervous tissue. Muscles vary significantly in size, shape, and arrangement of fibers. They range from tiny strands to large masses. Some muscles are broad in shape and some are narrow. Some are long and tapering and some are short and blunt. Some muscles are triangular, some quadrilateral, and some irregular. Several muscle groups form broad, flat, expanded sheets, like those that form the abdominal and thoracic walls, while others form bulky masses, as can be found in the upper and lower extremities.

The arrangement of fibers varies in different muscles. In some muscles, the fibers are parallel to the long axis of the muscle, in some they converge to a narrow attachment, and in some they are oblique. Muscle fibers may even be curved, as found in sphincter muscles. The direction of the composition of the fibers and the size and shape of the muscle groups are significant in relationship to function. For example, the arrangement of the muscle fibers in the rectus femoris (medial aspect of the thigh) are *bipennate* (double-feathered). A muscle with this type of arrangement can produce the strongest contraction. Muscles are divided into three types on the basis of their structure and function (Fig. 18-3):

Skeletal muscle (also called striated): predominantly under voluntary control

TABLE 18–1.
IMPORTANT MUSCLES OF THE BODY

Muscle	Location	Action	Notes
NECK AND SHOULDERS			
Sternocleidomastoid	Side of neck	Helps keep head erect	If diseased or injured, head is permanently drawn to one side (torticollis)
Deltoid	Shoulder	Moves upper arm outward from body	Site for intramuscular injections
ARM AND ANTERIOR CHEST			
Biceps	Front of upper arms	Flexes forearm	
Triceps	Posteriorly to biceps	Extends forearm	
Pectoralis major	Anterior upper portion of chest	Help to bring arms across chest	
Pectoralis minor			
Serratus anterior	Anterior chest, arising from ribs		
RESPIRATION			
Diaphragm	Between the abdominal and thoracic cavities	Assists in process of breathing	When it contracts it moves downward, making chest cavity larger, forming a partial vacuum around lungs, causing air to rush into them. When it relaxes it pushes upward, and air is forced out of lungs
Intercostal	Between the ribs	Help to enlarge the chest cavity	
ABDOMEN			
Internal oblique	Flat bands that stretch from ribs to pelvis, overlapping in layers from various angles	Support abdominal organs	An opening in muscle creates weakness where a hernia (rupture) may occur
External oblique			
Transversus abdominis			
Rectus abdominis			
BACK AND POSTERIOR CHEST			
Trapezius dorsi	Across back and posterior chest	Helps to lift shoulder	Also called "swimming muscle"
Latissimus dorsi and other back muscles	Across back and posterior chest	Work in groups; help to stand erect, balance when heavy objects are carried, and turn or bend body; adducts upper arm	
GLUTEAL			
Gluteus maximus	Form the buttocks	Help change from sitting to standing positions; help in walking	Frequently used as site for intramuscular injections
Gluteus medius			
Gluteus minimus			
THIGH AND LOWER LEG			
Quadriceps femoris	Anterior thigh	Extend leg and thigh	
Hamstring	Posterior thigh	Flexes and extends leg and thigh	
Gracilis	Thigh	Flexes and adducts leg; adducts thigh	
Sartorius	Thigh	Flexes and rotates thigh and leg	Called "tailor's muscle" because it allows sitting in cross-legged position
Tibialis anterior	Anterior lower leg	Elevates and flexes foot	

(continued)

TABLE 18–1.
IMPORTANT MUSCLES OF THE BODY (continued)

Muscle	Location	Action	Notes
THIGH AND LOWER LEG			
Gastrocnemius	Calf	Flexes foot and leg	Give calf rounded appearance
Soleus	Calf	Extends and rotates foot	
Peroneus longus	Calf	Extends, abducts, and everts foot	
Achilles tendon	Attaches calf muscle to heel bone	Allows extension of foot and gives "spring" to walk	Term derived from Greek mythology
HANDS			
Flexor carpi radialis	Humerus (medial epicondyle)	Flexes hand / Flexes forearm	
Extensor carpi radialis brevis	Humerus (lateral epicondyle)	Extends hand	
FEET			
Tibialis anterior	Tibia (lateral condyle)	Flexes foot / Inverts foot	
Soleus	Tibia (underneath gastrocnemius)	Extends foot (plantar flexion)	
Gastrocnemius	Femur (condyles)	Extends foot / Flexes lower leg	
HEAD			
Orbicularis oculi	Head	Moves eyes and wrinkles forehead	
Orbicularis oris	Head	Moves mouth and surrounding facial structures	
Masseter	Head	Assists in chewing by raising lower jaw	
Buccinator	Head	Moves fleshy portion of cheek for smiling	

(Rosdahl CB)

- **Smooth muscle** (also called visceral): primarily involuntary and comprises most of the muscular tissue of the digestive tract, bronchi, urinary bladder, and blood vessels
- **Cardiac muscle:** found only in the heart; has the unique property of generating its own electrical impulses (automaticity)

Skeletal Muscle

All voluntary muscles are controlled by a person's will. Thus, they make possible all deliberate acts. Examples include walking, chewing, swallowing, smiling, frowning, talking, or moving the eyeballs. Voluntary muscles are composed of skeletal (*striated*) tissue. Most of these muscles are attached to the skeleton by tendons at one or both ends. However, some muscles are attached to the skin, cartilage, and special organs, such as the eyeball, or to other muscles, like the tongue.

Muscles help to shape the body and to form its walls. As stated earlier, one function of muscles is to maintain the body's posture. The continued partial contraction of many skeletal muscles makes possible standing, sitting, and other maintained positions of the body.

Most voluntary muscles end in tough, whitish cords (**tendons,** also called leaders), by which they are attached to the bones that they move. Tendons run through layers of dense, fibrous tissue called **fascia,** which covers the muscle. The fascia, primarily, contains two layers: the superficial fascia, which lies directly under the skin, is a continuous sheet of loose connective tissue; the deep fascia, a strong, dense, fibrous tissue, lies directly under the superficial fascia. Extensions of the deep fascia become continuous with tendons. It serves as a protective barrier for the delicate structures of the body, such as the organ systems, glands, blood vessels, and nerves.

Smooth Muscle

Smooth muscle (*visceral*) is made up of fibers that are larger than most striated fibers. They are innervated by nerve fibers of the autonomic nervous system. Unlike

CHAPTER 18: Musculoskeletal Injuries   353

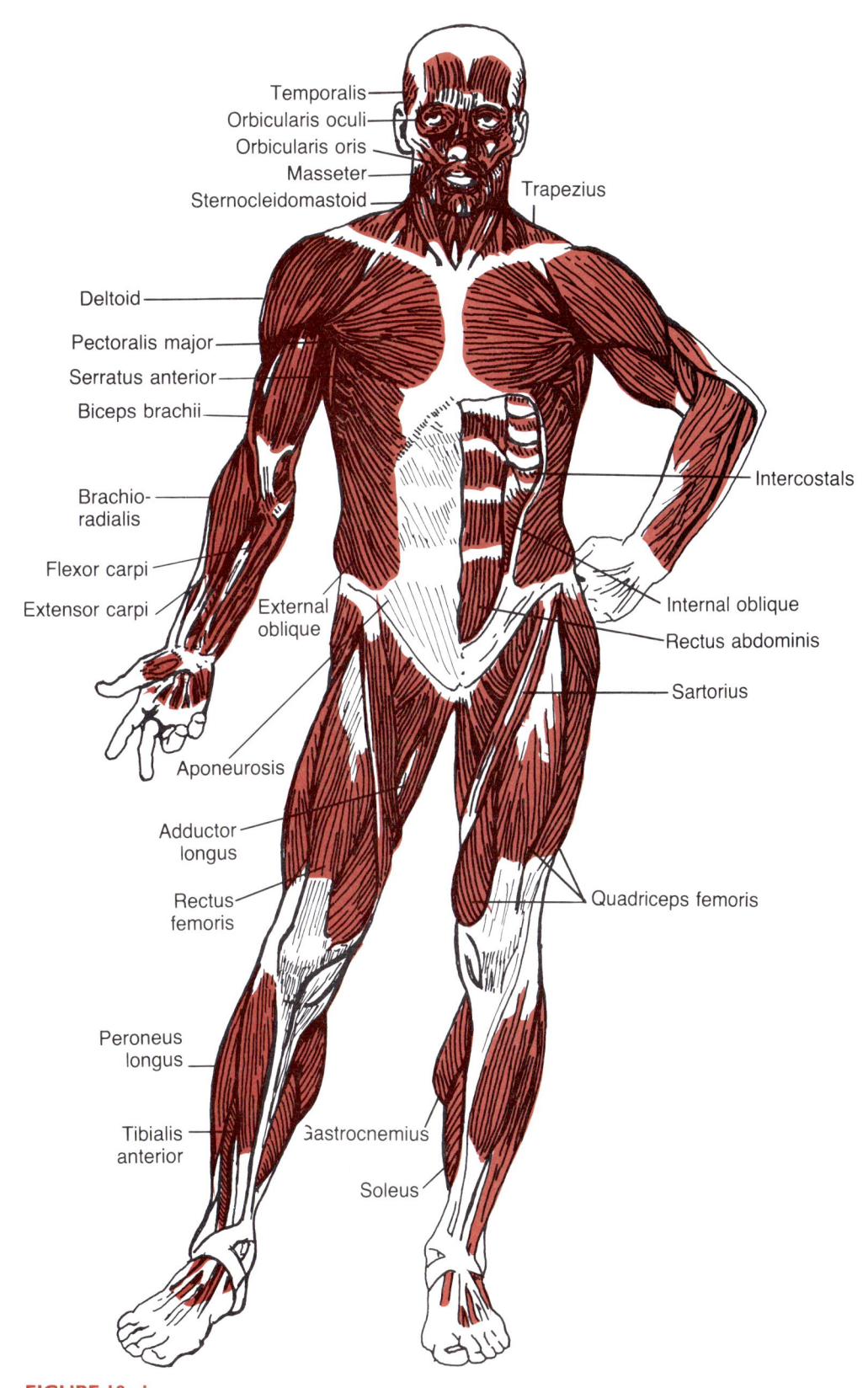

FIGURE 18-1.
Principal superficial skeletal muscles, anterior view. (Rosdahl CB)

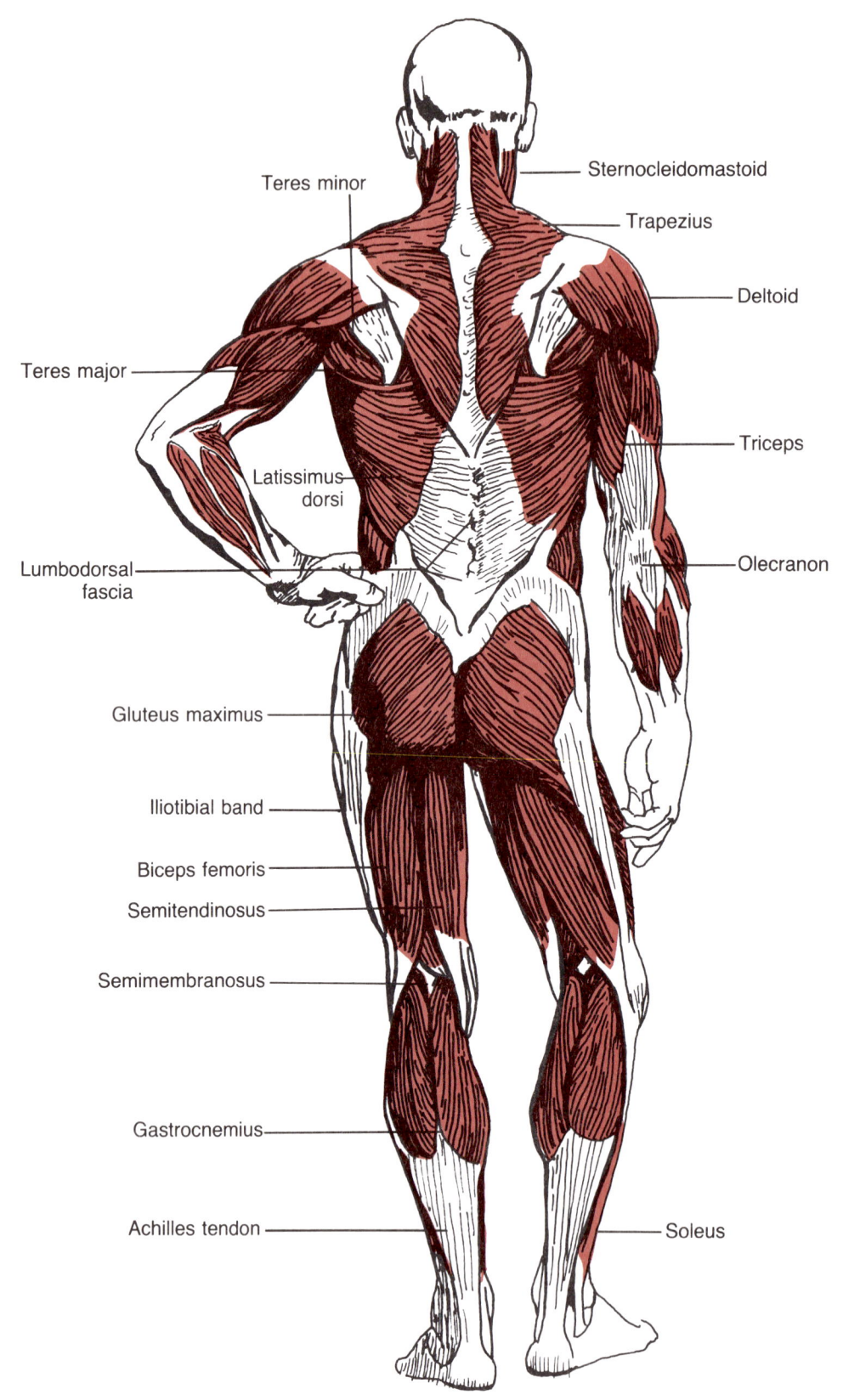

FIGURE 18–2.
Principal superficial skeletal muscles, posterior view. (Rosdahl CB)

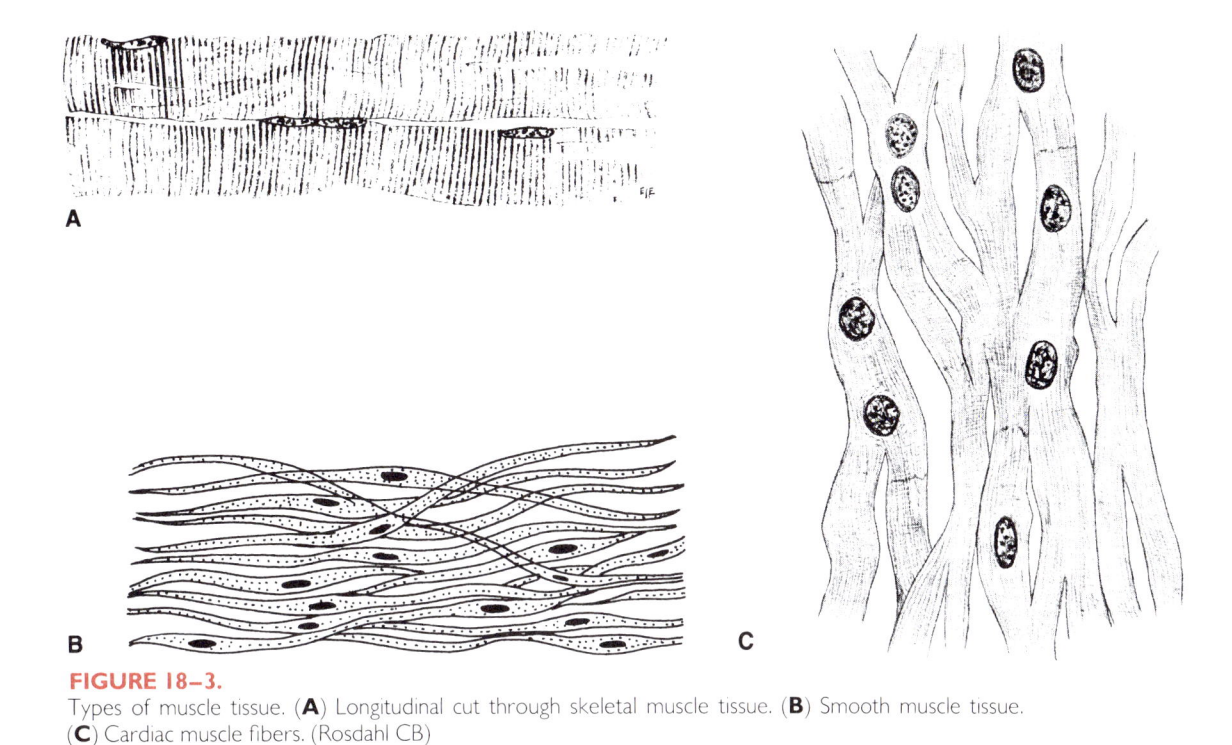

FIGURE 18–3.
Types of muscle tissue. (**A**) Longitudinal cut through skeletal muscle tissue. (**B**) Smooth muscle tissue. (**C**) Cardiac muscle fibers. (Rosdahl CB)

skeletal muscles, therefore, the actions of smooth muscles are not under voluntary control. Rather, they are involuntary and act in response to impulses sent from the various visceral motor centers in the brain. The internal organs of the body are predominantly composed of smooth muscle. It can be found in the walls of the digestive tract, trachea and bronchi, urinary bladder, and blood vessels. Some muscles are in two principal layers, circular and longitudinal. This specific arrangement supports the functional aspect of these organs by strengthening them and making possible their rhythmic, wavelike movements. For example, the peristaltic motion in the intestines propels food through the digestive tract.

Cardiac Muscle

Cardiac muscle is a special type of muscle found only in the heart. Although it is striated in appearance like skeletal muscle, it is involuntary. Cardiac muscle has the unique property of automaticity and is innervated by both sympathetic and parasympathetic nerve fibers. This muscle contracts and relaxes rapidly, continuously, and rhythmically about 60 to 80 times a minute (in the adult) without stopping. Because of the large energy expenditure, cardiac muscle requires a constant supply of oxygen.

Energy Production

The energy required for muscle contraction is derived from the metabolism of glucose. Muscle fibers must continually resynthesize *adenosine triphosphate* (energy) because they can store only small amounts of it. In normal metabolic pathways, the oxidization of glucose produces carbon dioxide and water. In the absence of oxygen, lactic acid is produced. Therefore, vigorous muscular activity is often followed by an increase in respiratory rate, thereby increasing oxygen delivery to and carbon dioxide removal from the tissues.

The sensation of muscle fatigue occurs when the energy supply to the muscle is inadequate or surpassed by the energy demands. It may also result from a deficiency of essential nutrients, electrolytes, or oxygen. For instance, in anemia the number of circulating red blood cells or hemoglobin is abnormally low. In some cases, both may be low. Therefore, less oxygen actually reaches the muscles, and they fatigue much more rapidly.

Energy is needed for muscles to do their work. However, only about one third of this energy is used for work. The remaining two thirds is released in the form of heat. Because skeletal muscle cells are both highly active and numerous, they produce a major share of total body heat. Skeletal muscle contractions, therefore, constitute one of the most important parts of the mechanism that maintains a balance of temperature. When the body is exposed to cold environmental temperatures, it can augment the production of heat through voluntary activity, such as walking, or through involuntary responses, such as shivering.

ANATOMY AND PHYSIOLOGY OF THE SKELETAL SYSTEM

Bone, like other tissue, consists of living cells and nonliving intercellular substance. The intercellular material, or matrix of bone, predominates. It is much more abundant than bone cells, and it contains many fibers of *collagen* (the body's most abundant protein). In these respects, bone's matrix resembles that of other connective tissues. However, it also differs strikingly from them. For one thing, it is hard and rigid, not soft and flexible. It is calcified. Calcium salts, notably calcium phosphate and calcium carbonate, impregnate the matrix of bone, thus giving bone its hard and rigid qualities.

There are four types of bones. Their names suggest their shapes: long bones, short bones, flat bones, and irregular bones. Each type of bone consists of many different structures, some visible to the naked eye (Fig. 18-4). The main, shaftlike portion of the bone is called the **diaphysis**. Its hollow, cylindrical shape and the thick compact bone that composes it adapt the diaphysis well to its function of providing strong support without cumbersome weight.

The **epiphyses** can be found at each end of the long bone. They have a bulbous shape that provides generous space near joints for muscle attachments and also gives stability to joints. Because of the innumerable small spaces in the bone of the epiphysis, it resembles a sponge. Therefore, it is commonly referred to as spongy, or cancellous bone. In most adult epiphyses, yellow marrow fills the spaces of cancellous bone except in the proximal epiphyses of the humerus and femur. These are filled with red marrow. The joint or articular surfaces of the epiphyses are covered by a thin layer of cartilage. This layer of tissue is called the **articular cartilage**. It functions as a cushion because of its resiliency against jars or blows.

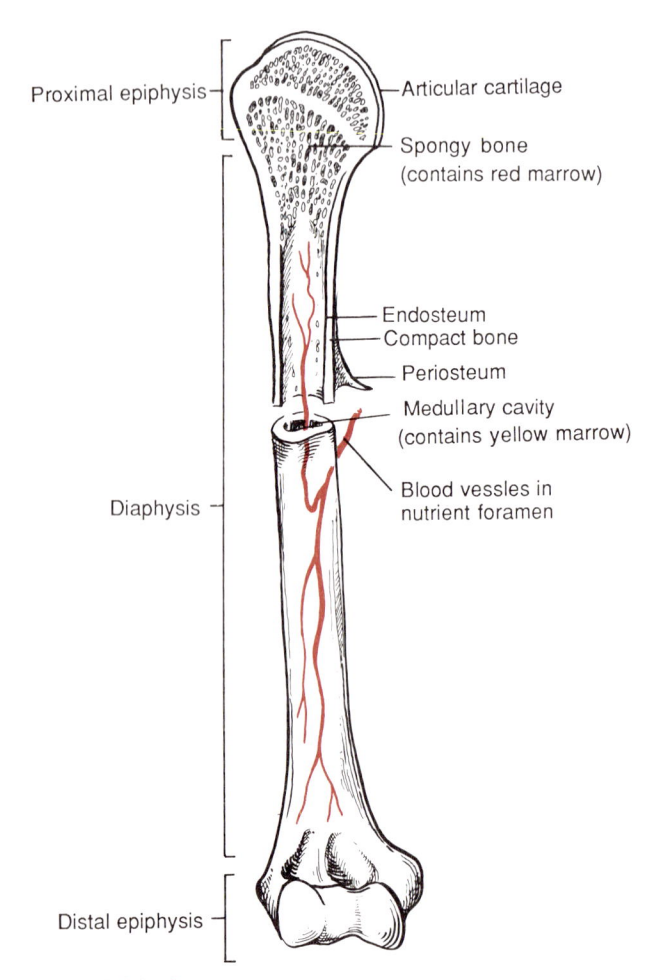

Covering the entire outer surface of the bone, except at joint surfaces where articular cartilage forms the covering, is a dense, white, fibrous membrane called the **periosteum**. Many fibers of the periosteum penetrate the underlying bone, thus welding the two structures together. Muscle tendon fibers interlace with periosteal fibers, thereby anchoring muscles firmly to bone. Further, the periosteal membrane contains many small blood vessels that send branches into the bone. Bone-forming cells, called **osteoblasts,** compose the inner layer of the periosteum. Because of these two factors, the blood vessels and osteoblasts, the periosteum functions essentially for bone cell survival and for bone formation, both of which are processes that continue throughout life.

Another important structure, the **medullary** (or marrow) **cavity,** is a tubelike hollow in the diaphysis (main shaft) of the bone. This cavity serves to manufacture blood cells. Bones are not lifeless structures. Rather, within this hard, seemingly lifeless material lie the many living bone cells. They must, like all living cells, continually receive food and oxygen and excrete their wastes. So blood supply to bone is important and abundant.

Functions

The human body is shaped by its bony framework. Without its 206 bones, the body would collapse. This bony framework is held together by **ligaments,** which connect bone to bone, layers of muscles, tendons, which connect muscles to bone or other structures, and various connective tissue. Bones and their adjacent tissues help to move, support, and protect the vital organs.

Bones perform the following five functions: support, protection, movement, hemopoiesis, and service as a mineral reservoir. Bones serve as the supporting framework of the body much as steel girders function as the supporting framework of modern buildings. Hard, bony "boxes" protect delicate structures enclosed by them. For example, the skull protects the brain, and the rib cage protects the lungs and the heart. Bones with their joints constitute levers. Muscles are anchored firmly to bones. As muscles contract and shorten, they pull on bones, thereby producing movement at a joint.

Hemopoiesis, which is the term for blood cell formation, is a vital process carried on by red bone marrow. In an infant's or child's body, virtually all of the bones contain red marrow; as the body ages, however, much

FIGURE 18-4.
Macroscopic appearance of a long bone that has been partially sectioned.

of it becomes transformed into yellow marrow, an inactive, fatty tissue. The main bones in an adult's body that contain red marrow are those of the chest, spinal column, base of the skull, upper arm, and thigh. The red marrow lies deeply hidden in bones, thus suggesting the importance of its function. Red marrow forms blood cells (red blood cells, some white cells, and platelets), and blood cells perform various functions essential for maintaining life.

Finally, bones serve as the major storage depot for calcium, phosphorous, and certain other minerals. Homeostasis of blood calcium concentration, which is essential for healthy survival, depends largely on changes in the rates of calcium movement between the blood and bones.

Skeletal System

The structural framework of the body, the skeleton, must be strong to provide support and protection, jointed to permit motion, and flexible to withstand stress. This structure can be separated into two main divisions, the axial and appendicular skeleton. Eighty bones make up the **axial skeleton**. These include 74 bones that form the upright axis of the body—the head, the neck, and the thorax—and 6 that form the tiny middle ear bones. The **appendicular skeleton** consists of 126 bones. The bones of the appendicular skeleton form the appendages to the axial skeleton, that is, the shoulder girdles, arms, wrists, hands, and the hip girdles, legs, ankles, and feet.

Axial Skeleton

SKULL. The skull rests on top of the spinal column. It contains the brain and the centers of special senses: sight, hearing, taste, and smell. Twenty-eight irregularly shaped bones form the skull. It consists of two major divisions: the *cranium* (brain case) and the face. The cranium is formed by eight bones: frontal, two parietal, two temporal, occipital, sphenoid, and ethmoid. The 14 bones that form the face are: two maxillary, two zygomatic (malar), two nasal, mandible, two lacrimal, two palatine, two inferior nasal conchae (turbinates), and vomer.

Thirteen of the 14 facial bones are immovable and interlocking. The immovable bones form the bony settings of the eyes, nose, cheeks, and mouth. The *lower jaw* (mandible) moves freely on hinge joints and is shaped like a horseshoe. The mandible is the largest and strongest bone of the face. Figure 18-5 shows the bones of the skull and face.

SPINAL COLUMN. The spinal column is the principal support system of the body. It constitutes the longitudinal axis of the skeleton. It is a flexible rather than rigid column because it is segmented. The spinal column consists of 24 irregularly shaped bones called **vertebrae** (the singular is "vertebra"), plus the sacrum and coccyx. Joints between the vertebrae permit forward, backward, and sideways movement of the column. To increase the carrying strength of the vertebral column and to make balance possible in the upright position, the spinal column is curved. Lying one vertebra on top of another forms a strong, flexible column, which is bound firmly by strong ligaments. Between each two vertebrae is a fluid-filled pad of tough cartilage, called the **intervertebral disc,** which acts as a shock absorber. These discs are extremely susceptible to injury from twisting, grinding, or improper lifting of heavy objects.

The first seven vertebrae, known as the cervical vertebrae (*or cervical spine*), constitute the skeletal framework of the neck. The skull is attached to the top of this section. The next twelve vertebrae are called thoracic vertebrae (*or thoracic spine*) because of their location in the posterior part of the chest or thoracic region. Further, this portion of the spine constitutes the upper back. Twelve pairs of rib bones are attached to these vertebrae and serve as support. The ribs form a cagelike structure that protects vital organs, such as the heart, lungs, aorta, and portions of the vena cava.

The lumbar vertebrae (*or lumbar spine*) is made up of the next five consecutive spinal bones. This portion of the spinal column is considered the lower back (also known as the "small" of the back). The cervical and lumbar vertebrae are the most frequently injured areas of the spinal column.

The sacrum (*or sacral spine*) comprises the next five vertebrae. These vertebrae are fused together, fashioning a single bone, which forms the posterior aspect of the pelvis. Like the sacral spine, the coccyx is formed by the fusion of four or five vertebrae. This portion of the spinal column, also called the *coccygeal spine*, is most commonly referred to as the "tail bone." This structure does not have the protrusions characteristic of the other vertebrae.

Vertebrae are designated by letters and numbers. Those in the cervical spine are referred to by the letter "C" with numbers one through seven, those in the thoracic region by the letter "T" with numbers one through twelve, and so on. In other words, if the third vertebra in the patient's lumbar spine is injured, the paramedic would report this fact as an injury to "L-3." The vertebral column is shown in Figure 18-6.

All the vertebrae resemble each other in certain features and differ in others (Fig. 18-7). Most of the vertebrae have a flat, rounded body placed anteriorly and centrally, a sharp or blunt spinous process that projects inferiorly in the posterior midline, and two transverse processes that project laterally. All except the sacrum and coccyx have a central opening, the **vertebral foramen**. This passage serves as a protective casing or tunnel, through which the spinal cord passes. Each thoracic vertebrae has articular facets for the ribs. The vertebral column as a whole articulates with the head, ribs, and iliac (pelvic) bones. Individual vertebrae articulate with each

358   UNIT THREE: TRAUMA

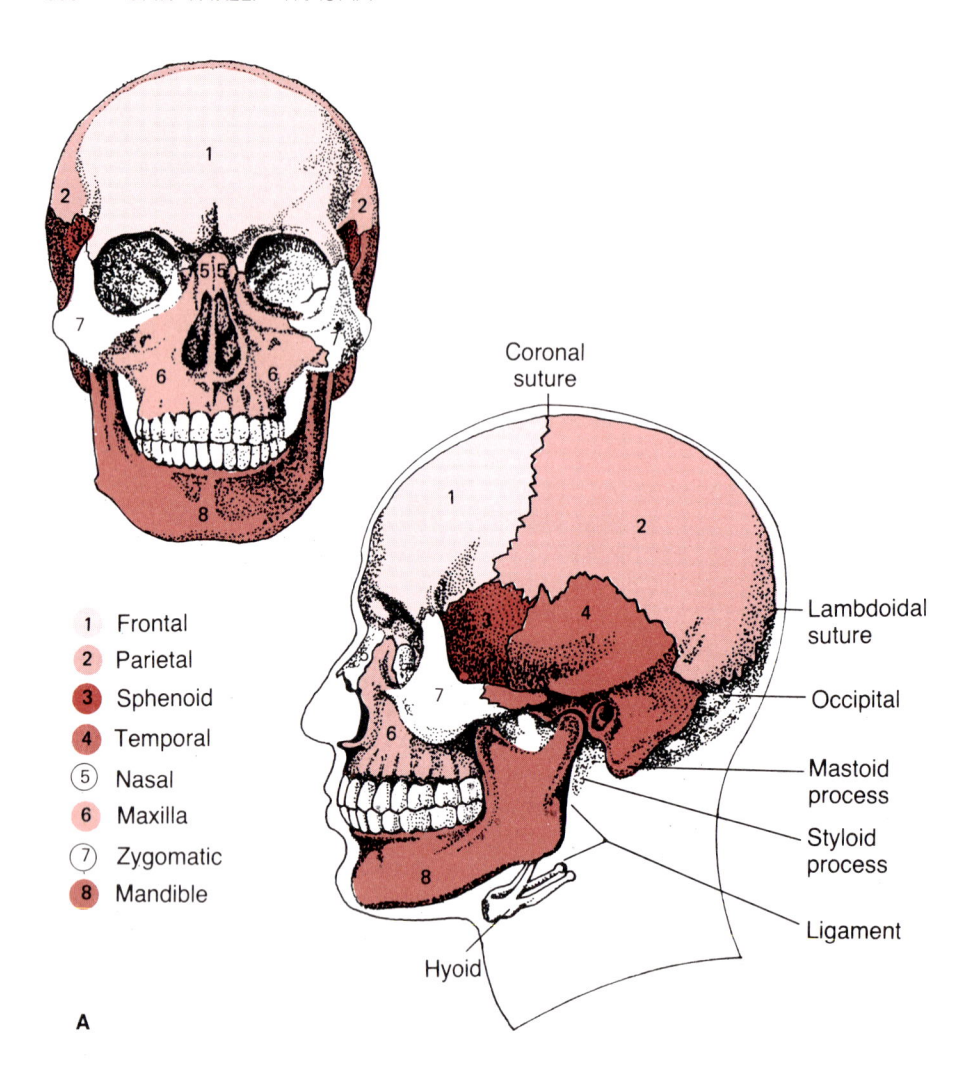

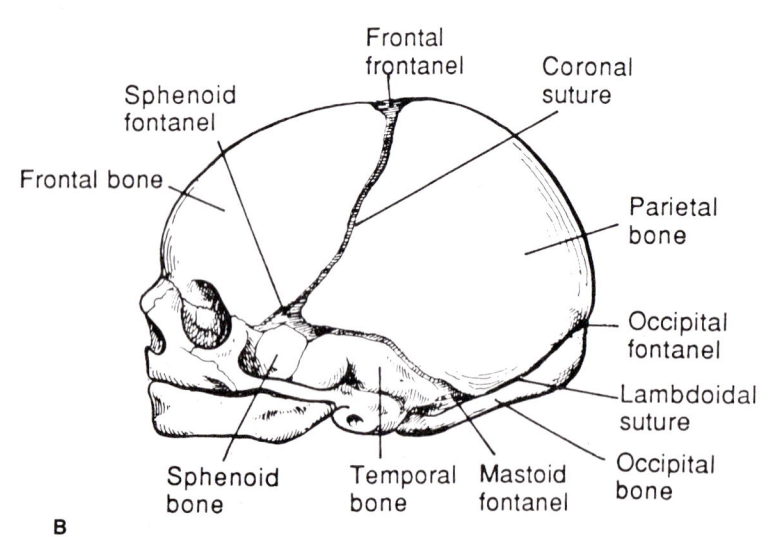

1. Frontal
2. Parietal
3. Sphenoid
4. Temporal
5. Nasal
6. Maxilla
7. Zygomatic
8. Mandible

FIGURE 18–5.
Bones of the skull and face. (**A**) Adult. (**B**) Infant. (Rosdahl CB)

arch of bone. Each one articulates with both the body and the transverse process of its corresponding thoracic vertebra. Strong ligaments bind the posterior ends of the ribs to the spinal column but allow slight gliding or tilting movements. This mechanical fact is important for breathing. The anterior ends of the top seven pairs of ribs are attached to the sternum by means of cartilage. They are considered the "*true*" ribs. The remaining five pairs are called "*false*" ribs, since each of the three pairs is attached anteriorly by cartilage to the pair of ribs above, thus indirectly to the sternum. The front ends of the last two pairs of ribs hang free and are called "floating" ribs.

Appendicular Skeleton

UPPER EXTREMITY. The upper extremity consists of the bones of the shoulder girdle, arm, forearm, wrist, and hand (Fig. 18-9). Two bones, the clavicle (collarbone) and scapula (shoulder blade) form the shoulder girdle. With the muscles that extend from it to the arms, thorax, neck, and head, the shoulder girdle helps to attach the arms to the trunk.

The humerus, or arm bone, is the largest bone in the upper extremity. Like other long bones, it consists of a shaft, or diaphysis, and two ends, or epiphyses. The upper end of the humerus (also called the head) is round; its distal end is flat. The round head articulates with the shallow cuplike structure of the scapula, forming a ball-and-socket joint. This is the most freely movable joint in the body and is easily dislocated. The humerus joins distally with both the radius and the ulna.

Two bones form the framework for the forearm: the radius on the thumb side and the ulna on the little finger side. The proximal end of the ulna forms most of the *olecranon process* (elbow joint). While the ulna can be palpated along its entire length, the upper two thirds of the radius is sheathed in muscle and cannot be palpated. Only the distal end of the radius, which enlarges to form most of the wrist joint, can be felt through the skin. The bony prominences on the distal ends of both the ulna and radius that form the socket for the wrist joint are referred to as styloid processes. The ulnar styloid is palpable on the little finger side of the wrist, and the radial styloid can be easily felt on the thumb side of the wrist.

Eight small, irregularly shaped bones, called carpal bones, form the wrist. Ligaments bind the carpals closely and firmly together in two rows of four each. The joints between the carpals and radius permit wrist and hand movement.

Five bones form the structural framework of the hands. Of the five metacarpal bones, which provide the hand its structural strength, the thumb forms the most freely movable joint with the carpals. This fact has great significance. Because of the wide range of movement possible between the thumb and the carpals—particularly,

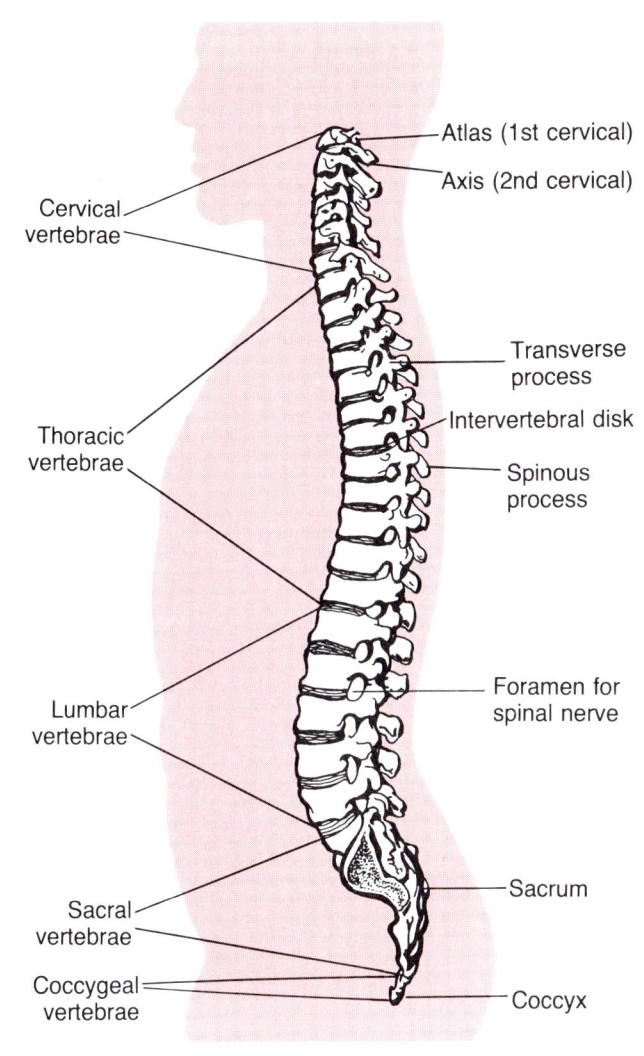

FIGURE 18-6.
Vertebral column, left lateral view. (Rosdahl CB)

other in joints between their bodies and between their articular processes.

STERNUM AND RIBS. The medial part (middle portion) of the anterior chest wall is supported by the **sternum**. This dagger-shaped structure can be divided into three parts (Fig. 18-8):

Manubrium: the upper handle part
Body: the middle "blade" portion
Xiphoid process: the lower tip, made up mostly of cartilage

The manubrium articulates with the clavicles and first pairs of ribs, whereas the next nine pairs of ribs join the body of the sternum, either directly or indirectly, by means of the costal cartilages.

The twelve pairs of ribs, together with the vertebral column and sternum, form the bony cage known as the thorax (see Fig. 18-8). Each individual rib is a semiflexible

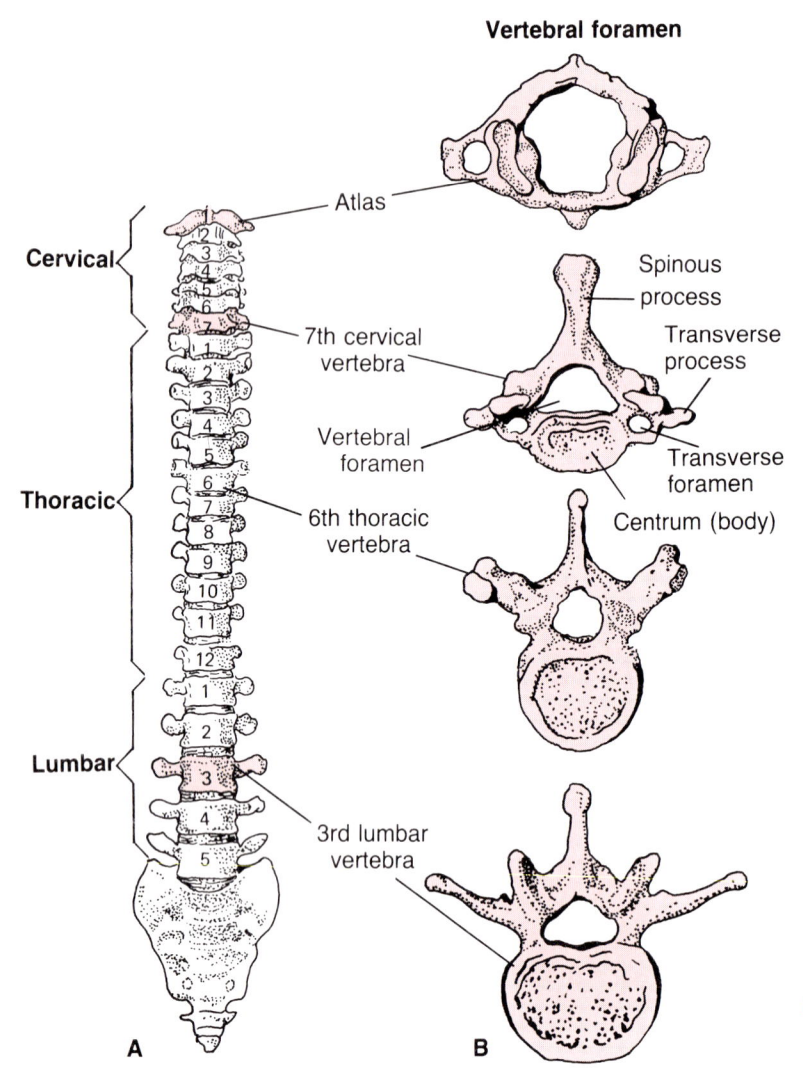

FIGURE 18-7.
Vertebral column with anterior view (**A**) and superior view (**B**) of vertebrae. (Rosdahl CB)

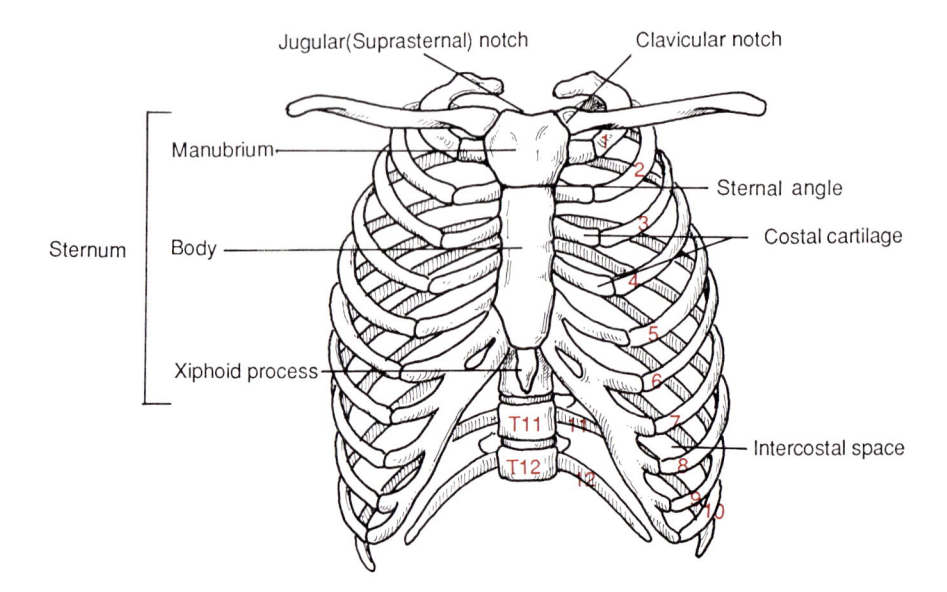

FIGURE 18-8.
Anterior view of the axial skeleton shows the sternum and ribs.

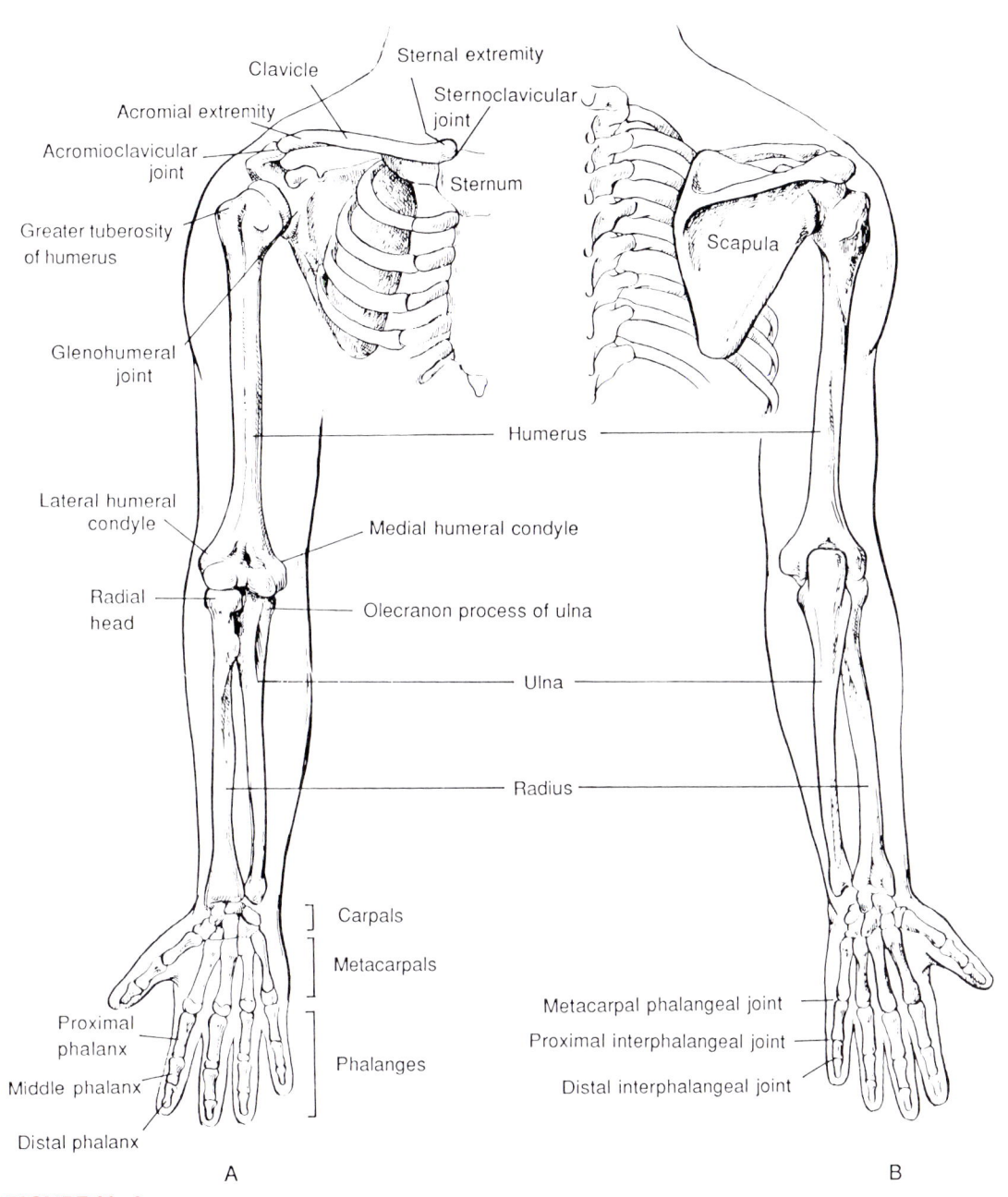

FIGURE 18-9.
Bones of the right upper extremity in the anterior view (**A**) and the posterior view (**B**).

the ability to oppose the thumb to the fingers—the human hand has much greater dexterity than the forepaw of any animal and has, thus, enabled human beings to manipulate their environment effectively. The phalanges are the bones that make up the fingers and thumbs. Each finger has three phalanges, and each thumb is composed of two.

LOWER EXTREMITY. Bones of the hip, thigh, leg, ankle, and foot constitute the lower extremity. Strong ligaments bind each hip bone to the sacrum posteriorly and to each other anteriorly to form the pelvic girdle. The pelvis is described as a stable, circular base that supports the trunk and attaches the lower extremities to it. The pelvic girdle is actually composed of three separate bones that, during the developmental periods, fuse together to form a single, massive irregular bone that is broader than any other bone in the body (Fig. 18-10). The largest and uppermost of the three bones is the ilium; the strongest and lowermost, the ischium; and the anteriormost, the pubis.

The entire pelvic girdle forms the floor of the abdominal cavity. The lower aspect of the cavity houses delicate organs, such as the bladder, the rectum, and internal portions of the reproductive system. The pelvic cavity is ex-

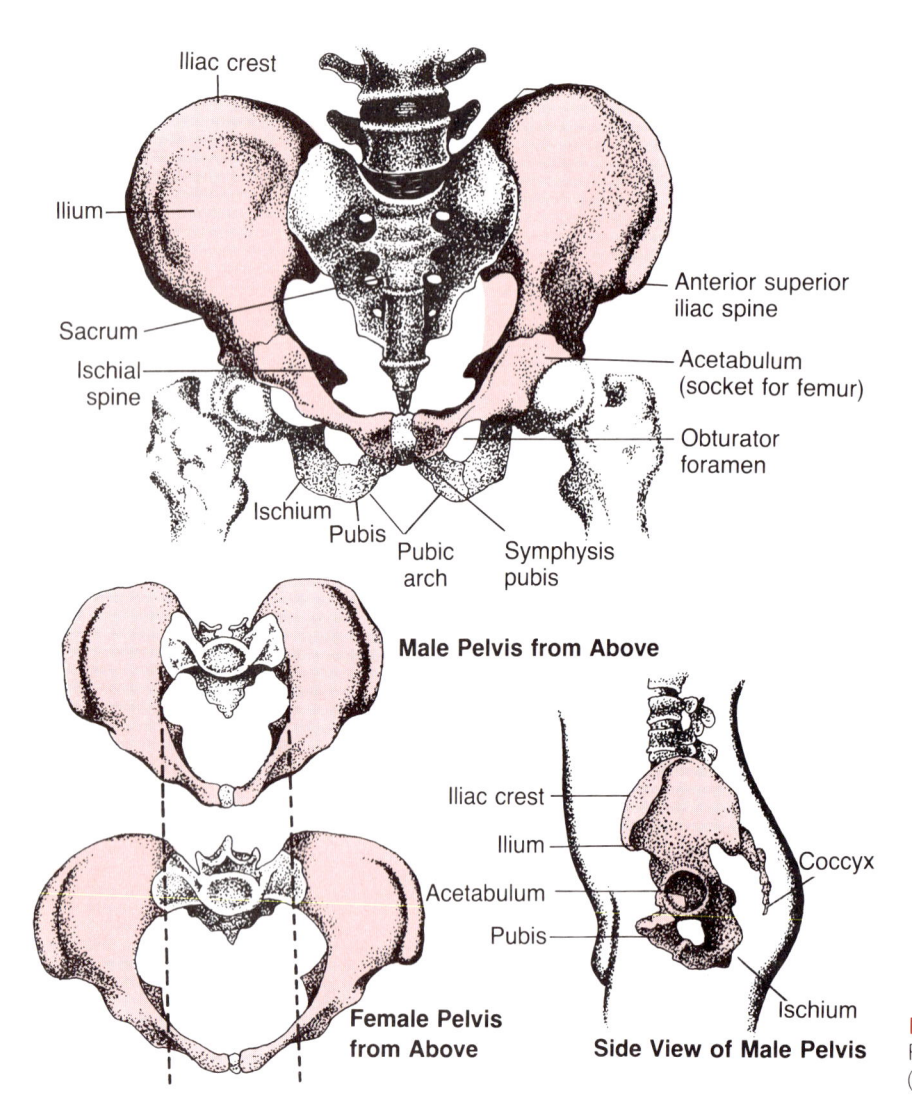

FIGURE 18-10.
Pelvic girdle with male and female pelvis. (Rosdahl CB)

tremely vascular, and a pelvic fracture may cause severe bleeding. The floor of the pelvic cavity helps to support the intestines.

The two thigh bones, called femurs, have the distinction of being the longest and heaviest bones in the body. They have several characteristic markings. For instance, proximally, the head and the greater and lesser trochanters are found, and the medial and lateral condyles lie distally. Both condyles and the greater trochanter can be palpated. Like the humerus, the distal end of the femur is flat, and the two condyles articulate with the tibia at the knee joint.

The knee joint is a strong hinge joint and, like the elbow, allows angular movement only. The joint is protected and stabilized in front by the **patella** (kneecap). The patella is a small, triangular-shaped bone in front of the large muscle of the front of the thigh. When the knee joint is extended, the patellar outline may be distinguished through the skin, but as the knee flexes, it sinks into the intercondylar notch of the femur and can no longer be delineated.

In anatomical terminology, the word "leg" is used only for that portion of the lower extremity between the knee and the ankle. Its two bones are the tibia and fibula. The tibia is the larger and stronger and more medially and superficially located of the two lower leg bones. The fibula is smaller and more laterally and deeply placed. The tibia's broad upper surface receives condyles of the femur to form the knee joint. The distal end, much smaller than the proximal aspect, forms the inner, rounded knob of the ankle. The fibula, more slender than the tibia, is not part of the true knee joint. Rather, it is attached at the top of the tibia.

The bony prominence at the ends of the tibia and fibula form the ankle joint socket; the talus, or ankle bone, fits inside the socket. The *calcaneus*, or heel bone, forms the prominence of the heel and fits against the undersurface of the talus. The structure of the foot is similar to that of the hand with certain differences that adapt it for supporting weight. One example is the much greater solidity and the more limited mobility of the great toe compared to the thumb. Also, the foot bones are held together in such a way as to form springy lengthwise and crosswise arches. It is these arches that furnish the supportive strength of the foot. Further, the two-way arch construction makes a highly stable base.

The talus, the calcaneus, and five other bones are referred to in a group as the tarsal bones. These constitute the rear portion of the foot. Five metatarsal bones form the substance of the foot, and 14 phalanges on each foot form the toes (two in the great toe, three in each other toe). Normally the tarsals and metatarsals play the major role in the functioning of the foot as the supporting structure, with the phalanges relatively unimportant. The reverse is true for the hand. Here, manipulation is the main function rather than support. Consequently, the phalanges are all important, and the carpals and metacarpals are subsidiary.

Figure 18-11 shows bones of the thigh, leg, ankle, and foot.

JOINTS. The skeletal system is made up of many separate bones that are held together by joints. All movements that change the positions of the bony parts of the body occur at joints. An **articulation** (joint) is a point of contact between bones, between cartilage and bones, or between teeth and bones. Joints are classified as to the degree of movement they permit. Functionally, joints may be classified as immovable, slightly movable, and freely movable. The structural classification of joints is based on the presence or absence of a synovial cavity (a space between articulating bones) and the kind of connective tissue that binds bones together. Structurally, joints are classified as **fibrous** (no synovial cavity and bones are held together by fibrous tissue), **cartilaginous** (no synovial cavity and bones are held together by cartilage), or **synovial** (synovial cavity in which bones that form the joints are surrounded by an articular capsule). Table 18-2 lists different types of joints.

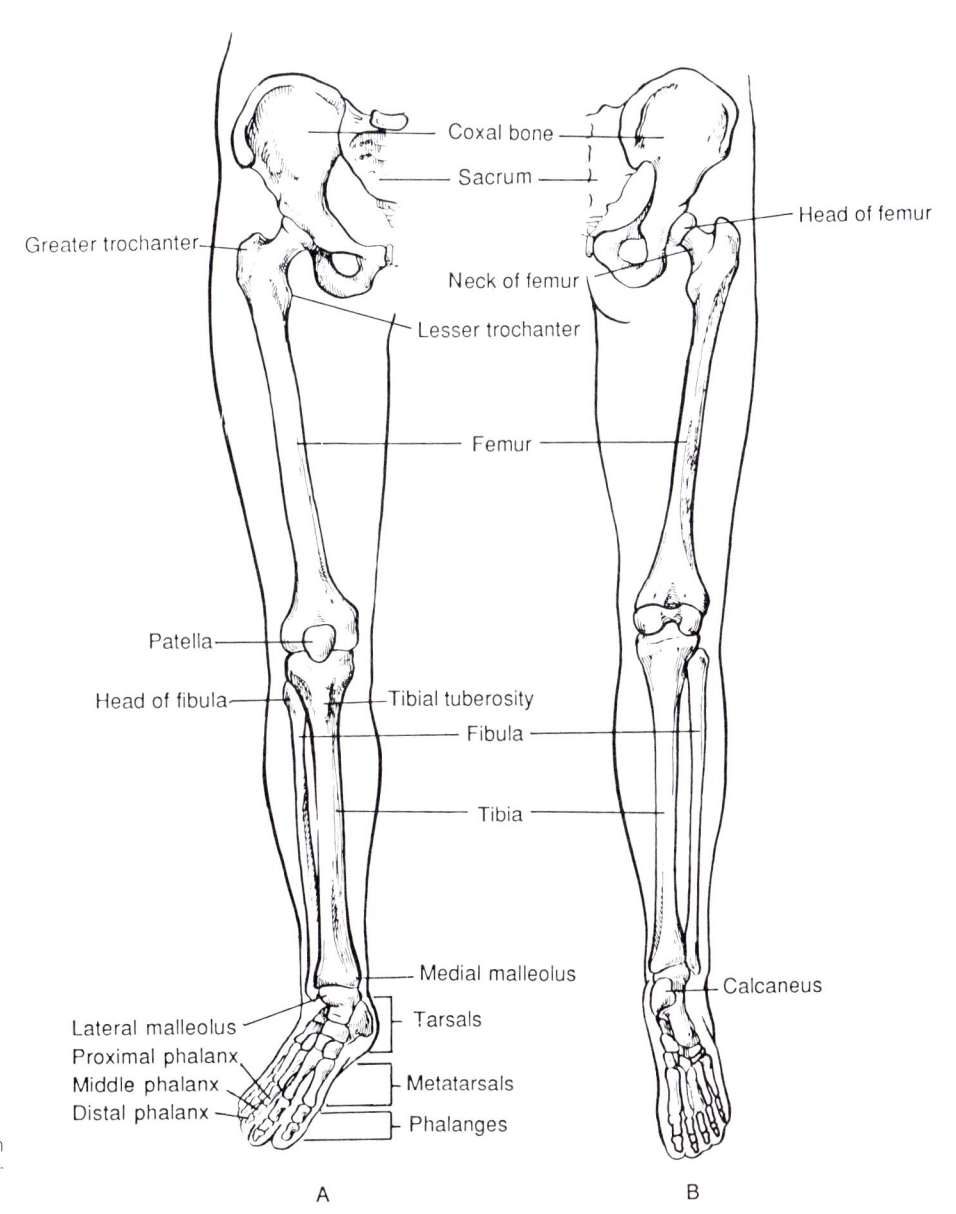

FIGURE 18–11.
Bones of the right lower extremity in the anterior view (**A**) and posterior view (**B**).

TABLE 18–2. TYPES OF JOINTS

Type	Description	Movement	Examples
FIBROUS (immovable)	No synovial cavity. Bones held together by fibrous tissue	No motion, or "give" only	Bones of skull fitted together with teethlike projections (sutures), roots of teeth in sockets of the maxillae and mandible
CARTILAGINOUS (slightly movable)	No synovial cavity. Bones held together by cartilage	Slight degree of flexibility	Intervertebral joints, costal cartilage, attachments of first 10 ribs to sternum, symphysis pubis
SYNOVIAL (freely movable)	Synovial cavity and articular cartilage present	Freely movable	Types of synovial joints listed below
Gliding	One bone slides over another. Surrounding structures restrict the motion	Gliding motion without any angular or circular movements	Joints between carpal bones, tarsal bones, the sternum and clavicle, and the scapula and clavicle
Hinge	Spool-shaped process fits into concave socket	Motion like a door on a hinge; permits flexion and extension	Finger, elbow, and knee
Pivot	Arch-shaped process fits around peglike process	Motion like turning a doorknob; permits rotation	Joint between the first and second cervical vertebrae allows rotation of the head from side to side; joint between the head of the radius and the radial notch of the ulna allows for supination and pronation of the palms
Condyloid	Oval-shaped condyle of one bone fits into an elliptical cavity of another bone	Allows motion in two planes at right angles, permits flexion, extension in one plane, abduction, adduction in another plane	Radiocarpal joint of wrist
Saddle	Articular surface of one bone is saddle-shaped and the articular surface of the other bone is shaped like a rider sitting in the saddle	Movements are side to side and back and forth; permits flexion, extension, abduction, adduction	Carpometacarpal joint of thumb, ankle
Ball-and-socket	Ball-like surface of one bone fitted into a cuplike depression of another bone	Rotating motions; permits widest range of motion: flexion, extension, abduction, adduction, rotation, circumduction	Shoulder and hip joints

Movable joints allow change of position and motion. Examples of joint movement (see Chapter 8) are as follows:

Flexion: decreases the angle between bones, such as bending
Extension: increases the angle between bones, such as straightening
Abduction: moves a bone away from the midline
Adduction: moves a bone toward the midline
Circumduction: moves a bone so its distal end describes a circle and the rest of the bone describes a cone
Pronation: turns the forearm so that the palm of the hand faces posterior or inferior
Supination: turns the forearm so that the palm of the hand faces anterior or superior
Gliding: slides one surface back and forth over the other

If a bone of a joint is capable of turning on its own long axis, the motion is called rotation. The motion of turning in toward midline of the body is called inward or internal rotation, and the motion of turning outward is called outward or external rotation. For instance, the humerus in the anatomical position is in external rotation.

Attempts to force joints to move beyond their normal limits can be disastrous. The structure of the joint determines the kind of movement that is possible, since the bone ends articulate, or fit into each other, at the joint. Examples of joint structures that permit certain kinds of joint movement are shown in Figure 18-12.

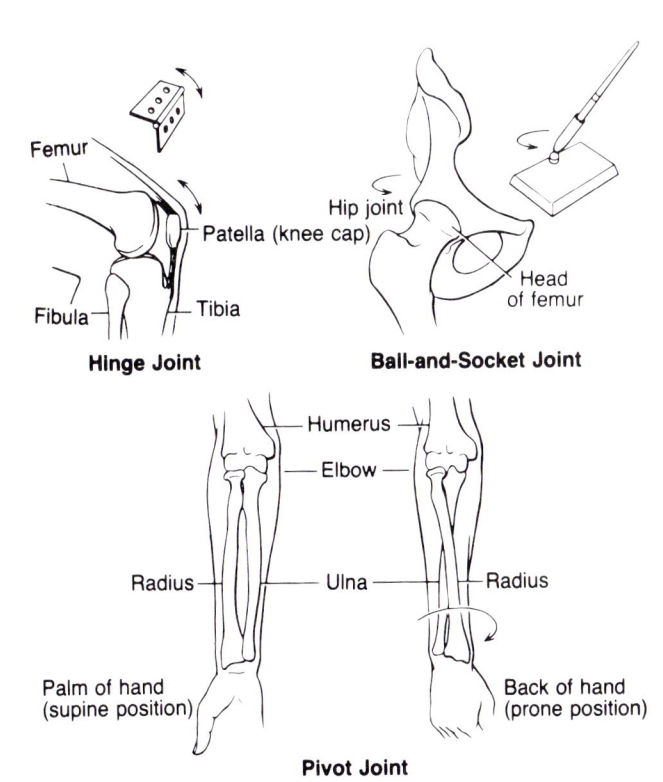

FIGURE 18–12.
Examples of three synovial joints. (Rosdahl CB)

INJURIES TO MUSCLE

Many rescuers anticipate that injuries to the musculoskeletal system will pose major problems, since the system is made up of 206 bones, six different types of joints, and more than 600 muscle groups. These injuries are among the most common faced by prehospital care providers. Muscles can be injured in a variety of ways. Overexerting a muscle may break fibers. Muscles subjected to trauma may be bruised, crushed, cut, torn, or otherwise injured, with or without a break in the skin. Muscles injured in any of these ways frequently become swollen, tender, painful, or weak.

Injuries to muscle, tendons, and ligaments occur when a joint or muscle is either torn or stretched beyond its normal limits. Primarily two types of injuries result from torn or stretched muscles, tendons, and ligaments. These are called strains and sprains.

Strain

A **strain** (also called a muscle pull) is a soft tissue injury or muscle spasm that occurs around a joint anywhere in the musculature. It is characterized by pain on active movement. No deformity or swelling is associated with a strain, and slow, gentle movement causes little, if any, pain. The muscle fibers involved are stretched and may be partially torn because of overexertion. The most common strain injuries occur in the back and are usually the result of lifting heavy objects or using improper lifting techniques.

Characteristics commonly associated with strains include the following:

- Acute "tearing"-type pain experienced at the time the injury occurred; people may state they heard or felt something "snap" at the time of injury
- Radiating or referred pain most commonly associated when people strain their back; pain may radiate downward to the leg muscles
- Pain with active movement of the joint involved
- Spasms in the area of the strain
- Disfigurement—either an indentation where tissues have separated or a swelling that indicates contracted tissue
- Severe weakness and loss of function

Sprain

A **sprain** is an injury in which ligaments are stretched, or even partially torn; it is usually precipitated by the sudden twisting of a joint beyond its normal range of motion. Sprains most commonly affect the knees and ankles and are characterized by pain, tenderness, swelling, and discoloration over the joint. Other associated characteristics include disability, loss of function of the joint, abnormal motion, and possible deformity.

Assessment

Most muscle injuries are not life-threatening. Though they are usually the most obvious type of injuries, attention should be focused first on the patient's vital functions. Only after the potential for life-threatening problems has been ruled out should focus be given to these other injuries.

An accurate history of the event should be obtained and the scene observed carefully to determine the mechanism of injury and forces involved. Most patients with injuries to the muscles complain of pain. Usually, the pain is localized to the area of injury. For a detailed history, it is important to determine how the injury occurred and the position the limb was in when it occurred. In assessing the patient, the paramedic needs to know the different types of forces involved, such as deceleration or direct impact. Also, it should be determined if the limb or joint had been injured previously. This information may provide a clue about the type of injury that is afflicting the patient.

The best way to assess the patient for strain and sprain injuries is to be familiar with the principal signs and symptoms that accompany them. Observe for swelling and ecchymosis (bruising). The patient frequently experiences tenderness in the joint, especially on palpation. Further, these patients tend to "guard" the area. Hence, they often hold the injured area in a comfortable position and avoid moving it. Determine the presence of distal pulses, the ability to move the joint, and if the patient has sensation below the point of injury.

Management

Strains are best cared for by avoiding stress on the injured area. It is often difficult to distinguish between the various musculoskeletal injuries—strains, sprains, dislocations, and fractures—in the field. Therefore, in most cases, assume that the area is fractured and immobilize it accordingly. If the exact nature of the injury is in question, the extremity should be immobilized, pending evaluation in the emergency department.

Specific care for strain injuries includes the following steps:

1. Place the patient in a comfortable position, such as reclining with the knees drawn up to take the pressure off the muscles.
2. Immobilize the area by splinting if needed.
3. Transport for definitive diagnosis.

Emergency care for sprains is best managed as if the injury were a fracture; it should be immobilized accordingly. The patient should not be allowed to walk or stand on a sprained knee or ankle. Before transport, the following "*RICE*" care should be provided:

R: Rest
I: Ice
C: Compression
E: Elevation

This care helps easy the pain and swelling often associated with sprains. It also facilitates healing of the injury by preventing any further aggravation of the involved tissues.

INJURIES TO BONE

Skeletal injuries are usually associated with external forces, though some may occur through disease, such as bone degeneration. Emergency care of fractures and dislocations is critical to prevent permanent disabilities.

Fracture

A *fracture* is a break in the continuity of a bone. It may be either closed, in which the overlying skin is intact, or open, in which the skin over the fracture site has been broken. Bone may or may not protrude through the wound. Open fractures are more serious than closed fractures because the risks of contamination and infection are greater.

Fractures are further classified according to their appearance by radiography. Although the paramedic does not have the luxury of radiographic equipment in the field, it is important to become familiar with the terminology and, based on the mechanism of injury, be able to estimate what the radiograph will reveal.

Examples of fractures shown on x-ray film are provided in Figure 18-13.

Fractures may be produced by the direct application of force to the bone, which causes the bone to break. They may also be caused by the indirect application of force to the bone, such as a fall with weight on an outstretched hand, which fractures the distal end of the radius, resulting in a Colles' fracture (the radius is displaced upward and backward). Many diseases of the bone, such as osteoporosis, and bone tumors can gradually weaken a bone until only slight stress can cause it to fracture. Fractures of this type are referred to as pathologic fractures.

Fractures unique to the midface, called **Le Fort's fractures,** can result from high-speed automobile trauma, in which the unrestrained driver or passenger is thrown through the windshield. About 150 times the force of gravity is required to fracture the midface; this force is significantly more than that needed to fracture any other facial bone. Classification of this type of fracture is based on the experiments of RenQee Le Fort, reported in 1901. He observed three general patterns of fracture that were caused by blunt trauma to the face (Fig. 18-14).

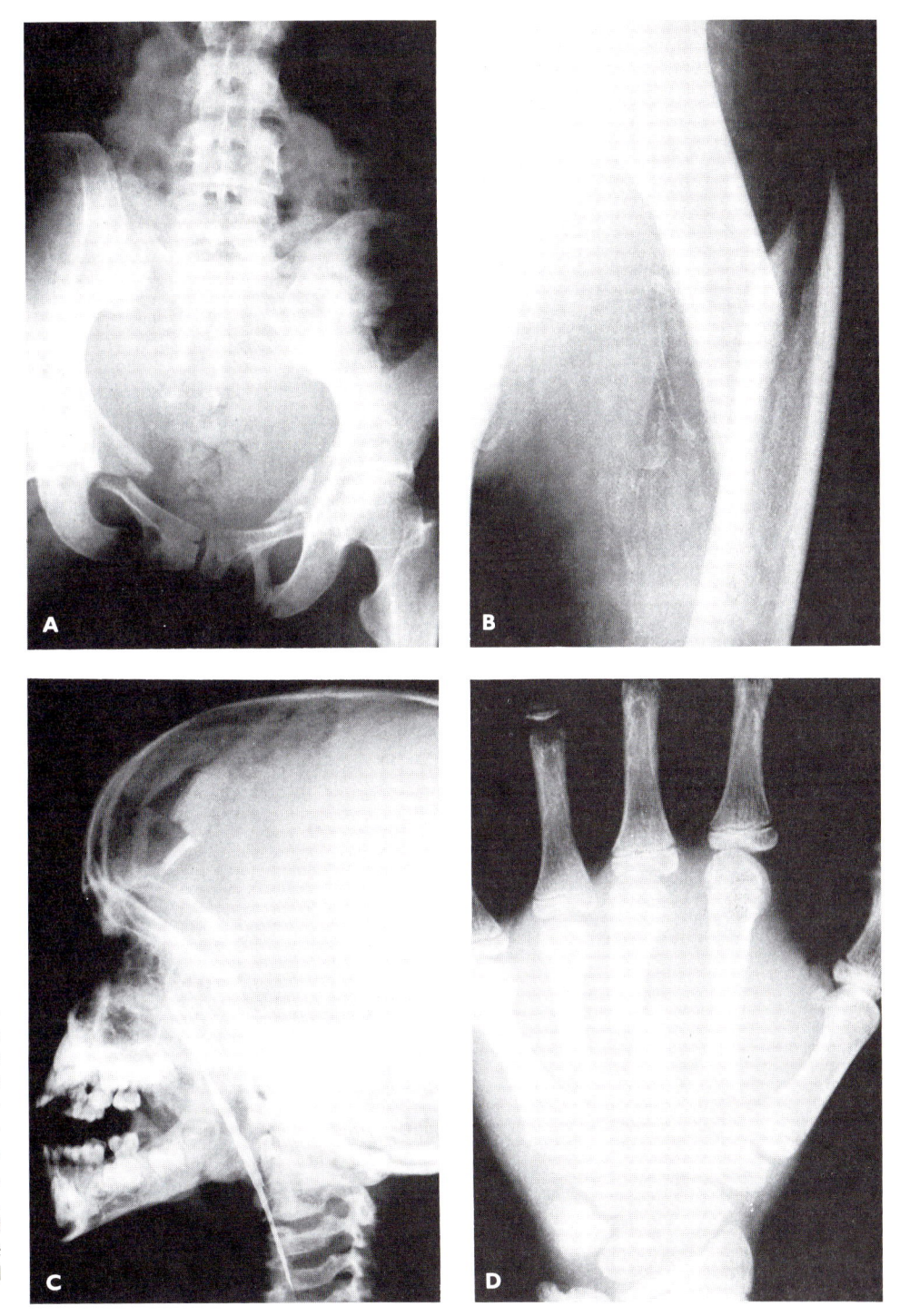

FIGURE 18–13.
X-ray film of various fractures. (**A**) Comminuted fracture of the pelvis caused by a motor vehicle accident. (**B**) Open spiral fracture of the femur caused by a cross-country skiing accident. (**C**) Depressed skull fracture to the frontal region, slightly left of mid-line, caused by a kick from a horse. (**D**) Oblique fracture of the third metacarpal and transverse fracture of the fourth metacarpal caused by a printing press accident.

Le Fort I: A transverse fracture that causes a separation of the alveolar portion of the maxilla at the level of the nasal floor

Le Fort II: A pyramidal fracture that causes a separation of the nasomaxillary complex from the zygomatic complexes

Le Fort III: Separation of the entire midface from the cranium

The primary concern in Le Fort's fractures is management of the airway.

Fractures of the sternum or the ribs usually result from crushing or squeezing of the chest. A fall, blow, or penetration of the chest wall by a weapon can have the same effect. The primary concern in such cases is that the lungs, heart, or major blood vessels may be punctured by the sharp ends of broken ribs.

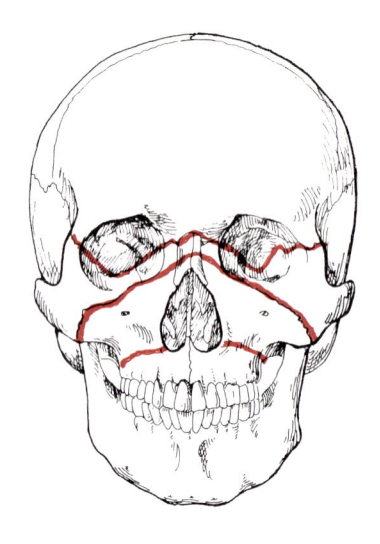

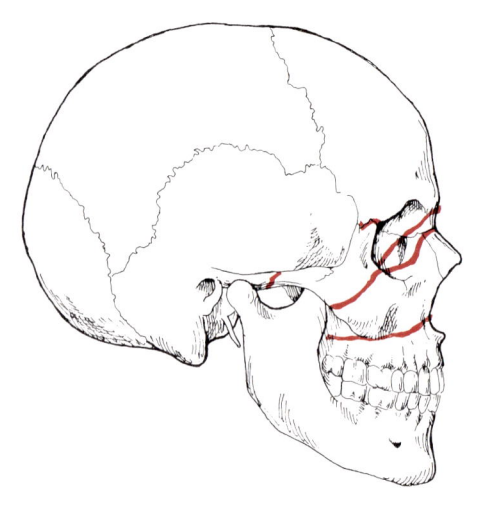

FIGURE 18–14.
Le Fort's classification of midface fractures.

CLASSIFICATION OF FRACTURES

Transverse
The fracture line is more or less at right angles to the long axis of the bone. It is usually produced by an angulation force.

Oblique
The fracture line extends obliquely across the bone, and fragments of the bone tend to slip by each other. It is usually caused by a twisting force.

Spiral
Usually results from twisting injuries; the fracture line has the appearance of a spiral or S shape. These injuries are commonly seen among skiers or from torsion produced by muscle contraction.

Greenstick
An incomplete fracture by a compression force in the long axis of the bone. Usually, the convex surface breaks while the concave surface remains intact. This type of fracture is most common among children, whose bones are more elastic than those of adults.

Compression
Damage to the bones with force from both ends. For example, one or more of the vertebrae of the spinal column may be compressed as a result of a blow or acceleration-deceleration accidents.

Depressed
A fragment is driven below the surface of the bone. This type of fracture occurs in flat bones, such as the skull.

Impacted
The broken ends are violently jammed together so that they telescope into each other.

Avulsion
A twisting motion causes part of the bone to be pulled away by a ligament or tendon.

Comminuted
Produced by a severe direct force. There are three or more fragments. Reduction is difficult to maintain in this type of fracture, and associated soft-tissue injuries are frequently severe.

Pathologic
Produced by minimal force through weak or diseased bone (bone cyst, Paget's disease, which produces localized areas of bone destruction, bony metastasis, tumor).

Epiphyseal
The epiphyseal plate can be separated from the diaphysis or epiphyses of a growing long bone if overstressed. Young children and preadolescent athletes are susceptible to this type of injury.

Fractures are also classified according to the position, number, and shape of the bone fragments, as shown in the box, "Classification of Fractures." Among these classifications are the *transverse fracture, oblique fracture, spiral fracture, greenstick fracture* (common among children), *compression fracture, depressed fracture, impacted fracture, avulsion fracture,* and the **comminuted fracture** (Fig. 18-15).

Assessment

With rare exceptions, fractures and other **orthopaedic** (or bone) injuries are not life-threatening. In the multiple-

CHAPTER 18: Musculoskeletal Injuries 369

injury patient, fractures may be the most obvious and dramatic injuries but may not necessarily be the most serious. Therefore, all life-threatening injuries must be ruled out before attention is turned to the evaluation and management of fractures.

Priorities for treating fractures are the following:

- Spinal fractures
- Fractures of the head and thoracic cage
- Pelvic fractures
- Fractures of the lower extremities
- Fractures of the upper extremities

If the force was strong enough to damage the pelvis or cause severe head and facial injuries, assume that the spine has also sustained injuries. Although life-threatening injuries must be dealt with first, examination of the extremities for fractures will most likely take place during the course of the secondary survey.

Common signs and symptoms often associated with fractures include: swelling, bruising, and hemorrhage from ruptured vessels in and around the fractured ends of bones. During the secondary survey, it is necessary to compare the injured extremity to the noninjured extremity to determine deformity of the limb. Also check to

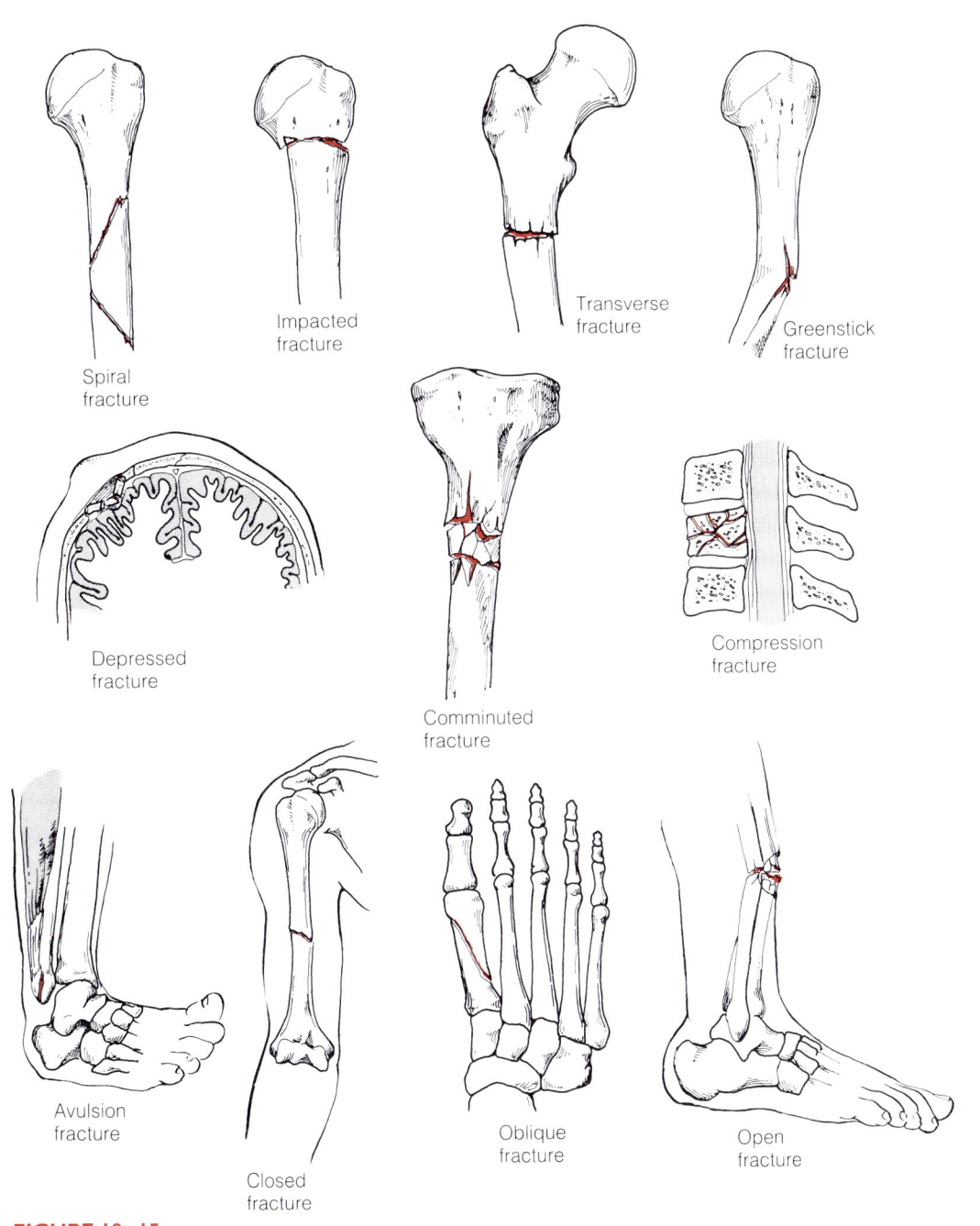

FIGURE 18–15.
Types of fractures.

see if the injured limb is shortened. This sign is a common one. Is it in an unnatural position? Is its motion false or unnatural? Can a difference in size or shape be seen? Is there ecchymosis on the skin? Is swelling found in an area that should not normally be swollen, particularly when compared to the other extremity? Is this swollen area pulsatile or is it rapidly growing? When inspecting the skull and thoracic cage, observe closely for depression-type fractures.

In addition to point tenderness, a grating sound, called **crepitus,** may be heard on palpation of the extremity. This is caused by broken bone fragments grinding against each other. A golden rule about crepitus advises not to attempt to elicit it in the field. This attempt can lead to further damage to nearby tissues and nerves and may exacerbate bleeding.

Examination of fractures should also include assessment of the nervous and circulatory systems. The primary symptom of fracture is pain, usually well localized to the fracture site. In addition, the pulses distal to the injury should be assessed carefully. Circulation and nerve function should be evaluated at least every 15 minutes. The patient should be asked to describe the sensation in the involved extremity. A prickling or tingling sensation is technically referred to as paresthesia. Sensory changes may indicate nerve or circulatory changes.

Assess the patient's ability to move the extremity. Inability to move the injured part (paralysis) may indicate peripheral nerve injury or circulatory impairment. Finally, check the color of the injured area. Note both the color and temperature of the fractured extremity. Pallor is another indicator that circulation and the nervous system network may be compromised.

Management

As has been emphasized throughout this chapter, management of potentially life-threatening problems should be identified and appropriately managed before treatment of musculoskeletal injuries is begun. If open fractures are found, the wounds should be dressed before splinting. This dressing helps to prevent further contamination and infection. An attempt should not be made to replace bone ends in open fractures. This action only complicates and increases infection. If possible, severely angulated fractures should be straightened or reduced. Caution should be used here, since prehospital personnel should never attempt to straighten fractures that involve joints.

Immobilization of any fracture requires that both the joint above and below the fracture be immobilized. Immobilization is accomplished by splinting and has several important purposes (Table 18-3). It prevents conversion of a closed fracture into an open one, which might occur if broken ends of bones are allowed to move freely as the patient is moved. Immobilization lessens damage to surrounding nerves, blood vessels, and other tissues by the broken bone ends. Proper immobilization above and below the fracture site helps to minimize bleeding and swelling. Finally, immobilization helps to diminish pain. Various types of splints are shown in Figure 18-16.

Dislocation

Bones that come together without a bony union form a joint. The body contains immovable joints, joints with limited motion, and freely movable joints. A **dislocation** is the displacement of a bone end from its articular surface, sometimes with associated tearing of the ligaments that normally hold the bone end in place. The shoulder, elbow, fingers, hips, and ankles are the joints most frequently affected.

The principal symptom of dislocation is pain or a feeling of pressure over the involved joint, as well as loss of motion of the joint. Other general signs and symptoms include rigidity, deformity, and moderate to severe swelling around the joint. If the dislocated bone end is pressing on a nerve, numbness or paralysis may also occur below the dislocation. If a blood vessel is being compressed, loss of pulse may occur below the dislocation. In any patient with a fracture or dislocation, the paramedic should check the strength of pulse and sensation on the side of the injury farthest from the heart. The absence of pulses means that the extremity is not receiving adequate blood. Transportation should then be instituted immediately.

Assessment

Assessment of dislocations is basically the same as for fractures, since these types of injuries are difficult to differentiate in the field. In any patient with a fracture or dislocation, the rescuer should always check the pulse, strength, and sensation distal to the injury. A person who is suffering from a dislocated joint most likely cannot move the extremity around the joint.

In the secondary survey, distal pulses and sensation should be checked after each immobilization and splinting. To check distal pulses, take following steps:

1. Palpate the pulse on the side of the injury away from the heart.
2. Check capillary refill by pressing a fingernail or toenail and observing the speed by which color returns to the area. Normal refill time is 2 seconds or less.
3. Absence of pulse or a prolonged capillary refill time means that either the injury itself or the splinting procedures are reducing circulation to the area. This condition must be corrected immediately by straightening the fractured or dislocated limb or by loosening the splint.

To check distal sensations, take the following steps:

1. Ask the patient to wiggle the fingers and toes.
2. Grasp a finger or toe and ask the patient if it can be felt.

TABLE 18-3.
MANAGEMENT OF SPECIFIC ORTHOPAEDIC INJURIES

Anatomical Region	Type of Injury	Immobilization Device
Neck (cervical vertebrae)	Fracture or dislocation	Cervical collar with long or short backboard or with a commercial spinal extrication device
Back (thoracic, lumbar, sacral, or coccygeal vertebrae)	Fracture or dislocation	Cervical collar with long backboard or with a commercial spinal extrication device
Chest (ribs, sternum)	Fracture	Sling and swath, secure pillow to chest with cravats
Clavicle	Fracture or dislocation	Sling and swath
Shoulder	Anterior dislocation	Splint in position found; sling, pillow, and swath
	Posterior dislocation	Sling and swath in position found
Arm (humerus)	Fracture	Sling and swath with padded board splint on posterolateral aspect of arm or padded wire-ladder splint
Elbow	Fracture or dislocation	Splint in position found; padded board splint or padded wire-ladder splint
Forearm (radius/ulna)	Fracture	Sling and swath with padded board splint on anterior aspect of forearm or air splint
Wrist	Fracture or dislocation	Splint in position found; sling and swath with padded board splint on anterior aspect of forearm and roller bandage placed in palm of hand to splint hand in position of function
Hand	Fracture or dislocation	Splint in position found; sling and swath with padded board splint on anterior aspect of forearm and roller bandage placed in palm of hand to splint hand in position of function
Finger	Fracture or dislocation	Padded tongue blade, aluminum splint, tape to adjacent (uninjured) finger, or wrap with bulky dressing
Pelvis	Fracture	Long backboard, or pneumatic anti-shock garment
Hip	Fracture	Long backboard, traction splint, padded long board splint, or secure injured leg to uninjured leg
	Dislocation	Long backboard with limb supported by pillows or rolled blankets
Thigh (femur)	Fracture	Traction splint
Knee	Fracture or dislocation	Splint in position found; padded long board splint or air splint
Leg (tibia/fibula)	Fracture	Padded long board splint or air splint
Ankle	Fracture or dislocation	Pillow or air splint
Foot	Fracture or dislocation	Pillow or air splint
Toe	Fracture or dislocation	Tape to adjacent (uninjured) toe or wrap with bulky dressing

TABLE 18-3.
MANAGEMENT OF SPECIFIC ORTHOPAEDIC INJURIES

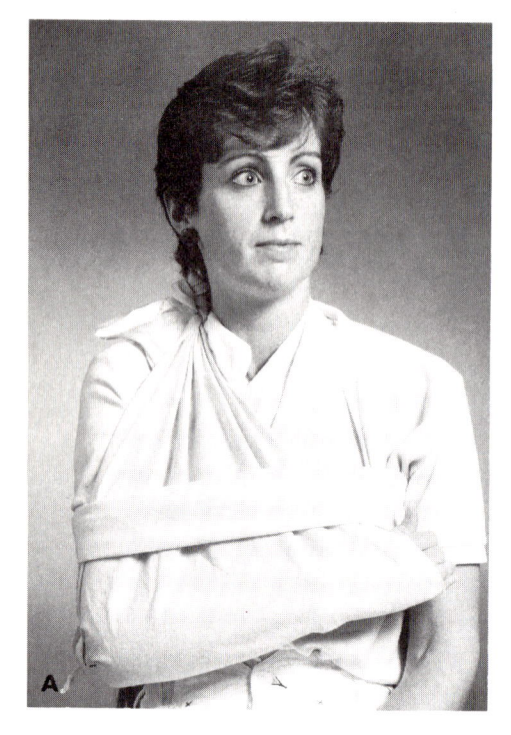

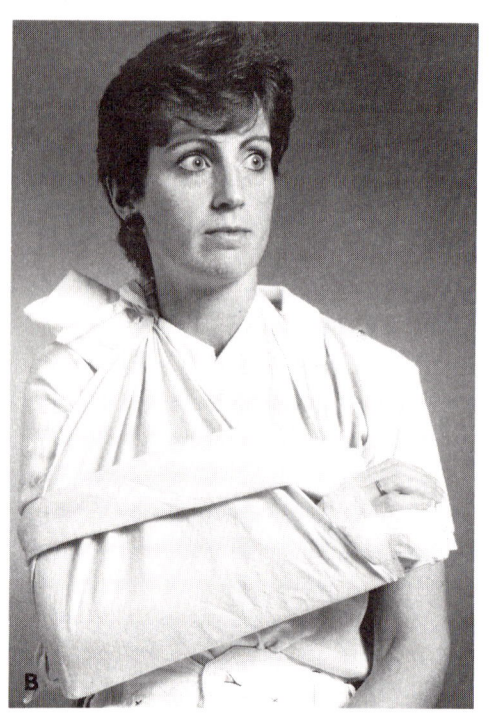

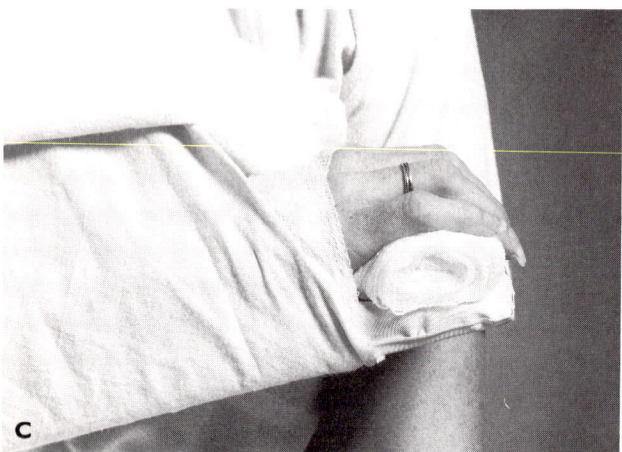

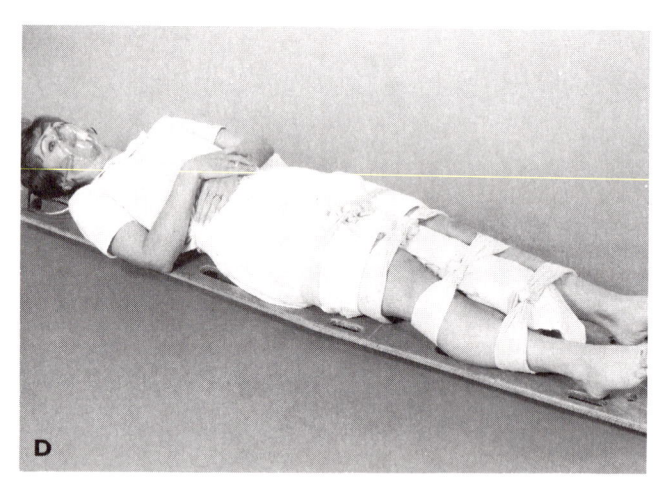

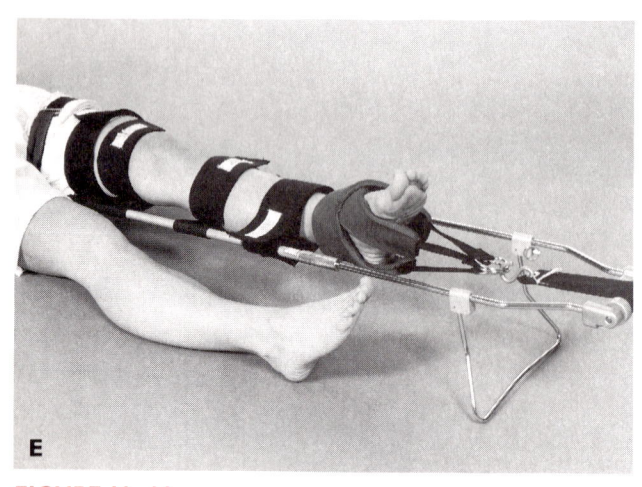

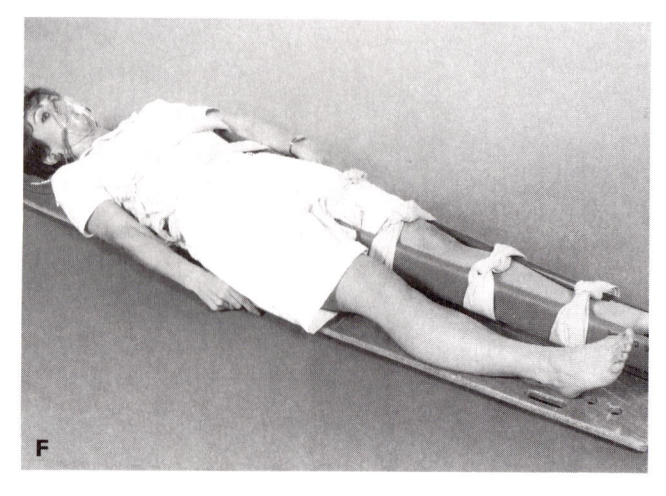

FIGURE 18-16.
Types of splints. (**A**) Sling and swath. (**B**) Sling and swath with padded board on anterior aspect of forearm. (**C**) Roller bandage placed in palm of hand to splint hand in position of function. (**D**) Long backboard with limb supported by pillows. (**E**) Traction splint. (**F**) Long backboard with padded long board splint. (**G**) Pillow splint. (**H**) Air splint.

FIGURE 18–16. (Continued)

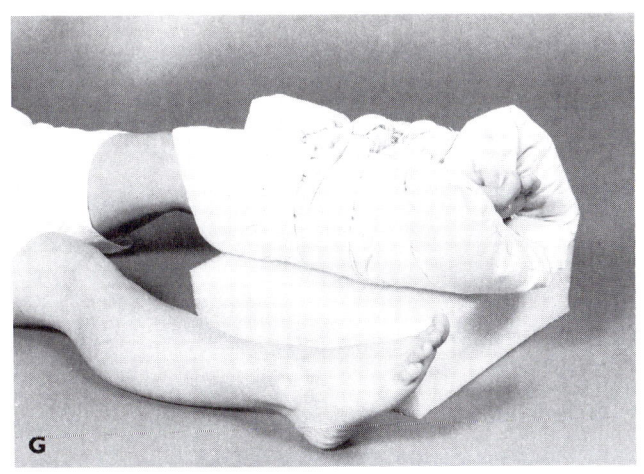

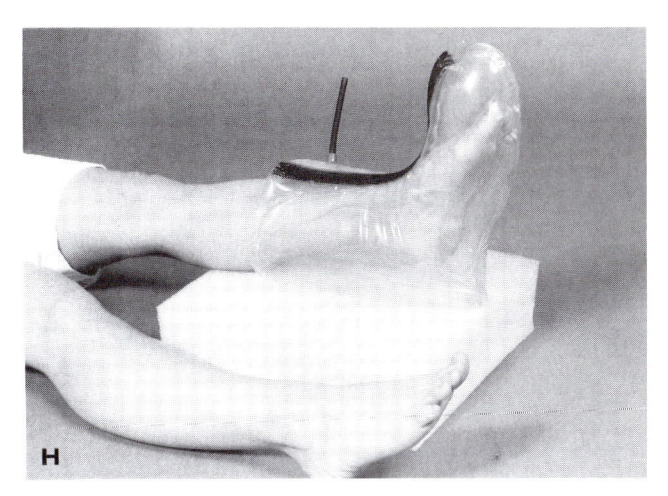

3. If the patient is unconscious, gently probe or pinch the skin and note any reactions to this mild pain.

Management

It is not always easy in the field to distinguish between a dislocation and a fracture that involves a joint. Furthermore, since dislocations involve joints and are often accompanied by fractures, emergency care is to immobilize all suspected dislocations in the position found. Proper splinting of dislocations is the same as for fractures: immobilize above and below the dislocated joint to maintain stability (see Table 18-3).

In the discussion of fractures, it was emphasized that an attempt should never be made to straighten or reduce fractures that involve joints. Therefore, since dislocations involve joints, reductions of dislocations should not be attempted, unless specifically ordered by the base physician. Perhaps the only dislocation that places the limb in immediate jeopardy is a dislocation of the knee. Dislocations of the wrist, elbow, shoulder, hip, and ankle can be tolerated for 2 to 3 hours without much risk of permanent damage. Dislocations of the knee and the absence of distal pulse, however, must be reduced within the first 2 hours after the injury occurs. In such cases, initiate early communications with the base hospital.

SUMMARY

Prehospital care providers see injuries that range from simple cuts and bruises to grossly disfiguring and dangerous multiple lacerations and fractures. Therefore, these professionals must be thoroughly prepared for every situation. Being prepared is much more than knowing simple bandaging and splinting techniques. An understanding of the basic anatomy and physiology of the part of the body affected by injury is crucial. Paramedics must be able to recognize the effect of injury and the mechanisms and forces involved, and they must appreciate what mishandling of an injured part can do. Finally, quick and efficient care should be provided in the absence of specialized supplies and equipment.

Musculoskeletal injuries usually do not pose life-threatening conditions. However, certain long bone injuries, such as femur fractures, can be true emergencies if hemorrhage occurs. The golden rule of care in any situation, but especially in dealing with injuries to the musculoskeletal system, is to rule out all life-threatening conditions before focusing on the more obvious types of injuries. This management involves a logical and detailed approach to patient care, with priority given to the patient's vital functions and a thorough secondary evaluation of the injuries to muscles, bones, and joints.

SUGGESTED READING

American Academy of Orthopaedic Surgeons: Emergency Care and Transportation of the Sick and Injured, 4th ed. Park Ridge, ORCO, 1987

Callahan ML: Current Therapy in Emergency Medicine. Philadelphia, BC Decker, 1987

Caroline NL: Emergency Care in the Streets, 4th ed. Boston, Little, Brown & Co, 1991

Kravis TC, Warner CG: Emergency Medicine: A Comprehensive Review, 2nd ed. Rockville, Maryland, Aspen Publishers, 1987

Polando G, Haverta C, Shall J et al: PASG use in pelvic fracture immoobilization. J Emerg Med Serv 15(3):48, 1990

Rosdahl CB: Textbook of Basic Nursing, 4th ed. Philadelphia, JB Lippincott, 1985

Tortora GJ, Anagnostakos NP: Principles of Anatomy and Physiology, 6th ed. New York, Harper and Row, 1990

US Department of Transportation, National Highway Traffic Safety Administration: Emergency Medical Technician—Paramedic: National Standards Curriculum. Washington, DC, US Government Printing Office, 1985

UNIT FOUR

Medical Emergencies

CHAPTER 19

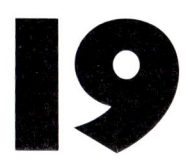

Respiratory Emergencies

Anatomy and Physiology of the Respiratory System
- **Upper Airway**
- **Lower Airway**
  - Trachea
  - Lungs
    - Bronchi
    - Bronchioles
    - Alveolar-capillary Interface
    - Alveoli
    - Exchange of Gases
    - Pleurae
- **Diaphragm and Chest Wall**
  - Muscles of Respiration and the Respiratory Process
    - Modified Forms of Respiration
    - Respiratory Volumes and Capacities
    - Innervation of the Respiratory Muscles
- **Neurologic Control of Breathing**

Assessment of the Patient in Respiratory Distress
- **Primary Survey**
- **Secondary Survey**
  - History
    - Medical History
  - Physical Examination
    - Inspection
    - Palpation
    - Auscultation
    - Pulsus Paradoxus

Respiratory Disorders
- **Upper Airway Obstruction**
  - Pathophysiology
  - Assessment
  - Management
- **Lower Airway Disorders**
  - Obstructive Lung Disease
    - Pathophysiology
    - Assessment
    - Management

Pneumonia
  Pathophysiology
  Assessment
  Management
Smoke and Toxic Product Inhalation
  Pathophysiology
  Assessment
  Management
Pulmonary Embolism
  Pathophysiology
  Assessment
  Management
Central Nervous System Disorders
  Pathophysiology
  Assessment
  Management
Hyperventilation Syndrome
  Pathophysiology
  Assessment
  Management

Summary

BEHAVIORAL OBJECTIVES
On successful completion of this chapter, the reader will be able to:

1. Identify and describe the function of the structures of the lower airway
2. Describe the process of gas exchange in the lungs
3. Identify the normal partial pressures of oxygen and carbon dioxide in the alveoli, venous blood, and arterial blood
4. Discuss the physiology of respiration and identify the systems involved
5. Describe the modified forms of respiration
6. Discuss respiratory volumes and capacities
7. Explain the process of neurologic control of breathing
8. Identify specific observations and physical findings to be evaluated in the patient with a respiratory complaint
9. Describe the techniques of inspection, palpation, and auscultation of the chest
10. Identify the basic principles of airway management
11. Describe the causes of upper airway obstruction, the pathophysiology, assessment, and management of each
12. Describe the pathophysiology, assessment, and management of patients in distress due to obstructive lung disease, pneumonia, smoke and toxic product inhalation, pulmonary embolism, central nervous system disorders, and hyperventilation syndrome
13. Define all of the key terms listed in this chapter

KEY TERMS

The following terms are defined in the chapter and glossary:

accessory muscles	central cyanosis	hiccup	nasal flaring	retractions
air trapping	chronic obstructive	hypercapnia	obstructive lung	rhonchi
alveoli	pulmonary disease	hyperpnea	disease	sighing
alveolar-capillary	(COPD)	hyperventilation	orthopnea	sneeze
interface	clubbing	hyperventilation	$PaCO_2$	status asthmaticus
alveolar ventilation	cough	syndrome	PaO_2	stridor
(V_A)	cyanosis	hypoventilation	$P\bar{v}CO_2$	surfactant
atelectasis	diaphoresis	hypoxemia	$P\bar{v}O_2$	tachypnea
apnea	diaphragm	hypoxia	peak flow meter	tidal volume (V_T)
auscultation	diffusion	inspiration	peripheral cyanosis	total lung capacity
breath sounds	dyspnea	inspiratory reserve	pleurae	(TLC)
bradypnea	elastic recoil	volume (IRV)	pleural friction rub	trachea
bronchi	eupnea	intercostal muscles	pleuritis	tracheal tugging
bronchioles	expiration	interstitial space	pulmonary embolism	wheezes
carbon dioxide	expiratory reserve	lower airway	pulsus paradoxus	vital capacity (VC)
carbon monoxide	volume (ERV)	lungs	rales	volume of dead space
carina	hemoptysis	metered dose inhaler	residual volume	gas (V_D)
carpopedal spasm			(RV)	

Patients who experience respiratory distress make up a significant portion of the paramedic's case load. While some of these situations may be of greater medical consequence than others, the paramedic must remember that the abrupt onset of dyspnea is of great concern to patients and their families.

To properly assess and manage respiratory distress, the paramedic must understand the underlying pathophysiology, based on a thorough knowledge of normal anatomy and physiology. Paramedics who possess such a firm theoretical base will be able to act confidently and correctly and provide appropriate treatment while allaying the fears of patients and their families.

ANATOMY AND PHYSIOLOGY OF THE RESPIRATORY SYSTEM

The respiratory system serves as a remarkably effective gas exchange device. Each day, more than 10,000 L of air enter the respiratory tract, where it is filtered, warmed, humidified, and pumped into the lower airway. Once in the lower airway, the air comes into contact with the pulmonary capillary system. Oxygen diffuses from alveolar air into the blood and is then transported in arterial blood to tissues to provide for metabolic needs in some 100 trillion cells. Carbon dioxide passes into the alveoli from the pulmonary capillaries. On expiration the carbon dioxide is returned to ambient air. In anatomical terms, this remarkable system is broken into four subsystems: upper airway, lower airway, alveolar-capillary interface, and the chest wall and diaphragm.

Upper Airway

As described in Chapter 10, the upper airway performs a number of important functions. The first is to serve as a passageway for air; all air that enters the lower airway must pass through the upper airway first. In addition to simply transmitting air into the lower airway, the upper airway serves to filter, warm, and humidify inspired air so that the air has reached body temperature 37°C (98.6°F) and about 95% relative humidity by the time it reaches the alveoli. Finally, the upper airway serves to protect the lower airway from foreign bodies that might damage or obstruct the delicate structures of the lung. Structures of the upper airway are shown in Chapter 10.

Lower Airway

The **lower airway**, shown in Figure 19-1, provides a route for air transmission from the larynx to the small airways just proximal to the alveoli. The lower airway functions to conduct air to the alveoli. In addition, the lower airway provides further warming and humidification of inspired air. Finally, the lower airway provides for removal of foreign particles via the mucus and ciliary escalator.

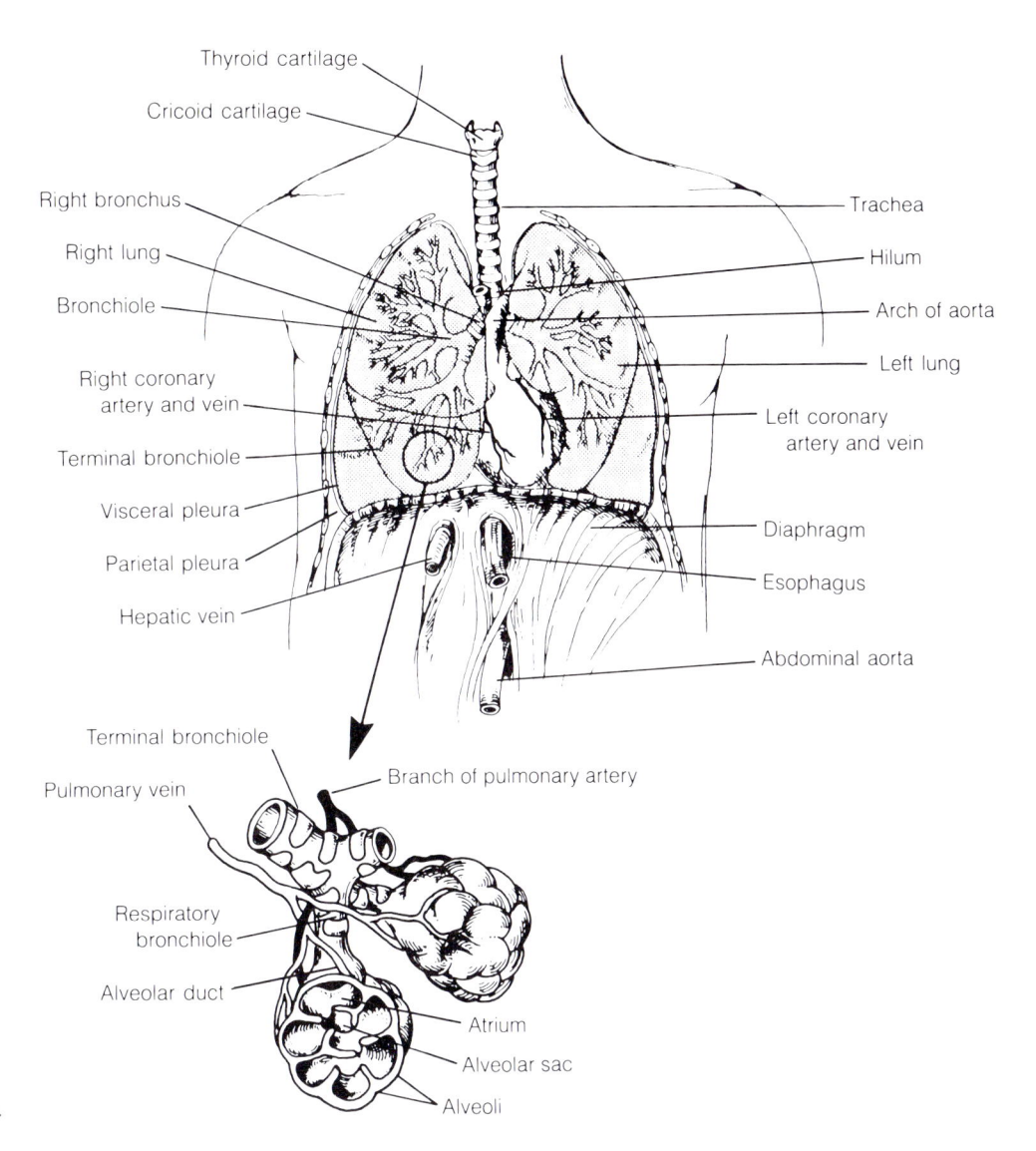

FIGURE 19-1.
Structures of the lower airway.

Trachea

The **trachea** is a tube, 1.5 to 2.5 cm in diameter, that extends from the larynx to the **carina** (point of bifurcation), where it divides into the left and right primary bronchi. The lining of the trachea is rich in *mucous glands* and is covered by cilia. A blanket of mucus is present on the tips of the cilia, which beat about 20 times per second. Foreign particles are caught in the mucus and moved up the *ciliary escalator* (at a rate of 2.3—3.5 mm/min) by the rhythmic movement of the cilia.

The trachea is constructed of C-shaped cartilaginous rings, with the open section of the "C" facing posteriorly. A cross section of the trachea is shown in Figure 19-2. The open portion of the "C" faces the esophagus.

Cigarette smoking decreases the function of the mucus and ciliary escalator, making the respiratory tract less able to remove foreign matter. Airway care for patients who smoke is, therefore, more difficult. Airway obstruction at the tracheal level may occur because of the pres-

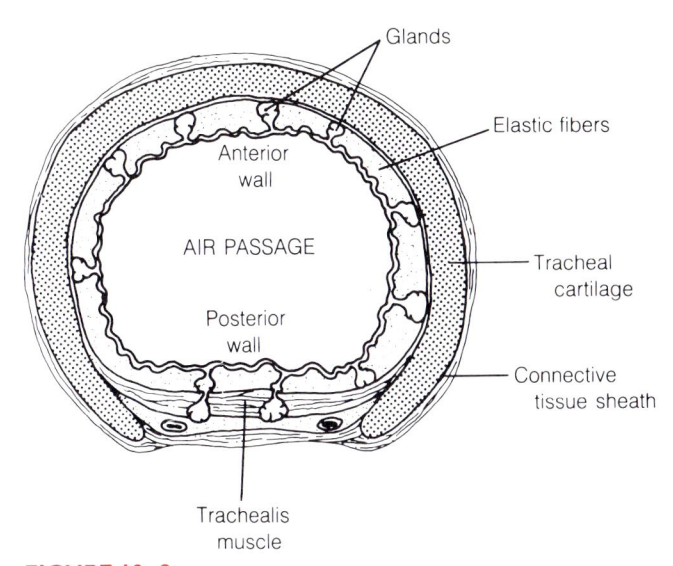

FIGURE 19-2.
Cross section of the trachea.

ence of a large object in the esophagus that distends the esophagus against the opening in the tracheal "C" cartilage.

Lungs

The **lungs** are the organs in which external respiration takes place. The two lungs, which sit side by side in the thoracic cavity, are composed of the components discussed in the following sections.

BRONCHI. The trachea *bifurcates* (splits) at the carina into two primary **bronchi,** of which the right bronchus is slightly larger and more vertical than the left. In structure, the bronchi resemble the trachea in that their walls contain incomplete cartilaginous rings and ciliated mucosa. The right primary bronchus and left primary bronchus divide further into the secondary, or lobar, bronchi that enter and supply air flow into the lobes of the lungs. The right lung has three lobar bronchi, and the left lung has two; the left lung has only two lobes because of the space taken up on the left by the heart. Figure 19-3 shows the relationship of the lobes of the lungs to the bronchi. The lobar bronchi are further divided to form tertiary bronchi and finally divide into the small bronchioles. As these subdivisions occur, the diameter of the airways decreases, with the smallest bronchioles having a diameter of less than 1 mm.

As can be seen in Figure 19-3, the left primary bronchus diverges from the trachea at a much more acute angle than does the right. Because of this difference in angles, endotracheal tubes frequently enter the *right* primary bronchus if advanced too far. This placement prevents the left lung from being ventilated. Fortunately, this condition usually is easy to identify by the prominence of breath sounds on the right and the absence of sound on the left. If this condition is found, the endotracheal tube is slowly pulled back until breath sounds are heard bilaterally.

BRONCHIOLES. The **bronchioles** are the final generation of airways before the alveoli are reached. By definition, bronchioles have no cartilage in their walls; bronchiolar walls consist solely of smooth muscle. This smooth muscle contracts in *bronchospasm* as in patients with asthma and other bronchospastic diseases. From the smallest bronchi, three to four more divisions form progressively smaller bronchioles before the terminal bronchiole is reached. The terminal bronchiole divides into respiratory bronchioles, the final bronchioles, which attach to an alveolar duct. The diameter of the respiratory bron-

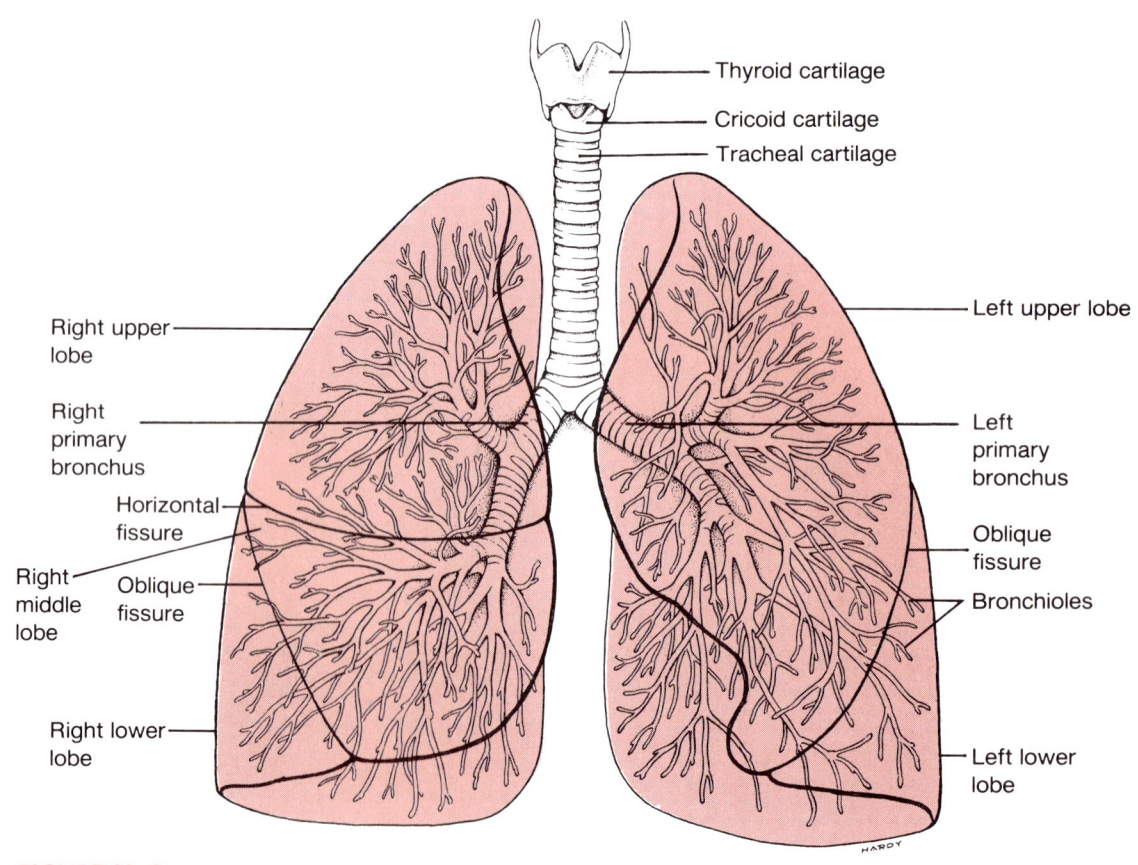

FIGURE 19–3.
Anterior view of the bronchial tree and lobes of the lungs. (Brunner LS, Suddarth DS)

chioles is about 0.5 mm. It is at this point in the lower airway that mucous glands and cilia become more scarce, until they eventually disappear. The alveolar ducts emerge from the respiratory bronchioles and form a cluster of air sacs known as alveoli (see Fig. 19-1).

ALVEOLAR-CAPILLARY INTERFACE. The function of the *alveolar-capillary interface* is to facilitate gas exchange between the lungs and the circulatory system. While many texts consider the capillary bed in a separate section, the alveoli and the capillary bed are intimately interrelated and are presented together in this chapter. Gases that enter this area are exchanged via diffusion, which is discussed in the section "Exchange of Gases."

ALVEOLI. The **alveoli** split off from the alveolar ducts in clusters. Each cluster of individual alveoli is known as a primary lobule and is about 3.5 mm in diameter. Each lobule contains about 2200 individual alveoli; each lung contains nearly 300 million alveoli. The walls of the alveoli are only one cell thick and are composed primarily of epithelium. Because of the thinness of these walls, they are prone to collapse. A fluid known as **surfactant** serves to prevent the alveoli from collapsing by lowering fluid surface tension ("pull") along the alveolar walls. Surfactant is important in cases of premature birth, as well as other diseases, in which a deficiency of surfactant allows alveoli to collapse.

Adjacent to the alveolus is the pulmonary capillary bed, which receives blood from the right heart via the pulmonary arteries. After gas transfer at the alveolar-capillary interface, the arterialized blood passes into the left atrium via the pulmonary veins (see Fig. 19-1). As with the alveolus, the wall of the capillary is thin. The space between the wall of the capillary and the wall of the alveolus is known as the **interstitial space,** and it is filled with fluid that is circulated via the lymphatic system. This interstitial space plays an important role in a number of disease states.

Several conditions involve the alveolar-capillary interface. A particular type of pneumonia, known as *interstitial pneumonitis*, causes swelling of the interstitial space. This swelling increases the distance between the capillary and alveolar walls, causing increased resistance to diffusion. If these diseases progress far enough, diffusion is impaired to the point at which equilibrium is not reached. In these cases, supplemental oxygen is needed to prevent hypoxia. **Hypoxia** is caused when sufficient oxygen is not available to meet the oxygen requirements of the cell of a particular tissue. The tissues most affected by hypoxia are the brain, lungs, heart, and liver. Left-sided heart failure can also affect gas diffusion. With left-sided failure, blood backs up from the left atrium into the pulmonary capillary bed. This backup of blood causes the capillaries to distend, and the pressure within these vessels increases. If the pressure increases enough, plasma is forced through the capillary walls into the interstitial space. As more fluid seeps into this space, the ability of gas to diffuse is impaired, causing hypoxia. Eventually, the pressure in the interstitial space may increase, causing a leakage of fluid into the alveoli. This mechanism is responsible for the hypoxia and pink, frothy sputum seen in pulmonary edema.

Pulmonary function can also affect the heart. In cases of air trapping in the lungs (such as in chronic obstructive pulmonary disease, discussed later), the alveoli are so overinflated that they compress the capillaries, narrowing their diameter. It is more difficult to pump blood through these narrower capillaries; this difficulty causes strain on the right side of the heart. In severe situations, this strain can be so pronounced as to cause blood to back up through the right heart into the major venous pools, including the liver, jugular veins, and ankles. Such patients present with apparent right-sided heart failure.

EXCHANGE OF GASES. The number of molecules of oxygen and carbon dioxide in the blood can be measured in terms of their partial pressure. In a person who is breathing *room air* (which normally contains 0.03% carbon dioxide, 21% oxygen, and 78.97% nitrogen), the partial pressure of oxygen in arterial blood (**PaO$_2$**) is 80 to 100 mm Hg, and the partial pressure of arterial carbon dioxide (**PaCO$_2$**) is 35 to 45 mm Hg. The venous blood has a partial pressure of O$_2$ (**P$\bar{v}$O$_2$**) of about 40 mm Hg and a partial pressure of CO$_2$ (**P$\bar{v}$CO$_2$**) of about 46 mm Hg. Gas exchange in the alveolus is shown in Figure 19-4.

Decreased PaO$_2$ (**hypoxemia**) can result from decreased alveolar ventilation, impaired oxygen diffusion, inadequate atmospheric O$_2$ (altitude), or from a mismatch of ventilation and perfusion due to pulmonary disease. Decreased PaO$_2$ also may be the result of cardiac disease. With normal lungs, the PaO$_2$ can be increased to values as high as 120 mm Hg through hyperventilation.

The PaCO$_2$ and P$\bar{v}$CO$_2$ represent a balance between the CO$_2$ produced in metabolism and eliminated in ventilation. The larger the volume of air that moves in and out of the lungs during each ventilation, the more CO$_2$ that is eliminated. This volume can be increased by increasing the rate and depth of breathing (*minute volume*). The minute volume is described in the section on the respiratory process.

Gases are exchanged following the laws of diffusion (Fig. 19-5). **Diffusion** means that gases continue to be exchanged until their concentrations are equal in both the alveolus and the capillary. This means that the oxygen never completely leaves the alveolus and the **carbon dioxide,** which is a waste product of cellular metabolism, never completely leaves the capillary. The greater the difference in gas concentration between the alveolus and the capillary, the more rapidly diffusion occurs. Increasing the concentration of oxygen in the alveolus (by giving supplemental oxygen), for example, increases the amount

Alveolus
$P_AO_2 = 100$ mm Hg
$P_ACO_2 = 40$ mm Hg

$P_vO_2 = 40$ mm Hg
$P_vCO_2 = 46$ mm Hg

Pulmonary artery
(mixed venous blood)

$P_aO_2 = 80-100$ mm Hg
$P_aCO_2 = 35-45$ mm Hg

Pulmonary vein
(arterial blood)

Capillary

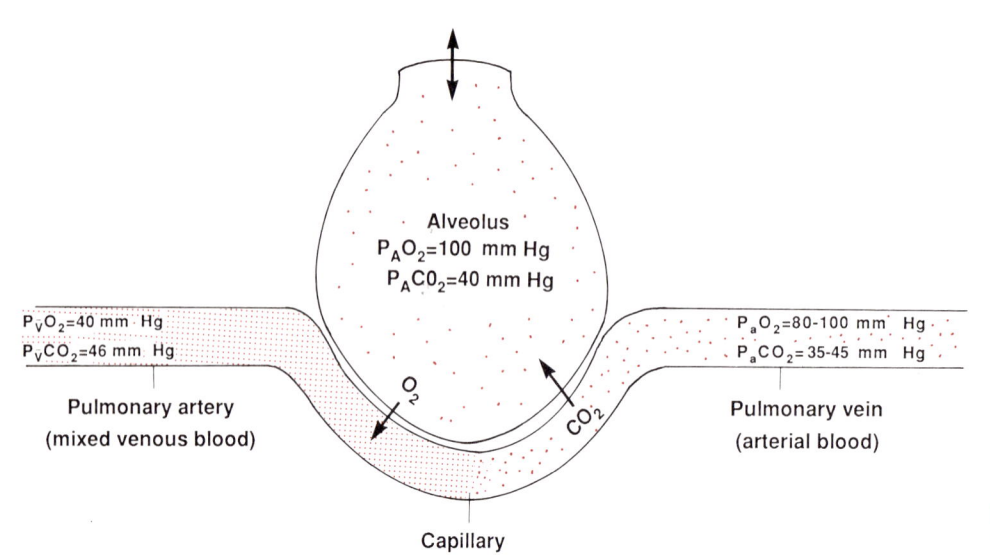

FIGURE 19–4.
Gas exchange in the alveolus.

of oxygen diffused into the bloodstream. This diffusion of gas is so efficient that, in the healthy person, equilibrium of concentrations is reached during the first one-third of the alveolar-capillary interface time. Air in the alveoli is constantly replaced by ventilation; on exhalation, the air that contains carbon dioxide is removed and replaced, on inhalation, by air fresh with oxygen.

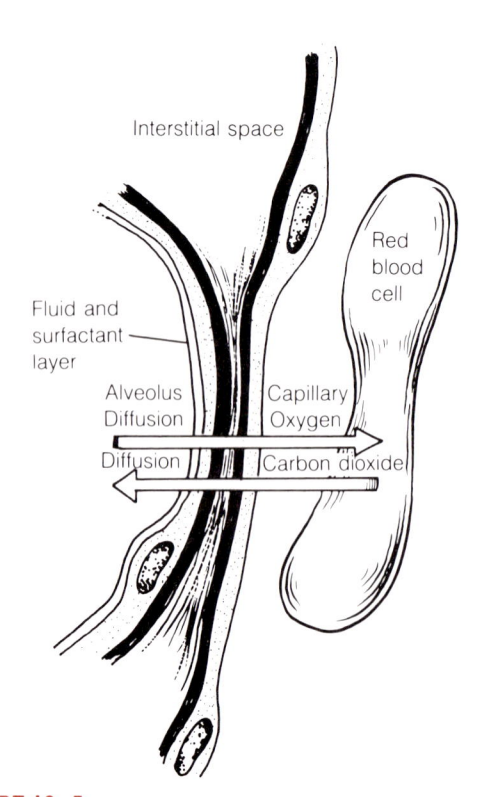

FIGURE 19–5.
Exchange of oxygen and carbon dioxide across the alveolar–capillary interface (diffusion).

PLEURAE. The *pleurae* are the membranes that cover the thoracic musculature and the lungs. The visceral pleura is the layer that covers the lungs, while the parietal pleura is the lining that covers the inner surface of the ribs and intercostal muscles. Because the lungs are positioned directly against the chest wall, no real space is between the two pleurae; rather, the space between the parietal pleura and the visceral pleura is referred to as a potential space. To prevent friction as the pleurae are rubbed against one another, a thin layer of pleural fluid serves as a lubricant. This lubricant allows the pleurae to slide silently on one another during breathing.

A number of conditions affect the pleura. In trauma, a hemothorax or pneumothorax occurs when blood or air, respectively, enters the pleural space, displacing lung tissue (see Chapter 16). Pleural pain, as can occur in pneumonia, is often caused by pleuritis. This condition is characterized by focal chest pain with breathing, due to the inflammation of the pleura.

Diaphragm and Chest Wall

The diaphragm and chest wall function by causing movement of air into and out of the lungs. This function is provided mainly by the diaphragm during normal quiet breathing, with the other thoracic muscles coming into play when the work of breathing increases.

Muscles of Respiration and the Respiratory Process

Ventilation is caused by changes in intrathoracic pressures. These changes are caused by the joint action of the muscles of respiration. To cause inspiration, the *diaphragm* (muscular structure that separates the thoracic and abdominal cavities) and the *intercostal muscles* (muscles between the ribs) must contract, causing the

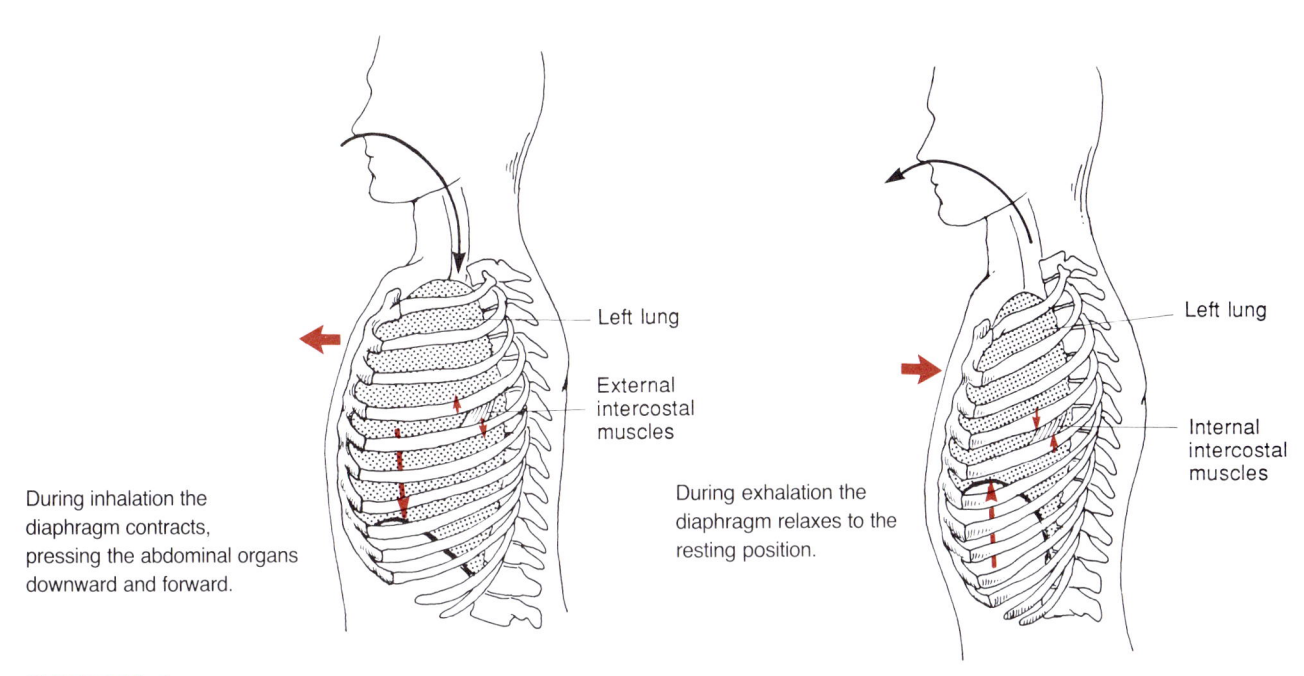

FIGURE 19-6.
Diagram of inspiration (left) and expiration (right).

chest to expand. The composite effect is to increase the volume of the thoracic cavity. As the volume increases, a subatmospheric pressure is created; air then enters the thorax in accord with the pressure difference. Air enters the lungs through the nose or mouth, a process known as **inspiration**. After inspiration, the intercostal muscles and diaphragm relax, and the walls of the alveoli rebound, because of the property of **elastic recoil**. These passive activities create an increase in intrathoracic pressure that causes air to exit the thorax through the nose or mouth, a process known as **expiration**. A diagram of inspiration and expiration is shown in Figure 19-6. The normal respiratory rate in the adult is 12 to 20 breaths per minute. In children, the normal respiratory rate is 18 to 26 breaths per minute, and infants normally breathe at 25 to 36 breaths per minute.

Another group of muscles, known collectively as the **accessory muscles** (because of their innervation by the spinal accessory nerve), play a role in respiratory distress. This muscle group, which includes the sternocleidomastoid and trapezius muscles, becomes active in increasing the intrathoracic volume during periods of respiratory insufficiency. Use of the accessory muscles is a clinical sign of respiratory decompensation.

MODIFIED FORMS OF RESPIRATION. Several forms of respiration act as protective mechanisms for the respiratory system. The **cough** mechanism consists of an initial irritation followed by a deep inspiration. After inspiration, a rapid closure of the glottis occurs while intercostal and abdominal muscles contract forcibly. As the intrathoracic pressure increases, the diaphragm pushes up, producing an explosive movement of air when the glottis is suddenly opened. A cough serves to expel foreign materials from the airway. A **sneeze** is a forceful exhalation from the nose, usually caused by nasal irritation. A **hiccup**, which serves no useful purpose, is a sudden inspiration against a closed glottis, caused by spasmodic contraction of the diaphragm. **Sighing** is a slow, deep inspiration followed by prolonged expiration. A sigh hyperinflates the lungs and may serve to re-expand atelectatic areas.

RESPIRATORY VOLUMES AND CAPACITIES. Respiratory volumes and capacities are measured by inhalation and exhalation into a spirometer that records a change in lung volume. Volume is measured in liters. The **total lung capacity (TLC)** is the volume of air in the lungs after a maximum inhalation. The TLC may be decreased in edema, pulmonary congestion, pneumothorax, hemothorax, or thoracic restriction and bronchiolar obstruction and emphysema. The **tidal volume (V_T)** is the volume of air normally inhaled or exhaled during each respiratory cycle. Decreased values of V_T occur in many types of pulmonary disorders and in neuromuscular diseases, such as myasthenia gravis. Decreased tidal breathing is almost always accompanied by an increased respiratory rate to maintain alveolar ventilation. A decreased V_T and rate usually is associated with respiratory center depression from drugs or brain stem lesions. Minute volume is a measurement of the V_T times the respiratory rate. The **inspiratory reserve volume (IRV)** is the maximum volume of air that can be inhaled after a normal inhalation. The **expiratory reserve volume (ERV)** is the maximum volume of air that can be exhaled after a normal exhalation. Reductions in IRV and ERV are typical in patients with restrictive disorders.

The *residual volume (RV)* is the volume of air that remains in the lungs at the end of a maximum expiration. An increase in RV indicates that, although maximum expiratory attempts were made, the lungs still contain an abnormally large volume of air. Increases in RV (known as *air trapping*) are characteristic of emphysema, asthma, and bronchial obstruction. As the RV becomes larger, more ventilation is required to adequately replenish the gas concentrations normal to the lung. This need usually causes an increase in V_T or rate, or both, and at the same time the work of breathing is increased. The RV may be decreased in diseases that occlude many alveoli, such as pneumonia. The *vital capacity (VC)* is the largest volume measured during complete expiration after the deepest inspiration. The VC is equal to IRV plus V_T plus ERV. The VC in adults varies directly with height and inversely with age and is generally smaller in females than in males. Decreases in VC can be caused by loss of distensible lung tissue, as in bronchiolar obstruction, pulmonary edema, pneumonia, or pulmonary congestion. A normal spirogram, which indicates lung volumes, is shown in Figure 19-7.

Two other components of respiratory function not shown on a spirogram are the *volume of dead space gas (V_D)* and *alveolar ventilation (V_A)*. The V_D is the volume, approximately 150 mL, that does not participate in pulmonary gas exchange. The V_D is larger in men than in women and becomes even larger in diseases that impede blood flow to the pulmonary capillaries. It may be decreased in asthma or in diseases characterized by bronchial obstruction. The V_A is the volume of air, approximately 350 mL, that comes into contact with the alveolar-capillary interface and is equal to V_T minus V_D. Decreased V_A associated with acute respiratory acidosis ($PaCO_2$ greater than 45 mm Hg and pH less than 7.35) represents *hypoventilation*. Increased V_A ($PaCO_2$ less than 35 mm Hg and pH greater than 7.45) is *hyperventilation*. Chronic hypoventilation and hyperventilation are associated with near-normal pH values but abnormal $PaCO_2$ values.

INNERVATION OF THE RESPIRATORY MUSCLES. The innervation of the respiratory muscles plays a role in a number of processes, especially trauma. The diaphragm is innervated by the right and left phrenic nerves, which exit the spinal column between the third and fifth cervical vertebrae. The intercostal muscles are innervated by the spinal nerves that exit the spinal column successively from the first to the twelfth thoracic vertebrae. Trauma patients who receive spinal injuries may have impaired respiratory status depending on the level of injury. If a cervical fracture crushes or severs the spinal cord above C-3, C-4, or C-5, nerve impulses from the brain can no longer reach the phrenic nerves, and, therefore, the diaphragm stops contracting. If artificial ventilation is not started, the patient will die. Cervical cord injuries that are below the C-3, C-4, or C-5 level affect rib expansion and its function in ventilation. Patients with thoracic spinal lesions have intact diaphragmatic function in addition to the use of some of the intercostal muscles.

Neurologic Control of Breathing

The overall control of respiration is held by the respiratory center, located in the medulla of the brain stem. This center is influenced by several factors. Most prominent, the pH of the cerebrospinal fluid, coupled with the $PaCO_2$, provides about 80% of the control of respiration.

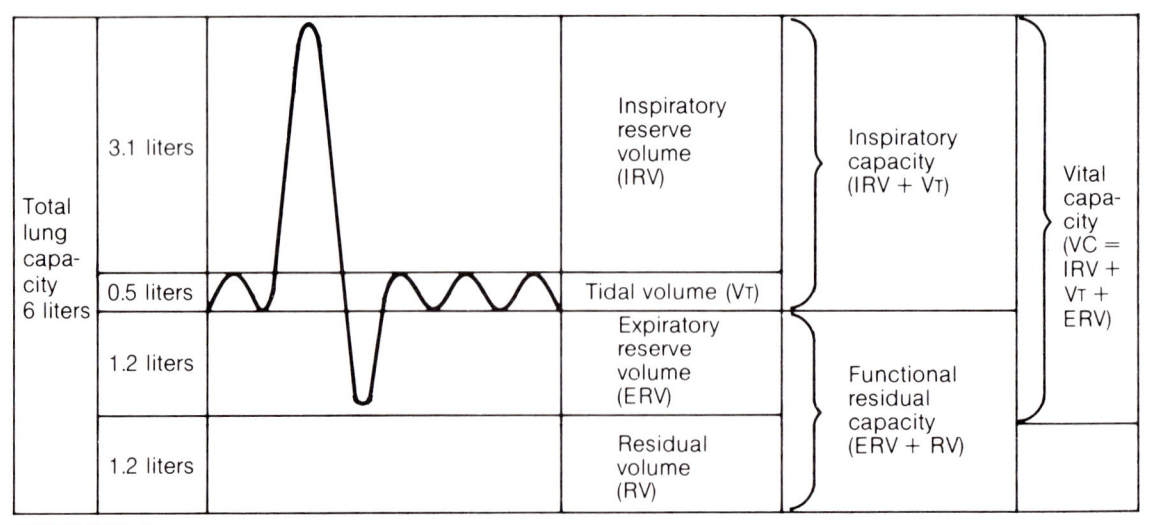

FIGURE 19-7.
Respiratory volumes and capacities. (Brunner LS, Suddarth DS)

As the cerebrospinal fluid becomes more acidic, as when carbon dioxide ($PaCO_2$ levels greater than 40 mm Hg) begins to build up in the bloodstream, the respiratory center is driven to increase the respiratory rate and depth. A secondary drive occurs via the PaO_2, which is sensed by peripheral baroreceptors located in the aortic arch and the carotid artery. A low PaO_2 (below 60 mm Hg) activates these receptors, which in turn stimulate the respiratory center, and impulses are sent to the muscles of respiration, increasing the rate and depth of breathing. Patients with chronic obstructive lung disease are unable to eliminate CO_2 normally, and their respiratory center gradually becomes accustomed to high $PaCO_2$ levels. In these patients, the PaO_2 becomes the dominant drive for respiration. The patient's respiratory rate and depth respond to PaO_2 levels below 60 mm Hg. Because of the low levels of PaO_2 required to maintain respiration, the patient is said to operate on a hypoxic drive. When a high level of oxygen is administered, the patient's respiratory drive may stop.

The control of breathing can be affected by conditions that affect either the central nervous system or the pH. Specifically, cerebrovascular accidents, head injuries, or central nervous system depressants may all alter respiratory status. In addition, processes that change the acid-base status, such as diabetic ketoacidosis or aspirin overdose, also produce changes in respiratory status. See Chapter 11 for a review of acid-base balance.

ASSESSMENT OF THE PATIENT IN RESPIRATORY DISTRESS

Assessment of the patient in respiratory distress can be a frustrating experience. External evidence of the degree of distress is frequently absent. Compounding the situation, the patient's and family's response to this crisis is frequently so hysterical as to make information from these sources appear unreliable. However, when performed systematically, the conventional primary and secondary surveys can provide the paramedic with a useful amount of information. In addition, a professional examination frequently allays some of the anxiety in the patient and family members, providing access to further information and bringing control to a previously chaotic scene.

Primary Survey

A primary survey is performed initially to allow any immediately life-threatening emergencies to be identified. Adequacy of airway and breathing is ensured in the unconscious patient by checking for the presence of normal quiet respiration. These normal findings should include a normal respiratory rate (**eupnea,** in the adult between 12 to 20 breaths per minute) and depth of respiration, as well as the absence of any extraneous sounds, such as snoring or gurgling, which would indicate an upper airway obstruction. In the conscious, speaking patient, the initial airway and breathing assessment is made by listening to the speech pattern. Patients who can speak in full sentences and who do not exhibit noisy respirations (indicating upper airway obstruction) have adequate airway and breathing function to allow the paramedic to move on to the final phase of the primary survey. The patient with **apnea** (no respiration) would require immediate resuscitative efforts. See Chapter 10 for airway management techniques and Appendix B for cardiopulmonary resuscitation protocols.

The primary survey is concluded with a check for adequate circulation. This part includes checking for the presence of a pulse and obvious hemorrhage. The patient who has a strong radial pulse (suggesting a blood pressure of at least 80 mm Hg systolic) has adequate circulatory function. Any abnormalities found in the primary survey must be managed satisfactorily before moving on to the secondary survey.

Secondary Survey

After the primary survey, the more extensive secondary survey is performed. During this survey, the patient's chief complaint is explored with the goal of discovering the nature of the problem. Ideally, management follows as a logical extension of this examination. The secondary survey includes the history and physical examination.

History

The first part of the patient history begins with the patient's chief complaint. The importance of the chief complaint cannot be overemphasized. Many patients have chief complaints that are different from apparent, visible problems. In addition, some subjective descriptions are classic for particular problems. For these reasons, it is crucial that the paramedic ask patients what the problem is and why they called for help.

Patients with respiratory problems have a number of chief complaints. Considered together, they are often called the cardinal signs of respiratory distress. One sign is **dyspnea** (difficult or labored breathing), which is frequently the reason that the patient called for help. Dyspnea can be caused by a number of physiologic processes. Asking the patient about activities at the onset of the dyspnea often clarifies the nature of the problem. Patients who describe dyspnea that begins only with exertion and whose dyspnea goes away immediately after exertion may be describing dyspnea of cardiac origin. In addition, dyspnea that is related to lying down (**orthopnea**), especially at night, is often of cardiac origin. This paroxysmal nocturnal dyspnea is a result of congestive heart failure. These types of dyspnea require a thorough cardiac examination.

Another cardinal sign is chest pain. Chest pain may be caused by a variety of diseases. Classic cardiac pain is substernal and often radiates to the shoulders, jaw, or arm. Chest pain may also be caused by trauma, pleuritis, esophageal disease, chest wall (musculoskeletal) disease, dissecting thoracic aneurysms, or pulmonary embolism. Pleuritis is often accompanied by a **pleural friction rub**, which can be heard by listening directly over the point of pain. The sound produced is nonmusical and has been compared to the creaking sound of old leather. It is commonly present during both inspiration and expiration. A pleural friction rub may accompany acute pleuritis or pulmonary embolism. The differential diagnosis of chest pain may be difficult. Often additional tests are needed to establish the diagnosis. It is important for the paramedic to understand that there are many causes and types of chest pain, and an accurate clinical history provides the most useful information for diagnosis.

The presence of a cough is the next cardinal sign. Despite the beliefs of many people, chronic cough is not normal. In the patient with a cough, it is important to find out about sputum production. Is sputum produced? If so, approximately how much? The color should be investigated to determine if the patient has a pulmonary infection. Yellow to green sputum is associated with infection. The presence of **hemoptysis**, or blood in the sputum, must also be determined. "*Coughing up blood*" is a frequent complaint of patients in respiratory distress. Blood-streaked sputum is usually from the upper airway and poses no significant problem. Patients who cough up bright red blood are either bleeding from the lungs or from the gastrointestinal tract. In either case, serious risk of exsanguination exists.

Another cardinal sign of respiratory distress is the presence of wheezing. Unfortunately, wheezing alone is not a useful diagnostic sign; wheezing is caused by airways narrowed from any cause. Included in causes of wheezing are exercise (which causes airway muscle spasm in some people), pulmonary edema, asthmatic attack, and pneumonia. The critical questions to ask are whether the patient chronically wheezes and whether this wheezing is worse than or different from normal.

The presence of signs of infection is the final cardinal sign that is assessed during the chief complaint. Shortness of breath associated with signs of infection may be due to pneumonia. A patient's complaint of fever, chills, or sweats may be useful in clarifying the cause of dyspnea.

Another aspect of the patient history is the history of the current episode. It is crucial to ask about the time of onset and duration of the episode. While these two questions may seem similar, they are very different. Time of onset means when a particular problem, such as shortness of breath, began. Because so many respiratory problems are chronic or long lasting, many patients answer this question with a time that is days or even years in the past.

When this response is given, the second question about the duration of the specific episode should be asked. For example, the patient may have had an upper respiratory infection for the past 2 weeks but developed an acute deterioration 4 hours before calling for help. It is also important to inquire about the activity at onset. A rapid onset of shortness of breath can be caused by a variety of factors. Cardiac causes are a particular concern in cases in which the onset occurred during exertion. Classically, cardiac shortness of breath occurs during exertion or stress and resolves almost immediately after the exertion or stress stops. Respiratory problems may develop with exercise but rarely resolve so quickly.

Because so many respiratory signs and symptoms are chronic, it is important to find out if the problem has happened before. Ask the patient what happened the last time and what the diagnosis was if medical treatment was sought. Taking the time to ask these questions can save time in rediagnosing a problem that the patient has already identified. If the problem is chronic, the paramedic can use this point in the evaluation to learn more about the medical history, which is discussed below. It is also important to ask the patient how bad this attack is in comparison to previous episodes. In chronic respiratory disease, the patient's subjective report is the most accurate indicator of acuity available on the scene. Regardless of chronicity, it is important to ask the patient what attempt was made to help the problem and if it was successful. Successful treatments, such as nitroglycerin or inhaled bronchodilators, often give a clue to the cause of the problem. Sometimes, the attempted treatments explain other signs and symptoms, such as a headache and flushing in a patient who took five nitroglycerin tablets to alleviate chest pain.

MEDICAL HISTORY. As stated before, it is important to learn if the patient has experienced previous episodes of similar problems. If respiratory problems are chronic, the known pulmonary diagnosis is important information to obtain. In many cases, the patient reports a diagnosis that the paramedic recognizes. Frequently, this information simplifies further assessment and management. Another crucial point is a history of previous intubation. Patients who have required intubation for respiratory symptoms are in a special, critical class of patients who should be observed and managed with great care. Intubation equipment should be quickly checked; these patients frequently deteriorate rapidly.

Another key aspect of the medical history is medication. Frequently, patients with chronic respiratory disease take a variety of pulmonary and cardiac medications. The paramedic should find out what medications, including over-the-counter preparations, the patient is currently taking. It is helpful to transport all of the medications with the patient. This action allows the attending physician to have a full medication history and to evaluate for outdated or inappropriate medications. Patients should also be asked if they are allergic to any medications.

Since certain pulmonary drugs are commonly prescribed, a brief discussion about medications used to manage respiratory distress is appropriate. These medications fall into four basic classes. The first and most often used are the *methylxanthines*. The most frequently used methylxanthine is theophylline, which is a bronchodilator that works by relaxing the smooth muscle in the bronchioles. Side effects include tachycardia, nausea and vomiting, headache, and, at toxic levels, ventricular tachycardia and grand mal seizures. Toxicity is a special concern since prehospital personnel frequently administer theophylline products. If the patient has been taking these agents at home, the potential for significant toxicity is very real. Table 19-1 lists common respiratory drugs, including theophylline preparations.

Another class of drugs used to manage respiratory conditions is the *sympathomimetics*, which are drugs that mimic the sympathetic nervous system. Stimulation of the sympathetic nervous system causes dilation of the airways at the bronchiolar level. Side effects of these drugs include other sympathetic signs and symptoms, especially tachycardia, muscle tremor, diaphoresis, and anxiety. As with the theophylline products, a careful history of these agents is crucial, since epinephrine, a sympathomimetic drug, is often given in prehospital medical care. Table 19-1 lists a number of sympathomimetics.

A third class of medications is *corticosteroids*. Corticosteroids are synthetic variations of the naturally occurring substance hydrocortisone. Although their mechanism is unclear, they exert an anti-inflammatory, antiallergic action. These two responses help prevent bronchospasm and open the airways after bronchospasm has occurred. On an acute basis, toxicity is not a problem. Table 19-1 lists some common corticosteroid preparations.

The final medication that merits inclusion in the medical history is *cromolyn sodium*, which exerts an antiallergic action by blocking the receptors for specific allergens. Competitive site binding prevents allergens from triggering these receptors, thus preventing the allergic responses of bronchospasm or mucous production (see Table 19-1).

In addition to learning the respiratory history and medication history, other medical problems are important to note. A history of cardiac, seizure, or diabetic problems is especially important, because medications the paramedic may give are potentially cardiotoxic, lower the seizure threshold, and cause a release of sugar into the blood, causing hyperglycemia. Another part of the medical his-

TABLE 19–1.
COMMON HOME PULMONARY MEDICATIONS

Class	Generic Name	Brand Name
Methylxanthine	aminophylline	Aminodur
	theophylline	Quibron
		Slo-bid
		Slo-Phyllin
		Somophyllin
		Tedral
		Theo-Dur
	oxtriphylline	Choledyl
Sympathomimetic	epinephrine	Adrenalin
	isoproterenol hydrochloride	Isuprel
	isoproterenol sulfate	Alupent
		Metaprel
	phenylephrine hydrochloride and isoetharine mesylate	Bronkometer
	terbutaline sulfate	Brethine
		Bricanyl
Corticosteroid	hydrocortisone sodium succinate	Solu-Cortef
	methylprednisolone sodium succinate	Solu-Medrol
	prednisone	Deltasone
	beclomethasone dipropionate	Vanceril
		Beclovent
	dexamethasone	Decadron
Cromolyn	cromolyn sodium	Intal
		Aarane

Patterns of Respiration	Description	Significance
One Minute		
Eupnea 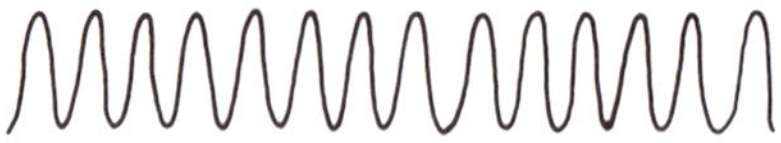	Normal rate and depth of respiration.	Normal respiratory function.
Apnea 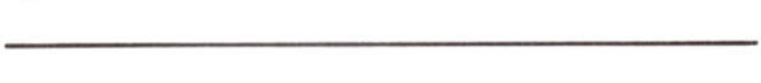	Complete cessation of respiration.	Respiratory arrest.
Bradypnea 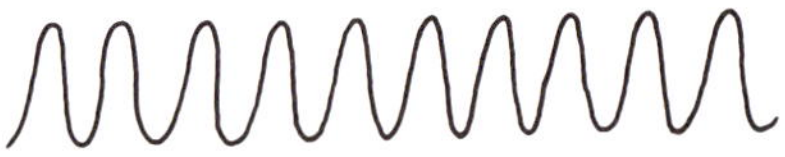	Rate less than 12 respirations per minute.	Neurologic disturbance. Electrolyte disturbance. Infection.
Tachypnea 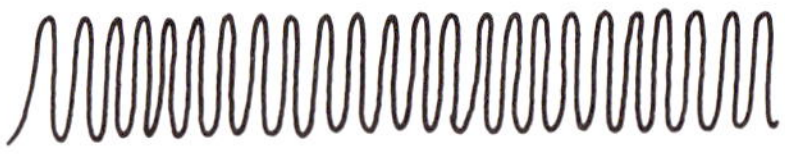	Rate greater than 20 respirations per minute.	Fear, pain, or injury.
Central Neurogenic Hyperventilation 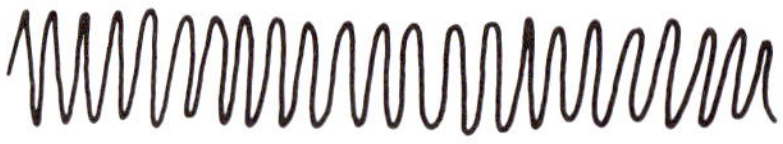	Sustained regular, rapid respirations, with forced inspiration and expiration.	May indicate a lesion of the low midbrain or upper pons areas of the brain stem.
Apneustic 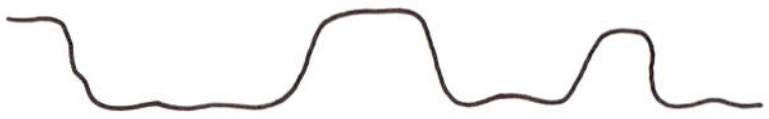	Prolonged inspiratory spasms with a pause at full inspiration. There may also be expiratory pauses.	May indicate a lesion of the mid or lower pons.
Ataxic (Biot's breathing) 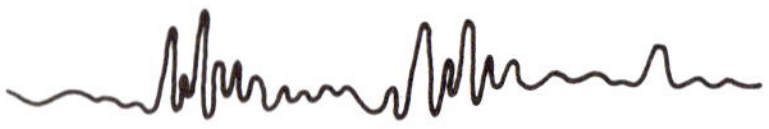	Gasping, irregular pattern with random deep and shallow respirations. Irregular pauses may also appear.	May indicate a lesion of the medulla.
Cheyne–Stokes 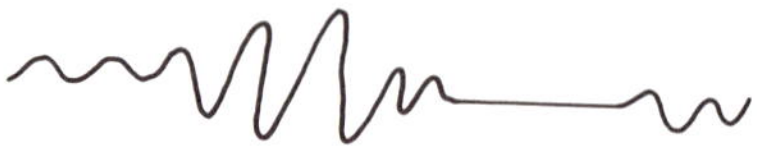	Cyclic increase and decrease in rate and depth of respiration followed by a period of apnea.	Increased intracranial pressure. Deep cerebral or cerebellar lesions. Congestive heart failure.
Kussmaul 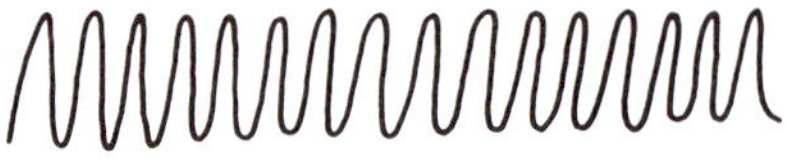	Fast respirations characterized by deep sighing.	Diabetic ketoacidosis. Metabolic acidosis. Renal failure.
Obstructive 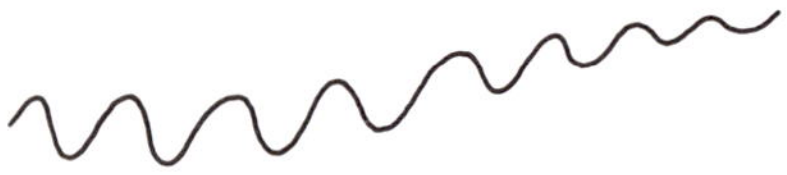	Prolonged expiration.	Chronic obstructive pulmonary disease.

FIGURE 19–8.
Patterns of respiration.

tory is the toxic exposure and smoking history. A number of conditions that present with respiratory symptoms are caused by exposure to toxic substances or by smoking. While it is difficult to determine certain toxic exposures, determination of smoking history is relatively easy. The most accepted means of taking a smoking history is to determine the number of packs per day and the years of smoking. When multiplied together, these yield the "pack-years" of smoking.

Physical Examination

The history is a critical feature of the assessment of the patient with respiratory insufficiency, particularly when the problem is chronic. An accurate history should enable the paramedic to determine the cause of the distress and, to a lesser extent, the acuity. The physical examination enables the paramedic to focus on assessing the acuity of the condition.

INSPECTION. The physical examination begins with inspection. Patients are observed for their general level of distress. A patient who is reclining in a chair appears to be in less distress than one who is sitting bolt upright. Is the patient confused, agitated, or combative? These conditions frequently indicate hypoxemia or **hypercapnia** (increased amount of carbon dioxide in the blood). Color is another important visual finding. **Cyanosis** (bluish discoloration of the skin and mucous membranes from lack of oxygen) is indicative of hypoxemia, although it is a late sign. **Central cyanosis** (cyanosis found around the lips and tongue) is a more accurate and useful finding than **peripheral cyanosis** (cyanosis of the skin and nail beds), which can be caused by fractures, poor circulation, or a variety of other problems. **Diaphoresis** (profuse sweating) is another useful sign. Diaphoresis is caused by increased sympathetic nervous system discharge and may be indicative of a compensatory response to a major acute illness.

Early in the patient examination the respiratory rate, pattern, and depth should be assessed. While **tachypnea** (rate greater than 20 breaths per minute in the adult) alone is not a particularly useful sign, the presence of rapid, deep respirations (**hyperpnea**) suggests a physiologic drive such as acidosis or hypoxia. **Bradypnea** (rate less than 12 breaths per minute in the adult) may be caused by a variety of factors and must be managed aggressively. A number of respiratory patterns, shown in Figure 19-8, are also significant.

Another visual clue is the presence of **retractions**, or use of the accessory muscles of respiration. The chest must be exposed to see these signs. Retractions and use of the accessory muscles are caused by breathing against obstruction; they are recognized by the way the skin is pulled in during inspiration. Retractions may be seen in between the ribs, at the sternum, or above the clavicles,

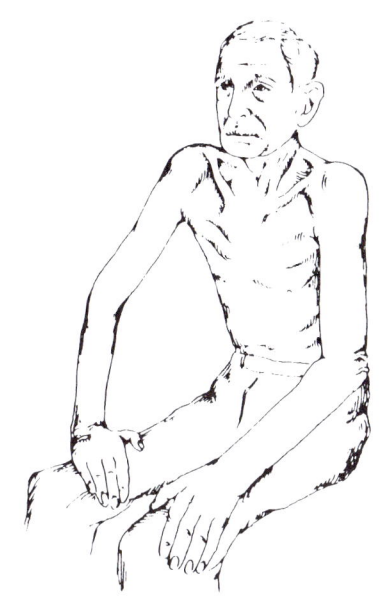

FIGURE 19–9.
The use of accessory muscles in a patient with retractions.

while use of the accessory muscles exposes the sternocleidomastoid and trapezius muscles in the neck. A patient with retractions is shown in Figure 19-9.

The presence of jugular venous distension is also assessed. When the patient is sitting up, the jugular veins should not be visible. The presence of jugular venous distension is either due to right-sided heart failure or to increased intrathoracic pressure, like that caused by tension pneumothorax. **Nasal flaring** (widening of the nostrils on inspiration) and **tracheal tugging** (pulling inward on tissue at the neck) are indications of airway obstruction. A final visual clue is the presence of clubbing. **Clubbing** is an enlargement and change in shape of the tip of one or more fingers or toes. While the causes of clubbing are not clear, the condition can be used to help deduce a history in the unconscious or uncooperative patient. The vast majority of patients who present with clubbing have some chronic pulmonary or cardiac disease, including bronchogenic carcinoma, advanced chronic obstructive pulmonary disease, cystic fibrosis, or cardiac disease that causes hypoxia, such as cyanotic congenital heart disease.

PALPATION. Palpation follows inspection in the physical examination. Initially, the skin should be palpated for *turgor* (fullness). Because of insensible losses of fluid during hyperventilation, patients in respiratory distress are frequently dehydrated. Also included in this portion of the examination is the pulse rate. In addition to simply counting the pulse, it should be examined for quality or strength and for regularity. Especially significant in the patient with respiratory distress is tachycardia, which often indicates hypoxia. Irregular pulses may be due to arrhythmias or pulsus paradoxus, which is discussed later.

In addition to palpating the pulse, the chest wall should be palpated. Initial palpation is performed to assess the presence of tenderness or pain around the ribs that might accompany broken ribs or chest wall trauma. In addition, uniformity of chest wall movement should be assessed by placing the hands low on the chest and asking the patient to breathe deeply. The hands should be watched for symmetry of motion; asymmetry may indicate major chest wall damage, such as that caused by a flail chest, or a volume loss in one lung, such as that caused by atelectasis. The paramedic should also palpate for *tracheal deviation*. This procedure is performed by placing the index finger in the sternal notch and pressing firmly toward the spine. The trachea is identified as a somewhat tubular structure that occupies about two thirds of the notch. Tracheal deviation is generally caused by tension pneumothorax, although tumors or past thoracic surgery may also cause this condition.

AUSCULTATION. After palpation, the chest is auscultated. **Auscultation** is listening to the chest to detect abnormalities in air flow through the major airways, bronchi, or bronchioles. While the chest can be adequately auscultated from either the front (anterior) or back (posterior), there are a number of advantages to auscultating posteriorly. The sounds heard over the front of the chest are usually quieter, because of the presence of the breasts and increased fat deposits. In contrast, sounds heard posteriorly tend to be clearer and louder. Posterior auscultation offers an additional advantage: the lower lobes of the lungs can only be heard when listening from the back or sides because of their wedge shape, as shown in Figure 19-10. Placement of the stethoscope should allow a comparison of breath sounds in all lobes of both lungs; the placements shown in Figure 19-11 allow this assessment. Because of changes in airway diameter with inspiration and expiration, breath sounds should be evaluated during both phases in each location.

The actual assessment of **breath sounds** is not difficult. However, confusion frequently occurs over what terms relate to what sounds and what those sounds mean. Uniform terms should be used within a given system to ensure clarity of communication. Normal breath sounds are quiet and clear where inspiration and expiration are approximately equal. Because they are so quiet, it is often necessary to ask the patient to take a deep breath to be able to hear any sound at all. Absent breath sounds are frequently mistaken for normal and may indicate a serious condition, although absence in one lobe does not mean absence in all lobes. To differentiate absent from

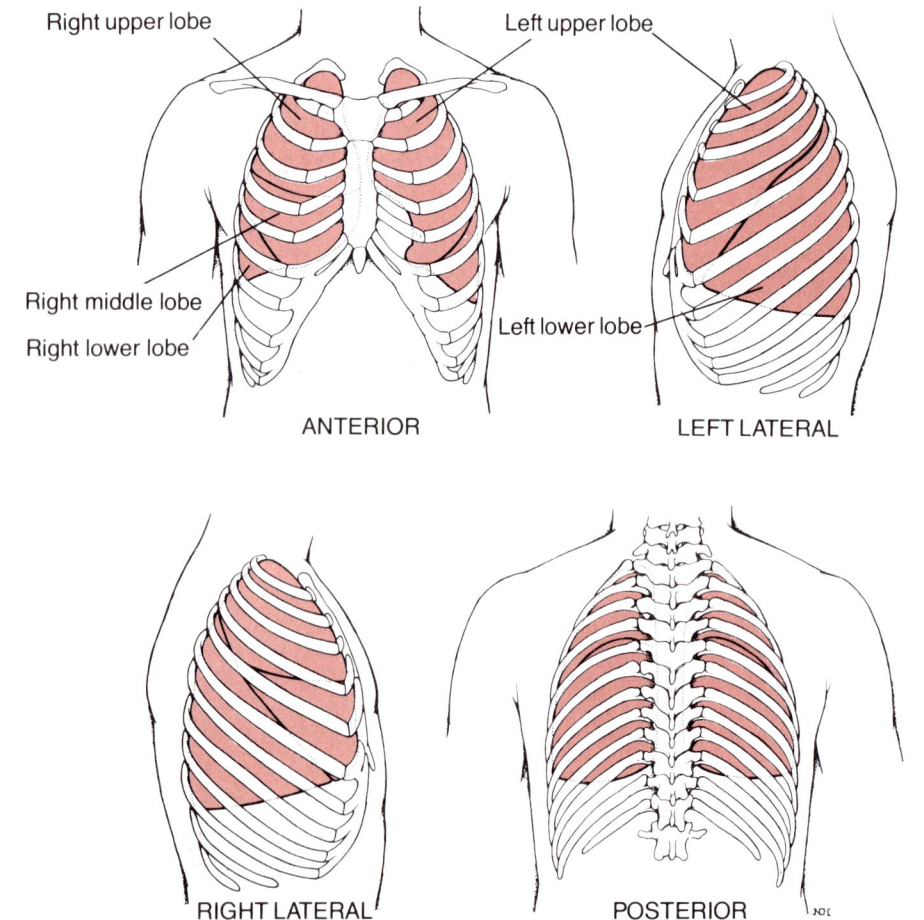

FIGURE 19-10.
Relationship of the lobes of the lung by topography. (Brunner LS, Suddarth DS)

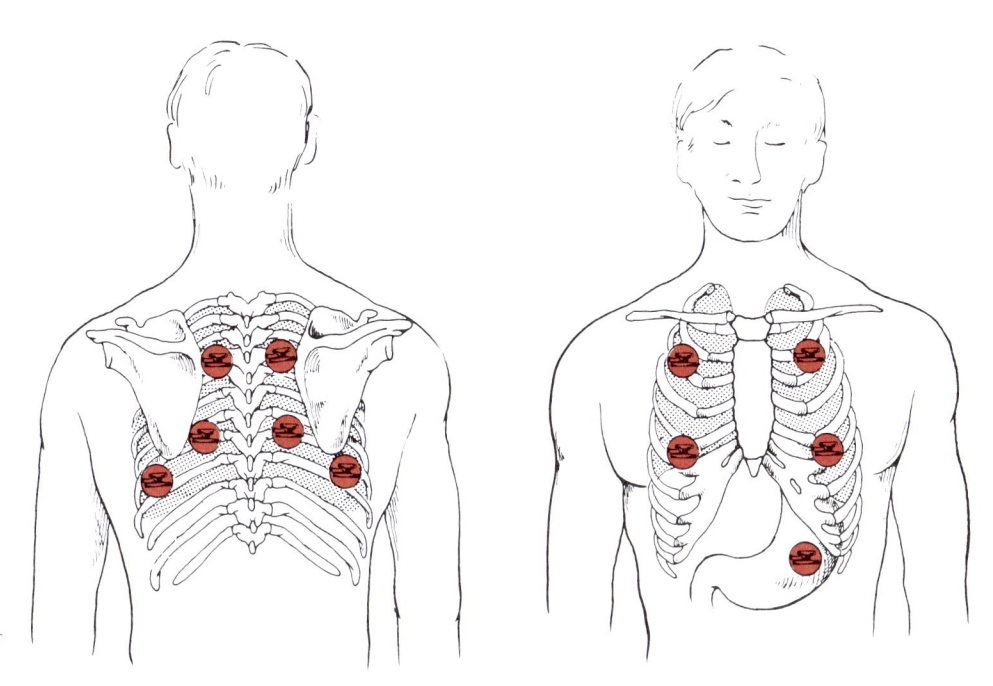

FIGURE 19–11.
Placement of the stethoscope for auscultation of breath sounds.

normal breath sounds, the patient should breathe deeply. In normal respiration, some sound should be heard; if nothing can be heard, absent breath sounds are probably the correct assessment. An additional clue comes from the patient's presentation. If the patient is in significant distress and has retractions, it is unlikely that the breath sounds are normal.

Normal breath sounds vary depending on the area of auscultation. As shown in Figure 19-12, the sounds have been divided into three types: bronchial or tubular, bronchovesicular, and vesicular. The normal air-filled lung acts as a filter to sound. Diminished breath sounds may result from decreases in sound generation with shallow breathing patterns.

Wheezes are high-pitched musical sounds that indicate narrowing of the airways from any cause. Because the airways naturally narrow somewhat during expiration, wheezes frequently start during expiration. As the patient's condition deteriorates, the wheezes may also become evident during inspiration. When documenting wheezes, the paramedic must note whether they were present during inspiration, expiration, or in both phases.

Stridor, like wheezes, is caused by airway narrowing. However, stridor, which often sounds like the barking of a seal, is caused by narrowing of the upper airway rather than the bronchi and bronchioles. Causes of stridor include croup, fractured larynx, or swelling in the airway caused by anaphylaxis. Because of the importance of upper airway integrity, patients with stridor should be handled with great care.

Rhonchi are low-pitched rumbling sounds that are caused by air moving through mucus. Pneumonia, upper respiratory tract infections, and bronchitis are three common disorders that cause rhonchi. Identification of this sound is aided greatly by a history of mucus production.

Rales make a crackling or bubbling sound and come in varying degrees of coarseness. Although their exact cause is not known, one theory holds that the sound is caused by air moving through fluid. Recognition of rales is important, because pulmonary edema is one of the disorders in which they are found. Chest pain, congestive heart failure, and significant respiratory distress often accompany rales. Rales and rhonchi frequently can be difficult to differentiate. However, the easiest way to distinguish between the two is to determine if the sound is continuous or if it is made up of a series of short discrete sounds. Rhonchi are continuous sounds that are often described as "*snoring.*" Rales are discontinuous; that is, they are made up of a series of discrete sounds that are described as "*crackling*" or "*popping*" in nature.

Competence in breath sound interpretation is important, particularly in difficult cases of differentiation between pulmonary edema and other disorders. Breath sounds are an important key to correct diagnosis and management.

PULSUS PARADOXUS. In addition to auscultating the chest, the blood pressure is auscultated. While determining the blood pressure, the pulsus paradoxus should be measured. ***Pulsus paradoxus*** refers to an accentuated decline in systolic blood pressure that coincides with inspiration. Normally, the systolic pressure decreases 5 to 10 mm Hg during inspiration. However, in a number of pathologic processes, which are discussed in a later section, the systolic pressure decreases abnormally, 10 to 20 mm Hg or more, during inspiration.

Bronchial or Tubular

Blowing, hollow sounds auscultated over the trachea

Ratio of inspiration to expiration

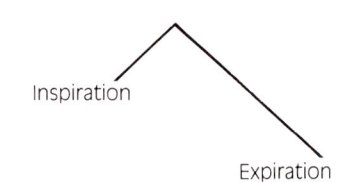

Inspiration is shorter than expiration
Expiration is longer, lower, and higher-pitched than inspiration

Bronchovesicular

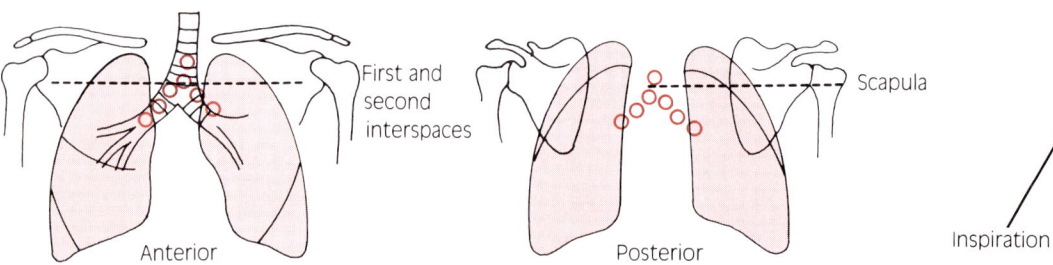

First and second interspaces

Scapula

Medium-pitched, medium intesity, blowing sounds auscultated over the first and second interspaces anteriorly and the scapula posteriorly

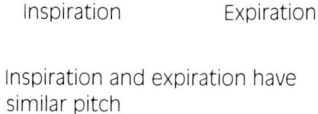

Inspiration and expiration have similar pitch

Vesicular

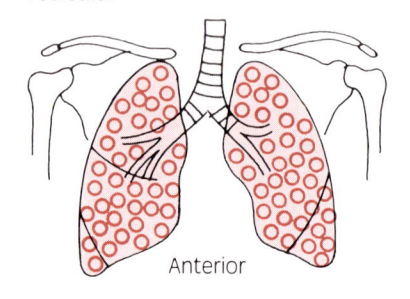

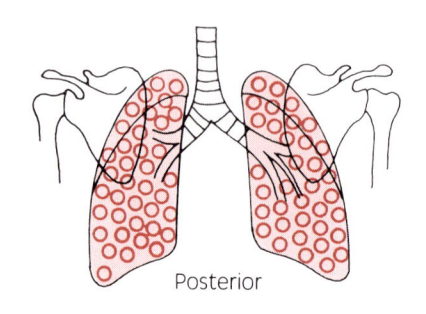

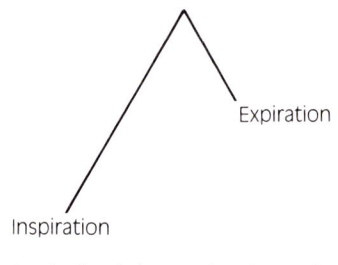

Soft, low-pitched sounds auscultated over the lung periphery

Inspiration is longer, louder, and higher-pitched than expiration

FIGURE 19–12.
Normal breath sounds. (Taylor C, Lillis C, LeMone P)

The ideal way to measure pulsus paradoxus is to ask the patient to hold a breath at inspiration and again at expiration while the blood pressure is taken. However, few patients in respiratory distress can tolerate such breath-holding. Instead, the pulsus paradoxus is measured by inflating the blood pressure cuff as usual and deflating the cuff slowly. As air is released from the cuff, the first sound heard typically is the systolic blood pressure. As the cuff is further deflated, a dulling or muffling of the sound may be heard when the conventional "*thump-thump*" is changed in character. The manometer reading should be noted when this change in character occurs. As the cuff is further deflated, the sound changes back to the normal "*thump-thump*"; again, the manometer reading should be noted.

Finally, the sound disappears entirely, marking the diastolic blood pressure. The pulsus paradoxus is the distance (in mm Hg) during which the sounds were muffled. It should be noted that the muffling may be anywhere in the total range between the systolic and diastolic pressures. In fact, it is common for the muffling to occur right at the systolic pressure, creating a sound that is frequently mistaken for patient movement. Because of the faintness of the sounds being listened for, pulsus paradoxus cannot be heard in a moving ambulance or noisy environment. While measuring pulsus paradoxus is not a skill that is used daily, it is worth learning and practicing since it is found in a number of conditions, including asthma, cardiac tamponade, hypovolemic shock, pulmonary embolism, and tension pneumothorax. The pathophysiology of pulsus paradoxus is discussed later in this chapter.

RESPIRATORY DISORDERS

A number of disease and traumatic states may affect the respiratory system. Many of these problems possess similarities based on whether they affect the upper airway, lower airway, alveoli, or chest wall. This section presents a number of common respiratory dysfunctions with a discussion of pathophysiology, pertinent assessment findings, and management.

Upper Airway Obstruction

Upper airway obstruction involves either partial or complete obstruction of the respiratory system. Chapter 10 presents a detailed discussion of upper airway disorders; only a brief review is presented here.

Pathophysiology

Obstruction of the upper airway can be caused by a number of factors. Most common is obstruction by the tongue in the comatose patient, although obstruction can also be caused by foreign bodies, spasm or edema (as in anaphylaxis), or trauma. In each case, obstruction creates a partial or complete restriction of air flow through the upper airway. This inability to ventilate leads to hypoxia and hypercapnia.

Assessment

A number of general indicators of respiratory distress may be present in the patient with an upper airway obstruction. Alterations in the level of consciousness, including unconsciousness, combativeness, or drowsiness may be indicative of hypoxemia or hypercarpnia.

In addition to these general findings, a number of specific indications of upper airway obstruction may be identified. Snoring or noisy respiration is diagnostic of an upper airway obstruction, as is stridor. The presence of retractions and the use of the accessory muscles of respiration are indicators of airway obstruction, although they cannot be used to differentiate between upper and lower airway obstruction. The presence of a pulsus paradoxus may indicate obstruction, although it is not specific. Finally, visible trauma to or swelling of the neck indicates the presence of airway trauma or edema.

Management

Management of airway obstruction begins with head position. Oropharyngeal or nasopharyngeal airways should be used to overcome obstruction by the tongue. Patients with foreign material in the airway require suction.

More secure airway control can be achieved a number of ways. Endotracheal intubation is the technique of choice, with the PtL airway, Combi-tube, esophageal obturator airway, or esophageal gastric tube airway as secondary options. In patients with airway trauma, cricothyroidotomy may be required to secure the airway adequately.

Patients who are not ventilating well require supplemental ventilation with oxygen. A pocket face mask may be used and generally provides better V_T than the bag-valve-mask device. However, the bag-valve-mask device allows the delivery of 100% oxygen, while the pocket mask is limited to approximately 40%. A positive-pressure oxygen-powered ventilator may also be used. This device permits the delivery of adequate V_T and 100% oxygen.

Lower Airway Disorders
Obstructive Lung Disease

The term **obstructive lung disease** refers to several diseases that have obstruction of the lower airway in common. Included in this group are asthma, chronic bronchitis, and emphysema; this group of diseases is known collectively as **chronic obstructive pulmonary disease (COPD)**. Taken together, obstructive lung disease results in a large number of ambulance calls, emergency department visits, and hospital admissions and results in more than 60,000 deaths per year.

PATHOPHYSIOLOGY. The common bond that unites these respiratory diseases is obstruction in the bronchi and bronchioles. This obstruction may be due to many factors. Mucus is frequently responsible for the obstruction seen in patients with chronic bronchitis. Smooth muscle spasm in the bronchioles causes obstruction in many disease states, including asthma. Airway edema results in airway obstruction in patients with allergies or anaphylactic reactions. It is important to remember that most patients have more than one cause of obstruction. These individual causes of obstruction are extremely important, as they form the basis of management.

Physiologically, the airways change diameter during respiration; the diameter increases on inspiration and decreases on expiration. This naturally occurring phenomenon must be appreciated to understand a pathologic component of obstructive lung disease: air trapping. A single obstructed airway can be viewed in the diagram in Figure 19-13. An obstruction blocks the lumen of the airway.

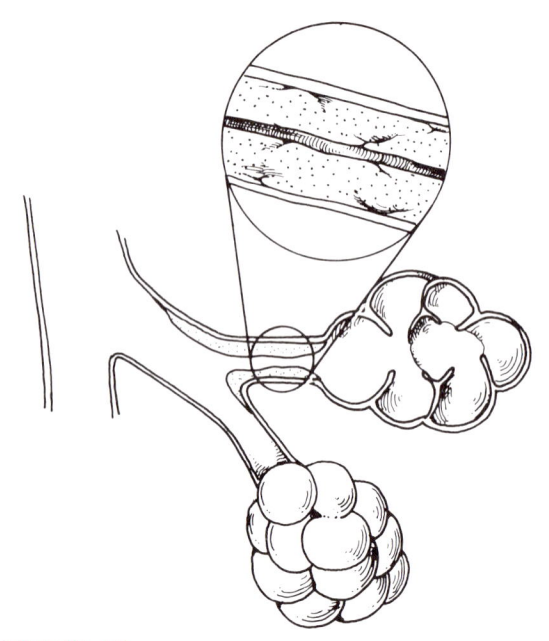

FIGURE 19–13.
Obstruction of the lumen of an airway.

During inspiration, the airway dilates, allowing air to flow into the alveolus. On expiration, the diameter of the airway decreases, trapping air behind the obstruction. This air trapping leads to hyperinflated alveoli because, with each inspiration, more air is squeezed into the alveolus. On a larger scale that involves many alveoli, this condition can lead to hypoxemia and hypercapnia because of the inability of the alveoli to provide fresh oxygen and remove carbon dioxide. This hyperinflation also leads to some secondary effects.

Air trapping is a feature shared by all obstructive lung diseases. However, the way in which the lung reacts to chronic air trapping varies somewhat from disease to disease. One frequent result of chronic hyperinflation is loss of elastic recoil. Elastic recoil, as discussed earlier in this chapter, is the elastic property in the walls of the alveoli that squeezes air out during exhalation. In some patients, chronic hyperinflation of the alveoli causes a loss of this elasticity, necessitating active exhalation. These patients must forcibly exhale, using the intercostal and abdominal muscles. This forceful exhalation significantly increases the work of breathing, thus decreasing the patient's tolerance for even mild exercise. Loss of elastic recoil is a permanent change.

Another change that may occur from chronically hyperinflated alveoli is the formation of blebs. Hyperinflated alveoli are thin walled because of the stretching of the alveolar walls (like blowing up a balloon; the fuller it gets, the thinner the walls). In addition, these alveoli are larger than normal, forcing alveolar walls to be pressed together, as shown in Figure 19-14. In some people with chronic pulmonary disease, the walls between these alveoli are destroyed, creating blebs. Blebs are large, ineffective, nonelastic alveoli made up of many alveoli that have blended together. The problem with blebs is that the gas exchange capability is lost because of a loss of alveolar-capillary interface. Figure 19-14 shows the amount of surface area that is lost when two alveoli form a *bleb*. This change is irreversible and frequently results in a need for supplemental oxygen to compensate for the patient's inability to exchange enough gas through the ineffective alveoli.

A number of other effects may be caused by air trapping. Hyperinflated alveoli may compress pulmonary capillaries as shown in Figure 19-15. This abnormality causes a number of effects. First, the compression of capillaries becomes more pronounced during inspiration, when the alveoli get slightly larger. If hyperinflation is present throughout the chest, this compression of pulmonary capillaries may actually impede blood flow from the right heart to the left heart, especially during inspiration. This impedance to flow from right to left causes a backup of blood through the right heart and may result in the classic signs of right-sided heart failure: jugular venous distension and pedal edema. These findings may present in patients with no cardiac disease and may be due solely to the degree of obstruction.

The impedance to flow from the right heart to the left also is responsible for creating pulsus paradoxus. As explained earlier, in pulsus paradoxus, the normal decline in systolic blood pressure during inspiration is accentuated. As alveoli become hyperinflated, the flow of blood through the lungs is impeded and is further impeded during inspiration. This decreased blood flow results in a decreased volume of blood that enters the left heart and that is then ejected by it. This causes the accentuated decrease in systolic pressure seen in pulsus paradoxus. Pulsus paradoxus is a sign not unique to this clinical cir-

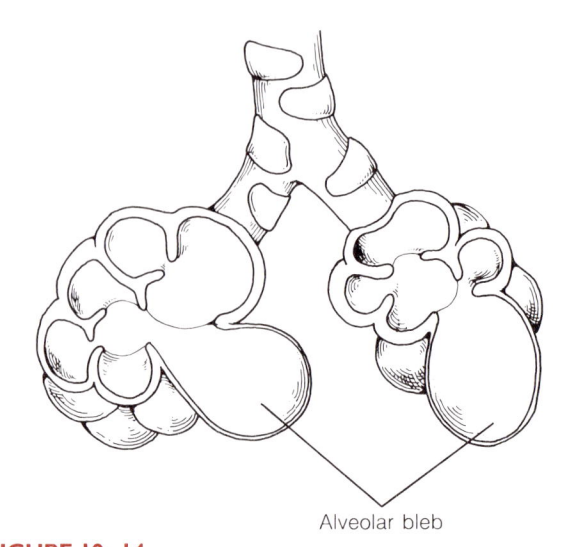

FIGURE 19–14.
Alveolar blebs.

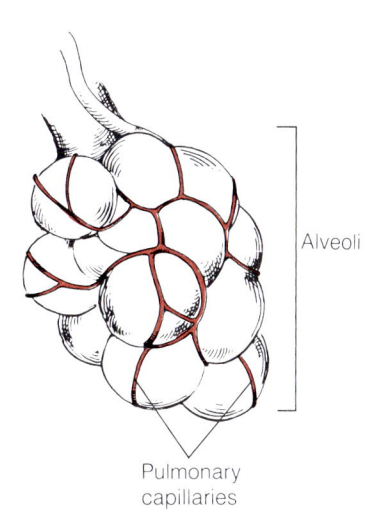

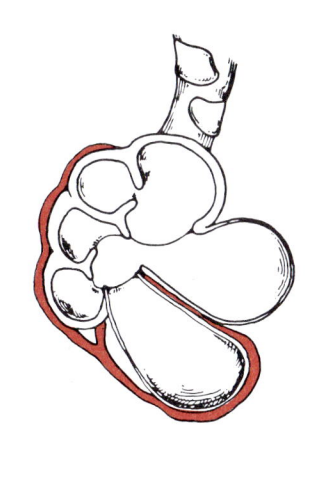

FIGURE 19–15.
Compressed pulmonary capillaries.

cumstance; it may be observed in other situations encountered by paramedics, most commonly acute cardiac tamponade. Unlike the loss of elastic recoil and the formation of blebs, the cardiac effects of hyperinflation are generally reversible with proper treatment.

Not all patients with obstructive lung disease possess all of the described characteristics. While every patient exhibits obstruction, the distribution of other lung changes varies according to the patient's disease process. Asthma, for example, is characterized by reversible airway obstruction; patients have temporary air trapping and may have signs of right-sided heart failure. However, the patient with asthma usually does not have a permanent loss of elastic recoil or bleb formation; these are irreversible changes. The obstruction in asthma may be due to a number of factors. In children, airway obstruction is frequently due to allergies or other external factors.

Adults, on the other hand, often have airway obstruction that is not associated with any external factors. ***Status asthmaticus*** is defined as a severe prolonged asthmatic attack that does not respond to therapy. While acute therapy for children and adults is identical, long-term therapy in children frequently revolves around treating allergies. Adults, generally, do not benefit from this treatment. In some patients, asthma attacks may be associated with emotional stress. However, an important point to remember is that these are real attacks. Whether the trigger for the attack is an allergy or an emotion, the bronchospasm is real and the patient needs immediate care.

Long-term cigarette smoking causes a number of permanent changes in the airway and alveolar structure. Included in these changes are increased mucus production, bleb formation, and loss of elastic recoil. It is important to note that even patients with severe airway destruction have some degree of reversible airway obstruction. It is this degree of reversibility that is treated.

Upper respiratory tract infections and pneumonia may cause significant mucus production and, hence, airway obstruction. In both cases, however, the airway obstruction is reversible, like asthma. Any condition that causes mucus production, as well as edema or smooth muscle spasm, can produce air trapping with signs and symptoms of obstructive lung disease, even if only for a brief time.

ASSESSMENT. Assessment of the patient with obstructive lung disease includes a complete patient history. Because of the chronicity of many of these diseases, it is frequently difficult to determine how acutely ill the patient is at the present time. A number of observations may assist in increasing the accuracy of the management. The level of consciousness is important. Any patient who demonstrates an alteration in level of consciousness due to airway obstruction is clearly acute. In addition, the patient's subjective assessment of the acuity of the attack is important.

Three physical findings are indicators of airway obstruction in the adult. The first is tachycardia; a pulse rate greater than 100 is associated with extreme airway obstruction. A second indicator is the presence of retractions and accessory muscle use. Finally, the presence of pulsus paradoxus greater than 10 to 20 mm Hg may be indicative of extreme airway obstruction. The presence of one, two, or all three of these signs is a good indication of degree of obstruction and the acuity of the attack.

Bronchoconstriction is often a problem in obstructive lung disease. An excellent way to determine the severity of bronchoconstriction is to measure the patient's peak flow. The peak flow is a measurement of how rapidly the patient can exhale. A patient who has bronchoconstriction exhales slowly. The measurement is made by asking the patient to inhale deeply and then exhale as quickly as possible through the peak flow meter. In general, an adult with a peak flow less than 150 L/min requires immediate treatment. Small, inexpensive devices that measure peak flow using a flow gauge are available for field use and are sometimes found in the patient's home. The peak flow measured by these portable devices is most useful for fol-

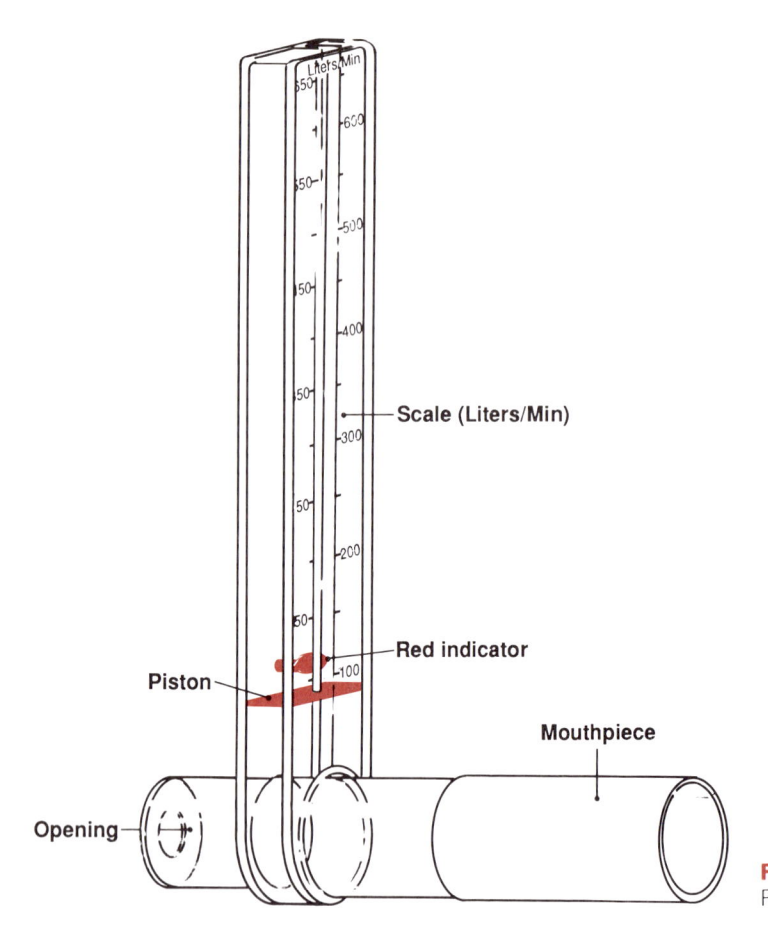

FIGURE 19-16.
Peak flow meter.

lowing gross changes in airway function. A portable *peak flow meter* is shown in Figure 19-16.

MANAGEMENT. Management of the patient with acute obstructive lung disease is based on airway management, oxygenation, and bronchodilation. If inadequate ventilation is present, the airway must be controlled and ventilation assisted. Intubation is indicated in patients who have an altered level of consciousness, a decreased gag reflex, or extremely poor air movement. After the airway and ventilation are managed, oxygen is administered. Because obstructive lung diseases cause hypoxia, oxygen is a critical aspect of management.

The initial dose of oxygen is 2 to 3 L/min by nasal cannula unless the patient is cyanotic, has cardiac arrhythmias, or is in respiratory arrest. The use of oxygen in the COPD patient is a topic of considerable controversy. The chronically high $PaCO_2$ in many patients with COPD causes the normal drive to breathe, based on $PaCO_2$, to be dulled. These patients instead rely on the PaO_2 to drive respiration. If given high-flow oxygen, some COPD patients may become lethargic, bradypneic, and, if not monitored, may become apneic. It is essential to understand that this syndrome only applies to selected patients. Most COPD patients and all asthmatics have no adverse reaction to oxygen therapy. Denial of adequate oxygen therapy in the hypoxic patient may lead to continued deterioration, myocardial infarction, and cerebral vascular accident. For these reasons, oxygen should be administered at a flow rate that prevents or resolves central cyanosis. If the patient develops lethargy or respiratory depression during this treatment, the airway must be managed and ventilation assisted or controlled. Never deprive a patient of oxygen for fear of depressing the respiratory drive.

After airway management and oxygen administration, the patient should be attached to the cardiac monitor and intravenous (IV) therapy started. Selection of IV fluid is largely based on the patient's hydration status. If signs of dehydration, such as poor skin turgor, dry mucous membranes, or hypotension are present, a volume expander such as normal saline or lactated Ringer's solution is appropriate via a large bore catheter. If signs of dehydration are not present, the fluid of choice is D_5W, administered at a keep open rate. This line is in place to facilitate medication administration.

Two classes of medications are available for administration. The first is the *sympathomimetic drugs*, so named because they mimic the sympathetic nervous system. Included in this group are epinephrine, terbutaline, and the inhaled sympathetic agents. The second group of drugs are the *methylxanthine preparations*. Both classes produce bronchodilation.

Sympathomimetic drugs stimulate the sympathetic nervous system. They are classified according to the type of receptor site they act on (see Chapter 12). Peripheral vasoconstriction is caused primarily by α agonists; β_1 agonists increase the heart's chronotropic and inotropic state; and β_2 agonists primarily cause bronchodilation as well as pulmonary vasodilation. Epinephrine is the most commonly used sympathomimetic drug; it stimulates all three types of sympathetic receptors. Use of epinephrine in the tachycardic patient, however, may result in hypertension with a significant increase in myocardial oxygen demand. For that reason, relatively selective β_2 agonists (e.g., terbutaline sulfate, albuterol, isoetharine, metaproterenol sulfate) that place less stress on the heart than epinephrine are the drugs of choice for patients with bronchospasm, particularly those who are elderly or who have a history of cardiac disease.

Epinephrine is the most commonly used parenteral sympathomimetic agent and may be given subcutaneously, intravenously, or endotracheally. Each route has advantages and disadvantages. The subcutaneous route (using a 1:1000 solution) is simple and has a fairly rapid onset. Subcutaneous epinephrine starts to work within 5 to 10 minutes and is gradually absorbed, causing few side effects. An additional advantage is its relatively short half-life (less than 30 minutes). Half-life refers to the time required for half of the drug to be metabolized by the body. Because it is metabolized so quickly, side effects caused by the drug subside rapidly. However, patients in extreme crisis do not absorb subcutaneous injections well because of peripheral shutdown; another route may be required. The adult subcutaneous dose is 0.1 to 0.5 mg.

The intravenous route for epinephrine (using a 1:10,000 solution) is fast acting and effective but can also be extremely cardiotoxic; high doses may cause ventricular arrhythmias and severe hypertension. Acute cerebral bleeds have also been caused by the severe increase in blood pressure. These side effects make this route of administration exceptionally risky. For this reason, intravenous epinephrine is usually not recommended for the management of obstructive lung disease in the field.

For the patient who requires intubation, endotracheal administration of epinephrine provides a rapid and effective means of delivery. Epinephrine is well absorbed across bronchial mucosa, and its direct action on bronchial smooth muscle makes endotracheal administration ideal when managing bronchospasm. A 1:10,000 solution should be used rather than the 1:1000 solution. The 1:10,000 solution is more dilute and allows for a higher volume to be used, causing less drug to adhere to the endotracheal tube and more to enter the bronchial tree. The dosage for adults is 0.3 to 0.5 mg, sprayed down the endotracheal tube. Holding the lungs inflated for several seconds after injection may enhance drug distribution to the terminal airways.

Terbutaline sulfate (Bricanyl, Brethine) is another sympathomimetic drug that can be used parenterally or by nebulization. Terbutaline sulfate is primarily a β_2 agonist. Because it does not have α effects, it tends to cause less of an increase in myocardial workload than epinephrine, a fact that makes it useful in patients who have a cardiac history. Side effects of terbutaline include anxiety and fine muscle tremors. Terbutaline sulfate is administered in a dose of 0.25 mg subcutaneously or, by aerosol from a metered dose inhaler with two inhalations separated by a 60-second interval.

Inhaled sympathomimetic agents provide an excellent therapy for acute bronchospasm in the prehospital setting. These agents are generally effective, safe, and easy to use. Application of bronchodilating drugs directly into the lungs allows a much lower dosage, thus minimizing side effects. In addition, bronchodilation with these agents is equal or superior to that achieved by subcutaneous therapy, except in cases of extreme respiratory distress when the patient is unable to cooperate with the treatment. Metaproterenol sulfate (Alupent, Metaprel) is one agent often used in the prehospital setting. The exact dose of bronchodilator varies with the drug used; the dosage of metaproterenol sulfate for nebulization is 2.5 mL of an 0.4% or 0.6% unit dose (10 or 15 mg of drug, respectively). Administration is via an oxygen-powered nebulizer, such as that shown in Figure 19-17. The oxygen flow rate usually is adjusted to 6 to 8 L/min to produce a

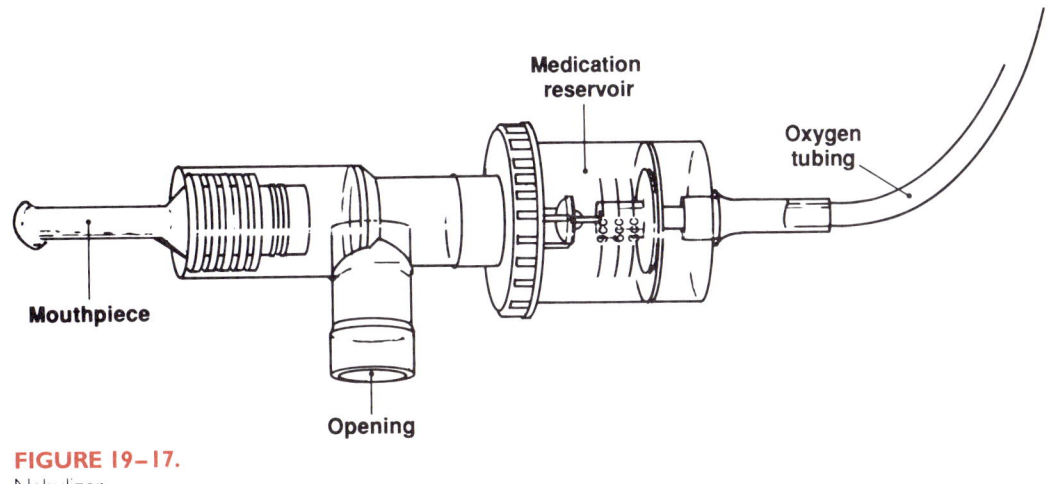

FIGURE 19-17.
Nebulizer.

> ### USE OF A NEBULIZER
>
> The proper use of a nebulizer depends on good technique. For patients older than 5 years of age, a mouthpiece is more effective than a mask. Use a mask for very young children. The process of administering the mist is as follows:
>
> 1. Explain process to the patient.
> 2. Have the patient exhale as much air as possible.
> 3. Place mouthpiece in patient's mouth (or mask over nose and mouth) and have patient slowly inhale.
> 4. After patient has maximally inhaled, remove the mouthpiece (or mask) and instruct patient to hold breath for 1 to 2 seconds, then slowly exhale.
> 5. Repeat process until mist is gone.

fine mist. Technique is paramount to the administration of inhaled medications. The paramedic should control the nebulizer and the inhalation of the drug. The optimal technique for use of nebulized drugs is described in the box, "Use of a Nebulizer." Therapy should be discontinued if the patient's heart rate increases more than 15 to 20 beats per minute or if cardiac arrhythmias appear.

Other common β agonists used via inhalation to produce bronchodilation are isoetharine (Bronkosol, Bronkometer) and albuterol (Proventil, Ventolin) (see Appendix E). Metaproterenol sulfate, isoetharine, and albuterol can be administered by **metered dose inhaler,** an alternative form of inhalation administration. Metered dose inhalers contain a canister of liquid medication that does not require dilution or mixing. The canister fits into a mouthpiece device; when squeezed, the inhaler delivers a measured amount of medication, called a metered dose. A spacing device acts as a holding area for medication and attaches to the mouthpiece portion of the canister. The medication is first squirted into one end of the spacing device. The medication is breathed in from the opposite end. Spacing devices come in many shapes and sizes, but they all work in the same manner. Using a spacing device with the metered dose inhaler ensures that the correct dose of medication is received and makes administration easier for the patient. Metered dose inhalers are frequently used by patients for self-administration but may also be used by the paramedic as a form of drug administration. Figure 19-18 shows the use of a metered dose inhaler.

Theophylline ethylenediamine (Aminophylline) is another drug that can be used to manage acute bronchospasm in the field, usually after the use of sympathomimetic agents. Theophylline ethylenediamine's effect is due to its action as a smooth muscle relaxant; relaxation of the smooth muscle that lines the bronchioles results in bronchodilation. Theophylline ethylenediamine also acts as a mild diuretic, providing a therapeutic advantage to the management of patients with mild congestive heart failure. Adverse cardiovascular actions include tachycardia, palpitations, and hypertension. Muscle tremors are another common side effect, as is anxiety. As the dose of the drug is increased, the patient often experiences nausea, vomiting, and headache. If the dose is increased still further, to a toxic level, grand mal seizures and ventricular tachycardia can occur. A significant disadvantage to the use of theophylline ethylenediamine is its long half-life, which in adults is several hours. However, the time required to eliminate half of the dose from the body is considerably shorter in smokers and children.

During the patient assessment, the paramedic should determine if the patient has taken any theophylline-containing compounds and record the amount and time of the last dose and the duration of therapy. Theophylline products include Marax, Primatene, Quibron, Slo-Phyllin, Slo-bid, Somophyllin, Tedral, and Theo-Dur. The loading dose of theophylline ethylenediamine is 6 mg/kg diluted in 100 mL of D_5W or normal saline and placed in a calibrated volume set (see Chapter 29, Fig. 29-9). This mixture is administered IV over a 20-minute period if the patient has not received theophylline products in the last 36 hours. A loading dose of 1 mg/kg diluted in 100 mL D_5W or normal saline is administered IV over a 20-minute period if the patient has taken theophylline products in the last 36 hours.

Because theophylline ethylenediamine is metabolized in the liver and is not distributed into fatty tissues, significant dosage alterations must be made for elderly patients or those who have liver disease or congestive heart failure, are cigarette smokers, or are significantly obese.

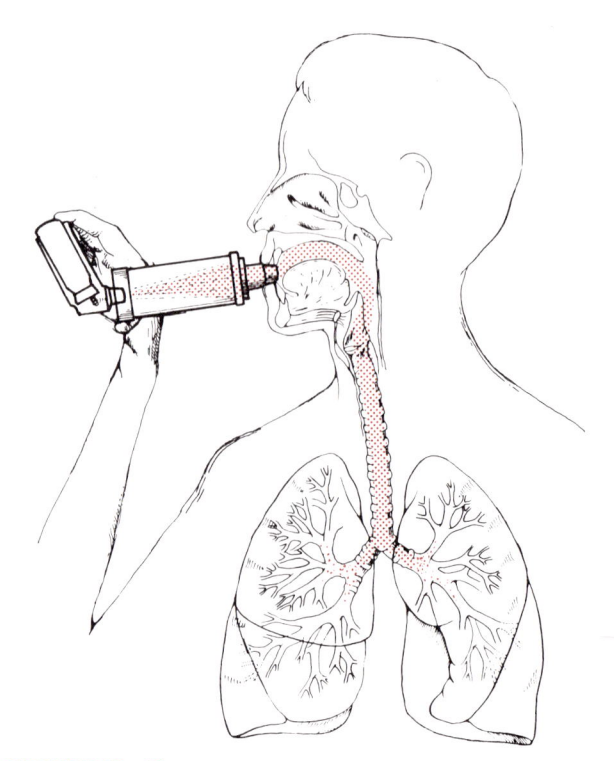

FIGURE 19-18.
Metered dose inhaler.

TABLE 19-2. BRONCHODILATORS

Drug	Class	Field Use	Dose
Albuterol	Sympathomimetic	Asthma Emphysema	Give 2.5 mg; dilute 0.5 mL of the 0.5% solution for inhalation with 2.5 mL of normal saline
Ephinephrine	Sympathomimetic	Bronchiolitis Asthma	1:1000 solution, give 0.1–0.5 mg subcutaneously or intramuscularly
Isoetharine	Sympathomimetic	Bronchospasm	1–2 inhalations with metered-dose inhaler
Metaproterenol sulfate	Sympathomimetic	Asthma COPD	2.5 mL of a 0.4% or 0.6% unit dose in nebulizer over a 10–15-minute period
Terbutaline sulfate	Sympathomimetic	Bronchospasm	2 inhalations separated by a 60-second interval with a metered dose inhaler
Theophylline ethylenediamine	Methylxanthine	Asthma Bronchospasm	Loading dose of 6 mg/kg IV infusion diluted in 100 mL D_5W or normal saline over a 20-minute period if patient has had no theophylline products in the last 36 hours
			Loading dose of 1 mg/kg IV infusion diluted in 100 mL D_5W or normal saline over a 20-minute period if patient has had theophylline products in the last 36 hours

These factors must be communicated to the base hospital when requesting a theophylline ethylenediamine order to ensure that the correct dose is selected. Whether a loading or maintenance dose is used, infusion should be slowed if the patient develops significant nausea and vomiting; these are symptoms that indicate moderate toxicity. If the drip is allowed to continue, seizures and ventricular arrhythmias may occur. The advent of nebulized bronchodilators such as metaproterenol for field use will lead to a decreased need for IV theophylline ethylenediamine. Nebulized sympathomimetic bronchodilators are the drugs of first choice in the treatment of bronchospasm in terms of both efficacy and safety. Table 19-2 summarizes the bronchodilators.

The evaluation of successful treatment after administering the bronchodilators should include a maximum peak flow of 150 L/min, clearer breath sounds, improved level of consciousness, improved skin color, and improved ability of the patient to converse. Pulse oximetry should reflect improved peripheral oxygen saturation in the initially desaturated patient. If these factors are not observed, administration of bronchodilators should be repeated.

Pneumonia

Pneumonia is a common disease entity found in prehospital emergency care. Despite its relative frequency, pneumonia remains a serious condition that is the fifth leading cause of death in the United States. It is most threatening in patients who are very young or very old.

PATHOPHYSIOLOGY. Pneumonia is an inflammation of the lungs. Although most frequently caused by bacterial organisms, pneumonia can also be caused by viral or fungal organisms, as well as aspiration or chemical exposure. Inflammation of the lungs causes edema of the alveoli and small airways, as well as changes in permeability of cell walls in the alveoli. These changes in membrane permeability allow *purulent exudate* (pus) and fluid to flow between the alveoli, enabling the infection to spread easily. The interstitial space may also be affected, thus inhibiting the diffusion of oxygen into the capillaries. Bronchiolar obstruction by mucus prevents adequate air exchange in the alveoli. If this poor air exchange is allowed to continue, the pulmonary capillaries remove all the air from the affected alveoli, causing them to collapse. Collapse of the alveoli, known as **atelectasis,** is a common result of pneumonia.

Another condition found with pneumonia is **pleuritis,** which is an inflammation of the pleura. Pleuritis is usually caused by the same organisms that caused the pneumonia. If the pneumonia is caused by a bacterial invasion, an overwhelming systemic infection, or sepsis, may also occur. Pneumonia is the most common cause of sepsis.

ASSESSMENT. A number of assessment findings, in addition to the classic signs of respiratory distress described earlier, are useful in the evaluation of the patient with pneumonia. The patient is frequently very old and often presents with a history of exposure to cold, cigarette smoking, or alcoholism. Cold exposure decreases the lung's ability to filter bacteria in the upper airway, while smoking diminishes the function of the cilia. Sputum production is frequently increased, especially in bacterial pneumonias. Sputum may be brown or rust in color, because of a combination of blood and purulent exudate (pus). Fever, with accompanying chills, is frequently present. Signs of dehydration are also present because of the fever. Chest pain due to pleuritis may be present. This pain is classically focal and increases with inspiration. If listened for, a pleural friction rub may be heard beneath the area of chest pain.

MANAGEMENT. Management of the patient with pneumonia is based on providing adequate oxygenation, hydration, and bronchodilation. Adequate oxygen must be administered to eliminate central cyanosis and to relieve subjective shortness of breath. Patients who present with fever and dehydration also require infusion of a volume expander, such as normal saline or lactated Ringer's solution, through a large bore catheter. In older patients with an accompanying history of congestive heart failure, care must be exercised to prevent fluid overload. Finally, the use of bronchodilators may be considered if bronchospasm is noted (see Table 19-2).

Besides the fundamental management modalities, the patient should be placed in a position of comfort, usually sitting upright. Cardiac monitoring is prudent. No efforts should be made to enhance mucus removal, such as postural drainage or clapping. These maneuvers increase bronchospasm and shortness of breath and are reserved until the patient's condition is stabilized. Care should be taken to avoid contamination of the emergency team members when caring for the patient who is coughing frequently. Masks should be worn by either the patient or the paramedic, or both, to prevent the spread of infection.

Smoke and Toxic Product Inhalation

A significant portion of the annual 8000 deaths from fires is due to problems associated with inhalation of smoke and toxic products of combustion rather than from burns. The rapid growth of synthetic products has produced a myriad of new, deadly products of combustion.

PATHOPHYSIOLOGY. The syndrome of smoke inhalation is actually made up of three separate entities. The first, and most insidious, is carbon monoxide poisoning. **Carbon monoxide** is an odorless, colorless gas that is produced by combustion. When it enters the tissues it causes depression of cellular function. The brain is especially sensitive to the effects of carbon monoxide. This effect is the result of hypoxia, which is due to carbon monoxide's strong affinity for hemoglobin; carbon monoxide is 200 times more attracted to hemoglobin than is oxygen. The effect of this affinity is the occupation of all available hemoglobin by carbon monoxide, making the hemoglobin unavailable to carry oxygen. This problem is further worsened by carbon monoxide's long half-life. In room air, 4 to 5 hours are required for one half of the carbon monoxide to be eliminated.

Pulmonary thermal injury is the second component of smoke inhalation. Actual burns to the lungs are rare, because of the upper airway's phenomenal ability to exchange heat. However, this heat exchange takes its toll on the upper airway, causing edema and airway obstruction. The risk of pulmonary burns increases in hot fires and with the release of steam, which carries heat 2000 times more efficiently than does dry air. Symptoms can occur as long as 18 hours after exposure to thermal inhalation.

The final component of smoke inhalation is smoke or toxic product poisoning. As is true of any poisoning, the response of the body to toxic products varies depending on the poison involved. This response is compounded further by the fact that substances release many different products of combustion depending on the heat, availability of oxygen, and speed of burning. As a result, management of smoke poisoning is frequently based on management of symptoms because of the unavailability of precise information about what product was inhaled.

Regardless of which of the above syndromes is present, the body demonstrates a consistent response. Immediate laryngospasm accompanies exposure to smoke unless the patient is unconscious; in the unconscious patient, this vital protective mechanism is lost. As the exposure continues, ciliary function is depressed, decreasing the lungs' ability to remove foreign substances. In cases of severe exposure, alveolar surfactant is damaged, causing atelectasis. Finally, in advanced stages, the cell walls are damaged, allowing fluid to flow into the alveoli and the tracheal wall to slough off; these changes result in pulmonary edema and hemoptysis.

ASSESSMENT. The history of the exposure is one of the most important assessment findings in the smoke inhalation patient. A history of loss of consciousness during exposure indicates a serious condition because of the loss of the laryngospastic response. Entrapment in a closed space indicates a heavy exposure to both heat and smoke. A history of release of steam during the fire increases the suspicion of airway burns. In addition, a history of previous cardiac or pulmonary disease, as well as cigarette smoking and alcoholism, help identify high-risk patients.

The initial examination also yields valuable information. The presence of smoking, burned clothing makes the degree of exposure obvious. Singed facial and nasal hairs and facial burns are suggestive of airway burns. Visible swelling and blistering of the pharynx confirms the presence of airway burns. Stridor indicates upper airway obstruction. Skin color may be cyanotic or red from carbon monoxide poisoning. The cherry-red skin color associated with carbon monoxide poisoning frequently is not clinically evident, and cyanosis may be present instead because of hypoxia.

The examination must also include a search for associated findings. Explosions and falls in fires create traumatic injuries. Medical problems, such as intoxication, overdose, and cardiac disease, are also found quite often. The examination must be thorough to identify such hidden diagnoses.

MANAGEMENT. Management of the smoke inhalation patient requires a high index of suspicion, based on the above findings. Specific steps include removal from the toxic environment, aggressive management of the airway, adequate ventilation, and oxygenation. Management begins with removal of the patient from the environment without endangering the paramedic. After removal, intubation should be performed in any patient with severe respiratory distress, visible edema of the pharynx, or significant facial burning. It is imperative to intubate early, as signs of respiratory distress often appear late, occurring immediately before total airway obstruction. If obstruction has already occurred and intubation is impossible, cricothyroidotomy should be considered. After the airway is established, meticulous airway care should be exercised, including suctioning and positive-pressure ventilation as required. High-flow oxygen is vital in managing the smoke inhalation victim. Administration of 100% oxygen decreases the half-life of carbon monoxide from 5 hours to 30 minutes.

Rapid transport to the appropriate facility and management of associated conditions are indicated. Burned clothing must be removed and burns dressed. Intravenous access must be established and volume replaced if shock or burns are present. Bronchodilators may also be appropriate if bronchospasm is present (see Table 19-2).

Pulmonary Embolism

Pulmonary embolism is a frequent and sometimes fatal condition that is rarely recognized in the field. Identification of this condition is based on a thorough history and careful assessment.

PATHOPHYSIOLOGY. A pulmonary embolus is a foreign body that lodges in the pulmonary capillary bed. The severity of symptoms and mortality depend on the location and size of the embolus; the more lung tissue distal to the embolus, the graver the condition. Massive pulmonary thromboembolism results in cardiovascular collapse or cardiorespiratory arrest. *Emboli* are most commonly blood clots that have migrated from the deep veins of the legs. However, emboli may also be clots released from pelvic fractures, fat emboli from long bone fractures, or amniotic fluid emboli in pregnant women.

Regardless of the origin of the embolus, when it lodges in the pulmonary arteries, the results are the same. Blood flow distal to the embolus ceases, causing constriction of the bronchioles supplied by that branch of the pulmonary artery. Hypoxia may occur because of the inability of blood in the affected artery to be oxygenated. In cases that involve large emboli, the embolus causes a backup of blood in the right side of the heart, resulting in right heart strain and classic signs of right-sided heart failure.

ASSESSMENT. One of the reasons why pulmonary emboli are rarely recognized in the field is the absence of a clear combination of signs and symptoms unique to the condition. The history provides one of the strongest factors to correctly identify the patient with a pulmonary embolus. Factors that are associated with the highest risk of developing pulmonary emboli include a recent period of immobilization, vascular disease, such as varicose veins or phlebitis, and recent surgery. Other risk factors include pregnancy, smoking, and cardiac disease.

Dyspnea is the most frequently reported sign in patients with pulmonary embolism. Chest pain may be present, most commonly pleuritic pain. Substernal chest pain indistinguishable from angina pectoris may also occur. The onset of signs and symptoms often is sudden. Patients may complain of anxiety, nausea, and vomiting. The most common sign of pulmonary embolism is tachypnea, with cyanosis and diaphoresis present in serious cases. Breath sounds are variable, and a pleural friction rub is common. The cardiac rhythm should be monitored, although it is valuable only to rule out other causes of the chest pain. These nonspecific findings place the emphasis on the history for correct assessment of pulmonary embolism.

MANAGEMENT. Correct management of pulmonary embolism is straightforward and does not depend on correct identification of the problem. Oxygen is administered at a rate that eliminates central cyanosis, and ventilation and airway control are exercised as appropriate to the patient's condition. Other supportive management is undertaken as indicated by patient presentation.

Central Nervous System Disorders

The central nervous system (CNS) plays a vital role in respiratory function. Disease or trauma to the CNS has predictable effects on pulmonary function.

PATHOPHYSIOLOGY. As discussed earlier in this chapter, the respiratory process depends on the movement of the diaphragm and, to a lesser extent, the accessory muscles. These muscles are in turn directed by the medulla, located in the brain stem. A number of conditions alter either the ability of the medulla to direct the respiratory process or the ability of the chest cage to respond. An overdose of CNS depressants, such as barbiturates, narcotics, and alcohol, impairs the medullary function, generally leading to a slowing of respiratory rate. Stimulants of the CNS, such as amphetamines and cocaine, cause the opposite effect, leading to tachypnea. Head trauma and cerebral vascular accidents frequently impair brain stem function, leading to alterations in ventilatory function.

Spinal injuries may also cause respiratory impairment. Injuries above the third cervical vertebra generally cause respiratory arrest. Injuries below C-3 but high in the thorax impair function of the intercostal muscles, causing the diaphragm to perform all of the work of breathing.

Neuromuscular diseases, such as myasthenia gravis, also have an effect on respiratory function. These diseases, which impair neurotransmission across the synapse, frequently result in diminished respiratory depth or respiratory arrest.

ASSESSMENT. History plays a major role in correct recognition of neurologic causes of respiratory insufficiency. A history of overdose or drug paraphernalia on-scene is suggestive. A history of rapid loss of consciousness without respiratory symptoms points to a neurologic etiology. A history of recent head or spine trauma may be related to presentation in patients with slowly developing neurologic lesions.

The neurologic examination is essential to identify the patient with CNS-induced respiratory compromise. The presence of new symptoms, such as facial droop, weakness in the extremities, or pupillary changes, should alert the paramedic to a neurologic cause. Visible trauma to the head or spine is an obvious sign.

Finally, the respiratory examination provides valuable information for the diagnosis of CNS-related pulmonary disorders. Deep breaths that move the abdomen but not the chest wall are known as diaphragmatic respirations; these are caused by cervical lesions below C-3. Patients who are not initiating respiratory efforts and who are easy to ventilate may have a CNS lesion. The absence of retractions and other signs of respiratory distress helps to confirm this assessment, as do clear breath sounds. That is, patients who are not ventilating well but demonstrate no typical signs of respiratory distress are frequently suffering from neurologic problems.

MANAGEMENT. Management of the patient with neurologically caused respiratory dysfunction focuses on providing adequate ventilation and managing the causative problem. Intubation is appropriate when airway control is required. Ventilation should be assisted or controlled, and additional oxygen should be provided. High-flow oxygen is rarely required since the lungs themselves are not diseased.

Hyperventilation Syndrome

Some people have what are commonly called "*anxiety attacks.*" During these episodes, they may hyperventilate (increase the rate or depth of breathing). This hyperventilation produces a number of physiologic effects that, when considered together, are known as **hyperventilation syndrome**.

PATHOPHYSIOLOGY. In the acute situation, hyperventilation produces a rapid decline in $PaCO_2$ and a rise in pH. These changes in the blood are responsible for the symptoms associated with hyperventilation syndrome. A rapid fall in $PaCO_2$ causes constriction of blood vessels in the brain. This decrease in blood flow to the brain frequently causes dizziness and, infrequently, may precipitate seizure activity. The alkalosis associated with hyperventilation syndrome causes a decrease in the serum ionized calcium level. This decrease, in turn, may cause spasms of the hands and feet, a condition known as **carpopedal spasm**.

ASSESSMENT. It is extremely important that the patient assessment differentiate between hyperventilation syndrome and other disease states that cause an increase in the rate or depth of ventilation. Often, a patient suddenly hyperventilates as a way to compensate for a metabolic acidosis (as in diabetic ketoacidosis) or hypoxemia (as in pulmonary embolism). To treat such patients for anxiety-induced hyperventilation would be disastrous. On the other hand, failure to treat anxiety-induced hyperventilation is unlikely to have any dire consequences.

A tentative diagnosis of hyperventilation syndrome can be made only after the possibility of more serious conditions has been eliminated. Patients who experience hyperventilation syndrome often complain of dizziness and fatigue. They appear nervous and may tell the paramedic that they cannot catch their breath. Some patients also complain of numbness or a tingling sensation (paresthesia) in their hands and feet and around their mouth.

When performing the physical examination, the paramedic should look for tachypnea, or an exaggerated depth of breathing. However, deep breathing may also indicate that the patient is suffering from diabetic ketoacidosis. Carpopedal spasm may be found on physical examination in hyperventilation syndrome, and in some cases seizure activity may be present.

MANAGEMENT. In the treatment of the patient who is experiencing hyperventilation syndrome, psychological management is preferred over medical management. A little hand holding and calm reassurance may be all that is required to handle these situations. Patients may not be aware that they are overbreathing, and they may be able to control their respiratory pattern with a little coaching from the paramedic. Encouraging patients to hold their breath for a few seconds at a time may be all that it takes to break the pattern of hyperventilation.

The traditional method of treating anxiety-induced hyperventilation is to have the patient breathe into a paper bag. While this technique allows the $PaCO_2$ to rise (and the pH to decline), its application can be dangerous if the paramedic has made an incorrect diagnosis.

SUMMARY

The respiratory system is a complex, efficient system that serves to provide fresh oxygen to the tissues while removing waste gases. The system can be divided into four subsystems that include the upper airway, lower airways, alveolar-capillary interface, and diaphragm and chest wall. Each subsystem has specific disorders that are important for the paramedic to be able to recognize.

Assessment of the patient with respiratory complaints begins when the primary survey is performed to recognize the immediate, life-threatening disorders. The secondary assessment is focused on patient history and the presence of signs of respiratory distress. These signs include cyanosis, alterations in level of consciousness, tachycardia, retractions or use of accessory muscles, and pulsus paradoxus.

Regardless of the etiology, management of respiratory complaints must be based on airway control, adequate oxygenation, and adequate ventilation. After these basic requirements are met, bronchodilation and management of associated conditions may be undertaken.

SUGGESTED READING

Cherniack RM: Drugs for the Respiratory System. Orlando, Grune & Stratton, 1986

Dismuke SE, Wagner EH: Pulmonary embolism as a cause of death: The changing mortality in hospitalized patients. JAMA 255:2039, 1986

Downie RL: Obstructive airway disease: Respiratory emergencies. Top Emerg Med 8:13, 1987

Eitel DR, Meador SA, Drawbaugh R et al: Prehospital administration of inhaled metaproterenol. Ann Emerg Med 19:1412, 1990

Hoellerich VL, Wigton RS: Diagnosing pulmonary embolism using clinical findings. Arch Intern Med 146:1699, 1986

Littenberg B, Gluck EH: A controlled trial of methylprednisolone in the emergency treatment of acute asthma. N Engl J Med 314:150, 1986

Ruple JA, Geronimo P: Inspiring Confidence in Oxygen Therapy. J Emerg Med Serv 15(11):24, 1990

Schneider SM: Effect of a treatment protocol on the efficiency of care of the adult acute asthmatic. Ann Emerg Med 15:703, 1986

US Department of Transportation, National Highway Traffic Safety Administration: Emergency Medical Technician—Paramedic: National Standards Curriculum. Washington, DC, US Government Printing Office, 1985

Wilkins RL, Hodgkin JE, Lopez B: Lung Sounds: A Practical Guide. St. Louis, CV Mosby, 1988

CHAPTER 20

Cardiovascular Emergencies

Anatomy and Physiology of the Cardiovascular System
  Systemic Circulation
  Pulmonary Circulation
  Anatomy of the Heart
  Physiology of the Heart
    Regulation of Cardiac Function
    Electrophysiology

Patient Assessment for Cardiac-related Problems
  Patient History
  Physical Examination

Cardiovascular Disease States: Recognition and Management
  Atherosclerosis
  Angina Pectoris
  Myocardial Infarction
  Heart Failure
    Left Ventricular Failure and Pulmonary Edema
    Right Ventricular Failure
  Cardiogenic Shock
  Cardiac Arrest and Sudden Death

Other Acquired and Congenital Diseases of the Cardiovascular System
  Valvular Heart Disease
  Pericardial Disorders
  Lung Disorders That Affect the Heart
  Blood Pressure Disorders
  Peripheral Vascular Disease

Prehospital Interventions for Specific Cardiac Conditions
  Oxygen
  Nitroglycerin
  Morphine Sulfate
  Nitrous Oxide
  Furosemide
  Theophylline Ethylenediamine
  Dopamine
  Epinephrine
  Sodium Bicarbonate

Arrhythmias: Interpretation and Therapeutic Intervention
  Basic Concepts of EKG Monitoring
  P Wave, QRS Complex, and T Wave
  Rhythm Strip Analysis
  Etiology and Mechanism of Arrhythmias
  Arrhythmias That Originate in the SA Node
    Sinus Bradycardia
    Sinus Tachycardia
    Sinus Arrhythmia
    Sinus Arrest
  Arrhythmias That Originate in the Atria
    Wandering Atrial Pacemaker
    Premature Atrial Complex
    Paroxysmal Supraventricular Tachycardia
    Atrial Flutter
    Atrial Fibrillation
  Arrhythmias That Originate in the AV Junction
    Junctional Escape Complexes and Rhythms
    Premature Junctional Complex
    Accelerated Junctional Rhythm
    Paroxysmal Junctional Tachycardia
  Arrhythmias That Originate in the Ventricles
    Ventricular Escape Complexes and Rhythms
    Accelerated Idioventricular Rhythm
    Premature Ventricular Complex
    Ventricular Tachycardia
    Ventricular Fibrillation
    Asystole

Arrhythmias That are Disorders of Conduction
  First Degree AV Block
  Second Degree AV Block
    Type I (Mobitz I or Wenckebach)
    Type II (Mobitz II)
  Third Degree AV Block
Artificial Pacemaker Rhythms
Prehospital Intervention: EKG Monitoring
Prehospital Intervention for Arrhythmias That Result From Increased Automaticity or Reentry
  Carotid Sinus Massage
  Valsalva's Maneuver
  Verapamil
  Lidocaine
  Bretylium Tosylate
  Precordial Thump
  Manual Defibrillation

Skill 20-1. Defibrillation and Synchronized Cardioversion
  Automated Defibrillation
  Emergency Synchronized Cardioversion

Prehospital Intervention for Arrhythmias That Result From Decreased Automaticity or Conduction Disturbances
  Atropine Sulfate
  Isoproterenol
  Noninvasive Cardiac Pacing

Summary

BEHAVIORAL OBJECTIVES

On successful completion of this chapter, the reader will be able to:

1. Describe the systemic and the pulmonary circulations
2. Label the anatomical structures of the heart
3. Describe the fundamentals of cardiac physiology
4. Describe the assessment of a patient for cardiac problems
5. Identify and describe the prehospital management of angina pectoris, myocardial infarction, left ventricular failure, right ventricular failure, cardiogenic shock, and cardiac arrest
6. Identify and state the prehospital management of valvular heart disease, pericardial disorders, cor pulmonale, hypertension, and peripheral vascular disorders
7. State the dosage and describe the prehospital use of oxygen, nitroglycerin, morphine sulfate, nitrous oxide, furosemide, theophylline ethylenediamine, dopamine, epinephrine, and sodium bicarbonate
8. Identify EKG waves and intervals
9. Evaluate EKG rate and rhythm
10. Explain the causes of arrhythmias
11. Identify and describe the management of the four arrhythmias that originate in the SA node
12. Identify and describe the management of the five arrhythmias that originate in the atria
13. Identify and describe the management of the four arrhythmias that originate at the AV junction
14. Identify and describe the management of the six arrhythmias that originate in the ventricles
15. Identify and describe the management of four variations of AV block
16. Describe the placement and function of artificial pacemakers
17. Given the proper equipment, demonstrate the procedure for manual defibrillation
18. Explain the prehospital management of arrhythmias that result from increased automaticity, reentry, decreased automaticity, and conduction disturbances
19. Define all of the key terms listed in this chapter

KEY TERMS

The following terms are defined in the chapter and glossary:

accelerated idioventricular rhythm
accelerated junctional rhythm
acetylcholine
acute arterial occlusion
adventitia
anastomoses
angina or angina pectoris
arrhythmias
arterioles
arteriosclerosis
artificial cardiac pacemaker
asystole
atherosclerosis
atherosclerotic heart disease
atria
atrial fibrillation
atrial flutter
atrioventricular (AV) blocks
atrioventricular (AV) node
atropine sulfate
automaticity
bretylium tosylate
bruit
bundle branches
bundle of His
capillaries
cardiac output
cardiac tamponade
cardiogenic shock
carotid sinus massage
chordae tendineae
congestive heart failure
conductivity
coronary artery disease
cor pulmonale
defibrillation
delta wave
depolarization
diastole
dissecting aortic aneurysm
dopamine
ectopy
electrocardiogram (EKG or ECG)
EKG monitoring
electromechanical dissociation
endocardium
epicardium
epinephrine
excitability
external or transcutaneous pacing
first degree AV block
furosemide
internodal and interatrial tracts
intima
isoproterenol
joules
junctional escape complexes and rhythms
lead II
left ventricular failure
lidocaine
media
mitral valve
Mobitz I
Mobitz II
modified chest lead 1 (MCL$_1$)
morphine sulfate
multifocal atrial tachycardia (MAT)
myocardial infarction
myocardial ischemia
myocardium
nitroglycerin
nitrous oxide
norepinephrine
oxygen
paroxysmal junctional tachycardia
paroxysmal nocturnal dyspnea
paroxysmal supraventricular tachycardia (PSVT or SVT)
pericarditis
pericardium
PR interval
precordial thump

(continued)

CHAPTER 20: Cardiovascular Emergencies

KEY TERMS (continued)

premature atrial complex (PAC)	*Q wave*	*sodium bicarbonate (NaHCO₃)*	*thrombophlebitis*	*ventricular escape complexes and rhythms*
premature junctional complex (PJC)	*right ventricular failure*	*ST segment*	*torsades de pointes*	*ventricular fibrillation*
premature ventricular complex (PVC)	*R wave*	*stroke volume*	*tricuspid valve*	*ventricular tachycardia*
pulmonary edema	*second degree AV block*	*syncope*	*type I second degree AV block*	*verapamil*
pulse deficit	*semilunar valves*	*S wave*	*type II second degree AV block*	*wandering atrial pacemaker*
pulsus paradoxus	*sinoatrial (SA) or sinus node*	*synchronized cardioversion*	*T wave*	*Wenckebach*
Purkinje system	*sinus arrest*	*systole*	*vagus nerve*	*Wolff—Parkinson—White syndrome*
P wave	*sinus arrhythmia*	*theophylline ethylenediamine*	*Valsalva's maneuver*	
QRS complex	*sinus bradycardia*	*third degree AV block*	*valvular heart disease*	
	sinus tachycardia		*ventricles*	

In the United States, nearly half of all deaths are due to cardiovascular disease. The majority of these deaths occur outside of the hospital setting, usually within an hour or two after the onset of symptoms. Often in the case of a cardiovascular emergency, the paramedic's actions make the difference between life and death.

The skilled paramedic must be prepared to make a rapid, accurate assessment of the patient during a cardiovascular emergency. The assessment often includes not only taking a history and a physical examination but also interpreting an electrocardiogram.

Prehospital intervention in cardiovascular emergencies requires that the paramedic be prepared to employ a vast array of knowledge and techniques. Drug therapy in these situations may range from the simple use of oxygen to the complex titration of vasopressors. The patient may be reasonably stable or in full cardiopulmonary arrest. Defibrillation or cardioversion may be required at a moment's notice.

This chapter includes cardiovascular anatomy and physiology, a thorough knowledge of which is necessary before the paramedic can correctly manage a cardiovascular emergency. The pathophysiology that underlies the more common cardiovascular diseases is discussed, along with the appropriate prehospital management. A great deal of the chapter is devoted to the identification and management (chemical and electrical) of arrhythmias.

ANATOMY AND PHYSIOLOGY OF THE CARDIOVASCULAR SYSTEM

Systemic Circulation

The systemic or peripheral circulation is comprised of a circuit of blood vessels that transport needed substances for cellular metabolism to body tissues and remove the waste products of metabolism from those same body tissues. With the exception of the interconnecting capillaries, the anatomy of all blood vessel walls is a similar three-layer design (Fig. 20-1). The **intima** is the smooth single-cell layer that lines the inside of all blood vessel walls. The middle layer of elastic fibers and muscle, the **media**, gives strength and recoil to blood vessels. Contraction or relaxation of this muscle layer serves to vary the diameter of the blood vessel lumen, the cavity within the vessel through which blood flows. Finally, the **adventitia**, a tough outer layer of fibrous tissue, protects the blood vessel. The systemic circulation is considered to have an arterial (*delivery*) side and a venous (*return*) side (Fig. 20-2).

Arteries, by definition, are blood vessels that carry blood away from the heart and, with the exception of the pulmonary artery, transport oxygenated blood. Arteries carry blood under high pressure and, therefore, are equipped with a much thicker medial layer than other

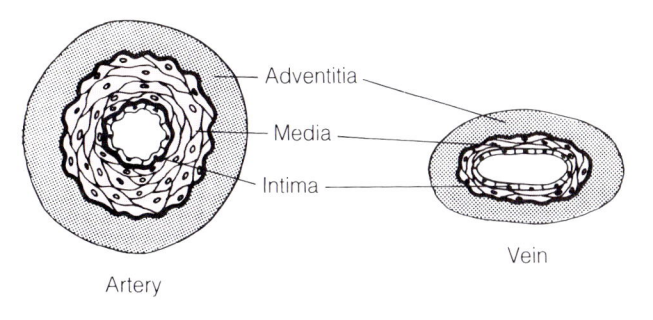

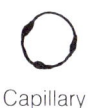

FIGURE 20-1.
Blood vessels in cross section.

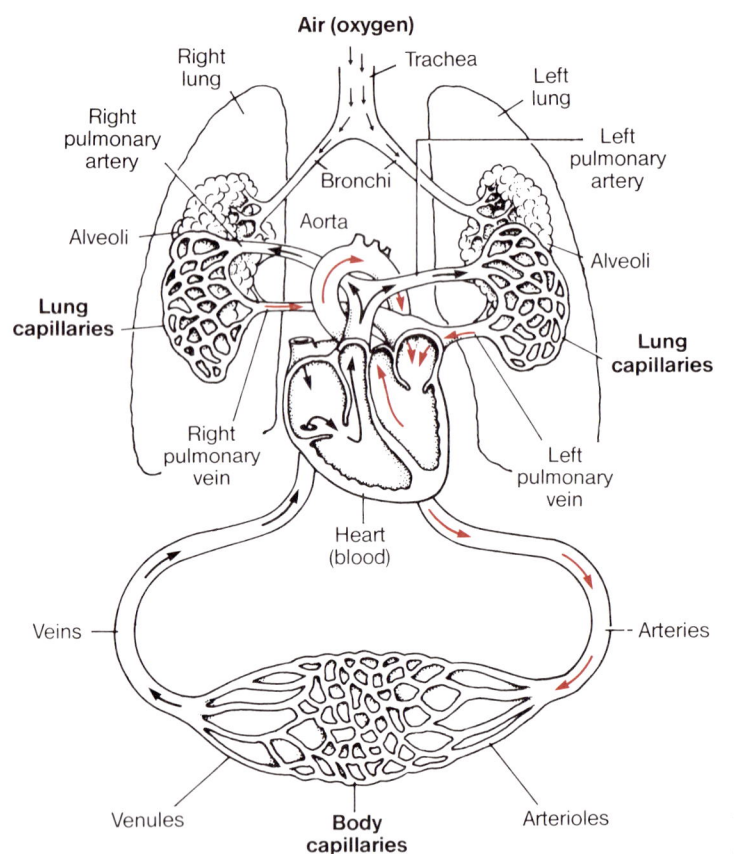

FIGURE 20-2.
Schematic drawing of systemic circulation. (Start at bottom of diagram.) Loaded with carbon dioxide, blood from the tissue capillaries goes through venules and veins into the right atrium and ventricle of the heart (black arrows), from which it is pumped into the lungs. Having excreted carbon dioxide and picked up oxygen, it flows into the left atrium and the left ventricle (color arrows). From there it is pumped through the aorta into the systemic circulation (arteries and arterioles) until it reaches the body capillaries, where it gives up oxygen and picks up carbon dioxide. (Brunner LS and Suddarth DS)

blood vessels. Major arteries of the body to recognize include the aorta, subclavian, internal and external carotids, axillary, brachial, radial, common iliac, and femoral arteries (Fig. 20-3).

Arterioles are the smallest branches of the arterial tree and have the capability to control blood flow to organs by their degree of constriction or dilation. The structures that are found at the termination of arterioles and that form a connection between the arterial and venous systems are the **capillaries** (Fig. 20-4). These are microscopic, intertwined vessels of single-cell thickness. While all other blood vessels are responsible merely for the transport of blood, the capillaries actually exchange nutrients, fluid, and gas with the cells. This process is facilitated by diffusion, osmosis, and the thinness and large surface area of the capillary walls.

Blood flow through the capillaries culminates in the venules, the first and smallest vessels on the venous side of the circulation. The convergence of venules creates veins, the vessels that carry blood back to the heart. With the exception of the pulmonary veins, veins carry blood that is low in oxygen and high in carbon dioxide content. Veins carry blood under much lower pressure than arteries. Movement of this low-pressure blood, often against gravity, is aided by the negative intrathoracic pressure created during the inspiratory phase of ventilation, the "*milking*" action of large muscles that surround veins, particularly in the legs, and a series of intermittent one-way valves in the veins to prevent back flow of blood between heart contractions. Major veins of the body include the superior and inferior vena cava, internal and external jugular, subclavian, axillary, innominate, iliac, and femoral veins (Fig. 20-5).

Pulmonary Circulation

Like the systemic circulation, the pulmonary circulation consists of a continuous circuit of blood vessels. In this circuit, blood flows out of the heart through the pulmonary artery, which branches off into pulmonary capillaries that surround the pulmonary alveoli (Fig. 20-6). Gas exchange occurs across the thin walls of the alveoli, allowing release of carbon dioxide from the blood and absorption of oxygen. The pulmonary capillaries then converge into pulmonary veins and return oxygenated blood back to the heart.

An important feature of the pulmonary circulation is its great capacity to regulate blood flow through the lungs. Pulmonary vessels are capable of directing blood flow to the best-ventilated areas of the lung, if the need arises. They are also capable of accommodating large fluctuations in blood flow without overburdening the heart.

CHAPTER 20: Cardiovascular Emergencies 409

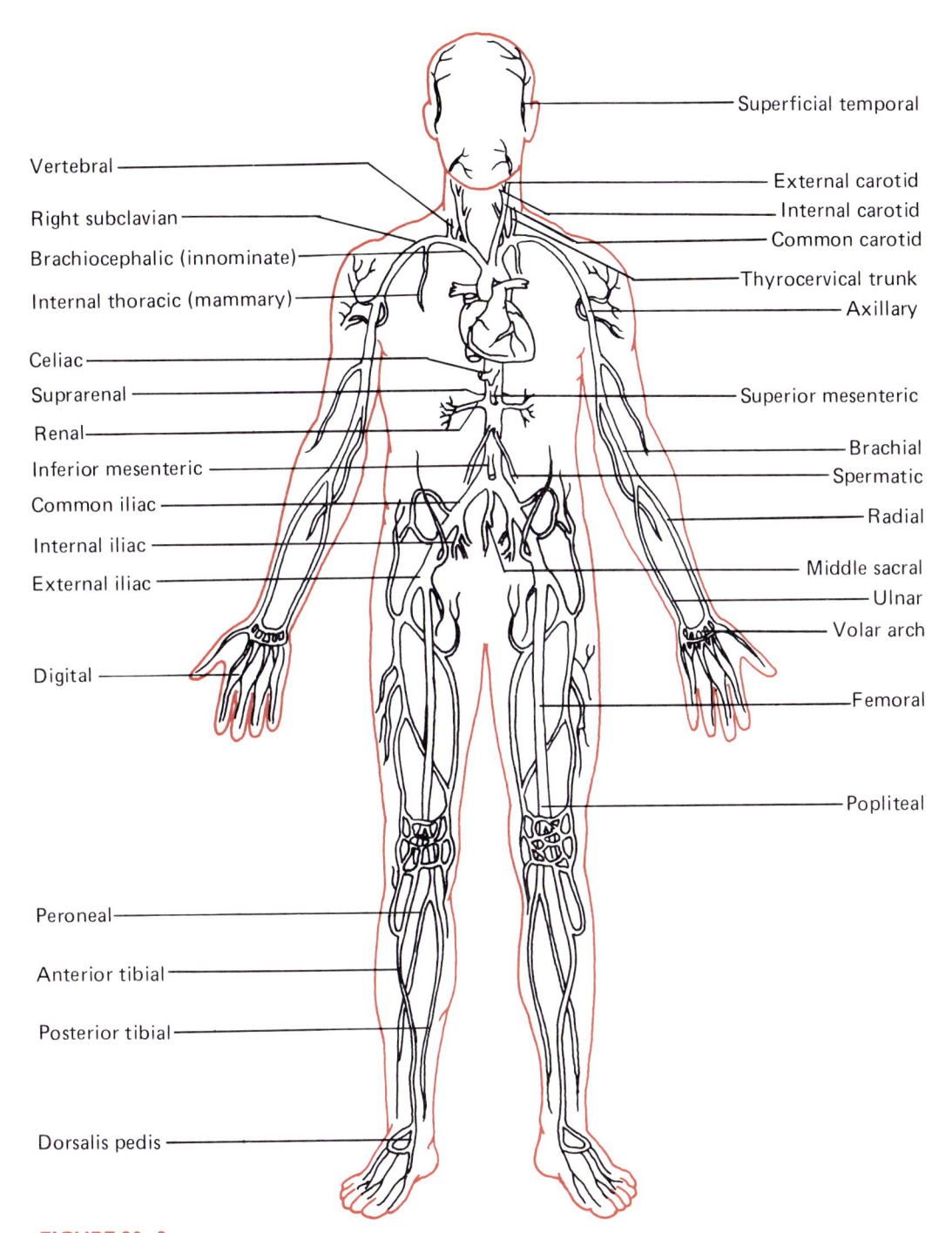

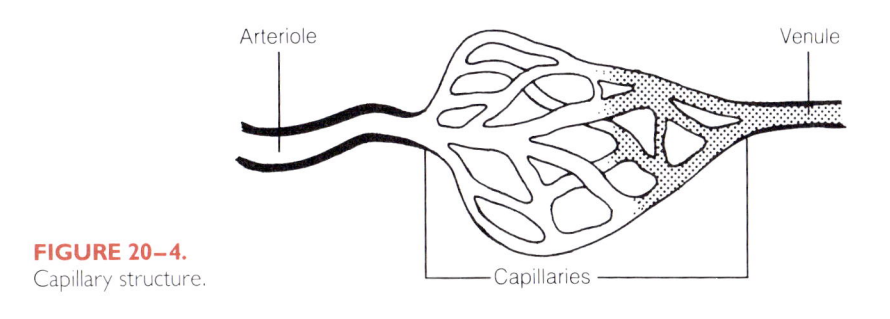

FIGURE 20–3.
Principal arteries that carry blood away from the heart. (Rosdahl CB)

FIGURE 20–4.
Capillary structure.

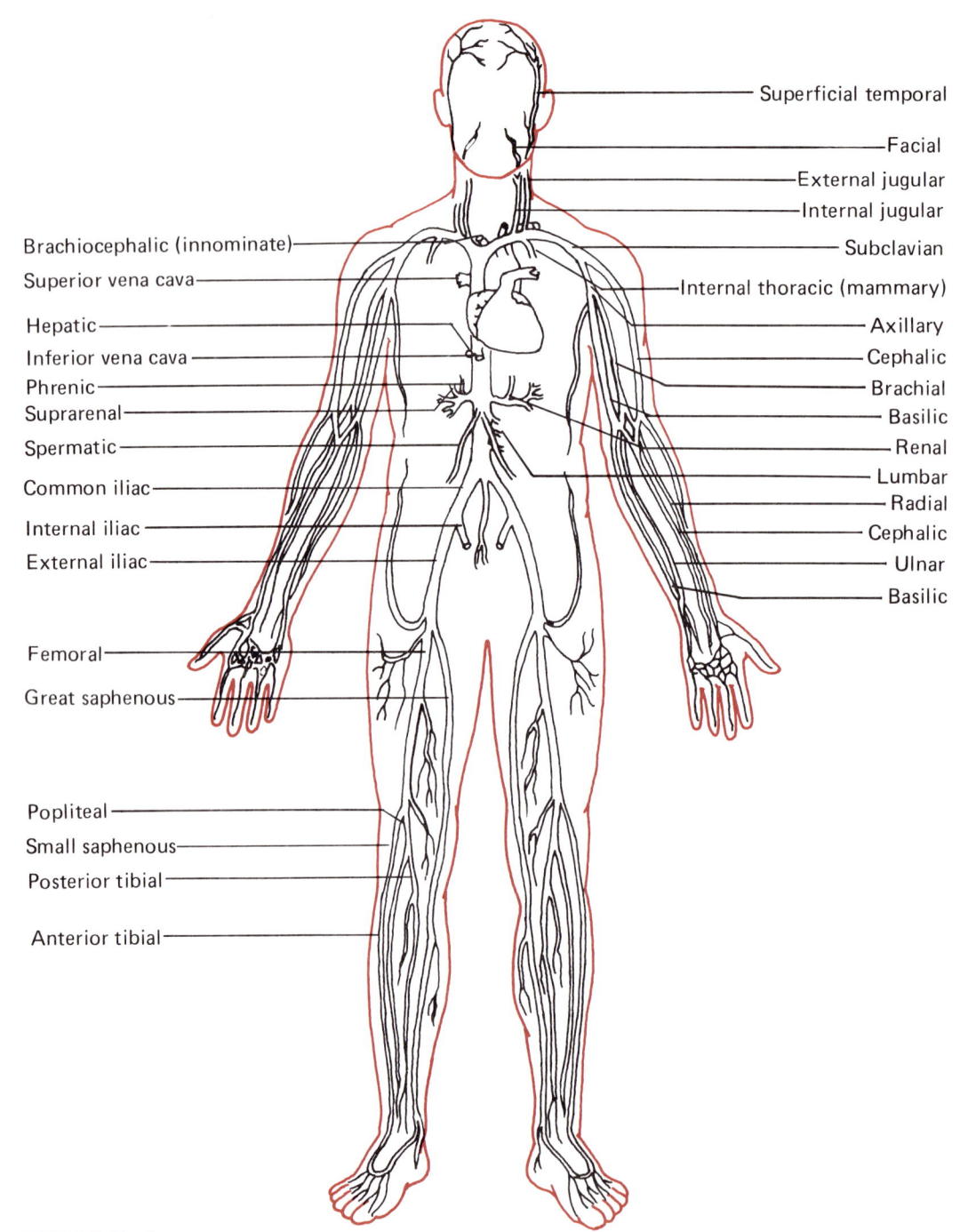

FIGURE 20–5.
Principal veins that carry blood toward the heart. (Rosdahl CB)

Anatomy of the Heart

The central structure of the cardiovascular system, the pump, is located in the mediastinum. The heart is protected in the thorax by the bony structures of the sternum anteriorly, the spinal column posteriorly, and the rib cage. This fist-sized muscular organ is conical in shape. The base of the cone is at the top of the heart, and the apex, the pointed part, is at the bottom. The heart lies in the chest rotated slightly counterclockwise, with the apex tipped anteriorly so that the back surface of the heart actually lies over the diaphragm. The pulmonary artery, the aorta, the superior and inferior vena cava, and the pulmonary veins are all large vessels that attach to the base of the heart and anchor it in the thoracic cavity. These vessels are often referred to collectively as the great vessels.

The heart, like the blood vessels, is composed of sev-

CHAPTER 20: Cardiovascular Emergencies 411

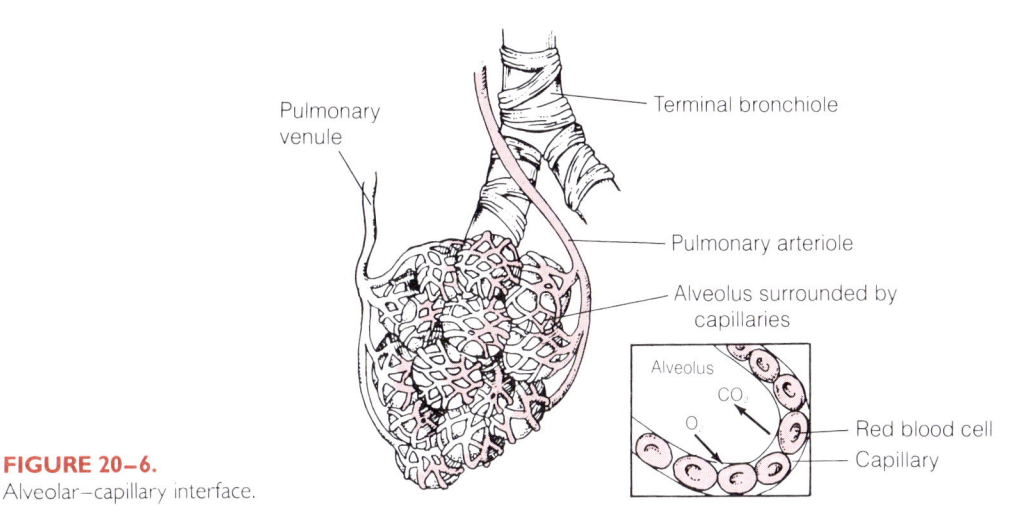

FIGURE 20–6.
Alveolar–capillary interface.

eral different layers of tissue. Surrounding the heart itself is a protective sac called the **pericardium.** This double-walled sac has an inner, serous (*visceral*) layer and an outer, fibrous (*parietal*) layer. Between these layers is found the pericardial space, which contains a small amount of pericardial fluid, a lubricant to prevent friction during heart contraction. The layers of the heart wall itself include the **epicardium** or outermost layer; the **myocardium,** the thick middle layer of cardiac muscle; and the **endocardium,** the smooth layer of connective tissue that lines the inside of the heart (Fig. 20-7).

Myocardial tissue is a special type of contractile tissue found only in the heart. Although it is similar in appearance to skeletal muscle, myocardial tissue has some structural and electrical properties that are unique. These properties are described more fully in the discussion of electrophysiology.

The heart is a hollow muscle with an internal skeleton of connective tissue that creates four separate chambers (Fig. 20-8). The superior chambers of the heart are the right and left **atria.** These chambers primarily collect blood as it enters the heart and help fill the lower chambers. The more thickly muscled lower chambers of the heart are called **ventricles.** These are the primary pumping chambers of the heart, the left having a thicker myocardial layer than the right. Vertical walls composed of connective and muscle tissue that separates the two atria and two ventricles are called the interatrial septum and the interventricular septum, respectively.

In addition, the atria and ventricles are separated from each other by two sets of valves composed of endocardial and connective tissue. These valves prevent back flow of blood during and after cardiac contraction. The first set, the atrioventricular (AV) valves, are located between each atrium and ventricle. The **tricuspid valve,** which is between the right atrium and ventricle, derives its name from its construction of three feathery cusps or leaflets. The left AV valve, which has only two cusps, is called

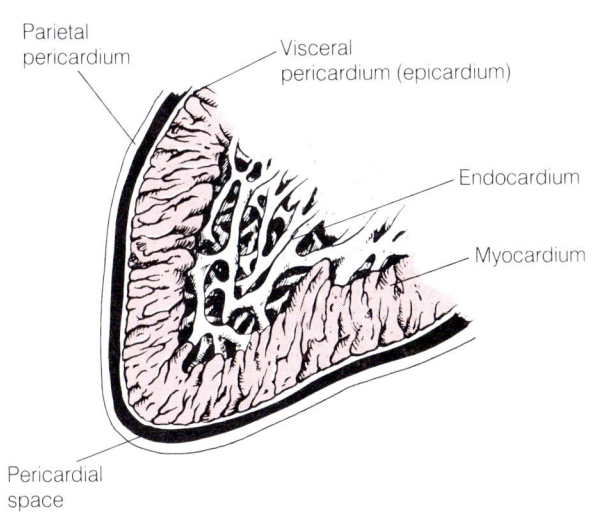

FIGURE 20–7.
A diagram of the layers of the heart wall that shows the components of the outer pericardium, muscle layer (myocardium), and inner lining (endocardium).

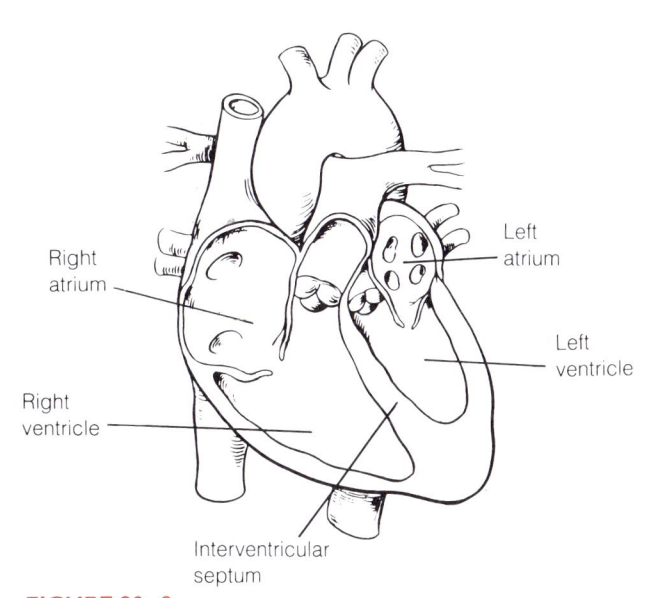

FIGURE 20–8.
Chambers of the heart.

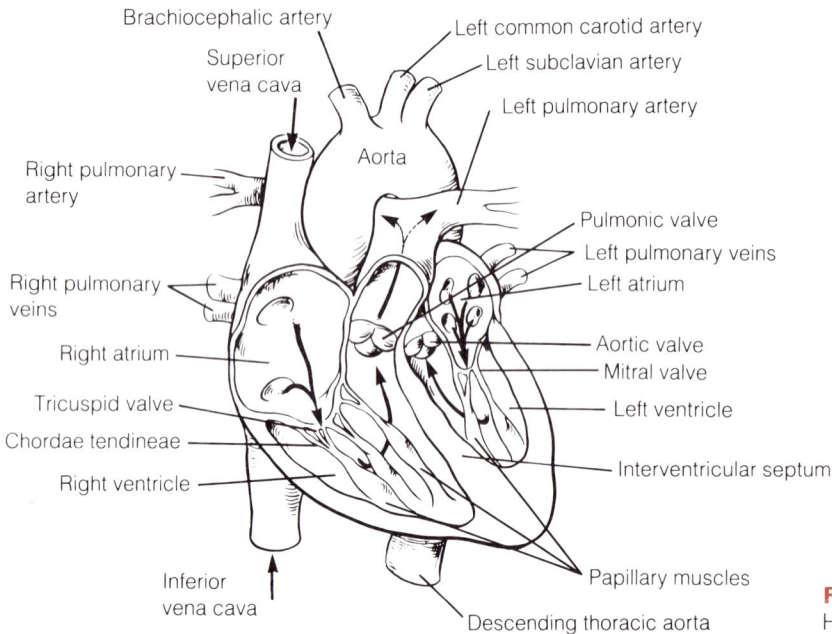

FIGURE 20-9.
Heart valves, great vessels, and normal blood flow.

the *mitral valve.* Both are connected by stringlike fibers called *chordae tendineae* to the papillary muscles at the apex of the ventricles (Fig. 20-9). The AV valves open to allow ventricular filling when the intra-atrial pressure exceeds the intraventricular pressure during atrial contraction. The onset of ventricular contraction creates pressure to close the AV valves. The papillary muscles and chordae tendineae prevent ballooning of the AV valve leaflets back into the atria at this time. The other set of valves, called *semilunar valves,* function by similar pressure changes and prevent the flow of blood back into the ventricles after contraction. The two semilunar valves are the pulmonic valve, located in the outflow tract from the right ventricle to the pulmonary artery, and the aortic valve, situated between the left ventricle and the aorta.

No discussion of heart anatomy is complete without addressing the coronary arteries and veins. These vessels provide the blood supply to the heart muscle and electrical conduction system. The coronary arteries, left and right, are the first to branch off the aorta, just above the

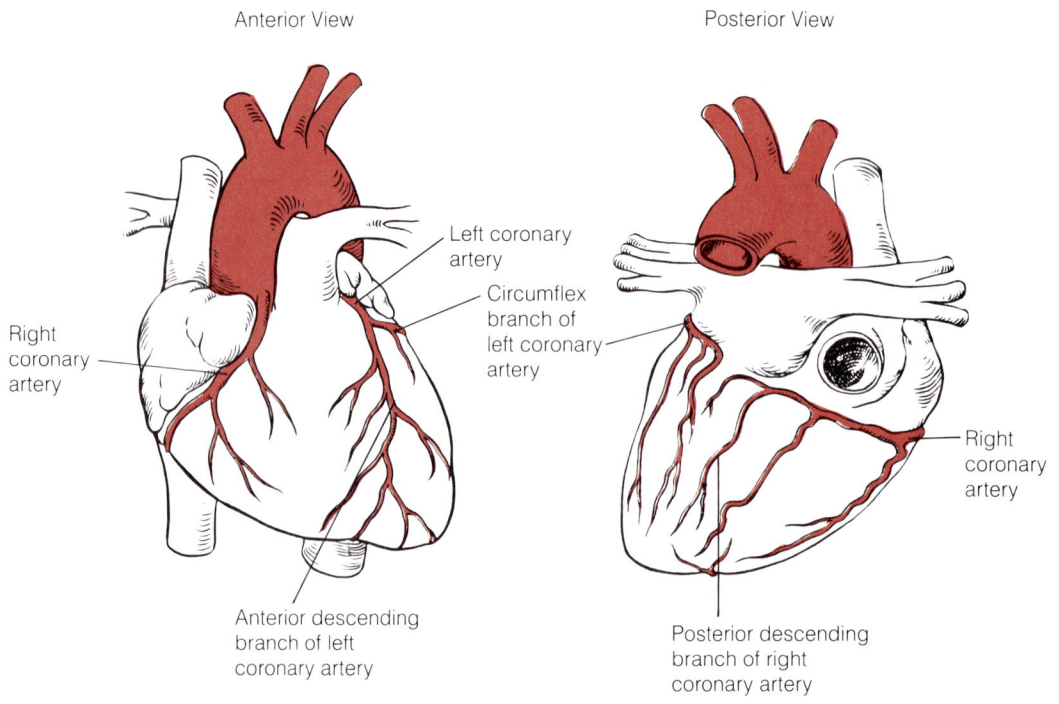

FIGURE 20-10.
Coronary arterial circulation.

leaflets of the aortic valve (Fig. 20-10). The left coronary artery has two major branches. The anterior descending branch runs along the anterior surface of the heart, while the circumflex branch courses in the groove between the left atrium and ventricle (left AV groove) to the posterior surface of the heart. These two branches supply arterial blood to the left ventricle, interventricular septum, and part of the right ventricle, in addition to certain electrical conduction structures in those areas. The right coronary artery arises from the aorta and courses along the right AV groove to the posterior surface of the heart. This artery supplies arterial flow to the right atrium, right ventricle, and part of the left ventricle, in addition to certain electrical conduction structures in those areas. The heart's arterial anatomy is such that the left ventricle has a dual blood supply, from both coronary arteries. Another protective feature is that many interconnections, or **anastomoses,** exist between the arterioles of the coronary arteries, allowing for development of collateral circulation, if needed. The coronary veins correspond in distribution to the arteries described above. They drain venous blood into the right atrium. The largest of these veins, the coronary sinus, provides venous drainage of the left ventricle.

Physiology of the Heart

Normal blood flow through the heart begins at the right atrium, which receives systemic venous blood from the superior and inferior venae cavae (see Fig. 20-9). Blood passes from the right atrium, across the tricuspid valve, to the right ventricle. It is then pumped across the pulmonary valve into the pulmonary artery. Outside the heart, the two branches (left and right) of the pulmonary artery distribute blood to the lungs for gas exchange in the pulmonary capillaries. Oxygenated blood returns to the heart's left atrium via four pulmonary veins. After passing across the mitral valve, blood enters the left ventricle, where it is pumped across the aortic valve and then enters the coronary arteries and the peripheral circulation via the aorta.

The complete cycle of mechanical pumping of blood through the heart and pulmonary circulation is referred to as the cardiac cycle (Fig. 20-11). In this cycle, right and left atria contract just before the beginning of right and left ventricular contraction. Much of the flow of blood from atria to ventricles occurs by gravity, but atrial contraction is necessary to fill the ventricles to maximum. The simultaneous contraction of the right and left ventricles while the atria relax creates pressure to close the AV valves, open the aortic and pulmonary valves, and propel blood into the pulmonary and systemic circulation.

The contraction phase of the cardiac cycle is called **systole** (a term generally used to refer to ventricular contraction vs. atrial contraction). **Diastole** is the relaxation phase of the cardiac cycle, when the ventricles are filling. This phase lasts much longer than systole (0.52 second

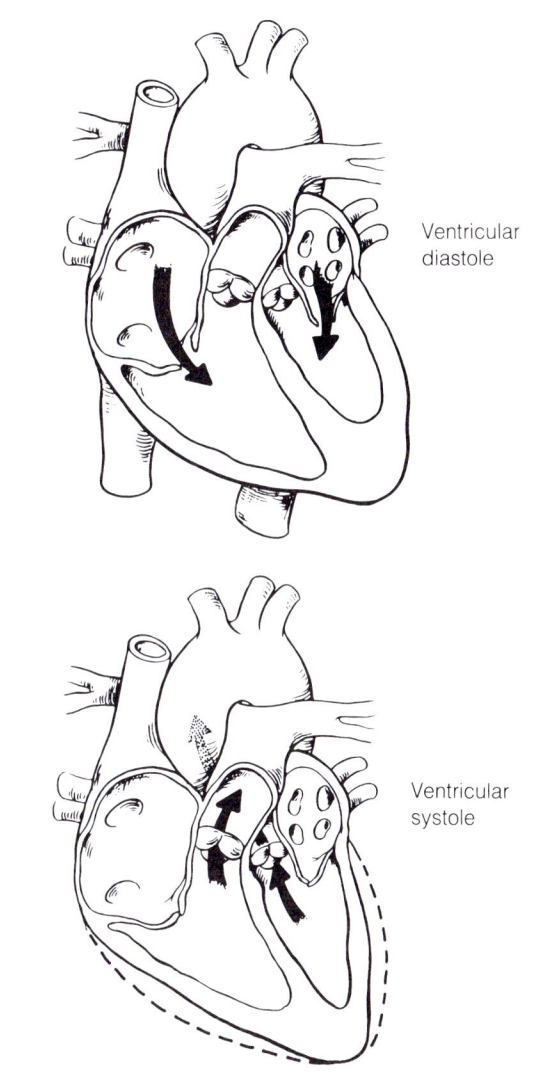

FIGURE 20–11.
The mechanical cardiac cycle.

vs. 0.28 second at a heart rate of 75 beats per minute). Increases in heart rate more significantly reduce the length of diastole than of systole. The duration of the diastolic phase is important, as this is when about 70% of coronary artery flow occurs and complete filling of the ventricles takes place.

In addition to the relationship of the atria to the ventricles in the cardiac cycle, the pumping action of the heart should also be understood from the standpoint of a right and left pump. The right pump, the right atrium and ventricle, normally has low pressure because it works only against the resistance of the pulmonary vascular bed. The left atrium and ventricle, however, form a hardworking, high-pressure pump to move blood against systemic resistance. This difference in function accounts for the anatomical feature of a left ventricular wall that is three times thicker than the right.

The amount of blood that is ejected from either ventricle with a single contraction is called the **stroke volume.** This volume is about 60 to 100 mL, although a healthy adult heart has a great capability to increase this amount.

Stroke volume is determined and affected by three factors: preload, afterload, and cardiac contractility. Preload can be thought of as the pressure with which the ventricle fills. This pressure is influenced by the amount of venous blood return. A feature of myocardial muscle is that the more it is stretched (up to a limit), the greater its force of contraction. Therefore, stroke volume can be increased considerably by increasing the blood volume that fills the ventricles and, thus, increasing the amount of myocardial muscle fiber stretch. This concept is known as Starling's law of the heart. Afterload, or the resistance against which the ventricles contract, also influences stroke volume. Afterload is determined by systemic arterial resistance. Cardiac contractility is the third major determinant of stroke volume. It is the intrinsic state of the heart muscle's force of contraction, also called the heart's contractile (or inotropic) state.

Stroke volume (S.V.) and heart rate (H.R.) determine the heart's **cardiac output** (C.O.), the amount of blood pumped through the circulatory system per minute (S.V. x H.R. = C.O.). As discussed, the capability to increase stroke volume alone can improve the cardiac output. However, heart rate also has great impact. Rate increases in the healthy heart can improve the cardiac output up to threefold. Cardiac output, along with systemic vascular resistance, are the determinants of systemic blood pressure.

Regulation of Cardiac Function

Mechanical and electrical activity of the heart are controlled by the autonomic nervous system. The heart is innervated by fibers of both the sympathetic and parasympathetic systems. These influence cardiac rate, conductivity, and contractility (Fig. 20-12).

Parasympathetic innervation via the large **vagus nerve** is primarily to the atria, although some vagal fibers are also in the ventricles. When the parasympathetic chemical mediator, **acetylcholine,** is released, heart rate and conduction are slowed. The parasympathetic system can be stimulated through carotid sinus pressure and Valsalva's maneuver.

Sympathetic nerve fibers, which arise in the thoracic and lumbar ganglia, innervate both atria and ventricles. The sympathetic chemical mediator, **norepinephrine,** acts on both α- and β-adrenergic receptor sites in the cardiovascular system. Stimulation of α receptors, while having no direct effect on the heart, causes peripheral vasoconstriction. Effects of β stimulation include increased heart rate, enhanced conduction and contractility, and peripheral vasodilation.

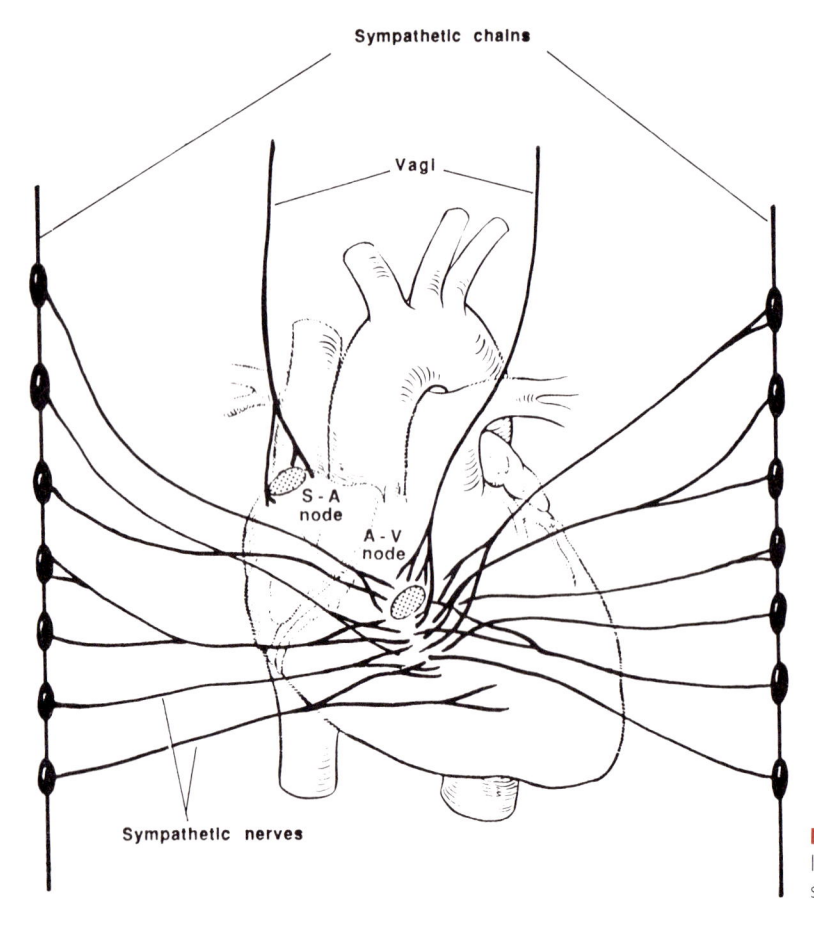

FIGURE 20-12.
Innervation of the heart by sympathetic and parasympathetic nerves.

The heart's mechanical and electrical functions are also influenced by proper electrolyte balance. The major electrolytes involved in cardiac function—sodium, calcium, and potassium—are addressed in the next section.

Electrophysiology

An understanding of the normal anatomy and physiology of the electrical conduction of the heart is the basis for learning arrhythmia interpretation and management. Myocardial fibers possess highly specialized electrical properties in addition to the mechanical property of contractility. **Automaticity,** the ability to generate an electrical impulse independent of stimulation by the nervous system or any other source, is the property of a certain number of special cardiac cells called pacemaker cells. Two other electrical properties, excitability and conductivity, are possessed by all myocardial cells. **Excitability** is the ability of cells to respond to electrical stimulation. **Conductivity** is the ability to pass or propagate an electrical impulse from cell to cell through the heart. These three properties are constantly involved in the electrical conduction system of the heart.

The heart's electrical conduction system is a network of structures that allows electrical impulses to spread through the heart with much greater speed than if they had to spread through muscle cells alone. The structures of the conduction system, in sequence of normal electrical conduction, are the following (Fig. 20-13):

Sinoatrial (SA) or sinus node: This grouping of specialized cells, located in the right atrium near the entrance of the superior vena cava, is normally the dominant pacemaker of the heart.

Internodal and interatrial tracts: Although some controversy exists, these tracts are thought to consist of a number of pathways that route electrical impulses between the SA node and the AV node and that spread them across the atrial muscle.

Atrioventricular (AV) node: This node is part of an area called AV junctional tissue, which includes some surrounding tissue plus the connected bundle of His. Although AV junctional tissue contains pacemaker cells, none are thought to exist in the AV node itself. The AV node slows conduction, creating a slight delay before electrical impulses are carried to the ventricles.

Bundle of His (common bundle or AV bundle): Located at the top of the interventricular septum, this bundle of fibers extends directly from the AV node and connects the atria and ventricles electrically.

Bundle branches: The bundle of His splits into two conduction paths called the right and left bundle branches. The left branch bifurcates again to create two fascicles. These bundles carry electrical impulses at high speed to the tissue of the interventricular septum and to each ventricle simultaneously.

Purkinje system: The bundle branches terminate with this network of fibers. They spread electrical impulses rapidly throughout the ventricular walls.

The creation of electrical impulses and the spread of impulses through the electrical conduction system occur through a process called **depolarization.** During depolarization, the electrical charge of a cell is altered by the shifting of electrolyte concentrations on either side of the cell membrane. This change in electrical charge stimulates the muscle fiber to contract. Depolarization involves alteration of the precise concentration of electrolytes maintained inside and outside the cell by chemical pumps in the cell walls. A resting, or "polarized," cell is normally more electrically negative on the inside of the cell wall than on the outside (Fig. 20-14). Electrical stimulation, however, changes the permeability of the cell wall and allows movement of positively charged ions, particularly sodium (Na^+), into the cell. The rush of sodium, along with the slower influx of calcium (Ca^{++}), causes the inside of the cell to change from negative to positive. The cell is then said to be depolarized. The response of the

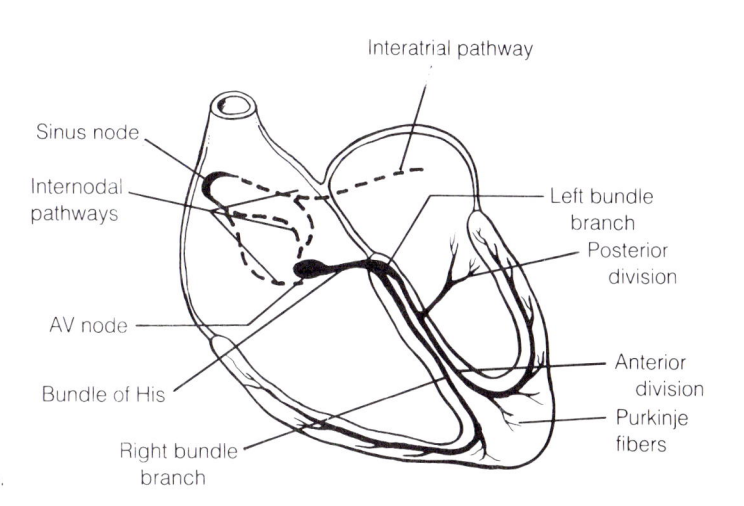

FIGURE 20-13.
Structures of the electrical conduction system.

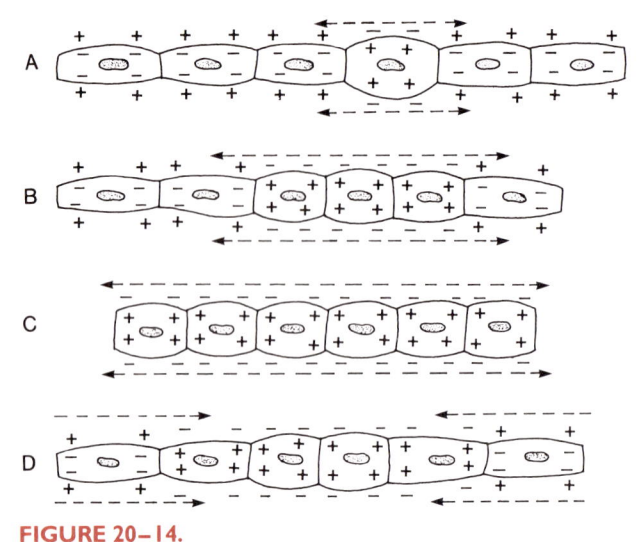

FIGURE 20-14.
The depolarization process. A single cell has depolarized (**A**). A wave propagates from cell to cell (**B**) until all are depolarized (**C**). Repolarization then restores each cell's normal polarity (**D**).

muscle to this electrical change is contraction. Because of the property of conductivity, this process of depolarization moves rapidly from cell to cell in the conduction pathway and throughout the muscle cells of the heart (Fig. 20-15).

Some myocardial cells do not have to wait to be reached by a spreading depolarization wave but are capable of self-initiating depolarization. These special cells, called *pacemaker cells*, possess the property of automaticity and are found throughout the conduction system with the exception of the AV node itself. Pacemaker cells are not inactive during diastole as are nonpacemaker cells, but they spontaneously become less and less negative until a certain threshold is reached, allowing them to depolarize. Depending on their location in the heart, pacemaker cells have different rates of spontaneous discharge, which is referred to as their *inherent* or *intrinsic* rate. The SA node has an intrinsic rate of 60 to 100 per minute, compared to an AV junctional tissue rate of 40 to 60 per minute, and a ventricular intrinsic rate of 20 to 40 per minute. Each of these areas has the capability to act as the pacemaker of the heart. However, the SA node is the usual pacemaker because it has the fastest rate of discharge and, therefore, is able to suppress all slower pacemaker sites.

After depolarization, myocardial cells must return to their resting state of internal negativity for further depolarization to occur. The proper distribution of electrolytes is reestablished by the cell wall chemical pumps, which pump sodium (Na^+) out of the cell and return potassium (K^+) into the cell. This process of reestablishing the internal negative charge of the cell is called repolarization. Depolarization and repolarization can be seen on an ***electrocardiogram (EKG or ECG).*** For purposes of this text, the term EKG wil be used. It is important to keep in mind that the EKG gives information only about electrical activity; it tells us nothing about how well the heart is working mechanically. The last part of this chapter fully discusses the interpretation of normal EKGs and a variety of EKG rhythm disturbances.

Regulation of the heart's electrical activity, like mechanical activity, is influenced by the autonomic nervous system. Sympathetic stimulation of α-adrenergic receptor sites has no effect on cardiac electrical activity, but β stimulation increases automaticity, conduction velocity, and excitability in both the atria and ventricles. Parasympathetic (or vagal) stimulation causes slower firing of the SA node and decreased AV conduction, with probably no major effect on the ventricles.

PATIENT ASSESSMENT FOR CARDIAC-RELATED PROBLEMS

The process of identifying and managing a patient's cardiovascular problems begins with the paramedic's ability to recognize cardiac-related symptoms, obtain a patient history, and perform an appropriate physical examination. The prehospital diagnosis of cardiac problems is

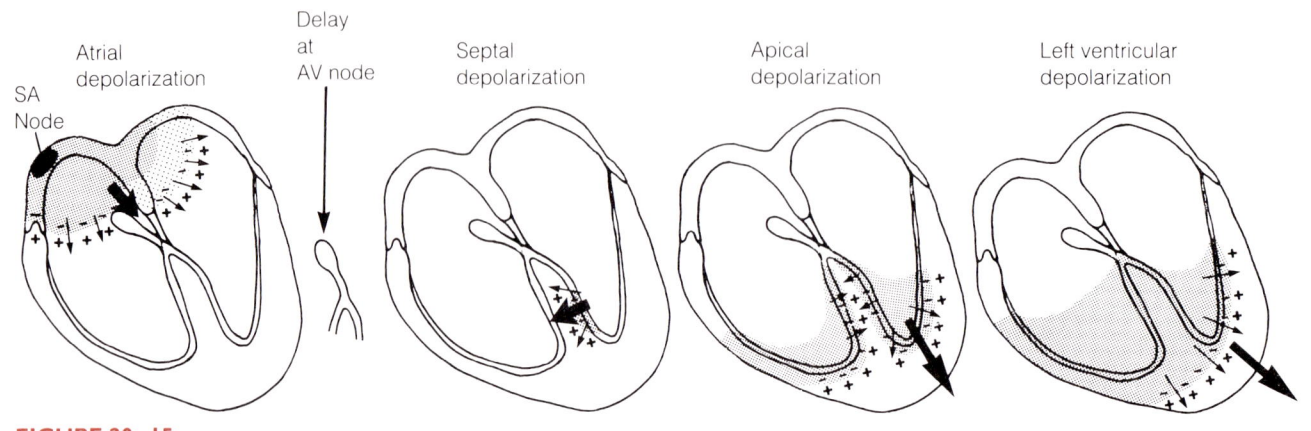

FIGURE 20-15.
Progression of depolarization through the heart.

based primarily on patient history, including the patient's chief complaint and history of the present illness. A medical history may help create a high index of suspicion for cardiac problems and may help modify the therapeutic intervention for a given patient. A physical examination, although less helpful in diagnosing cardiac problems, provides needed information about the current status of the cardiovascular system.

Patient History

A patient history is the first necessary step to assess the patient's problem and formulate a management approach. The patient's chief complaint, that is, what caused the call for assistance, should be determined immediately in the interview. The chief complaint is the patient's perceived physical and mental changes, and it should be reported and documented in the patient's own words. The most common cardiac-related chief complaints include the following:

- Chest or epigastric pain, discomfort, or pressure
- Shoulder, arm, jaw, or neck pain or discomfort
- Difficulty breathing or shortness of breath
- Fainting
- Abnormal heartbeat or palpitations

Chest or epigastric pain is the most common symptom of myocardial infarction. Obtaining a history of the present illness is important because there are many causes of chest pain other than cardiac. The paramedic should try to find out primary location of the chest pain, radiation of the pain, duration, quality or character of the pain, factors that precipitated the pain, measures that relieve or increase the pain (including medications), other associated symptoms, and any history of similar episodes.

Pain or discomfort in the area of the shoulders, arms, neck, or jaw commonly occurs in myocardial infarction in conjunction with chest pain. However, this type of pain occasionally occurs without any chest pain at all and may be the patient's sole chief complaint. Significant history to obtain includes the same factors listed above for chest pain.

Dyspnea, although a common associated symptom of myocardial infarction, may also be the primary symptom of pulmonary congestion due to acute heart failure. It is a subjective symptom, making its severity difficult to judge. The history of the present illness to obtain in dyspnea includes duration, circumstances of onset, anything that aggravates or alleviates it (including medications), associated symptoms, previous similar episodes, and history of cardiac problems. Like chest pain, dyspnea may have many noncardiac causes. Therefore, it is necessary to inquire about any recent history of cold, infections, fever, or history of chronic obstructive pulmonary disease (COPD) or other lung disease.

The chief complaint of fainting, called **syncope,** may be the sole symptom of a cardiac problem, especially in elderly patients. *Cardiac syncope* is caused by a decrease in cardiac output and cerebral perfusion that may be either transient or prolonged. This decrease may occur because of sudden pump damage or because of abnormal heart rhythms. The paramedic should try to determine the following information to help differentiate cardiac syncope from other possible causes: circumstances of occurrence (including the patient's presyncopal position), symptoms before syncope, duration of loss of consciousness, other associated symptoms, and previous similar episodes.

A patient's perception of an abnormal heartbeat may prompt the chief complaint of palpitations, irregular heartbeat, fluttering, or skipping beats. These complaints are usually related to irregularities in heart rhythm or rapid heart rates. Pertinent history of the present illness includes: circumstances of occurrence, duration of symptoms, associated symptoms (especially dizziness, lightheadedness, or chest pain), and previous similar episodes.

The medical history of a cardiac patient usually does not greatly alter prehospital management of that patient. Management is based on the current symptoms regardless of the history. However, a medical history may contribute to better definition of the patient's problem and create a higher index of suspicion for cardiac etiology of some of the chief complaints. Time should not be consumed obtaining family, personal, and social history since these will be investigated fully in-hospital. Instead, a quick determination should be made of the following medical history:

Is the patient currently being treated for any serious medical illness?
Does the patient have any chronic serious illness or ever been known to have had heart attack or angina, heart failure, hypertension, diabetes, stroke, or chronic lung disease?
Is the patient taking any prescription medications, particularly cardiac medications, such as nitroglycerin, digitalis, propranolol, or other β-blocking drugs, diuretics, antihypertensives, or other "heart medications"?
Does the patient have any allergies?

Physical Examination

The next step in patient assessment is the physical examination, conducted to collect objective data about the patient's complaints to correlate with the history. A complete head-to-toe secondary examination, such as would be done in a trauma patient, usually is not indicated in the assessment of cardiac patients. Rather, the physical examination should be directed toward specific organ systems and guided by the patient's complaints and symptoms.

Once the primary survey has been accomplished, vital signs should be measured, and a mini-neurologic examination should be performed. This examination includes evaluation of systolic and diastolic blood pressure, respiratory rate, pulse rate and regularity (which may provide the first indication of arrhythmias), and determination of the patient's general level of consciousness. Alterations in level of consciousness may indicate decreased cerebral perfusion due to poor cardiac output and must be assessed in light of what is the normal mental status for individual patients.

The secondary survey, like any, is performed by looking, listening, and feeling for abnormalities, but with specific attention to the cardiovascular and respiratory systems. In addition to the general observations made by looking at the patient and the surroundings, several specifics areas should be examined closely:

Look at skin color and check for adequate capillary refill. These observations indicate red blood cell oxygenation and the adequacy of pump action.

Look at the jugular veins for distention, which indicates back pressure in the systemic venous circulation due to acute or chronic pump failure. Examination for jugular venous distention should be done with the patient's head elevated approximately 45°. This condition may be difficult to assess in obese patients.

Look for peripheral edema caused by chronic congestion in the systemic venous circulation. This edema may range from mild to pitting. Pitting edema is that which leaves a prolonged indentation of the tissue when finger pressure is applied. Edema is most obvious in the patient's dependent parts. These are legs and feet in ambulatory patients and the sacral area in bedridden patients.

Look for other indicators that a patient is being treated for cardiac problems, such as the presence of a nitroglycerin patch on the skin or a cardiac pacemaker implanted under the skin.

Listening, as part of the cardiovascular examination, primarily involves auscultation with a stethoscope for sounds produced by the lungs, heart, and blood vessels. The lungs should be auscultated to assess for type and equality of breath sounds and the presence of any adventitious sounds that may indicate pulmonary congestion or edema. Detailed auscultation of the heart for abnormal heart sounds is often not performed in the field. It is a difficult assessment to make even under ideal conditions and the results of this examination do not drastically alter patient management. However, the paramedic may auscultate the heart to identify the two normal heart sounds, S_1 and S_2. S_1 is the first heart sound, produced by closure of the AV valves during ventricular contraction. The second heart sound, S_2, is produced by closure of the aortic and pulmonary valves during ventricular diastole. In certain patients, auscultating the heart to count the apical pulse may reveal a **pulse deficit,** the difference between the apical and peripheral pulse rates. Pulse deficit occurs in a number of abnormal heart rhythms. At times, it may also be appropriate to auscultate blood vessels. Arteries are normally silent when auscultated with a stethoscope but may produce a pulse-related blowing sound, called a **bruit,** if partially occluded by atherosclerosis. The carotid arteries should always be auscultated for bruits before performing carotid artery massage.

The final skill the paramedic uses in the cardiovascular examination is palpation. As mentioned previously, peripheral edema may be felt, as well as seen, in the extremities or sacral region of heart failure patients. Peripheral pulses should be palpated with special attention to rate, regularity, side-to-side equality, and the presence of a pulse deficit. Finally, the patient's skin is felt for temperature, dryness or dampness, and resiliency.

CARDIOVASCULAR DISEASE STATES: RECOGNITION AND MANAGEMENT

Atherosclerosis

Coronary artery disease and its complications are the leading cause of death in the Western Hemisphere. The primary etiology, **arteriosclerosis,** is a chronic disease of arteries that causes abnormal thickening and hardening of vessel walls, resulting in loss of elasticity. The coronary arteries are particularly prone to a common type of arteriosclerosis, called *intimal atherosclerosis*, which is present to some degree in most people older than 20 years of age. **Atherosclerosis** affects the intima of arteries in a number of stages over a period of years. The disease begins with an injury to the intima of a coronary artery, resulting in adherence of blood platelets and other plasma parts to the injury site. Smooth muscle cells proliferate and lipids accumulate abnormally in the artery's intima, producing a fatty streak in the early stage. With further progression of the disease, hard atherosclerotic plaques may actually form from lipid deposits, along with scar formation (fibrosis) and calcification. Plaque growth is usually slow and gradual as more fats are deposited and scar tissue develops, but it may be hastened by the rupture of small blood vessels into the plaque. The results of atherosclerosis are roughening of the intimal wall, loss of vessel elasticity, and progressive obstruction of the lumen of the coronary artery (Fig. 20-16). The final disease stage, the occurrence of clinical symptoms, may not occur for many years until obstruction sufficiently interferes with arterial blood supply to the myocardium. If the obstruction has progressed gradually, symptoms may be further delayed or may never occur if the heart is able to develop new vessels, called *collateral circulation*, in the affected area. The clinical manifestations of coronary atherosclerosis include angina pectoris, myocardial infarction, and sudden death, any of which may present as the first evidence of coronary artery disease.

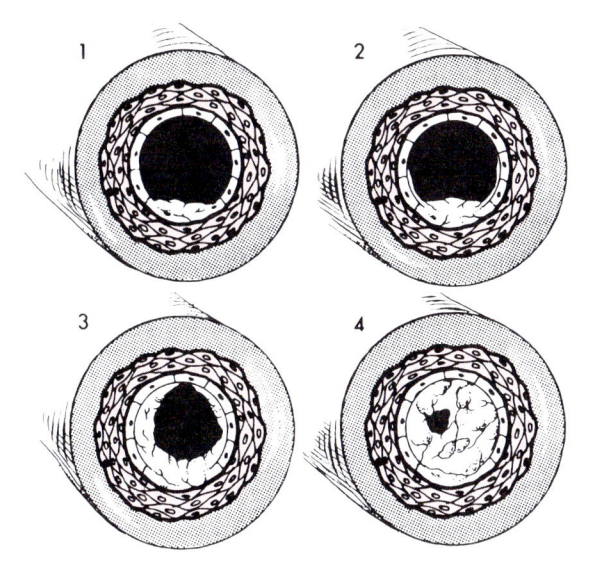

FIGURE 20–16.
Stages of atherosclerosis.

It is estimated that more than 4 million Americans have coronary artery disease and more than half a million people die annually from heart attacks. A decline in the mortality rate since 1960 has been attributed to the recognition of the factors that increase the risk of the development and progression of atherosclerosis. The primary risk factors are hypertension, elevated serum cholesterol, cigarette smoking, and diabetes mellitus. Other factors that are associated to varying degrees with increased risk are the following:

- Advanced age
- Sex (male)
- Race (nonwhite)
- Physical inactivity
- Obesity
- Personality (Type A)

Some of the above risk factors may be determined by genetic makeup, some may be modifiable, and some may not. It is important to recognize that the risk of developing coronary atherosclerosis is determined not just by the existence of a risk factor, but by the number of risk factors an individual has, the degree of abnormality of any factor, and the length of time the factor has existed. The paramedic should be aware of risk factors in terms of personal prevention of coronary artery disease and recognition of those patients most likely to have the disease.

Coronary artery atherosclerosis is the leading cause of cardiac emergencies that the paramedic will encounter in the field. To do its work of pumping blood to all body tissues, the heart muscle must have a good flow of oxygenated blood that can increase when cardiac work increases, such as with physical or emotional exertion. Even during normal activity, the heart muscle extracts about 70% of the oxygen supplied to it, as compared with about 25% extraction by other body organs. Because the oxygen reserve of the myocardium (i.e., the additional amount of oxygen available to the heart from arterial blood) is limited, the heart must rely on increased flow in times of stress. A deficiency of blood supply to the heart to meet myocardial oxygen needs results in a condition called **myocardial ischemia.** Prolonged ischemia or complete obstruction of blood flow causes necrosis, or cell death (Fig. 20-17).

Angina Pectoris

Angina pectoris, characterized by chest discomfort, occurs when the oxygen demands of the heart exceed blood supply for a short period of time, causing myocardial ischemia without any actual cell death. Although most commonly caused by coronary atherosclerosis, angina may also be the result of spasm of coronary arteries. Angina is most frequently precipitated by physical activity or emotional stress that temporarily increases the heart's metabolic rate and need for oxygen. This predictable form

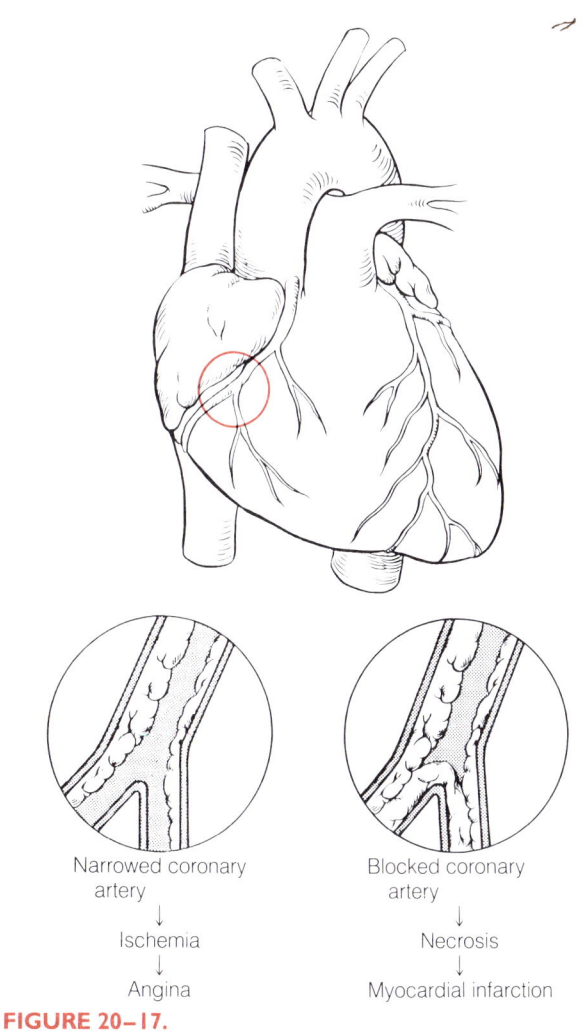

FIGURE 20–17.
Results of coronary atherosclerosis.

of angina, brought on by exertion, is termed "*stable*" angina. However, in the later stages of atherosclerosis, angina may occur less predictably, occurring at rest and with greater frequency, duration, or severity, and is referred to as "*unstable*" angina.

Coronary artery obstruction is generally well advanced when angina begins to occur. The signs and symptoms of angina result from a build-up of lactic acid and carbon dioxide in the ischemic myocardium. The primary symptom is discomfort or pain substernally. This myocardial pain is characteristically described as pressure, heaviness, tightness, or squeezing and most commonly occurs at the time of exertion or stress. Because anginal discomfort may also be experienced in the epigastric area, it is frequently mistaken for indigestion, and the patient may fail to recognize it as a cardiac symptom at its first occurrence. Although approximately one third of angina patients feel discomfort only in the chest, pain may also be experienced or spread (*radiate*) to one or both shoulders, arms, neck, jaw, or through to the back. Other associated symptoms that may or may not be present include anxiety, diaphoresis, and shortness of breath.

Stable angina is usually of short duration, lasting 3 to 5 minutes, although occasionally longer. Because no actual myocardial cell death occurs, the condition is reversible. Relief is generally obtained when the patient rests or, if the patient is receiving medical management for this condition, when nitroglycerin is taken. Although no permanent heart damage occurs, the patient may be at risk for arrhythmias during the period of myocardial ischemia.

Because of the transient nature of this condition, the patient may not even activate the emergency medical services (EMS) system for an angina attack. However, when paramedics are called, management of this patient includes recognition of symptoms of myocardial ischemia and adequate history taking to confirm the diagnosis. Stable angina usually responds to physical rest, emotional reassurance, oxygen administration, and the administration of nitroglycerin sublingually. If the patient has a history of angina, the paramedic should determine and convey to the medical control physician if nitroglycerin has already been taken, how much, and if there was any response. Whenever symptoms persist despite intervention, the paramedic must presume something more serious than angina is occurring and recognize that more extensive prehospital management and hospitalization are indicated.

Myocardial Infarction

Myocardial infarction is a condition in which actual death (*necrosis*) of a portion of heart muscle occurs because of severe, prolonged ischemia. It is most often associated with coronary artery occlusion due to atherosclerosis but, like angina, has also been attributed to coronary artery spasm with or without coronary artery disease. Other events that may precipitate an myocardial infarction include microemboli, acute volume overload, hypotension, or acute respiratory failure and hypoxia.

Permanent, irreversible myocardial damage occurs with a myocardial infarction. The location and size of the infarct depend on the site of the obstruction in the coronary arteries. The majority of infarctions are of the left ventricle, although the right ventricle is occasionally involved. Damage to the anterior, lateral, or septal myocardial walls is usually due to left coronary artery obstruction, while right coronary artery obstruction usually results in inferior wall infarction. Myocardial infarctions may extend through the full thickness of the myocardial wall (*transmural*) or may extend only part way through the muscle (*subendocardial*).

Myocardial infarction carries a high mortality rate because of several serious complications. The most common and earliest cause of death is the development of sudden, fatal arrhythmias. These arrhythmias often originate from the ring of ischemic myocardium that surrounds the site of actual necrosis (Fig. 20-18). The second cause of death from myocardial infarction is pump failure, usually due to extensive myocardial damage. Recognition of the signs and symptoms of myocardial infarction and prompt management are important to prevent these fatal complications.

Chest pain is the presenting symptom in the majority of patients with myocardial infarction. Although frequently severe, it may also be moderate, minimal, or, on occasion, absent. This myocardial pain has the same characteristics as the pain of angina. It is most often felt substernally, although it may also be located in the epigastric

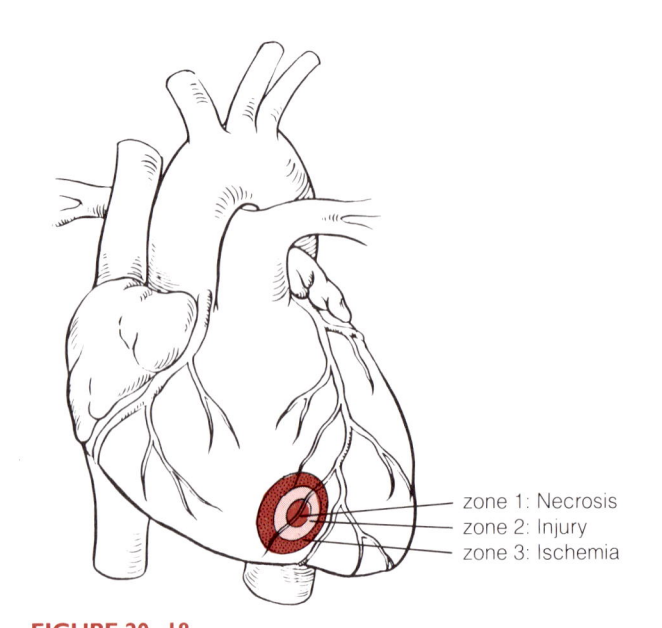

FIGURE 20-18.
Heart muscle damage in acute myocardial infarction.

zone 1: Necrosis
zone 2: Injury
zone 3: Ischemia

region. The pain is usually described as heavy, tight, squeezing pressure, or sometimes burning in nature. Even more commonly than with angina, the pain may radiate into either shoulder or arm (frequently the left), the neck, jaw, or through to the back. Unlike stable angina, however, pain from myocardial infarction often occurs at rest without any precipitating factors. It is a long-lasting pain, although it may wax and wane, and is not altered or relieved by nitroglycerin, antacids, other medications, or anything else the patient may do to attempt relief.

Although the classic presentation of symptoms of myocardial infarction differs in severity and duration from angina, it is important to recognize that myocardial infarction may present with subtle symptoms that are indistinguishable from those of prolonged angina. Also, some patients present with atypical pain, such as shoulder, arm, neck, or jaw pain in the absence of chest pain. Other patients, particularly the elderly, may only complain of general malaise, sweating, or an episode of syncope. A certain percentage of patients have "*silent*" myocardial infarctions without any symptoms and are only diagnosed at a later date by EKG changes. It is, therefore, essential to be familiar with all the possible indicators of myocardial ischemia, along with compatible patient history, to recognize those patients who warrant management for myocardial infarction.

Other symptoms and signs commonly associated with myocardial infarction besides pain are the following:

- Diaphoresis
- Anxiety and apprehension
- Shortness of breath
- Nausea or vomiting
- Pallor
- Generalized weakness

Vital signs may be variable depending on the extent of pump damage and the degree of autonomic nervous system response that occurs. The blood pressure may be entirely normal, elevated in response to sympathetic discharge, or low in response to parasympathetic discharge or pump failure. Pulse rate may vary for the same reasons; however, rate and rhythm may also be affected by the presence of arrhythmias. Respirations may be normal or increased.

Arrhythmias, as mentioned earlier, are the most common complication of myocardial infarction in the first few hours, occurring in 90% of all victims. Ventricular fibrillation is the most common life-threatening arrhythmia that requires immediate intervention. Other arrhythmias, although not immediately life-threatening, may be warning arrhythmias or forerunners of more serious disturbances and require early prehospital intervention. Still other arrhythmias of myocardial infarction are non–life-threatening and require no prehospital intervention. These complications are fully discussed in the last part of this chapter.

The management of myocardial infarction has three goals: relief of pain and apprehension, prevention of life-threatening arrhythmias, and limitation of infarct size. All of the prehospital interventions to be discussed are performed to accomplish one or more of these goals within the first few critical hours of myocardial infarction. After recognizing the patient's chief complaint and the history of the present illness as indicative of myocardial infarction, the paramedic should not delay the initiation of management. Further history should be obtained while conducting the physical examination and beginning intervention.

Physical rest and verbal reassurance are important to reduce the heart rate, thereby reducing myocardial oxygen demand. The patient should be placed in a position of comfort, ideally reclining on the stretcher with the head elevated at least 30°. Oxygen administration should be initiated as early as possible to increase oxygen delivery to ischemic myocardial tissue. Vital signs should be measured for a baseline reading, and measurement should be repeated frequently thereafter. The pulse check may give an early indication of arrhythmias if it is very slow, very fast, or irregular. As soon as possible, an intravenous (IV) solution of dextrose and water should be started, using a microdrip to minimize fluid infusion. Establishing the IV should be a high priority. The greatest threat to life in the first few hours are the arrhythmias that can be prevented or treated with IV medications. The EKG leads should be applied and a rhythm strip obtained to document the patient's initial rhythm and evaluate any arrhythmias. A 12-lead EKG is obtained in those systems that use or prepare for thrombolytic therapy. At this point, any further history taking and physical examination, including lung auscultation for early signs of heart failure, should be completed.

Medications are now administered either according to written protocols or following communication with the medical control physician to obtain verbal orders. Drugs routinely used in prehospital care for the management of myocardial infarction fall into two categories: drugs to relieve pain and myocardial ischemia and drugs for the management of arrhythmias.

Drugs for relief of pain and myocardial ischemia include nitroglycerin and morphine sulfate. Nitroglycerin dilates peripheral arteries and veins to reduce preload, afterload, and myocardial oxygen demand. It is also a coronary artery vasodilator and may increase flow in collateral coronary vessels. Because it can be administered sublingually, nitroglycerin may be ordered even before the IV is established and is the one drug that can be used when an IV cannot be started. Morphine sulfate is a narcotic analgesic that is administered in small IV increments until pain relief is obtained. In addition, morphine sulfate is a vasodilator, reducing myocardial oxygen demand by reducing venous return and systemic arterial resistance. Blood pressure must be monitored closely before, during, and after administration of either of these drugs, as hypotension could be catastrophic for an already compromised myocardium. Nitrous oxide is another effective analgesic that is used in certain EMS systems.

Drugs for the management of arrhythmias are addressed fully in the last part of this chapter. The most common of these drugs, lidocaine, is used to abolish the "*warning*" arrhythmia of premature ventricular contractions. It may also be given in the absence of any actual arrhythmias as a preventative measure. Other drugs that may be ordered for the patient with acute myocardial infarction include those for the management of slow heart rates, usually atropine. Drugs for the management of severe tachycardia (rapid heart rates) include lidocaine, bretylium, and, in some instances, verapamil.

Heart Failure

Heart failure is a condition that occurs when cardiac output is inadequate to meet the metabolic needs of the body. The basic problem in heart failure is a decrease in the pumping capacity of the heart. The term **congestive heart failure** reflects the circulatory congestion that occurs in heart failure with resulting fluid retention and edema formation. The left and right sides of the heart may develop pump failure independently of each other, resulting in different signs, symptoms, and prehospital management. However, it is helpful to remember that because the heart is comprised of two pumps in series, most patients with congestive heart failure have some degree of failure of both ventricles.

Left Ventricular Failure and Pulmonary Edema

Left ventricular failure is the inability of the left ventricle to pump blood adequately into the systemic circulation. This ineffective forward pumping causes a pressure of blood to be backed up into the pulmonary circulation, ultimately resulting in a condition called **pulmonary edema.** Left ventricular failure may be caused by various types of heart disease, including myocardial infarction, chronic hypertension, mitral valve disease, and certain arrhythmias. Myocardial infarctions can cause left ventricular failure when a large area of left ventricle is damaged acutely or when cardiac reserve is limited because of previous infarctions. Arrhythmias, particularly very rapid heart rates, are an etiology of left-sided heart failure when the shortening of the diastolic period prevents adequate ventricular filling and emptying and compromises coronary artery filling for oxygenation of the heart muscle. Slow heart rates, likewise, can compromise coronary artery perfusion and pump performance. Acute failure and pulmonary edema can also occur because of cessation of medication taken to control chronic heart failure.

In left ventricular failure, an imbalance in the output of the two sides of the heart occurs: the left ventricle is unable to eject all the blood delivered to it from the right. Left ventricular, followed by left atrial, pressure rises and is transmitted back to the pulmonary veins and capillaries. When pressure in the pulmonary vessels becomes too high, blood serum is forced into the alveoli, resulting in pulmonary edema. Patients with early left ventricular failure may have no symptoms at all at rest, but progressive fluid accumulation in the alveoli interferes with gas exchange and leads to death from hypoxia unless intervention occurs.

The cardinal sign of pulmonary edema is severe respiratory distress. The patient is dyspneic and orthopneic. Coughing spasms are not unusual because of the fluid irritation of the alveoli, and the patient may cough up a characteristic pink, frothy sputum. The patient may relate a previous history of paroxysmal nocturnal dyspnea. In **paroxysmal nocturnal dyspnea,** a form of transient pulmonary edema, the patient suddenly awakens at night with extreme shortness of breath and air-hunger. This episode usually resolves after the patient sits or stands up for a period of time, but it is a specific sign of left ventricular failure.

In pulmonary edema, the patient is frequently apprehensive, agitated, or even confused and uncooperative because of the frightening sensation of drowning and, possibly, because of inadequate cerebral perfusion. In the late stages, the patient may be lethargic and unresponsive. The skin is usually diaphoretic and may be cyanotic if hypoxia is severe.

Another sign of pulmonary edema is conveyed by the breath sounds heard on lung auscultation. Rales (crackles), rhonchi (bubbling), or wheezing may be present. Fine rales, indicating fluid in the alveoli, usually are heard bilaterally and do not clear with coughing. They may be auscultated in the lung bases only or extend all the way up to the scapulae. The presence of rhonchi indicates fluid in the larger airways and may mask the sound of rales. Wheezing may also occur in pulmonary edema because of a reflex spasm of the airways and should not be falsely attributed to asthma or COPD.

The external jugular veins should be observed. Obvious distention or pulsation of these veins may be present if severe pressure build-up has been transmitted all the way back through the right heart to the venous system.

The vital signs are characteristically elevated in pulmonary edema because of the body's attempt to compensate for the failing pump with intense sympathetic discharge. Marked hypertension, tachycardia, and tachypnea are all frequent findings. In addition, the pulse may be irregular if arrhythmias, either primary or secondary to hypoxia, are present. The length of time that cardiovascular compensatory mechanisms can prevail in a given patient is unknown. As these compensatory mechanisms fail, hypotension, bradycardia, and eventual respiratory arrest occur.

Chest pain may or may not be a symptom of pulmonary edema, depending on whether or not myocardial ischemia is present or whether any pain is masked by the patient's respiratory distress. Because myocardial infarction is such a common cause of left ventricular failure, all patients with pulmonary edema must be considered to also have had a myocardial infarction.

Pulmonary edema is a critical condition in which the patient can decompensate rapidly and unpredictably. Immediate emergency management is demanded. The goals of management are to improve oxygenation and ventilation, decrease venous return to the heart, and decrease the heart's oxygen demands.

Because time is of the essence, management should be initiated while obtaining the full history and performing the physical examination. Rest and reassurance are crucial to reduce myocardial oxygen needs. The patient should be placed in an upright position with feet dangling to maximize ventilation and enhance venous pooling. The patient should not lie flat at any time. A high concentration of oxygen should be administered by mask if it can be tolerated. Ideally, 100% oxygen by positive-pressure ventilation should be used if the patient is able to cooperate or if the level of consciousness is decreased significantly enough to permit assisted ventilation. Priority should be given to establishing an IV of D_5W for administration of medication. Microdrip tubing and an infusion rate just high enough to keep the vein open should be used, as additional fluid volume will worsen the patient's condition. Attach EKG electrodes and document the patient's initial rhythm. It is important to recognize and institute management for arrhythmias, which may be the primary cause of pulmonary edema, such as severe bradycardia and supraventricular or ventricular tachycardia.

Medications, administered according to written protocols or verbal orders, include drugs to decrease venous return, reduce circulating fluid volume, reduce anxiety, and counteract bronchospasm. Nitroglycerin and morphine sulfate, as previously mentioned, are potent peripheral vasodilators. By causing peripheral blood pooling, they reduce the volume of blood that returns to the failing left ventricle (preload), and they also decrease the resistance against which the heart muscle must pump (afterload). In addition, morphine is effective in reducing the patient's anxiety. Furosemide, in addition to reducing circulating blood volume by diuresis, acts as a vasodilator when administered IV. Theophylline ethylenediamine may be ordered for those pulmonary edema patients with significant wheezing due to bronchospasm, although it must be administered cautiously because of the cardiac arrhythmia side effects. Full information on administration of these drugs is found in the section "Prehospital Interventions for Specific Cardiac Conditions."

Right Ventricular Failure

Right ventricular failure is the inability of the right side of the heart to effectively pump blood, resulting in a pressure of blood backed-up into the systemic venous circulation and, thus, venous congestion. Although not usually a life-threatening emergency condition in itself, right ventricular failure should be recognized because of its frequent association with left ventricular failure and its need for medical management. Indeed, the most common cause of right ventricular failure is the overload from left ventricular failure. However, other etiologies that may result in isolated right ventricular failure include chronic obstructive pulmonary disease, acute pulmonary embolism, and infarction of the right atrium or ventricle.

Failure of the right ventricle to match stroke volume with venous return first causes right heart pressures to rise, followed by transmission of this pressure back to the venae cavae and the rest of the systemic venous system. When venous pressure becomes too high, blood serum is forced out into the interstitial spaces of the body, resulting in tissue edema. Venous congestion and fluid accumulation are the cardinal signs of right-sided congestive heart failure. Venous congestion is evidenced by jugular vein distention and complaints of pain or tenderness in certain organs, such as the liver. Fluid accumulation is evidenced by peripheral edema, usually of dependent body parts. In the ambulatory patient, swelling of the ankles and legs occurs, while, in bedridden patients, edema of the sacral region may be noted. Fluid accumulation may also occur in serous body cavities, such as the abdomen (*ascites*), pleural space (*pleural effusion*), or pericardium (*pericardial effusion*). Patients with chronic right-sided congestive heart failure may be able to tolerate large amounts of fluid accumulation without any real compromise of organ function.

The patient's medical history may be helpful, as right-sided heart failure is often a chronic condition. If previously diagnosed, these patients may use such lay terms as "enlarged heart" or "water build-up" to describe their heart failure. Frequently, a history of myocardial infarction is present, and the patient is often taking digitalis and some form of diuretic to control the chronic heart failure.

In terms of management, right ventricular failure causes no life-threatening emergencies. However, the patient with evidence of right ventricular failure may also have left ventricular failure and the potential for acute decompensation. Management of right ventricular failure includes the following:

- Placing the patient at rest to reduce metabolic demands of the body
- Administering oxygen in high concentration
- Measuring vital signs
- Establishing an IV of D_5W with a microdrip to keep the vein open
- EKG monitoring

Definitive management is conducted in the hospital, although the paramedic should be alert for any symptoms of left-sided heart failure that may warrant prehospital intervention.

Cardiogenic Shock

Cardiogenic shock is the most extreme form of pump failure, occurring when the function of the left ventricle is so compromised that the heart can no longer adequately perfuse body tissues. It is most often due to extensive myocardial infarction, involving about 40% or more of the left ventricle. Hypotension can be caused by a number of cardiac-related conditions, including bradyarrhythmia and tachyarrhythmia, severe dehydration, pain, and vasovagal reactions (action of stimuli from the vagus nerve on blood vessels). However, true cardiogenic shock is discussed here as pump failure and shock symptoms that persist when the aforementioned conditions either do not exist or have been corrected.

Cardiogenic shock should be suspected when the signs and symptoms of acute myocardial infarction are accompanied by severe hypotension and signs of poor tissue perfusion. The systolic blood pressure is usually less than 90 or at least 30 mm Hg lower than the patient's normal blood pressure. Impaired cerebral perfusion may alter the patient's level of consciousness, causing restlessness, apprehension, confusion, or even unconsciousness. Sinus tachycardia, a compensatory mechanism in any type of shock, is the most common heart rhythm in cardiogenic shock. When serious arrhythmias do exist, it is often impossible to know if the arrhythmia is the cause of the hypotension or if it is the result of the cardiogenic shock. In any case, all major arrhythmias should be corrected as soon as possible. Cardiogenic shock is also evidenced by other signs of impaired perfusion, such as cool, clammy, possibly dusky, or cyanotic skin, and compensatory mechanisms, such as tachypnea.

Cardiogenic shock due to extensive pump damage carries a high mortality rate (80%–90%), even with aggressive in-hospital management. Because of the need for hemodynamic monitoring devices and complicated drug therapy for these patients, prolonged attempts at stabilization in the field are not recommended. Management should be supportive and symptomatic while expediting transport. The patient's airway should be secured, using an oropharyngeal airway if the patient is unconscious, and a high concentration of oxygen administered. The patient should be positioned supine to maximize cerebral blood flow. Establishing an IV may be difficult because of cardiovascular collapse but should be attempted with D_5W to keep the vein open for possible drug therapy. The EKG should be monitored and major arrhythmias treated. Physical examination should include observation of jugular veins for distension and lung auscultation for evidence of pulmonary edema. Medications may be administered to enhance cardiac contractility according to written protocols or on direct physician order. Dopamine is the most commonly used prehospital drug because, in low IV doses, it increases renal blood flow in addition to improving contractility. As mentioned previously, rapid transport is indicated for the patient in cardiogenic shock because of the need for aggressive in-hospital management. Prolonged observation in the field for response to drug therapy is not appropriate.

Cardiac Arrest and Sudden Death

Sudden death is one of the major clinical syndromes of **atherosclerotic heart disease** and may be defined as death within 1 hour of the onset of symptoms. It accounts for 60% of all deaths from atherosclerotic heart disease and, in a significant number of patients, is the first manifestation of cardiac disease. In many cases of cardiac arrest, actual myocardial infarction is not present, but severe atherosclerotic disease is common. The risk factors for sudden death are obviously the same as for coronary artery disease.

Ventricular fibrillation is the arrhythmia responsible for the majority of cardiac arrests (60%–70%). Ventricular fibrillation may be a primary arrhythmia caused by myocardial ischemia or a secondary arrhythmia caused by other conditions, such as hypothermia, drug toxicity, and drowning. Other less common but also lethal arrhythmias associated with cardiac arrest include ventricular tachycardia, asystole, severe bradycardia, and electromechanical dissociation. Interpretation of these various arrhythmias is addressed fully in the last part of this chapter; at this point, however, a discussion of management is pertinent to the subject of sudden death.

No matter what arrhythmia is involved, some general considerations in the management of cardiac arrest are applicable. Basic life support is essential, so the paramedic must continually monitor the performance of cardiopulmonary resuscitation (CPR) if this responsibility is delegated to others. Airway management is also a high priority in resuscitation. The airway and ventilation can be managed by a number of methods. The most sophisticated is not always needed immediately if it delays institution of other high-priority management procedures. A third management consideration concerns cardiac arrest that results from conditions other than atherosclerotic heart disease. Arrests due to drowning, hypothermia, and trauma are all managed somewhat differently, particularly with regard to time spent at the scene and persistence in resuscitation attempts. Likewise, cardiac arrest in infants and children is rarely due to a primary arrhythmia but more frequently associated with hypoxia. In all these examples, recognition of the etiology of the arrest is important, as it may alter the approach to management.

Ventricular fibrillation is the most common and most correctable of the lethal arrhythmias that cause cardiac arrest. Primary ventricular fibrillation is somewhat easier to remove than ventricular fibrillation due to secondary causes. It has been demonstrated repeatedly that the best chance for resuscitation of the patient in ventricular fibrillation lies in early defibrillation. The paramedic must identify ventricular fibrillation and deliver the first shock as soon as possible on reaching the patient. Other techniques in the management of a ventricular fibrillation arrest should follow the American Heart Association's advanced cardiac life support protocols for ventricular fibrillation (Fig. 20-19). Nonperfusing ventricular tachycardia, the forerunner of ventricular fibrillation, must be treated with electrical intervention with the same expediency as ventricular fibrillation.

Management of bradycardia (slow rates) and asystole (absence of electrical activity) as presenting rhythms in cardiac arrest is invariably less successful than treatment of ventricular fibrillation and ventricular tachycardia. In addition to drug therapy to stimulate electrical activity, external pacing may be attempted, although this intervention has not yet been shown to be effective in prehospital arrest situations. Asystole is usually the end result of prolonged ventricular fibrillation or the primary result

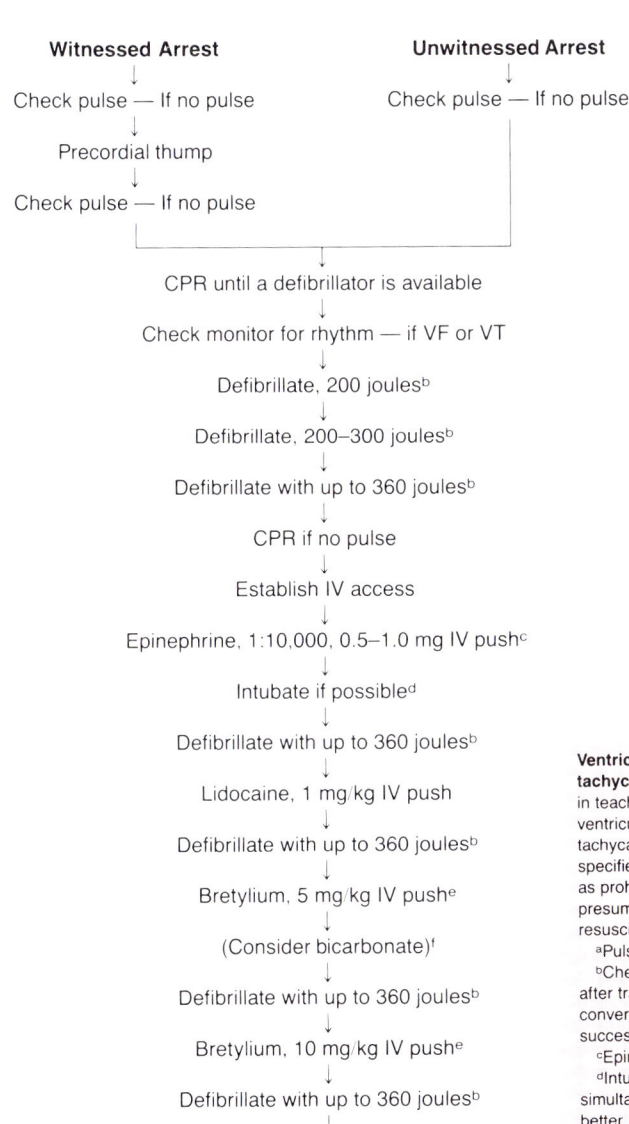

Witnessed Arrest
↓
Check pulse — If no pulse
↓
Precordial thump
↓
Check pulse — If no pulse

Unwitnessed Arrest
↓
Check pulse — If no pulse

↓
CPR until a defibrillator is available
↓
Check monitor for rhythm — if VF or VT
↓
Defibrillate, 200 joules[b]
↓
Defibrillate, 200–300 joules[b]
↓
Defibrillate with up to 360 joules[b]
↓
CPR if no pulse
↓
Establish IV access
↓
Epinephrine, 1:10,000, 0.5–1.0 mg IV push[c]
↓
Intubate if possible[d]
↓
Defibrillate with up to 360 joules[b]
↓
Lidocaine, 1 mg/kg IV push
↓
Defibrillate with up to 360 joules[b]
↓
Bretylium, 5 mg/kg IV push[e]
↓
(Consider bicarbonate)[f]
↓
Defibrillate with up to 360 joules[b]
↓
Bretylium, 10 mg/kg IV push[e]
↓
Defibrillate with up to 360 joules[b]
↓
Repeat lidocaine or bretylium
↓
Defibrillate with up to 360 joules[b]

Ventricular fibrillation (and pulseless ventricular tachycardia).[a] This sequence was developed to assist in teaching how to treat a broad range of patients with ventricular fibrillation (VF) or pulseless ventricular tachycardia (VT). Some patients may require care not specified herein. This algorithm should not be construed as prohibiting such flexibility. The flow of the algorithm presumes that VF is continuing. CPR = cardiopulmonary resuscitation.

[a]Pulseless VT should be treated identically to VF.
[b]Check pulse and rhythm after each shock. If VF recurs after transiently converting (rather than persists without ever converting), use whatever energy level has previously been successful for defibrillation.
[c]Epinephrine should be repeated every 5 minutes.
[d]Intubation is preferable. If it can be accompanied simultaneously with other techniques, then the earlier the better. However, defibrillation and epinephrine are more important initially if the patient can be ventilated without intubation.
[e]Some may prefer repeated doses of lidocaine, which may be given in 0.5-mg/kg boluses every 8 minutes to a total dose of 3 mg/kg.
[f]The value of sodium bicarbonate is questionable during cardiac arrest, and it is not recommended for routine cardiac arrest sequences. Consideration of its use in a dose of 1 mEq/kg is appropriate at this point. Half of the original dose may be repeated every 10 minutes if it is used.

FIGURE 20–19.
Advanced cardiac life support treatment protocol for ventricular fibrillation and pulseless ventricular tachycardia. (© American Heart Association: Textbook of Advanced Cardiac Life Support, 2nd ed, p 238. Dallas, American Heart Association, 1987)

```
Continue CPR
    ↓
Establish IV access
    ↓
Epinephrine, 1:10,000, 0.5–1.0 mg IV push[a]
    ↓
Intubate when possible[b]
    ↓
(Consider bicarbonate)[c]
    ↓
Consider hypovolemia,
cardiac tamponade,
tension pneumothorax,
hypoxemia,
acidosis,
pulmonary embolism
```

Electromechanical dissociation. This sequence was developed to assist in teaching how to treat a broad range of patients with electromechanical dissociation. Some patients may require care not specified herein. This algorithm should not be construed to prohibit such flexibility. The flow of the algorithm presumes that electromechanical dissociation is continuing. CPR = cardiopulmonary resuscitation; IV = intravenous.

[a]Epinephrine should be repeated every 5 minutes.

[b]Intubation is preferable. If it can be accomplished simultaneously with other techniques, then the earlier the better. However, epinephrine is more important initially if the patient can be ventilated without intubation.

[c]The value of sodium bicarbonate is questionable during cardiac arrest, and it is not recommended for routine cardiac arrest sequences. Consideration of its use in a dose of 1 mEq/kg is appropriate at this point. Half of the original dose may be repeated every 10 minutes if it is used.

FIGURE 20–20.
Advanced cardiac life support treatment protocol for electromechanical dissociation. (© American Heart Association: Textbook of Advanced Cardiac Life Support, 2nd ed, p 240. Dallas, American Heart Association, 1987)

of extensive myocardial damage. As such, the prognosis is universally poor no matter what management is used. It is important to be aware that the distinction between asystole and a fine ventricular fibrillation may be difficult to make on surface EKG. Therefore, defibrillation is indicated if any question of ventricular fibrillation exists, as that is the greatest hope for resuscitation.

Electromechanical dissociation is any organized EKG rhythm that has an adequate rate but produces no pulse. Some of the common causes of electromechanical dissociation include massive myocardial infarction, cardiac rupture and tamponade, hypovolemia, tension pneumothorax, and acute pulmonary embolism. Although the prognosis is poor, the paramedic should keep these etiologies of electromechanical dissociation in mind, as some are treatable in-hospital. Transport should be considered much earlier than usual if there is a possibility of a treatable etiology of electromechanical dissociation, such as hypovolemia. In such cases, the pneumatic anti-shock garment and IV volume loading may be indicated. Management of electromechanical dissociation is outlined in advanced cardiac life support protocols (Fig. 20-20).

OTHER ACQUIRED AND CONGENITAL DISEASES OF THE CARDIOVASCULAR SYSTEM

No discussion of cardiac disease states would be complete without including some of the other less common cardiovascular conditions that may present as prehospital emergencies or at least cause the patient to summon emergency assistance.

Valvular Heart Disease

Problems with the mechanical functioning of heart valves may be a congenital condition or may be acquired as the result of such problems as rheumatic heart disease, acute bacterial infections that attack and destroy the valves, or myocardial infarction that damages the valves' papillary muscles. **Valvular heart disease** may be an acute event or a chronic condition and most often affects the valves on the left side of the heart, the mitral and aortic valves. The three most common problems that develop with these valves are the following:

Stenosis: narrowing and failure of the valve to open easily

Regurgitation (or insufficiency): failure of the valve to close completely

Prolapse: a collapsing of the valve into the chamber behind it

It is important to recognize that patients with valvular disease may develop a number of serious complications, including various pulmonary problems, arrhythmias, syncope, angina, and systemic emboli. The symptoms and signs with which the patient presents may be attributed to other cardiac conditions unless the history of valvular heart disease is known. Acute pulmonary edema is likely to occur because of the backed-up pressure created in the left heart by a stenotic valve that is obstructing good forward blood flow or by the backward flow of blood through an incompetent valve. While most other etiologies of pulmonary edema are associated with older patients, severe valvular disease may precipitate this emergency in young adults.

Pericardial Disorders

Pericarditis is a term used to describe inflammation of the pericardial sac that surrounds the heart. This condition has a great number of causes, some of which are bacterial, viral, or fungal infections, chest trauma, uremia from kidney failure, and myocardial infarction. Pericarditis may produce chest pain, dyspnea, tachycardia, and fluid accumulation in the pericardial sac. Although the symptoms differ somewhat from those of acute myocardial infarction, pericarditis may be difficult to distinguish in the prehospital setting.

Pericarditis is not usually life-threatening in itself, but extensive pericardial fluid accumulation may lead to a potentially life-threatening condition called **cardiac tamponade.** This is a condition in which abnormal fluid accumulation in the pericardial sac restricts diastolic filling of the heart and leads to severe compromise of the cardiac output. In addition to all types of pericarditis, common causes of cardiac tamponade are bleeding into the pericardium from blunt or penetrating trauma, dissecting aortic aneurysm, ventricular rupture, or clotting disorders and tumors. Symptoms and signs include severe dyspnea, tachycardia, hypotension and narrow pulse pressure, and elevated central venous pressure as evidenced by jugular vein distension. Another sign that is almost always present in cardiac tamponade (but may also occur in other conditions) is a paradoxical pulse or **pulsus paradoxus.** This is a blood pressure drop of greater than 10 mm Hg on inspiration and can be detected while taking the blood pressure or palpating a pulse through several respiratory cycles. The presence of a paradoxical pulse, along with other symptoms and history, may help to confirm cardiac tamponade.

Although not a common prehospital emergency, cardiac tamponade must be considered in the presence of a compatible history, as rapid management and transport are necessary to reverse the disastrous consequences of this condition. Oxygen therapy and IV volume loading should be administered during rapid transport to the hospital for removal of the pericardial fluid by pericardiocentesis.

Lung Disorders That Affect the Heart

Certain pathologic conditions of the lung increase the resistance of the lungs to blood flow and may cause the right ventricle to fail in its attempt to perfuse pulmonary tissue. Right-sided heart failure that occurs as a result of increased lung resistance, independent of left ventricular function, is termed **cor pulmonale.** Cor pulmonale may be an acute event or a chronic condition.

The most common cause of chronic cor pulmonale is COPD. These patients have all the symptoms of right-sided heart failure in addition to COPD symptoms, and both conditions may be successfully managed with medications. When occasional decompensation occurs, it may be impossible for the paramedic to determine if the patient's respiratory symptoms are due to heart failure or COPD.

Acute cor pulmonale occurs when the right heart is faced with a sudden increase in lung vascular resistance due to obstruction of major pulmonary vessels. This condition usually is attributed to a pulmonary embolus, a blood clot that originates in the peripheral venous circulation or right heart and becomes lodged in the pulmonary arterial system. Although blood clots are most common, vessel obstruction occasionally is caused by air, fat, amniotic fluid, or clumps of bacteria. The degree of obstruction, the site of obstruction, and the patient's previous cardiovascular status determine the severity of symptoms and the outcome. A large clot that occludes a major pulmonary artery causes a sudden rise in pulmonary artery pressure, which the right ventricle is unable to overcome to maintain adequate lung perfusion. This state leads to poor blood return to the left heart, decreased cardiac output, and subsequent shock or cardiac arrest.

The most common predisposing factors for pulmonary embolism are prolonged immobilization, **thrombophlebitis** (inflammation in veins, particularly in the lower extremities), congestive heart failure, COPD, use of oral contraceptives, and malignancies. Presence of deep vein thrombophlebitis in a patient with suspected pulmonary embolism may help confirm the diagnosis. Pulmonary embolism is a difficult diagnosis to make in the field, and sometimes in the emergency department, as presenting symptoms and signs may be nonspecific and associated with a number of other disorders. Chest pain, dyspnea, and tachypnea are the most common signs and symptoms. Cough, hemoptysis, cyanosis, rales, diaphoresis, and shock may also be present; no one set of signs and symptoms for pulmonary embolism is found. If making a definitive diagnosis in the field is difficult or if a high index of suspicion for pulmonary embolism exists, prehospital management should be symptomatic, aimed at the relief of pulmonary edema and myocardial ischemia, with minimal delay of transport if the patient is in shock. Therapy includes a high concentration of oxygen, IV infusion to keep the vein open, and vasopressors, such as dopamine, to maintain blood pressure.

Blood Pressure Disorders

Chronically elevated blood pressure creates an increased workload for the heart as it attempts to eject blood against an increased afterload. Over time, this increased workload may lead to enlargement of the left ventricle, accelerated progression of atherosclerosis, myocardial ischemia if coronary artery disease is already present, and pulmonary edema due to left ventricular failure. Hypertension is also a major risk factor for strokes and aortic aneurysm. Therefore, diagnosis and control of hypertension are important to all patients.

Acute hypertensive emergency is defined as a rapid elevation of the diastolic blood pressure, usually to 130 mm Hg or more, accompanied by serious complications, such as hypertensive encephalopathy, hemorrhage into the brain, toxemia of pregnancy, pulmonary edema, or aortic dissection. Hypertensive encephalopathy is characterized by central nervous system (CNS) changes that develop over 24 to 48 hours, such as focal neurologic deficits, headache, blurred vision, confusion, stupor, and, possibly, seizures or coma. Although true hypertensive emergencies are relatively uncommon, they call for rapid, aggressive management, usually in-hospital. When obtaining a history from the severely hypertensive patient, the paramedic should determine if the patient is taking medication for hypertension and has neglected to take it, as hypertensive emergencies often occur as a result of poorly controlled hypertension. Prehospital management of a true hypertensive emergency is supportive rather than definitive. Oxygen therapy, a quiet environment, and symptomatic management for such problems as chest pain or pulmonary edema are indicated, with rapid transport to the hospital for carefully monitored drug therapy to lower the blood pressure.

Transient elevations of blood pressure are frequently seen as the result of other medical conditions, such as severe anxiety, transient cerebral ischemic attacks and thrombotic stroke, delirium tremens, and acute hypoxic states, such as those due to cardiogenic pulmonary edema, decompensated COPD, or asthma. Hypertension in these conditions is usually the result of the primary problem and resolves when that primary problem is corrected. Aggressive attempts to lower the blood pressure in these situations should not be made without first correcting the underlying problem, or severe hypotension could result. The difficulty of determining in the field whether severe hypertension is a primary or secondary event is another reason that drug management of blood pressure is usually done in-hospital. Thorough history taking by the paramedic remains important to help the emergency department physician formulate a management approach.

Peripheral Vascular Disease

The paramedic must be aware of a number of conditions that affect the peripheral vascular system to recognize those that are critical and require rapid intervention.

Noncritical peripheral vascular conditions include chronic, progressive diseases of both the arterial and venous vessels. Venous conditions include varicose veins and deep vein thrombophlebitis. The only emergency associated with varicose veins is severe bleeding into leg tissue if a vein ruptures. This bleeding is controlled by direct pressure during transport to the hospital. Deep vein thrombophlebitis is an inflamed clot that occurs commonly in the calf or leg vein, causing leg pain, redness, and swelling. Although in itself this condition is not a medical emergency, patients with thrombophlebitis may be prone to develop pulmonary emboli. The paramedic should not allow patients with this disorder to walk, should elevate the leg, and should only use gentle palpation when examining the site. The arterial side of the circulation may also be affected by a chronic, noncritical condition, called peripheral arterial atherosclerotic disease. This is a gradual, progressive obstruction of the peripheral arteries that creates pain on exercising, called intermittent claudication. These patients have a high incidence of atherosclerosis of other vital arteries, such as the aorta, coronary, and cerebral arteries, and may be prone to acute peripheral arterial occlusion. Both chronic venous and arterial diseases may result in skin ulcers on the lower extremities due to poor circulation.

Acute arterial occlusion is a somewhat more emergent condition. It is the sudden occlusion of arterial flow in an extremity or the abdomen as a result of trauma, clot formation, or an embolus. Signs and symptoms are sudden severe pain and, in an extremity, pulselessness, decreased temperature, and cyanosis, mottling, or pallor. Although serious, extremity occlusion is not life-threatening, as 4 to 8 hours are available to reestablish flow. The paramedic should protect the affected limb and not allow the patient to walk. Occlusion of the mesenteric artery in the abdomen may result in excruciating abdominal pain and shock, calling for prehospital management with oxygen, IV crystalloid infusion, and, possibly, analgesia with morphine sulfate.

The critical, life-threatening peripheral vascular conditions include aneurysms of the thoracic and abdominal aorta. An aneurysm is a nonspecific term that means dilation of a vessel. Aortic aneurysms are most commonly caused by atherosclerotic weakening of the wall of the aorta, causing it to balloon out. Aneurysms of the abdominal aorta, the most frequent site, are usually located below the renal arteries but may involve the renal and iliac arteries (Fig. 20-21). This aneurysm produces a pulsatile mass that may be palpated at or below the umbilicus when it reaches a size greater than 5 cm (Fig. 20-22). The life-threatening complication of abdominal aneurysm is rupture, which may present as shock or cardiac arrest. In addition to a pulsatile abdominal mass, signs and symptoms of a leaking or ruptured aneurysm in the non-arrested patient may include back (flank) pain, abdominal

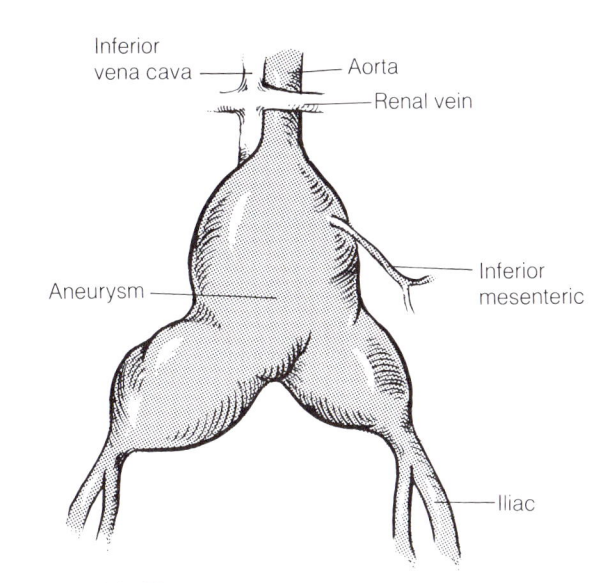

CHAPTER 20: Cardiovascular Emergencies 429

FIGURE 20-21.
Aneurysm of the abdominal aorta.

pain, hypotension, decreased femoral pulse, and the urge to defecate (if retroperitoneal leak). In the absence of these classic symptoms and signs, or in cardiac arrest, it may be impossible to diagnose this condition in the field unless the patient has a history of diagnosed abdominal aneurysm. The paramedic should have a high index of suspicion in any elderly patient with unexplained cardiovascular collapse and should be alert for compatible signs, symptoms, and medical history. Shock should be managed with oxygen, volume replacement with IV normal saline or lactated Ringer's solution, and pneumatic anti-shock garment according to protocols or orders. Prolonged field management is not warranted, as surgical intervention is necessary.

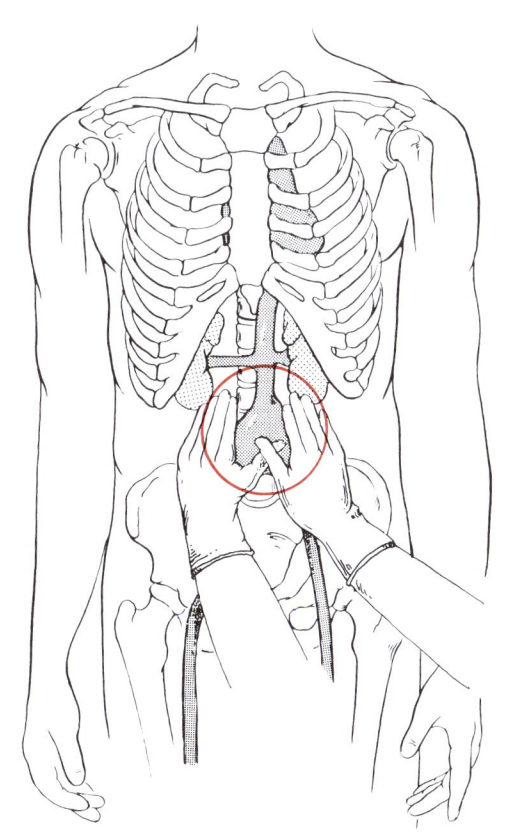

The most critical situation that involves aneurysm of the thoracic aorta is the development of a ***dissecting aortic aneurysm***. This is a hemorrhage into the middle layer (*media*) of the thoracic aorta that creates a false passage and hematoma (Fig. 20-23). This dissection may extend throughout the thoracic aorta to interrupt arterial flow through vital branches or may rupture into pericardial or pleural cavities (Fig. 20-24). Signs and symptoms of aortic dissection include severe ripping or tearing substernal chest pain or back pain and elevated blood pressure despite clinical appearance of shock. Other findings due to involvement of other arteries and structures include absent pulse or pulse deficit, side-to-side differences in blood pressure, neurologic changes, such as syncope, stroke or coma, or signs and symptoms of left-sided heart failure, acute myocardial infarction, or cardiac tamponade. Once again, a high index of suspicion is necessary to recognize this condition in the field, aided by physical examination findings and medical history. Prehospital management should include oxygen, IV normal saline or lactated Ringer's solution, and, possibly, morphine sulfate if the diagnosis is fairly certain. Transport of the patient should be expedited with most management performed en route,

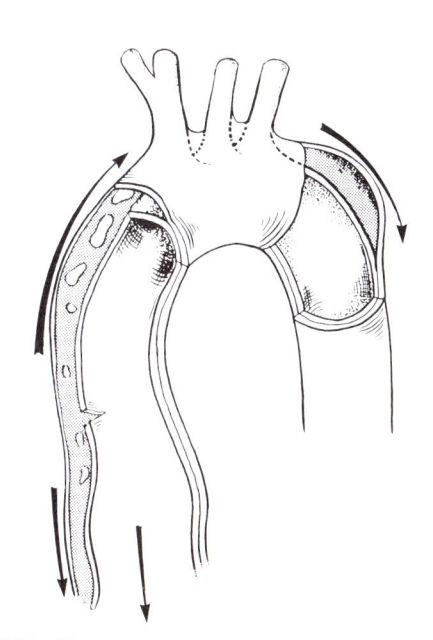

FIGURE 20-22.
Gentle palpation of the abdomen to identify an aneurysm.

FIGURE 20-23.
Dissecting thoracic aortic aneurysm.

FIGURE 20–24.
Types of thoracic aneurysm.

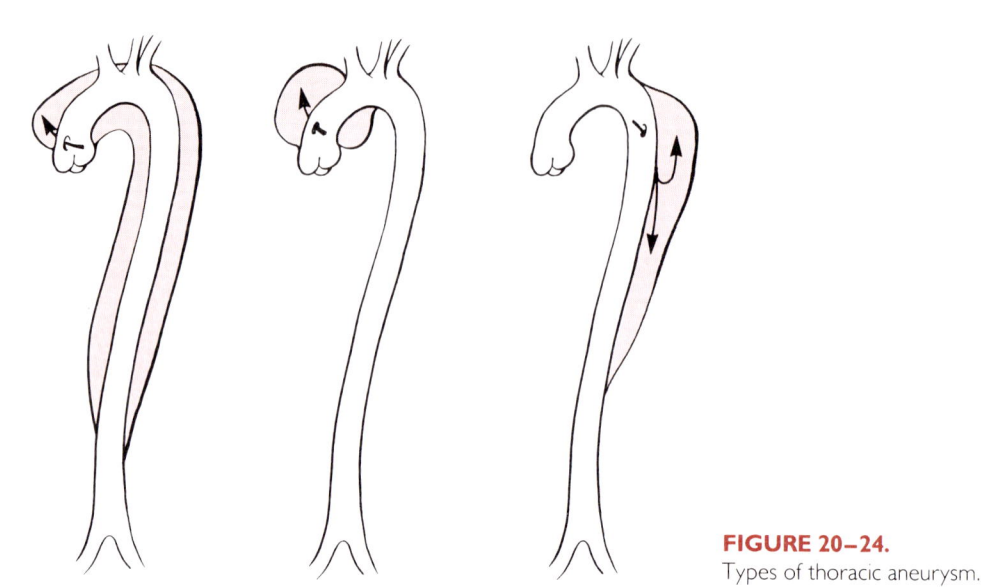

as survival from aortic dissection is possible if the condition is treated promptly.

PREHOSPITAL INTERVENTIONS FOR SPECIFIC CARDIAC CONDITIONS

The primary prehospital intervention for cardiac emergencies is pharmacologic therapy. With the exception of specific arrhythmia management, which is covered in the last part of this chapter, the following outline addresses drugs that are most commonly used to treat cardiac emergencies:

Myocardial ischemia and pain: oxygen, nitroglycerin, morphine sulfate, nitrous oxide
Pulmonary edema: oxygen, morphine sulfate, nitroglycerin, furosemide, theophylline ethylenediamine
Cardiogenic shock: oxygen, dopamine
Cardiac arrest: oxygen, epinephrine, sodium bicarbonate

Oxygen

Pharmacology and Actions. **Oxygen** is an odorless, tasteless gas that is necessary for all cellular life and proper metabolism. Supplementing the oxygen content of inspired air raises the amount of oxygen in the blood and, therefore, the amount delivered to tissues to counteract cellular hypoxia.

Cardiac Indications. Any situation in which generalized or localized hypoxia exists or is likely to develop, including cardiac arrest, symptoms of myocardial ischemia and necrosis, congestive heart failure, pulmonary edema, cardiogenic shock, peripheral vascular obstruction, and pulmonary embolism.

Precautions. Do not withhold oxygen from patients with a history of COPD, but possibly elect to begin administration of a lower FiO_2 (fraction of inspired oxygen) in these patients. Increase administration as needed based on the patient's clinical response.

Administration and Dosage. Administered by inhalation. A high FiO_2 is usually indicated for cardiovascular problems. This may be administered by simple face mask, partial rebreathing mask, or nonrebreathing mask, all at high-liter flow settings (10–15 L/min), or by positive-pressure ventilation in conjunction with a face mask, esophageal obturator airway, or endotracheal tube. Positive-pressure ventilation may also be beneficial in pulmonary edema, if the patient can tolerate it. Lower amounts of FiO_2 are delivered by nasal cannula at flow rates up to 6 L/min, and a cannula may be used for COPD patients or those who cannot tolerate a face mask.

Side Effects and Special Considerations.

1. There is no danger of oxygen toxicity from short-term prehospital administration.
2. Patients who are in need of high FiO_2 oxygen administration are often anxious about face masks. Attempt to reassure them before reverting to a nasal cannula.
3. Dry or irritated mucous membranes may result from nonhumidified oxygen, but this result usually is not a problem with short-term administration.
4. A patent airway must be maintained in both spontaneously breathing and assisted ventilation patients for oxygen therapy to be beneficial.

Nitroglycerin

Pharmacology and Actions. **Nitroglycerin** relaxes vascular smooth muscle, decreasing venous return to the heart, decreasing the arterial resistance against which the heart must pump, and also producing coronary artery dilation. The reduction in preload and afterload decreases the workload and, therefore, the oxygen consumption of the left ventricle, while the oxygen supply to the myocardium is improved.

Cardiac Indicators. Ischemic myocardial pain for stable and unstable angina and pulmonary edema due to left ventricular failure, for which nitroglycerin is used primarily for its peripheral venous dilation effect. Dilation of veins permits blood to pool in the venous circulation, slowing its return to the heart and lungs.

Precautions. Nitroglycerin is contraindicated in shock. Blood pressure should be monitored closely after administration, as hypotension may occur, further compromising myocardial perfusion.

Administration and Dosage. The usual dose is 0.3 mg (grain 1/200), 0.4 mg (grain 1/150), or 0.6 mg (grain 1/100) tablet allowed to dissolve sublingually or 0.4 mg administered by oral spray. This dose may be repeated in 3 to 5 minutes if needed.

Side Effects and Special Considerations.

1. Common side effects include headache, dizziness, and flushing.
2. Hypotension and reflex tachycardia may be a serious side effect in a patient with myocardial infarction. Hypotension usually responds to elevating the patient's feet or lowering the head.
3. Infrequently, nitroglycerin may produce a paradoxical slowing of heart rate.
4. Burning under the tongue indicates potency of the drug. Nitroglycerin is fairly unstable and deteriorates more rapidly with exposure to air, temperature extremes, and light. This quality necessitates storage in dark bottles, observation of expiration dates, and limiting opening and closing of bottles as much as possible.
5. Nitroglycerin may be particularly useful in cases of chest pain or pulmonary edema when it is not possible to establish an IV to administer IV medications.
6. For home use, patients may use long-acting nitroglycerin preparations, such as ointments and time-released capsules.

Morphine Sulfate

Pharmacology and Actions. **Morphine sulfate** is a potent narcotic analgesic that also dilates peripheral arteries and veins. This vasodilation reduces preload and afterload, thereby reducing cardiac work and oxygen consumption. Other narcotic actions include reduction of anxiety, lowered respiratory rate, and pupil constriction.

Cardiac Indications. Chest pain or other pain associated with myocardial infarction and pulmonary edema due to left ventricular failure.

Precautions. Morphine is contraindicated in shock and severe bradycardia. The blood pressure, pulse, and respiratory rate must be monitored closely before and after administration. Morphine must be used cautiously, if at all, in patients with COPD, respiratory depression, or history of use of other depressant drugs (e.g., alcohol, barbiturates).

Administration and Dosage. Morphine should be administered IV, slowly, in increments of 2 to 5 mg until pain relief or, in pulmonary edema, until the desired hemodynamic effect is obtained. This dose may be repeated every 5 to 30 minutes as necessary.

Side Effects and Special Considerations.

1. Side effects include respiratory depression, hypotension (common if the patient is hypovolemic or has decreased cardiac output), nausea and vomiting, decreased level of consciousness, or bradycardia due to increased vagal tone.
2. Slow IV administration helps to minimize hypotension and other side effects.
3. All effects of morphine can be reversed with IV naloxone.

Nitrous Oxide

Pharmacology and Actions. **Nitrous oxide** is an analgesic gas commonly used in combination with other drugs in general anesthesia. Used as a 50–50 mixture of nitrous oxide and oxygen, it is available for prehospital administration for pain relief (Nitronox). Its effects dissipate within minutes of terminating administration.

Cardiac Indications. Pain from acute myocardial infarction.

Precautions. Contraindications to nitrous oxide administration are the following:

- Any altered level of consciousness
- Chest trauma
- Abdominal distension
- Any respiratory problems or cyanosis that occurs with administration
- Early pregnancy
- *Inebriation* (alcohol intoxication)
- Inability to comply with instructions (e.g., senility, mental retardation, young children)

Administration and Dosage. Nitrous oxide must be self-administered by the patient. It is intermittently inhaled through a demand valve as needed until pain relief occurs or until drowsiness causes the patient to drop the administration mask or mouthpiece.

Side Effects and Special Considerations.

1. Side effects include drowsiness, nausea, slurred speech, and headache, light-headedness, euphoria, or confusion.
2. The ambulance must be well ventilated to prevent drug effects on the paramedic; use of an exhalation scavenger is recommended.
3. Patients with cardiac pain must be given oxygen during intervals when nitrous oxide is not being administered.
4. The exact role of nitrous oxide as an analgesic in prehospital care has not yet been well defined. While reports of its use in that environment indicate both efficacy and safety, many are concerned about possible side effects, both short-term and long-term.

Furosemide

Pharmacology and Actions. **Furosemide** is a rapid-acting drug that promotes urine excretion by inhibiting sodium reabsorption in the kidney. It also causes increased potassium excretion. In addition, IV administration is thought to cause venous dilation that results in decreased venous return or preload.

Cardiac Indications. Acute pulmonary edema.

Precautions. Furosemide is contraindicated in hypovolemic states and in pregnancy. Blood pressure should be monitored closely after administration, as hypotension could result from combined vasodilation and diuretic effects.

Administration and Dosage. The usual dosage of furosemide for management of acute pulmonary edema is 40 mg (normal range 0.5–2.0 mg/kg) administered IV over a 2-minute period.

Side Effects and Special Considerations. Immediate side effects include hypotension, nausea, and vomiting. With diuresis, dehydration and hypokalemia with associated cardiac arrhythmias can occur.

Theophylline Ethylenediamine

Pharmacology and Actions. **Theophylline ethylenediamine** (Aminophylline) acts primarily as a bronchodilator by its direct relaxant effect on the smooth muscle of the bronchial airways. Other effects include dilation of peripheral blood vessels, mild diuresis, and stimulation of cardiac, cerebral, and skeletal muscle tissues.

Cardiac Indications. Theophylline ethylenediamine may be useful for patients who experience respiratory distress secondary to bronchospasm in pulmonary edema of cardiac origin. More common use, however, is for patients with bronchospasm secondary to anaphylaxis, asthma, or COPD.

Precautions. This drug must be used with caution in patients with suspected myocardial infarction, hypotension, or arrhythmias because of its cardiac effects. In addition, patients with heart failure or hepatic disease may warrant a reduced drug dosage. Theophylline ethylenediamine should be administered slowly, usually by IV drip, to lessen risk of toxic and side effects, and the EKG should be monitored closely for arrhythmias during administration. The paramedic should determine if the patient is taking oral theophylline preparations and report this information to the base physician for reduction of theophylline ethylenediamine dosage.

Administration and Dosage. For pulmonary edema, 250 to 500 mg of theophylline ethylenediamine is usually added to 50 to 100 mg of D_5W and administered by IV infusion over at least a 20-minute period.

Side Effects and Special Considerations.

1. Cardiovascular side effects, particularly arrhythmias, are the most serious.
2. Hypotension, nausea and vomiting, and CNS disturbances, such as headache, dizziness, agitation, and light-headedness, are common side effects.

Dopamine

Pharmacology and Actions. A chemical precursor of epinephrine, **dopamine** exerts its cardiovascular effects from stimulation of dopamine receptors in the renal and mesenteric arteries and also from action on β- and α-adrenergic receptors. At low dosages (2–10 μg/kg/min), dopamine increases cardiac output and increases renal blood flow and, therefore, kidney function, with little or no peripheral vasoconstriction. However, drug effects are dose-related. At dosages of 10 to 20 μg/kg/min, the α effect of vasoconstriction occurs and may cause renal vasoconstriction. At dosages higher than 20 μg/kg/min, the α effect predominates, and renal and mesenteric blood flow decreases.

Cardiac Indications. Dopamine is the initial drug of choice for management of cardiogenic shock to increase cardiac output while maintaining renal function.

Precautions. Dopamine is contraindicated in the presence of uncontrolled arrhythmias, severe hypovolemia, or history of *pheochromocytoma* (tumor of the adrenal gland).

The IV site must be monitored closely, as dopamine infiltration may cause tissue necrosis. Administration must be precisely controlled to obtain desired results and avoid toxicity; therefore, meticulous monitoring of the IV infusion and patient vital signs is needed. An IV infusion pump is the preferred method of regulation. The patient who is taking potentiating monoamine oxidase inhibitors (e.g., Parnate, Marplan, Nardil) must be given reduced dosages of dopamine.

Administration and Dosage. Dopamine is administered by continuous IV infusion only, using a microdrip administration tubing. Mixing 200 mg of dopamine in 250 mL of D_5W yields a concentration of 800 $\mu g/mL$. The infusion usually is started at 2 to 5 $\mu g/kg/min$ and adjusted according to the patient's clinical response.

Side Effects and Special Considerations. Side effects of dopamine are tachyarrhythmia and ectopic beats, nausea and vomiting, headache, and angina, especially at higher doses.

Epinephrine

Pharmacology and Actions. **Epinephrine** acts directly on β-adrenergic receptors of the heart to increase rate and contractility and on α-adrenergic receptors in blood vessels to increase systemic vascular resistance. The results of these actions are increased cardiac output and blood pressure. The major benefit of epinephrine use in cardiac arrest is thought to be improved coronary and cerebral blood flow during CPR. Epinephrine also causes bronchodilation by β stimulation.

Cardiac Indications. Cardiac arrest secondary to ventricular fibrillation, asystole, or electromechanical dissociation, to improve perfusion during CPR and to stimulate or enhance cardiac electrical activity, and bradyarrhythmia that is refractory to other therapy.

Precautions. The use of epinephrine for cardiac arrest has no contraindications except, in some instances, for cardiac arrest due to ventricular tachycardia. Intracardiac injection in the field is not recommended because of numerous complications, including production of intractable ventricular fibrillation if injected into the myocardium.

Administration and Dosage. In cardiac arrest, epinephrine 1:10,000 solution is administered IV in a dose of 0.5 to 1.0 mg. This dose may be repeated at 5-minute intervals as necessary. Larger doses (5–10 mg) are being investigated and may be recommended in the near future. When an IV route cannot be established or is delayed, 1.0 mg of 1:10,000 epinephrine can be administered through an endotracheal tube.

Side Effects and Special Considerations. Epinephrine has no side effects in a nonperfusing cardiac arrest patient. Side effects encountered when epinephrine is used for perfusing bradyarrhythmia is discussed in the last part of this chapter.

Sodium Bicarbonate

Pharmacology and Actions. **Sodium bicarbonate ($NaHCO_3$)** is an alkalinizing agent sometimes used to treat acidosis that results from metabolism by hypoxic body tissues during cardiac arrest. Sodium bicarbonate raises arterial blood pH by combining with excess hydrogen ions:

$$HCO_3^- + H^+ \rightleftharpoons H_2CO_3 \rightleftharpoons CO_2 + H_2O$$

A result of this buffering reaction is the formation of carbon dioxide, which must be eliminated by the lungs. Although previously thought to improve the outcome from cardiac arrest by reversing the adverse effects of acidosis, sodium bicarbonate, current data indicate, has many detrimental effects that outweigh its possible benefits in most situations (see side effects).

Cardiac Indications. Sodium bicarbonate should be used, if at all, for cardiac arrest only after more proven interventions, such as defibrillation, support of ventilation including intubation, and pharmacologic therapies such as epinephrine and antiarrhythmic drugs, have been employed. For this reason, sodium bicarbonate is not indicated during approximately the first 10 minutes of management of a routine cardiac arrest.

Precautions. Sodium bicarbonate may inactivate catecholamines and, therefore, should not be administered or allowed to mix with drugs such as epinephrine and dopamine.

Administration and Dosage. When used for cardiac arrest, 1 mEq/kg should be given as the initial dose, and no more than half this dose should be given every 10 minutes thereafter.

Side Effects and Special Considerations. Current laboratory and clinical data indicate that sodium bicarbonate may have the following effects:

1. May produce an acidosis from carbon dioxide generation; rapidly diffusible carbon dioxide enters myocardial and brain cells and may depress their function
2. May worsen central venous (and therefore generalized tissue) acidosis as a consequence of carbon dioxide retention
3. May induce hyperosmolality and hypernatremia
4. May cause extracellular alkalosis and lead to such

adverse effects as acute hypokalemia and cardiac arrhythmias
5. May impair the release of oxygen from hemoglobin

For all of these reasons, in addition to the fact that this drug has not been shown to improve survival from cardiac arrest, sodium bicarbonate is no longer standard initial treatment in cardiac arrest.

ARRHYTHMIAS: INTERPRETATION AND THERAPEUTIC INTERVENTION

As described in the first part of this chapter, the normal electrical conduction pathway of the heart consists of the SA node, the internodal and interatrial tracts, the AV node, the bundle of His, the right and left bundle branches, and the Purkinje system. Depolarization of the heart muscle via this conduction pathway can be graphically displayed on an EKG. Each wave of an EKG recording can be related to an electrical activity that occurs in the heart. The purpose of this section is to provide a full explanation of the normal EKG and the various abnormal rhythms, or **arrhythmias,** that can create complications for the cardiac patient. Recognition of these arrhythmias must be combined with knowledge of their physiologic effects and appropriate emergency intervention.

Basic Concepts of EKG Monitoring

Movement of electrolytes across the membranes of myocardial cells (depolarization and repolarization) results in a flow of electrical current and the creation of an electrical field. The body acts as a giant conductor of electrical current. Electrical activity that originates in the heart can be detected on the body surface by applying skin electrodes to measure voltage changes of the cells between them. These voltage changes are amplified and visually displayed on an oscilloscope and graph paper. The resulting EKG is a series of continuous waves and deflections that reflect the heart's electrical activity from a certain "view." Many views, each called a lead, can be obtained by monitoring the voltage changes between electrodes placed in a variety of positions on the body. A *bipolar lead* is merely a combination of two electrodes, one negative and one positive. Any electrical impulse that is moving directly toward the positive electrode of a bipolar lead creates the largest upright (positive) deflection possible on EKG. An impulse that is moving directly away from the positive electrode creates the largest downward (negative) deflection (Fig. 20-25). No deflection, called an *isoelectric line,* means that either no electrical impulse is present or it is moving perpendicular to the electrodes.

A full 12-lead EKG is normally inspected in-hospital to obtain a more complete view of cardiac electrical ac-

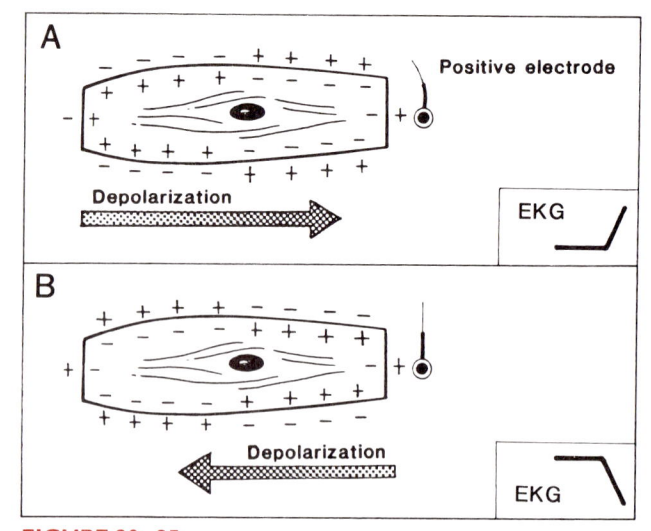

FIGURE 20-25.
Influence of electrical flow direction on EKG deflections.

tivity. A 12-lead EKG may be necessary to make a definitive diagnosis of some arrhythmias, such as a wide-complex tachycardia. Field 12-lead EKGs may also be used more commonly if thrombolytic intervention is shown to be beneficial and feasible in the prehospital setting. However, for basic arrhythmia interpretation in prehospital care, it is usually sufficient to use a single bipolar lead. This single lead, sometimes referred to as a monitoring lead, usually is noncalibrated in respect to the EKG machine and is chosen because it displays clear wave forms. The two most commonly used leads for prehospital EKG monitoring are **lead II** and **modified chest lead 1 (MCL$_1$)**. A monitoring lead uses three skin electrodes, a positive, negative, and ground. Figure 20-26 illustrates the placement of electrodes for both lead II and MCL$_1$. In lead II, the summation of the heart's electrical current flows directly toward the positive electrode. This flow produces the best view of the EKG waves, a fact that accounts for the frequent use of this lead for monitoring. The MCL$_1$ is used in some systems and helps determine the site of origin of some abnormal complexes. This text only examines how various EKG waves relate to each other in a single lead and only refers to lead II interpretation.

Paper tracings of the EKG patterns from a monitoring lead inscribed on graph paper are called rhythm strips. Rhythm strips are valuable because they permit analysis of the EKG in more detail. A number of factors can be measured and compared because the graph paper moves past a heated stylus at a standard, constant speed, usually 25 mm/second (Fig. 20-27).

The vertical lines on the graph measure time—one small box equals .04 second, one large box equals .20 second—and can be used to measure the duration of various events. Horizontal lines on the graph paper measure voltage—0.1 mV per each small box. Voltage measurement,

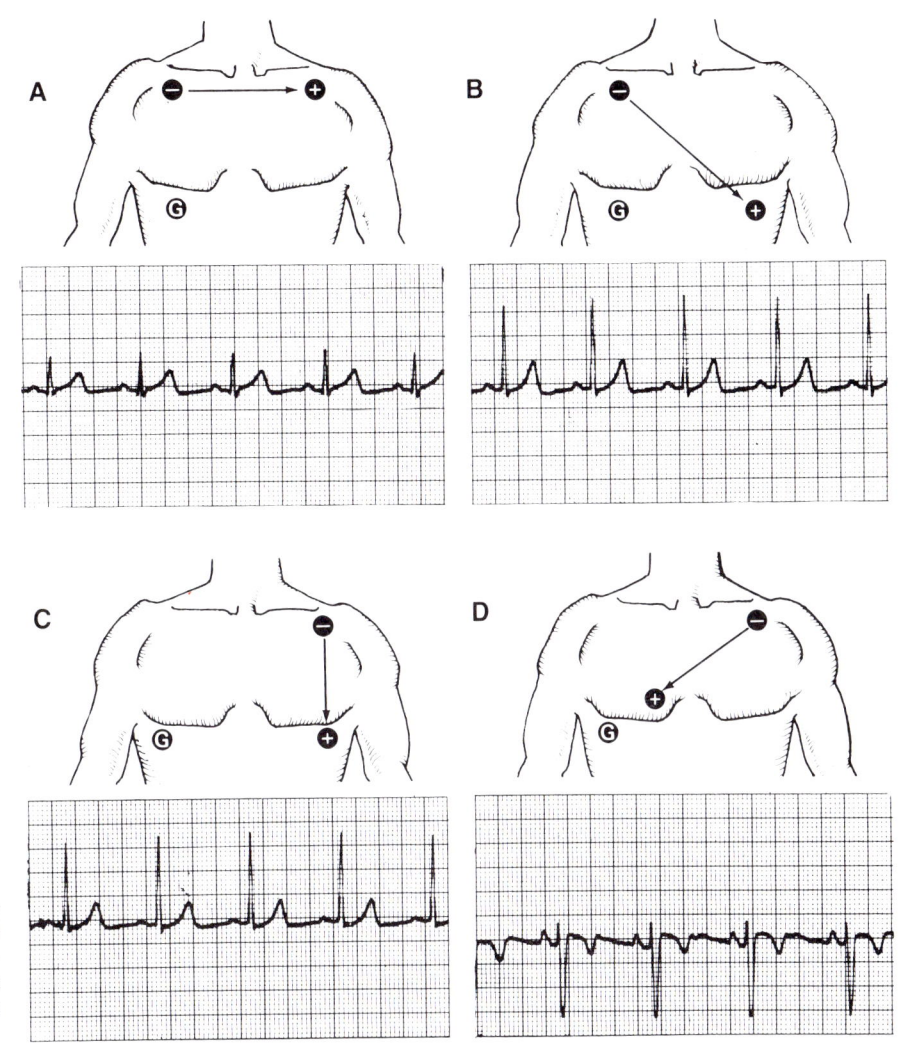

FIGURE 20-26.
Electrode placement for monitoring leads. Lead I (**A**), lead II (**B**), lead III (**C**), lead MCL₁ (**D**). (© American Heart Association: Textbook of Advanced Cardiac Life Support, 2nd ed, p 52. Dallas, American Heart Association, 1987)

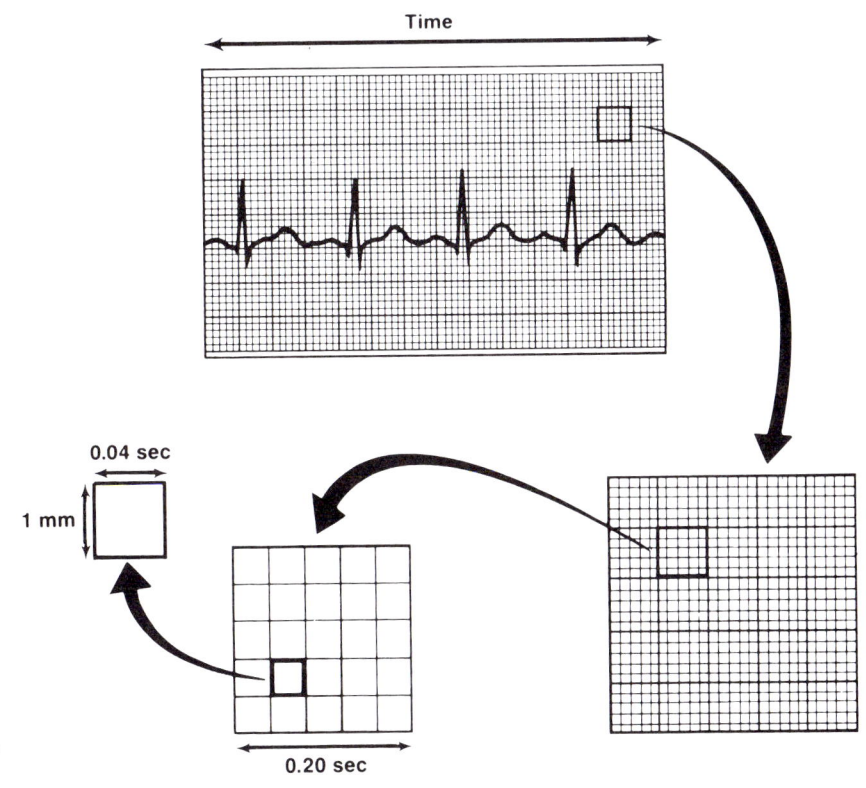

FIGURE 20-27.
EKG graph paper values. (Bunting–Blake L, Parker J, Weigel A, White RD)

435

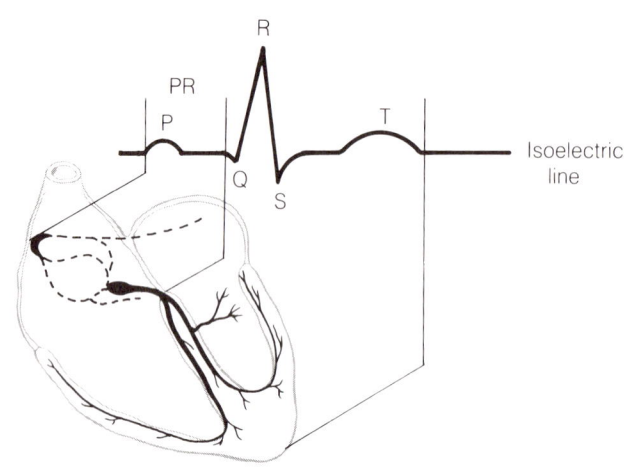

FIGURE 20-28.
Relationship of electrical events in the heart to surface EKG.

however, is only relevant when considering calibrated tracings, such as with a 12-lead EKG.

P Wave, QRS Complex, and T Wave

With these basic concepts in mind, this section examines how an EKG tracing specifically reflects cardiac electrical activity. A single cardiac cycle inscribes waves on the EKG that correspond to each electrical event in the heart from the beginning of depolarization of the atria, up to and including repolarization of the ventricles. The waves of a single cardiac cycle are labeled the P wave, QRS complex, and T wave (Fig. 20-28). Between waves and cycles, the EKG records an isoelectric line, which indicates absence of net electrical activity.

The **P wave**, usually the first wave seen, is a small, rounded upright (positive) wave that indicates depolarization of the atria has occurred. The **QRS complex** is a collective term for three deflections that follow the P wave: the **Q wave**, the first downward (negative) deflection after the P wave; the **R wave**, the first positive deflection after the P wave; and the **S wave**, the first negative deflection after the R wave. Although all three waves are not always seen, and the QRS line can have a variety of shapes, it is always referred to as a QRS complex. It indicates that depolarization of the ventricular muscle has occurred.

The **T wave**, the rounded wave that follows and is usually in the same direction as the QRS complex, corresponds with repolarization of the ventricles. No wave is normally visible to indicate atrial repolarization, as it is overshadowed by the QRS complex. Two intervals are also frequently considered on the EKG (Fig. 20-29). The **PR interval** is the distance between the beginning of the P wave and the beginning of the QRS complex. This interval measures the time it takes a depolarization wave to travel from the atria to the ventricles, including the delay at the AV node. The other interval, the **ST segment**, is the distance between the S wave of the QRS complex and the beginning of the T wave. This interval, which is usually an isoelectric line, indicates the length of time between ventricular depolarization and the beginning of repolarization.

A final event that can be recorded on surface EKG is the heart's refractory period. This is the recovery period of the heart, the period of time when cells have been depolarized but have not yet returned to their polarized state, and, thus, they are unable to respond to stimulation. On an EKG, this period includes the QRS complex and T wave and may be further defined as absolute and relative refractory periods (Fig. 20-30). The absolute refractory period, from the beginning of the QRS complex to the apex of the T wave, is the time during which electrical stimulation produces no depolarization at all. However, during the *relative refractory period* (vulnerable period), on the down slope of the T wave, depolarization may occur if the electrical stimulus is sufficiently strong.

In addition to the EKG waves produced by the heart's electrical activity, deflections are occasionally produced by other influences and are referred to as *EKG artifact*.

Since artifact in the EKG tracing can make interpretation difficult, the paramedic needs to recognize and eliminate it whenever possible. Some of the common causes of *artifact* are loose electrodes, patient movement

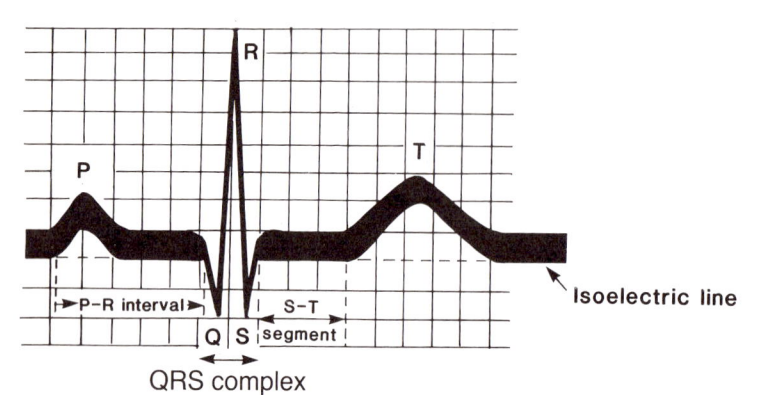

FIGURE 20-29.
The electrical pattern of the cardiac cycle shows waves and intervals.

CHAPTER 20: Cardiovascular Emergencies 437

and muscle tremors, EKG calibration marks, 60-cycle (electrical) interference, and malfunction of the EKG machine, patient cable, or lead wires (Fig. 20-31).

Despite the heavy emphasis of this section on EKG interpretation, it is important to keep in mind that an EKG rhythm strip only provides limited information about the heart's electrical activity and virtually no information about the adequacy of cardiac contraction. Information that cannot be obtained with certainty from an EKG monitoring lead includes the presence or location of a myocardial infarction, enlargement of heart chambers, and side-to-side changes in conduction or location of impulse formation. It is usually necessary to record a full 12-lead EKG to obtain this information. Important information the paramedic can derive from a monitoring lead includes heart rate, regularity, *ectopy* (abnormal im-

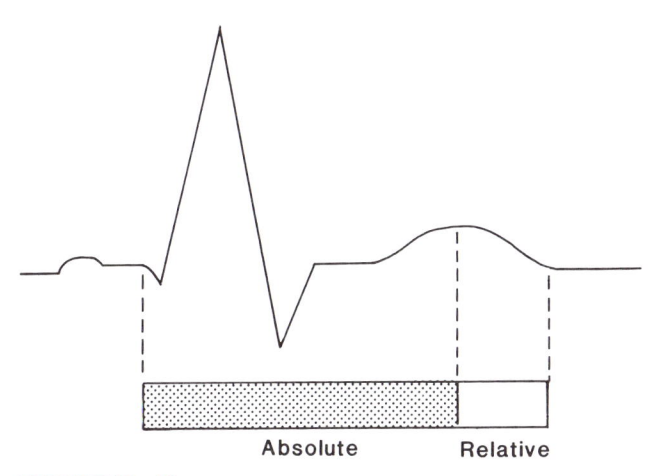

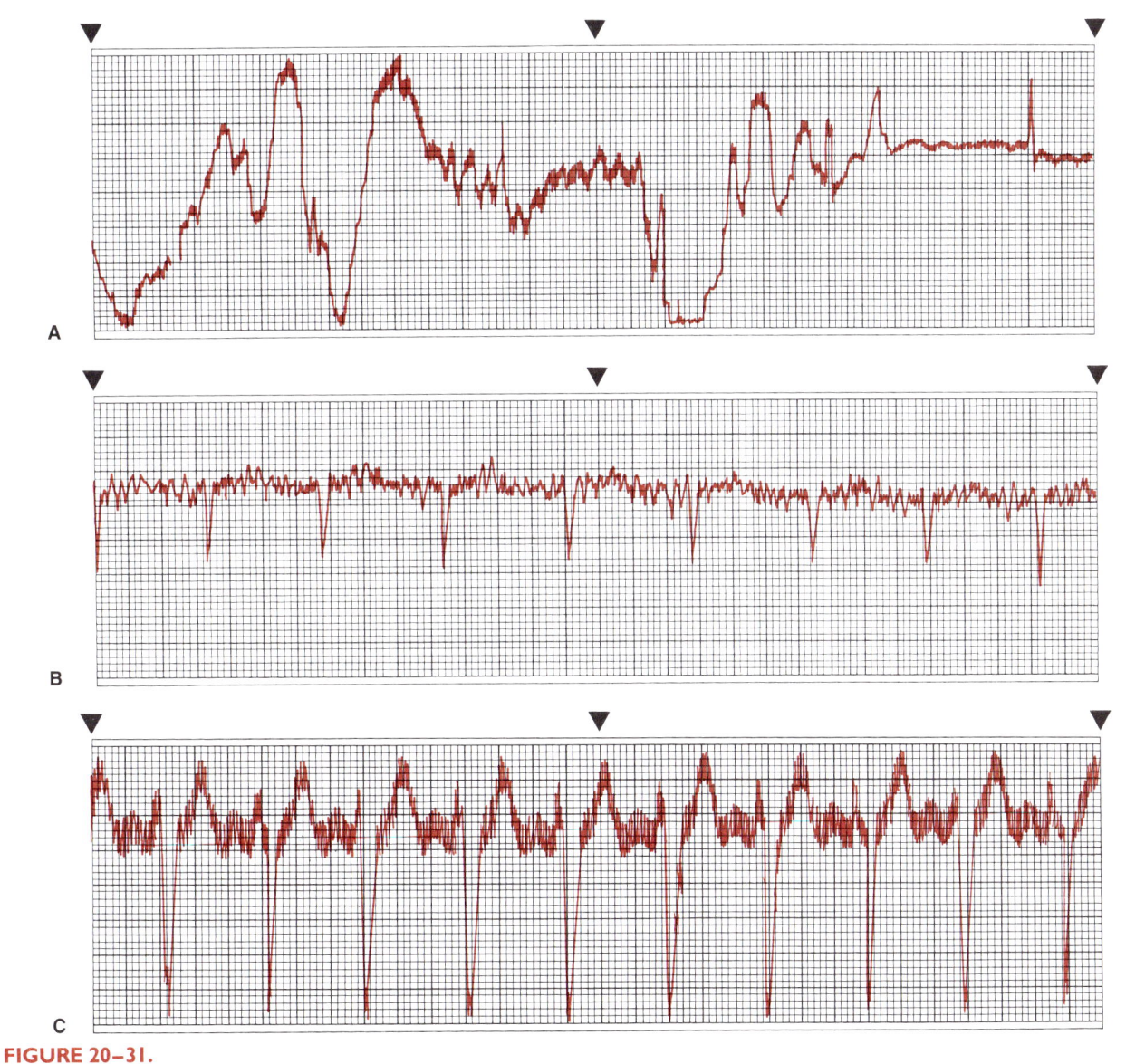

FIGURE 20-30
Refractory period.

FIGURE 20-31.
Artifact. Loose electrodes (**A**), muscle tremor (**B**), and 60-cycle interference (**C**). (Bunting–Blake L, Parker J, Weigel A, White RD)

pulses), and conduction time in various parts of the heart. This information, however basic, is what the paramedic and medical control physician consider along with clinical findings to determine prehospital intervention.

As previously suggested, some EMS systems may use field 12-lead EKGs to obtain information indicative of acute myocardial infarction, such as ST segment elevation, either in preparation for in-hospital administration of thrombolytic drugs or for the prehospital administration of such drugs. These diagnostic and therapeutic interventions are investigational at this time. If their feasibility and efficacy are established, 12-lead EKG recording in the field will become more common.

Rhythm Strip Analysis

Arrhythmia interpretation is most easily accomplished when a consistent approach or format is used in the analysis process. Each of the many possible arrhythmias can be described according to the chosen format, and the "rules" for known arrhythmias can be used as a comparison for analysis of an unknown arrhythmia. Although any number of formats can be used, the paramedic should strive to use one approach consistently and perform all steps in the analysis process to avoid interpretation errors. The format that is used in this text is to analyze rate, rhythm, P waves, PR interval, and QRS complex.

The first step is to *analyze the rate*. In most cases, this step calculates the ventricular rate, but both atrial and ventricular rates should be examined if they differ. The rate of most regular rhythms can be quickly determined by counting the number of graph boxes between two R waves on the rhythm strip. The number of large boxes divided into 300 or the number of small boxes divided into 1500 yields the rate per minute. Although it is easiest to memorize the values for large boxes (Table 20-1), it may at times be necessary to count small boxes, especially if the rate is rapid. Another way to estimate rate is to count the number of R waves that occur in a 6-second strip, using time markers on the EKG graph paper and multiplying that number by 10 (Fig. 20-32). Although this calculation is less accurate, it is the best method to use to obtain an average rate for irregular rhythms that have varying intervals between the R waves. A normal heart rate is 60 to 100 complexes per minute. Any rate less than 60 per minute is termed bradycardia, and a rate greater than 100 is called tachycardia.

Step 2 in the analysis format is to *analyze the rhythm*. This analysis is accomplished by measuring the intervals between the R waves across an entire rhythm strip to determine regularity or irregularity (Fig. 20-33). If the rhythm is irregular, it should be noted whether the irregularity has any pattern, whether the irregularity is just occasional in one or two R-

TABLE 20-1.
HEART RATE CALCULATION BY COUNTING NUMBER OF LARGE BOXES

Number of Large Boxes	Rate/Min.
1	300
2	150
3	100
4	75
5	60
6	50
7	43
8	37
9	33
10	30
11	27
12	25
13	23
14	21
15	20

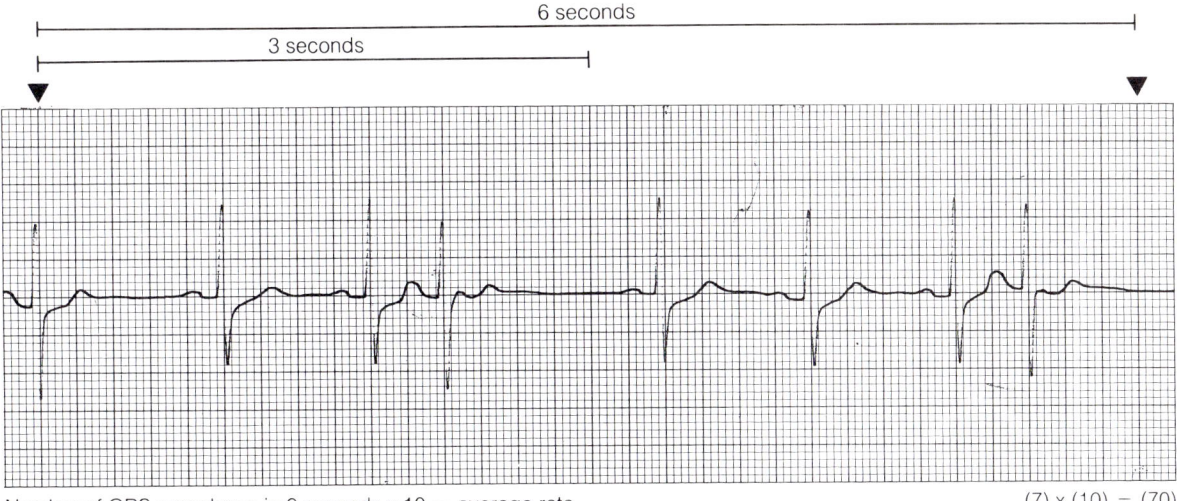

Number of QRS complexes in 6 seconds x 10 = average rate   (7) x (10) = (70)

FIGURE 20–32.
Rate calculation using EKG paper time markers (Huff J, Doernbach DP, White RD)

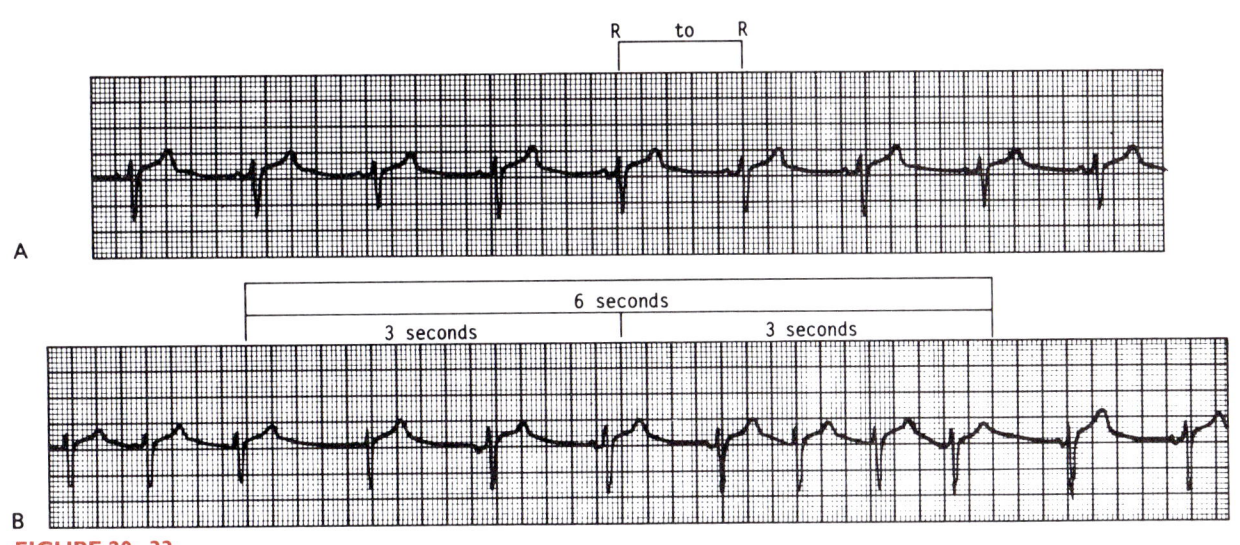

A

B

FIGURE 20–33.
Determining rhythm or irregularity. (Brunner LS and Suddarth DS)

to-R intervals, or whether the rhythm is totally irregular. Rhythms that vary less than 0.16 second (4 small boxes) between the longest and shortest R-to-R intervals are generally considered to be regular. An analysis of the atrial rhythm, the regularity of P-to-P intervals, should also be performed and leads to Step 3.

Step 3, *analyzing the P wave*, requires several additional observations. It should be determined if each QRS complex has one P wave and the P wave's position in relationship to the QRS complex, if P waves are upright or inverted, and, finally, if all P waves look alike.

Step 4, which is related to *P wave analysis*, is measurement of the PR interval. The measurement begins where the P wave first leaves the isoelectric line and ends with the first deflection of the QRS complex, whether it goes in a negative or positive direction. A normal PR interval is 0.12 to 0.20 per second, 3 to 5 small boxes, and should be constant for all complexes in the strip.

Step 5, the final step, is to *analyze the QRS complexes* in appearance and duration. Measurements are made from the first deflection of the QRS complex to where the S wave stops and begins the ST segment. If these points are above or below the baseline, an imaginary line can be dropped from the point to the baseline to help measure. All QRS complexes in a normal rhythm should look alike and measure 0.10 second or less (less than 3 small boxes) from the first to the last deflection (Fig. 20-34). Some references state that a duration of up to 0.12 second may be normal. This number may be used as an acceptable upper limit, or the borderline of normal.

440 UNIT FOUR: MEDICAL EMERGENCIES

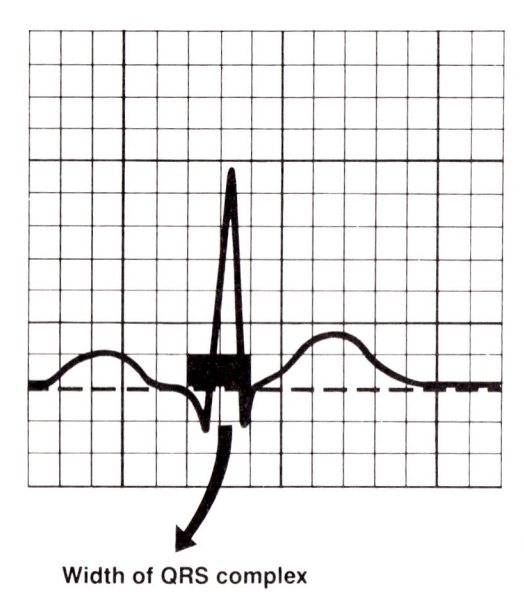

Width of QRS complex

FIGURE 20–34.
Measuring QRS complex duration. (Bunting–Blake L, Parker J, Weigel A, White RD)

Using the above format, we are now able to describe the heart's normal EKG rhythm, that is, the normal sinus rhythm, as it would appear on a lead II rhythm strip:

RATE: *60–100/min*
RHYTHM: *Regular, both atrial and ventricular*
P WAVES: *One before each QRS complex; all upright and uniform*
PR INTERVAL: *0.12–0.20 sec and constant*
QRS COMPLEX: *0.10 or less sec and all alike*

Immediately following, there is a reproduction of an actual rhythm strip showing a variation of normal sinus rhythm, accompanied by a description of its characteristics.

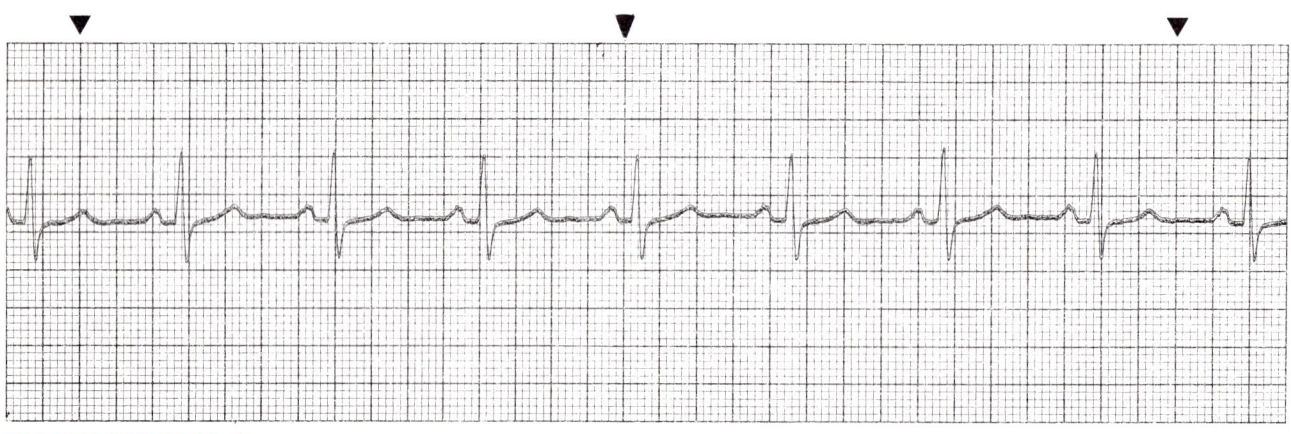

RHYTHM STRIP 20–1.
(Huff J, Doernbach DP, White RD)

STRIP #: *1*
RATE: *75/min*
RHYTHM: *Regular*
P WAVE: *One per QRS complex; upright and uniform*
PR INTERVAL: *0.16 sec and constant*
QRS COMPLEX: *0.08 sec and all alike*
RHYTHM INTERPRETATION: *Normal sinus rhythm*

Etiology and Mechanism of Arrhythmias

Arrhythmias have numerous causes, including the following:

- Myocardial ischemia or infarction
- Distention of heart chambers (often caused by congestive heart failure)
- Hypoxia
- Acid-base imbalance
- Electrolyte imbalance
- Autonomic nervous system imbalance
- Drug side effects and toxicity
- CNS damage
- Hypothermia
- Electrocution

In certain instances, arrhythmias may be a normal occurrence. They may have little significance in a healthy heart and not require the same management as arrhythmias that occur in the setting of myocardial ischemia. No matter what the cause or type of arrhythmia, it must be continuously emphasized that patients should be treated according to their symptoms, not merely their EKG.

Two mechanisms basically are responsible for the occurrence of arrhythmias. The first is a disorder of impulse formation or *automaticity*, which was previously discussed in relation to the heart's pacemaker cells. When automaticity is enhanced, electrical impulses may be initiated in cardiac cells other than those that usually possess the capability to spontaneously depolarize. Increased or enhanced automaticity is often the mechanism that creates tachycardia and premature complexes. Conversely, depressed automaticity leads to bradycardia.

The other mechanism responsible for arrhythmias is a disorder of conduction called *reentry*. Reentry occurs when conductivity is altered in the various branches of a conduction pathway. For reentry to occur, one branch of a conduction path must have slowed conduction while the other branch has a one-way block (Fig. 20-35). As an advancing depolarization wave is able to move forward slowly through one branch but not the other, it may circle back and conduct "backward" (*retrograde*) through the branch that was originally blocked (block is unidirectional). By the time the impulse arrives back at the origin of the branch, the depolarized tissue has sufficiently repolarized to respond to stimulation, and the process repeats itself. This phenomenon is sometimes referred to as circus reentry and can

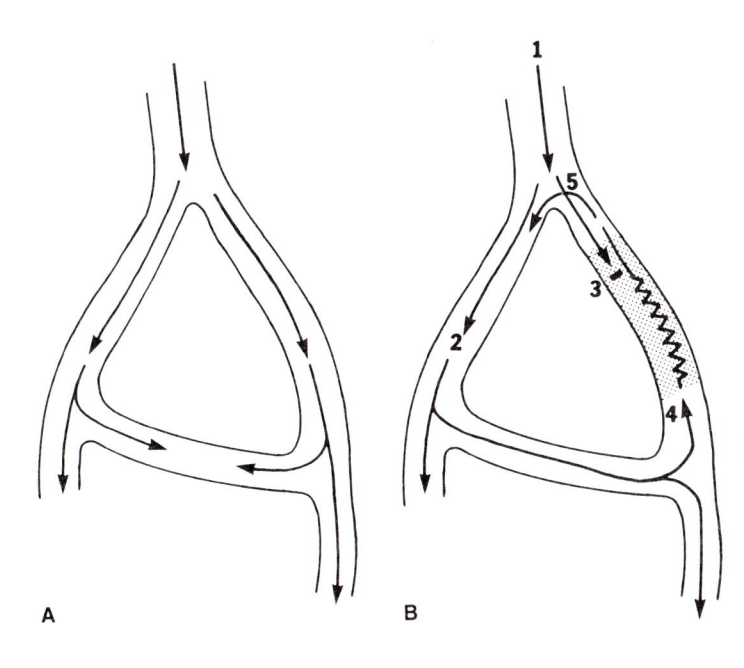

FIGURE 20-35.
(**A**) The conduction velocity is uniform through normal terminal Purkinje fibers. (**B**) A severely depressed segment of terminal Purkinje causes the impulse (1) to travel normally (2), be blocked at the depressed segment (3), return through this tissue from the opposite direction (4), and initiate reentry phenomenon (5).

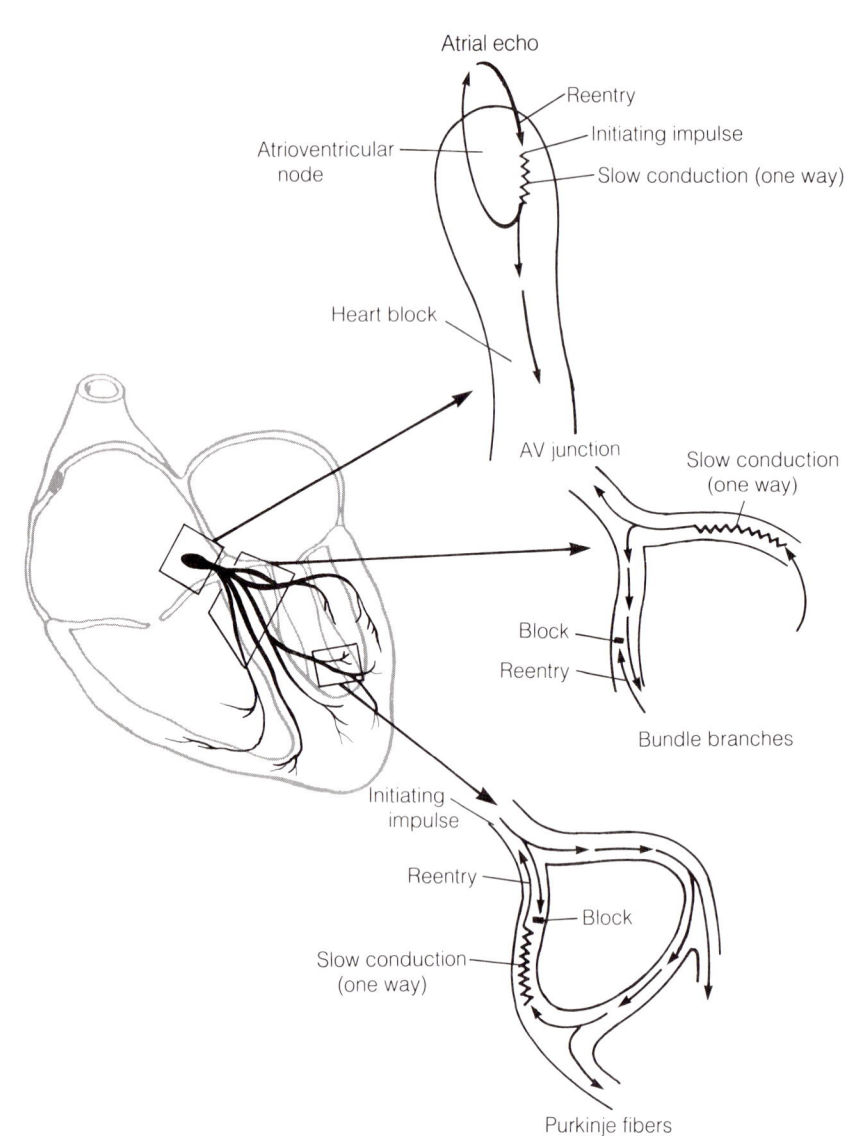

FIGURE 20-36.
Reentry in various areas of the heart.

either create rapid rates or isolated premature complexes. Reentry may occur in any part of the myocardium or conduction network (Fig. 20-36).

Of the arrhythmias discussed here, some are caused by changes in automaticity, some by reentry, and some by a combination of these two mechanisms. Although it is often impossible to distinguish between these two mechanisms on surface EKG, understanding the concepts helps to master EKG interpretation and the rationale for various therapeutic modalities. In addition to reentry, other disorders of conduction are discussed later in this section.

Arrhythmias That Originate in the SA Node

The EKG features common to all cardiac rhythms that originate in the SA node (the sinus rhythms) are upright P waves that are all similar in appearance, normal duration PR intervals, and normal duration QRS complexes, assuming no ventricular conduction disturbances are present. Sinus rhythms to be described, in addition to normal sinus rhythm, are sinus bradycardia, sinus tachycardia, sinus arrhythmia, and sinus arrest.

Sinus Bradycardia

Sinus bradycardia is the rhythm that results when SA node discharge is less than 60 per minute. Etiology of this rhythm includes increased vagal tone, SA node disease or ischemia, and certain drug effects, such as digitalis and β blockers. The EKG characteristics for a lead II rhythm strip are the following:

RATE: *Less than 60/min*
RHYTHM: *Regular*
P WAVES: *One before each QRS complex; all upright and uniform*
PR INTERVAL: *Constant and normal (0.12–0.20 sec)*
QRS COMPLEX: *Normal (0.10 sec or less)*

Clinical Significance. Sinus bradycardia is normal in athletes and during sleep. In acute myocardial infarction, it may be protective and beneficial, or the slow rate may compromise cardiac output, resulting in further ischemia, hypotension, or CNS symptoms. It may also predispose to premature ectopic complexes and rhythms.

Management. None is indicated if the patient is asymptomatic. If hypotension or premature beats are present, atropine is the drug of choice.

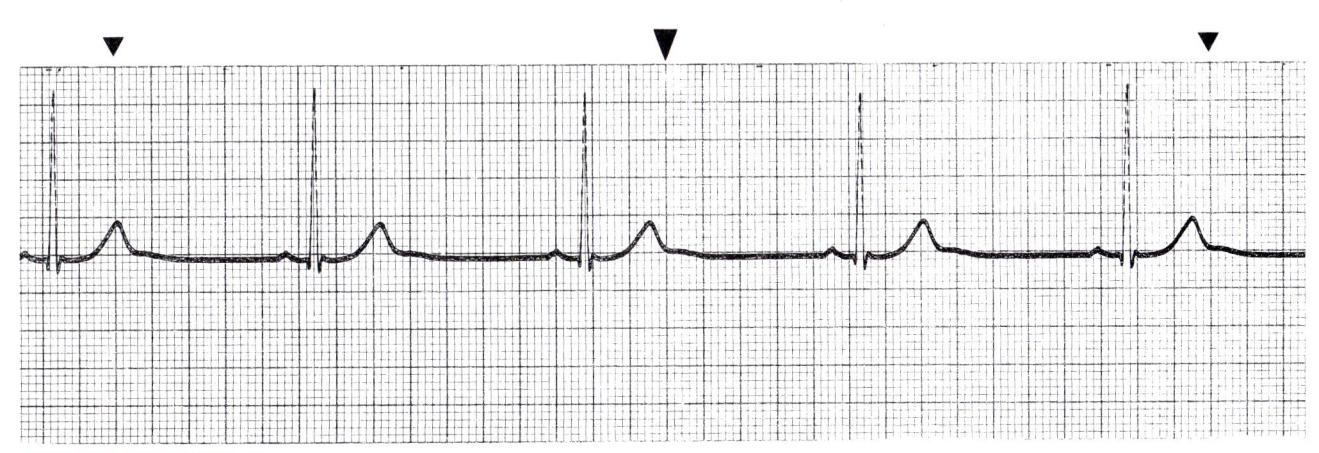

RHYTHM STRIP 20–2.
(Huff J, Doernbach DP, White RD)

STRIP #: *2*
RATE: *40/min*
RHYTHM: *Regular*
P WAVE: *One per QRS complex; upright and uniform*
PR INTERVAL: *0.14–0.16 sec*
QRS COMPLEX: *0.08 sec and all alike*
RHYTHM INTERPRETATION: *Sinus bradycardia*

Sinus Tachycardia

Sinus tachycardia results when the SA node discharges at a rate greater than 100 per minute. Upper limits of sinus discharge at rest are about 150 to 160, although the sinus discharge is capable of pacing faster than this with exercise. The etiology of this arrhythmia includes a number of physiologic stresses, including exercise, anxiety, fever, anemia, hypovolemia, and pump failure. The EKG characteristics for a lead II rhythm strip are the following:

RATE: *Greater than 100*
RHYTHM: *Regular*
P WAVES: *One before each QRS complex, all upright and uniform*
PR INTERVAL: *Constant and normal (0.12–0.20 sec)*
QRS COMPLEX: *Normal (0.10 sec or less)*

Clinical Significance. Sinus tachycardia may be of no physiologic significance. However, it may reflect compensation for a decreased stroke volume, and the increased rate may cause detrimental increases in myocardial oxygen demand, especially in patients with coronary artery disease.

Management. Place the patient at rest and attempt to determine and correct underlying disease state or condition.

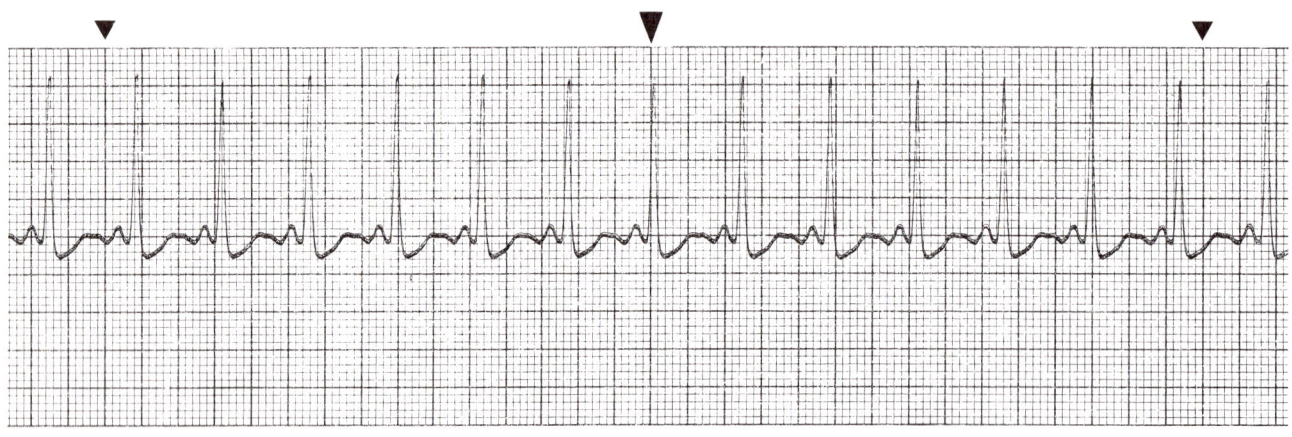

RHYTHM STRIP 20–3.
(Huff J, Doernbach DP, White RD)

STRIP #: *3*
RATE: *125/min*
RHYTHM: *Regular*
P WAVE: *One per QRS complex; upright and uniform*
PR INTERVAL: *0.12 sec and constant*
QRS COMPLEX: *0.06–0.08 sec and all alike*
RHYTHM INTERPRETATION: *Sinus tachycardia*

Sinus Arrhythmia

Sinus arrhythmia occurs when irregular discharge of the SA node manifests itself by a cyclical variation of the R-to-R interval. The most common etiology is the influence of the inspiratory and expiratory phases of the respiratory cycle. There is also a form of sinus arrhythmia that is not influenced by respiration. The EKG characteristics for a lead II rhythm strip are the following:

RATE: *Usually normal (60–100/min); frequently increases with inspiration and decreases with expiration*
RHYTHM: *Irregular by 0.16/sec or more between the longest and shortest R-to-R intervals; rhythm variation is cyclical*
P WAVES: *One before each QRS complex; all upright and uniform*
PR INTERVAL: *Constant and normal (0.12–0.20 sec)*
QRS COMPLEX: *Normal (0.10 sec or less)*

Clinical Significance. This phenomenon is normal, particularly in the young and old.

Management. None required.

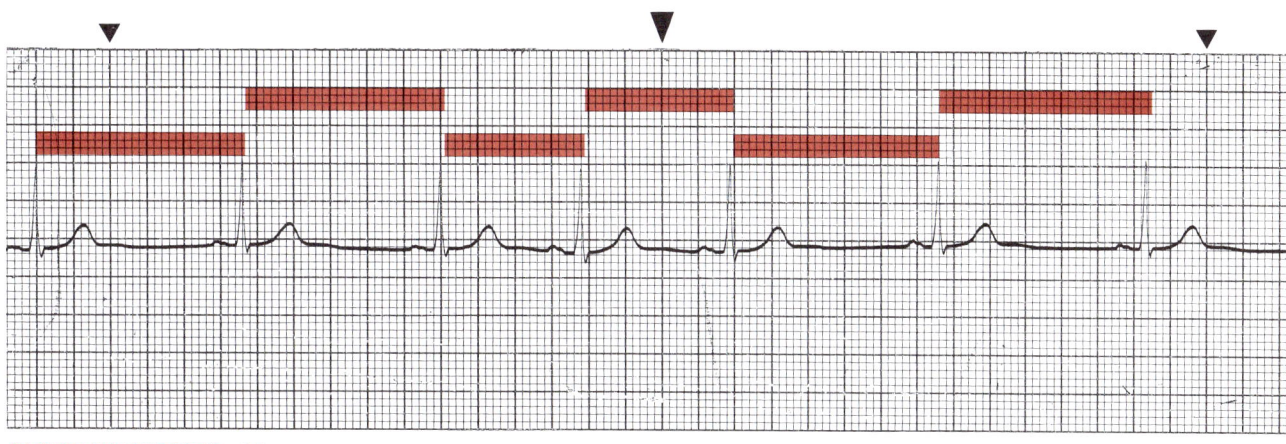

RHYTHM STRIP 20–4A.
(Huff J, Doernbach DP, White RD)

STRIP #: *4A*
RATE: *60/min*
RHYTHM: *Irregular; speeds and slows*
P WAVE: *One per QRS complex; upright and uniform*
PR INTERVAL: *0.12 sec and constant*
QRS COMPLEX: *0.06–0.08 sec and all alike*
RHYTHM INTERPRETATION: *Sinus arrhythmia*

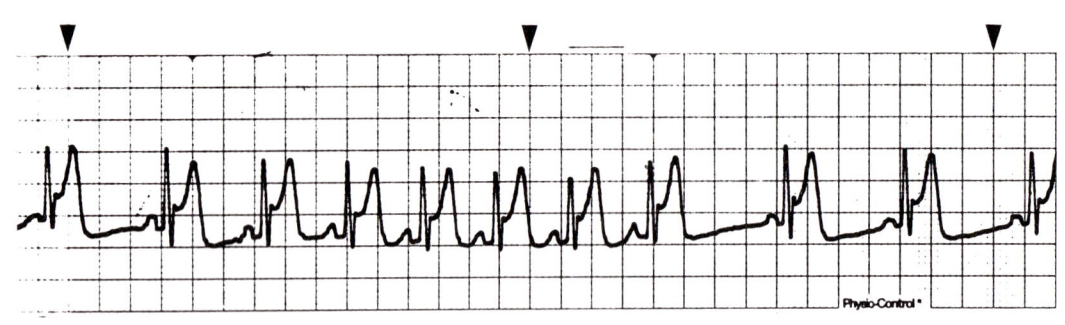

RHYTHM STRIP 20–4B.
(White RD: Paramedic EKG Collection)

STRIP #: *4B*

RATE: *90/min*

RHYTHM: *Irregular; speeds and slows*

P WAVE: *One per QRS complex; upright and uniform*

PR INTERVAL: *0.12 sec and constant*

QRS COMPLEX: *0.06 sec and all alike*

RHYTHM INTERPRETATION: *Marked sinus arrhythmia in a 60-year-old male with an acute inferior wall myocardial infarction. Hyperacute T waves and ST segment elevation are also present.*

Sinus Arrest

Sinus arrest results from failure of the SA node to discharge for a period of time and is manifested by the absence of any EKG waves for one or more cardiac cycles. Electrical activity is resumed when either the SA node resets itself and resumes discharge or when a lower latent pacemaker begins to discharge, creating an escape complex or rhythm. The etiology of sinus arrest includes ischemia of the SA node, digitalis toxicity, degenerative fibrotic disease in the SA node, or excessive vagal tone. EKG characteristics for a lead II rhythm strip are the following:

> **RATE**: *Normal to slow, depending on duration and frequency of sinus arrest*
> **RHYTHM**: *Irregular*
> **P WAVES**: *Normal but absent for one or more cardiac cycles*
> **PR INTERVAL**: *Normal but absent for one or more cardiac cycles*
> **QRS COMPLEX**: *Normal but absent for one or more cardiac cycles*

Clinical Significance. Sinus arrest may cause no symptoms if escape rhythm occurs promptly. However, frequent or prolonged sinus arrest may compromise cardiac output because of decreased rate. Slow rates may also precipitate other arrhythmias.

Management. If the patient is asymptomatic, only observation is necessary. The patient who is bradycardic and symptomatic or who is having ventricular ectopy should receive atropine to increase the sinus rate.

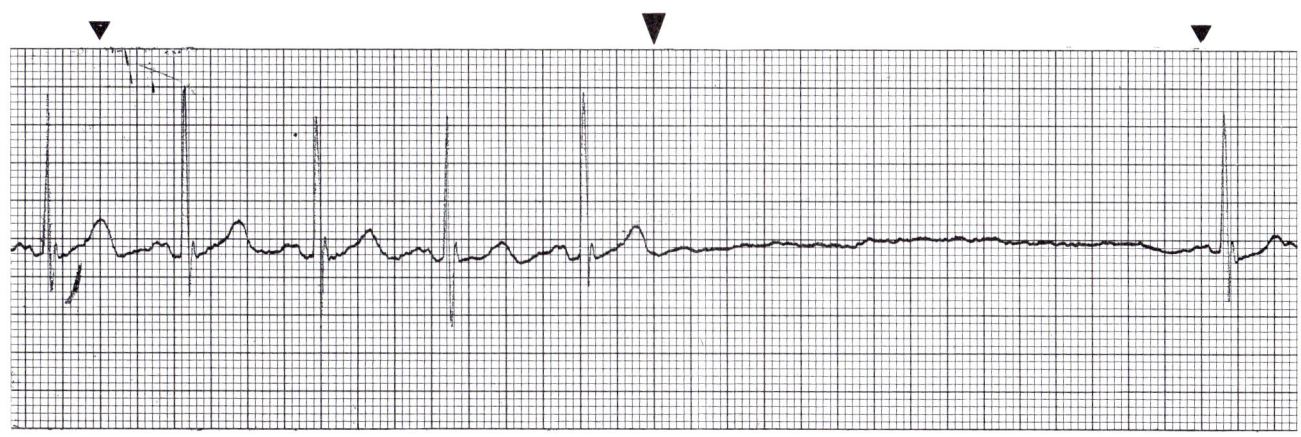

RHYTHM STRIP 20–5.
(Huff J, Doernbach DP, White RD)

STRIP #: *5*
RATE: *83/min, dropping to 17/min*
RHYTHM: *Irregular*
P WAVE: *One per QRS complex; upright and uniform; absent for 3½ secs*
PR INTERVAL: *0.16 sec and constant*
QRS COMPLEX: *0.06–0.08 sec and all alike*
RHYTHM INTERPRETATION: *Normal sinus rhythm with period of sinus arrest*

Arrhythmias That Originate in the Atria

The EKG features common to all cardiac rhythms that originate in the atria are P waves that differ in appearance from sinus P waves, and normal duration QRS complexes, provided no ventricular conduction disturbances are present. Atrial rhythms to be described are wandering atrial pacemaker, premature atrial complexes, paroxysmal supraventricular tachycardia, atrial flutter, and atrial fibrillation.

Wandering Atrial Pacemaker

Wandering atrial pacemaker occurs when the pacemaker site transfers from the SA node to other latent pacemaker sites in the atria and AV junction and then moves back to the SA node. The result of this activity is that the appearance of the P waves gradually changes over the course of several cardiac cycles. This arrhythmia, like sinus arrhythmia, is often a normal phenomenon in young and old patients but may, at times, be associated with underlying heart disease. The EKG characteristics for a lead II rhythm strip are the following:

RATE: *Normal (60–100/min)*
RHYTHM: *Usually irregular*
P WAVES: *Size and shape vary from complex to complex and may become inverted or disappear completely*
PR INTERVAL: *May vary and become less than 0.12 sec*
QRS COMPLEX: *Normal (0.10 sec or less)*

Clinical Significance. No detrimental effect.

Management. None required.

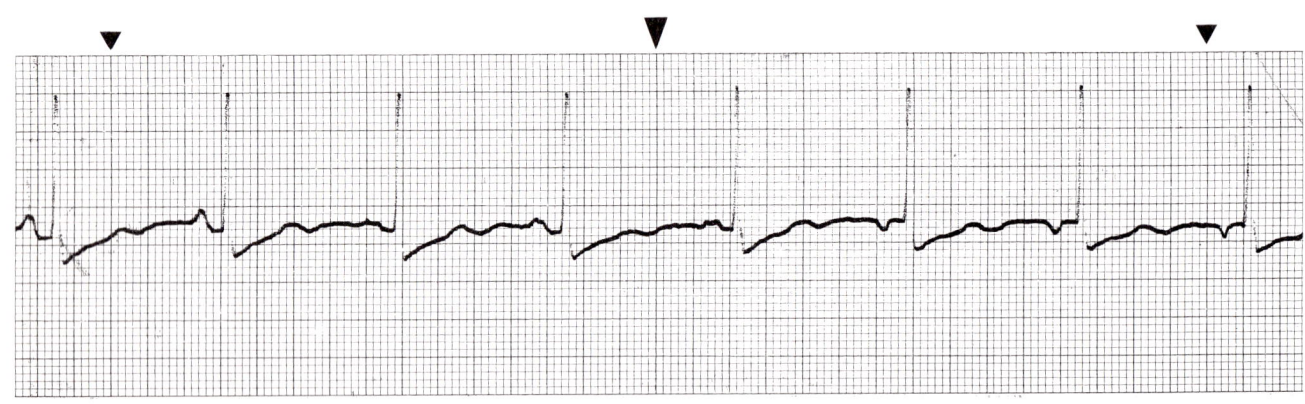

RHYTHM STRIP 20–6.
(Huff J, Doernbach DP, White RD)

STRIP #: *6*
RATE: *65/min*
RHYTHM: *Regular*
P WAVE: *One per QRS complex; vary in size and shape*
PR INTERVAL: *0.16–0.18 sec*
QRS COMPLEX: *0.04–0.06 sec and all alike*
RHYTHM INTERPRETATION: *Wandering atrial pacemaker*

Premature Atrial Complex

A ***premature atrial complex (PAC)*** is a single complex that occurs during sinus rhythm earlier than the next expected sinus complex. It is created by premature discharge of an ectopic focus located somewhere in the atria other than the SA node. It frequently depolarizes the SA node prematurely, creating a pause in the EKG as the SA node resets its cycle. This pause is termed "*noncompensatory*," meaning that the interval between the two normal complexes that flank the PAC is less than twice the normal R-to-R interval. Less commonly, a "*compensatory*" pause of twice the normal R-to-R interval occurs if the SA node is refractory to depolarization by the PAC. Among the various etiologies of PACs are use of caffeine, tobacco, or alcohol, stress, hypoxia, digitalis toxicity, certain drugs that stimulate the sympathetic nervous system, and organic heart disease. Premature atrial complexes may occur in normal hearts and have no apparent cause. The EKG characteristics for a lead II rhythm strip are the following:

RATE: *Depends on rate of underlying rhythm*
RHYTHM: *Irregular whenever PAC occurs*
P WAVES: *Premature and different shape from the sinus P waves; may be buried in the preceding T wave*
PR INTERVAL: *May be normal, prolonged, or short*
QRS COMPLEX: *Usually normal but may be greater than 0.10 sec if the PAC is abnormally conducted through ventricles or absent if the PAC is blocked because of refractory ventricles*

Clinical Significance. Isolated PACs are of little consequence. However, in patients with heart disease, frequent PACs may precede or precipitate more serious atrial arrhythmias, such as paroxysmal supraventricular tachycardia, atrial fibrillation, or atrial flutter.

Management. No prehospital management is indicated, but the patient with frequent PACs should be monitored closely for other atrial arrhythmias. See Rhythm Strips 20-7A–20.7D on the following pages.)

450 UNIT FOUR: MEDICAL EMERGENCIES

RHYTHM STRIP 20–7A.
(Huff J, Doernbach DP, White RD)

STRIP #: 7A
RATE: *Basic rate 58/min (average, 60/min)*
RHYTHM: *Irregular, due to premature complex*
P WAVE: *One per QRS complex; upright; one premature*
PR INTERVAL: *0.16 sec and constant*
QRS COMPLEX: *0.04–0.06 sec and all alike*
RHYTHM INTERPRETATION: *Sinus bradycardia with one premature atrial complex (with a noncompensatory pause)*

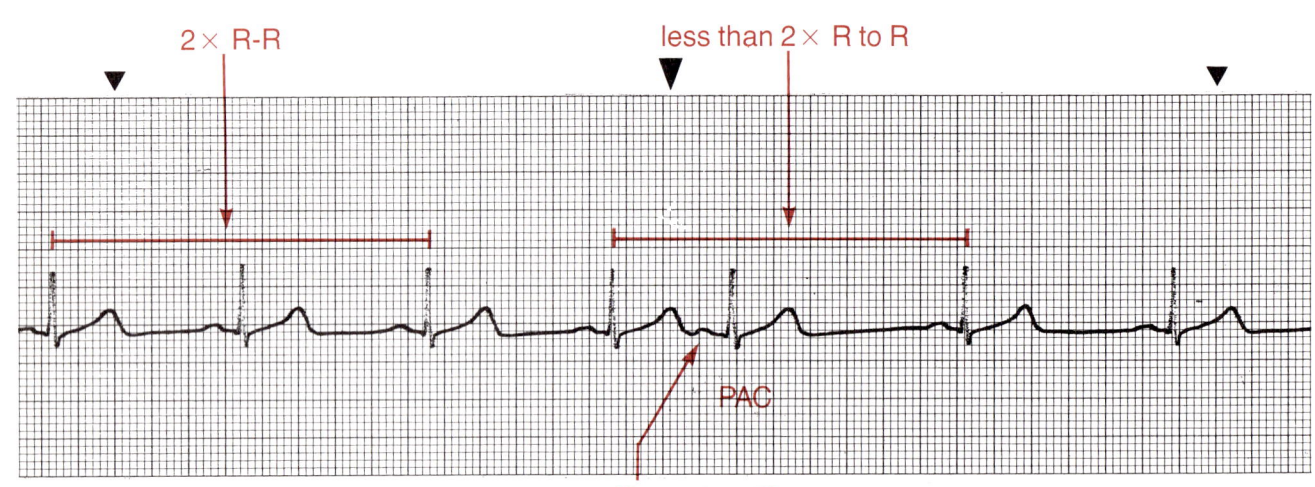

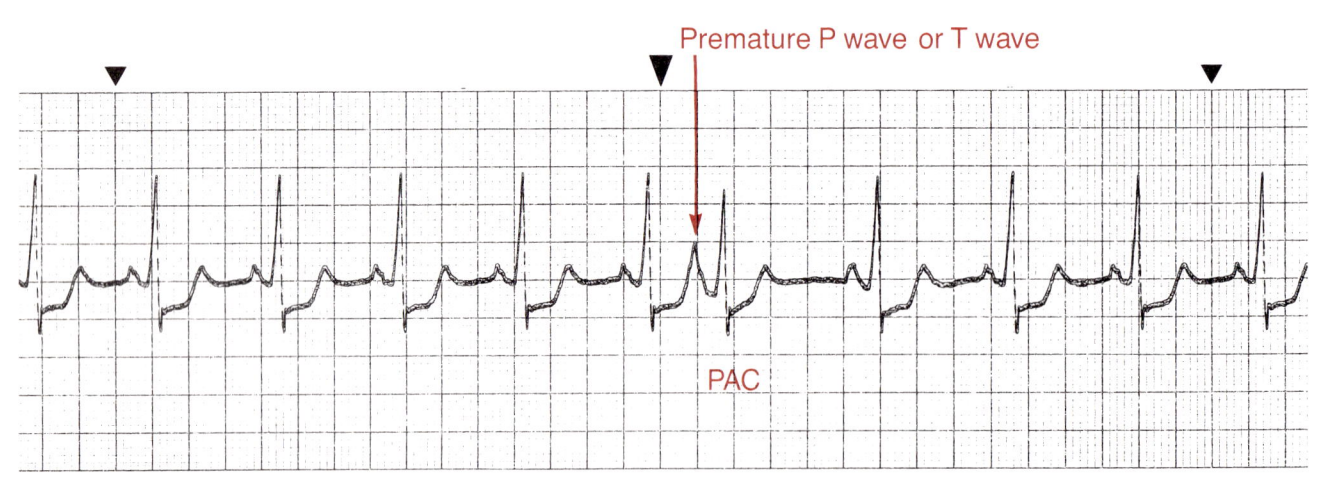

RHYTHM STRIP 20–7B.
(Huff J, Doernbach DP, White RD)

STRIP #: 7B
RATE: *Basic rate 88/min (average, 90/min)*
RHYTHM: *Irregular, due to premature complex*
P WAVE: *One per QRS complex; upright; one premature with different shape*
PR INTERVAL: *0.12 sec and constant except for premature complex*
QRS COMPLEX: *0.08 sec and all alike*
RHYTHM INTERPRETATION: *Sinus rhythm with one premature atrial complex*

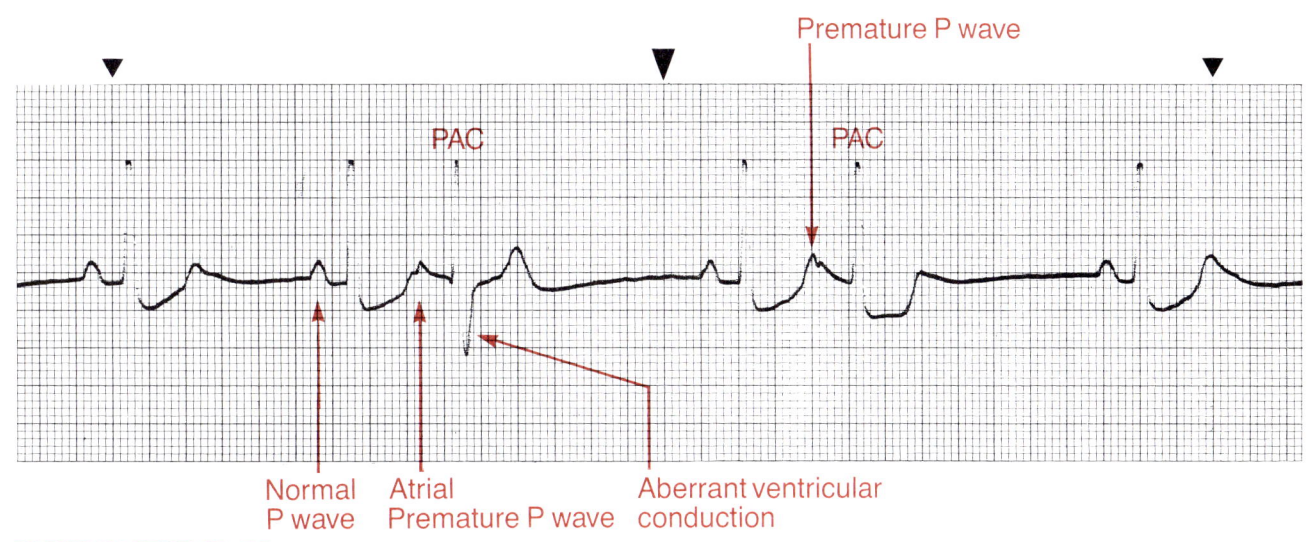

RHYTHM STRIP 20–7C.
(Huff J, Doernbach DP, White RD)

STRIP #: 7C
RATE: *Basic rate 50/min (average, 60/min)*
RHYTHM: *Irregular, due to premature complexes*
P WAVE: *One per QRS complex; upright; two premature with different shapes*
PR INTERVAL: *0.20 sec and constant*
QRS COMPLEX: *0.08 sec; one 0.12 sec with different shape*
RHYTHM INTERPRETATION: *Sinus bradycardia with premature atrial complexes, one with aberrant (abnormal) ventricular conduction*

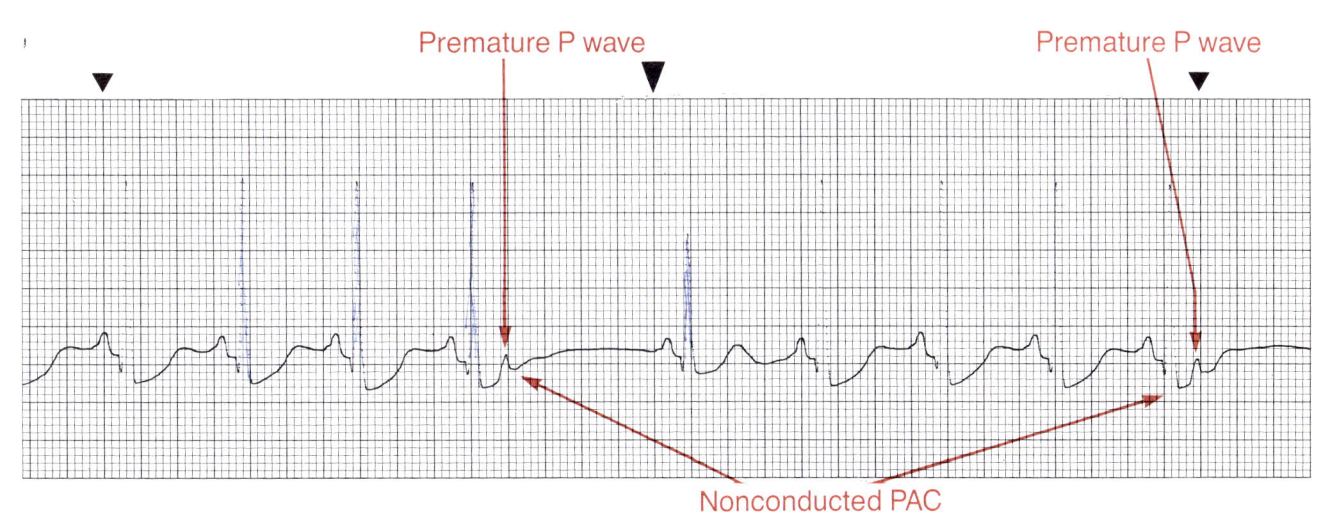

RHYTHM STRIP 20–7D.
(Huff J, Doernbach DP, White RD)

STRIP #: 7D
RATE: *Basic rate 94/min (average, 90/min)*
RHYTHM: *Irregular, due to two pauses*
P WAVE: *One per QRS complex; upright; two premature not followed by QRS complexes*
PR INTERVAL: *0.12 sec and constant*
QRS COMPLEX: *0.08 sec and all alike*
RHYTHM INTERPRETATION: *Sinus rhythm with two nonconducted premature atrial complexes*

Paroxysmal Supraventricular Tachycardia

Paroxysmal supraventricular tachycardia (PSVT or SVT), formerly called atrial tachycardia, is a rhythm initiated by a premature impulse from the atria or ventricles that is recycled by a reentry circuit, most commonly in the AV node. (Reentry also occurs in the SA node or atrial muscle but much less frequently.) The resultant rhythm overrides the SA node with a rate generally between 150 to 250 complexes per minute, is very regular, and occurs in paroxysms with sudden onset and abrupt termination. This tachycardia may last for minutes to hours. Although rarely seen in the setting of acute myocardial infarction, PSVT is frequently associated with underlying atherosclerotic heart disease or rheumatic heart disease. Conduction through accessory pathways (AV accessory connections), most frequently found in a congenital condition called Wolff-Parkinson-White syndrome, is another mechanism for PSVT in addition to AV nodal reentry.

Paroxysmal supraventricular tachycardia may occur at any age and may also be unassociated with heart disease. Factors that may precipitate PSVT are stress, smoking, caffeine, and overexertion, although it may be unrelated to any particular cause. The EKG characteristics for a lead II rhythm strip are the following:

RATE: *150–250/min*
RHYTHM: *Characteristically regular*
P WAVES: *Frequently buried in preceding T waves and difficult to see; if visible, different shape than sinus P waves*
PR INTERVAL: *Usually not possible to measure*
QRS COMPLEX: *Usually normal (0.10 sec or less) but may be wide if abnormally conducted through ventricles*

Wolff-Parkinson-White syndrome may be identified by an abnormally short PR interval (less than 0.12 second) and a "slurring" effect at the beginning of the QRS complex. This "slurring" effect is known as a **delta wave** (Fig. 20-37), and it usually results in an abnormally wide QRS complex. When these EKG changes are present, they confirm the presence of ventricular pre-excitation along an accessory AV connection. Such connections can become participants in the reentry tachycardia that may occur in patients with Wolff-Parkinson-White syndrome. It is also important to note that patients who have this syndrome with a history of episodes of PSVT may have normal EKGs when in sinus rhythm.

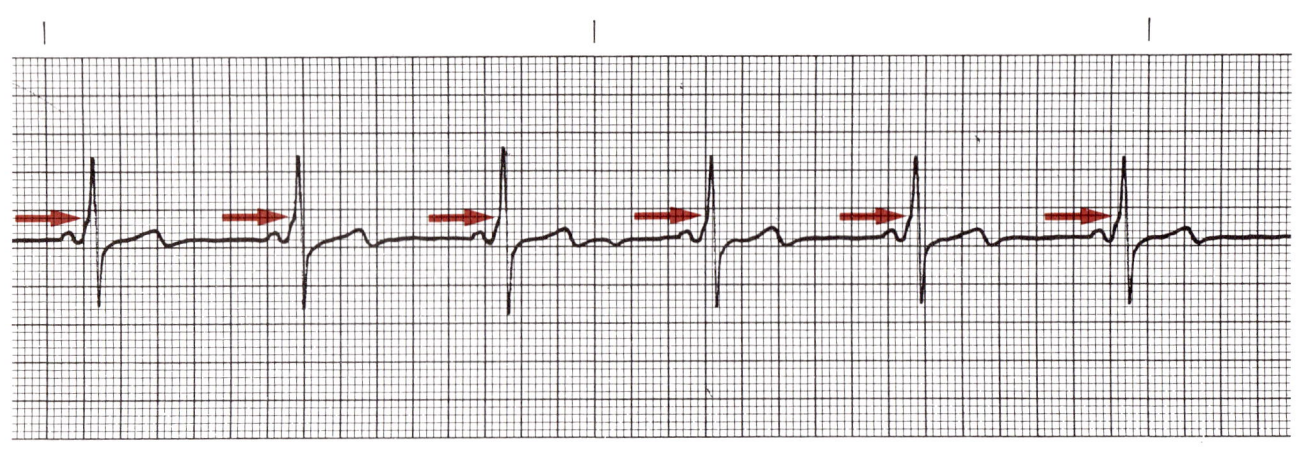

FIGURE 20–37.
EKG pattern in Wolff–Parkinson–White syndrome.

Clinical Significance. Patients frequently have the sensation of palpitations during episodes of tachycardia and may feel anxious or nervous. Although PSVT may be well tolerated for short periods of time or in healthy hearts, the rapid rates frequently compromise cardiac output in patients with underlying heart disease. Reduced filling time, stroke volume, and coronary artery perfusion may lead to syncope, angina, hypotension, or congestive heart failure.

Management. Prehospital intervention depends on the degree of decompensation that is occurring. Vagal maneuvers, such as Valsalva's maneuver (bearing down) or carotid sinus massage, are often effective and should be attempted according to local medical protocols. A calcium-channel blocking drug, such as verapamil, is the drug of choice if simple vagal maneuvers fail. The advent of the drug adenosine (see Appendix D) makes it likely that this drug will be used instead of, or in addition to, verapamil for treating PSVT. Adenosine effectively terminates PSVT and has the distinct advantage of a short duration of action. A bolus of 6 mg is given rapidly through an antecubital venous catheter. If necessary a second dose of 12 mg can be given two minutes later. Adenosine slows conduction through the AV node. Because its half-life is less than 10 seconds there are no prolonged adverse effects. Transient side effects include facial flushing, dyspnea, and chest pressure. If signs and symptoms of cardiac decompensation occur, synchronized cardioversion is indicated and is frequently successful at low-energy (less than 100 J) settings (Fig. 20-38).

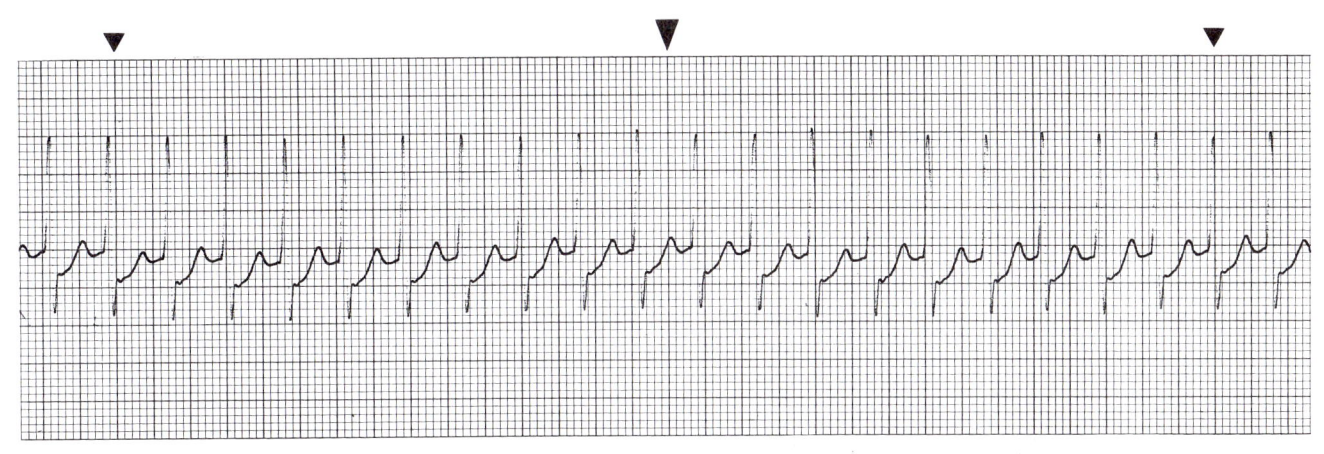

RHYTHM STRIP 20–8A.
(Huff J, Doernbach DP, White RD)

STRIP #: *8A*
RATE: *188/min*
RHYTHM: *Regular*
P WAVE: *Not visible*
PR INTERVAL: *Unmeasurable*
QRS COMPLEX: *0.06–0.08 sec and all alike*
RHYTHM INTERPRETATION: *Paroxysmal supraventricular tachycardia*

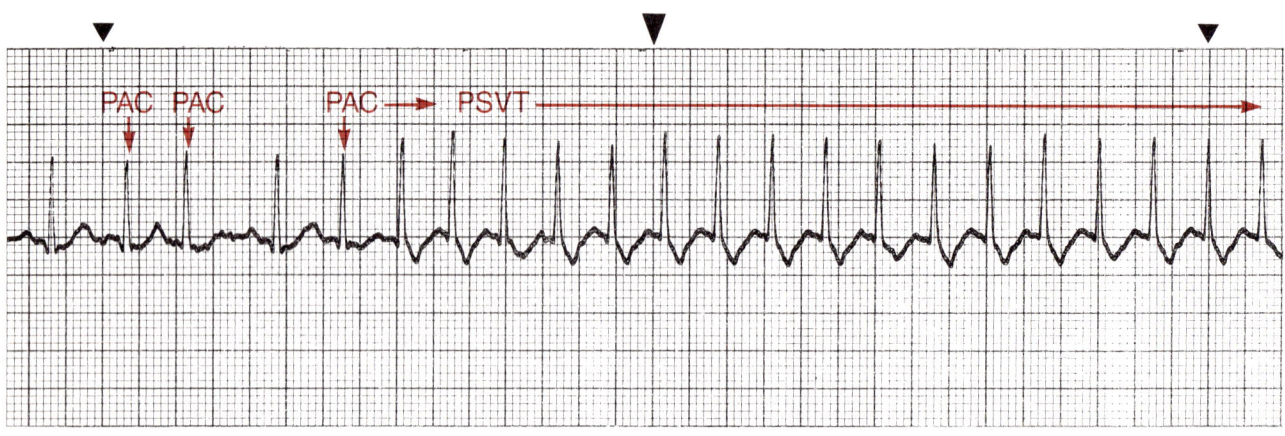

RHYTHM STRIP 20–8B.
(Huff J, Doernbach DP, White RD)

STRIP #: *8B*
RATE: *214/min*
RHYTHM: *Irregular, changing to regular*
P WAVE: *Only three clearly visible; upright with varying shapes*
PR INTERVAL: *0.12 sec and constant*
QRS COMPLEX: *0.04 sec*
RHYTHM INTERPRETATION: *Beats 1 and 4 are sinus beats; beats 2, 3, and 5 are premature atrial complexes; the fifth beat precipitates a paroxysmal supraventricular tachycardia.*

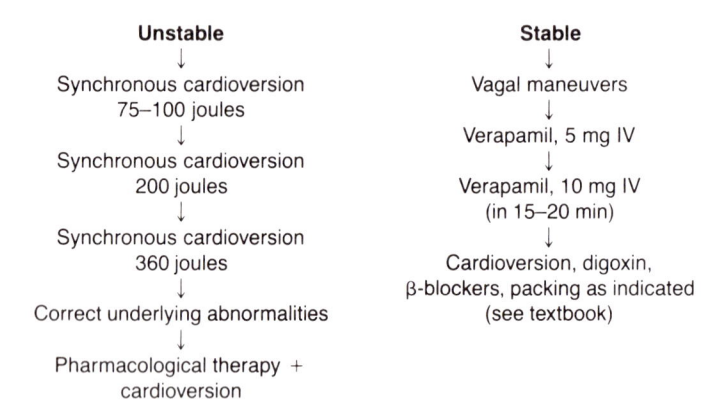

Unstable	Stable
↓	↓
Synchronous cardioversion 75–100 joules	Vagal maneuvers
↓	↓
Synchronous cardioversion 200 joules	Verapamil, 5 mg IV
↓	↓
Synchronous cardioversion 360 joules	Verapamil, 10 mg IV (in 15–20 min)
↓	↓
Correct underlying abnormalities	Cardioversion, digoxin, β-blockers, packing as indicated (see textbook)
↓	
Pharmacological therapy + cardioversion	

If conversion occurs but PSVT recurs, repeated electrical cardioversion is *not* indicated. Sedation should be used as time permits.

Paroxysmal supraventricular tachycardia (PSVT). This sequence was developed to assist in teaching how to treat a broad range of patients with sustained PSVT. Some patients may require care not specified herein. This algorithm should not be construed as prohibiting such flexibility. The flow of the algorithm presumes that PSVT is continuing. IV = intravenous.

FIGURE 20–38.
Advanced cardiac life support treatment protocol for paroxysmal supraventricular tachycardia. (© American Heart Association: Textbook of Advanced Cardiac Life Support, 2nd ed, p 244. Dallas, American Heart Association, 1987)

Atrial Flutter

Atrial flutter is the arrhythmia that results from atrial impulses generated at a rate of 250 to 350 per minute by an area of enhanced automaticity or reentry within the atria. The AV node usually cannot conduct at these high rates and, therefore, conducts impulses to the ventricles at a two-to-one, three-to-one, four-to-one, or greater ratio (but rarely a one-to-one ratio). A discrepancy results between atrial and ventricular rates. The degree of AV block may be consistent or variable. Although atrial flutter is rarely a direct result of acute myocardial infarction, it is usually associated with cardiac disease. The EKG characteristics for a lead II rhythm strip are the following:

RATE: *Atrial, 250–350/min; ventricular, varies*

RHYTHM: *Atrial rhythm regular; ventricular rhythm usually regular but may be irregular if AV conduction ratio varies*

P WAVES: *Two or more flutter waves before each QRS complex resemble a "saw-toothed" or "picket-fence" pattern and appear inverted; may be difficult to identify in the two-to-one flutter, but suspect when rhythm is regular and rate is 140–160/min*

PR INTERVAL: *Flutter-to-R interval may be constant or variable*

QRS COMPLEX: *Normal (0.10 sec or less)*

Clinical Significance. Atrial flutter with high conduction ratios that result in normal ventricular rates are usually well tolerated. However, rapid ventricular rates may compromise cardiac output and precipitate all the associated symptoms.

Management. Prehospital intervention is indicated for atrial flutter only for rapid ventricular rates with hemodynamic compromise. Synchronized cardioversion is the preferred management, as atrial flutter often responds to low-energy (25 J) settings. Intravenous verapamil can slow the ventricular response but does not necessarily convert the flutter to normal sinus rhythm. Vagal maneuvers rarely convert atrial flutter but, rather, create a brief slowing of ventricular rate by increasing AV block. This effect may help distinguish a two-to-one atrial flutter from PSVT, but it has no therapeutic benefit. (See Rhythm Strips 20-9A and 20-9B on the following page.)

456 UNIT FOUR: MEDICAL EMERGENCIES

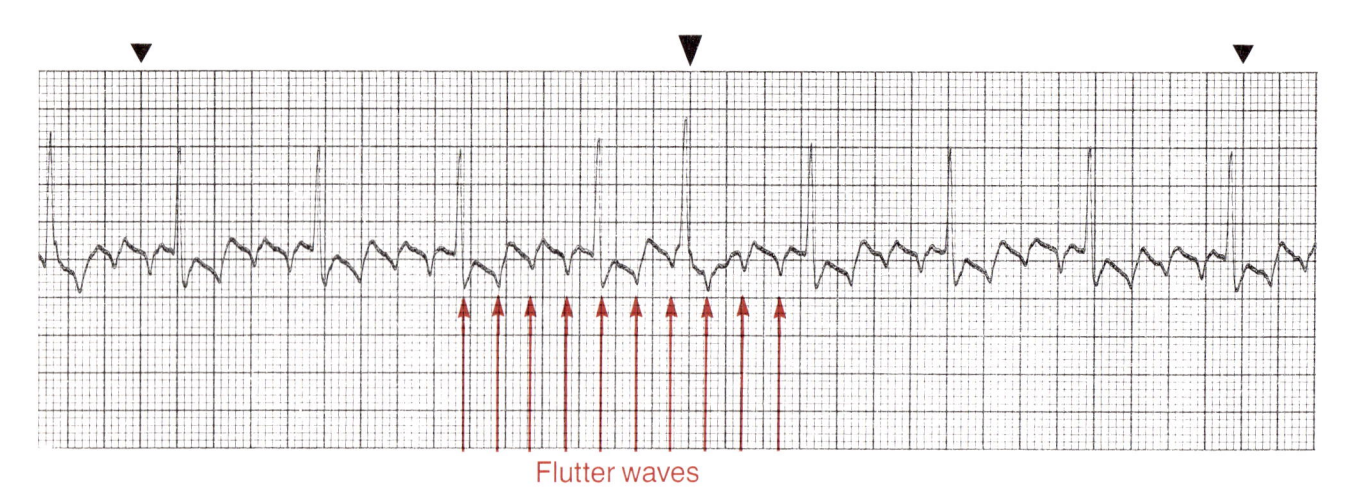

RHYTHM STRIP 20–9A.
(Huff J, Doernbach DP, White RD)

STRIP #: *20-9A*
RATE: *Atrial, 300/min; ventricular, 90/min*
RHYTHM: *Regular atrial; irregular ventricular*
P WAVE: *Flutter waves*
PR INTERVAL: *Unmeasurable*
QRS COMPLEX: *0.06 sec and all alike*
RHYTHM INTERPRETATION: *Atrial flutter with variable AV conduction (4:1 and 2:1)*

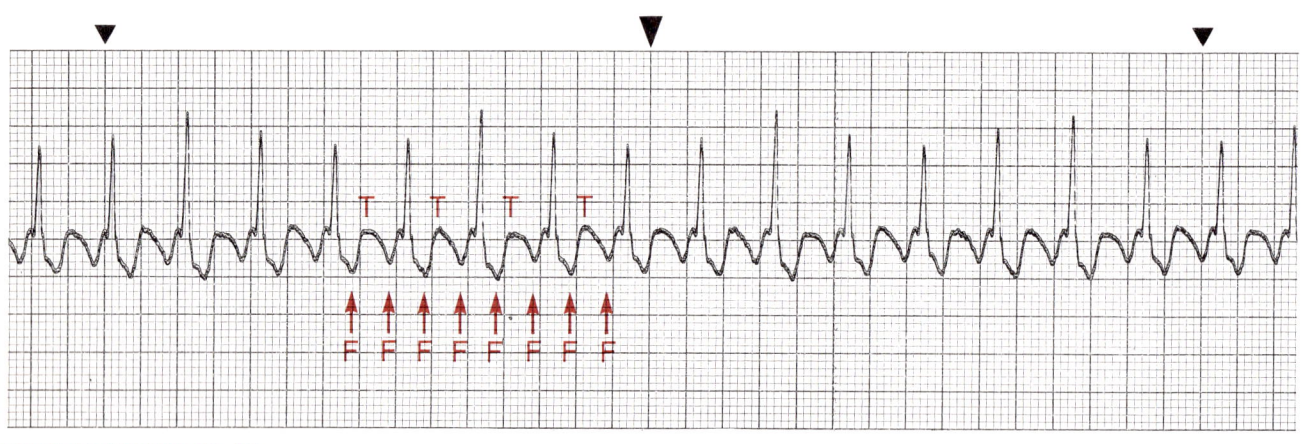

RHYTHM STRIP 20–9B.
(Huff J, Doernbach DP, White RD)

STRIP #: *9B*
RATE: *Atrial, 300/min; ventricular, 150/min*
RHYTHM: *Regular*
P WAVE: *Not visible; flutter waves (F) present*
PR INTERVAL: *Unmeasurable*
QRS COMPLEX: *0.06 sec and all alike*
RHYTHM INTERPRETATION: *Atrial flutter with 2:1 AV conduction*

Atrial Fibrillation

Atrial fibrillation occurs when there is rapid, erratic electrical discharge from multiple atrial ectopic foci or from multiple reentry circuits within the atria, generating 350 to 600 impulses per minute. The AV node, overwhelmed by this number of impulses, conducts whatever it can to the ventricles in a random, highly variable manner. Although atrial fibrillation may be paroxysmal and occur in normal hearts, it is more often a chronic arrhythmia associated with underlying heart disease, such as congestive heart failure and atherosclerotic and rheumatic valvular heart disease. The EKG characteristics for a lead II rhythm strip are the following:

RATE: *Atrial, 350/min or greater (cannot be counted); ventricular, varies greatly*

RHYTHM: *Irregular*

P WAVES: *No true P waves; wavy, irregular deflections called fibrillatory waves may be seen; very fine, low amplitude fibrillatory waves may appear isoelectric*

PR INTERVAL: *None*

QRS COMPLEX: *Usually normal (0.10 sec or less) but may be wide if abnormally conducted through the ventricles*

Clinical Significance. The total irregularity of atrial fibrillation causes varying degrees of ventricular filling. This variation is commonly manifested by a pulse deficit, the difference between the patient's apical and peripheral pulse rates. Cardiac output may be decreased by as much as 20% to 25% because of lack of coordinated atrial contraction. In chronic atrial fibrillation treated with digitalis to slow AV conduction, the ventricular response may be within normal range (controlled atrial fibrillation) and the arrhythmia well tolerated. Slow ventricular response of less than 60 per minute may compromise cardiac output and, frequently, is caused by digitalis toxicity. Rapid ventricular response (uncontrolled), usually in new atrial fibrillation, may compromise cardiac output. These patients may develop angina, myocardial infarction, congestive heart failure, or shock.

Management. For rapid ventricular rates that cause hemodynamic compromise, synchronized cardioversion is indicated to convert the arrhythmia to sinus rhythm. Verapamil administration may be considered to slow AV conduction but is contraindicated in patients with Wolff-Parkinson-White syndrome with atrial fibrillation (or flutter) because the drug may cause dangerous acceleration of the ventricular rate (see discussion of verapamil). (See Rhythm Strips 20-10A–20-10C on the following pages.)

458 UNIT FOUR: MEDICAL EMERGENCIES

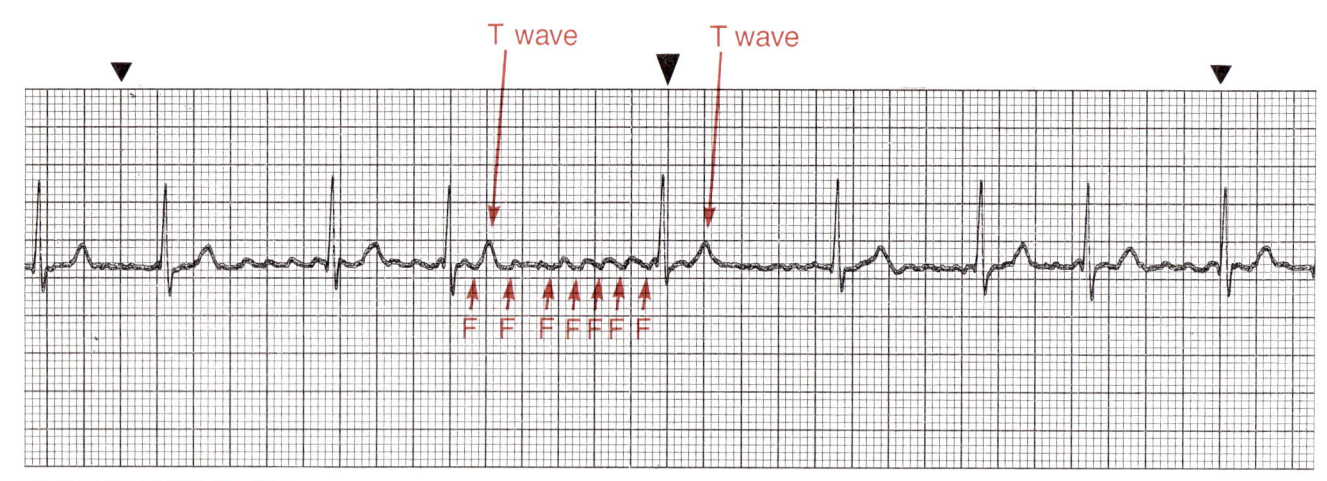

RHYTHM STRIP 20–10A.
(Huff J, Doernbach DP, White RD)

STRIP #: *10A*
RATE: *Atrial 400/min or greater; ventricular, 80/min*
RHYTHM: *Totally irregular*
P WAVE: *Not visible; fibrillation (F) waves present*
PR INTERVAL: *Unmeasurable*
QRS COMPLEX: *0.06–0.08 sec and all alike*
RHYTHM INTERPRETATION: *Atrial fibrillation with normal ventricular response (controlled)*

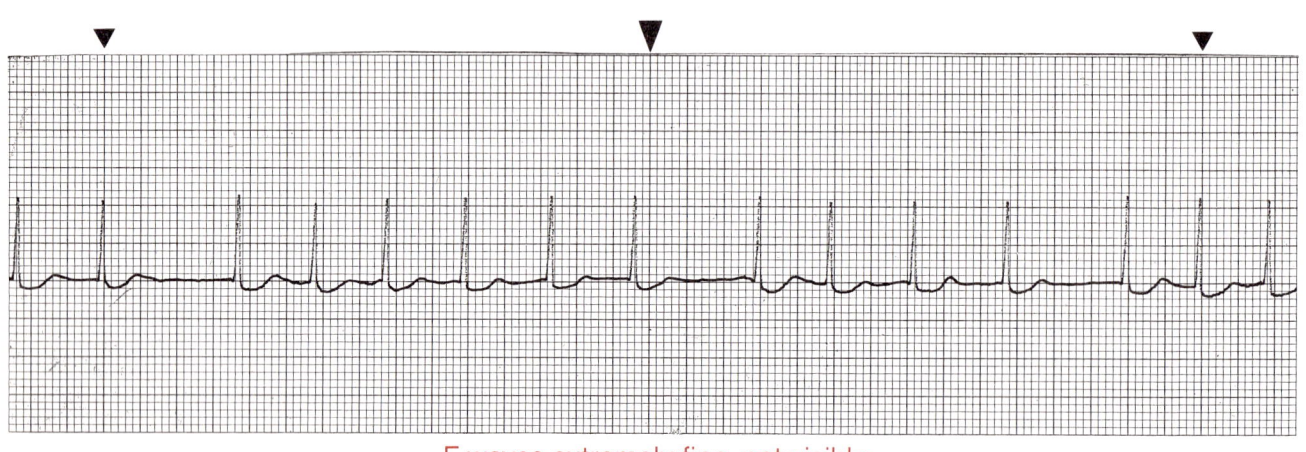

RHYTHM STRIP 20–10B.
(Huff J, Doernbach DP, White RD)

STRIP #: *10B*
RATE: *130/min*
RHYTHM: *Totally irregular*
P WAVE: *Not visible; fibrillation (F) waves extremely fine*
PR INTERVAL: *Unmeasurable*
QRS COMPLEX: *0.04 sec and all alike*
RHYTHM INTERPRETATION: *Atrial fibrillation with rapid ventricular response (uncontrolled)*

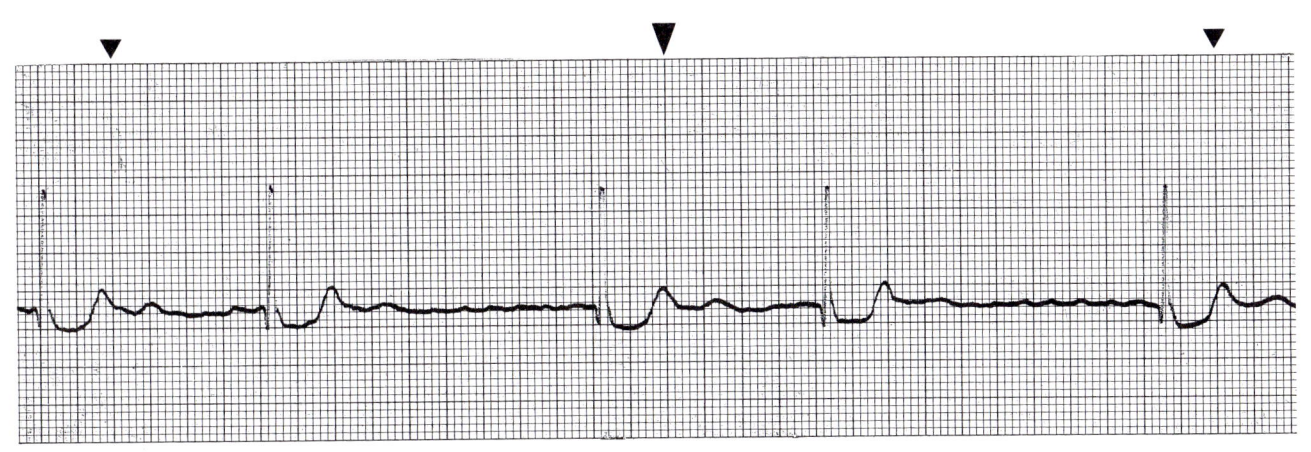

RHYTHM STRIP 20–10C.
(Huff J, Doernbach DP, White RD)

STRIP #: *10-C*
RATE: *40/min*
RHYTHM: *Totally irregular*
P WAVE: *Not visible; fibrillation waves present*
PR INTERVAL: *Unmeasurable*
QRS COMPLEX: *0.06 sec and all alike*
RHYTHM INTERPRETATION: *Atrial fibrillation with slow ventricular response*

Multifocal atrial tachycardia (MAT) is an arrhythmia that may closely resemble atrial fibrillation on the EKG. It is a disorder of automaticity characterized by atrial rates greater than 100 per minute, P waves of at least three different morphologies (shapes) in the same lead, and irregular P-to-P, PR, and R-to-R intervals. It is commonly seen in patients with COPD but may also occur in other medical emergencies, such as acute myocardial ischemia or infarction. It is not an uncommon arrhythmia in out-of-hospital patients, though it is typically not recognized as such and instead is diagnosed as atrial fibrillation. A high index of suspicion and a careful examination of the EKG will confirm the diagnosis in these situations.

While it is satisfying to make the correct rhythm diagnosis it also has important therapeutic implications. Cardioversion is ineffective in terminating MAT, as is digoxin. If the ventricular rate is rapid and treatment warranted verapamil can be used. It is safe and effective, consistently slowing heart rate, and sometimes restoring sinus rhythm.

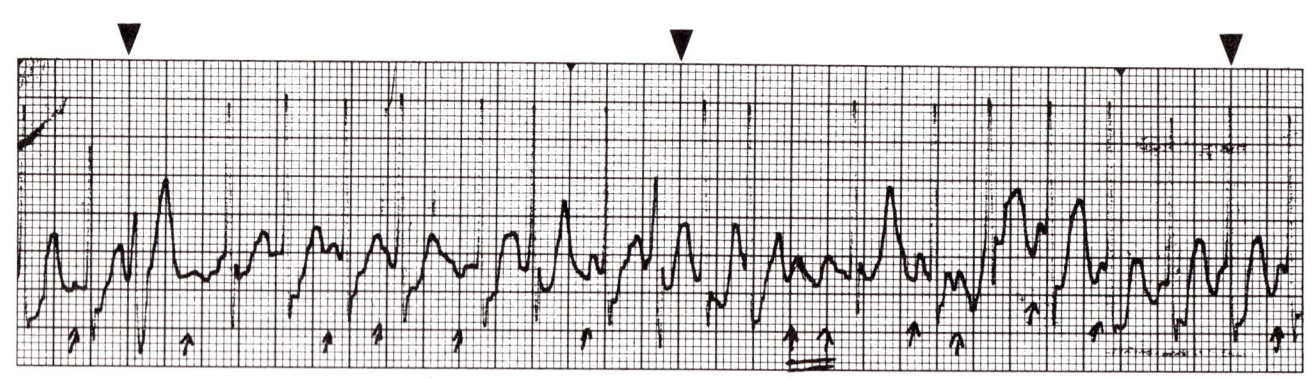

RHYTHM STRIP 20–10D.
(White RD: Paramedic EKG Collection)

STRIP #: *10-D*

RATE: *Atrial, variable, greater than 200/min; ventricular, 180/min*

RHYTHM: *Irregular, atrial and ventricular*

P WAVE: *Not visible for all QRS complexes; varying shapes and numbers per QRS complex*

PR INTERVAL: *Variable*

QRS COMPLEX: *0.08–0.12 sec and all alike except complex #2*

RHYTHM INTERPRETATION: *Multifocal atrial tachycardia (MAT) recorded in the field in a patient with chronic obstructive lung disease on theophylline medication. Verapamil, 5 mg, reduced the ventricular rate.*

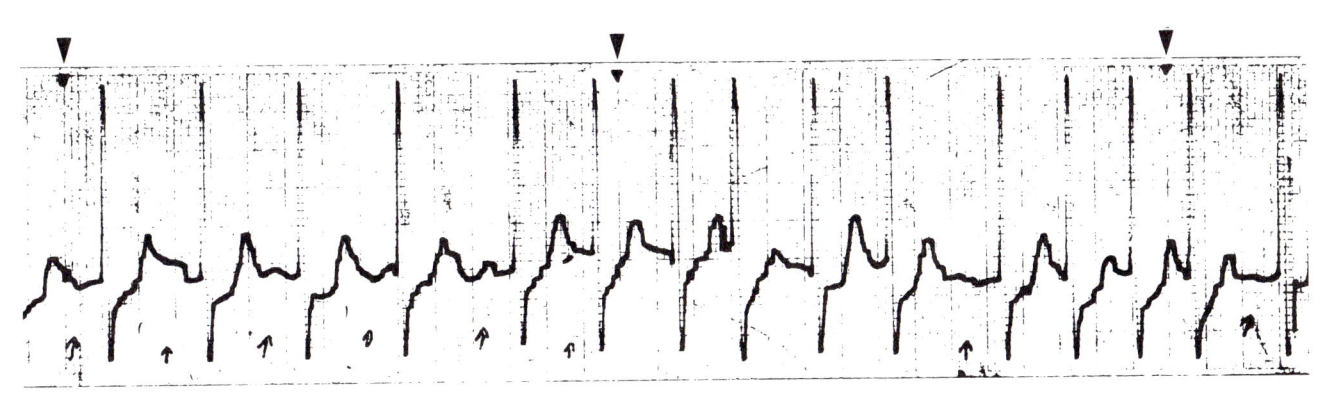

RHYTHM STRIP 20–10E.
(White RD: Paramedic EKG Collection)

STRIP #: *10-E*

RATE: *Atrial and ventricular 130/min*

RHYTHM: *Irregular, both atrial and ventricular*

P WAVE: *Several different morphologic configurations (examples marked with arrows)*

PR INTERVAL: *Variable*

QRS COMPLEX: *Narrow (0.08 sec), all alike*

RHYTHM INTERPRETATION: *Multifocal (multiform) atrial tachycardia (MAT), recorded by paramedics in a 71-year-old man experiencing an acute inferior wall myocardial infarction. No history of chronic pulmonary disease. Following admission, "atrial fibrillation" was diagnosed and cardioversion attempted, followed by ventricular fibrillation, which was defibrillated. Cardioversion is ineffective in MAT.*

Arrhythmias That Originate in the AV Junction

The tissue of the AV junction, with the exception of the AV node itself, has pacemaker capabilities and can act as a back-up to the SA node. At other times, various factors create increased automaticity or reentry in the AV junction, resulting in abnormal complexes and rhythms. The EKG features common to all junctional rhythms include P waves that are inverted in lead II because the impulse initiated in the AV junction depolarizes the atria in a retrograde fashion, in a direction away from the positive electrode (Fig. 20-39). The relationship of the P wave to the QRS complex depends on the timing of atrial depolarization to ventricular depolarization. The P wave appears before the QRS complex if atria are depolarized first, after the QRS complex if ventricles are depolarized first, and during the QRS complex and not visible if atria and ventricles are depolarized simultaneously. PR intervals are frequently shortened. QRS complexes are of normal duration provided no ventricular conduction disturbance is present. Junctional rhythms to be described are junctional escape complexes and rhythm, premature junctional complex, accelerated junctional rhythm, and paroxysmal junctional tachycardia.

Junctional Escape Complexes and Rhythms

Junctional escape complexes and rhythms occur when impulses from the SA node cannot penetrate the AV node or when the sinus rate drops to less than that of the AV junction, allowing it to take over as pacemaker for one or more cardiac cycles. The resulting complex or rhythm (if a series of complexes is seen) is called an escape complex or escape rhythm and has a rate within the inherent rate of the AV junction, 40 to 60 per minute. By definition, the distance from the last normal complex to an escape complex is greater than the normal R-to-R interval, or, in other words, an escape complex comes later than the next expected sinus complex. Escape complexes may be caused by sinus slowing from enhanced vagal tone or by disease, such as damage to the SA node or AV node above the site of the escape focus. The EKG characteristics for a lead II rhythm strip are the following:

RATE: *40–60/min*
RHYTHM: *Irregular if a single escape complex occurs, regular if escape rhythm persists*
P WAVES: *Inverted preceding or following QRS complex or absent (hidden in QRS complex)*
PR INTERVAL: *If P wave precedes QRS complex, usually less than 0.12 sec*
QRS COMPLEX: *Normal (0.10 sec or less)*

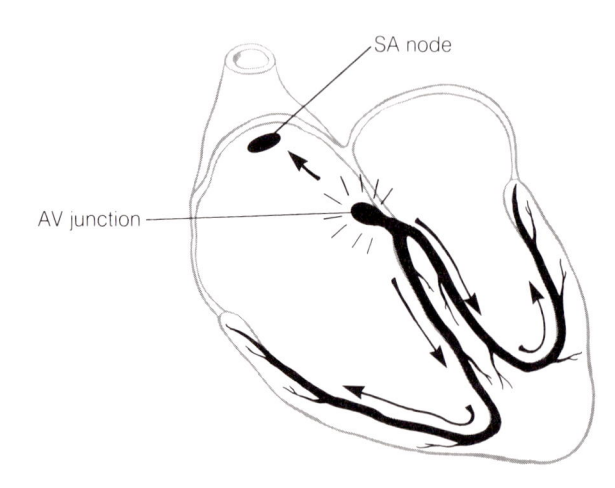

FIGURE 20–39.
Electrical flow in junctional rhythms.

Clinical Significance. The escape complex or rhythm serves as a safety mechanism and may be well tolerated. However, the slow rates generated by junctional escape rhythm often cause decreased cardiac output and all its associated symptoms.

Management. If the patient is stable, no management is required other than careful monitoring. Symptomatic patients should be treated with atropine to increase AV discharge rate or stimulate SA node discharge. Rhythms that do not respond to atropine may require management with a β-stimulating drug, such as isoproterenol, or with external pacing.

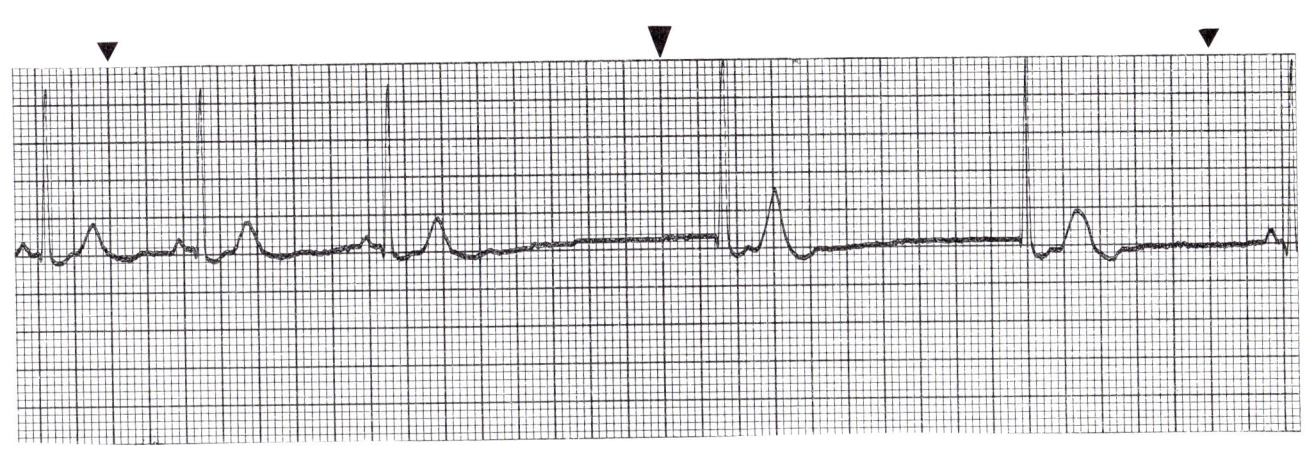

RHYTHM STRIP 20–11A.
(White RD: Paramedic EKG Collection)

STRIP #: *11A*
RATE: *60/min, dropping to 35/min*
RHYTHM: *Irregular*
P WAVE: *Upright and uniform; do not precede every QRS complex*
PR INTERVAL: *0.12 sec and constant*
QRS COMPLEX: *0.06 sec and all alike*
RHYTHM INTERPRETATION: *Sinus arrhythmia with sinus arrest (two junctional escape beats are present during the arrest)*

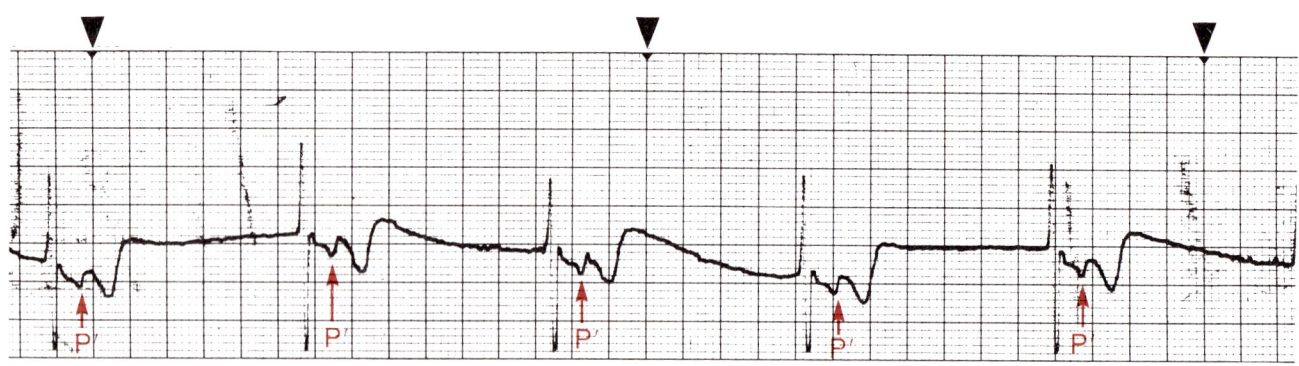

RHYTHM STRIP 20-11B.
(White RD: Paramedic EKG Collection)

STRIP #: *11-B*

RATE: *44/min*

RHYTHM: *Regular*

P WAVE: *Inverted and uniform; one after each QRS complex*

PR INTERVAL: *Unmeasurable*

QRS COMPLEX: *0.08 sec and all alike*

RHYTHM INTERPRETATION: *Junctional escape rhythm in a 59-year-old male whose chief complaint was a syncopal episode*

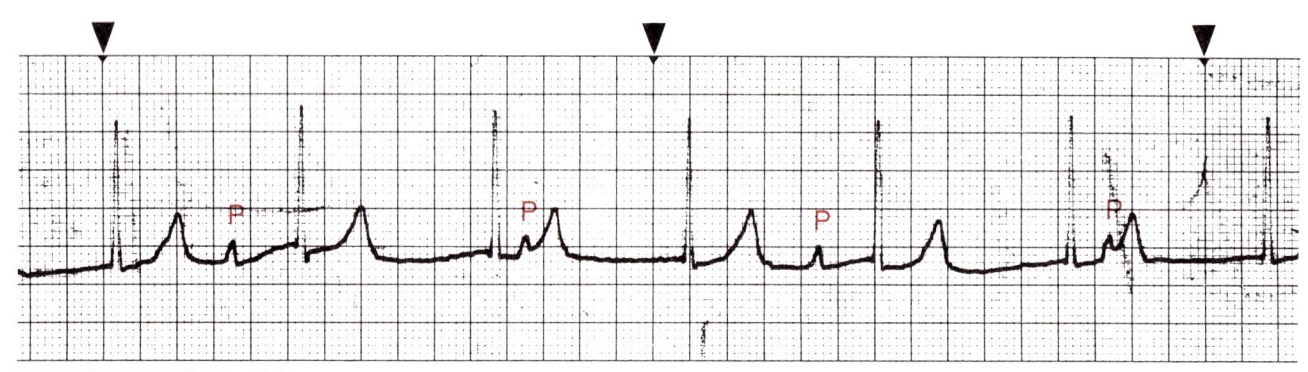

RHYTHM STRIP 20-11C.
(White RD: Paramedic EKG Collection)

STRIP #: *11C*

RATE: *Atrial, 38/min; ventricular, 55/min*

RHYTHM: *Regular, atrial and ventricular*

P WAVE: *Upright and uniform; do not precede every QRS complex*

PR INTERVAL: *Variable or absent*

QRS COMPLEX: *0.08 sec and all alike*

RHYTHM INTERPRETATION: *Marked sinus bradycardia with junctional escape rhythm causing AV dissociation. This rhythm was secondary to verapamil overdose in a 73-year-old female.*

Premature Junctional Complex

A *premature junctional complex (PJC)* is similar to a PAC in that it is a single complex that occurs during sinus rhythm earlier than the next expected sinus complex. It is created by premature discharge of an ectopic focus located somewhere in the AV junctional tissue. The pause that follows a PJC may be compensatory or noncompensatory, depending on whether or not the SA node was depolarized by the PJC before the next spontaneous sinus discharge. The etiology of PJCs is similar to that of PACs. The EKG characteristics for a lead II rhythm strip are the following:

RATE: *Depends on rate of underlying rhythm*
RHYTHM: *Irregular whenever PJC occurs*
P WAVES: *Inverted preceding or following QRS complex or absent (hidden in QRS complex)*
PR INTERVAL: *If P wave precedes QRS complex, usually less than 0.12 sec*
QRS COMPLEX: *Normal (0.10 sec or less)*

Clinical Significance. While isolated PJCs are of no consequence, frequent PJCs may be forerunners of tachycardiac junctional arrhythmias.

Management. None required prehospital.

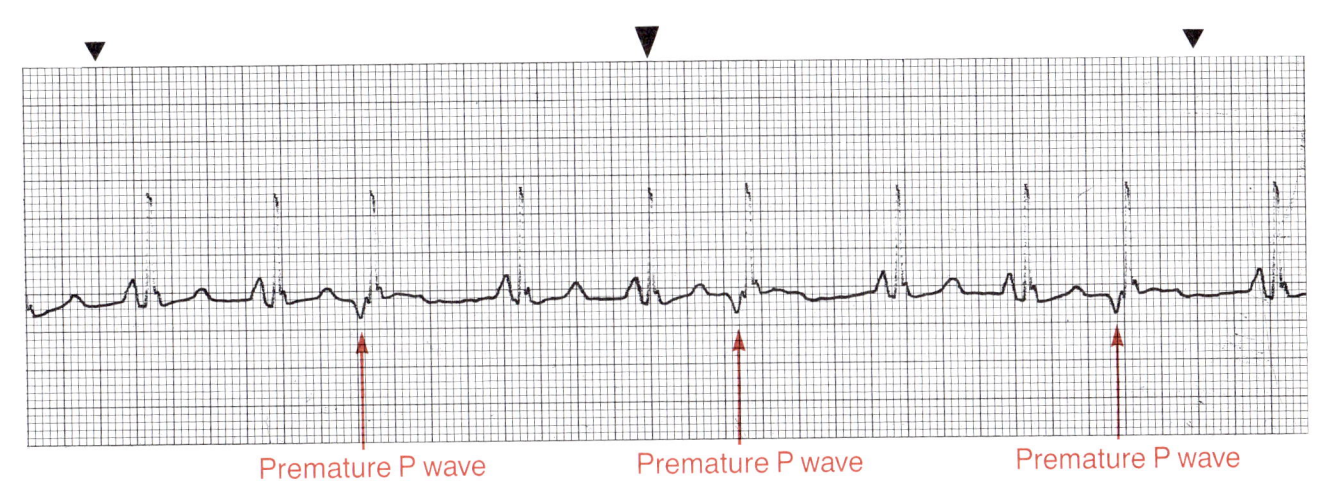

RHYTHM STRIP 20–12A.
(Huff J, Doernbach DP, White RD)

STRIP #: *12A*
RATE: *Basic rate 88/min (average, 90/min)*
RHYTHM: *Regularly irregular (every third complex is premature)*
P WAVE: *One per QRS complex; inverted before premature complexes*
PR INTERVAL: *0.12 sec for upright P waves; 0.06 sec for inverted P waves*
QRS COMPLEX: *0.06–0.08 sec and all alike*
RHYTHM INTERPRETATION: *Sinus rhythm with three premature junctional complexes*

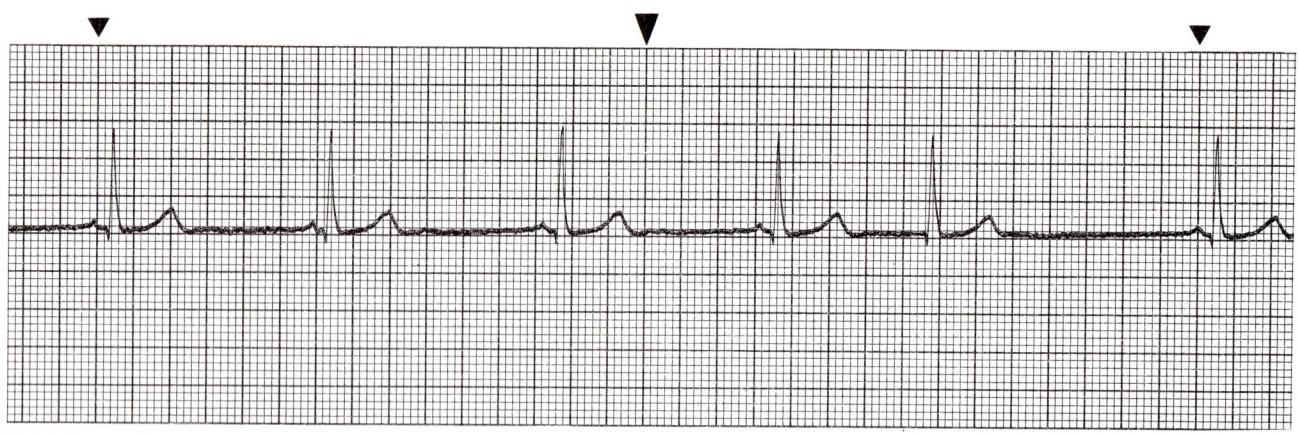

RHYTHM STRIP 20–12B.
(Huff J, Doernbach DP, White RD)

STRIP #: *12B*

RATE: *Basic rate 47/min (average, 50/min)*

RHYTHM: *Irregular, due to one premature complex*

P WAVE: *Upright and uniform; not visible before premature QRS complex*

PR INTERVAL: *0.10–0.12 sec*

QRS COMPLEX: *0.08 sec and all alike*

RHYTHM INTERPRETATION: *Sinus bradycardia with one premature junctional complex (P wave buried in QRS complex)*

Accelerated Junctional Rhythm

Accelerated junctional rhythm results from increased automaticity of the AV junction, causing it to discharge faster than its inherent rate and override the SA node. Because this condition technically is a tachycardia for the AV junction, some call this rhythm nonparoxysmal junctional tachycardia. The atria may be depolarized by the impulses that arise in the AV junction; more commonly, however, they are controlled independently by the SA node, and AV dissociation may be evident (P waves and QRS complex unrelated to each other). Etiology of this arrhythmia includes ischemia of the AV junction and digitalis toxicity. The EKG characteristics for a lead II rhythm strip are the following:

RATE: *60–100/min*
RHYTHM: *Same as for junctional escape rhythm*
P WAVES: *Same as for junctional escape rhythm*
PR INTERVAL: *Same as for junctional escape rhythm*
QRS COMPLEX: *Same as for junctional escape rhythm*

Clinical Significance. The normal ventricular rate that occurs with this rhythm means it is usually well tolerated.

Management. No prehospital intervention usually is required.

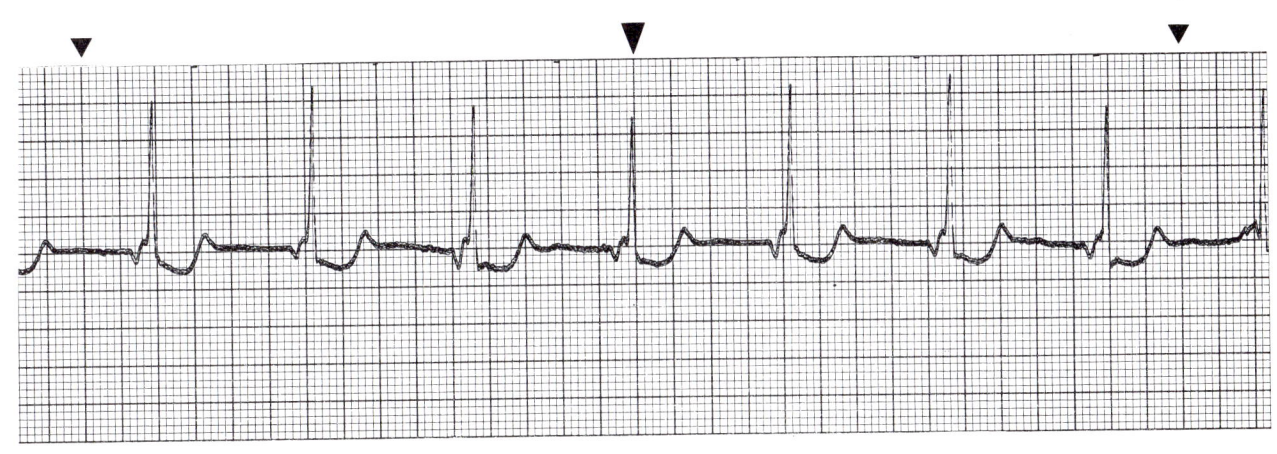

RHYTHM STRIP 20–13.
(Huff J, Doernbach DP, White RD)

STRIP #: *13*
RATE: *72/min*
RHYTHM: *Regular*
P WAVE: *One per QRS complex; inverted and uniform*
PR INTERVAL: *0.08 sec and constant*
QRS COMPLEX: *0.04–0.06 sec and all alike*
RHYTHM INTERPRETATION: *Accelerated junctional rhythm*

Paroxysmal Junctional Tachycardia

Paroxysmal junctional tachycardia occurs when automaticity of a site in the AV junction is greatly increased or when a reentry circuit in the AV junction stimulates the ventricles at a rate of 100 to 180 per minute. This arrhythmia is most commonly referred to as PSVT because the mechanism, etiology, EKG characteristics, significance, and management are the same as for a paroxysmal tachycardia originated by an atrial impulse. Refer to the previous discussion of PSVT in the section "Arrhythmias That Originate in the Atria."

Arrhythmias That Originate in the Ventricles

All arrhythmias that originate in the ventricles depolarize the ventricles in an abnormal manner, from side to side, and at a slower speed than if the ventricles were being simultaneously depolarized via the efficient bundle branch-Purkinje system. For this reason, the EKG feature that is common to all ventricular rhythms is a QRS complex that is greater than 0.10 second in duration. The P waves of ventricular arrhythmias are either absent or, if visible, have no consistent relationship to the QRS complexes (AV dissociation). The ventricular rhythms discussed are ventricular escape complex and rhythm, accelerated idioventricular rhythm, premature ventricular contraction, ventricular tachycardia, ventricular fibrillation, and asystole.

Ventricular Escape Complexes and Rhythms

Ventricular escape complexes and rhythms occur when impulses from higher pacemakers fail to reach the ventricles or when the rate of discharge of higher pacemakers becomes less than the inherent rate of the ventricles. The ventricle is then able to take over as pacemaker for one or more cardiac cycles and creates an escape complex or rhythm (if a series of complexes is seen) at the inherent rate of the ventricles, 20 to 40 per minute. Like any escape mechanism, a ventricular escape complex occurs later than the next expected normal complex. The etiology of ventricular escape is almost always underlying heart disease that causes slowing of SA and AV nodal pacemaker sites or a high degree of block at the AV node. Ventricular escape rhythm (also called idioventricular rhythm) is frequently the first organized electrical activity seen after electrical defibrillation or the last electrical activity in the dying heart. The EKG characteristics for a lead II rhythm strip are the following:

RATE: *20–40/min, occasionally less*
RHYTHM: *Irregular if a single escape complex occurs, usually regular if escape rhythm is present; however, low pacemaker sites may be irregular*
P WAVES: *None*
PR INTERVAL: *None*
QRS COMPLEX: *Wide (0.12 sec or greater)*

Clinical Significance. The escape complex or rhythm serves as a safety mechanism, but the slow rate of a ventricular escape rhythm severely compromises cardiac output and precipitates any of the associated symptoms. Ventricular escape rhythm may be a perfusing or nonperfusing rhythm so that close monitoring of the pulse is warranted in a decompensated patient with this rhythm.

Management. Occasional ventricular escape complexes may be treated with atropine to increase the discharge of higher pacemakers. With perfusing or nonperfusing ventricular escape rhythm (idioventricular rhythm), atropine may be administered to increase rate; however, it is frequently necessary to use a β stimulator, such as isoproterenol, to stimulate the ventricular pacemaker site. External pacing may also be used if available. Because the patient has no effective higher pacemaker, lidocaine should never be administered to a patient in a ventricular escape rhythm.

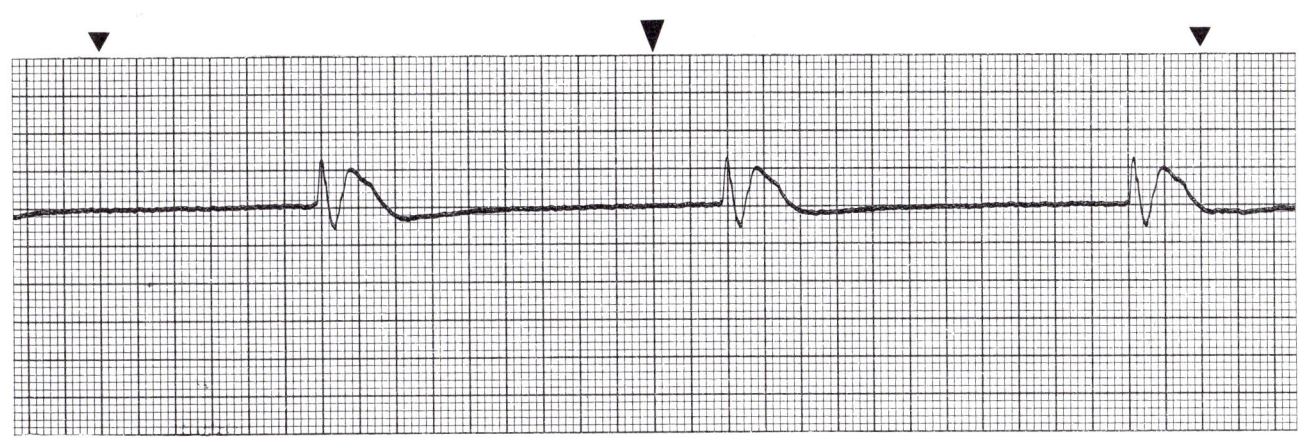

RHYTHM STRIP 20–14A.
(Huff J, Doernbach DP, White RD)

STRIP #: *14A*
RATE: *27/min*
RHYTHM: *Regular*
P WAVE: *Not visible*
PR INTERVAL: *Unmeasurable*
QRS COMPLEX: *0.16 sec and all alike*
RHYTHM INTERPRETATION: *Ventricular escape rhythm (idioventricular rhythm)*

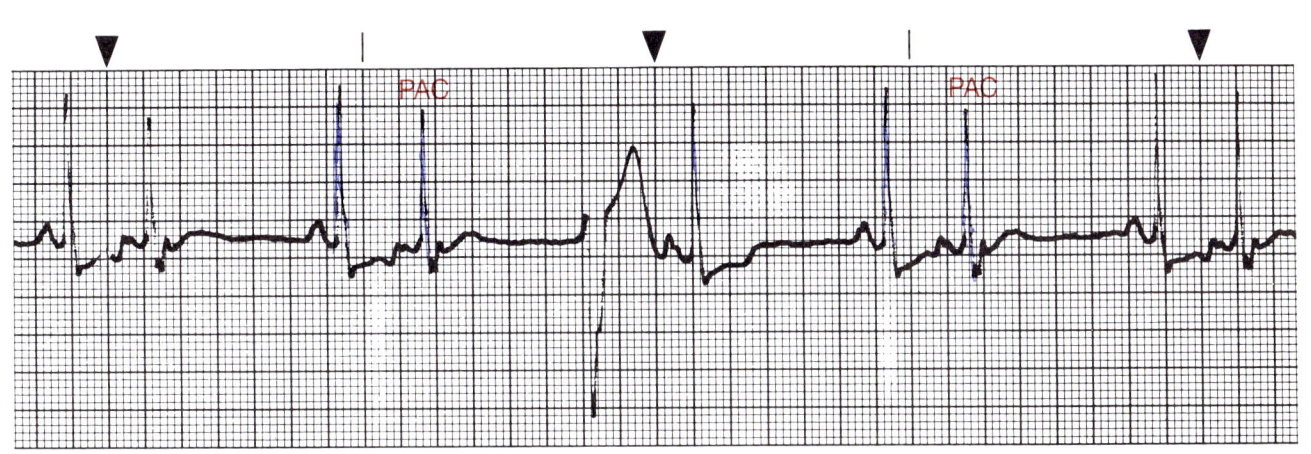

RHYTHM STRIP 20–14B.

STRIP #: *14B*
RATE: *Atrial, 55/min; ventricular, 80/min*
RHYTHM: *Irregular, atrial and ventricular*
P WAVE: *Change in shape before several premature complexes; absent before one complex*
PR INTERVAL: *0.12–0.16 sec*
QRS COMPLEX: *0.08–0.12 sec; one complex greater than 0.12 sec*
RHYTHM INTERPRETATION: *Sinus bradycardia with frequent premature atrial complexes and one ventricular escape complex*

Accelerated Idioventricular Rhythm

Accelerated idioventricular rhythm is evidence that ventricular pacemaker sites are capable of developing increased automaticity and discharging faster than the inherent ventricular rate. Because the rate of this arrhythmia rarely exceeds 100 but is faster than ventricular escape rhythm, the ventricles often compete with the SA node for control of the heart, and "*fusion*" complexes are common. The atria usually remain under the influence of the SA node, so AV dissociation may be present. A myocardial infarction is a common etiology of accelerated idioventricular rhythm. It is generally thought to be a benign arrhythmia, as it has not been shown to adversely affect the patient's recovery and rarely precipitates more rapid ventricular rhythms. A second etiology for accelerated idioventricular rhythm is digitalis toxicity. The EKG characteristics for a lead II rhythm strip are the following:

RATE: *40–100/min*
RHYTHM: *Regular*
P WAVES: *Absent or, if visible, not consistently related to QRS complex*
PR INTERVAL: *None or variable*
QRS COMPLEX: *Wide (0.12 sec or greater)*

Clinical Significance. This rhythm usually is well tolerated by the patient, as the rate is in a normal range. At times, loss of sequential AV contraction may decrease cardiac output.

Management. There is difference of opinion as to whether this arrhythmia requires management if the patient is asymptomatic. Close monitoring of the EKG and management of the underlying condition may be all that is required. If the patient is bradycardic or symptomatic or if the base physician wishes to treat, atropine may be used to speed the sinus rate or lidocaine used to suppress the ectopic ventricular focus.

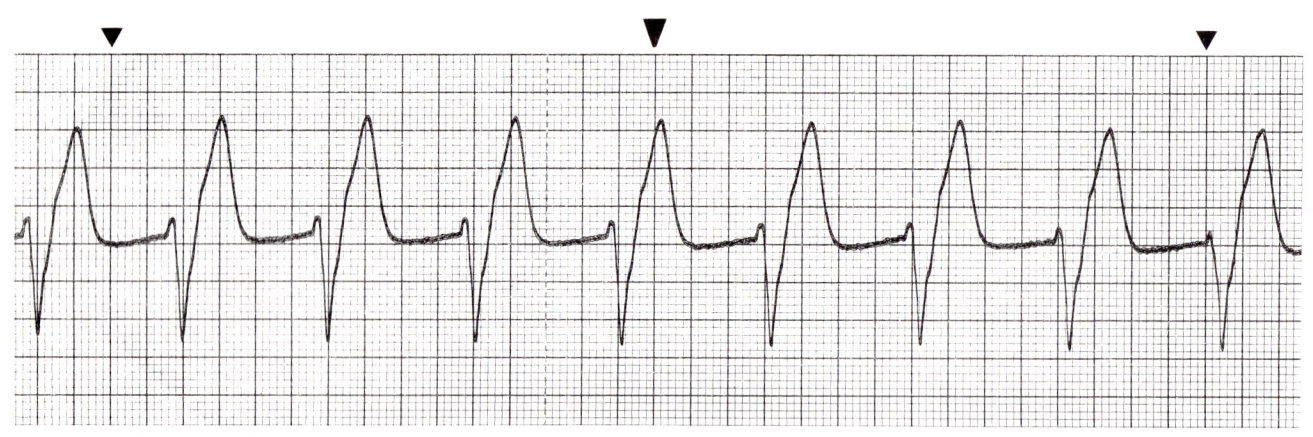

RHYTHM STRIP 20–15.
(Huff J, Doernbach DP, White RD)

STRIP #: *15*
RATE: *75/min*
RHYTHM: *Regular*
P WAVE: *Not visible*
PR INTERVAL: *Unmeasurable*
QRS COMPLEX: *0.16 sec and all alike*
RHYTHM INTERPRETATION: *Accelerated idioventricular rhythm*

Premature Ventricular Complex

Premature ventricular complex (PVC) occurs when an ectopic focus in either ventricle creates an impulse that depolarizes the heart earlier than the next expected sinus complex. The resulting premature complex has an abnormally wide, often bizarre-appearing QRS complex because of the altered sequence of ventricular depolarization and altered repolarization, reflected by a T wave in the opposite direction of the QRS complex. Because the PVC does not usually depolarize and reset the SA node, the pause that follows the PVC is usually, but not always, fully compensatory. Occasionally a PVC falls between two sinus complexes without interrupting the rhythm and is called an interpolated PVC. Premature ventricular complexes may be unifocal and uniform, arising from one focus and having the same appearance, or multifocal and multiformed, arising from many foci with different shapes. The distance between the preceding complex and the PVC, called the coupling interval, is usually constant for uniform PVCs but may vary with those that are multiformed. Premature ventricular complexes frequently occur in patterns or in repetition of complexes. The terms ventricular bigeminy, trigeminy, and quadrigeminy refer to PVCs that occur every second complex, every third complex, and every fourth complex, respectively. It is also not unusual to see two or more PVCs occurring in a row, creating couplets or triplets. A higher degree of ventricular ectopic activity is indicated by frequent PVCs, multiform PVCs, repetitive PVCs, and PVCs that occur during the relative refractory period of the ventricles, on the peak of the T wave. These latter R-on-T wave PVCs that occur during the heart's vulnerable period can trigger repetitive firing of the ventricles, leading to lethal tachycardia.

Premature ventricular complexes may be caused by increased automaticity or a reentry mechanism. They may also occur in apparently normal hearts and be of little consequence. They are, however, the most common ventricular arrhythmia caused by myocardial ischemia and infarction and, in this setting, may lead to more serious arrhythmias. Other etiologies of PVCs are hypoxia, acid-base imbalance, electrolyte imbalance, certain drug side effects or toxicity, and increased sympathetic tone. The EKG characteristics for a lead II rhythm strip are the following:

RATE: *Depends on rate of underlying rhythm*
RHYTHM: *Irregular whenever PVC occurs*
P WAVES: *Usually none associated with the PVC*
PR INTERVAL: *None*
QRS COMPLEX: *Wide (0.12 sec or greater), may be notched, may have increased amplitude*

Clinical Significance. In patients without heart disease and acute cardiac symptoms, PVCs are of little consequence. In the setting of myocardial ischemia or infarction, PVCs may trigger lethal ventricular arrhythmias. Patients may sense the occurrence of PVCs as skipped heartbeats. Because the ventricles are only partially filled at the time of a PVC, frequently no pulse is generated by the PVC, creating a pulse deficit. Frequent nonperfusing PVCs may compromise overall cardiac output.

Management. None is required if no history or symptoms of cardiac problems exist. In patients suspected of having myocardial ischemia or infarction, lidocaine administration should be instituted in the presence of any PVCs (Fig. 20-40). Premature ventricular complexes that occur because of slow heart rates may be suppressed by the administration of atropine and, if needed, pacing to increase the rate. Lidocaine should be used with caution, if at all, in the presence of bradycardia because of its action of suppressing escape pacemaker sites that may be needed.

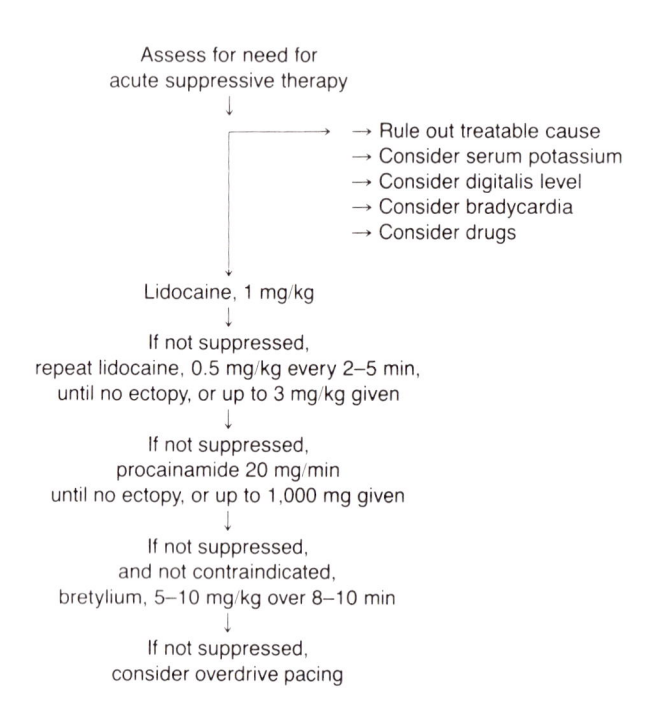

```
        Assess for need for
     acute suppressive therapy
                ↓
                ├──────→ → Rule out treatable cause
                │         → Consider serum potassium
                │         → Consider digitalis level
                │         → Consider bradycardia
                │         → Consider drugs
                ↓
         Lidocaine, 1 mg/kg
                ↓
            If not suppressed,
    repeat lidocaine, 0.5 mg/kg every 2–5 min,
       until no ectopy, or up to 3 mg/kg given
                ↓
            If not suppressed,
         procainamide 20 mg/min
     until no ectopy, or up to 1,000 mg given
                ↓
            If not suppressed,
          and not contraindicated,
     bretylium, 5–10 mg/kg over 8–10 min
                ↓
            If not suppressed,
        consider overdrive pacing
```

Once ectopy is resolved, maintain as follows:
  After lidocaine, 1 mg/kg . . . . .Lidocaine drip, 2 mg/min
  After lidocaine, 1–2 mg/kg . . . . .Lidocaine drip, 3 mg/min
  After lidocaine, 2–3 mg/kg . . . . .Lidocaine drip, 4 mg/min
  After procainamide . . . . .Procainamide drip, 1–4 mg/min
                                           (Check blood level.)
  After bretylium . . . . .Bretylium drip, 2 mg/min

Ventricular ectopy: acute suppressive therapy. This sequence was developed to assist in teaching how to treat a broad range of patients with ventricular ectopy. Some patients may require therapy not specified herein. This algorithm should not be construed as prohibiting such flexibility.

FIGURE 20–40.
Advanced cardiac life support treatment protocol for ventricular ectopy. (© American Heart Association: Textbook of Advanced Cardiac Life Support, 2nd ed, p 243. Dallas, American Heart Association, 1987)

Full compensatory pause
2 × R to R

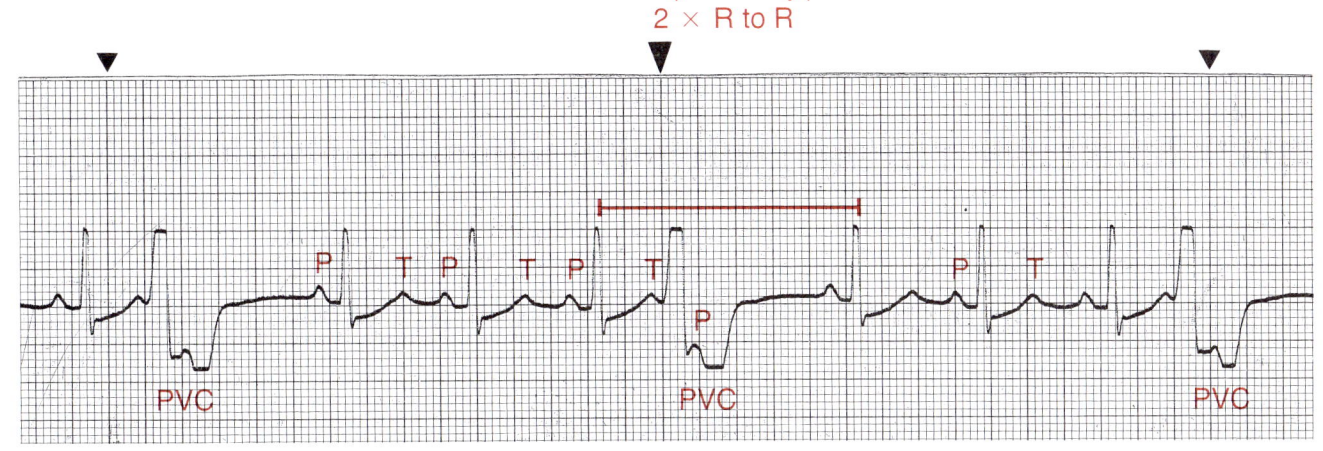

RHYTHM STRIP 20–16A.
(Huff J, Doernbach DP, White RD)

STRIP #: *16A*

RATE: *Basic rate, 88/min (average, 90/min)*

RHYTHM: *Regular atrial; regularly irregular ventricular*

P WAVE: *Upright and uniform; visible after each premature complex*

PR INTERVAL: *0.14–0.16 sec*

QRS COMPLEX: *0.06 sec, premature complexes greater than 0.12 sec and alike*

RHYTHM INTERPRETATION: *Sinus rhythm with three uniform premature ventricular complexes*

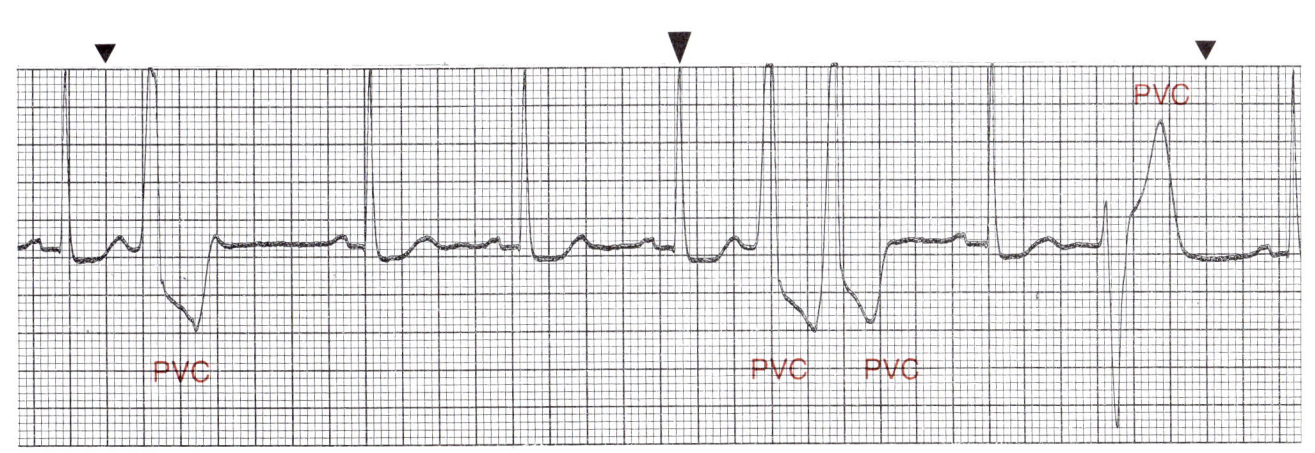

RHYTHM STRIP 20–16B.
(Huff J, Doernbach DP, White RD)

STRIP #: *16B*

RATE: *Basic rate, 72/min (average, 80/min)*

RHYTHM: *Irregular, due to premature complexes*

P WAVE: *Upright and uniform; not visible before premature complexes*

PR INTERVAL: *0.18–0.20 sec*

QRS COMPLEX: *0.06 sec; premature complexes 0.12 sec with varying shapes*

RHYTHM INTERPRETATION: *Sinus rhythm with multiform and coupled premature ventricular complexes*

474 UNIT FOUR: MEDICAL EMERGENCIES

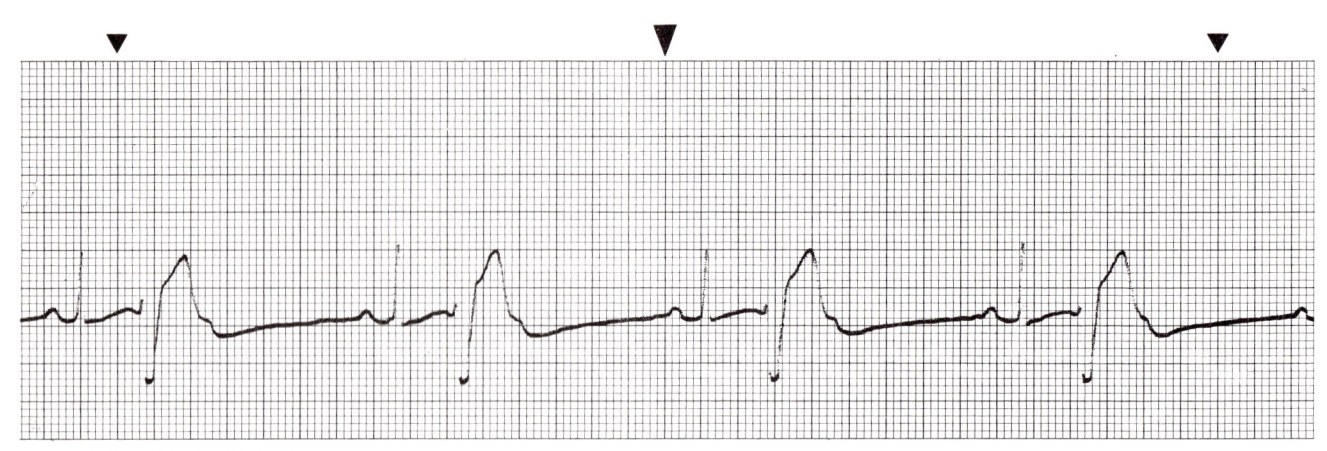

RHYTHM STRIP 20–16C.
(Huff J, Doernbach DP, White RD)

STRIP #: *16C*
RATE: *Average 70/min*
RHYTHM: *Regular atrial, regularly irregular ventricular*
P WAVE: *Upright and uniform; not visible before premature complexes*
PR INTERVAL: *0.20 sec and constant*
QRS COMPLEX: *0.04 sec; premature complexes 0.12 sec*
RHYTHM INTERPRETATION: *Sinus rhythm with premature ventricular complexes in a bigeminal pattern*

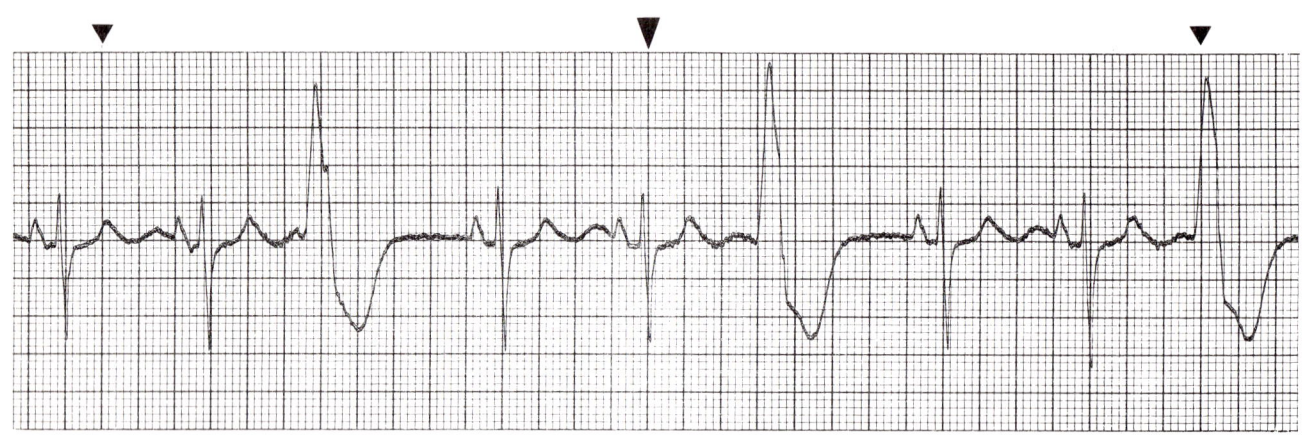

RHYTHM STRIP 20–16D.
(Huff J, Doernbach DP, White RD)

STRIP #: *16D*
RATE: *Basic rate, 75/min (average, 70/min)*
RHYTHM: *Regular atrial; regularly irregular ventricular*
P WAVE: *Upright and uniform; not visible before premature complexes*
PR INTERVAL: *0.12 sec and constant*
QRS COMPLEX: *0.08 sec; premature complexes 0.16 sec*
RHYTHM INTERPRETATION: *Sinus rhythm with premature ventricular complexes in a trigeminal pattern*

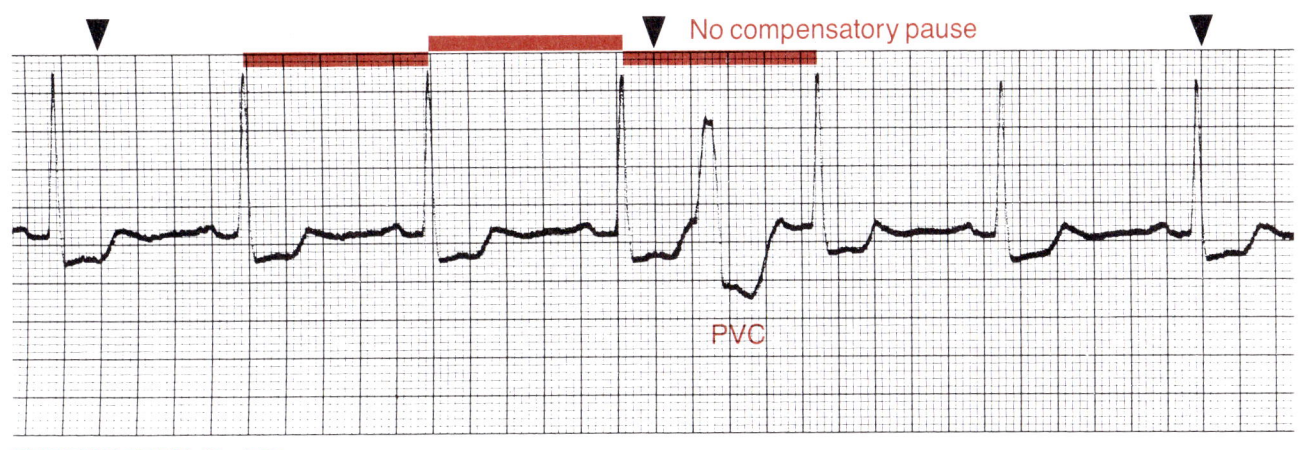

RHYTHM STRIP 20–16E.

STRIP #: *16E*

RATE: *Atrial, 60/min; ventricular, 70/min*

RHYTHM: *Regular except for one complex*

P WAVE: *Upright and uniform before narrow QRS complexes; none visible before one wide QRS complex*

PR INTERVAL: *0.20 sec and constant*

QRS COMPLEX: *0.10 sec; one complex greater than 0.12 sec*

RHYTHM INTERPRETATION: *Sinus rhythm with one interpolated premature ventricular complex*

Ventricular Tachycardia

Ventricular tachycardia occurs when there is a reentry circuit or a rapid discharge from a focus in the ventricles at a rate greater than 100 per minute that overrides the primary pacemaker. Atrioventricular dissociation (independent atrial and ventricular activity) may be evident if the atria continue to be under the control of the SA node. This state may result in uncoordinated contraction of the atria and the ventricles. Ventricular tachycardia rarely occurs in normal hearts. Its etiology is the same as that for PVCs. The EKG characteristics for a lead II rhythm strip are the following:

RATE: *100–250/min*

RHYTHM: *Regular or slightly irregular*

P WAVES: *None or not associated with the QRS complexes if AV dissociation is present; look for P waves indicative of AV dissociation, which is present in about 30% of patients with ventricular tachycardia*

PR INTERVAL: *None*

QRS COMPLEX: *Wide (0.12 sec or greater); QRS complex width greater than 0.14 sec is common; may be notched, have increased amplitude; look for intermittent narrower QRS complexes that represent fusion or capture complexes; if present, they strongly support the diagnosis of ventricular tachycardia*

Clinical Significance. Ventricular tachycardia may be perfusing or nonperfusing and well tolerated or poorly tolerated depending on its rate, duration, and the degree of underlying heart disease. It is a common and misleading perception that this arrhythmia always causes serious hemodynamic compromise. However, cardiac output and coronary artery perfusion often are decreased because of the rapid rate combined with poor stroke volume from loss of synchronized atrial-ventricular activity. Untreated, this rhythm may deteriorate to ventricular fibrillation.

Management. If the patient is perfusing and conscious, lidocaine administration may be attempted to terminate the arrhythmia. However, any patient who has signs of hemodynamic decompensation or who is in actual cardiac arrest should receive cardioversion as soon as possible (Fig. 20-41). Low-energy settings (50 J) may successfully convert ventricular tachycardia. This treatment may be followed by lidocaine or other antiarrhythmic drug administration to prevent recurrence of the tachycardia or to facilitate further cardioversion attempts. It should be noted that verapamil should never be administered for any wide QRS complex tachycardia. Ventricular tachycardia is the most common wide complex tachycardia (about 85%), and, in this situation, verapamil is likely to produce cardiovascular collapse. (See Rhythm Strips 20-17A and 20-17B on page 478.)

CHAPTER 20: Cardiovascular Emergencies 477

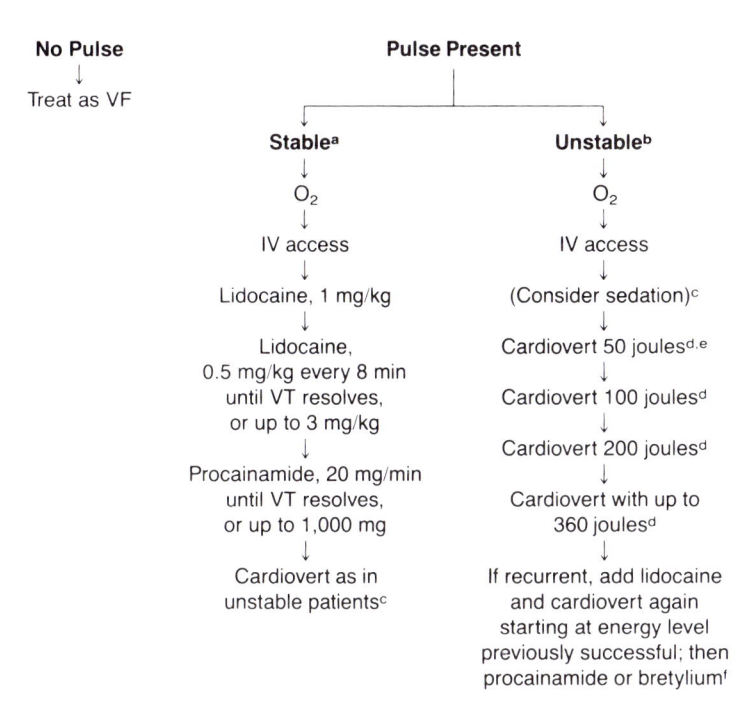

```
No Pulse                 Pulse Present
   ↓                  ┌──────┴──────┐
Treat as VF          ↓              ↓
                  Stableᵃ        Unstableᵇ
                    ↓              ↓
                   O₂             O₂
                    ↓              ↓
                 IV access      IV access
                    ↓              ↓
              Lidocaine, 1 mg/kg  (Consider sedation)ᶜ
                    ↓              ↓
                Lidocaine,      Cardiovert 50 joulesᵈ,ᵉ
            0.5 mg/kg every 8 min    ↓
             until VT resolves,  Cardiovert 100 joulesᵈ
              or up to 3 mg/kg      ↓
                    ↓           Cardiovert 200 joulesᵈ
             Procainamide, 20 mg/min  ↓
              until VT resolves,  Cardiovert with up to
              or up to 1,000 mg      360 joulesᵈ
                    ↓              ↓
               Cardiovert as in  If recurrent, add lidocaine
              unstable patientsᶜ  and cardiovert again
                                  starting at energy level
                                  previously successful; then
                                  procainamide or bretyliumᶠ
```

Sustained ventricular tachycardia (VT). This sequence was developed to assist in teaching how to treat a broad range of patients with sustained VT. Some patients may require care not specified herein. This algorithm should not be construed as prohibiting such flexibility. The flow of the algorithm presumes that VT is continuing. VF = ventricular fibrillation; IV = intravenous.

[a] If the patient becomes unstable (see footnote b for definition) at any time, move to "Unstable" arm of algorithm.

[b] Unstable indicates symptoms (e.g., chest pain or dyspnea), hypotension (systolic blood pressure <90 mmHg), congestive heart failure, ischemia, or infarction.

[c] Sedation should be considered for all patients, including those defined in footnote b as unstable, except those who are hemodynamically unstable (e.g., hypotensive, in pulmonary edema, or unconscious).

[d] If hypotension, pulmonary edema, or unconsciousness is present, unsynchronized cardioversion should be done to avoid the delay associated with synchronization.

[e] In the absence of hypotension, pulmonary edema, or unconsciousness, a precordial thump may be employed prior to cardioversion.

[f] Once VT has resolved, begin intravenous infusion of the antiarrhythmic agent that has aided resolution of VT. If hypotension, pulmonary edema, or unconsciousness is present, use lidocaine if cardioversion alone is unsuccessful, followed by bretylium. In all other patients, the recommended order of therapy is lidocaine, procainamide, and then bretylium.

FIGURE 20–41.
Advanced cardiac life support treatment protocol for ventricular tachycardia. (© American Heart Association: Textbook of Advanced Cardiac Life Support, 2nd ed, p 241. Dallas, American Heart Association, 1987)

478 UNIT FOUR: MEDICAL EMERGENCIES

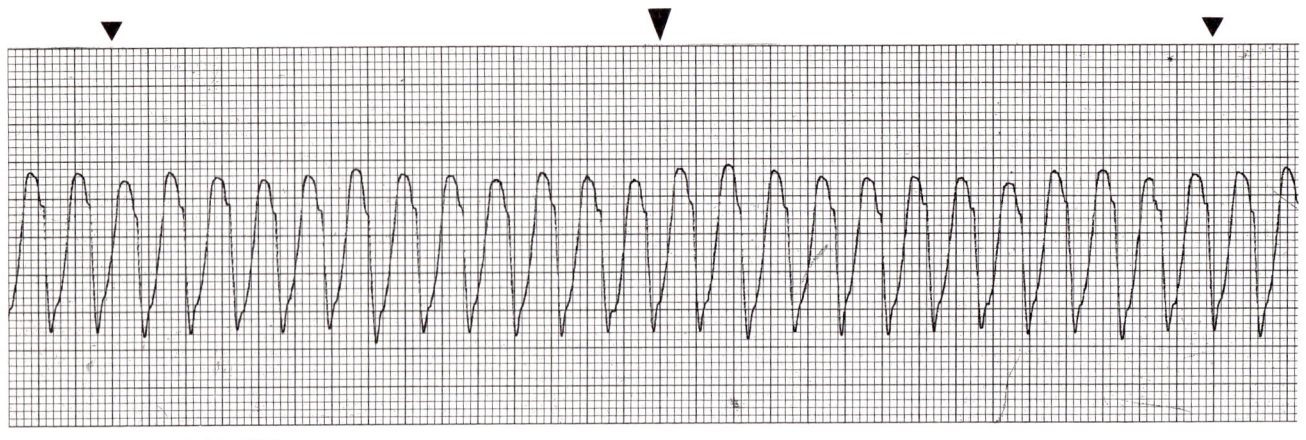

RHYTHM STRIP 20–17A.
(Huff J, Doernbach DP, White RD)

STRIP #: *17A*
RATE: *250/min*
RHYTHM: *Regular*
P WAVE: *Not visible*
PR INTERVAL: *Unmeasurable*
QRS COMPLEX: *0.16 sec and all alike*
RHYTHM INTERPRETATION: *Ventricular tachycardia with stable vital signs in a 63-year-old male with a history of a myocardial infarction 1 year before this episode*

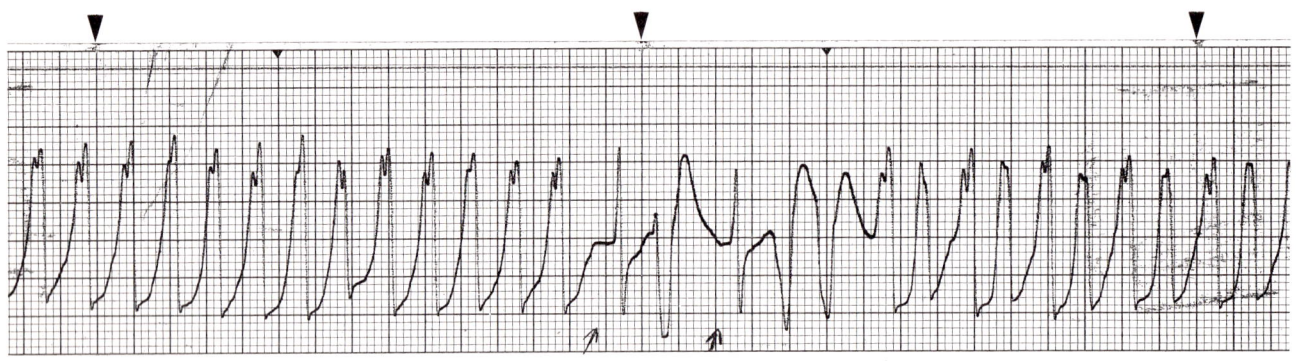

RHYTHM STRIP 20–17B.
(White RD: Paramedic EKG Collection)

STRIP #: *17B*
RATE: *240/min*
RHYTHM: *Slightly irregular*
P WAVE: *Not visible*
PR INTERVAL: *Unmeasurable*
QRS COMPLEX: *0.12–0.16 sec; two are 0.08 sec*
RHYTHM INTERPRETATION: *Ventricular tachycardia with two supraventricular capture complexes. The unusual alteration of QRS complex morphology after the capture complexes is secondary to a capture complex-induced alteration in the reentry circuit of the ventricular tachycardia.*

One unusual variant of ventricular tachycardia is known as **torsades de pointes** (literally "twisting of the points"). In torsades, the polarity of the complexes is constantly shifting, giving the rhythm strip a twisted appearance. Torsades may be caused by several disorders, including electrolyte imbalances and acute ischemia, and commonly is an effect of certain antiarrhythmic agents that increase the QT interval. These agents include disopyramide, procainamide, and quinidine. The term *polymorphous ventricular tachycardia* is applied to a torsadeslike arrhythmia that is not associated with QT interval prolongation. Torsades often converts to a sinus rhythm spontaneously, but it may degenerate into ventricular fibrillation. Management of diagnosed torsades de pointes is with bretylium, phenytoin, propranolol, or in-hospital pacing.

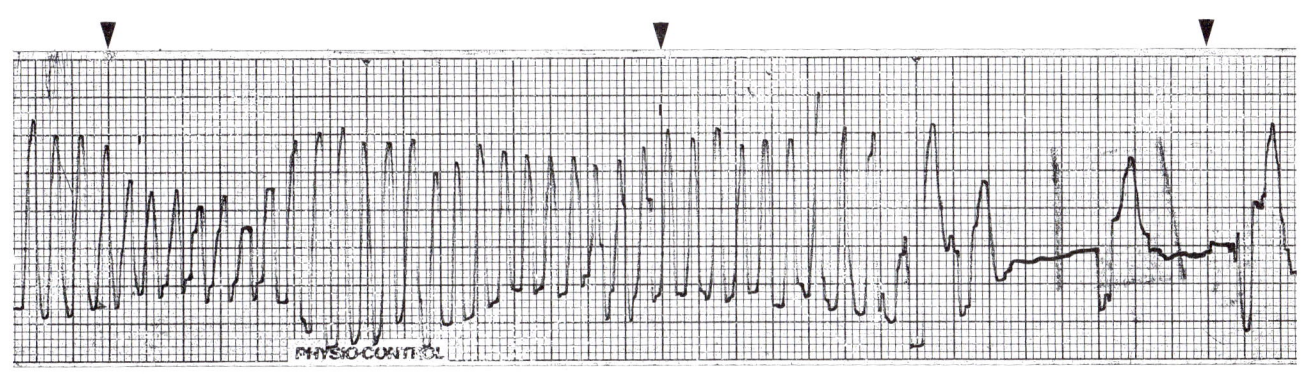

RHYTHM STRIP 20–17C.
(White RD: Paramedic EKG Collection)

STRIP #: *17C*

RATE: *Greater than 350/min, slowing to 75/min*

RHYTHM: *Generally regular*

P WAVE: *Not visible*

PR INTERVAL: *Unmeasurable*

QRS COMPLEX: *Wide and bizarre; varying amplitude and polarity ("twisting of the points")*

RHYTHM INTERPRETATION: *Polymorphous ventricular tachycardia (PVT) with spontaneous conversion in a 49-year-old male with acute myocardial ischemia*

Ventricular Fibrillation

Ventricular fibrillation is a chaotic, disorganized rhythm caused by numerous areas of electrical discharge or multiple reentry circuits in the ventricles, creating electrical havoc. Total absence of any organized electrical activity and only quivering of heart muscle fibers rapidly lead to death. Although ventricular fibrillation has a wide variety of causes, the most common etiology is coronary artery disease and acute myocardial infarction. The EKG characteristics for a lead II rhythm strip are not easily measurable and have undulations of varying amplitude and shape with no visible normal waves or complexes. The amplitude and frequency of the fibrillatory waves can be used to define the type of fibrillation as being coarse, medium, or fine in quality. This distinction is often used to assess the likelihood of successful elimination of ventricular fibrillation by electrical shocks.

Clinical Significance. Ventricular fibrillation results in cardiac arrest due to lack of organized cardiac contraction.

Management. Early defibrillation is the most important management for ventricular fibrillation as demonstrated in numerous research projects to date. Defibrillation should initially be attempted up to three times in rapid succession at energy settings of 200 to 300 J, increasing up to a maximum of 360 J. Other management modalities that should be instituted for ventricular fibrillation that is refractory to electrical defibrillation include CPR, definitive airway management, usually by endotracheal intubation, and IV drug administration before additional shocks. Drugs include epinephrine to improve perfusion of coronary arteries and other vital organs during CPR and lidocaine to help suppress ventricular ectopy and enhance defibrillation attempts. Other antiarrhythmic drugs, such as bretylium, may also be used. Patients who remain in cardiac arrest for more than 10 minutes may receive sodium bicarbonate according to medical protocols. Refer to Figure 20-19 for the American Heart Association's advanced life support protocols for ventricular fibrillation.

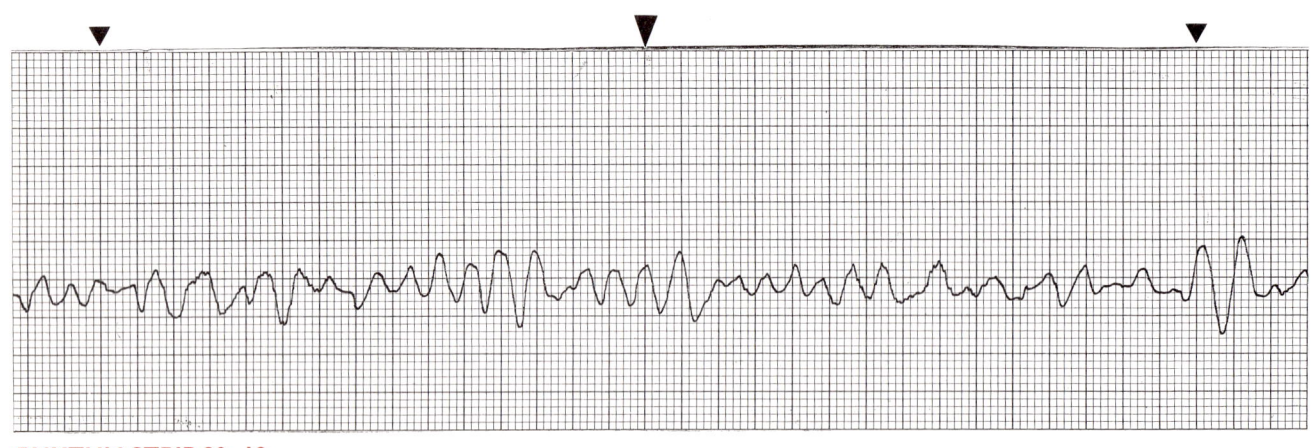

RHYTHM STRIP 20–18.
(Huff J, Doernbach DP, White RD)

STRIP #: *18*
RATE: *Unmeasurable*
RHYTHM: *Chaotic*
P WAVE: *Not visible; wave deflections are irregular and chaotic and vary in height, size, and shape*
PR INTERVAL: *Unmeasurable*
QRS COMPLEX: *Absent*
RHYTHM INTERPRETATION: *Ventricular fibrillation*

Asystole

Asystole occurs when electrical activity in the ventricles is completely absent. Asystole is the end result of ventricular fibrillation gone uncorrected. When it occurs as the initial rhythm in cardiac arrest, it is usually associated with massive myocardial damage. On EKG, there are no discernible waves or complexes but only an isoelectric line, although P waves may be present in ventricular standstill.

Clinical Significance. The absence of electrical and, therefore, mechanical function results in cardiac arrest. The prognosis for resuscitation from asystole is universally dismal to date.

Management. Asystole should be confirmed by checking the EKG in two different leads. Prehospital management consists primarily of CPR, definitive airway management usually with an endotracheal tube, and administration of epinephrine and, possibly, atropine. Prolonged cardiac arrest may warrant administration of sodium bicarbonate. External pacing may be attempted but has not been demonstrated to be very effective. It is important to keep in mind that it may be difficult to distinguish asystole from a low-amplitude ventricular fibrillation and that ventricular fibrillation is, at times, erroneously recorded on surface EKG as asystole. For these reasons, local medical protocols may include defibrillation of apparent asystole if any uncertainty remains after a lead search to identify underlying ventricular fibrillation. Advanced cardiac life support protocols for asystole are shown in Figure 20-42. (See Rhythm Strips 20-19A and 20-19B on the following page.)

If rhythm is unclear and possibly ventricular fibrillation, defibrillate as for VF.
If asystole is present,[a]
↓
Continue CPR
↓
Establish IV access
↓
Epinephrine, 1:10,000, 0.5–1.0 mg IV push[b]
↓
Intubate when possible[c]
↓
Atropine, 1.0 mg IV push (repeated in 5 min)
↓
(Consider bicarbonate)[d]
↓
Consider pacing

Asystole (cardiac standstill). This sequence was developed to assist in teaching how to treat a broad range of patients with asystole. Some patients may require care not specified herein. This algorithm should not be construed to prohibit such flexibility. The flow of the algorithm presumes asystole is continuing. VF = ventricular fibrillation; IV = intravenous; CPR = cardiopulmonary resuscitation.
[a]Asystole should be confirmed in two leads.
[b]Epinephrine should be repeated every 5 minutes.
[c]Intubation is preferable; if it can be accomplished simultaneously with other techniques, then the earlier the better. However, cardiopulmonary resuscitation (CPR) and the use of epinephrine are more important initially if the patient can be ventilated without intubation. (Endotracheal epinephrine may be used.)
[d]The value of sodium bicarbonate is questionable during cardiac arrest, and it is not recommended for routine cardiac arrest sequences. Consideration of its use in a dose of 1 mEq/kg is appropriate at this point. Half of the original dose may be repeated every 10 minutes if it is used.

FIGURE 20–42.
Advanced cardiac life support treatment protocol for asystole. (© American Heart Association: Textbook of Advanced Cardiac Life Support, 2nd ed, p 239. Dallas, American Heart Association, 1987)

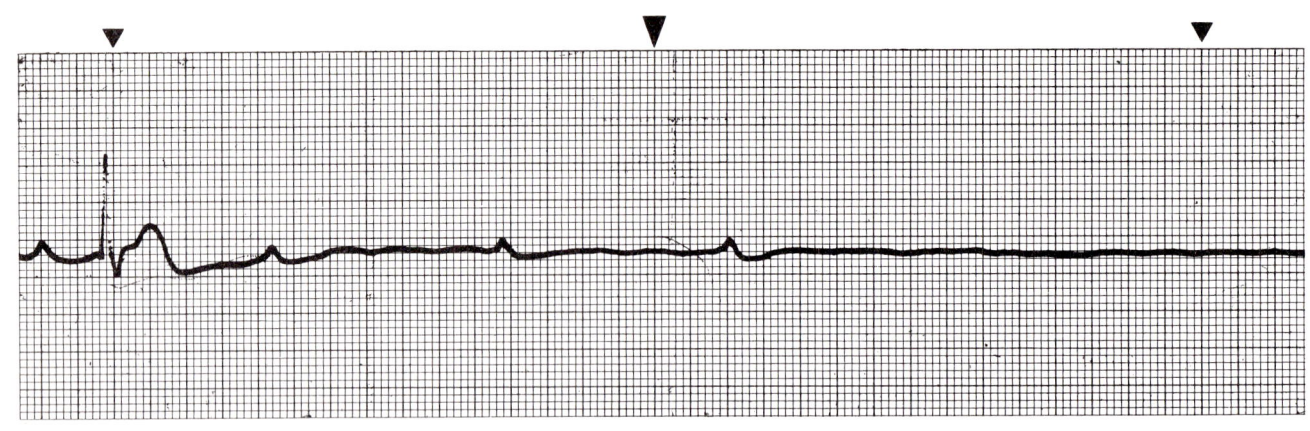

RHYTHM STRIP 20–19A.
(Huff J, Doernbach DP, White RD)

STRIP #: *19A*

RATE: *Atrial, less than 30/min; ventricular, essentially 0*

RHYTHM: *Irregular atrial*

P WAVE: *Upright and uniform; P waves present only at beginning of strip; most not followed by QRS complexes*

PR INTERVAL: *0.36 sec for single QRS complex*

QRS COMPLEX: *0.12 sec for single complex*

RHYTHM INTERPRETATION: *Single cardiac cycle that terminates in primary ventricular standstill and asystole*

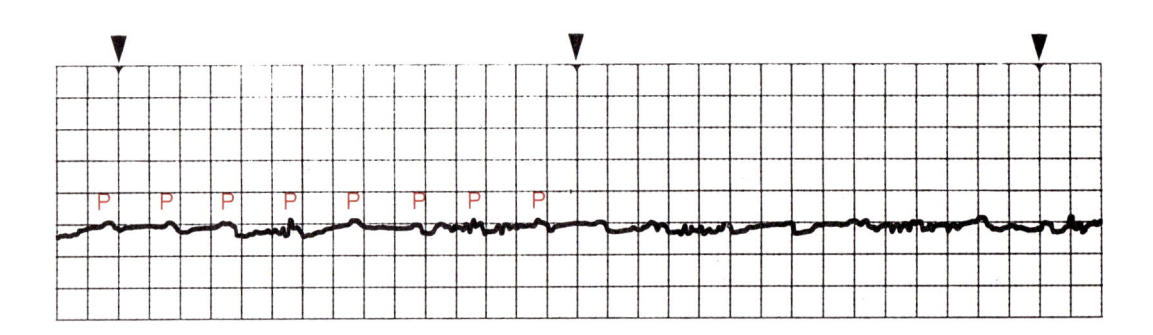

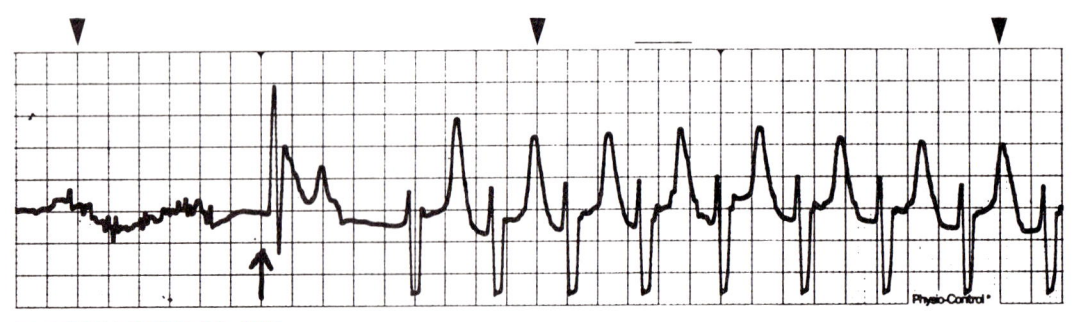

RHYTHM STRIP 20–19B.
(White RD: Paramedic EKG Collection)

STRIP #: *19B*

RHYTHM INTERPRETATION: *Ventricular asystole with sinus tachycardia in a 72-year-old female with repeated brief episodes of syncope, which prompted the EMS call. A 12-second period of standstill was terminated by a single precordial thump at arrow. Carotid sinus hypersensitivity was diagnosed and a permanent pacemaker inserted.*

Arrhythmias That Are Disorders of Conduction

Atrioventricular (AV) blocks reflect delay or interruption in conduction of impulses through the AV junction due to disease in this region. This pathologic block, due to such conditions as ischemia, necrosis, degenerative diseases of the conduction system, and certain drug toxicity, is quite different from the physiologic AV block that occurs in atrial flutter and fibrillation. Atrioventricular blocks traditionally have been divided into three categories: first, second, and third degree. Although this classification is used for discussion purposes, a more meaningful classification may be made according to location of the block. Various AV blocks may occur at the level of the AV node, at the level of the bundle of His, or below the bifurcation of the bundle of His (Fig. 20-43). The site of this block can often be determined on EKG and, along with clinical findings, may help determine urgency and management of the block. Blocks at the level of the AV node are usually reversible, while blocks below the bundle of His are usually irreversible and frequently progress to more serious degrees.

Advanced cardiac life support protocols for bradycardia (sinus and AV blocks) are shown in Figure 20-44.

First Degree AV Block

First degree AV block is a condition in which conduction of impulses through the AV junction is delayed, but no actual block occurs. The site of first degree block is usually at the level of the AV node and may be caused by acute ischemia or digitalis preparations, among other causes. The only alteration in the EKG is a PR interval prolonged for more than 0.20 second.

Clinical Significance. Since all atrial impulses are conducted to the ventricles, this block is not detrimental to the patient and frequently resolves when the ischemia resolves. However, a newly developed first degree block may be the forerunner of more advanced degrees of block.

Management. No definitive management is required, but the EKG should be monitored closely.

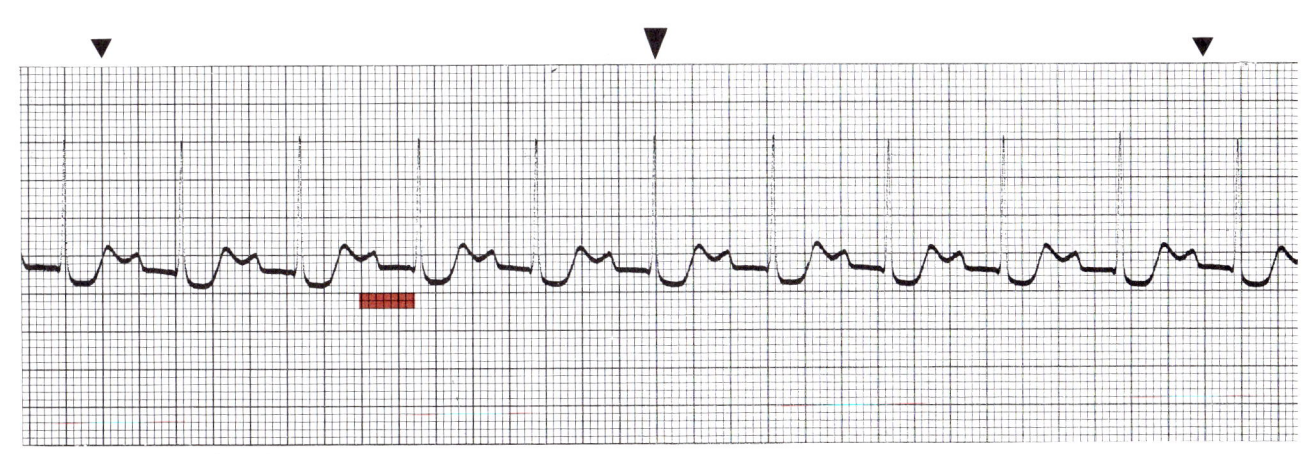

RHYTHM STRIP 20–20.
(Huff J, Doernbach DP, White RD)

STRIP #: *20*
RATE: *94/min*
RHYTHM: *Regular*
P WAVE: *One per QRS complex; upright and uniform*
PR INTERVAL: *0.28 sec and constant*
QRS COMPLEX: *0.04–0.06 sec and all alike*
RHYTHM INTERPRETATION: *Sinus rhythm with first degree AV block*

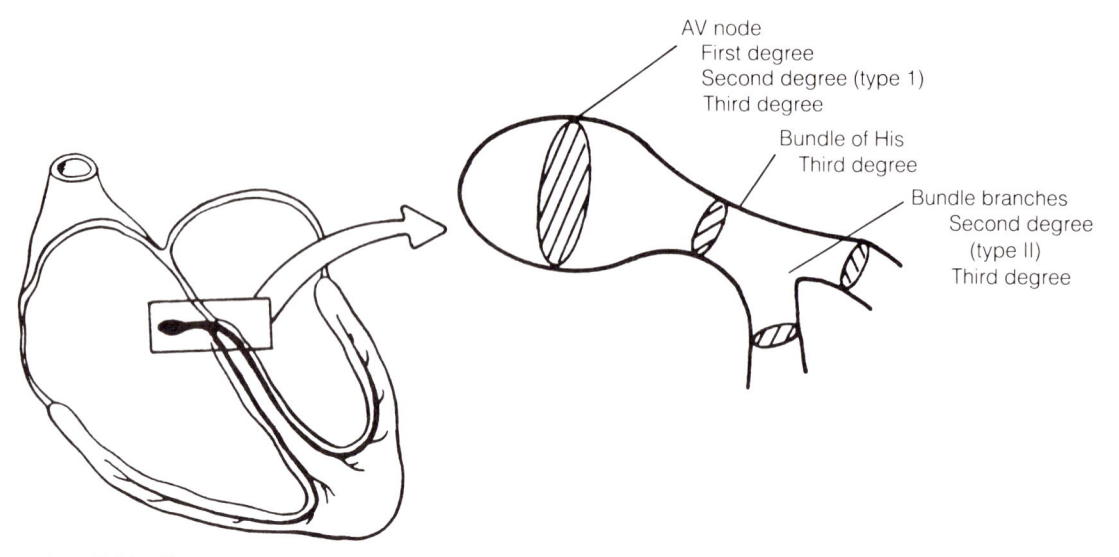

FIGURE 20–43.
Potential sites of AV block.

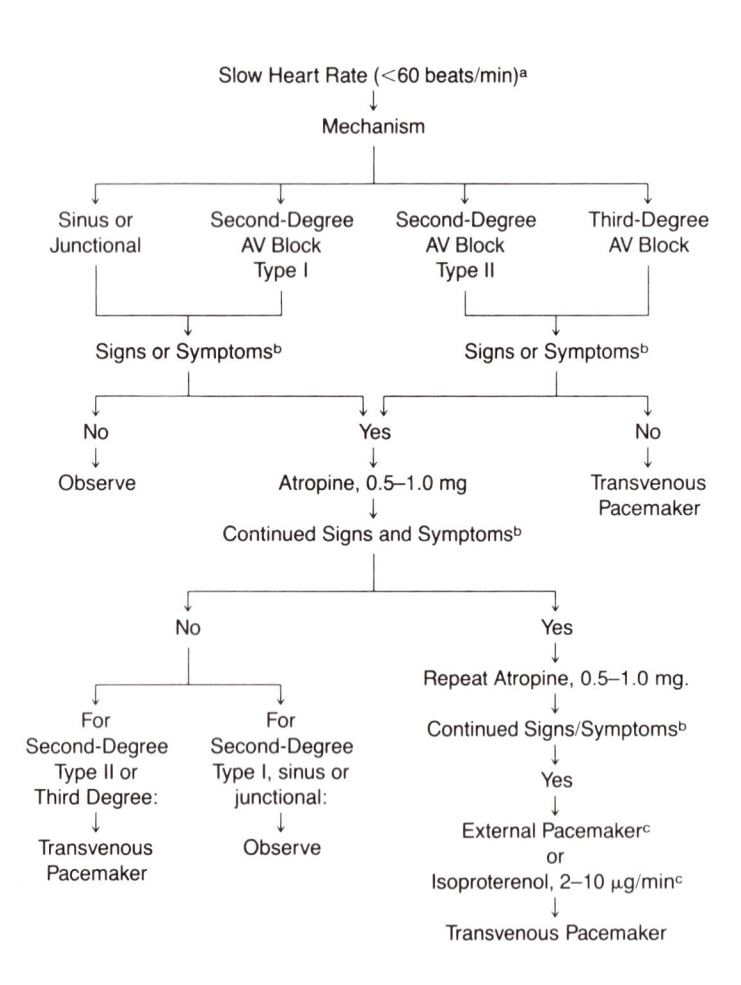

Bradycardia. This sequence was developed to assist in teaching how to treat a broad range of patients with bradycardia. Some patients may require care not specified herein. This algorithm should not be construed to prohibit such flexibility. AV = atrioventricular.
[a] A solitary chest (precordial) thump or cough may stimulate cardiac electrical activity and result in improved cardiac output. Either may be tried at this point.
[b] Hypotension (blood pressure <90 mmHg), premature ventricular contractions, altered mental status or physical symptoms (e.g., chest pain or dyspnea), ischemia, or infarction.
[c] Temporizing therapy.

FIGURE 20–44.
Advanced cardiac life support treatment protocol for bradycardia. (© American Heart Association: Textbook of Advanced Cardiac Life Support, 2nd ed, p 242. Dallas, American Heart Association, 1987)

Second Degree AV Block

Second degree AV block is divided into Type I (Mobitz I or Wenckebach) and Type II (Mobitz II).

TYPE I (MOBITZ I OR WENCKEBACH). **Type I second degree AV block,** also called **Mobitz I** or **Wenckebach,** is an intermittent block in which the AV junction becomes progressively slower in transmitting the sinus impulse over a series of cycles, until it finally blocks an impulse completely. This condition produces on EKG a characteristic cyclic pattern of PR intervals that become progressively longer until one P wave is totally blocked and produces no QRS complex. After a pause, during which the AV node recovers, this cycle is repeated. The ratio of conduction (or P waves to QRS complexes) may be constant or variable and is commonly two to one, three to two, four to three, or five to four. Although the P-to-P interval is constant in type I block, the R-to-R interval decreases if two or more complexes in a row are conducted before the dropped (blocked) complex. This pattern produces grouping of QRS complexes on a long EKG tracing, one of the important clues to interpretation. Type I block usually occurs at the level of the AV node. Its etiology may be increased vagal tone, certain drug effects, or AV junctional ischemia, often associated with inferior myocardial infarction. The EKG features for a lead II rhythm strip are the following:

RATE: *Atrial rate unaffected; ventricular rate may be normal or slightly slow*

RHYTHM: *Atrial regular; ventricular irregular with characteristic group complexes*

P WAVES: *More P waves than QRS complexes; all upright and uniform*

PR INTERVAL: *Progressively lengthening before nonconducted P wave (dropped complex) except when conduction ratio is two to one*

QRS COMPLEX: *0.10 sec or less, provided no other conduction disturbance is present*

Clinical Significance. Type I second degree AV block, because it is often associated with ischemia rather then necrosis, may only be a temporary conduction disturbance that resolves spontaneously. However, 50% of cases associated with a myocardial infarction progress to more advanced forms of AV block. If complete heart block develops, however, heart rate usually is sustained by a junctional escape pacemaker at 40 to 60 beats per minute, which may temporarily provide adequate cardiac output. There is also the potential for slow rates with type I second degree AV block caused by frequently dropped complexes and their accompanying pauses, leading to decreased cardiac output and its associated problems.

Management. If excessive slowing of the heart rate occurs, IV atropine is usually effective. (See Rhythm Strips 20-21A and 20-21B on the following page.)

486 UNIT FOUR: MEDICAL EMERGENCIES

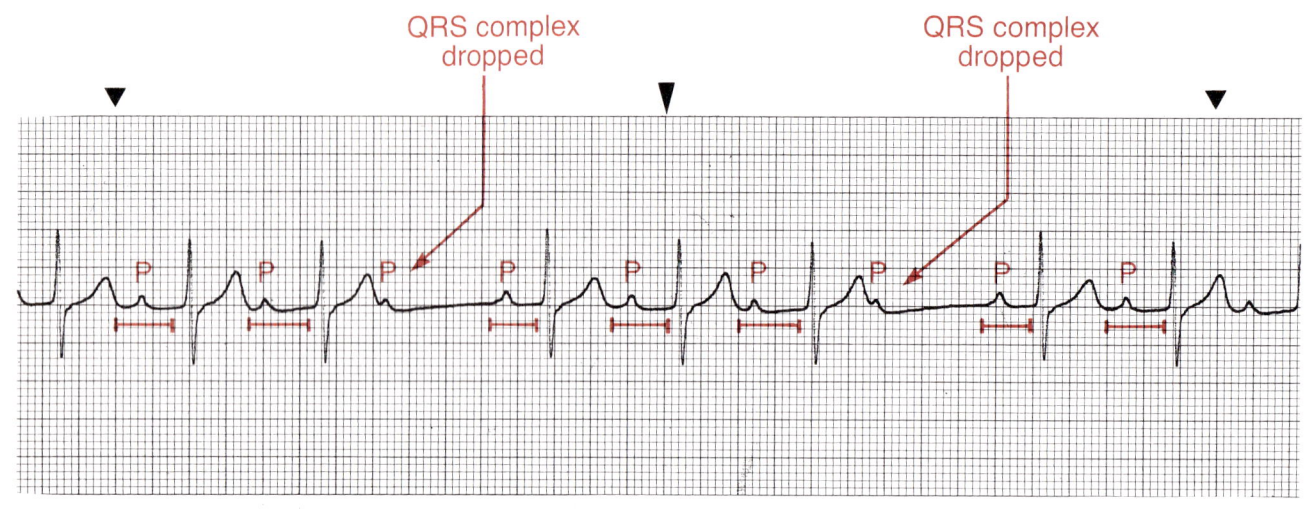

RHYTHM STRIP 20–21A.
(Huff J, Doernbach DP, White RD)

STRIP #: *21A*

RATE: *Atrial, 88/min; ventricular, 70/min*

RHYTHM: *Regular atrial; irregular ventricular*

P WAVE: *Upright and uniform; two not followed by QRS complexes (or more than one preceding some QRS complexes)*

PR INTERVAL: *Cyclical lengthening from 0.24 to 0.28 to 0.36 sec before "dropped" QRS complex*

QRS COMPLEX: *0.06–0.08 sec and all alike*

RHYTHM INTERPRETATION: *Sinus rhythm with second degree AV block, type I (4:3 conduction)*

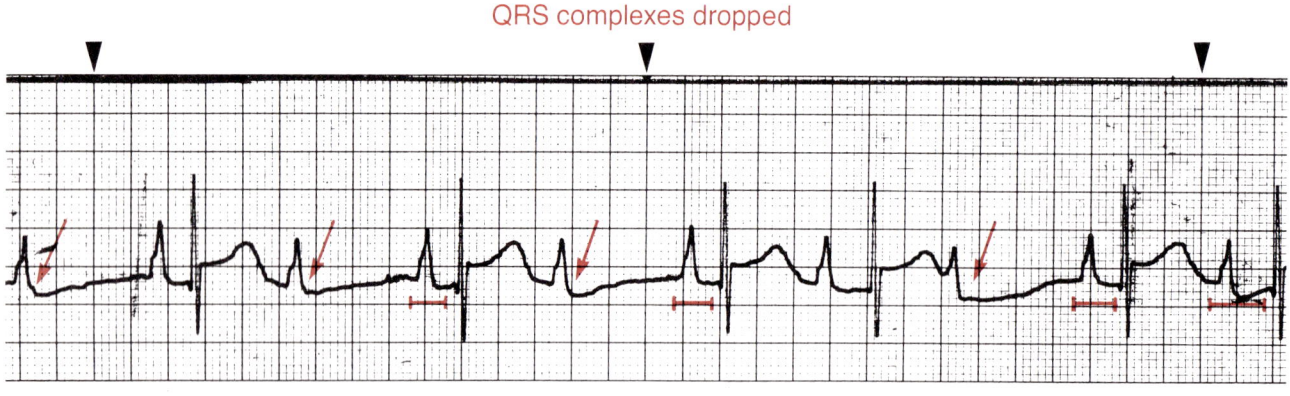

RHYTHM STRIP 20–21B.
(White RD: Paramedic EKG Collection)

STRIP #: *21B*

RATE: *Atrial, 83/min; ventricular, 50/min*

RHYTHM: *Regular atrial; irregular ventricular*

P WAVE: *Upright and uniform; more than one preceding some QRS complexes (or not all P waves followed by QRS complexes)*

PR INTERVAL: *Cyclical lengthening from 0.24 to 0.30 sec before "dropped" QRS complex*

QRS COMPLEX: *0.08 sec and all alike*

RHYTHM INTERPRETATION: *Sinus rhythm with second degree AV block, type I (2:1 and 3:2 conduction) in a 70-year-old female with an acute inferior wall myocardial infarction*

TYPE II (MOBITZ II). ***Type II second degree AV block,*** also called ***Mobitz II*** is an intermittent block that also produces P waves that are not conducted, but it does not have any prolongation of the PR interval before the dropped QRS complex. The PR intervals may be normal or prolonged but are usually constant. The conduction ratio, usually constant but sometimes variable, is commonly two to one, three to one, or four to one, producing two, three, or four P waves to every QRS complex. Type II block usually occurs below the level of the bifurcation of the bundle of His, involving both bundle branches. The QRS complexes are abnormally wide when one bundle branch is blocked and are absent when both bundle branches are blocked. In a two-to-one block, the QRS complex duration may be the only feature that suggests type II block, although even QRS complex prolongation does not assure this diagnosis. The etiology of type II second degree AV block is frequently necrosis of the interventricular septum due to anterior myocardial infarction. The EKG features for a lead II rhythm strip are the following:

RATE: *Atrial rate unaffected; ventricular rate usually slow*
RHYTHM: *Usually regular unless conduction ratio varies*
P WAVES: *More than one P wave for each QRS complex, all upright and uniform*
PR INTERVAL: *May be normal or prolonged but constant*
QRS COMPLEX: *Often wide (0.12 sec or greater)*

Clinical Significance. The slow rates associated with this block frequently compromise cardiac output and produce all the associated symptoms. Although less common than type I block, type II is considered more serious because of its association with extensive myocardial necrosis. It frequently progresses to third degree AV block and, when it does so, results in slow heart rates (20–40) sustained by a ventricular escape pacemaker.

Management. In the field, only temporizing measures are possible, as the patient usually requires pacemaker implantation. Therapeutic modalities to increase heart rate include IV atropine, β stimulators, such as isoproterenol, and external pacing, if available.

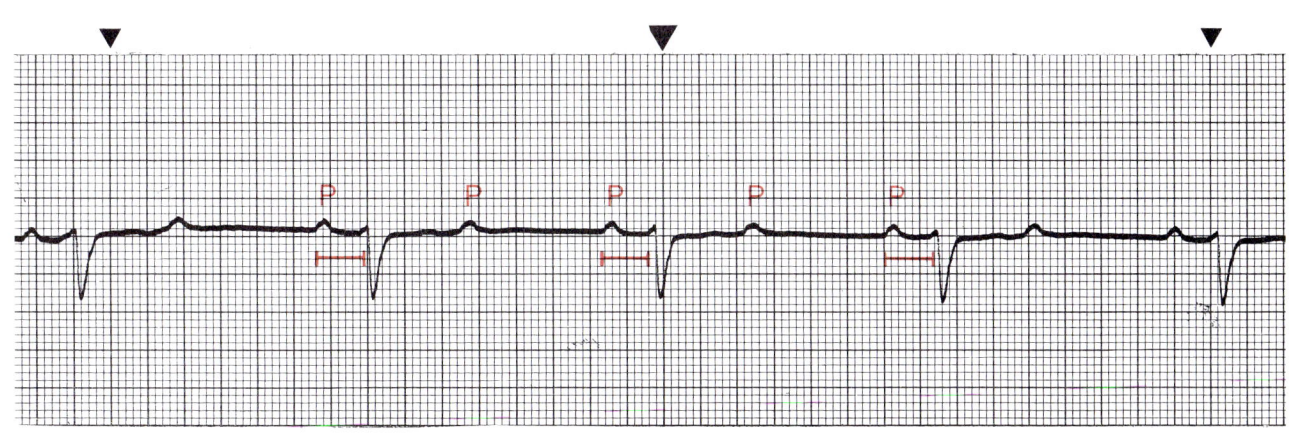

RHYTHM STRIP 20–22.
(Huff J, Doernbach DP, White RD)

STRIP #: *22*
RATE: *Atrial, 76/min; ventricular, 38/min*
RHYTHM: *Regular, atrial and ventricular*
P WAVE: *Upright and uniform; two P waves before each QRS complex (or not all P waves followed by QRS complexes)*
PR INTERVAL: *0.28 sec and constant*
QRS COMPLEX: *0.12 sec and all alike*
RHYTHM INTERPRETATION: *Sinus rhythm with 2:1 second degree AV block, type II*

Third Degree AV Block

In ***third degree AV block***, also called *complete heart block*, conduction between atria and ventricles is totally absent because of complete electrical block at or below the AV node. The atria remain under the influence of the SA node but are completely independent of the ventricles, which must rely on activation by an escape pacemaker somewhere below the level of the block. If the block is high in the AV junction, a junctional escape pacemaker with a relatively good rate assumes control; a block low in the bundle of His results in a slow ventricular escape rhythm. The two independent pacemakers are manifested by regular P-to-P intervals and regular R-to-R intervals but no relationship between the P waves and QRS complexes (AV dissociation). Etiology of third degree AV block includes a myocardial infarction, digitalis toxicity, and, particularly in the elderly, certain degenerative diseases of the conduction system. The EKG features for a lead II rhythm strip are the following:

RATE: *Atrial rate unaffected; ventricular rate 40 to 60 if escape focus is junctional, less than 40 if escape focus is ventricular*
RHYTHM: *Both atrial and ventricular usually regular (ventricular may be irregular if escape pacemaker is very low)*
P WAVES: *More P waves than QRS complexes; all upright and uniform; may be superimposed on QRS complexes or T waves*
PR INTERVAL: *Varies greatly*
QRS COMPLEX: *Normal if ventricles are activated by junctional escape focus, wide if escape focus is ventricular*

Clinical Significance. The slow heart rates that frequently occur with complete block along with loss of atrial and ventricular synchronization often cause severe compromise of cardiac output. Patients may develop hypotension, chest pain, or acute heart failure. Syncope is common, especially at the onset of block before an escape pacemaker has been activated (*Stokes-Adams syndrome*).

Management. Once again, prehospital management can only temporize this condition, as definitive management is pacemaker insertion. Atropine may be administered to attempt to stimulate some AV conduction or speed the rate of a junctional escape focus. Often, a β stimulator, such as isoproterenol, or external pacing is required to increase the ventricular rate. Transport should be expedited and the receiving hospital alerted for preparation for pacemaker insertion.

CHAPTER 20: Cardiovascular Emergencies

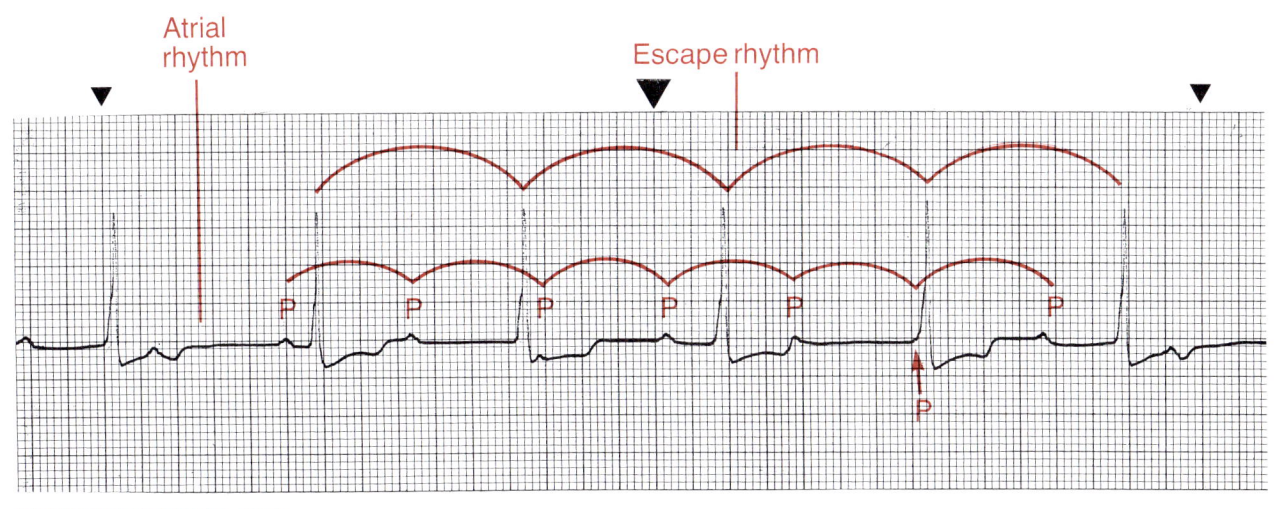

RHYTHM STRIP 20–23A.
(Huff J, Doernbach DP, White RD)

STRIP #: *23A*

RATE: *Atrial, 88/min; ventricular, 58/min*

RHYTHM: *Regular, atrial and ventricular*

P WAVE: *Upright and uniform; more than one preceding some QRS complexes (or not all P waves followed by QRS complexes)*

PR INTERVAL: *Varies greatly; P waves not relating to QRS complexes*

QRS COMPLEX: *0.08 sec and all alike*

RHYTHM INTERPRETATION: *Sinus rhythm with third degree complete AV block and junctional escape pacemaker*

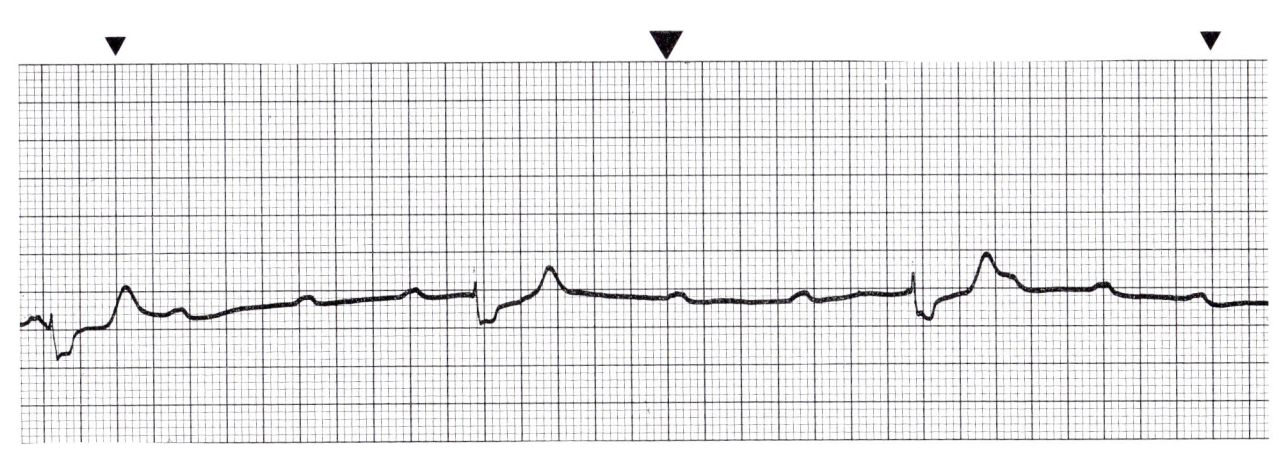

RHYTHM STRIP 20–23B.
(Huff J, Doernbach DP, White RD)

STRIP #: *23B*

RATE: *Atrial, 100/min; ventricular, 25/min*

RHYTHM: *Fairly regular, atrial and ventricular*

P WAVE: *Upright and uniform; more than one preceding each QRS complex (or not all P waves followed by QRS complexes)*

PR INTERVAL: *Varies greatly; P waves not relating to QRS complexes*

QRS COMPLEX: *0.12 sec and all alike*

RHYTHM INTERPRETATION: *Sinus rhythm with third degree (complete) AV block and ventricular escape pacemaker*

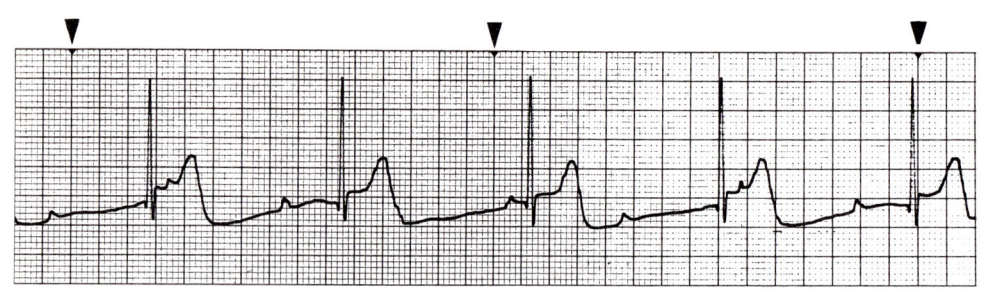

RHYTHM STRIP 20–23C.
(White RD: Paramedic EKG Collection)

STRIP #: *23C*

RATE: *Atrial, 75/min; ventricular, 45/min*

RHYTHM: *Regular, atrial and ventricular*

P WAVE: *Upright and uniform; more than one preceding some QRS complexes (or not all P waves followed by QRS complexes)*

PR INTERVAL: *Varies greatly; P waves not relating to QRS complexes*

QRS COMPLEX: *Less than 0.08 sec and all alike*

RHYTHM INTERPRETATION: *Sinus rhythm with complete AV block and junctional escape rhythm in a 57-year-old female with an acute inferior myocardial infarction*

In addition to AV block, other disorders of conduction that the paramedic will encounter include problems with conduction through the ventricles via the bundle-branch system. *Aberrant conduction* and *bundle-branch block* are two terms used to describe EKG complexes that originate above the ventricles but encounter some sort of problem with conduction through the ventricles.

The term aberrant conduction is used to describe supraventricular impulses that have normal atrial and AV conduction but that are conducted through the ventricles in a delayed manner. This phenomenon frequently is seen with premature impulses that, because of their prematurity, reach the ventricles when one of the bundle branches (usually the right) is still refractory and cannot conduct. Conduction through one ventricle is normal but delayed in the other, as the impulse must travel a slower route through muscle tissue to depolarize the blocked side. Aberrant conduction may occur with PACs or PJCs and is common in atrial fibrillation because of the extreme irregularity of the rhythm.

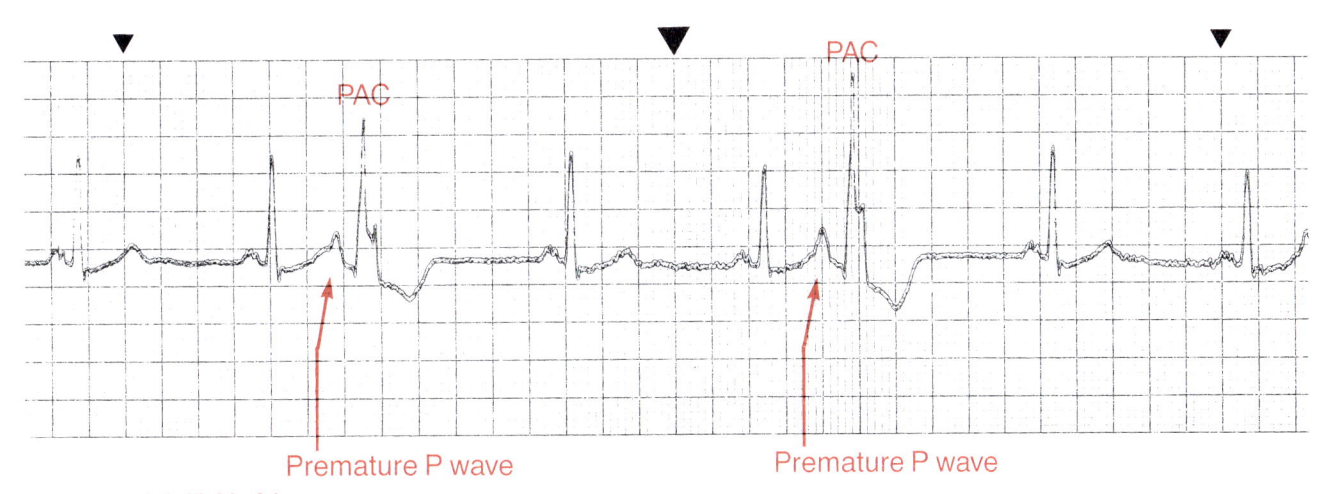

RHYTHM STRIP 20–24.
(Huff J, Doernbach DP, White RD)

STRIP #: *24*
RATE: *Basic rate 58/min (average, 60/min)*
RHYTHM: *Irregular, due to premature complexes*
P WAVE: *One per QRS complex; upright; two premature with different shape*
PR INTERVAL: *0.12–0.14 sec*
QRS COMPLEX: *0.06–0.08 sec; premature complexes 0.12–0.14 sec*
RHYTHM INTERPRETATION: *Sinus bradycardia with aberrantly conducted premature atrial complexes*

The term bundle-branch block is used to describe a rhythm that is supraventricular in origin, but all the impulses in the rhythm are conducted through the ventricles in a delayed manner. Bundle-branch block usually is caused by ischemia or necrosis of either the right or left bundle branch, making it unable to conduct impulses to the ventricle it supplies. In the prehospital setting, bundle-branch block may be a new occurrence or a chronic condition.

The EKG features of these ventricular conduction disturbances involve changes in the characteristics of the QRS complexes. The duration of the QRS complex becomes 0.12 second or greater because of slower conduction through myocardial muscle in the blocked ventricle (Fig. 20-45). The shape of the QRS complex may also be altered to appear notched or slurred. This notching is evidence of rapid depolarization of one ventricle via the normal bundle branch, followed by slower depolarization of the ventricle with the bundle-branch block.

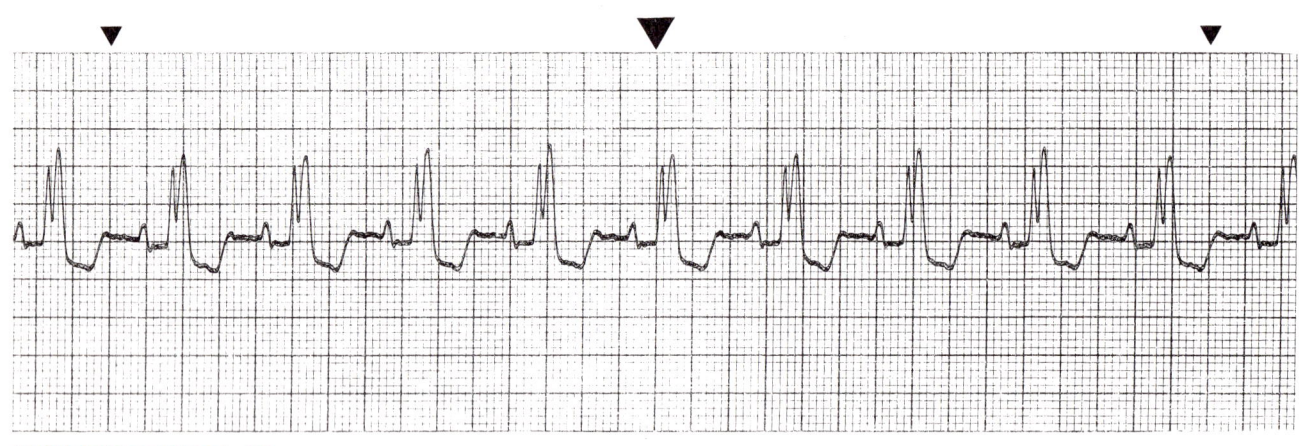

RHYTHM STRIP 20–25.
(Huff J, Doernbach DP, White RD)

STRIP #: *25*
RATE: *88/min*
RHYTHM: *Regular*
P WAVE: *One per QRS complex; upright and uniform*
PR INTERVAL: *0.16 sec and constant*
QRS COMPLEX: *0.12 sec; notched and all alike*
RHYTHM INTERPRETATION: *Normal sinus rhythm with bundle-branch block*

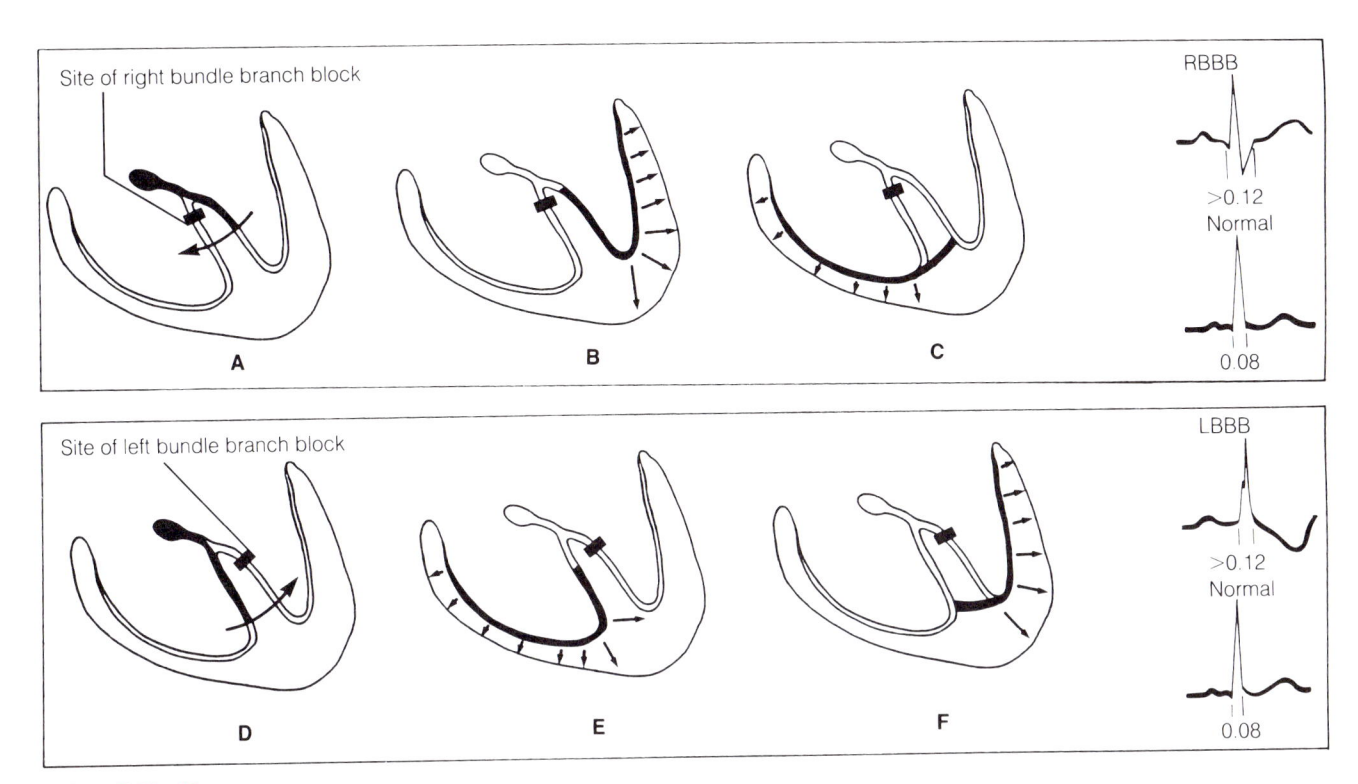

FIGURE 20-45.
Altered ventricular conduction due to right bundle-branch block (top) and left bundle-branch block (bottom). Arrows show direction of septal depolarization (**A**), left ventricular muscle depolarization (**B**), delayed right ventricular muscle depolarization (**C**), direction of septal depolarization (**D**), right ventricular muscle depolarization (**E**), and delayed left ventricular muscle depolarization (**F**).

Although the presence of aberrant conduction or bundle-branch block does not alter the management of patients, it may pose difficulties in rhythm interpretation. It may be impossible to distinguish with a lead II rhythm strip between PVCs and aberrantly conducted PACs or PJCs. Likewise, a PSVT with bundle-branch block or runs of successive aberrantly conducted complexes may closely resemble ventricular tachycardia.

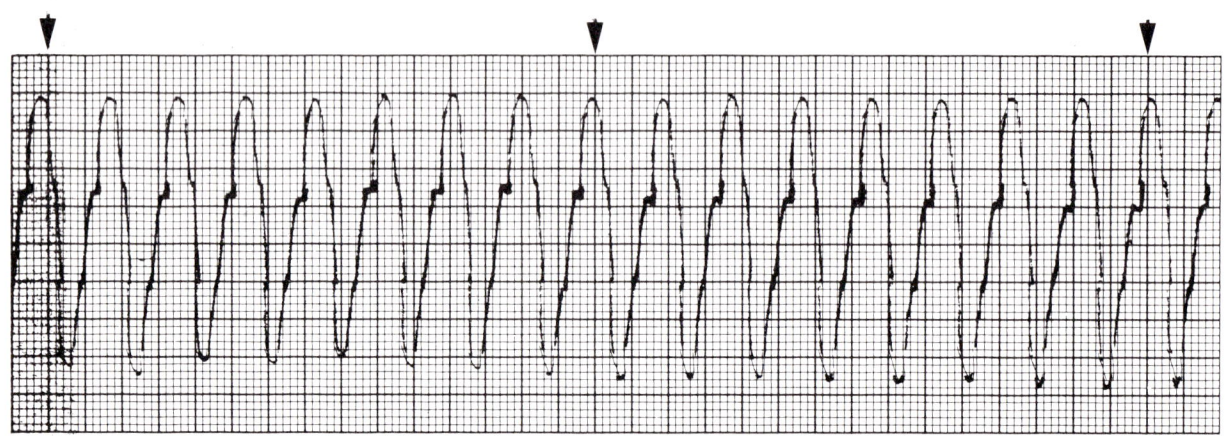

RHYTHM STRIP 20–26.
(Hurst C)

STRIP #: *26*
RATE: *150/min*
RHYTHM: *Regular*
P WAVE: *Not visible*
PR INTERVAL: *Unmeasurable*
QRS COMPLEX: *Greater than 0.12 sec and all alike*
RHYTHM INTERPRETATION: *Supraventricular tachycardia with aberration; not ventricular tachycardia*

Paramedics must be aware that supraventricular complexes or rhythms, at times, may have abnormally wide QRS complexes, and they must search for other features of the arrhythmia that may aid in the interpretation (e.g., the presence of normal P waves that precede each wide QRS complex). When doubt exists, it is safest to treat all premature complexes or rhythms with wide QRS complexes as though they are ventricular in origin until a more definitive interpretation can be made on 12-lead EKG. Failure to treat a rhythm that may be due to ventricular ectopy holds greater risk than failure to manage a more benign supraventricular rhythm.

Artificial Pacemaker Rhythms

An *artificial cardiac pacemaker* is a device used to electronically stimulate the heart in place of the heart's own natural pacemaker and conduction system. It is comprised of one or more electrodes implanted in the heart connected to a power source for generating regular, timed stimuli (Fig. 20-46). Some of the indications for insertion of a pacemaker are continuous or intermittent third degree AV block, second degree AV block type II, chronic atrial fibrillation with bradycardic ventricular response, and *sick sinus syndrome* (a condition manifested by sinus block, severe sinus bradycardia, or alternating periods of bradycardia and tachycardia). Several types of pacemakers exist, but the most common types used for the above conditions are the ventricular and the dual chambered pacemakers. Ventricular pacemakers stimulate only the ventricle, while dual chambered types stimulate both atrium and ventricle if needed. Dual chambered pacers are most beneficial for patients who require synchronized atrial-ventricular pumping to maintain cardiac output.

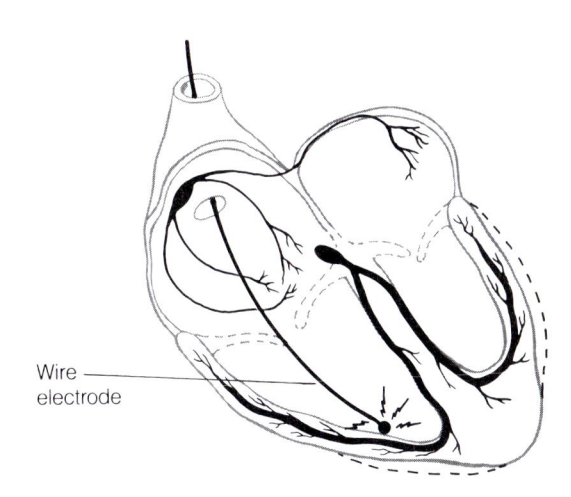

FIGURE 20–46.
Artificial ventricular pacemaker.

Pacemakers may be preset to stimulate the heart continuously or intermittently. A fixed-rate, or asynchronous, pacemaker fires continuously at a preset rate without regard to the patient's own electrical activity. A demand, or synchronous, pacemaker has a sensing device to detect the patient's electrical activity and acts as an escape mechanism, only firing if the patient's rate drops below the pacemaker's preset rate. Depending on the type of pacemaker, activation stimulates the atrium and the ventricle, thus artificially producing an EKG rhythm. A pacemaker spike, a mark on the EKG that projects upward or downward from the baseline, is the indication that the pacemaker has fired. Demand ventricular pacemakers have both a sensing and pacing device located in the ventricle, and a pacing spike normally is followed by a wide, "ventricular-looking" QRS complex.

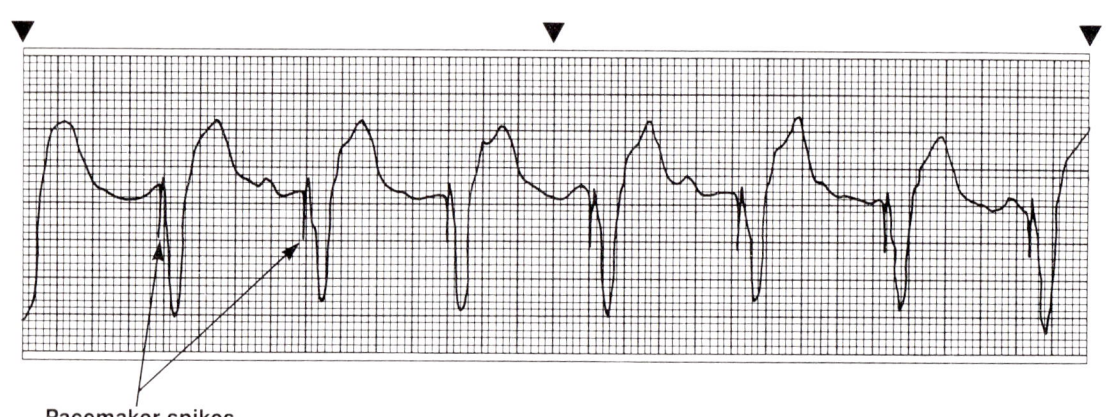

Pacemaker spikes

RHYTHM STRIP 20–27.
(Bunting–Blake L, Parker J, Weigel A)

STRIP #: 27
RATE: *Atrial, 100/min; ventricular, 75/min*
RHYTHM: *Regular, atrial and ventricular*
P WAVE: *Upright and uniform, not preceding all QRS complexes (some buried in QRS complexes)*
PR INTERVAL: *Variable or none; P waves not relating to QRS complexes*
QRS COMPLEX: *0.20 sec; and all alike; pacemaker spike preceding each QRS complex*
RHYTHM INTERPRETATION: *Ventricular pacemaker in capture with underlying sinus tachycardia*

Dual chambered pacemakers have sensing and pacing devices located both in the atrium and ventricle. The spike produced by the atrial electrode should be followed by a P wave, and the ventricular electrode generates a spike followed by a wide QRS complex.

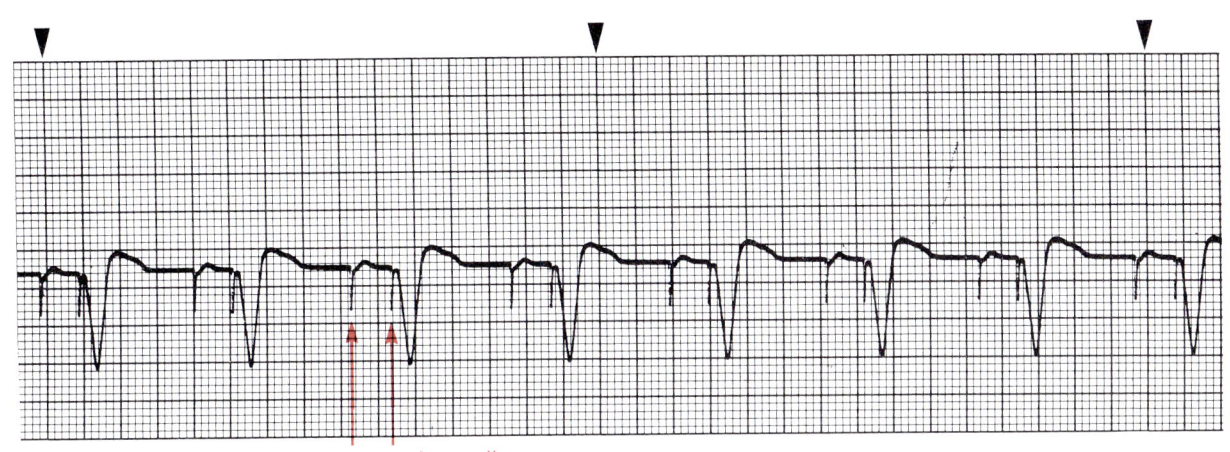

Pacemaker spikes

RHYTHM STRIP 20–28.
(Hurst C)

STRIP #: *28*

RATE: *68/min*

RHYTHM: *Regular*

P WAVE: *One per QRS complex; upright and uniform; each P wave preceded by pacemaker spike*

PR INTERVAL: *Pacemaker atrial–ventricular interval is 0.20 sec*

QRS COMPLEX: *0.16 sec and all alike; each QRS complex preceded by pacemaker spike*

RHYTHM INTERPRETATION: *Dual chambered (or atrial–ventricular sequential) pacer in capture*

498 UNIT FOUR: MEDICAL EMERGENCIES

A pacemaker is said to be in capture when a spike produces an EKG wave or complex. The EKG features of artificial pacemaker rhythms for a lead II rhythm strip are the following:

RATE: *Varies according to preset rate of pacemaker*

RHYTHM: *Regular if pacemaker is asynchronous or pacing constantly; irregular if pacing only on demand or synchronous*

P WAVES: *None produced by ventricular pacemaker—sinus P waves may be seen but are unrelated to QRS complexes; dual chambered pacer should have P waves after each atrial spike*

PR INTERVAL: *None for ventricular pacer; dual chambered pacer produces ventricular spike at constant interval from P wave*

QRS COMPLEX: *Wide (0.12 sec or greater) after each ventricular spike in paced rhythm; patient's own electrical activity may generate QRS complexes that are different from the paced QRS complexes*

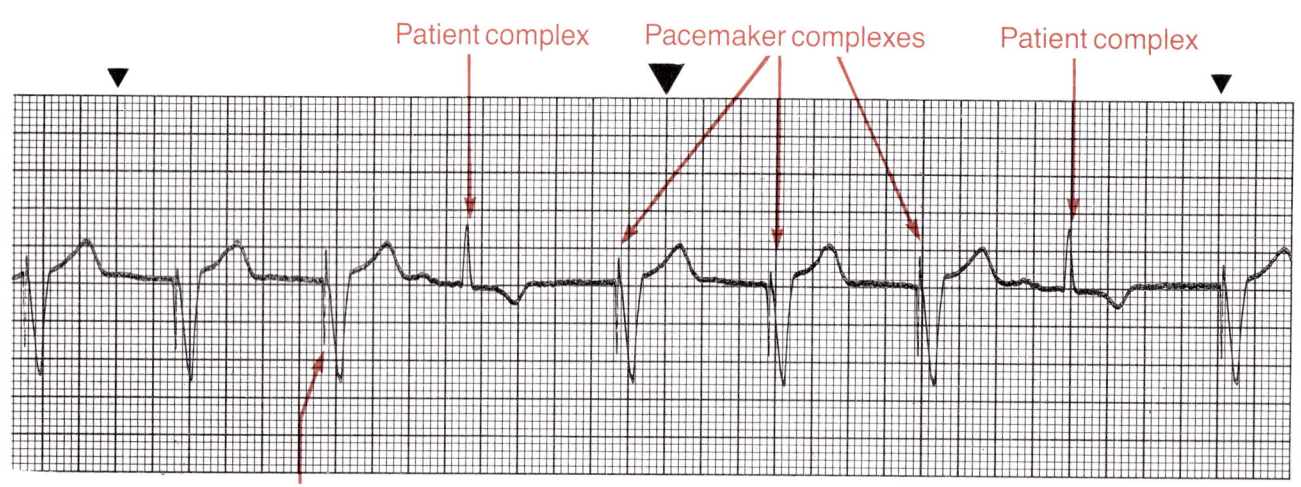

RHYTHM STRIP 20–29.
(Huff J, Doernbach DP, White RD)

STRIP #: *29*

AUTOMATIC INTERVAL RATE: *72/min*

ANALYSIS: *The first three complexes are paced complexes, followed by a patient complex, three paced complexes, a patient complex, and a paced complex*

INTERPRETATION: *Ventricular demand pacemaker set at rate of 72/min*

Problems that occur with artificial cardiac pacemakers and result in prehospital emergencies fall under the categories of failure to pace, failure to capture, and failure to sense. Failure to pace usually results in severe bradycardia or asystole and requires immediate intervention to sustain the patient until a new pacer can be inserted. Absence of pacemaker spikes may be due to a failure in any part of the pacemaker system and cannot be corrected in the field. Unlike older pacemakers, failure to pace (and runaway pacemaker) is usually not caused by low battery power. With the newer power sources, the pacing rate gradually increases as the battery runs low and is detected early by the patients, who regularly monitor their own pulse. The patient with a pacer that fails to pace must be rapidly transported to the hospital while receiving support with rate-stimulating drugs, CPR, or external pacing as appropriate.

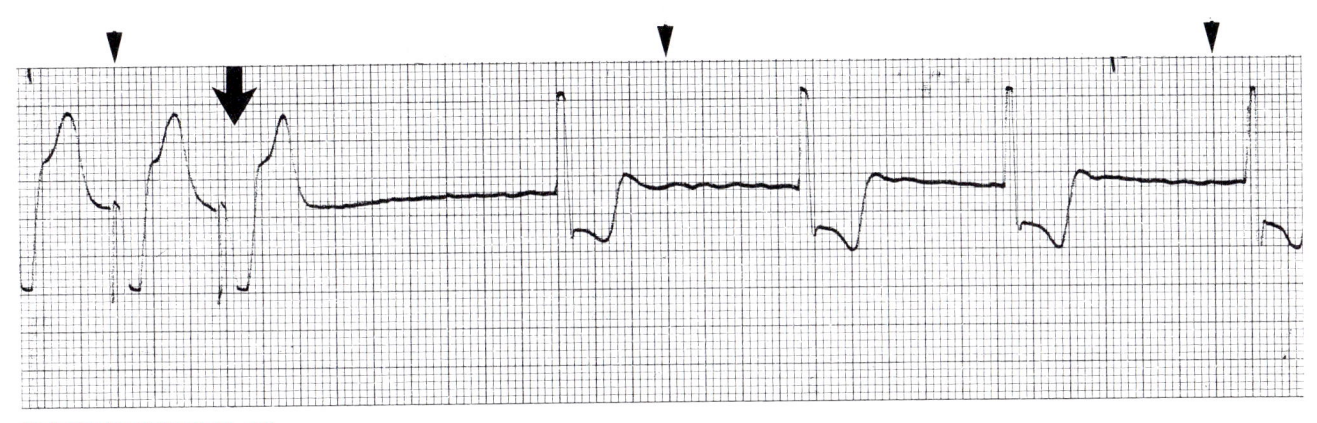

RHYTHM STRIP 20–30.
(Huff J, Doernbach DP, White RD)

STRIP #: 30

AUTOMATIC INTERVAL RATE: *100/min*

ANALYSIS: *The first three complexes are paced complexes. When the pacemaker malfunctions, the underlying patient rhythm (atrial fibrillation) is at a rate of only 20–30/min*

INTERPRETATION: *Failure to pace with resultant bradycardia*

The failure to capture (*no response to pacing stimuli*) is evidenced on EKG by pacemaker spikes that are not followed by QRS complexes. This problem has the same disastrous results as failure to pace, and the patient requires supportive measures and rapid transport for new pacemaker insertion.

Failure to sense occurs in demand (*synchronous*) pacemakers when they fail to stop pacing when patients have electrical activity of their own. The failure causes the pacemaker to perform essentially like a fixed-rate pacemaker, and it competes with the heart's natural pacemaker. This problem is frequently due to electrode dislodgment. Although not immediately life-threatening, the pacemaker could discharge during the vulnerable period of the cardiac cycle and produce dangerous tachycardia or fibrillation. This risk is increased in patients who are more susceptible to fibrillation because of myocardial infarction, electrolyte imbalance, or digitalis toxicity.

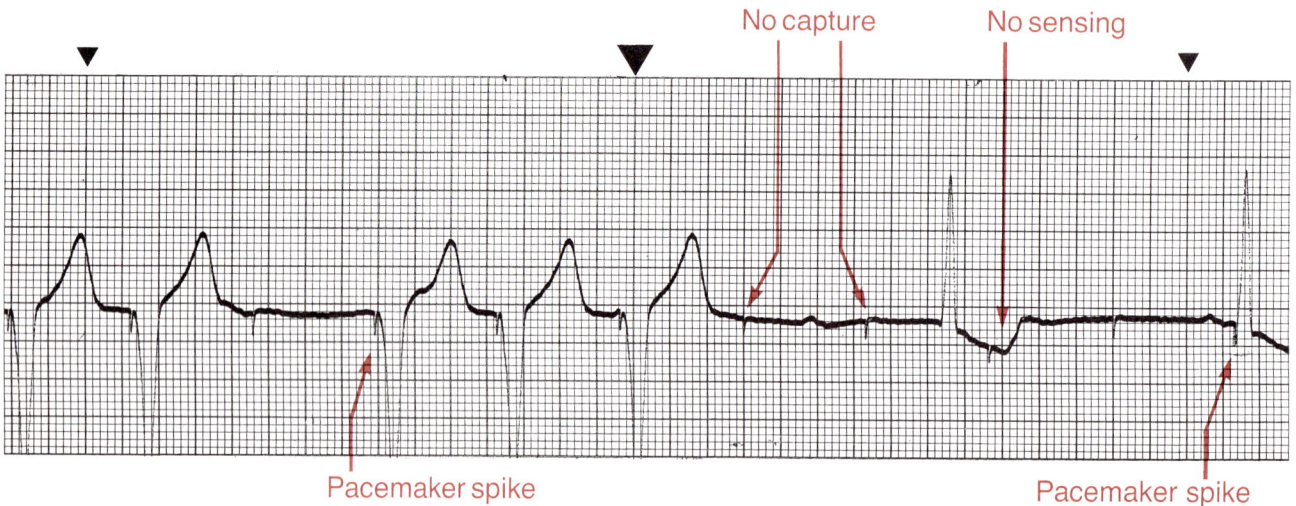

RHYTHM STRIP 20–31.
(Huff J, Doernbach DP, White RD)

STRIP #: *31*

AUTOMATIC INTERVAL RATE: *88/min*

ANALYSIS: *The first two complexes are paced complexes, followed by loss of capture, three paced complexes, two loss of capture complexes, a patient complex, a sensing malfunction, loss of capture, and a patient complex (a pacer spike is noted in the last QRS complex)*

INTERPRETATION: *Ventricular demand pacemaker with failure to capture and failure to sense*

Emergency management of patients with pacemakers is generally the same as for any cardiac patient. Ventricular ectopy can be treated in the usual manner, as lidocaine does not suppress response of the ventricles to pacemaker stimulation. Bradyarrhythmia, asystole, and ventricular fibrillation that result from pacemaker failure are treated in the usual manner, except that prolonged stabilization at the scene is not appropriate. Finally, pacemaker patients may be defibrillated as other patients are, but the defibrillator paddles should not be placed closer than 5 inches from the pacemaker battery pack.

Table 20-2 provides a summary chart of arrhythmias.

Prehospital Intervention: EKG Monitoring

The procedure of **EKG monitoring** is performed to detect all forms of arrhythmias and is indicated for any patient with signs and symptoms of myocardial ischemia, pump failure, respiratory compromise, possible myocardial trauma, or any other risk of developing cardiac arrhythmias. Paramedics must be familiar with the mechanism and controls of their particular monitor-defibrillator, as each brand is different. However, most portable monitor-defibrillators used by paramedics have in common the following components:

- Oscilloscope
- EKG monitor controls
- Patient cable and lead wires
- Paper strip recorder
- Paddle electrodes or defibrillation pads
- Defibrillator controls
- Synchronizer switch

The two most common leads used for prehospital EKG monitoring are lead II and MCL_1. Lead II is used widely, as it tends to produce the best view of EKG waves, particularly P waves. The MCL_1 lead is best when the site of origin of ectopic complexes needs to be determined, as when distinguishing PACs with aberrant conduction from PVCs.

The EKG may be monitored by holding electrodes contained in the defibrillator paddles against the chest or by attaching skin electrodes to the chest wall. The paddle electrodes produce more artifact on EKG and are generally used only in the cardiac arrest setting for a "*quick look*" at the rhythm before intervention. Paddle electrodes (dual function adhesive monitor-defibrillator pads have replaced paddles in many EMS systems for cardiac arrest management) also provide a back-up monitoring system in the event of patient cable–lead wire failure. To use paddle electrodes to monitor, the oscilloscope power must be turned on and the lead selector turned to "*paddles*." Saline or gel defibrillation pads should be positioned on the patient's chest or a liberal amount of conductive cream should be applied to the paddle surfaces to enhance electrode-skin contact and maximize the quality of the EKG tracing. The paddles are held firmly on the chest wall, the negative electrode on the right upper chest and positive electrode on the left lower chest, while the monitor is observed and a rhythm strip obtained.

The procedure for using disposable adhesive skin electrodes to monitor the EKG involves selection of appropriate electrode sites and skin preparation. Electrode sites are chosen based on the type of monitoring lead desired, using care to avoid placement over large muscle masses, large quantities of chest hair, bony structure, or any place that would prevent the electrode from lying flat against the skin. In addition, the electrodes should not be placed in the same location in which paddles would be placed if defibrillation were required. Chest electrode placement for a lead II monitoring lead is positive electrode on the left lower chest and negative electrode on the right upper chest. For an MCL_1 configuration, the positive electrode is placed on the right lower chest and negative electrode on the left upper chest. In both leads, placement of the ground electrode varies and is not crucial, as long as it is away from the other two electrodes (see Fig. 20-26).

The skin at the selected sites should be prepared by quickly rubbing with an alcohol pad. This action removes dirt and body oils, allowing for better adhesion and electrode contact and, thus, a clearer EKG tracing. The skin should be allowed to dry before electrode placement, as alcohol breaks down the electrode adhesive. If necessary, shave small areas of chest hair before placing the electrode. Apply electrodes to prepped sites, checking the adhesive side of the electrode to assure the electrode pad conductive cream is moist. The lead wires on the patient cable, which are frequently color coded to the electrode site, are then attached. The patient cable is plugged into the monitor, oscilloscope power turned on, and, if applicable, the lead selector set to the desired lead. Gain or sensitivity should be adjusted as needed for optimal visibility. The monitor may be calibrated by pushing the 1 mV calibration button while running a paper EKG tracing and observing for proper height of the calibration mark (1 mV = 10 mm). Calibration is necessary primarily for description of ventricular fibrillation as coarse, medium, or fine. Some monitors are equipped with an audio rate sensor. Use of this "beeper" is optional, and volume should be adjusted with consideration for the patient's anxiety level.

Problems with obtaining good quality EKG tracings can be both aggravating for the paramedic and dangerous for the patient if arrhythmias go undetected. The most common source of the problem is poor electrode contact with the skin. Reasons for poor electrode contact include excessive hair, an electrode loosened or dislodged because of diaphoresis or patient movement, dried conductive gel on disposable electrodes, and electrode placement over bony structures. Sometimes, an initially poor tracing improves over time as the conductive gel on the elec-

(text continues on page 506)

TABLE 20-2.
SUMMARY CHART OF ARRHYTHMIAS

Arrhythmia	Rate (complexes/ minute)	Rhythm	P Waves
NORMAL RATES			
Normal sinus rhythm	60–100	Regular	Normal, one preceding each QRS complex, same in configuration
Sinus arrhythmia	60–100, may be < 60 or > 100	Irregular; cyclic slowing and speeding with respirations	Normal
Wandering atrial pacemaker (WAP)	Usually normal, may be < 60	Usually irregular	Change in configuration, may become inverted or disappear
Accelerated junctional rhythm	60–100	Regular	Retrograde before or after QRS complex or none (buried in QRS complex)
Accelerated ventricular rhythm	40–100	Usually regular	None associated with the ventricular complexes
BRADYCARDIA			
Sinus bradycardia	< 60	Regular	Normal
Sinus arrest	< 60 because of pauses	Regular with pauses that are not multiples of the sinus cycle length	Present and normal but missing during pauses
Junctional rhythm	40–60	Regular	Retrograde before or after QRS complex or none (buried in QRS complex)
Idioventricular rhythm	20–40	Regular to slightly irregular	None associated with QRS complex
TACHYCARDIA			
Sinus tachycardia	> 100	Regular	Normal
Paroxysmal supraventricular tachycardia (PSVT) (includes atrial and junctional tachycardia)	100–250, usually > 150	Regular	Present, but abnormal in configuration; may be buried in preceding P wave
Multifocal atrial tachycardia (MAT)	> 100	Irregular	At least three different configurations in one lead
Ventricular tachycardia	100–250	Slightly irregular or regular	None associated with the ventricular complexes; sinus P wave may be visible in QRS complex

PR Interval	QRS Complex	Comments
Normal	Normal	A normal P wave is the hallmark of sinus rhythms.
Normal	Normal	Irregularity is caused by increase and decrease in vagal tone due to respirations that cause the SA node to depolarize faster, then slower in a cycle.
Normal; may change as the configuration of the P wave changes	Normal	Two or more different P waves may be seen as the atrial focus changes. Focus may move into AV junction.
None, or usually less than 0.12 second	Normal	Occurs when a focus in the junction with a faster rate than the SA node becomes the pacemaker.
Variable, if any	Wide, bizarre ventricular complexes; fusion complexes common	May occur when the sinus and ventricular pacemaker rates are nearly the same. When depolarizing faster than the sinus, the ventricular focus is in command. The pacemaker shifts back and forth from the sinus to the ventricle (two pacemakers compete for control of the heart).
Normal	Normal	May be normal physiologic response.
Normal	Normal, but missing during pauses	
None, or usually less than 0.12 second	Normal	Occurs when the SA node slows, allowing the junction to take over as pacemaker (an escape rhythm).
Variable, if any	Wide, bizarre ventricular complexes	Occurs when all higher pacemakers fail or are blocked (an escape rhythm).
Normal	Normal, but may widen at faster rates	
May not be measurable	Normal, but may be widened at faster rates owing to aberrant conduction through the ventricles	Begins abruptly with a PAC or PJC, which sets up a reentry circuit in the AV junction. Rapid rate often makes visualization of P waves impossible. Differentiation of atrial and junctional tachycardia is not important to management.
Varies	Normal, but may be widened at faster rates	May closely resemble atrial fibrillation.
None	Wide, bizarre QRS complex; some may be slightly different because of the sinus P wave that marches independently through the QRS complexes	Ventricular tachycardia is triggered by a PVC. May see fusion complexes associated.

(continued)

TABLE 20-2.
(Continued)

Arrhythmia	Rate (complexes/minute)	Rhythm	P Waves
ESCAPE COMPLEXES			
Junctional escape complexes	Underlying rate is usually slow	Irregular because of the pauses; escape complex is late	Retrograde before or after QRS complex or none (buried in QRS complex)
Ventricular escape complexes	Underlying rate is slow	Irregular because of pauses; escape complex is late	None preceding escape complex
PREMATURE COMPLEXES			
Premature atrial complexes (PACs)	Underlying rhythm plus PACs	Irregular because of premature complexes	P wave of premature complex is abnormal in configuration
Premature junctional complexes (PJCs)	Underlying rhythm plus PJCs	Irregular because of premature complexes	Normal in underlying rhythm; premature complex has: retrograde P wave preceding QRS complex; retrograde P wave after QRS complex; or no P wave visible (buried in QRS complex)
Premature ventricular complexes (PVCs)	Underlying rhythm plus PVCs	Irregular because of premature complexes	None preceding PVC
Fusion complexes	Underlying rhythm plus fusion complexes	*Atrial*, regular; *ventricular*, slightly irregular	Normal, with P-to-P interval regular
AV BLOCKS			
First degree AV block	Depends on underlying sinus rhythm	Depends on underlying sinus rhythm	Normal and all are conducted
Second degree AV block type I (Mobitz I, Wenckebach)	Atrial more than ventricular	*Atrial*, regular; *ventricular*, irregular because of changing PR interval and dropped complex	Normal, but not all are conducted
Second degree AV block type II (Mobitz II)	Ventricular less than atrial	*Atrial*, regular; *ventricular*, regular (if conduction ratio constant)	Normal, but not all are conducted
Third degree AV block or complete AV block	*Atrial*, normal; *ventricular*, slow	*Atrial*, regular; *ventricular*, regular but slower than the atria; may be irregular with ventricular escape pacemaker	Normal, but not related to the QRS complex; none conducted

PR Interval	QRS Complex	Comments
None, or usually less than 0.12 second	Normal	The junctional complexes occur after a long pause. They are not premature.
None	Wide, bizzare ventricular complex	Occurs when a pause in the underlying rhythm becomes long enough and no higher pacemaker escapes.
Normal, but may be different than the sinus PR interval	Normal; or wide and bizarre owing to aberrant conduction through the ventricles during partial refractory period; or missing owing to extreme prematurity of P wave that falls during the absolute refractory period of the ventricles	The amount of prematurity of the complex determines whether the QRS complex is normal, aberrant, or absent.
None, or usually less than 0.12 seconds with a retrograde P wave	Same as for PACs	The presence or absence of retrograde P waves is caused by a difference in conduction velocity through the AV node. This placement of P waves is true in all junctional rhythms.
None	Wide and bizarre	The rhythm may have a compensatory pause after the PVC or it may be interpolated.
PR interval of fusion complex is less than the normal complex	Varies from slightly widened to wide, bizarre complex; R-to-R interval is early on the fusion complex	Rhythm results from the combination of the sinus impulse and a premature ventricular complex that are occurring at nearly the same time and each is partially depolarizing the heart.
Greater than 0.20 seconds and constant	None missing	The AV node delays the impulse longer than normal.
Prolongs with each successive complex until a QRS complex is dropped	R-to-R interval is irregular; QRS complex is missing after some P waves	The AV node fatigues, and the PR interval gradually prolongs until the AV node blocks out one impulse. During the pause that follows, the AV node recovers, and the next beat is normal and the progression begins again.
Normal, or prolonged but constant if conducted	Not every P wave is followed by a QRS complex	The bundle branches block out every other or two or three P waves as they come down, until one branch recovers and one impulse is conducted.
Varies with each complex	Wide, slow, ventricular complexes, but may be normal if the ventricular pacemaker is in the AV junction	The AV node is completely fatigued, and it blocks out all impulses from the SA node and won't conduct to the ventricles. The ventricles are paced by a focus in the AV junction or ventricles.

(Continued)

TABLE 20-2.
(Continued)

Arrhythmia	Rate (complexes/ minute)	Rhythm	P Waves
TERMINAL RHYTHMS			
Primary ventricular standstill	Atrial, normal; ventricular, none	Regular	Normal
Agonal rhythm	Slow	Irregular	None
Asystole	None	None	None
FLUTTER AND FIBRILLATION			
Atrial flutter	Atrial, 250–350; ventricular, varies greatly with conduction ratio, less than atrial	Atrial, regular; ventricular, regular or irregular	None, but flutter waves (regular saw-toothed wave forms)
Atrial fibrillation	Atrial, >350; ventricular, >100 uncontrolled, <100 controlled	Totally irregular	None, but fibrillation waves (totally chaotic, irregular wave forms); may vary from coarse (wormy baseline) to fine (straight-line fibrillation) waves
Ventricular fibrillation	None	Totally irregular, chaotic	None

(Modified from Hurst C: Dysrhythmia Interpretation, p. 197. Philadelphia, JB Lippincott, 1986)

trode breaks down skin resistance. If poor electrode contact has been ruled out as the cause of a poor tracing, further trouble-shooting should include checking for patient movement or muscle tremors, broken patient cable, broken lead wire, faulty grounding, or malfunctioning oscilloscope.

Paper write-outs of EKG rhythms should be obtained as documentation of patient status, changes in condition, and response to management unless this documentation is done entirely by telemetry. Although governed by local medical protocol, EKG write-outs or rhythm strips are usually obtained to document the patient's initial rhythm, any changes in rhythm, EKG patterns during defibrillation or synchronized cardioversion, and rhythm changes while administering drugs.

Prehospital Intervention for Arrhythmias That Result From Increased Automaticity or Reentry

Carotid Sinus Massage

Carotid sinus massage is one of several techniques used to increase vagal tone to convert a PSVT to a sinus rhythm. This technique involves stimulation of pressure receptors (baroreceptors) in the carotid arteries, which causes increased parasympathetic discharge. The result is slowing of AV conduction, thereby interrupting AV reentry.

This procedure is primarily used for the patient with PSVT who does not have severe hemodynamic compromise that requires more drastic intervention. Before receiving carotid massage, the patient should be receiving oxygen therapy, have an IV line in place, and be EKG monitored. Patients should be placed on their backs with their necks hyperextended, and each carotid pulse should be separately palpated and auscultated with a stethoscope. Carotid massage is contraindicated if pulses are unequal, carotid bruits are heard, or if the patient has a history of cerebrovascular accident (CVA). To perform the massage, the patient's head is tilted to either side, and the index and middle fingers are placed over the artery below the angle of the jaw, as high on the neck as possible (Fig. 20-47). The artery is then firmly massaged by pressing it against the vertebral column and rubbing. The EKG should be monitored continuously, and massage should be terminated at the first signs of slowing of rate or heart block. A continuous EKG write-out should be obtained

PR Interval	QRS Complex	Comments
None	None	The AV node blocks all impulses, and no ventricular pacemaker escapes.
None	Multifocal ventricular complexes	A "dying heart."
None	None	A straight line.
None	May be two, three, four or more flutter waves for each QRS complex	Ventricular rhythm may be regular if a constant (e.g., 4:1) ratio of flutter waves to QRS complexes exists, but it is irregular if the ratio varies.
None	Usually normal; may be widened at faster rates and very irregular rhythms; or totally irregular	The ventricular rhythm is irregular because of the varying response of the AV node to constant irregular bombardment of the atrial impulses.
None	None but irregular wave forms	

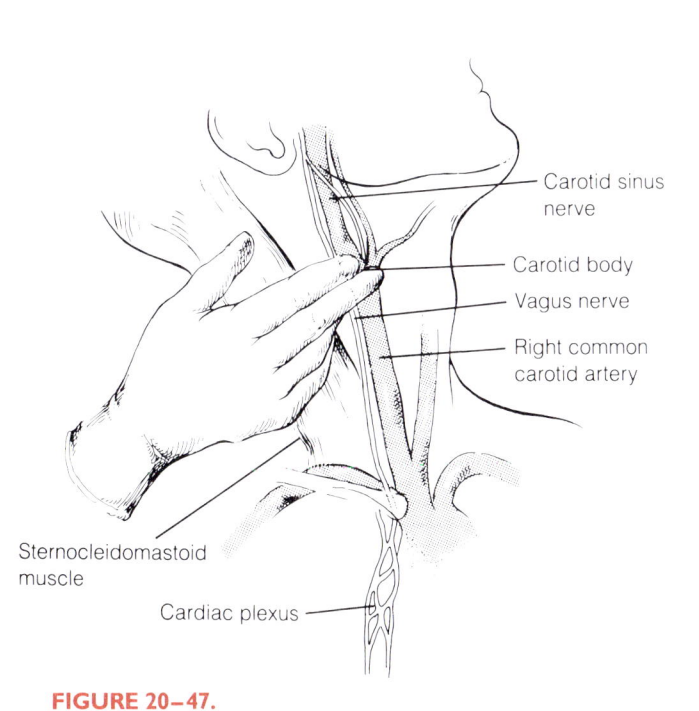

FIGURE 20-47.
Carotid sinus massage.

to document the procedure. Both carotids should never be massaged simultaneously and should not be massaged for longer than 15 to 20 seconds. The procedure may be repeated on the same or alternate side if it is initially ineffective, but numerous attempts, delaying other therapeutic interventions, are not appropriate.

Like all procedures, carotid massage may produce complications, including arrhythmias such as asystole, PVCs, and ventricular tachycardia or fibrillation. Another serious complication is the interruption of cerebral circulation that results in syncope, seizure, or stroke. Finally, increased parasympathetic tone may cause hypotension, nausea, or vomiting. These latter complications are transient but may have detrimental effects if, for example, airway compromise or aspiration occurs.

Valsalva's Maneuver

Reflex vagal discharge can also be obtained by having the patient perform **Valsalva's maneuver,** ideally in the supine position. This *"bearing-down"* action is rapid and easy for the patient to do and, in many EMS systems, is the preferred form of reflex vagal stimulation because of its uniform safety, rapidity, and ease of application.

Verapamil

Pharmacology and Actions. **Verapamil** is one of several drugs called calcium-channel blocking agents. It inhibits movement of calcium, vital for contraction, into cardiac and vascular smooth muscle during depolarization. This inhibition results in reduced cardiac contractility and, therefore, reduced myocardial oxygen consumption. It also dilates coronary and peripheral blood vessels, resulting in improved coronary blood flow and reduced systemic vascular resistance. Most important to prehospital use are the electrophysiologic properties of the drug. It slows AV nodal conduction and lengthens the refractory period of the AV node.

Cardiac Indications. Verapamil is used to terminate PSVT, a rhythm commonly caused by a reentry circuit in the AV node, when vagal maneuvers have been unsuccessful.

In addition, it helps slow the ventricular response in rapid atrial fibrillation or flutter.

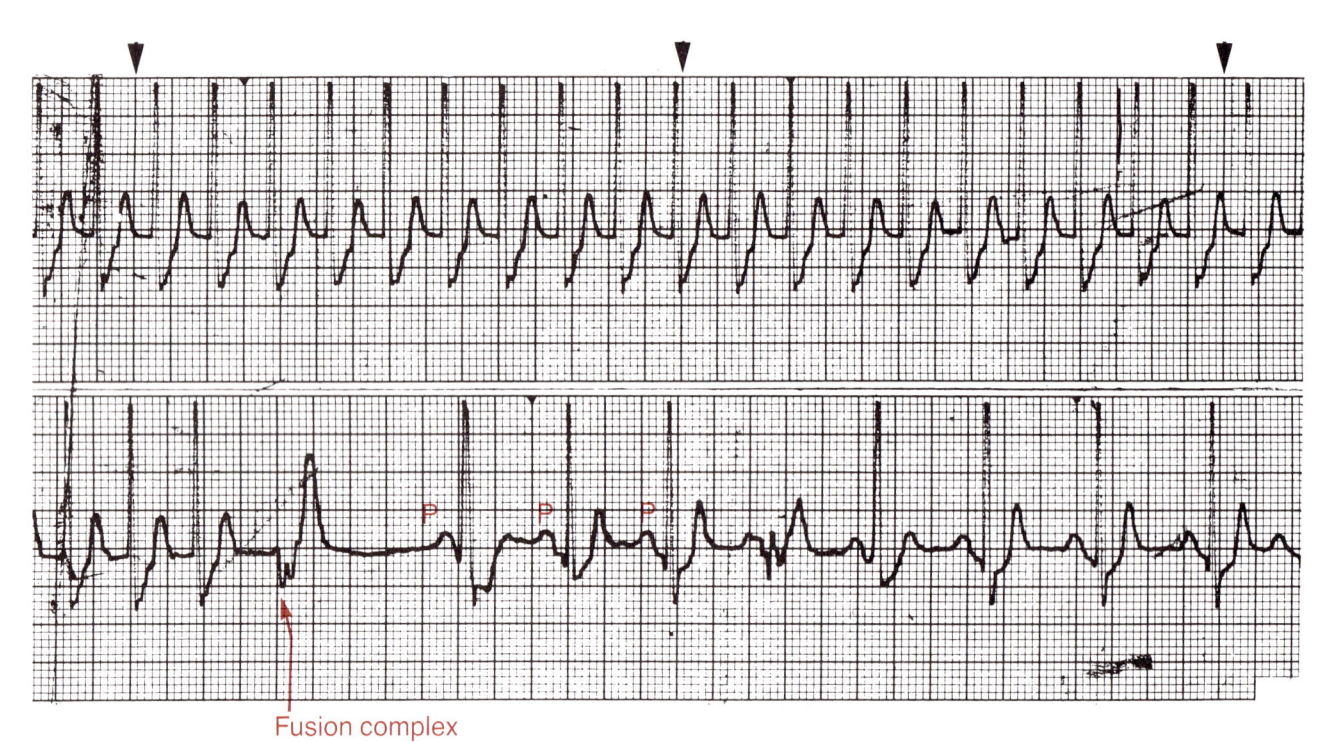

RHYTHM STRIP 20–32.
(White RD: Paramedic EKG Collection)

STRIP #: *32*
RATE: *188/min slowing to approximately 100/min*
RHYTHM: *Generally regular except transition between rates*
P WAVE: *Visible only at slower rate with one per QRS complex; upright and uniform*
PR INTERVAL: *0.16 sec and constant*
QRS COMPLEX: *Most less than 0.10 sec; two complexes 0.12 sec with different shapes*
RHYTHM INTERPRETATION: *Paroxysmal supraventricular tachycardia that converts to sinus tachycardia. Two fusion complexes are present. This conversion in a 60-year-old male occurred after the injection of 5 mg verapamil.*

Precautions. The blood pressure must be monitored closely during administration, as vasodilation may cause hypotension. It is important to obtain a medication history from the patient, as drugs such as digitalis or β-blockers (e.g., propranolol, metoprolol, atenolol) may potentiate verapamil's AV blocking action, creating severe AV block or asystole. Verapamil is contraindicated in patients with AV block or history of congestive heart failure or sick sinus syndrome and in patients with wide-complex tachycardia. If the rhythm is ventricular in origin cardiovascular collapse may ensue after verapamil injection. It should also be determined if the patient has known Wolff-Parkinson-White syndrome; although verapamil may be safely used for PSVT in these patients, it should not be used if patients with this syndrome are in atrial fibrillation or atrial flutter. In these situations, verapamil may dangerously accelerate the ventricular rate by increasing impulse conduction into the ventricles via the accessory pathway.

Administration and Dosage. A bolus injection of 5 mg is administered over a 1- to 2-minute period. This dosage may be followed in 15 to 30 minutes by a 10 mg bolus, but no more than 10 mg should be given in a single dose. Verapamil acts rapidly, and a peak effect occurs within 3 to 5 minutes.

Side Effects and Special Considerations. Intravenous administration frequently is followed by a transient fall in blood pressure. This hypotension may be treated by elevating the patient's legs and usually resolves in 10 to 20 minutes. Other serious side effects are congestive heart failure, severe bradycardia, and increased accessory pathway conduction in patients with Wolff-Parkinson-White syndrome, as described above.

As previously discussed, adenosine, which also slows AV conduction, may become the drug of choice in PSVT because of its efficacy and short duration of action.

Lidocaine

Pharmacology and Actions. **Lidocaine** is an antiarrhythmic drug that suppresses beats and rhythms of ventricular origin. It is thought to act primarily by depressing conduction in ischemic tissue, thus interrupting reentry pathways that may exist without significantly altering conduction or contractility in healthy tissue. Lidocaine also elevates the ventricular fibrillation threshold. Lidocaine is not effective in suppressing most atrial arrhythmias.

Cardiac Indications. Lidocaine is the drug of choice for suppressing PVCs and ventricular tachycardia that occur in the setting of myocardial ischemia or infarction.

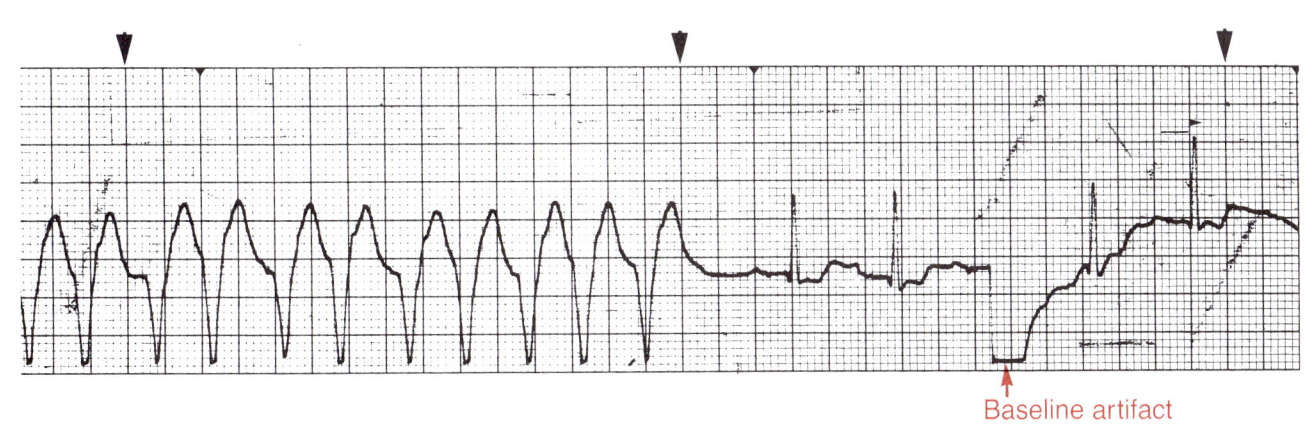

RHYTHM STRIP 20–33.
(White RD: Paramedic EKG Collection)

STRIP #: 33
RATE: *180/min slowing to approximately 100/min*
RHYTHM: *Slightly irregular, changing to regular*
P WAVE: *Only visible at slower rate; one per QRS complex; upright and uniform*
PR INTERVAL: *0.20 sec and constant*
QRS COMPLEX: *Greater than 0.12 sec changing to 0.08 sec*
RHYTHM INTERPRETATION: *Ventricular tachycardia that converts to sinus tachycardia. This conversion in an elderly male with chest pain and hypotension occurred after the injection of lidocaine.*

Lidocaine may also be administered in the absence of these arrhythmias to prevent their development when it is strongly suspected that the patient has a myocardial infarction. In cardiac arrest, lidocaine should be administered for ventricular tachycardia or fibrillation that is recurrent or that has been refractory to initial therapeutic intervention. Lidocaine should be administered after successful conversion of a lethal ventricular arrhythmia, provided no contraindications, such as severe bradycardia, AV block, or any kind or escape rhythm, are present.

Precautions. Because lidocaine is metabolized by the liver, doses should be reduced by half to prevent toxicity in any patient who has reduced hepatic blood flow, such as patients with congestive heart failure, liver cirrhosis or dysfunction, or shock from any cause. Orders for reduced dosage should also be expected for patients older than 70 years. Lidocaine should be used with caution, if at all, in the presence of conduction system disorders or bradycardia to avoid suppression of potential escape pacemaker sites. Toxic effects and side effects are more common when lidocaine blood levels rise too rapidly; therefore, IV bolus administration should be no faster than 50 mg/min.

Administration and Dosage. Lidocaine may be administered by multiple bolus injections alone or in combination with a continuous IV infusion; a number of regimens may be used for this administration. A common method administers a 1 mg/kg bolus (approximately 75 mg) over a 2-minute period, a dosage that may be followed by a continuous IV infusion at 2 mg/min. To maintain therapeutic blood concentrations, boluses of 0.5 mg/kg are then repeated every 8 minutes up to a total dose of 3 mg/kg. The IV infusion may be increased by 1 mg/min after each bolus, if necessary, but the maximum infusion rate should be 4 mg/min. This or a similar IV bolus-infusion regimen is appropriate both for suppression of ventricular arrhythmias and for prevention of ectopy, although the total bolus dose recommended for prophylaxis is 2 mg/kg. As noted previously, the total dose should be reduced by half for elderly patients and for patients with congestive heart failure, liver disease, or shock. For ventricular fibrillation resistant to defibrillation, only bolus therapy should be used at 8- to 10-minute intervals with a continuous infusion started after successful resuscitation. Lidocaine may also be administered via an endotracheal tube if establishment of an IV route is delayed or not possible.

Side Effects and Special Considerations. True hypersensitivity or allergy to lidocaine is rare, and known allergy to other "*caine*" drugs does not preclude lidocaine administration. Most adverse reactions to lidocaine are manifestations of toxicity and can be minimized by slow IV administration and consideration of the patient's age, liver function, and cardiac output when the dosage is being determined. Toxic effects are primarily CNS-related and include the following:

- Muscle twitching, tremors
- Slurred speech
- Altered level of consciousness
- Decreased hearing
- Numbness
- Seizures

Although not common, depression of cardiac automaticity and conduction and hypotension may occur. A final consideration for lidocaine is that, for emergency management, IV bolus administration must precede continuous infusion. Use of continuous infusion alone would take 30 to 60 minutes to obtain a therapeutic blood level.

Bretylium Tosylate

Pharmacology and Actions. The action of **bretylium tosylate** is complex and not totally understood, as it possesses both direct cardiac effects and effects on the autonomic nervous system. Although pharmacologically different from lidocaine, it also elevates the ventricular fibrillation threshold and terminates reentry pathways to suppress ventricular arrhythmias. Because the mechanisms by which bretylium disrupts reentry pathways are thought to be different from those of lidocaine, it may be useful if lidocaine in maximum dosage has not controlled ventricular arrhythmias. It initially causes a discharge of norepinephrine from sympathetic nerve endings, followed by a blockage of norepinephrine release. This effect may result in an initial increase in heart rate and arterial blood pressure when administered for ventricular tachycardia, followed by hypotension about 20 minutes after bolus injection (see side effects below).

Cardiac Indications. In prehospital care, the use of bretylium is limited to management of ventricular fibrillation and ventricular tachycardia that have been unresponsive to shocks and lidocaine or that have recurred despite lidocaine in maximum dosage.

Precautions. Bretylium has no contraindications when used for cardiac arrest. However, it should be used with caution if digitalis toxicity is suspected. The medical control physician may wish to reduce epinephrine dosages when bretylium is used. Also, because it is not significantly metabolized before excretion, toxic effects may be more likely in patients with renal failure.

Administration and Dosage. For ventricular fibrillation, the initial dosage is 5 mg/kg or 350 to 500 mg given by IV bolus injection and followed by attempted defibrillation. If there is no response to this administration, a dose of 10 mg/kg or 700 to 1000 mg is given and may be repeated at 15- to 30-minute intervals, usually until a maximum dose of 30 mg/kg has been given. For persistent, recurring ventricular tachycardia, the initial dose is 5 to 10 mg/kg administered over an 8- to 10-minute period. Dilution of the drug in 50 mL D_5W before injection facilitates slow administration and minimizes side effects.

Side Effects and Special Considerations. Although side effects are not a major consideration in the cardiac arrest patient, they may occur in the patient with perfusing ventricular tachycardia. Side effects include transient hypertension and increasing tachycardia after injection, later postural hypotension, and nausea and vomiting after rapid injection. Postural hypotension should be suspected about 20 minutes after a bolus injection. If clinically significant, it can be treated by leg elevation, IV fluid administration, calcium chloride injection, or dopamine infusion, the latter rarely required.

Precordial Thump

A **precordial thump** is a blow delivered to the sternum to generate a small amount of electrical current. The thump is sometimes effective in causing depolarization to interrupt a tachyarrhythmia and allow resumption of a more normal, organized rhythm. For prehospital use, it is recommended only in situations when the patient is being EKG monitored. A solitary precordial thump should be delivered at the onset of monitored ventricular fibrillation or ventricular tachycardia and may be successful in terminating these life-threatening arrhythmias. A thump may also be used in patients with asystole if fine ventricular fibrillation is suspected. For situations in which a defibrillator is unavailable, the precordial thump is recommended for any witnessed cardiac arrest. This procedure should only be used for adult patients.

The technique for precordial thump is to sharply strike the midsternal area of the chest with the fist (thumb side up) from a height of 10 to 12 inches. Positioning the fist and arm parallel to the long axis of the sternum helps to avoid injuring adjacent ribs. The patient who is still conscious should quickly be told what is to be done before the blow is delivered. Although this technique is appropriate immediately after ventricular tachycardia or fibrillation is noted, no more than one or two blows should be attempted before other management measures are initiated.

Manual Defibrillation

Defibrillation, reserved for the management of ventricular fibrillation, involves passing sufficient electrical current through the heart to depolarize fibrillating cells and allow them to repolarize uniformly, restoring organized, coordinated contractions. It has been demonstrated that it is not necessary to depolarize the entire heart to terminate fibrillation, but only a "*critical mass*" of myocardium. The requirements to defibrillate this critical mass vary with individual patients and situations.

The components of a portable defibrillator include an adjustable, high-voltage direct-current power supply, an energy storage capacitor, a connection to paddles or pads by a current-limiting inductor, and the paddle electrodes themselves. Alternating current defibrillators, the first type developed, are no longer in use. Direct current has been shown to be more effective and cause less myocardial muscle damage. The electrical charge delivered by the direct current defibrillator is several thousand volts over the brief time period of 4 to 12 milliseconds. The strength of the shock delivered is expressed in energy, called **joules** or watt seconds:

Energy (joules) = power (watts) × duration (seconds)

Because it is not possible to shock the heart directly (unless the chest is open), the amount of current that actually passes through the heart is reduced by the resistance of the chest wall. For this reason, it is important to lower the resistance pathway between defibrillator paddles as much as possible. (This discussion assumes that standard defibrillator paddles are being used; however, some of the same considerations also apply to disposable defibrillator pads.) Factors that influence chest wall (thoracic) resistance that must be considered in the technique used for defibrillation are the following:

Paddle size: Larger surface area paddles are thought to be more effective and cause less myocardial damage from the electrical current. Optimal size paddles for adult patients have a surface area of 10 cm diameter on the circular paddles. This size is used on all portable defibrillators. For infants, 4.5-cm diameter paddles are adequate, although 8-cm paddles may be appropriate for older children.

Paddle placement: Placement of both paddles on the anterior surface of the chest (*transthoracic placement*) is recommended for prehospital use for both adult and pediatric patients. One paddle is positioned to the right of the upper sternum just below the clavicle. The other paddle is positioned to the left of the left nipple in the anterior axillary line, over the apex of the heart (Fig. 20-48). Some defibrillator companies label the negative electrode paddle as "*sternum*" and the positive electrode paddle as "*apex*," but reversing these paddles has no effect on defibrillation, only on the appearance of the resulting EKG deflections. Under no circumstances should the "sternum" paddle be positioned directly over the less-conductive sternum. Anteroposterior placement, one paddle anteriorly over the precordium and the other behind the heart on the back, is an alternative to transthoracic placement. At this time, no evidence of the superiority

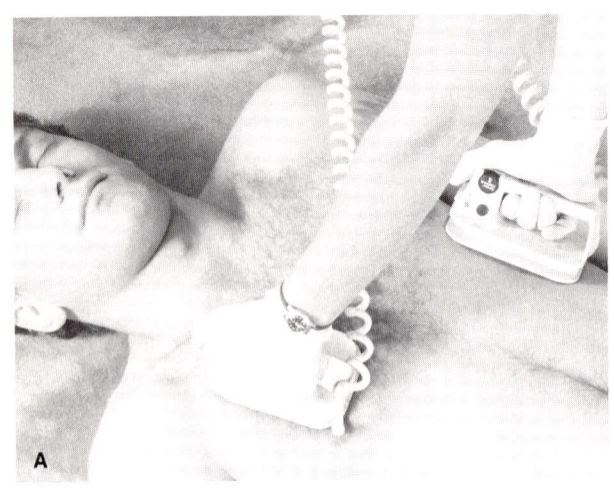

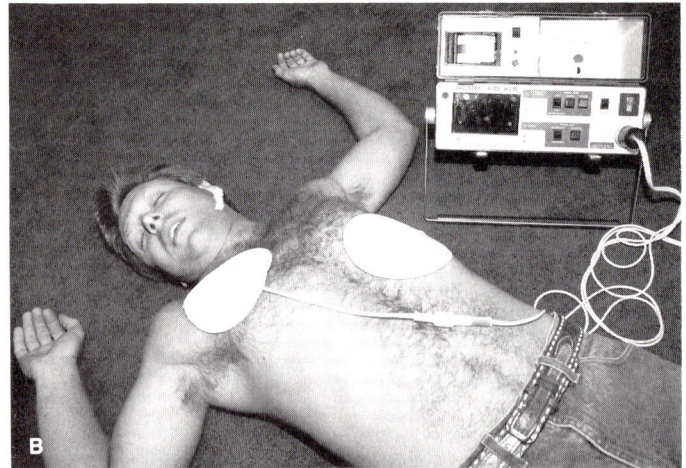

FIGURE 20–48.
Paddle (**A**) and electrode pad (**B**) placement for defibrillation. (Photo B: Bunting–Blake L, Parker J, Weigel A, White RD)

of this placement in emergency situations has been found. However, there are two situations in which anteroposterior placement may be warranted. In patients with automatic implantable cardioverter-defibrillators (AICDs) or pacemaker cardioverter-defibrillators (PCDs) the insulating effect of AICD or PCD ventricular patch electrodes may prevent externally applied current from traversing the heart during attempted antero–anterolateral defibrillation. If initial attempts by this placement are unsuccessful anteroposterior paddle or pad positioning should be considered. Secondly, in patients with implanted pacemakers anteroposterior placement may reduce the risk of transfer of defibrillating current to the pacemaker lead/electrode system, which can produce loss of capture from acute elevation of pacing threshold. In any case, when antero–anterolateral placement is used (the initially preferred method) the defibrillator paddles or pads should always be placed about 5 inches away from the implanted AICD, PCD, or pacemaker generator.

Paddle-skin interface: A conductive medium between the paddle surface and skin is important to reduce transthoracic resistance. Many materials are acceptable for this purpose, including creams, pastes, saline-soaked gauze pads, and prepackaged gelled pads. Studies to help choose a low-impedance substance are available, and some evidence suggests that commercially available electrode pastes may lower resistance more effectively than other conductive media. Care must be used with creams and saline pads to avoid "bridging" of the delivered charge due to smearing or running of the conductive medium.

Paddle pressure: Firm downward pressure, the equivalent of 25 lb, should be used to maximally decrease thoracic resistance. Care should be used to avoid leaning with body weight on the paddles because of the risk of slippage.

Number and time interval of previous shocks: Because transthoracic resistance decreases transiently with repeated shocks, rapid repetition of shocks may allow delivery of more energy to the heart without greatly increasing shock strength. The initial defibrillation shocks should be administered rapidly and consecutively without interruption for anything, including CPR. The only exception to this rule is if charging the paddles takes longer than 30 seconds, in which case CPR should be resumed.

Inspiratory vs. expiratory phase of ventilation: Evidence suggests that transthoracic resistance is higher when the lungs are filled with air during inspiration. It may be beneficial to time delivery of the shock to expiration and to use firm paddle pressure to assist deflation of the lungs.

In addition to the above considerations for decreasing transthoracic resistance, other factors influence the success of defibrillation:

Duration of ventricular fibrillation: Early defibrillation is the single most important factor in determining successful management and resuscitation in ventricular fibrillation. It has been demonstrated that initiating CPR in less than 4 minutes and defibrillation in less than 8 minutes yields a significantly higher resuscitation success rate.

Condition of the myocardium: It is generally agreed that it is more difficult to defibrillate the heart in the presence of acidosis, hypoxia, electrolyte imbalances, hypothermia, or drug toxicity. Likewise, secondary ventricular fibrillation from preexisting diseases, such as left ventricular failure, ventricular aneurysm, or hypovolemia, is much more difficult to correct than primary ventricular fibrillation.

It is clear that the amount of energy used for defibrillation influences its success. Shocks of inadequate strength fail to terminate fibrillation, while high energy shocks can result in myocardial damage. An overall relationship between energy requirements and size exists, as evidenced by the difference in pediatric and adult energy requirements. However, a direct size–energy relationship does not seem to exist for most adults of various weights. It is generally agreed that a maximum dose of 360 J is sufficient to terminate ventricular fibrillation in most patients.

Based on prospective studies of prehospital and in-hospital cardiac arrests, the American Heart Association has established recommendations for energy requirements for defibrillation of ventricular fibrillation and nonperfusing ventricular tachycardia. The initial defibrillation attempt should be at about 200 J. If this amount is unsuccessful, a second shock should be delivered at 200 to 300 J. Raising the shock energy may guarantee a greater and more predictable increase in current flow. If the first two shocks fail to defibrillate, a third shock should be immediately delivered at not more than 360 J. Recurring ventricular fibrillation during the course of the cardiac arrest should be shocked at whatever energy setting was previously successfully. Energy dose recommendations for pediatric patients are 2 J/kg initially, increased to 4 J/kg for the second and third attempts. Further energy increases should be made only after careful reassessment of patient oxygenation and acid-base status, as ventricular fibrillation is rarely a primary event in pediatric patients.

Defibrillation should be accomplished as soon as possible on identifying cardiac arrest, and nothing, including CPR, should take priority. The procedure for defibrillation is shown in Skill 20-1.

A final consideration in this discussion of defibrillation relates to its use for asystole. Ventricular fibrillation on surface EKG at times may mimic asystole in a single monitor lead or in very low-amplitude fibrillation. When asystole is seen using "quick look" paddles, defibrillation pads, or chest electrodes in the lead II configuration, changing the electrode placement 180° to MCL_1 (right lower and left upper chest) may yield a clearer picture of fibrillation. Obviously, the patient must still be defibrillated with paddles or pads in the lead II position. If any question exists as to whether a rhythm is ventricular fibrillation or asystole, it is probably best to defibrillate the patient, as there is potentially much to gain by attempting defibrillation and little to gain by omitting it.

Automated Defibrillation

The importance of early defibrillation to the success of resuscitation from ventricular fibrillation cannot be overstated. Technological advances in recent years have made possible the safe and effective use of defibrillators by prehospital personnel who either do not have, or do not need, the extensive education of paramedics in rhythm recognition and intervention. The advent of automated defibrillators has allowed the placement of these lifesaving devices in the hands of those emergency personnel who are strategically located to most rapidly respond to cardiac emergencies.

All automated defibrillators on the market use a computer microprocessor to determine the EKG rhythm. Various algorithms evaluate different characteristics of the EKG pattern to determine the presence or absence of ventricular fibrillation or rapid ventricular tachycardia. Automated defibrillators are safe and reliable because most use a sampling technique by which several sequential analyses are made and must agree with each other before the device confirms ventricular fibrillation and allows delivery of a shock. Most devices do not shock asystole and are unable to differentiate very fine ventricular fibrillation from asystole. Automated defibrillators include those devices that are fully automatic, requiring no intervention by the operator after initial activation, or semiautomatic, requiring the operator to interact with the device to deliver a shock.

The physical components common to both fully automatic and semiautomatic defibrillators include the following:

- Battery power source
- Dual function monitor-defibrillator pads and cable
- EKG and voice tape recorder and computer memory module
- Visual display and audible operational prompts
- Loose electrode prompt or indicator

Other components of automated defibrillators that may vary with brand and degree of automaticity include the following:

- Press-to-shock button
- EKG display screen
- Heart rate indicator
- EKG printer
- Capability to print out postevent report

The automated defibrillator is attached to the patient by two adhesive electrodes that are designed both to detect the cardiac rhythm and to deliver the defibrillatory shock. The placement of these pads on the patient's chest is the same as for manual defibrillation with paddles or pads. When the device is turned on and the appropriate button pushed, the machine analyzes the patient's rhythm in a matter of seconds. It is imperative during this analysis phase that rescuers stop CPR and any other movement of the patient that might interfere with the machine's ability to interpret the EKG. If the defibrillator interprets the

(text continues on page 517)

514 UNIT FOUR: MEDICAL EMERGENCIES

SKILL 20-1.
DEFIBRILLATION AND SYNCHRONIZED CARDIOVERSION

ACTIVITY	HOW PERFORMED	WHY PERFORMED
1. Check: Responsiveness Airway Breathing Circulation	Establish responsiveness Stabilize neck, open the airway Assess breathing Check for a pulse Check for hemorrhage	The primary survey is a rapid evaluation, less than 45 seconds, to identify and correct any life-threatening problems.
2. Assemble and check: Primary equipment (Activity 2A): ■ Monitor-defibrillator ■ Electrode paste or defibrillation pads Accessory equipment and supplies: ■ Gloves	Turn monitor on (Activity 2B) and put on gloves.	Defibrillation or cardioversion must be accomplished rapidly. Having all equipment ready reduces time delays during the procedure.

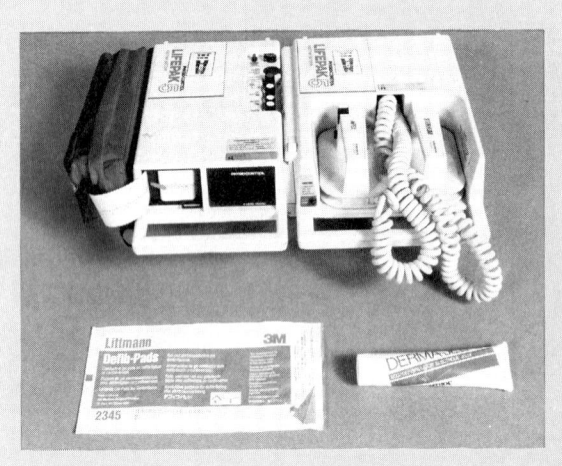

ACTIVITY 2A.
Primary equipment.

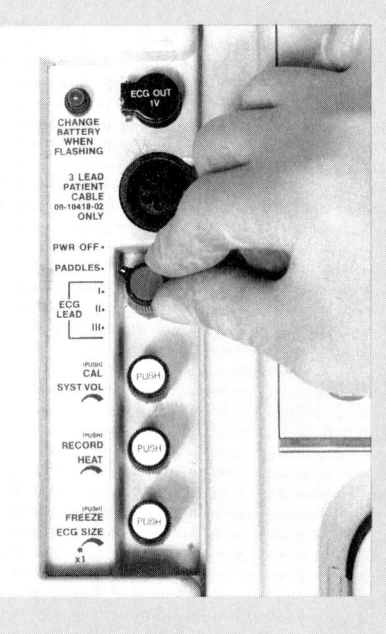

ACTIVITY 2B.
Turn on monitor.

3. Establish rhythm diagnosis	Perform a "quick look" by placing paddles or defibrillation pads on the patient's chest: one inferior to the clavicle on the right side and one on the left side, midaxillary line over the apex of the heart (Activity 3).	The "quick look" allows a rapid rhythm assessment without the delay of applying electrodes. This procedure also allows defibrillation, if indicated, to be performed immediately.

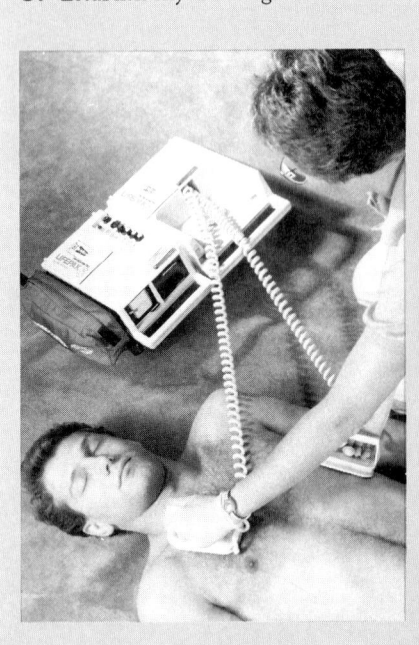

ACTIVITY 3.
Establish rhythm diagnosis.

(continued)

SKILL 20–1.
DEFIBRILLATION AND SYNCHRONIZED CARDIOVERSION (continued)

ACTIVITY	HOW PERFORMED	WHY PERFORMED
4. Determine need for defibrillation or cardioversion	Identify ventricular fibrillation, ventricular tachycardia without a pulse, or ventricular tachycardia that has a pulse but is causing severe hemodynamic compromise.	Correct rhythm diagnosis is essential to avoid possible harm to the patient from unnecessary electrical defibrillation. *Ventricular tachycardia without a pulse is treated like ventricular fibrillation. Ventricular tachycardia with a pulse requires synchronized cardioversion.*
5. Prepare defibrillator and patient	Set energy level to joules desired (Activity 5A). Apply electrode paste on paddles or place defibrillation pads on the chest (Activity 5B). Charge defibrillator. If synchronized cardioversion is indicated, set unit on synchronized mode (Activity 5C) and consider sedating the patient if time and patient condition allow.	Rapid, organized completion of these steps allows immediate defibrillation as soon as the defibrillator reaches full charge. Sedation may help relax conscious patients and ease the discomfort of cardioversion, provided their condition is such that they can tolerate the delay for administering the medication.

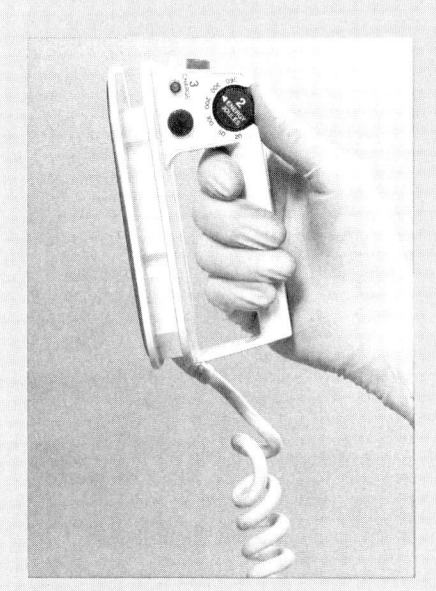

ACTIVITY 5A. Prepare defibrillator; set joules.

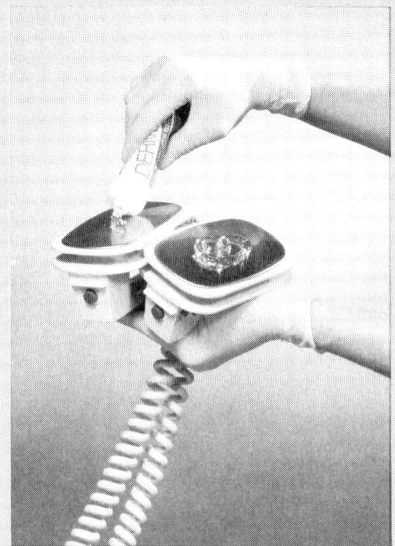

ACTIVITY 5B. Apply electrode paste on paddles.

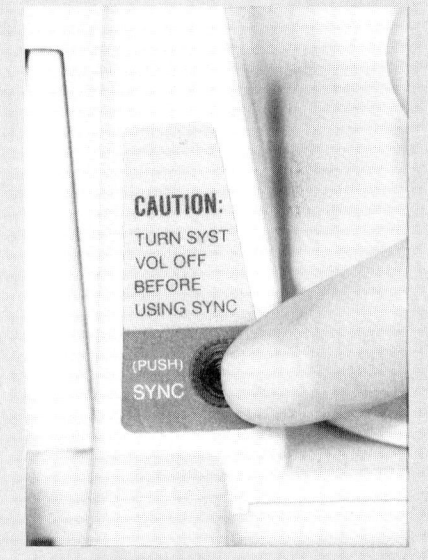

ACTIVITY 5C. Set unit on synchronized mode if indicated.

(continued)

SKILL 20–1.
DEFIBRILLATION AND SYNCHRONIZED CARDIOVERSION (continued)

ACTIVITY	HOW PERFORMED	WHY PERFORMED
6. Reassess pulse and EKG	Palpate for carotid pulse. Reconfirm rhythm. (Activity 6).	Rhythms frequently change in unstable patients. Accurate rhythm diagnosis is essential to avoid possible harm to the patient from unnecessary electrical shock.

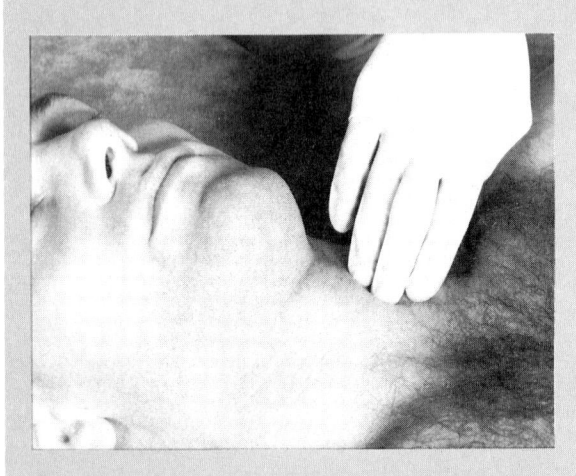

ACTIVITY 6.
Reassess pulse and EKG.

7. Defibrillate or cardiovert	If using paddles, position as described above. Apply firm pressure on paddles, about 25 lb of pressure.	Proper paddle placement and proper pressure is needed to deliver maximum energy and minimize thoracic resistance.
	Reconfirm rhythm again and shout "CLEAR" (Activity 7A). Make sure no personnel are directly or indirectly in contact with the patient. Depress the discharge buttons on the paddles simultaneously or depress button on defibrillator (Activity 7B).	The necessity of shouting "CLEAR" cannot be overemphasized. Anyone in contact with the patient may also receive an electrical shock.

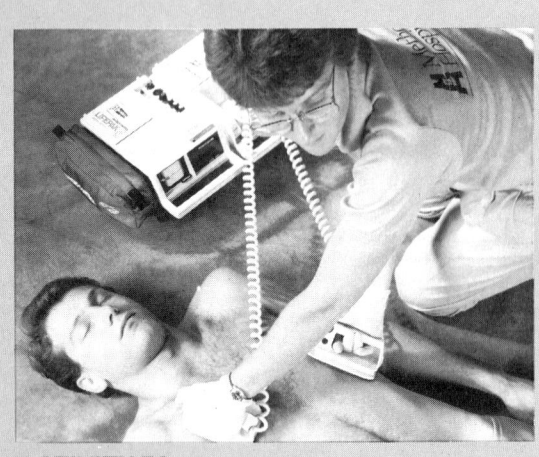

ACTIVITY 7A.
Reconfirm rhythm again and shout "CLEAR."

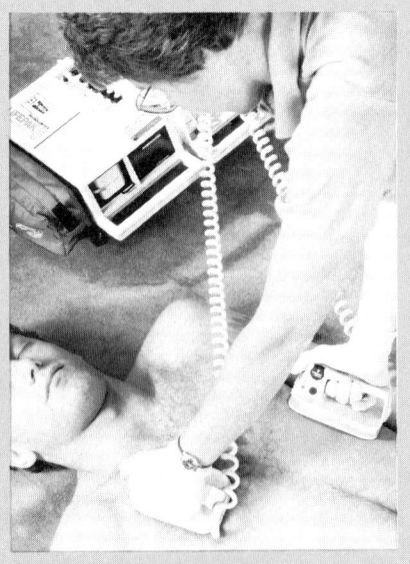

ACTIVITY 7B.
Depress discharge buttons on paddles simultaneously.

(continued)

CHAPTER 20: Cardiovascular Emergencies 517

SKILL 20-1.
DEFIBRILLATION AND SYNCHRONIZED CARDIOVERSION (continued)

ACTIVITY	HOW PERFORMED	WHY PERFORMED
8. Reassess pulse and EKG	Palpate for carotid pulse. Reconfirm rhythm. (Activity 8).	Rapid determination of the success or failure of the shock is essential to minimize delays in delivering further shocks if indicated or to otherwise stabilize the patient's corrected rhythm.

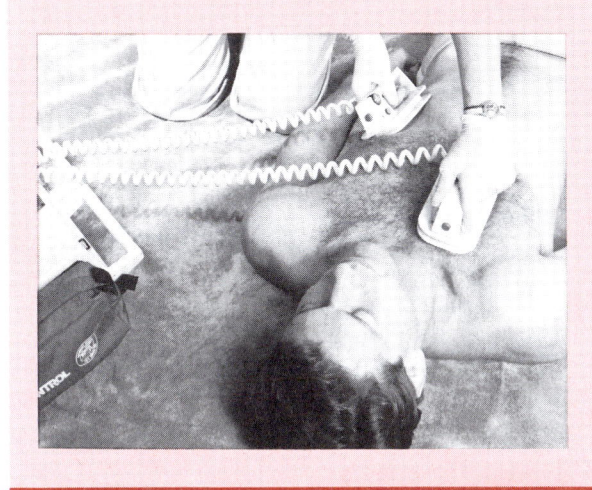

ACTIVITY 8.
Reconfirm rhythm by placing paddles on chest.

---

rhythm as ventricular fibrillation, a fully automatic device independently delivers a shock to the patient after advising personnel to stand back. An interpretation of ventricular fibrillation by a semiautomatic device results in a visual and audible prompt to the rescuer to activate a button to deliver the shock. In this situation, the operator must take responsibility for clearing all personnel from contact with the patient before defibrillation. After delivery of the shock and a pulse check, the automated defibrillator may be reactivated to repeat the analysis or shock sequence. Automated defibrillators can be programmed to deliver the first several shocks at predetermined energy levels in accordance with local medical protocols or may allow the operator to select from alternative settings. Unless a device is designed to allow adjustment of energy settings to low levels in the field, automated defibrillators should not be used on pediatric patients. The automated defibrillator can be left on the patient until advanced life support personnel arrive or during transport to the hospital in case of recurrence of a lethal arrhythmia.

General considerations for use of an automated defibrillator include the following:

1. Remember the basic skills of patient assessment to determine if a patient is in cardiac arrest.
2. The operator of the defibrillator should attach the device and deliver a shock as soon as possible after reaching the patient (ideally in less than 2 minutes). Do not delay defibrillation to perform airway management and chest compressions if these can be done by other personnel.
3. Stop CPR and assure that no one is touching or moving the patient while the defibrillator is analyzing the rhythm.
4. Have the machine reanalyze the rhythm after each and every defibrillation.
5. When no further shock is indicated by the device after defibrillation and no pulse is present, continue CPR for 1 minute, then repeat pulse check and rhythm analysis. Patients often have no rhythm or a slow rhythm after defibrillation, which improves with time and oxygenation.

Emergency Synchronized Cardioversion

Synchronized cardioversion uses the same concepts and techniques as defibrillation to deliver an electrical current to the heart. In cardioversion, however, the shock is timed to the heart's existing electrical activity to avoid stimulation during the relative refractory, or vulnerable, period. A synchronizing circuit built into the defibrillator allows delivery of the shock to be programmed to occur during a specific part of the QRS complex, often during the R wave. Synchronization is thought to be beneficial in reducing the energy requirements and the incidence of postshock arrhythmias.

The most common prehospital indication for synchronized cardioversion is perfusing ventricular tachycardia, although nonsynchronized defibrillation should be used in the setting of cardiac arrest if synchronization will cause any delay in management. Other rhythms treated with synchronized cardioversion are supraventricular tachycardia that causes severe hemodynamic compromise including PSVT, atrial fibrillation with rapid ventricular response, and two-to-one atrial flutter.

Energy requirements for synchronized cardioversion are determined by the type of arrhythmia and the urgency to terminate the arrhythmia based on the patient's clinical condition. Not more than 50 J should be used for ventricular tachycardia unless the patient is pulseless or unconscious. Initial cardioversion attempts of supraventricular tachycardia should not be greater than 25 to 100 J (i.e., 25 J for atrial flutter, 75–100 J for PSVT and atrial fibrillation). Local protocols should define exact energy doses.

The procedure for synchronized cardioversion is the same as described for defibrillation (see Skill 20-1) with the following exceptions:

1. Sedation with diazepam or similar amnesic drug may be indicated before cardioversion for conscious patients.
2. A synchronizer switch or button must be used to activate the synchronizer circuitry.
3. Chest electrodes should be applied to obtain a high-quality EKG tracing. Lead placement and gain should be adjusted to obtain maximum height of the R wave to ensure sensing by the synchronizer. Proper sensing can be observed on most oscilloscopes by the appearance of a marker artifact on each R wave or by a flashing QRS complex detector light.
4. Discharge buttons must be pressed and held down until the shock is delivered.
5. If ventricular fibrillation occurs after cardioversion, the synchronizer switch must be manually turned off on some machines before it is possible to proceed with defibrillation.

Prehospital Intervention for Arrhythmias That Result From Decreased Automaticity or Conduction Disturbances

Atropine Sulfate

Pharmacology and Actions.. **Atropine sulfate** is a potent parasympathetic (vagal) blocking agent. Its actions are to increase the rate of SA node discharge and improve AV conduction. By increasing sinus rate, it also helps inhibit ventricular ectopic activity. Finally, atropine has been shown to occasionally restore a cardiac rhythm in cardiac arrest patients with asystole.

Cardiac Indications.. Atropine is indicated to increase heart rate in any type of bradycardia accompanied by hemodynamically significant hypotension, ventricular ectopic complexes, and any other signs or symptoms of hemodynamic decompensation. Atropine may also be indicated for ventricular asystole.

Precautions.. Atropine should not be administered to a bradycardic patient who is hemodynamically stable; unnecessarily increasing the heart rate may be detrimental to an ischemic myocardium by creating increased myocardial oxygen demand. The same danger exists when patients have an excessive rate acceleration in response to atropine administration.

Administration and Dosage.. For bradycardia, a bolus injection of 0.5 mg is administered IV. This dose may be repeated at 5-minute intervals as needed, the total dose usually not to exceed 2 mg. Atropine is one of the few drugs for which rapid IV bolus administration is recommended. Administering slowly or in doses less than 0.5 mg may result in a paradoxical slowing of the heart rate. The initial dose for management of asystole is 1 mg repeated in 5 minutes if asystole persists. When an IV cannot be established, atropine may also be administered via an endotracheal tube.

Side Effects and Special Considerations.. Side effects include decreased gastrointestinal motility, urinary retention, and pupillary dilation. Atropine may be less effective than β-stimulating drugs in the management of third degree AV block, but it should be attempted as the first-line drug to increase AV conduction.

Isoproterenol

Pharmacology and Actions.. **Isoproterenol**, a potent β-stimulating drug, is related to epinephrine but lacks the α-stimulating properties of epinephrine. Isoproterenol affects both the electrical and mechanical functions of the heart, increasing heart rate and contractility. Because of these effects, it also significantly increases oxygen demand and may worsen myocardial ischemia.

Cardiac Indications.. The only indication for isoproterenol is for immediate, temporary control of any hemodynamically compromising bradycardia that has not responded to atropine administration. It is only recommended for perfusing rhythms, as epinephrine is more appropriate in the setting of cardiac arrest.

Precautions.. Because β stimulation increases cardiac automaticity, patients should be monitored closely for the development of arrhythmias, and this drug should be administered with caution when ventricular arrhythmias preexist.

Dosage and Administration.. Isoproterenol is administered for bradycardia by continuous IV infusion and is titrated according to heart rate and blood pressure response. One milligram of drug is diluted in 250 mg of D_5W for a concentration of 4 μg/mL. It can be administered using a microdrip infusion set at a rate of 2 to 10 μg/min.

Extreme care must be used to monitor drug administration to avoid excessive increases in heart rate and blood pressure.

Side Effects and Special Considerations.. Tachycardia and extension of infarct size due to increased oxygen demand are the most serious side effects. The infusion should be slowed or stopped if ventricular arrhythmias develop. Transport of the patient who requires isoproterenol should be expedited, as definitive management is pacemaker insertion.

Noninvasive Cardiac Pacing

Noninvasive cardiac pacing, also called **external or transcutaneous pacing,** is a temporary, noninvasive method of cardiac pacing performed by delivering electrical impulses to the heart via large body surface electrodes. It is most helpful in patients whose primary problem is heart rate but whose myocardial mechanical function is good. External pacing is indicated for any bradycardia that causes severe hemodynamic compromise that has not responded to pharmacologic intervention. It has also been used after successful defibrillation of ventricular fibrillation until the patient's own cardiac electrical activity has normalized. External pacing has not proven to be effective in cardiac arrest.

The type of external pacemaker and local medical protocols govern the specific operation of the device, but general steps in the procedure for external pacing are the following:

- Application of chest electrodes
- Selection of current output
- Selection of pacing rate
- Selection of pacing mode (i.e., asynchronous vs. demand)
- Activation of pacer
- Observation of EKG for pacing capture
- Adjustment of current output (if necessary) until capture obtained
- Documentation by EKG write-out

Some chest muscle contraction may be expected with external pacing. These contractions may make it difficult to palpate a carotid pulse during pacing when peripheral pulses are absent because of cardiovascular collapse. Although muscle contractions are generally not painful, they may be uncomfortable for the patient who is conscious or who regains consciousness during pacing, and sedation may be indicated.

SUMMARY

In a cardiovascular emergency, a skilled paramedic is often the difference between life and death for the patient. The paramedic makes the first assessment of the patient and arrives at the conclusion that the problem is cardiac related. Often, the clues that the problem is of cardiac origin are subtle, and it takes a high index of suspicion on the paramedic's part to interpret them correctly. Familiarity with cardiovascular anatomy and physiology, both normal and abnormal, creates a firm foundation on which to construct a management plan.

Proper management of a cardiac-related problem begins with the patient assessment. It may also call on the paramedic's ability to make a swift, accurate interpretation of the patient's EKG. Prehospital intervention for the condition might require the administration of cardiac drugs or the institution of electrical therapy. In the most serious situations, CPR is required. It is of paramount importance that the paramedic be prepared to act swiftly and correctly during a cardiac emergency.

SUGGESTED READING

American Heart Association: Instructor's Manual for Advanced Cardiac Life Support, 2nd ed. Dallas, American Heart Association, 1988

American Heart Association: Textbook of Advanced Cardiac Life Support, 2nd ed. Dallas, American Heart Association, 1987

American Heart Association: Standards and guidelines for cardiopulmonary resuscitation (CPR) and emergency cardiac care (ECG). JAMA 255:2905, 1986

Andreoli KG, Zipes DP, Wallace AG, Kinny MR, Fowkes VK: Comprehensive Cardiac Care, 6th ed. St. Louis, CV Mosby, 1987

Baerman JM, Morady F, DiCarlo LA: Differentiation of ventricular tachycardia from supraventricular tachycardia with aberration: Value of the clinical history. Ann Emerg Med 16:40, 1987

Bunting–Blake L, Parker J, Weigel A, White RD: Defibrillation: A Manual for the EMT. Philadelphia, JB Lippincott, 1985

Codini MA: Management of acute myocardial infarction. Med Clin North Am 70:769, 1986

Conan S, Taigman M: Recognition of acute myocardial infarction. J Emerg Med Serv 12(10):49, 1987

Cummins RO:Encouraging early defibrillation: The American Heart Association and Automated External Defibrillators.Ann Emerg Med 19:1245, 1990

Eisenbery MS, Cummins RO: Code Blue: Cardiac Arrest and Resuscitation. Philadelphia, WB Saunders, 1987

Erickson B: Heart Sounds and Murmurs: A Practical Guide. St. Louis, CV Mosby, 1987

Ferguson RK, Vlasses PH: Hypertensive emergencies and urgencies. JAMA 255:1607, 1986

Grauer K, Cavallaro D: ACLS Mega Code Review Study Cards. St. Louis, CV Mosby, 1988

Grauer K, Curry RW Jr: Clinical Electrocardiography: A Primary Care Approach. Oradell, Medical Economics Books, 1987

Haddad A, Dean DG: Interpreting ECGs: An Advanced Self-test Guide, 2nd ed. Oradell, Medical Economics Books, 1987

Huff J, Doernback DP, White RD: ECG Workout: Exercises in Arrhythmia Interpretation. Philadelphia, JB Lippincott, 1985

Huszar RJ: Basic Dysrhythmias: Interpretation and Management. St. Louis, CV Mosby, 1988

Ruggie N: Congestive heart failure. Med Clin North Am 70:829, 1986

Stein E: Interpretation of Arrhythmias: A Self-study Program. Philadelphia, Lea & Febiger, 1988

Stults KR, Cummins RO: Fully automatic vs. shock advisory defibrillators. J Emerg Med Serv 12(9):71, 1987

Thaler MS: The Only EKG Book You'll Ever Need. Philadelphia, JB Lippincott, 1988

US Department of Transportation, National Highway Traffic Safety Administration: Emergency Medical Technician–Paramedic: National Standards Curriculum. Washington, DC, US Government Printing Office, 1985

Wharton JM, Goldschlager N: Interpreting Cardiac Dysrhythmias. Oradell, Medical Economics Books, 1987

Wiederhold R: Electrocardiography: The Monitoring Lead. San Diego, Harcourt Brace Jovanovich, 1988

CHAPTER 21

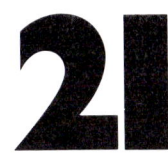

Endocrine Emergencies

Anatomy and Physiology of the Endocrine System
  Hormones
    Hormone Regulation
  Endocrine Glands
    Pituitary Gland
      Anterior Pituitary
      Posterior Pituitary
    Thyroid Gland
      Hyperthyroidism
      Hypothyroidism
    Parathyroid Glands
      Hyperparathyroidism
      Hypoparathyroidism

    Adrenal Glands
      Adrenal Cortex
      Adrenal Medulla
    Pancreas
      Glucagon
      Insulin
      Diabetes Mellitus
    The Ovaries
    The Testes
Assessment of Endocrine Emergencies

Diabetic Emergencies
  Diabetic Ketoacidosis
    Assessment
    Management
  Hyperosmolar Hyperglycemic Nonketotic Coma
    Assessment
    Management
  Hypoglycemia
    Assessment
    Management
Summary

BEHAVIORAL OBJECTIVES

On successful completion of this chapter, the reader will be able to:

1. Discuss hormone production and regulation
2. Describe the structures and functions of the pituitary gland, thyroid gland, parathyroid glands, adrenal glands, pancreas, ovaries, and testes
3. Discuss the pathophysiology of hyperthyroidism, hypothyroidism, hyperparathyroidism, and hypoparathyroidism
4. Describe the role of insulin and glucagon and their effects on blood glucose levels
5. Explain primary and secondary diabetes mellitus
6. Describe the proper assessment of the patient with known or suspected endocrine problems
7. Explain the differences between diabetic ketoacidosis, hyperosmolar hyperglycemic nonketotic coma, and hypoglycemia
8. Describe the assessment and management of diabetic ketoacidosis, hyperosmolar hyperglycemic nonketotic coma, and hypoglycemia
9. Define all of the key terms in this chapter

KEY TERMS

The following terms are defined in the chapter and glossary:

*adenohypophysis
adrenal cortex
adrenal glands
adrenal medulla
adrenocorticotropin (ACTH)
androgens
antidiuretic hormone (ADH)
calcitonin
catecholamines
Cushing's syndrome
diabetes mellitus
diabetic ketoacidosis
endocrine
follicle-stimulating hormone (FSH)
glucagon
glucocorticoids
growth hormone (GH)
hormones
hyperglycemia
hyperthyroidism
hyperparathyroidism
hypoglycemia
hyperosmolar hyperglycemic nonketotic coma
hypoparathyroidism
hypothalamus
hypothyroidism
insulin
luteinizing hormone (LH)
mineralocorticoids
neurohypophysis
ovaries
oxytocin
pancreas
parathyroid glands
parathyroid hormone (PTH)
pituitary gland
polydipsia
polyphagia
polyuria
prolactin
sella turcica
testes
thyroid gland
thyroid-stimulating hormone (TSH)
thyroxine (T_4)
triiodothyronine (T_3)*

The human **endocrine** system is a complex and integrated network that functions to maintain homeostasis, promote growth and sexual development, and allow adaptation to the physiologic stresses placed on the organism. The primary components of this system are the endocrine glands and their respective hormones.

Because of the complexity of this system, problems can arise at numerous points. Inadequate hormone production, abnormal hormonal structure, impaired receptor function, and loss of proper regulatory mechanisms are but a few of the factors that may produce endocrine system dysfunction. In some cases, the resulting disorder may be a slow process that develops over the course of many years, while, in other instances, impaired endocrine function may manifest as an acute life-threatening condition.

Basic anatomy and physiology of the endocrine system is followed by a more in-depth discussion of the individual endocrine glands. Endocrine emergencies, their pathophysiology, clinical presentation, and management is examined with emphasis placed on those areas most frequently seen in the field.

ANATOMY AND PHYSIOLOGY OF THE ENDOCRINE SYSTEM

Hormones

Simply stated, **hormones** are chemical substances that are released into the bloodstream and exert an effect at distant target organs. Hormones belong to different chemical classes including amines (e.g., thyroxine), polypeptides (e.g., insulin), glycoproteins (e.g., thyrotropin), and steroids (e.g., progesterone).

Although the mechanism by which hormones bring about their biologic effects is complex, the fundamental feature involves the binding of the hormone with a specific receptor. Two general patterns of hormone-receptor action have been well defined, based largely on the location of the hormone. In the case of steroid hormones, the receptor is located within the cytoplasm of the cell. The steroid hormone travels to its target organ, crosses the cell membrane, and binds to a cytoplasmic receptor, at which point the hormone-receptor complex travels to the cell nucleus where it brings about its characteristic actions. In the case of polypeptide hormones, the receptor is located within the cell membrane itself. The polypeptide hormone again travels to its target organ, but, instead of entering the cell, it binds to a receptor in the cell membrane and initiates a series of intracellular chemical reactions, which, in turn, bring about the hormone's characteristic biologic actions. Although the location of the receptor varies as described above, the common feature in each case is the interaction between the hormone and its specific receptor.

Hormone Regulation

Hormone production and release in the various endocrine organs is under a variety of control mechanisms. A major regulatory mechanism involves the interaction of the hypothalamic-pituitary-target organ system. Understanding this system requires that one distinguish between "*tropic hormones*" and "*effector hormones*."

The tropic hormones are released from the hypothalamus and pituitary gland. The **hypothalamus** lies directly beneath the cerebral hemispheres of the brain and along with regulating water balance and body temperature, it secretes tropic hormones, which then stimulate the release of pituitary tropic hormones. Tropic hormones have minimal direct biologic effects themselves, and are primarily regulatory hormones that stimulate or inhibit release of hormones from the various endocrine glands. The effector hormones, on the other hand, are released by the target endocrine glands and are responsible for producing biologic effects in the organism.

In a typical case, hypothalamic tropic hormones (i.e., thyrotropin releasing hormone) are directed to the pituitary gland, where they act to stimulate pituitary tropic hormone release. The released pituitary hormone (i.e., thyrotropin) then travels to its target organ (i.e., thyroid gland), where it stimulates production and release of the effector hormone (i.e., thyroxine). Once released, the concentration of the hormone in the blood is naturally increased. The increased blood hormone concentration acts to mediate the biologic effects of the hormone, while at the same time signalling the higher regulatory centers (e.g., hypothalamus and pituitary gland) to stop release of their tropic hormones. Without the stimulus from these tropic hormones, the target organ ceases production of its hormone and the blood concentration falls. This process is called the "*negative feedback system*" (Fig. 21-1); "negative" because increased blood concentrations of the effector hormone inhibit the hypothalamic-pituitary system, and "feedback" because of the interrelation between the target organ and the hypothalamic-pituitary system.

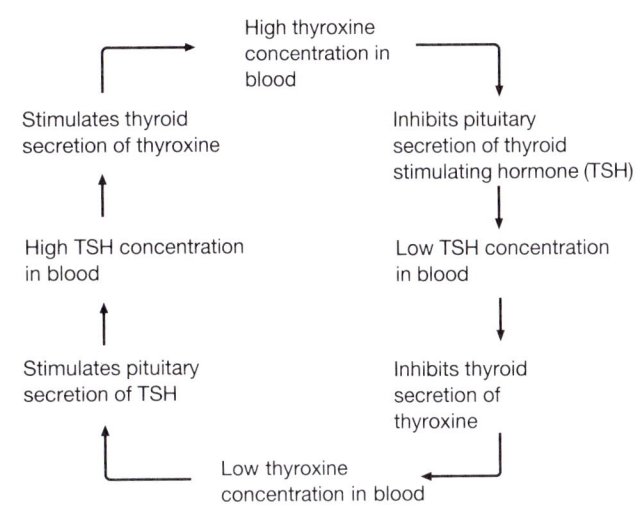

FIGURE 21–1.
Negative feedback control of TSH and thyroxine secretion, a homeostatic mechanism that tends to keep the blood level of thyroxine within a narrow range.

Endocrine Glands

Endocrine glands are distinguished from other glands (*exocrine*) by the fact that they do not possess ducts but, instead, secrete their products directly into the systemic circulation. The major endocrine glands of the human body are shown in Figure 21-2 and include the pituitary

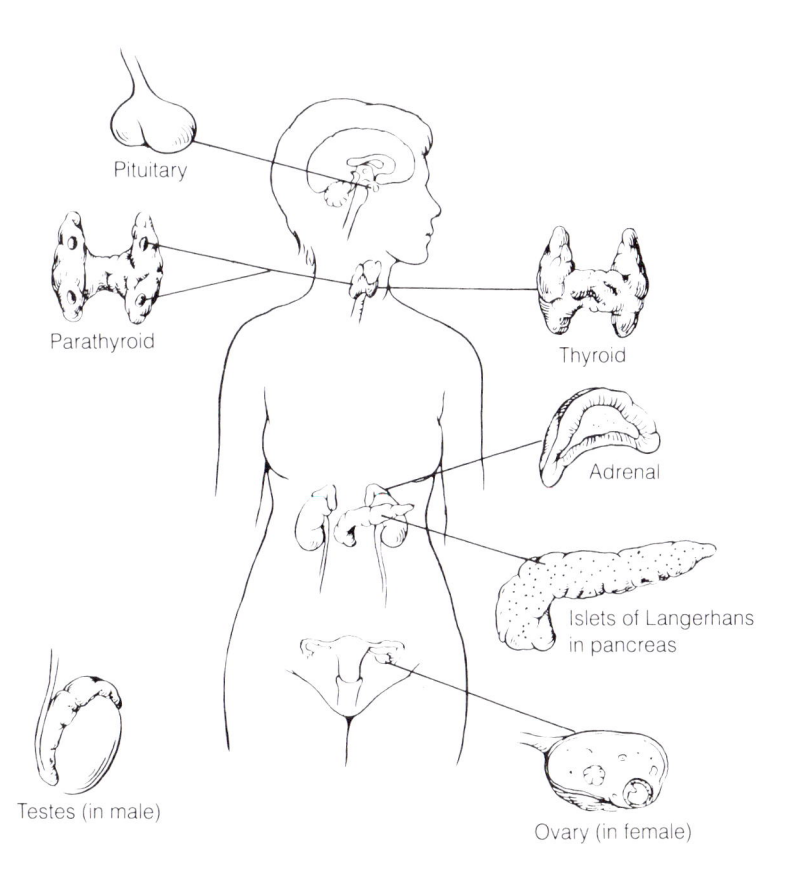

FIGURE 21–2.
Glands of the endocrine system.

TABLE 21-1.
THE ENDOCRINE GLANDS AND THEIR HORMONES

Endocrine Glands	Hormones	Effects
Anterior pituitary	Adrenocorticotropin (ACTH)	Stimulates adrenal cortex to produce cortical hormones
	Growth hormone (GH; somatotropin)	Promotes growth of all body tissues
	Thyroid stimulating hormone (TSH)	Stimulates thyroid gland to produce thyroid hormones
	Prolactin	Stimulates milk production
	Luteinizing hormone (LH)	Controls ovulation and menstruation in women
	Follicle-stimulating hormone (FSH)	Stimulates growth of ovarian follicles and testes; promotes development of sperm cells
Posterior pituitary	Antidiuretic hormone (ADH; vasopressin)	Promotes reabsorption of water in kidney tubules; stimulates smooth muscle of blood vessels to constrict
	Oxytocin	Stimulates milk production; causes contraction of muscle of uterus
Thyroid	Triiodothyronine (T_3)	Regulates metabolic rate
	Thyroxine (T_4)	Regulates metabolic rate
	Calcitonin	Decreases calcium level in blood
Parathyroid	Parathyroid hormone (PTH)	Regulates amount of calcium and phosphorus in blood
Adrenal cortex	Glucocorticoids	Aids in metabolism of carbohydrates, proteins, and fats; anti-inflammatory properties
	Mineralcorticoids	Aids in regulating electrolytes and water balance
	Androgens	Promotes sexual growth
Adrenal medulla	Epinephrine	Increases blood pressure and heart rate; speeds up many body processes
	Norepinephrine	Similar actions to epinephrine
Pancreas	Glucagon	Stimulates liver to release glucose
	Insulin	Aids transport of glucose into cells
Ovaries	Estrogen	Stimulates growth of female sexual organs
	Progesterone	Stimulates development of secretory parts of mammary glands; aids in maintaining pregnancy
Testes	Testosterone	Stimulates growth of male sexual organs

gland, thyroid gland, parathyroid glands, adrenal glands, pancreas, ovaries, and testes.

In each of these organs, chemical substances called hormones are released directly into the bloodstream, where they travel to specific target organs to exert their biologic effects (Table 21-1).

Pituitary Gland

The **pituitary gland** is a small pea-shaped structure that weighs about 0.5 g and is located at the base of the brain in a small depression in the sphenoid bone known as the ***sella turcica***. Here, it receives input from the central nervous system (via the hypothalamus) above and, in turn, secretes hormones into the bloodstream, which in many cases act to regulate the function of the body's endocrine glands. Because of the pituitary's role as a linkage between the central nervous system and the body's endocrine system and its regulatory control over the major endocrine glands, it is often referred to as the body's "*master endocrine*" gland (Fig. 21-3).

The pituitary gland is divided structurally and func-

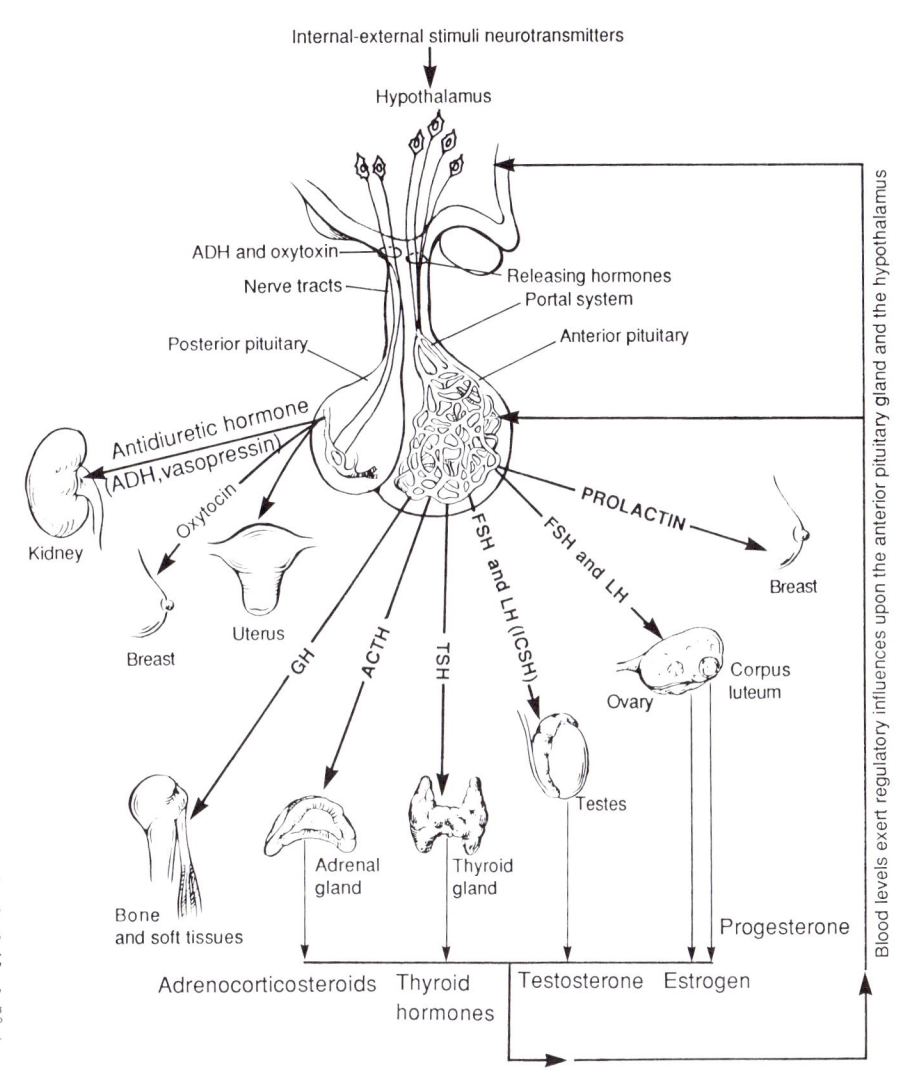

FIGURE 21-3.
The pituitary gland and its interrelationships with the heart and target tissues. ADH indicates antidiuretic hormone; GH, growth hormone; ACTH, corticotropin; TSH, thyroid-stimulating hormone; FSH, follicle-stimulating hormone; LH, luteinizing hormone; and ICSH, interstitial cell-stimulating hormone (in males)

tionally into an anterior pituitary lobe (*adenohypophysis*) and a posterior pituitary lobe (*neurohypophysis*).

ANTERIOR PITUITARY. The anterior pituitary synthesizes and secretes six polypeptide hormones: corticotropin, growth hormone, thyrotropin, prolactin, luteinizing hormone, and follicle-stimulating hormone. These are, for the most part, tropic hormones in that their primary action is to mediate the release of effector hormones from the various endocrine glands.

Adrenocorticotropin (ACTH), also known as corticotropin, travels to its target organ, the adrenal glands (adrenal cortex), where it stimulates the release of mineralocorticoids, glucocorticoids, and androgenic steroids. **Growth hormone (GH)**, also known as somatotropin, is secreted into the bloodstream, where it has a variety of effects on multiple body tissues, the overall effect being to stimulate body growth. **Thyroid-stimulating hormone (TSH)**, also known as thyrotropin, acts on the thyroid gland, promoting growth of the gland as well as increased synthesis and release of thyroid hormones. **Prolactin** has its major role during pregnancy, when it enhances milk production and, in conjunction with other hormones, stimulates breast development. The gonadotropins, which influence the sexual glands, include both **luteinizing hormone (LH)** and **follicle-stimulating hormone (FSH)** and act on the ovary and testis, causing growth and stimulating both sex hormone production and *spermatogenesis* (development of sperm cells).

POSTERIOR PITUITARY. The posterior pituitary secretes two polypeptide hormones, antidiuretic hormone and oxytocin. Both hormones are actually synthesized in the hypothalamus and transported down along nerve axons to the posterior pituitary, where they are stored until needed. After an appropriate stimulus, they are released into the bloodstream and travel to their respective sites of action.

Antidiuretic hormone (ADH), also known as vasopressin, has its primary actions in the kidney, where it stimulates increased water reabsorption. **Oxytocin** has effects both on the breast, where it stimulates milk ejection, and in the uterus, where it causes muscular contraction.

Thyroid Gland

The **thyroid gland** is a highly vascular endocrine gland that lies in front and to the side of the trachea in the lower part of the neck. It consists of right and left lobes that lie on either side of the trachea and are joined across the midline anteriorly, at the level of the second to fourth tracheal rings, by a thin band of tissue called the isthmus. In addition to the two lobes and the isthmus, a significant number of people have an extra lobe, the pyramidal lobe, which is a narrow, elongated band of tissue that ascends in the midline from the isthmus (Fig. 21-4). The extensive blood supply to the thyroid gland and its close proximity to the cricoid cartilage make a complete understanding of its anatomy critical to cases in which emergency airway management calls for a cricothyroidotomy, so that the serious complications of hemorrhage and damage to the gland can be avoided. Varying greatly in size, it ranges in weight from 18 to 31 g and tends to be larger in women, young people, and in well-nourished people. It tends to increase in size during menstruation and pregnancy, and it shrinks with age.

The thyroid gland plays a major role in the regulation of metabolism, growth and development, and calcium balance. The three hormones secreted by this gland are triiodothyronine, thyroxine, and calcitonin.

Both **triiodothyronine** (T_3) and **thyroxine** (T_4) are iodine-containing amino acid derivatives that are stored in saclike regions of the gland known as follicles. In response to activation by the pituitary hormone TSH, the follicles of the thyroid gland release both T_3 and T_4 directly into the bloodstream, where the hormones are distributed to tissues and organs throughout the body. They act to increase oxygen consumption and generate heat, with the overall effect of an increase in metabolic activity. In younger people, these hormones are also essential for proper skeletal growth and for maturation of the nervous system.

Calcitonin, also a polypeptide hormone, is produced by a discrete group of cells ("C-cells") located within the thyroid gland. Its primary function is to regulate serum calcium, to prevent this substance from reaching excessive levels.

HYPERTHYROIDISM. Abnormal thyroid function may result in the release of either too much or too little thyroid hormone into the bloodstream. In **hyperthyroidism** (thyrotoxicosis), the excess thyroid hormone results in a hypermetabolic state characterized by the following:

- Weight loss
- Diarrhea
- Heat intolerance
- Tremor
- *Exophthalmos* (abnormal protrusion of the eyeball)
- Anxiety
- Palpitations
- Fatigue
- Dyspnea
- Irritability

Physical examination often shows an anxious patient whose skin is warm and moist. Systolic blood pressure may be increased and diastolic pressure decreased (i.e., increased pulse pressure). Neurologic examination often reveals increased deep tendon reflexes. Cardiac monitoring is likely to reveal an arrhythmia, frequently sinus tachycardia or atrial fibrillation. If symptoms are severe, the patient is said to be having a "*thyroid storm*" or "thy-

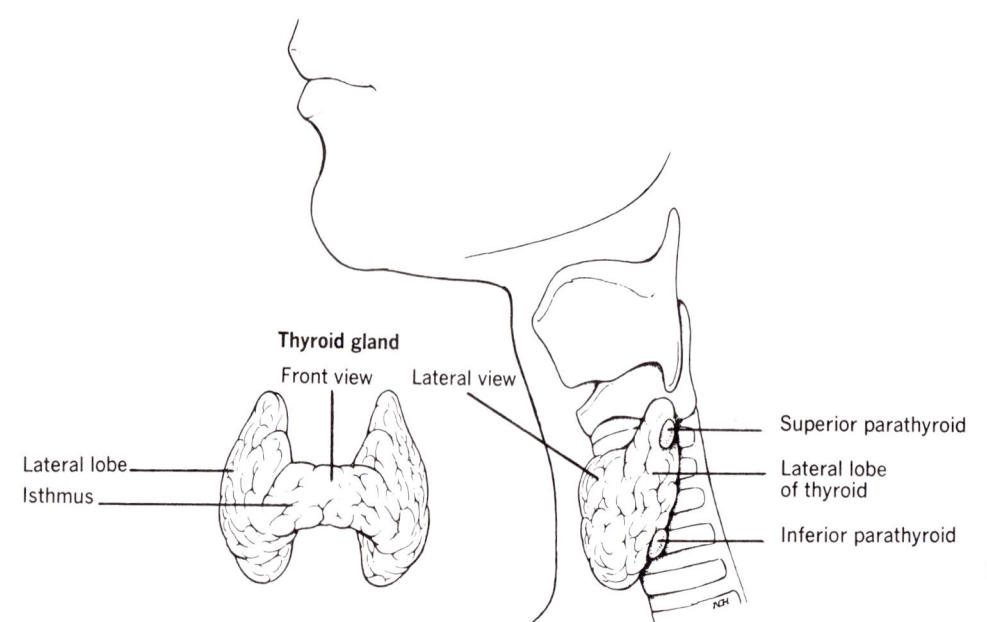

FIGURE 21-4.

The thyroid and parathyroid glands. (Rosdahl CB)

rotoxic crisis." Field treatment for symptomatic hyperthyroid patients is nonspecific and calls for monitoring of vital signs, careful cardiac monitoring, supportive treatment, and transport to a medical facility.

HYPOTHYROIDISM. In **hypothyroidism** (myxedema), the deficiency of thyroid hormone results in a hypometabolic state characterized by the following:

- Weight gain
- Cold intolerance
- Constipation
- Depression
- Muscle cramps
- Lethargy (drowsiness)

Physical examination often reveals a lethargic person. Skin may be dry, cool, and thickened. Neurologic examination may reveal an ataxic (muscular incoordination) gait in a person with an altered mental state. Heart sounds may be slow and distant, and cardiac monitoring may reveal a cardiac arrhythmia, commonly sinus bradycardia. Examination of the neck may show a scar from a prior thyroid operation. Because severe cases of hypothyroidism, known as "*myxedema crisis,*" carry a high risk of mortality, it is important to recognize these patients. Treatment is largely supportive with monitoring of vital signs and cardiac rhythm and transport to a medical facility.

Parathyroid Glands

The **parathyroid glands** consist of four pea-shaped glands that are situated in the neck in close proximity to the thyroid gland. Two of the glands lie, one on each side, just behind the upper pole of the right and left thyroid lobes and are called the superior parathyroid glands; while the other two glands lie, one on each side, just behind the lower pole of the right and left thyroid lobes and are called the inferior parathyroid glands (see Fig. 21-4).

The parathyroid glands are largely responsible for maintaining proper calcium levels in the bloodstream through the secretion of a polypeptide hormone, known appropriately as **parathyroid hormone (PTH)**. Parathyroid hormone has effects at three sites: the kidney, the bone, and the intestine. In each of these places, the hormone acts to increase blood calcium levels. In the kidney, it acts directly to increase calcium reabsorption and stimulates excretion of phosphate and bicarbonate. In addition, it stimulates the production of the active form of vitamin D. In bone, it directly stimulates reabsorption, with the net release of calcium and phosphate into the blood. In the intestine, it acts indirectly by stimulating renal production of vitamin D, which in turn causes increased intestinal reabsorption of calcium.

The key factor that regulates PTH release is the concentration of the blood calcium. When blood calcium is low, PTH is released, and *hypocalcemia* (low blood calcium) is prevented through increased reabsorption of calcium in the kidney, bone, and intestine. Conversely, when blood calcium is high, PTH release is inhibited, and *hypercalcemia* (high blood calcium) is prevented through decreased reabsorption of calcium in the kidney, bone, and intestine.

Disorders of parathyroid function may result from either deficient secretion of PTH, producing the clinical syndrome of hypoparathyroidism, or from excess secretion of PTH, with the resulting syndrome of hyperparathyroidism.

HYPERPARATHYROIDISM. In **hyperparathyroidism**, the patient may exhibit problems related to high levels of blood calcium (hypercalcemia). Signs and symptoms are nonspecific and often involve the gastrointestinal tract (nausea and vomiting) and the central nervous system (altered mental state and impaired cognitive functions). Physical examination is also variable and often of little help, though at times cardiac arrhythmias and altered deep tendon reflexes may be found. The electrocardiogram often shows a characteristic shortening of the QT interval. Management is essentially supportive, with monitoring of vital signs and support of cardiovascular and respiratory functions.

HYPOPARATHYROIDISM. In **hypoparathyroidism**, one finds abnormally low levels of blood calcium (hypocalcemia) along with high levels of blood phosphate. Clinically, these biochemical abnormalities result in neuromuscular irritability and instability characterized by *paresthesia* (numbness and tingling), muscle cramps and spasms (*carpopedal spasms*), and convulsions. On physical examination, the deep tendon reflexes are often found to be abnormal, being either hyperactive or hypoactive, depending on the degree of hypocalcemia. Skin changes may be present, including eczema, dry skin, and uneven hair distribution, if the condition is longstanding. On the electrocardiogram, the QT interval, characteristically, is prolonged, without associated U waves. Management again is supportive, basically, and includes monitoring of vital signs and cardiac rhythm and support of cardiovascular and respiratory functions. Transport to a medical facility is mandatory.

Adrenal Glands

The **adrenal glands** are small, pyramidal-shaped organs with a combined weight of approximately 10 g. They are located retroperitoneally and lie in close association with the upper part of each kidney. Each of the two glands consists of a cortex, which composes 90% of the gland, and a medulla, which makes up the remaining 10%. Although these two parts of the gland secrete different hormones and regulate different metabolic functions, the overall job of the adrenal glands can be viewed as an adaptive one, in which homeostasis is maintained despite day-to-day stresses.

ADRENAL CORTEX. The *adrenal cortex,* which makes up the bulk of each adrenal gland, secretes three functionally distinct groups of steroid hormones: glucocorticoids, mineralocorticoids, and androgens. The *glucocorticoids* have their primary effects on carbohydrate metabolism; they help maintain proper blood glucose levels by decreasing peripheral glucose uptake while at the same time stimulating increased liver glucose production. Increased lipolysis (breakdown of fats) and muscle breakdown occur, and the resulting products are sent to the liver help increase glucose production.

In addition to their effects on carbohydrate metabolism, the glucocorticoids also have important anti-inflammatory properties, which serve as the basis for their clinical use in many circumstances (e.g., the use of dexamethasone in head trauma). The *mineralocorticoids,* the most common of which is aldosterone, have their principal actions on water and electrolyte balance. They act primarily in the kidney, where they stimulate sodium and water reabsorption and facilitate potassium and hydrogen secretion. Insufficient production of mineralocorticoids results in dehydration secondary to decreased sodium and water reabsorption. Excessive production of mineralocorticoids can cause increased fluid retention secondary to increased sodium and water retention, hypokalemia (low blood potassium) secondary to increased secretion of potassium, and a metabolic alkalosis from increased hydrogen secretion.

The adrenal *androgens* (sex hormones) have a variety of functions, the most important of which is their role in the promotion of sexual growth and development.

ADRENAL MEDULLA. The *adrenal medulla,* which makes up about 10% of the entire adrenal gland, secretes as its primary hormones the *catecholamines* epinephrine and norepinephrine. Although not important in the fine regulation of body functions, the adrenal medulla serves an important homeostatic function in the face of stress. Release of adrenal catecholamines results in the typical "fight or flight" response, with increased heart rate, cardiac output, and systemic blood pressure.

Although a variety of problems may result from abnormal adrenal gland function, among the most important is that of adrenocortical insufficiency. This condition results when production of adrenal glucocorticoids or mineralocorticoids is inadequate. The clinical features often involve multiple systems: gastrointestinal system (nausea, vomiting, and abdominal pain), central nervous system (lethargy, depressed level of consciousness, or coma), and cardiovascular system (hypotension and tachycardia). The patient may be extremely ill and be in a state of hypovolemic shock when first encountered. Because adrenocortical insufficiency may be a life-threatening condition, rapid recognition and management is necessary. Vital signs and cardiac rhythm should be carefully monitored. An intravenous (IV) line should be inserted, and fluid replacement should be guided to maintain an adequate blood pressure. Respiratory status should be watched carefully and supplemental support provided if necessary. Rapid transport to a nearby medical facility is mandatory.

Pancreas

The *pancreas* is a solid tongue-shaped organ that measures 15 to 20 cm in length and weighs about 85 g. It is located retroperitoneally in the upper portion of the abdomen behind the stomach and in close proximity to the duodenum and spleen.

The pancreas serves as both an exocrine and endocrine gland. The bulk of the pancreas aids digestion; made up of acinar cells that secrete digestive enzymes into the duodenum via the pancreatic duct, it is the exocrine portion of the organ.

The endocrine portion of the pancreas is made up of small groups of hormone-producing cells that are scattered throughout the organ and known collectively as the *islets of Langerhans.* Cells within the islets of Langerhans produce and secrete their hormones directly into the bloodstream and, hence, are classified as being endocrine cells. The two major cell types that make up the islets of Langerhans are alpha cells, which secrete glucagon, and beta cells, which secrete insulin.

GLUCAGON. *Glucagon* is also a polypeptide hormone that is produced and secreted directly into the bloodstream by the alpha cells of the endocrine pancreas. Its release is, like insulin, largely regulated by blood glucose levels, but in a reciprocal manner; it is inhibited by *hyperglycemia* (increased blood glucose levels) and stimulated by *hypoglycemia* (decreased blood glucose levels). The overall effects of glucagon tend to be opposite those of insulin; its most important action is to increase blood glucose levels.

INSULIN. *Insulin* is a polypeptide hormone produced and secreted directly into the bloodstream by the beta cells of the endocrine pancreas. The most important stimulator of insulin release is the concentration of blood glucose. When blood glucose levels are high, such as after a meal, the pancreas increases its release of insulin. Conversely, when blood glucose levels are low, insulin release is diminished.

The primary role of insulin is to encourage storage of ingested nutrients. It has important effects on carbohydrate, protein, and lipid metabolism. With respect to carbohydrate metabolism, insulin promotes uptake of glucose from the bloodstream, while at the same time it inhibits the liver from releasing glucose. The net effect is to lower plasma glucose levels and increase intracellular glucose levels. In protein metabolism, insulin acts on muscle tissue to stimulate both the uptake of amino acids and their subsequent conversion into protein. Lastly, insulin influences lipid metabolism by increasing *adipose* (fatty) tissue uptake of *lipids* (triglycerides) from the blood and preventing the breakdown and release of free fatty acids into the bloodstream.

In summary, insulin promotes the uptake of blood glucose into body tissues, amino acids into muscle tissue, and triglycerides into fat tissue. The clinical results are lowered blood glucose, increased muscle protein synthesis, and increased fat deposition.

DIABETES MELLITUS. Pancreatic disorders result from a number of factors and may affect either the exocrine or endocrine portion of the gland. From a clinical point of view, the most important pancreatic endocrine disorder is **diabetes mellitus**. This is a metabolic disorder due to insulin deficiency that results in impaired carbohydrate metabolism, which, in turn, leads to persistent hyperglycemia. Diabetes mellitus may be broken down into primary diabetes mellitus and secondary diabetes mellitus.

In the majority of cases where there is no clear explanation for the cause of the diabetes, the term primary diabetes mellitus is applied. Within this category, two forms may be distinguished: type I or insulin-dependent diabetes mellitus, also known as juvenile diabetes, and type II or non–insulin-dependent diabetes mellitus, also referred to as adult-onset diabetes. Type I is distinguished by its onset during childhood or early adulthood, minimal to no pancreatic production of insulin, a tendency toward development of ketosis (abnormally large amounts of ketone bodies in the tissues and fluids), and the need for treatment with insulin. Type II is characterized by its later onset, usually after age 40, the presence of pancreatic-produced insulin, infrequent development of ketosis, and treatment that may require diet control and oral medications but rarely insulin.

In secondary diabetes mellitus, an underlying cause for the persistent elevation in blood sugar is found. Pancreatic destruction from alcohol, tumors, or cystic fibrosis, drugs such as steroids, diuretics, and adrenergic agents, hormonal disturbances such as **Cushing's syndrome** (excessive production of glucocorticoids from the adrenal cortex) and acromegaly, and genetic diseases, including Turner's syndrome, may all produce low effective insulin levels and result in hyperglycemia. Because the hyperglycemia is the result of a preexisting condition, the term secondary diabetes mellitus is used.

In both primary and secondary diabetes mellitus, a relative or absolute insulin deficiency results in a persistent hyperglycemia that causes an osmotic diuresis with dehydration, thirst, and **polyuria** (frequent urination). Weakness and fatigue are common, as is blurred vision. A history of frequent skin infections or itching may also be found. The clinical history and presentation often vary depending on the type of diabetes mellitus present. In type I, the onset is abrupt, with the patient presenting clinically with polyuria, **polydipsia** (increased thirst), and **polyphagia** (pathologic overeating). Often a paradoxical history of weight loss is seen despite an increased appetite. In type II, the onset is more insidious, developing over weeks to months, with a progressive history of polyuria and polydipsia, often associated with chronic fatigue, weakness, blurred vision, and frequent skin infections.

The complications of diabetes mellitus may reflect acute problems, such as diabetic ketoacidosis, hyperosmolar hyperglycemic nonketotic coma, and hypoglycemia, or the long-term degenerative changes of the disease process, which include blindness, renal damage, atherosclerosis, and nerve damage.

The Ovaries

The adult female **ovaries** consist of two spheroidal structures that each weigh about 6 g. They are located posterior to the peritoneum and are in close association to both the fallopian tubes and the uterus, to which they are attached by the ovarian ligament. The ovaries secrete a number of hormones, the most important of which are the steroid hormones estrogen and progesterone. These hormones play important roles in both sexual development and maturation and in the menstrual cycle. Abnormalities in ovarian hormone production may be manifested by altered sexual development, infertility, and alterations in the normal menstrual cycle.

The Testes

The adult male **testes** are approximately 4.5 by 2.5 cm in size and are housed outside the body proper in the scrotal sac. In structure, they are made up of two functionally distinct components, the Leydig cells (interstitial cells) and the seminiferous tubules. The former act as the endocrine component of the testes and secrete the hormone testosterone, which is responsible for sexual differentiation in the fetus, secondary sex characteristics in the pubertal male, and maintenance of potency and libido during adulthood. The seminiferous tubules are responsible for production of the male spermatozoa during adulthood. Abnormal functioning of the testes or the hypothalamic-pituitary–regulating system may result in diminished development of the secondary sex characteristics (e.g., high-pitched voice, decreased axillary and pubic hair, small penis and testes) or infertility.

ASSESSMENT OF ENDOCRINE EMERGENCIES

Proper assessment of the patient with a known or suspected endocrine problem is vital if an accurate field diagnosis and adequate management are to be provided. In some cases, an endocrine emergency may be suspected based on the medical history or particular findings on physical examination. Because many of the serious endocrine emergencies result in an altered mental state or a shocklike state, the paramedic often is faced with an unconscious or semiconscious person who is unable to provide a clear medical history. For this reason, it is crucial that the possibility of an endocrine emergency be considered in any patient who presents with shock or an unexplained alteration in mental status.

If obtainable, the medical history may be of great assistance in providing clues that point to an endocrine problem. Does the patient's chief complaint have an obvious etiologic basis (i.e., the cause is known), or, as in the case of many endocrine problems, are the complaints general and nonspecific? Keep in mind the classic symptoms of diabetes mellitus, which include polyphagia, polydipsia, and polyuria. Remember that many of the endocrine disorders can present with multiple complaints that refer to several body systems, such as the central nervous system (e.g., altered mental status), the gastrointestinal system (nausea, vomiting, constipation), or the musculoskeletal system (numbness, tremors, weakness). Is there an unexplained loss of consciousness, as can be seen with diabetic ketoacidosis, hypoglycemia, hypothyroidism (e.g., myxedema coma), hyperosmolar hyperglycemic nonketotic coma, and acute adrenal crisis? Does the history of the present illness reveal an acute onset, as is typical with hypoglycemia, or has development been more gradual, as with diabetic ketoacidosis?

Obtain information about the medical history and inquire specifically about any endocrine problems, such as diabetes, pancreatic disease, or thyroid problems. Does the patient take any medications that suggest an underlying endocrine disorder, such as insulin or chlorpropamide for diabetes mellitus, thyroxine for hypothyroidism, or steroids for adrenal insufficiency? Has the patient had any prior operations that might have involved the endocrine glands and resulted in hormone deficiency?

As always, the initial physical assessment should start with the primary survey. Airway, breathing, circulation, and an intact cervical spine must be insured before proceeding further. The secondary survey and additional physical examination should involve a complete set of vital signs, along with a systematic assessment of the major body systems. Vital signs should be monitored repeatedly, and, if suggested by the patient's condition, *orthostatic* (postural) changes should be checked for. The head and neck examination should check for any signs of trauma, airway obstruction, or tracheal displacement. The lungs are auscultated to insure adequate respiratory excursion, air exchange, and the absence of rales, rhonchi, or wheezes. Cardiac examination should include palpation for the apical impulse and auscultation for the normal and clear S_1 and S_2 heart sounds. The abdomen is evaluated for any signs of trauma, pulsating masses, tenderness, or rigidity. Extremities are examined for fractures, deformity, impaired capillary refill and cyanosis, clubbing, or edema. Finally, a brief neurologic examination is important to document the patient's mental status, examine pupillary reflexes, and ascertain any focal neurologic findings.

DIABETIC EMERGENCIES

The three types of diabetic emergencies are summarized in Table 21-2.

Diabetic Ketoacidosis

Diabetic ketoacidosis is an acute metabolic complication of diabetes that results from the combined effects of an inadequate supply of insulin in association with elevated levels of glucagon.

This hormonal imbalance has the net effect of preventing the uptake and use of glucose as an energy substrate in several body tissues (e.g., muscle tissue) with resulting hyperglycemia and a shift to the breakdown and use of fats and protein as the primary body fuel. The altered metabolism results in the generation of large quantities of *ketone bodies* (i.e., beta-hydroxybutyric acid and acetoacetic acid), which accumulate in the bloodstream. The major clinical findings can be traced to the two hallmark biochemical features of diabetic ketoacidosis just mentioned: hyperglycemia and hyperketonemia. The high concentration of glucose in the blood is filtered by the kidney, but, unable to be fully reabsorbed, it passes into the urine (*glycosuria*), pulling large amounts of water with it and accounting for the frequent finding of polyuria. The resulting osmotic diuresis causes both dehydration, which manifests itself as polydipsia, and a depleted intravascular volume, which may present clinically as hypotension.

The hyperketonemia produces a metabolic acidosis that may cause a combination of *tachypnea* (rapid respiratory rate) and *hyperpnea* (increased respiratory volume), a respiratory pattern known as Kussmaul's breathing. This breathing pattern attempts to "blow off" carbon dioxide and normalize the blood pH. Other more diffuse clinical findings that may result include abdominal pain, nausea, vomiting, and an altered mental state.

Diabetic ketoacidosis may arise in three basic settings. It may be the initial presentation of type I diabetes mellitus in an unknowing and apparently healthy person. In instances in which a history of diabetes is established, the two most common precipitants are decreased insulin administration or increased physiologic stresses. Decreased insulin dosages may be the result of noncompliance, forgetfulness, or improper medication adjustment. Increased

TABLE 21–2.
THREE TYPES OF DIABETIC EMERGENCIES

Findings	Diabetic Ketoacidosis	Hyperosmolar Hyperglycemic Nonketotic Coma	Hypoglycemia
Insulin history	Insufficient or absent	Insufficient or absent	Excessive
Onset	Gradual, over several days	Gradual, over several days	Usually rapid, over a period of minutes
Sugar intake	Excessive	Excessive	Insufficient
General findings	Restlessness, merging into unconsciousness; weakness; dehydration; muscle aches; dry, red, warm skin	Stuporous, comatose; weakness; weight loss; usually elderly	Abnormally aggressive, merging into unconsciousness; weakness; pale, cold, clammy skin
Respiratory	Air hunger; Kussmaul's breathing; fruity (acetone) odor on breath; rapid respirations	No odor on breath	No odor on breath; normal or shallow respirations
Cardiovascular	Weak, rapid pulse; normal or low blood pressure	Weak, rapid pulse; low blood pressure	Normal or rapid and full pulse; normal blood pressure
Nervous	Headache	Seizures	Headache; dizziness; tremors
Gastrointestinal	Intense thirst; anorexia; nausea and vomiting; abdominal pain	Intense thirst; intense hunger; nausea and vomiting rare; absent abdominal pain; increased quantities of urine	Absent thirst; intense hunger; nausea and vomiting rare; absent abdominal pain; drooling

physiologic stresses are an important and often overlooked cause of diabetic ketoacidosis. These may be physical (i.e., trauma), emotional (i.e., psychosocial stressors), or medical (i.e., infection) conditions that act to effectively increase the body's insulin requirements so that a previously therapeutic dosage of insulin becomes ineffective in the face of these additional stresses.

Often, the development of diabetic ketoacidosis has a multifactorial etiology. A typical example can be seen in the case of a diabetic who becomes ill with an infection. The associated fever, nausea, vomiting, *anorexia* (loss of appetite), and general malaise often prompt patients to decrease their normal insulin dosage in the mistaken belief that because they are "sick" and "eating less" they need less insulin. On the contrary, the presence of infection is a major physiologic stress that acts to increase the body's insulin requirements. The combination of the stress placed on the body by infection and the lowered dosage of insulin administered by the patient is often enough to decompensate a previously stable diabetic and precipitate severe diabetic ketoacidosis.

Assessment

Evaluation of the patient suspected of having diabetic ketoacidosis should start with a search for a predisposing factor. Is the patient a known diabetic? If so, has the insulin dosage changed recently? Has the patient had a recent infection or suffered any other physiologic stresses? If the patient is not a known diabetic, then careful questioning for the recent development of polyuria, polydipsia, polyphagia, weight loss, and weakness may indicate the new onset of diabetes mellitus. Patients should also be asked if they have taken insulin or eaten recently. For cases in which a history is not available (e.g., an unconscious patient), a quick look in the refrigerator or medicine chest may yield a bottle of insulin or box of syringes that suggest underlying diabetes mellitus.

Physical examination often shows a clinical picture dominated by dehydration, altered mental state, and abnormal respiratory pattern. Vital signs may, in severe cases, show hypotension, tachycardia, and deep, rapid, and labored respirations (Kussmaul's breathing). The breath has a characteristic "fruity" odor (acetone) to it, often likened to the smell of nail-polish remover. Orthostatic changes may be present if dehydration is significant. The skin is often warm, flushed, and dry. Examination of the heart and lungs is usually unremarkable, except perhaps for a compensatory tachycardia if dehydration is severe. Though unclear why, abdominal pain may be present and the abdomen tender to palpation. The neurologic examination may reveal an altered mental status that ranges from an alert person to one who is comatose, depending on the severity of the underlying metabolic derangement.

In summary, a history of polyuria, polydipsia, and polyphagia, along with physical findings of warm, dry, and flushed skin with a "fruity" odor to the breath and Kussmaul's breathing, is highly suggestive of diabetic ketoacidosis.

Management

Management of the patient with suspected diabetic ketoacidosis calls for supportive measures and transport to a medical facility where definitive treatment can be carried out. A patent airway should be insured and careful positioning maintained to prevent aspiration in the event of vomiting. Supplemental oxygen administration is indicated to help maintain tissue oxygenation. Ventilatory status should be carefully monitored because severe metabolic acidosis can result in respiratory depression, necessitating assisted ventilation. Cardiac monitoring should be instituted to detect and correct any cardiac arrhythmias that result. If feasible, a baseline blood sample should be drawn for transport to the hospital. At the same time, a rapid blood sugar level can be determined in the field with a glucose reagent test strip (e.g., Detrostix). An IV line should be placed with infusion of lactated Ringer's solution, normal saline, or plasma expanders, depending on the severity of dehydration.

When the patient is unconscious, diabetic ketoacidosis may be difficult to distinguish from insulin-induced hypoglycemia or any of the numerous other causes of an altered mental state. In such cases, administration of a bolus of 50 mL of 50% dextrose may be indicated in the event that underlying hypoglycemia is present; and, if narcotic ingestion is suspected, then naloxone, 0.8 mg is indicated. Thiamine, 100 mg administered intramuscularly (IM), is indicated if there is a history of alcohol abuse. Once the above measures have been carried out, vital signs should be monitored and transport to a receiving hospital undertaken.

A note of caution is needed here, applicable to assessment and treatment of all patients with altered states of consciousness or in coma of unknown etiology. If cerebral ischemia is present hyperglycemia may worsen cerebral injury by increasing cerebral intracellular acidosis from anaerobic metabolism of glucose. Therefore, whenever possible, blood glucose should be measured with reagent strips or ideally with a glucometer before administering dextrose to such patietns.

Hyperosmolar Hyperglycemic Nonketotic Coma

Hyperosmolar hyperglycemic nonketotic coma is a clinical entity principally characterized by severe hyperosmolality, often secondary to extreme hyperglycemia. Plasma glucose concentration is frequently greater than 600 mg/100 mL (normal is about 100 mg/100 mL), and serum osmolarity may exceed 350 mOsm/L (normal is about 280 mOsm/L). In the majority of instances, ketosis or acidemia is minimal, hence the designation of hyperosmolar hyperglycemic "nonketotic" coma. The problem occurs more frequently in older people who have some precipitating cause, such as cerebrovascular accident, infection, or trauma.

Assessment

Although this condition can be seen in a variety of clinical settings, it is most commonly seen in type II diabetes mellitus, either as the presenting symptom of a previously healthy person or in the poorly controlled condition of a middle-aged person. Clinically, a history of polyuria and polydipsia may be present, along with gradual changes in mental state. Often, the paramedic is faced with a patient who presents only with a coma of unknown etiology. A history of diabetes mellitus should immediately raise the possibility of hyperosmolar hyperglycemic nonketotic coma. Because diagnosis of hyperosmolar hyperglycemic nonketotic coma relies on in-hospital documentation of blood glucose and serum osmolality, it is frequently difficult to distinguish in the field between hypoglycemia, diabetic ketoacidosis, and hyperosmolar hyperglycemic nonketotic coma.

Management

Field management should include managing the airway and administering oxygen, drawing baseline blood samples for transport to the hospital, and establishing an IV line with subsequent administration of fluids. If the patient is comatose, administration of 50 mL of 50% dextrose in an IV bolus is necessary to protect against the possibility of hypoglycemia as an inciting cause. Whenever possible blood glucose should be measured first, as discussed above. If the patient is unconscious for unknown reasons, and if narcotic ingestion is suspected, then naloxone, 0.8 mg, is indicated. Thiamine, 100 mg IM, is indicated if there is a history of alcohol abuse. Once the above measures have been carried out, vital signs should be monitored and transport to a receiving hospital undertaken.

Hypoglycemia

Hypoglycemia results when blood glucose levels fall below that required for normal body functioning. Since glucose is the primary energy source of the brain and various other tissues, hypoglycemia can produce a serious and potentially life-threatening condition. Although insulin administration is a leading cause of hypoglycemia ("*insulin shock*"), it should not be forgotten that this problem can arise from fasting, pancreatic tumors, oral antidiabetic medications, and a wide variety of other conditions that act to lower blood sugar levels.

The clinical features of patients who suffer from hypoglycemia are the combined effects of a decreased energy supply to the central nervous system and a hyperadrenergic state that results from a compensatory increase in catecholamine secretion. The inadequate energy supply, caused by the low levels of blood sugar that reach the brain, alters the patient's mental state. Mental status changes span the spectrum from irritability and mild confusion to stupor and coma, depending on the degree of hypoglycemia. In some cases, neurologic signs, such as seizures, may accompany the alteration in mental state. The compensatory release of increased quantities of the catecholamines, epinephrine and norepinephrine, produces a generalized "fight or flight" response with tremors, diaphoresis, palpitations, tachycardia, and cool, pale skin.

Assessment

Assessment of the patient with suspected hypoglycemia often reveals a predisposing factor. A history of diabetes mellitus, prolonged fasting, and alcoholism should, in the appropriate clinical setting, raise the suspicion of hypoglycemia. If a history is available, it often reveals the sudden onset of such symptoms as weakness, irritability, hunger, confusion, anxiety, or bizarre behavior. Patients should be asked if they have taken insulin or eaten recently. Physical examination, in severe cases, reveals a stuporous or unconscious person in moderate distress. The pulse is rapid, and respirations are normal or shallow. The skin is often cool, pale, and diaphoretic. Pulmonary findings are usually unremarkable. The cardiac examination shows normal S_1 and S_2 heart sounds, significant only perhaps for an increased rate. The extremities are often cool, pale, and diaphoretic.

The neurologic examination may show a variety of nonspecific findings. Mental status is invariably altered and may range from mild confusion to coma. Deep tendon reflexes may be increased and neurologic findings such as facial grimacing, paresis, and paralysis may be present. In some cases, seizures may be present. Two points must be kept in mind: the possibility of hypoglycemia ("insulin shock"; "hypoglycemic coma") should always be considered in any unconscious patient for whom an explanation is not self-evident; and mild or early stages of hypoglycemia may present with only subtle changes, such as irritability, difficulty concentrating, or bizarre behavior. These findings should not be overlooked, since failure to recognize them may be critical.

Management

Management of suspected hypoglycemia is directed at supporting vital body functions and rapidly raising blood glucose levels. As in all medical emergencies, the first priorities are to insure a patent airway, satisfactory ventilation, adequate circulation, and an intact cervical spine. Supplemental oxygen may be provided to insure good tissue oxygenation. After these priorities, an IV line should be placed with infusion of a glucose-containing solution, such as D_5W. A baseline blood sample should be drawn and brought to the hospital for analysis. If a glucose reagent strip is available, a quick approximation of the blood glucose level should be determined in the field. Portable glucometers are available for quantitative glucose measurement and their use is recommended before administration of dextrose. For cases in which the patient's mental state is significantly altered, an IV bolus of 50 mL of 50% dextrose should be given. Depending on the patient's response, repeat administration of dextrose may be carried out. If the patient is unconscious and the etiology unclear, then the administration of naloxone, 0.8 mg IV, and thiamine, 100 mg IM, is indicated in the event that an underlying opiate intoxication or a history of alcohol abuse is present. In all cases, both vital signs and the cardiac rhythm should be monitored and transport to a medical facility undertaken.

SUMMARY

Endocrine emergencies stem from a variety of disorders. Since the body has a number of endocrine glands, the process of investigation into the medical problem can be quite complex. A thorough knowledge of the endocrine glands and their function will benefit the paramedic in the assessment process. A medical history of endocrine disorders helps the assessment process.

SUGGESTED READING

Bourn S: Diabetic ketoacidosis. J Emerg Med Serv 13(5):61, 1988

Frohman LA: Neuroendocrine regulation and its function. In Wyngaarden JB, Smith LH (eds): Textbook of Medicine, 17th ed. Philadelphia, WB Saunders, 1985

Larsen PR: The thyroid. In Wyngaarden JB, Smith LH (eds): Textbook of Medicine, 17th ed. Philadelphia, WB Saunders, 1985

Meehan J: Prehospital Care: Administrative and Clinical Management. Rockville, Aspen, 1987

Olefsky JM: Diabetes mellitus. In Wyngaarden JB, Smith LH (eds): Textbook of Medicine, 17th ed. Philadelphia, WB Saunders, 1985

Service FJ: Hypoglycemic disorders. In Wyngaarden JB, Smith LH (eds): Textbook of Medicine, 17th ed. Philadelphia, WB Saunders, 1985

Slovis CM, Mork VC, Slovis RJ et al: Diabetic ketoacidosis and infection: Leukocyte count and differential as early predictors of serious infection. Am J Emerg Med 5:1, 1987

US Department of Transportation, National Highway Traffic Safety Administration: Emergency Medical Technician–Paramedic: National Standards Curriculum. Washington, DC, US Government Printing Office, 1985

CHAPTER 22

Neurologic Emergencies

Anatomy and Physiology of the Nervous System
  Neuron
    Axon
    Dendrites
    Myelin Sheath
    Neurilemma
  Brain
    Meninges
    Blood Supply
    Divisions
      Cerebrum
      Diencephalon
      Cerebellum
      Brain Stem

Spinal Cord
Peripheral Nervous System
  Autonomic Nervous System
    Sympathetic Division
    Parasympathetic Division
Assessment of Nervous System Emergencies
  Primary Survey
  Secondary Survey
    History
    Vital Signs
    Neurologic Evaluation
    Physical Examination

Types of Nervous System Disorders
  Coma
    Pathophysiology
    Assessment
    Management
  Seizure
    Pathophysiology
    Assessment
    Management
  Status Epilepticus
    Pathophysiology
    Assessment
    Management
  Stroke
    Pathophysiology
    Assessment
    Management
Summary

BEHAVIORAL OBJECTIVES
On successful completion of this chapter, the reader will be able to:

1. Identify the parts of a neuron and describe their function
2. Identify and describe the protective mechanisms of the brain
3. Describe the arterial and venous circulation to the brain
4. Locate the major functional areas in the brain for speech, vision, personality, balance and coordination, sensory and motor functions
5. Name and locate on a chart or model the six divisions of the brain
6. List the functions of the spinal cord
7. Describe the protective mechanisms for the spinal cord
8. State the functions of the peripheral nervous system, name the two divisions, and describe the actions of each
9. Identify specific observations and physical findings to be evaluated in the patient with a nervous system disorder
10. Describe the rating system for the Glasgow Coma Scale
11. Describe the pathophysiology, assessment, and management of coma, seizure, status epilepticus, and stroke
12. Define all of the key terms listed in this chapter

KEY TERMS

The following terms are defined in the chapter and glossary:

AVPU
acetylcholine
afferent neurons
arachnoid
autonomic nervous system
axon
brain stem
central nervous system (CNS)
cerebellum
cerebral cortex
cerebrovascular accident
cerebrospinal fluid
cerebrum
cervical spine
circle of Willis
coccyx
coma
cranial nerves
Cushing's reflex
decerebrate posturing
decorticate posturing
dendrites
dermatomes
diencephalon
dura mater
efferent neurons
epidural space
epilepsy
epinephrine
fight or flight syndrome
ganglia
Glasgow Coma Scale
homeostasis
hypothalamus
interneurons
Jacksonian seizure
lumbar spine
medulla oblongata
meninges
midbrain
myelin sheath
neurilemma
neuron
nodes of Ranvier
norepinephrine
parasympathetic division
peripheral nervous system
pia mater
pons
postganglionic neurons
preganglionic neurons
sacral spine
seizure
soma
spinal cord
spinal nerves
status epilepticus
stroke
subarachnoid space
subdural space
sympathetic division
synapses
thalamus
thoracic spine
vertebrae

In the field, paramedics encounter various emergencies that affect neurologic function. Building a foundational understanding of the structure and function of the nervous system and of the types of disorders that often disrupt it will better prepare the paramedic to provide care to patients with neurologic disorders.

ANATOMY AND PHYSIOLOGY OF THE NERVOUS SYSTEM

Survival of the human body depends on the maintenance of a relatively constant internal environment known as **homeostasis**. A multitude of complex events must function properly for the body to maintain homeostatic levels. The nervous system plays a key role in homeostasis because it functions as the body's control center. Along with the endocrine system, it controls all of the communication channels throughout the body.

Survival of the human body also depends on its ability to interact with the external environment. Being able to sense stimuli from the outside, the body can initiate a series of mechanisms that protect it from environmental extremes and immediate threats to life.

Since the nervous system is highly complex, it is divided into two major parts: the central nervous system, and the peripheral nervous system. The **central nervous system (CNS)** is composed of the brain and spinal cord. It functions as the body's communication control center and is directly responsible for all aspects of cognitive (act of knowing) and voluntary nervous function.

The **peripheral nervous system** includes all nerve fibers outside the brain and spinal cord. The peripheral nervous system sends messages in the form of nerve impulses, which it receives from tissues and organs, to the CNS. Once there, impulses are processed by the CNS. The peripheral nervous system then sends these messages back to the tissues and organs, producing certain actions such as glandular secretion.

The peripheral nervous system is further divided into the cranial nerves, the spinal nerves, and the autonomic nervous system. The autonomic nervous system plays an essential role in maintaining homeostatic levels. It supplies smooth muscle, cardiac muscle, and glandular epithelial tissue. The autonomic nervous system has sympathetic and parasympathetic divisions. These divisions are discussed in further detail later in the chapter. To obtain a better understanding of the nervous system, paramedics must first learn about the different anatomical structures within it and their basic functions.

Neuron

The basic unit of the nervous system is the individual nerve cell called the **neuron**. The body has literally billions of neurons, and each is composed of a cell body, called the **soma**. The cell body is the largest part of the neuron. Like other cells found throughout the body, the structure of the soma consists of a plasma membrane, a nucleus, and various organelles, notably mitochondria and Golgi apparatus. Groups of neurons in the CNS are called nerves. Groups of nerves located outside the CNS, in the periphery, are called **ganglia**.

CHAPTER 22: Neurologic Emergencies **537**

Structures that specifically characterize the neuron include axons, dendrites, a myelin sheath, and neurilemma. To provide a better understanding of the arrangement and function of these aspects of the neuron, they are considered individually.

Axon

An ***axon*** is a fiber that extends from the cell body (Fig. 22-1). Each neuron contains only one axon fiber. Both its length and diameter vary among neurons. The velocity of impulse conduction is specifically related to the diameter of the axon. The velocity of impulse conduction is faster with an increase in diameter. The primary function of the axon is to carry the nerve impulse away from the soma. The axon may connect to a muscle or sense organ, or it may terminate at another neuron's dendrites.

Dendrites

Dendrites are also fibers that extend from the cell body of the neuron (see Fig. 22-1). Unlike the single axon, which carries impulses away from the cell, dendrites are composed of many branching fibers that carry impulses to the soma. The distal ends of the dendrites' branches receive stimuli from the axons of other nerve cells. Thus, they are often referred to as receptors.

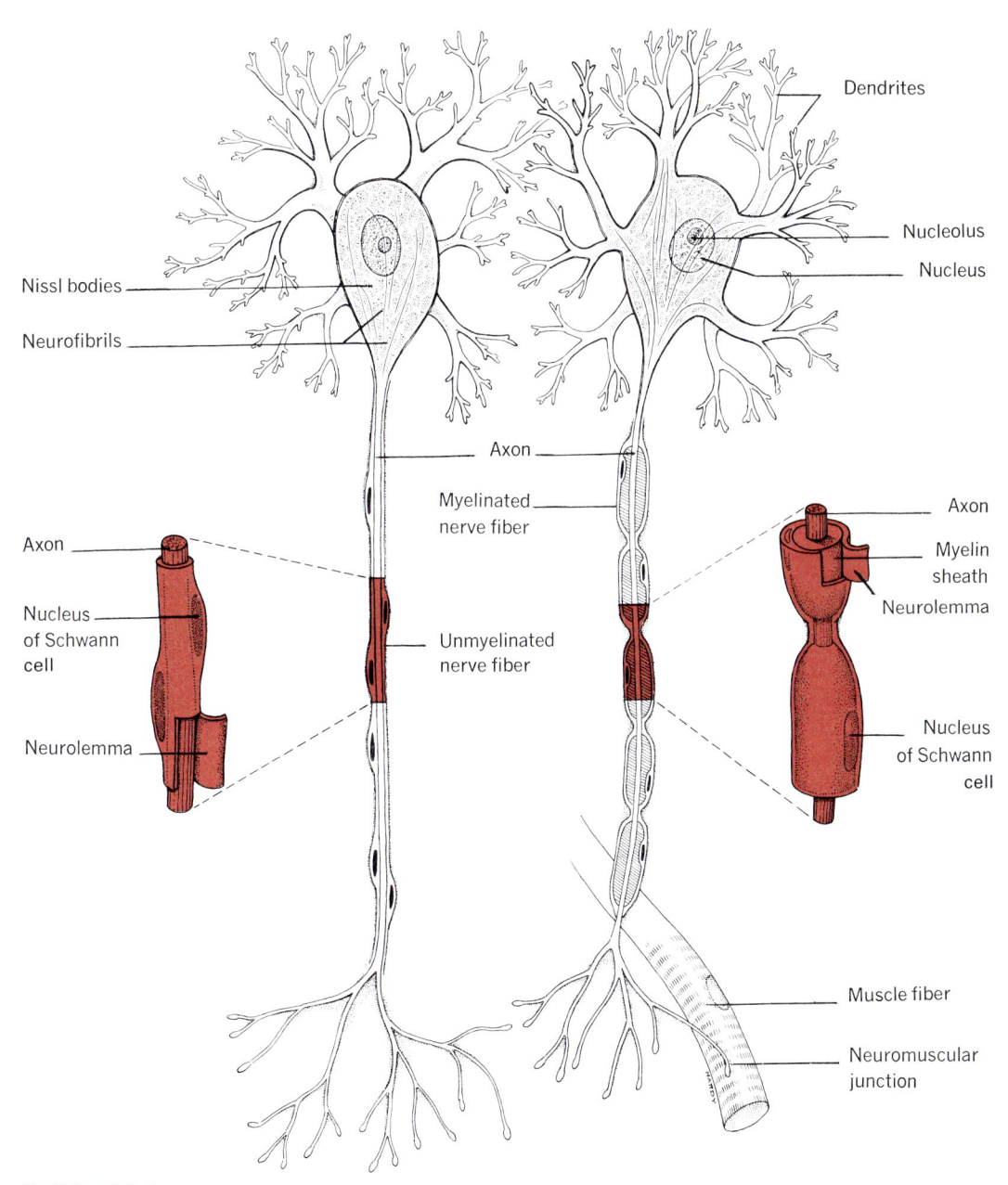

FIGURE 22-1.
Structure of a typical unmyelinated and myelinated neuron. (Rosdahl CB)

Myelin Sheath

Around the axon fiber are two sheaths: the ***myelin sheath*** and the neurilemma (see Fig. 22-1). The myelin sheath is a segmented cover that wraps around some of the axons. It is composed of a fatty tissue (myelin), which serves a protective function for the nerve fiber. The spaces between each segment of the myelinated axon are referred to as ***nodes of Ranvier***. As the impulse conduction moves across the fiber it "jumps" from one node to the next. Thus, the myelin sheath further serves to increase the rate at which impulses can be conducted. Because this sheath is composed of fatty tissue, it takes on a characteristic whitish color. Myelinated fibers are often referred to as *white matter,* whereas unmyelinated fibers are called *gray matter,* since they are grayish in appearance.

Neurilemma

The ***neurilemma,*** also called the sheath of Schwann, is a continuous sheath that covers both the myelinated and unmyelinated nerve fibers. Nerve fibers covered with both the myelin sheath and neurilemma are found in peripheral nerves. Peripheral nerves are those that lie outside the brain and spinal cord. This sheath is thought to function in the regeneration of diseased or injured axons in the periphery. Damage to the nerves in the brain and spinal cord usually is permanent, since they do not possess this outer covering and, therefore, are unable to regenerate.

Three types of neurons exist: afferent (sensory), efferent (motor), and interneurons (connecting neurons). ***Afferent neurons*** send nerve impulses from all parts of the body by means of receptors to the CNS. These impulses or messages are then processed by the brain, which sends a response back to the organs in the periphery (Fig. 22-2). If action is required after a stimulus is received, nerve impulses travel from the brain and spinal cord to organs by ***efferent neurons*** to bring about the proper response. Afferent and efferent neurons are connected by a group of nerve fibers called ***interneurons***. Thus, sensory neurons are stimulated and send stimuli or impulses to the CNS. These impulses then move from the sensory or afferent fiber to the motor or efferent fiber via the connecting interneuron, and the impulse is carried to specific tissues or organs.

Brain

The brain is one of the largest organs in the human body. It weighs about 3 lb in the average adult male. The tissue of the brain is extremely delicate and, thus, easily injured. The brain is provided with two protective coverings: an outer covering, which consists of a bony shell called the cranium, and an inner covering, which is composed of three distinctive membranes referred to as meninges.

The entire skull is composed of 28 bones. It is divided into two parts, the cranium and the face. Eight bones fashion the cranium, and fourteen make up the face. The eight bones of the cranium are held together by immovable joints, called *sutures*. The hard, immovable structure of the cranium helps to protect the brain from injury caused by forces that strike the head; however, forces can be great enough to cause the bones of the skull to fracture and, thus, possibly injure the brain. Injuries of the brain are discussed in Chapter 15.

Meninges

The three inner coverings that protect the brain are known as the ***meninges*** (membranes). Each layer is uniquely different in composition, but all function as protective barriers to the delicate tissue of the brain. The innermost layer is called the ***pia mater***. It derives its name from Latin and literally means, "gentle mother." It is a thin, almost translucent, layer of tissue that is continuous with the brain tissue itself. The pia mater is highly vascular and thus provides a generous blood supply to the brain. The membranous layer that lies above the pia mater is called the arachnoid membrane. ***Arachnoid,*** which means "spider web," is so named because of its weblike composition. Like the pia mater, this layer is extremely thin and delicate. The outermost protective layer within the skull is known as the ***dura mater***. Unlike the other membranes that line the brain tissue, the dura mater is a tough, white fibrous material. It is a thick, nonelastic tissue that encapsulates both the pia mater and arachnoid membranes. Further, the dura mater tightly adheres to the inner lining of the bony cranium, thus forming a tight seal around the delicate tissues of the brain. The meninges are shown in Figure 22-3.

The meningeal layers form a tight bond between themselves, thus prohibiting any actual space for fluid or blood. However, in discussions about the meninges reference is often made to "potential" spaces that lie between the three layers. The term potential is used because in the normal, healthy person no actual space exists. When injury or trauma occurs and the brain is consequently damaged, blood vessels may tear, and blood may leak between the meninges and occupy the potential spaces, making them real or actual spaces. These types of injuries and their effects on human systems are discussed in Chapter 15.

The names given to these potential spaces are determined by their actual location. For example, the space between the dura mater and the *periosteum* (lining) of the skull is referred to as the ***epidural space***. An epidural bleed often causes the dura mater to separate from the cranium. The area between the dura mater and the arachnoid membrane is known as the ***subdural space***. Large amounts of blood from a ruptured vessel can accumulate in this space. This type of injury is known as a subdural hematoma (localized collection of blood in the tissues as

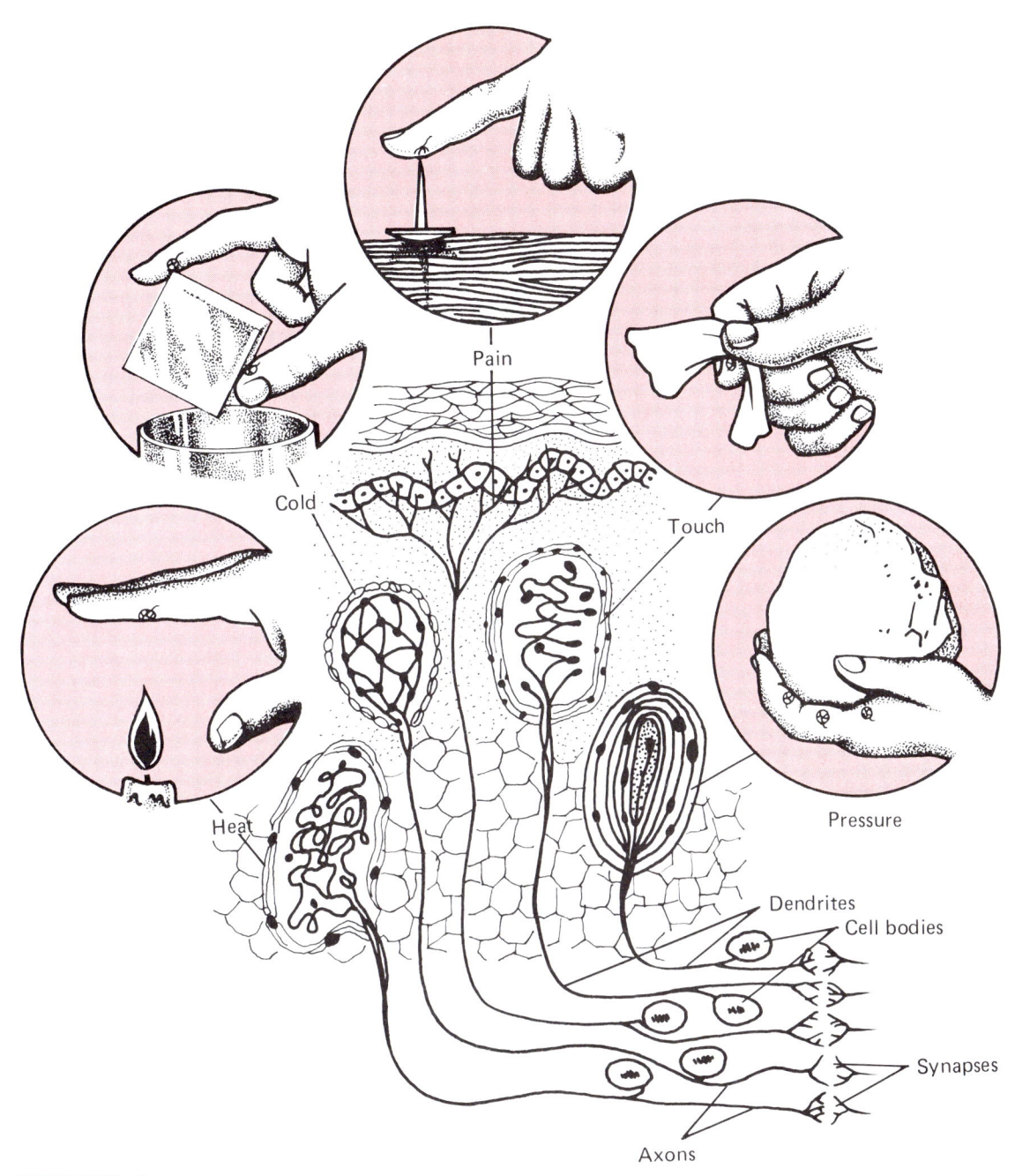

FIGURE 22–2.
Receptors in the skin receive stimuli and bring information to afferent neurons, which carry impulses to the brain or spinal cord. (Rosdahl CB)

a result of injury or a broken blood vessel). The *subarachnoid space* is that area below the arachnoid membrane but above the pia mater. In the healthy person, cerebrospinal fluid is found in this space. *Cerebrospinal fluid* is a thin, watery fluid that bathes the brain and spinal cord. It is often referred to as the "*shock absorber*" for the brain. It further functions as a fortifying substance for the brain because it contains certain nutrients, including glucose. It is important for the paramedic to become familiar with these divisions or spaces when treating the head-injured patient (see Fig. 22-3). A further examination of the pathophysiology and treatment of head injuries is given in Chapter 15.

Blood Supply

Since 25% of the circulating blood volume is directed to the brain, it is highly vascularized. Two vertebral arteries emerge from the subclavian artery and eventually join to become the basilar artery, which feeds the posterior brain. The internal carotid arteries branch into the opthalmic and posterior communicating arteries. These fur-

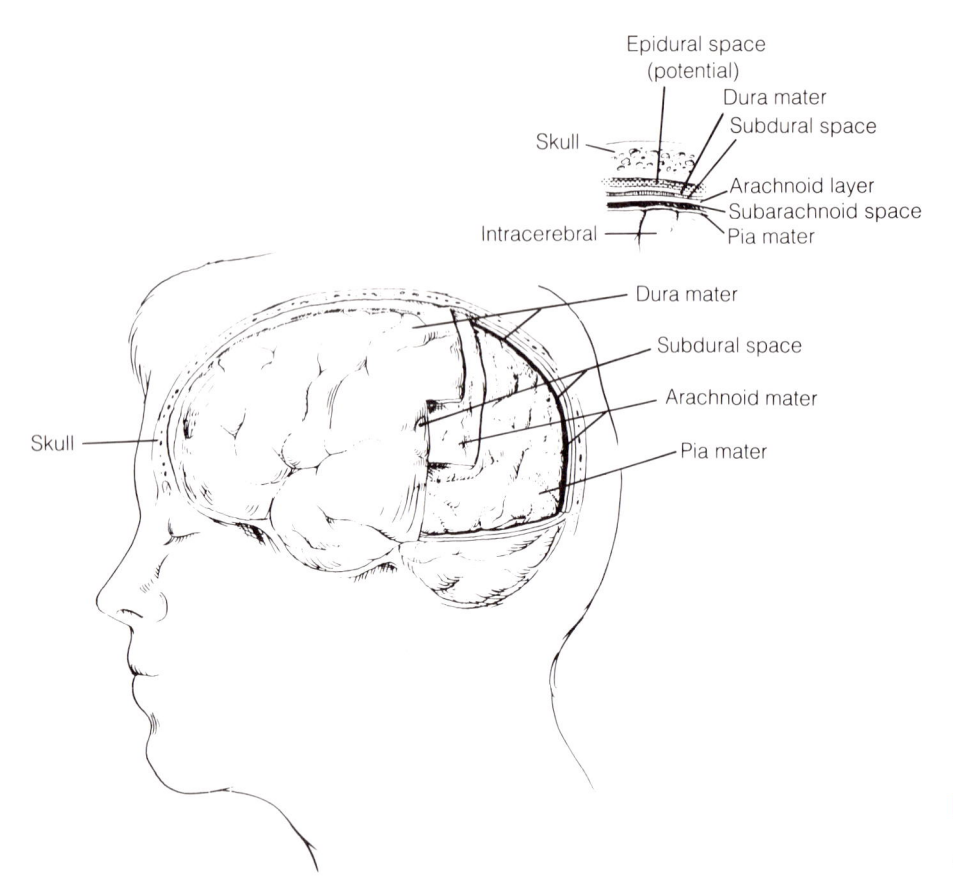

FIGURE 22–3.
Meningeal layers and their potential spaces.

ther divide into the anterior and middle cerebral arteries, which supply the anterior and middle brain. The vertebral and carotid arteries communicate with each other at the base of the brain in an area called the **circle of Willis**. If one of these main vessels becomes occluded, the circle of Willis allows one of the other vessels to supply the blocked area of the brain (Fig. 22-4). Blood leaves the brain primarily through the venous sinuses, which drains into the internal jugular veins. Blood from the face, neck, and scalp drains into the external jugular veins.

Divisions

The brain is only one organ. For the purpose of study and examination, it is separated into six divisions: the cerebrum, diencephalon, cerebellum, the medulla oblongata, pons, and midbrain. The medulla oblongata, pons, and midbrain are collectively thought of as the brain stem. Together they constitute the inferior portion of the brain, which is also the upper aspect of the spinal cord. Figure 22-5 shows the divisions of the brain.

CEREBRUM. The **cerebrum** is the largest division of the brain. It is also the most superiorly located. The cerebrum is further divided into right and left symmetrical halves, called hemispheres. The right hemisphere coordinates the left half of the body, and the left hemisphere coordinates the right half of the body. The surface of the cerebrum, which resembles a continuous series of sausagelike convolutions, is called the **cerebral cortex**. The cerebral cortex is a thin layer composed of gray matter (unmyelinated fibers). The cerebral cortex, though extremely thin, has six layers. Each one is composed of millions of neurons and nerve fibers. Thus, an immense amount of potential information can be processed by the human brain because of this structure. White matter (myelinated fibers) can be found deeper within the cerebrum, underneath the layers of the cerebral cortex. The cerebrum controls sensory and motor functions and also houses the centers for memory, speech, emotions, and thought processes (Fig. 22-6).

DIENCEPHALON. Located just inferior to the cerebrum is a division of the brain known as the **diencephalon**. The two structures that primarily form the diencephalon are the thalamus and the hypothalamus. Some researchers support the theory that the cerebral cortex, during the course of evolutionary development, emanated as an outgrowth of the thalamus. This idea is supported structurally because the cerebral cortex is closely connected to corresponding areas of the thalamus. In function, many nerve impulses from the spinal cord, brain stem, and even certain areas of the brain are conducted into the thalamus before they reach the cerebrum. Axons within the thalamus conduct these impulses to virtually all areas of the

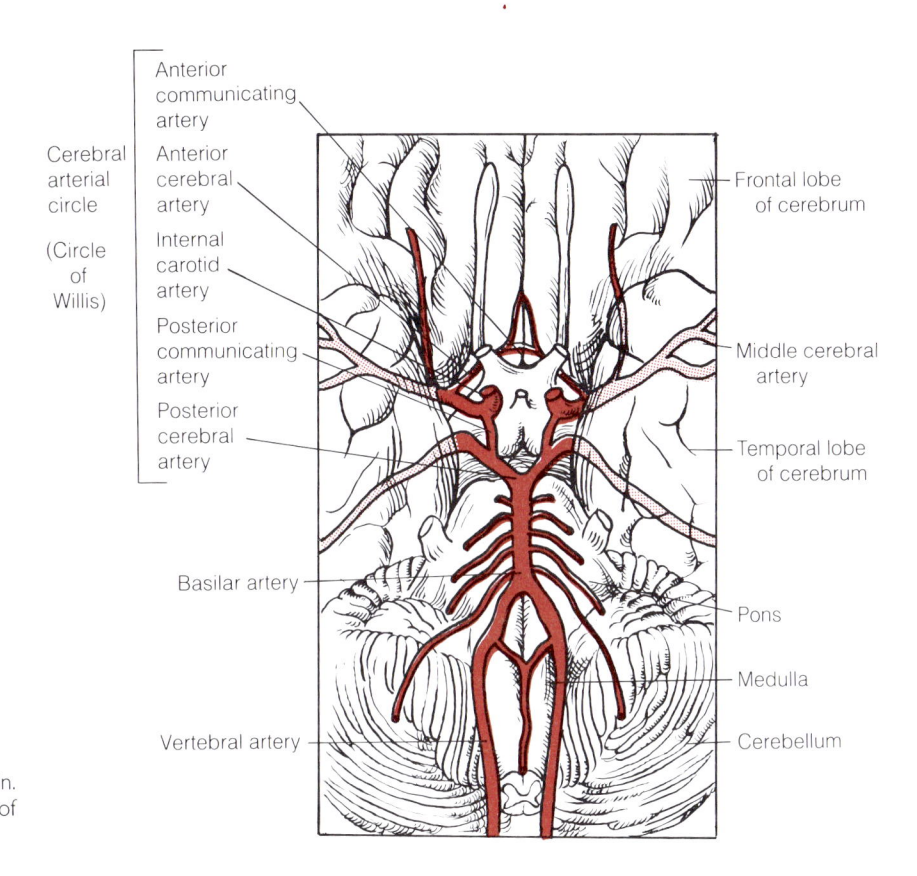

FIGURE 22-4.
Principal arteries of the base of the brain. Note the arteries that make up the circle of Willis.

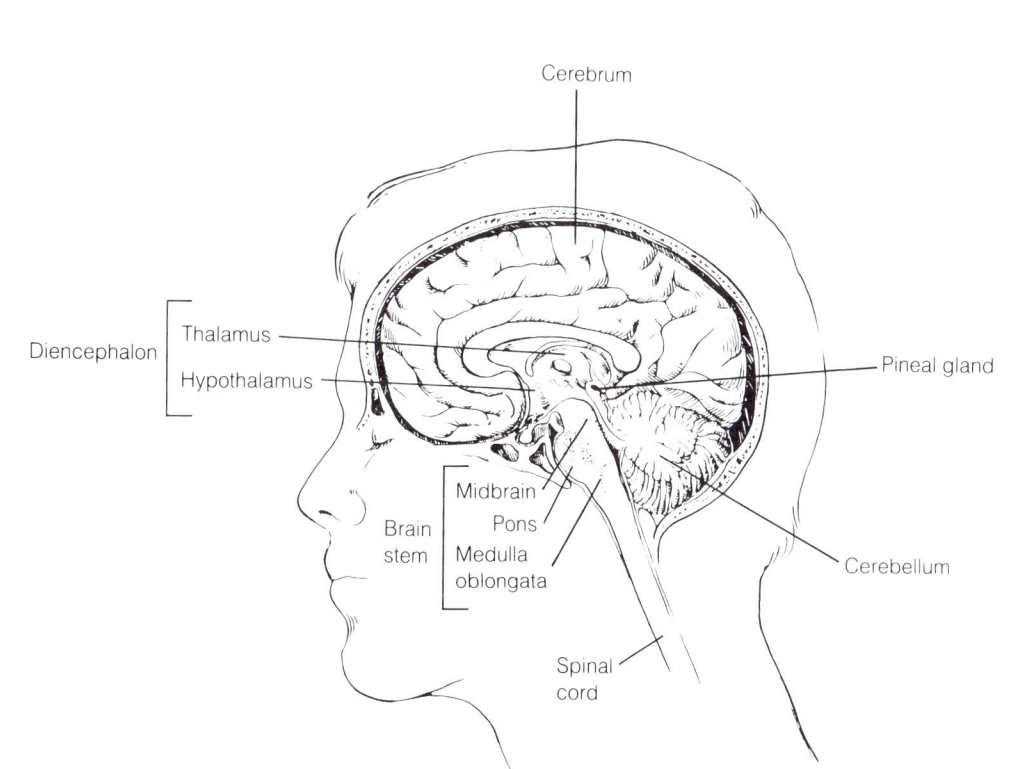

FIGURE 22-5.
Divisions of the brain.

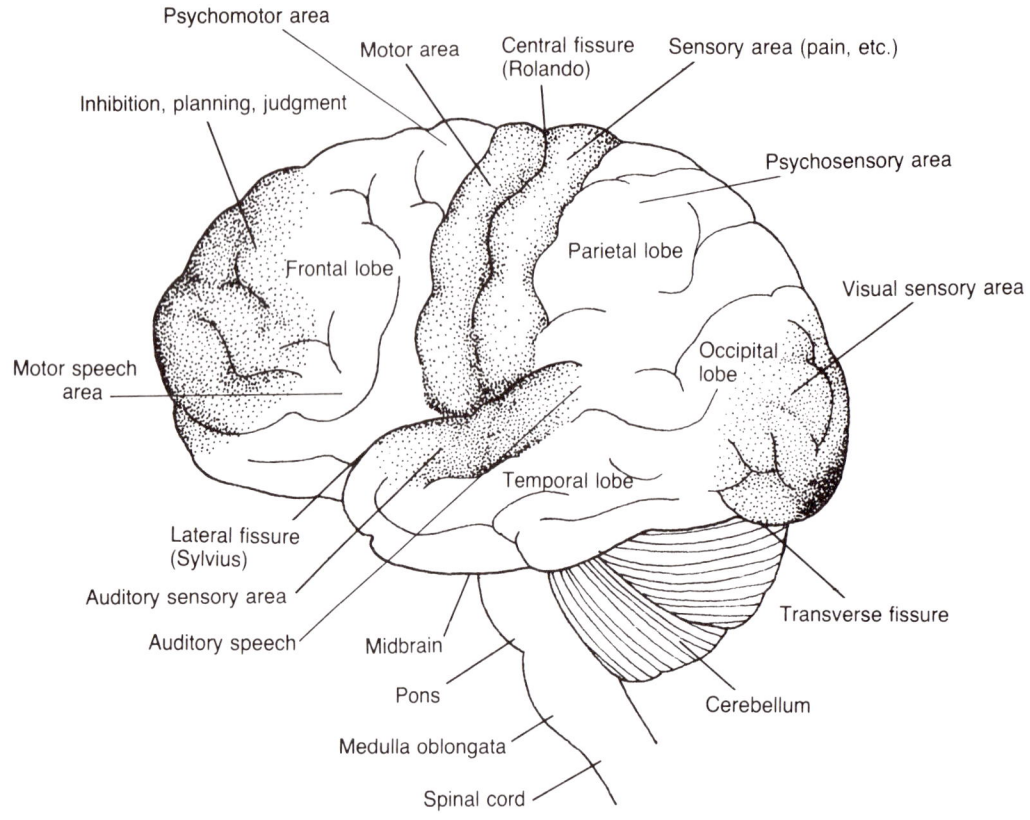

FIGURE 22–6.
Lobes, fissures, and major functional areas of the cerebrum. (Rosdahl CB)

cerebral cortex. Hence, it acts as a "relay station" for sensory impulses en route to the cerebral cortex.

The **thalamus** has several functions in addition to relaying various sensory impulses to the cerebrum. On reaching the thalamus, receptors recognize crude, less critical sensations of pain, temperature, and touch. The thalamus also plays a role, to some extent, in the brain's perception of pleasantness and unpleasantness and arousal or alertness; it also helps to facilitate complex reflex movements.

The **hypothalamus,** the other predominant division of the diencephalon, is a small structure. Though it weighs only 7 g, its performance is vital for human survival and enjoyment of life. Similar to the thalamus, the hypothalamus has several specific functions. For example, it adjoins the psyche (mind) to the body (also referred to as the soma). It serves as a bridge between two separate communication systems, the nervous system and the endocrine system. Certain areas of the hypothalamus regulate and coordinate autonomic activities, such as changes in heart rate and blood pressure; these functions are discussed in further detail later in this chapter. By secreting specific chemicals into the blood, it can influence appetite and food intake, sleep and arousal states, water and other chemical balances, and the development of mating and certain sex cell characteristics. The hypothalamus also plays a crucial role in the mechanism that maintains normal body temperature. The paramedic may encounter a patient with a marked elevation in body temperature. Frequently, this condition is secondary to injuries or other abnormalities of the hypothalamus.

CEREBELLUM. After the cerebrum, the next largest section of the brain is the **cerebellum** (little brain). It is located below the posterior aspect of the cerebrum. The cerebrum and the cerebellum both share common anatomical and physiologic attributes. For example, both are composed of gray matter in the outer surfaces and white matter in the inner tissue layers. Another common characteristic is the "groovelike" pattern on their outer surfaces. However, the grooves or convolutions of the cerebellum are thinner and less pronounced than those of the cerebrum. Like the cerebrum, the cerebellum also has right and left hemispheres.

The cerebellum functions in the synergistic (cooperative) control of skeletal muscle movements. That is, it governs coordinated movement. Normal muscular movement involves groups of muscles that function as a unit. As the primary muscles contract, other groups of muscles relax, thus producing certain types of movement. In a way, the system is one of checks and balances. This coordinated group action makes possible movements that are smooth, steady, and precise, according to the force and extent of movement required for certain conditions. The cerebellum also functions to help control posture and to maintain equilibrium.

BRAIN STEM. The **brain stem** is a compilation of the ***medulla oblongata, pons,*** and ***midbrain***. The pons is located between the medulla oblongata and midbrain. The medulla forms the inferior aspect of the brain stem, and the midbrain the superior aspect. The brain stem is inferior to the cerebrum and anterior to the cerebellum. Thus, it forms both the middle and lower aspects of the brain.

The functional activity of the brain stem is associated closely with that of the spinal cord. It is not only the lower portion of the brain but also the superior aspect of the spinal cord. It is responsible for sensory, motor, and reflex functions. The different divisions of the brain stem house certain special nerve centers. For example, the pons accommodates the pneumotaxic centers, which help regulate respiratory rhythms. The midbrain contains many reflex centers that coordinate pupillary reflexes and eye movements. The medulla oblongata, considered by many to be the most vital part of the brain, contains important reflex centers, such as the cardiac, vasomotor, and respiratory centers. These centers are often called the "vital centers" because their proper functioning is essential for survival. Injury or disease that directly affects the functioning of these centers is often fatal. Therefore, rapid and thorough patient assessment and early initiation of aggressive treatment is essential, especially with head-injured patients.

Spinal Cord

The **spinal cord** functions in two ways. First, it acts as a two-way path for conducting impulses to and from the brain. Some reflexes, however, do not require the brain's input. Thus, the second function of the spinal cord is that of a reflex center. Reflexes are natural protective measures for the body. For instance, one does not have to literally think about moving a hand away after placing it on a hot surface, but rather, immediately pulls it away in a jerking type of motion. This reflex action is mediated by the spinal cord.

The spinal cord is approximately 18 inches in length. It extends from the brain stem, through the foramen magnum (hole at the base of the skull through which the cord passes), to a level between the first and second lumbar vertebrae. It is 10 mm in diameter and is contained in a cavity called the spinal canal. This canal is approximately 15 mm in diameter. As with the brain itself, the cord is protected by the three meninges: dura mater, arachnoid membrane, and the pia mater. Also, cerebrospinal fluid helps to protect the cord from injury. Because the neurons in the spinal cord cannot be regenerated, much like the neurons in the brain, a further protective structure is provided.

Strong, bony coverings called **vertebrae** protect the spinal cord in the same fashion that the skull protects the brain. Each vertebra includes several components. The vertebral body is the solid, anterior portion. Projecting posteriorly from the body are two pedicles that unite with two *laminae* (thin layers of bone). The two laminae fuse at the midline. The opening created by the pedicles and laminae allows the spinal cord to travel through the vertebrae. At the point where the laminae join, the spinous process projects posteriorly and inferiorly. The transverse process extends laterally from the junction of each pedicle and lamina. Muscles and ligaments attach to these processes, which allow for movement of the spine. See Chapter 18 for illustrations of the spinal vertebrae.

The spinal column is divided into five sections. The cervical vertebrae (***cervical spine***) include the top seven bones. Eight of the thirty-one spinal nerve roots originate in this section of the spinal column. Below the cervical vertebrae are twelve thoracic vertebrae (***thoracic spine***) and the corresponding twelve nerve roots. The lumbar vertebrae (***lumbar spine***) are the next five bones of the spinal column. They also have five corresponding nerve roots. The lower portion of the cervical spine and the upper portion of the lumbar vertebrae are the most commonly damaged vertebrae in the trauma patient. After the lumbar region of the column is the sacrum (***sacral spine***). The sacrum is composed of four to five bones fused together and five nerve roots. Finally, the ***coccyx*** (tail bone) possesses three to four fused bones and one nerve root. See Chapter 18 for illustrations of the spinal column.

Peripheral Nervous System

The CNS is composed of the brain and spinal cord. All other nervous system organs, namely, the cranial nerves, spinal nerves, autonomic nerves, and ganglia make up the peripheral nervous system. The primary function of the peripheral nervous system is to connect various parts of the body to the CNS.

The twelve pair of nerves that arise from the undersurface of the brain are called ***cranial nerves*** (Fig. 22-7). They are responsible for the functioning of the facial organs and head. Each nerve pair is numbered and assigned a name. For the names and specific functions of each pair of the cranial nerves, refer to Table 22-1. Just as the head and face are innervated by the cranial nerves, the remainder of the body is innervated by the peripheral nervous system, which originates from the spinal nerve roots located in the spinal canal.

Each of the 31 spinal nerve roots yields a pair of ***spinal nerves***. The dorsal (posterior) nerve contains afferent fibers and the ventral (anterior) nerve contains efferent fibers. These spinal nerves extend branches to the skin

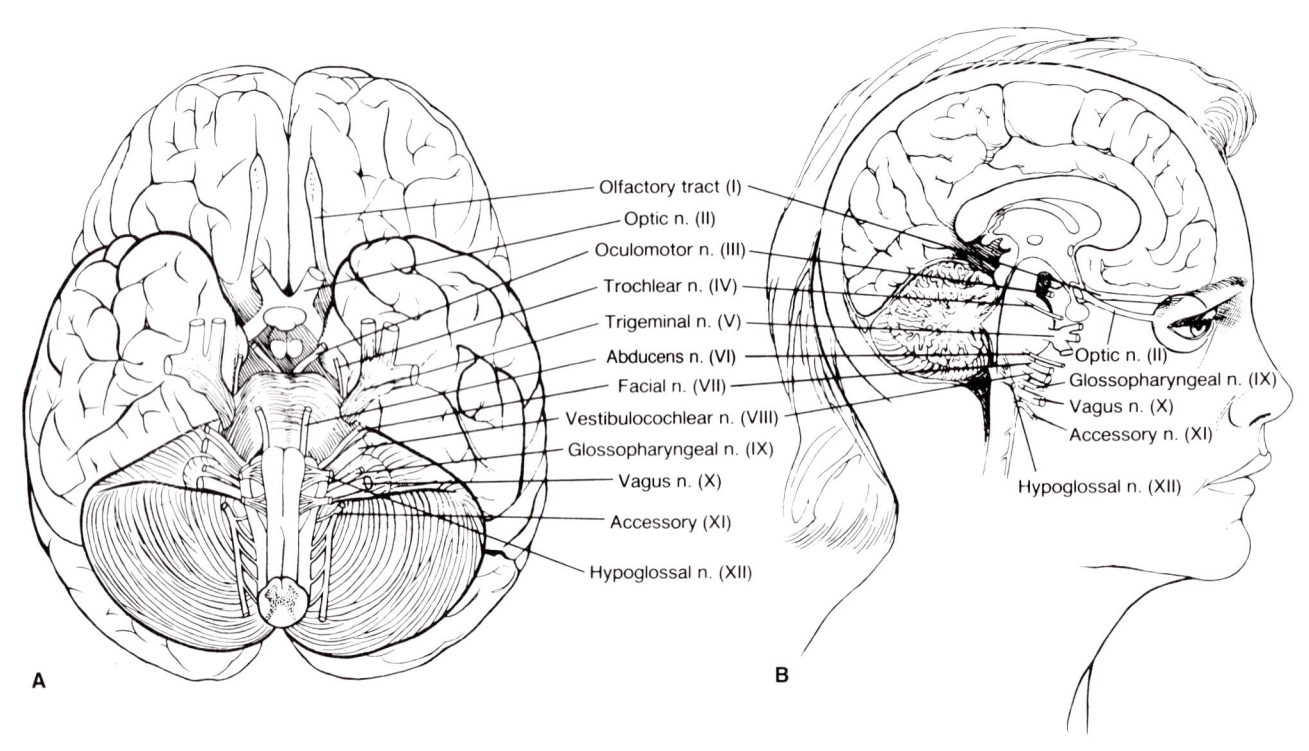

FIGURE 22-7.
The cranial nerves. (**A**) Inferior view of the brain shows the cranial nerves. (**B**) Lateral view of the brain shows a schematized version of the cranial nerves. (Brunner LS, Suddarth DS)

TABLE 22-1.
THE CRANIAL NERVES AND THEIR FUNCTIONS

Number	Name	Functions	Distribution
I	Olfactory	Smell	Nasal mucous membrane
II	Optic	Vision	Retina
III	Oculomotor	Eye movements	Most ocular muscles
IV	Trochlear (smallest cranial nerves)	Voluntary eye movements	Superior oblique muscle of eye
V	Trigeminal (largest cranial nerves)	Sensations of head and face; movement of mandible	Skin of face; tongue; teeth; muscles of mastication
	Ophthalmic branch	Sensations from front of head and face, eye sockets, and upper nose	
	Maxillary branch	Sensations from nose, mouth, and upper jaw, cheek, and upper lip	
	Mandibular branch	Sensations of tongue, lower teeth, chin	
VI	Abducent	Eye movements	Lateral rectus muscle of eye
VII	Facial	Taste; facial expressions	Muscles of expression
VIII	Vestibulocochlear (acoustic)	Hearing and balance	Internal auditory meatus
	Cochlear division	Conducts impulses related to hearing	
	Vestibular division	Conducts impulses related to equilibrium (balance)	
IX	Glossopharyngeal	Controls swallowing; gives information on pressure and oxygen tension of blood	Pharynx, posterior third of tongue, parotid
X	Vagus ("wanderer") (Only cranial nerve not restricted to head and neck)	Somatic motor function; parasympathetic functions; speech	Pharynx, larynx, heart, lungs, esophagus, stomach, abdominal viscera
XI	Accessory	Rotation of head; raising of shoulder	Arising from medulla and spinal cord
XII	Hypoglossal	Movement of tongue	Intrinsic muscle of tongue

(Rosdahl CB)

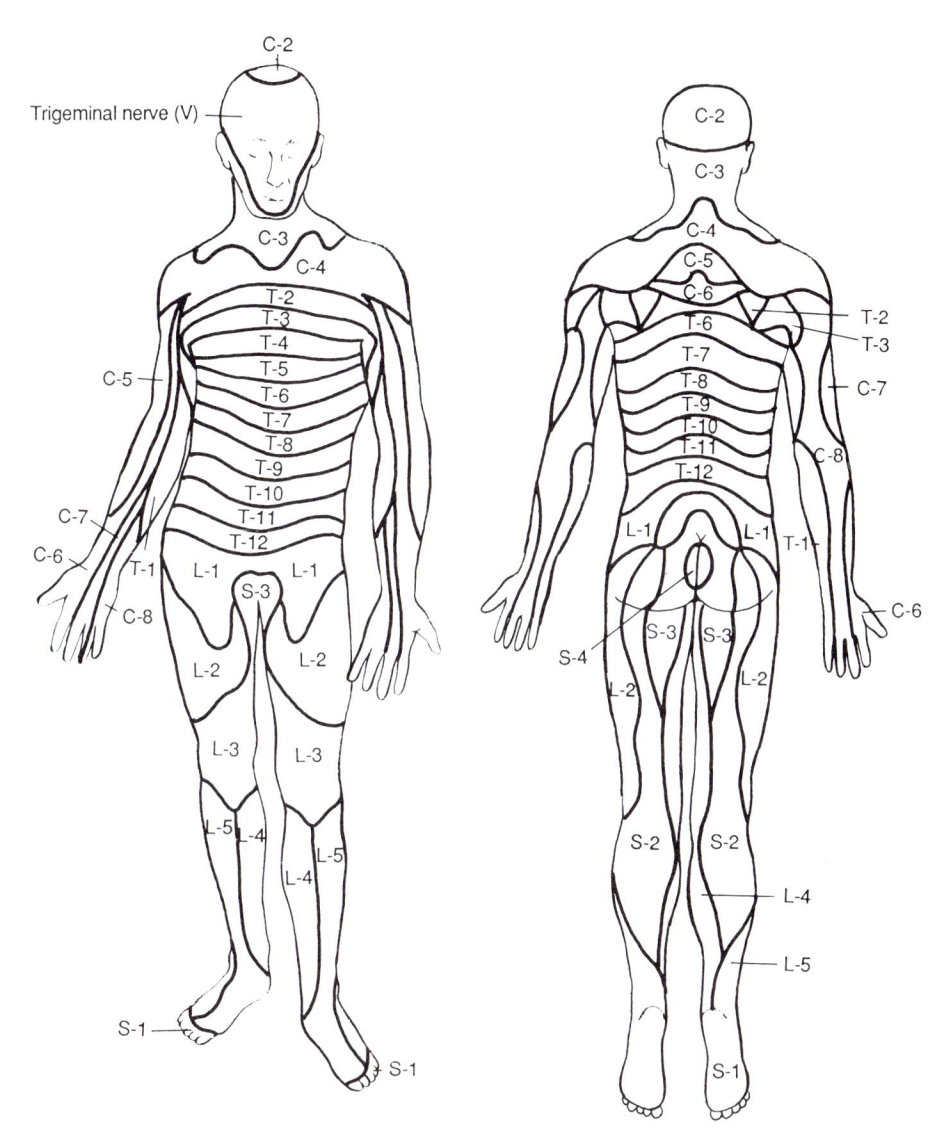

FIGURE 22–8.
Distribution of spinal nerves to dermatomes, showing an anterior and posterior view. C, indicates cervical segments; T, thoracic segments; L, lumbar segments; S, sacral segments.

so that they can transmit signals of pain, temperature, and touch to the spinal cord. The "*zones*" created by the 31 pairs of spinal nerves around the body are called **dermatomes**. Through the use of a dermatome chart (Fig. 22-8), the level at which neural dysfunction begins can be determined and assessed for altered or decreased sensation. The shoulder girdle, for example, is controlled by nerves that emanate from C-5, C-6, and C-7. Loss of sensation that begins at the nipple line indicates damage at T-4, while loss of sensation at the umbilicus level results from damage at T-10. Hip extension is controlled by L-5, S-1, and S-2. In general, the closer the damage is to the brain stem, the more severe the injury and the resulting incapacity.

The peripheral nervous system can be further divided into the somatic and the visceral systems. The latter is most commonly referred to as the autonomic nervous system. The somatic nervous system innervates skeletal muscle tissue, whereas the autonomic nervous system innervates all smooth muscle, cardiac muscle, and glandular tissue. The somatic nervous system is primarily responsible for conscious, voluntary movement. A person can control movement of the arms and legs. Since this system is made up of both sensory nerves, which carry nerve impulses to the CNS, and motor nerves, which carry the impulses from the CNS back to the skeletal organs, it has the capacity to function not only in movement but also in the detection of various sensations. Thus, the somatic system sends information about pain, temperature, touch, and pressure to the brain, and one can voluntarily act on these sensory perceptions.

Many activities in the body take place by involuntary movement, over which a person has no control. An example of this type of movement is peristalsis, the "wave-like" motion of the intestinal walls, which propels food through the intestinal tract. Involuntary movement is under the control of the autonomic nervous system, which is explained in the next section.

Autonomic Nervous System

The *autonomic nervous system* consists specifically of motor nerve fibers. It is responsible for carrying nerve impulses from the brain and spinal cord to smooth muscle throughout the body, including the heart and various glands. This system helps regulate many activities, including arterial blood pressure, gastrointestinal motility and secretion, urinary bladder emptying, sweating, body temperature, and heart rate.

The paramedic needs to be familiar with this division of the nervous system not only because of its vital functioning but, also, because many signs and symptoms detected in patients in the field are, in essence, the effects of the autonomic nervous system. Furthermore, as was explained in Chapter 12, many of the drugs used in prehospital advanced life support have a profound influence on the autonomic nervous system. Therefore, a sound understanding of the autonomic nervous system is paramount to the assessment and treatment of patients in the prehospital setting.

The autonomic nervous system is controlled by autonomic "centers." These centers are actually groups of neurons located in the CNS, specifically in the hypothalamus, brain stem, and spinal cord. They function to control autonomic performance. Stimulation of the hypothalamus regulates many of the autonomic features through release of various hormones. The autonomic nervous system is composed of efferent neurons that conduct nerve impulses from the CNS to visceral effectors. Visceral effectors are classified in terms of tissues and organs. The types of tissues affected are smooth muscle, cardiac muscle, and glandular tissue. In the organs, visceral effectors include the heart, blood vessels, iris, ciliary muscles, hair muscles, many of the organs located in the thoracic and abdominal areas, and numerous glands throughout the body.

The conduction pathway in the autonomic nervous system, from the CNS to visceral effectors, is composed of two successive neurons: preganglionic neurons and postganglionic neurons (Fig. 22-9). The term ganglia denotes groups of nerve cell bodies located outside the CNS. **Preganglionic neurons** are groups of neurons that conduct impulses from the CNS to autonomic ganglia. After the nerve impulses reach the ganglia, **postganglionic neurons** conduct the impulses to the visceral effectors (organs). Points of contact between neurons are called **synapses**. The axon of one neuron is closely associated with the next successive neuron's dendrites. Nerve impulses move from the axon of one neuron to the dendrites of another neuron.

The autonomic nervous system can be further divided into the sympathetic and parasympathetic divisions. Stimulation from these two divisions has opposing effects

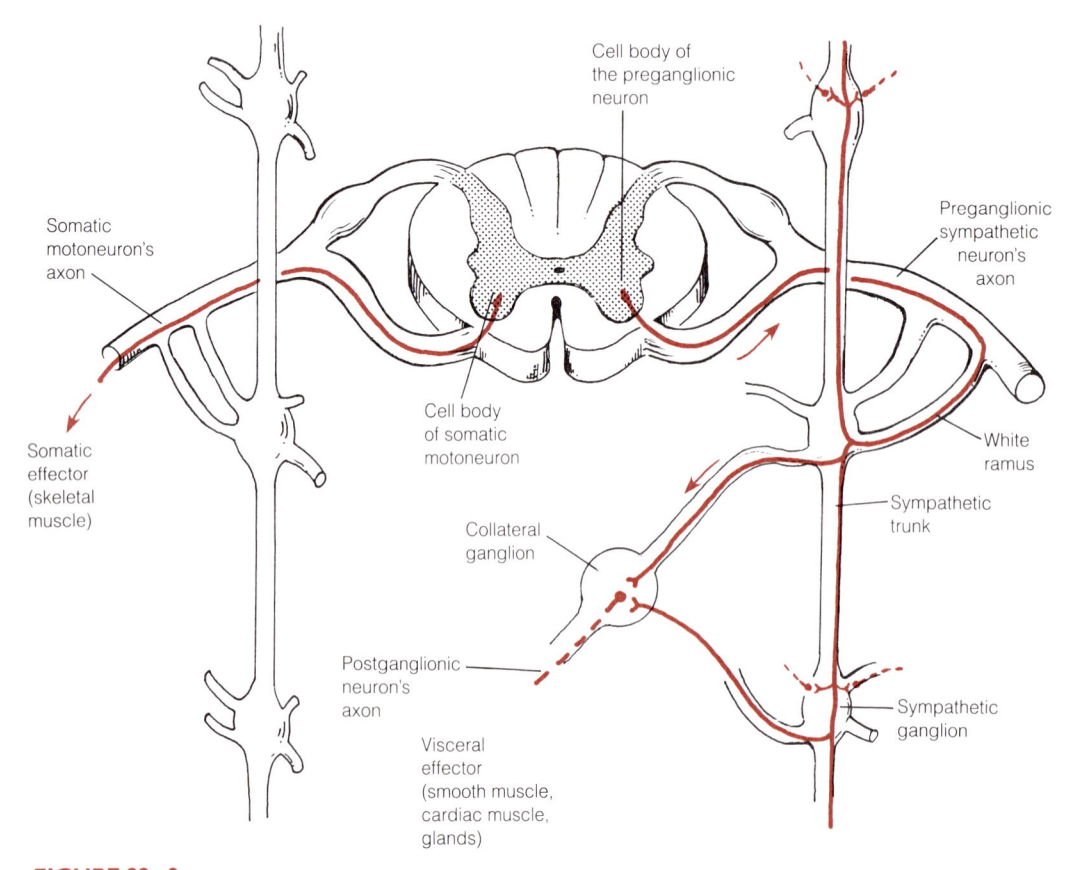

FIGURE 22-9.
The difference is shown between the sympathetic pathway from the spinal cord to visceral effectors and the pathway from the cord to somatic effectors.

on the organs that they supply. For instance, the effect of the sympathetic division on the heart is an increase in rate, whereas that of the parasympathetic division is a decrease in the heart rate. Most of the tissue and organs affected by the autonomic nervous system are innervated by both sympathetic and parasympathetic fibers. In addition, both the sympathetic and parasympathetic divisions continuously conduct impulses to the individual organs. Based on this concept, using the example above, a relatively constant heart rate is maintained.

SYMPATHETIC DIVISION. Ganglia of the **sympathetic division** are located bilaterally on the anterior surface of the spinal column. They are connected by short fibers that run through them, casting the appearance of two chains extending down the spinal column. The sympathetic ganglia are often referred to as the "sympathetic chain ganglia." This chain is composed of approximately 22 ganglia. It extends from the level of the second cervical vertebra (C-2) to the coccyx.

Preganglionic neurons of the sympathetic division leave the spinal column at the level of the first thoracic (T-1) and the second lumbar (L-2) spinal nerves. They have their cell bodies in the anterior roots of T-1 and L-2. For this reason, the sympathetic division is also known as the thoracolumbar division.

The effects or actions of the sympathetic division are systemic, that is, they affect the entire body. In the healthy person, under normal conditions, the sympathetic division functions to maintain the regular balance and functioning of autonomic organs and tissues. As stated above, this function is accomplished by antagonizing the effects exerted on the specific organs by the parasympathetic division. In so doing, homeostatic levels are maintained.

The sympathetic division also performs another role. It functions as the body's "emergency" system, often referred to as the ***fight or flight syndrome***. This reaction is often induced by various degrees of stress. The sympathetic division prepares the body for action by predominating impulse conduction to the visceral organs. Thus, the organs manifest more sympathetic than parasympathetic effects. Examples of sympathetic effects include an increase in heart rate, increase in myocardial contractility, blood vessel dilation in skeletal muscles (vasodilation), blood vessel constriction in smooth muscle (vasoconstriction), bronchial dilation, pupillary dilation, stimulation of sweat glands, and an increase in blood glucose levels. A summary of the effects of sympathetic stimulation on organs is shown in Chapter 12. People are able to use the additional energy made available from sympathetic stimulation to engage in intense physical and mental activities.

These effects are produced by the release of epinephrine from the adrenal glands and norepinephrine from sympathetic nerve endings during sympathetic division stimulation. As was described in Chapter 12, **norepinephrine** is a chemical neurotransmitter for the sympathetic division. The electrical impulse travels along conduction pathways across the synapses, between axons and dendrites (nerve fibers). Neurotransmitters, such as **acetylcholine**, facilitate movement of electrical impulses across synaptic junctions. They are stored in the presynaptic neurons, the neurons located before the synapse or junction. Specifically, they are stored in the terminal end of the axon of the presynaptic neuron, known as synaptic knobs.

Norepinephrine is released from the postganglionic neurons of the sympathetic division. Hence, it is released at the synapse between the axon and the organ that is affected. An aggregate of microscopic sacs, called vesicles, make up synaptic knobs. In the sympathetic division, each vesicle contains approximately 10,000 molecules of norepinephrine. If an intense or stressful situation confronts a person, massive amounts of norepinephrine can be released from the synaptic knobs of postganglionic neurons. The impact on the body from the release of norepinephrine into the system lasts only a short period of time. Therefore, **epinephrine**, also known as adrenaline, is released from the adrenal glands. Epinephrine functions to prolong the sympathetic effects of norepinephrine.

PARASYMPATHETIC DIVISION. As stated above, organs of the autonomic nervous system continuously receive nerve impulses from both the sympathetic and parasympathetic divisions. The normal function of these organs is determined by the summation of the two opposing factors on the organs. Under most conditions, the ***parasympathetic division*** predominates the viscera. It manifests vegetativelike effects on organs in the body.

Cell bodies of the parasympathetic preganglionic neurons are located in the brain stem and in the sacral aspect of the spinal cord. Therefore, the parasympathetic division is often referred to as the craniosacral division. As noted above, sympathetic ganglia are located near the spinal column. Parasympathetic ganglia, on the other hand, are located close to the visceral effectors. Usually, they form a synapse with a single effector. Therefore, the parasympathetic division manifests local effects, as opposed to the systemic actions seen with the sympathetic division.

Acetylcholine, the primary neurotransmitter for the parasympathetic division, is released from the synaptic knobs of preganglionic sympathetic and parasympathetic neurons and from postganglionic parasympathetic neurons (see Chapter 12). As noted above, norepinephrine is the primary neurotransmitter for the sympathetic division, and it is specifically released from postganglionic sympathetic neurons.

An integral component of the parasympathetic division is the vagus nerve. The vagus nerve (10th cranial nerve) is responsible for about 75% of the actions of parasympathetic stimulation. It controls certain actions of the heart, stomach, and gastrointestinal tract. Stimulation of the vagus nerve produces a characteristic slowing of heart rate.

The release of acetylcholine on visceral effectors, enhanced by vagus stimulation, produces other effects. Digestive glands are stimulated to release enzymatic juices, such as saliva, and hormones, such as insulin, which enhance digestion and absorption of food substances. Stimulation of parasympathetic fibers also increases peristalsis. This action, in turn, promotes not only the absorption and use of foods but also the elimination of waste products from the body.

ASSESSMENT OF NERVOUS SYSTEM EMERGENCIES

Primary Survey

Patient assessment always begins with the primary survey. A rapid, thorough performance of this survey yields evidence of immediate, life-threatening problems. In the primary survey of the neurologic patient, the patient's responsiveness and respiratory status are the most serious concerns. Subtle changes in the patient's mental status should alert the paramedic to potential unseen complications that result from disease or injury. As was already noted, damage to the CNS often results in a decline in overall respiratory performance. This condition, in turn, is followed by poor gas exchange, hypoxia, and, ultimately, death.

In the unconscious patient, the paramedic should always assume cervical spine injury and coordinate care of the patient accordingly. To open the unconscious person's airway, the jaw-thrust maneuver should be used rather than hyperextending the neck with the head-tilt/chin-lift technique. Oropharyngeal and nasopharyngeal airways work well as an initial stabilization of the unconscious patient's airway. Unconscious people cannot protect their airways from blood or vomitus.

Many complications can arise from head injuries and diseases that affect the respiratory control centers in the brain. Increases in intracranial pressure often lead to respiratory arrest. Since intracranial pressure cannot be measured in the field, the paramedic needs to learn the signs and symptoms associated with it, suspect it, and begin treatment in the early stages. Furthermore, the paramedic should anticipate vomiting in these patients and be ready to suction aggressively in an attempt to prevent aspiration of gastric contents.

Secondary Survey

History

As with any medical or traumatic crisis faced by the paramedic, obtaining an accurate and thorough history may be the deciding factor in providing appropriate prehospital and follow-up care. This history is especially important in nervous system disorders, because patients may be confused or paralyzed, and the information obtained at their home or from bystanders may not be available at the hospital.

When obtaining the history, the paramedic should ascertain if the problem is medical or trauma related. If trauma is suspected, the paramedic must take into consideration the mechanisms of injury and the kinematics involved. Incorporating these aspects into the overall assessment and history of the patient offers clues to underlying complications. Also, mental status needs to be critically evaluated in the trauma patient. The paramedic should discern if the patient had any loss of consciousness before the paramedic's arrival on the scene. If the patient did lose consciousness, it is important to determine if this loss preceded the traumatic event or if it was caused by the event. This information needs to be documented accurately and communicated to the emergency physician. If a change in the level of consciousness is noticed at any time during the patient's prehospital care, the base (hospital) physician should be immediately notified.

As with any other patient, the paramedic needs to determine the patient's chief complaint. The chief complaint is what the patient states is wrong rather than what the paramedic on the scene perceives the problem to be. This information should be obtained soon after making contact with the patient. The paramedic should encourage the patient to elaborate on this problem.

Any associated signs and symptoms should be evaluated carefully. This process is an integral part of putting the puzzle together. Noting characteristic signs and symptoms helps to clarify the whole picture and, thus, helps to determine the underlying problem. If neurologic damage is suspected, it is especially important to note any loss of sensation or paresthesia.

Finally, both the immediate history of the situation and the medical history should be taken into account. Factors such as drug or alcohol abuse, hypertension, diabetes, or past neck or spine injuries can complicate the presenting problem, especially in the seriously injured patient.

In the nontraumatic patient who presents with neurologic difficulties, the paramedic should obtain a detailed, chronological account of the problem. Again, this includes understanding the chief complaint, details of the present illness, and any underlying medical problems. For example, if the patient complains of "dizziness and passing out," the paramedic needs to ascertain the circumstances that accompanied onset of the experience, including the patient's position (standing, sitting, or lying down) and when they "passed out" (syncope). In addition, it should be noted if the patient has been experiencing peculiar headaches, and the duration and intensity of the pain should be noted. It should be determined if the patient has experienced this problem previously, if the present problem is worse than before, and if anything makes the problem better or worse.

Important clues are often gained by taking into account the immediate environment. This survey includes the atmosphere of the room or home, the presenting circumstances or situations, such as extremely stressful or hostile feelings being exhibited, and the presence of medications, medic alert tags, and bottles of alcohol or drug paraphernalia.

A variety of neurologic complications can affect patients. Some of them are obvious, such as loss of sensation in an extremity, and others are subtle. Patients may present with what appears to be a normal mental status, and then, gradually, their condition deteriorates; others experience changes in level of consciousness immediately. The paramedic should convey, as with any emergency, a professional attitude in dealing with neurologic patients. Time should be devoted to a thorough investigation of the presenting complaint, which should be supplemented with an accurate, detailed account of the event, past medical problems, and any outstanding aspects noted during the run, whether during transport or on the scene. This information helps both prehospital and in-hospital care providers determine treatment.

Vital Signs

Vital signs should be assessed frequently in all patients, but especially patients suspected of having neurologic complications. It is important that the paramedic recognize any changes in the vital signs. They provide a baseline evaluation of the patient's present condition and help indicate if this condition is improving or deteriorating.

The respiratory system is often affected by neurologic impediments. Respiratory patterns may be normal or may fall under one of several variations, such as Cheyne-Stokes respiration, central neurogenic hyperventilation, ataxic breathing, or apneustic breathing. These abnormal breathing patterns are described in Chapter 19. Furthermore, in providing care for these patients, the paramedic should observe for signs of poor intercostal muscle effort and diaphragmatic breathing.

In addition to causing respiratory fluctuations, intracranial pressure changes may also affect the patient's heart rate, blood pressure, and body temperature. Many factors can lead to an increase in intracranial pressure. In head-injured patients, since the bony cranium tightly encases the brain, no room is available to accept the blood and fluid that may leak from the vasculature into the bony cavity. This state results in an elevation of the pressure inside the cranium. Classically, in the early stages of increasing intracranial pressure, the heart rate slows and the blood pressure and temperature rise. This phenomenon is called **Cushing's reflex**. As pressure increases in the cranial vault, blood flow to the brain decreases.

As intracranial pressure continues to rise, pressure is often put on the third cranial nerve, which is responsible for pupillary dilation. Thus, the classic "blown pupil" often is seen. In the later stages of increasing intracranial pressure, the heart rate begins to increase and the blood pressure drops. Hypotension, therefore, is a late sign in head-injured patients, and death is most often imminent. It is common to note cardiac arrhythmias during this time. Management should be aimed at reducing the intracranial pressure by aggressive hyperventilation rather than treating the arrhythmias.

Neurologic Evaluation

The level of consciousness is one of the most reliable diagnostic signs in the evaluation of neurologic status. The mnemonic device **AVPU** provides a rapid and convenient way to determine baseline neurologic condition:

A: Alert
V: Responds to verbal stimuli
P: Responds only to painful stimuli
U: Unresponsive

The patient's level of consciousness must be reassessed frequently throughout transport to the hospital. Rapid and severe changes in mental state are likely to occur, since neurologic complications often affect intracranial pressure.

When reporting findings on the radio or run reports, descriptive terms should be used to help abate confusion and misinterpretation between the paramedic and base physician. For example, the term "semiconscious" can be interpreted many ways by different people. The paramedic should rely on devices such as AVPU to communicate, for example, that the patient is responsive only to painful stimulus.

Physical Examination

In addition to evaluating the state of consciousness in the neurologic exam, patient assessment also includes the position in which the patient was found, speech patterns, movement of extremities, pupillary size and reaction, extraocular (eye) motions, and posturing.

The position in which the patient was found is an important consideration. Often, certain positions can suggest or indicate underlying problems. Seizure patients are frequently found in bizarre or unusual positions immediately after the event. Also, it is common to find them *incontinent* (uncontrolled bladder or bowel movement). Patients who have had a stroke might display hemiparesis (one-sided weakness) or hemiplegia (paralysis on one half of the body). Also, one corner of the mouth may droop downward.

The patient's speech may also be affected in neurologic emergencies and, therefore, must be examined. Note if the speech is slurred. Are the words and word patterns appropriate or incomprehensible? Does the patient repeat a word or word phrase over and over again? Has the patient lost the ability to understand? This information can be obtained by noting if the patient follows simple commands like, "squeeze my hand," or "nod your head."

Note if the patient can move the extremities. Then determine whether this movement is *purposeful* (smooth, coordinated movement) or *nonpurposeful* (uncoordinated, sporadic). It is important to note whether or not the patient can localize pain and withdraw from a painful stimulus.

Further, determine the patient's proprioception. This is the ability to determine motion, position, and sensation. Ask the patient to move both arms, both legs, and the fingers and toes of each extremity. Have the patient push and pull the toes and fingers against resistance. Also, wiggle the patient's toe to see if the patient can distinguish which toe is being touched and in which direction it is being moved. It is appropriate at this stage in the examination to ask the patient to squeeze both of your hands to evaluate equal or bilateral grip strength. Ask the patient to grasp the middle three fingers of your hand and squeeze while you gradually pull away. If you offer your entire hand, the patient may not be able to effect a firm grasp, either because your hand is much larger than the patient's or because the patient's condition is generally weakened as a result of injury or illness.

Next, observe the pupils. Are they equal in size? Unequal pupils are normal for only about 5% of the total population. Do they react to light? Is this reaction brisk or sluggish? Note if the pupils are abnormally constricted or dilated. Again, care should be taken to use descriptive language and to be as exact as possible when reporting these observations.

While noting the patient's pupils, take care also to observe any extraocular movements. Patients should be able to move their eyes in full directional ranges. This ability can be checked by having patients follow a moving finger or object with their gaze.

When significant damage occurs as a result of a head trauma and in some types of CNS disorders, patients may begin to display posturing. Decorticate and decerebrate are two types of posturing. Usually, after these two stages, the patient no longer responds to any type of noxious or painful stimuli. In **decorticate posturing**, the legs and feet extend and the arms flex. However, this extension and flexion is nonpurposeful in nature; that is, the patient does not localize the origin of the noxious stimulus. This type of movement is suggestive of significant head trauma. Though prognosis is extremely poor for patients who exhibit either of these two movements, decerebrate posturing conveys a worse prognosis than decorticate posturing. In **decerebrate posturing**, both legs extend and also both arms extend, and the upper extremities rotate inward. This movement usually is indicative of damage to the brain stem.

Examples of decorticate and decerebrate posturing are shown in Figure 22-10.

If trauma is suspected, then further assessment is needed. The spine should be inspected for injury. When

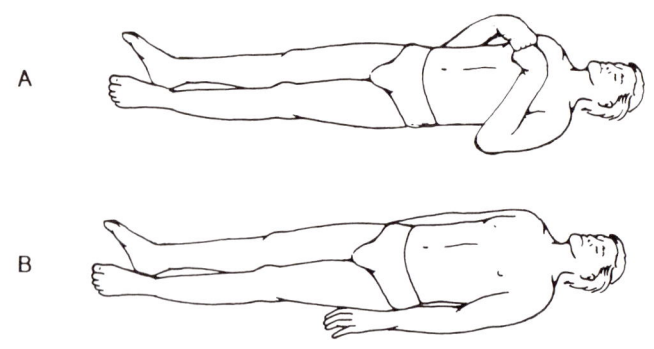

FIGURE 22-10.
Decorticate (**A**) and decerebrate (**B**) posturing.

preparing the patient to be log-rolled onto a long backboard, palpate the patient's back. Note any deformity or bruising, and determine if the patient experiences any pain or a point of tenderness along the spine. If the patient experiences any loss of sensation or movement, note at what level on the spinal column this loss begins. Also, note if sensation and movement is lost below this point. Any neurologic deficit noted in the spinal exam should be communicated to the base physician.

The **Glasgow Coma Scale** is used as a guide to assess the baseline degree of brain dysfunction from one point in time to another. It assesses to what degree the patient can control opening the eyes, verbal capacity, and motor responses. This scale is used universally among both prehospital and in-hospital care providers. Therefore, when reporting the Glasgow Coma Score, the paramedic should state both the sum total and the breakdown of each category. For a further explanation of the Glasgow Coma Scale, refer to Chapter 9 and Appendix C.

TYPES OF NERVOUS SYSTEM EMERGENCIES

Coma

Coma is an abnormally deep state of unconsciousness from which the patient cannot be aroused by external stimuli. Many conditions, including acute injury and drug overdose, can cause coma. Management of the comatose patient can be difficult, since an accurate and detailed history of the event frequently is unobtainable. Helpful clues as to the cause of the comatose state are sometimes found in the immediate surrounding environment. The paramedic needs to develop a keen sense of perception when dealing with coma.

Pathophysiology

The cerebral cortex and the reticular activating system control consciousness. The cerebral cortex controls content or "intake data" received from the environment. Under normal circumstances, one can think about and understand this data. Human activity is a result of this understanding. The functions of the cerebral cortex are best manifested in the ability to perform various motor tasks and exchange ideas.

The reticular activating system, on the other hand, functions as the "*arousal center*" for the body. It is responsible for "keeping the brain awake." The reticular activating system is not a distinct anatomical structure but, rather, is an indiscriminate formation that extends from the lower aspect of the brain stem up to the thalamus and throughout the cerebral cortex. Dysfunction of either of these two structures results in coma.

For coma to ensue, either both right and left cerebral cortexes have to be affected or the reticular activating system has to be damaged. Various conditions can readily affect the functioning of both the cerebral cortex and the reticular activating system. These conditions are categorized as being "structural" or "metabolic" in nature. Conditions such as head trauma, tumors, and intracranial hemorrhage are examples of structural lesions that can lead to coma. Metabolic conditions that can produce coma include hypoxia, hypoglycemia, drug and alcohol overdose, acid-base derangements, and electrolyte imbalance.

As a general rule, structural lesions affect the reticular activating system, whereas the cerebral cortex is most affected by metabolic problems. Signs and symptoms that characterize structural coma include a sudden onset, usually preceded by some type of *prodrome* (warning sign), and unequal pupils. Also, the secondary exam often reveals problems on one side, such as hemiparesis. Metabolic coma, on the other hand, is usually preceded by fever and is of slower onset, and the secondary exam is often symmetrical. In addition, many of these patients have a history of seizure disorders, diabetes, or recurrent drug or alcohol abuse.

One easy way to remember the various conditions that can lead to coma is to memorize the mnemonic *AEIOU TIPS*:

A : Acidosis or Alcohol
E : Epilepsy
I : Infection
O : Overdose
U : Uremia
T : Trauma
I : Insulin
P : Psychosis
S : Stroke

Assessment

After a patent airway is secured and the paramedic is comfortable with the patient's respiratory and circulatory status, the cause of the problem should be sought. When patients are truly comatose, they are not able to verbally communicate any information. Thus, close attention is required to notice any nonverbal clues during the secondary survey.

During a thorough head-to-toe exam, the head should be inspected for deformity, depressions, or lacerations that would suggest any type of head trauma. Note any obvious signs of rising intracranial pressure, such as "blown" or unequal pupils or the presence of Cushing's reflex. Note if decerebrate or decorticate posturing is present.

The paramedic may notice a characteristic "fruity" odor on the patient's breath, which could indicate ketoacidosis. Blood may be seen in the mouth from a tongue laceration that might have occurred during the course of a seizure. The color of the patient's skin might provide important insight into the cause of the coma. Is jaundice present? Are there any indications of hypoxia, such as cyanosis around the lips and mouth? The paramedic should inspect the nail beds for cyanosis.

Inspection of the patient's body, especially the arms for needle tracks, which would suggest drug overdose, is important. Finally, determine if the extremities are more flaccid on one side than the other. This type of important information can be obtained if the paramedic develops a skillful "hands on" approach to assessment.

In addition to the information gained by the secondary exam, pertinent information about the nature of the problem can also be obtained from the family, on-scene bystanders, and the environment itself. For example, try to determine the length of time the patient has been in a coma. Did the coma come on suddenly, or was it a gradual progression? Also, elicit whether the patient has a recent history of head trauma.

Management

Airway management is the first priority. If it is compromised, then it must be attended to immediately. Early recognition and management of airway complications increase the chances of reversing these often lethal events. However, it is important to maintain a high degree of suspicion about possible cervical spine injury with comatose patients. The goal is to protect the airway while preventing further harm or aggravation to the cervical spine. Frequently, a simple chin-lift or jaw-thrust maneuver is sufficient. The head-tilt/chin-lift maneuver is not recommended until potential cervical spine complications can be ruled out.

If these steps are not adequate, then an oropharyngeal or nasopharyngeal airway may be required. The gag reflex may still be present in the conscious or semiconscious patient. Vomiting is a common hazard that is difficult to manage, especially in the spine-injured patient. Definitive airway control is accomplished by endotracheal intubation. The paramedic needs to be proficient in this skill to effectively control the airway. This control is especially important in the presence of cervical spine injury. Other ventilatory adjuncts, such as bag-valve-mask devices, should be used as necessary. In addition, oxygen should be administered to all comatose patients regardless of the cause.

These patients often require intravenous (IV) therapy. Once a vein is accessed, the paramedic should draw blood (10–30 mL) and place it in blood tubes to be evaluated at the hospital. The blood-glucose level should also be determined. Prehospital tests, however, normally only provide a baseline status level. This information should be communicated to the hospital once it is obtained.

An IV solution of 0.9% NaCl or lactated Ringer's solution should be infused at a keep-open rate. These solutions can be used to fluid-challenge the patient if necessary, and they also are compatible with almost all IV medications. This point is critical in managing coma, since the specific underlying abnormality is often unclear in the prehospital setting.

Common medications administered to comatose patients, depending on the underlying cause, include 50% dextrose (25 g), naloxone (0.4–0.6 mg), thiamine (100 mg), and sodium bicarbonate (50–100 mEq). Since disturbances in cardiac rhythm can be lethal, most coma patients need to have their cardiac status monitored throughout transport to the hospital. In addition, if the patient's eyes are open, the paramedic may want to take steps to protect them by gently taping the eyelids shut. This action prevents the eyes from becoming excessively dry because of decreased tear flow. Furthermore, if injuries permit, the patient should be transported in the lateral recumbent position. This position facilitates suctioning and helps prevent aspiration of blood, vomit, or secretions if the patient is not already intubated.

Seizure

A *seizure* is a manifestation of a massive electrical discharge of one or more groups of neurons in the brain. During a seizure attack, bizarre muscle movements, strange sensations and perceptions that precede the attack (prodrome), and a complete loss of consciousness can occur. These uncontrollable aspects reflect the specific area of the brain involved. A seizure is not a disease but a manifestation or symptom of an underlying disorder.

The terms epilepsy and seizure are often so closely associated with one another that many people use them interchangeably. Pathologically, they are not the same. **Epilepsy** is defined as recurrent seizures from an unknown cause thought to be irreversible. Treatment, therefore, is aimed at suppressing the abnormal activity of the neurons in the brain rather than at reversing the cause. Seizures, on the other hand, are mostly thought to be caused by some type of reversible underlying condition or disorder. Treatment in this case is aimed at correcting the abnormality.

Various conditions can cause seizures. Like comas, these conditions can be the result of either structural or metabolic complications. Examples of these include stroke, head trauma, toxins (including alcohol and other drugs), hypoxia, hypoglycemia, infections, other metabolic disorders (including diabetes and high fevers), brain tumors, vascular disorders, eclampsia, and idiopathy (specific etiology unknown; the majority fall into this category).

Pathophysiology

To the inexperienced eye, all seizures may seem much alike. However, several types of seizures exist. They can be categorized as either partial or focal complex seizures or general complex seizures. They are grouped according to their site of origin in the brain.

Partial complex seizures, also referred to as *focal seizures*, arise from a localized area in the brain. They may be caused by either a structural lesion, such as an intracranial hemorrhage from head trauma, or a metabolic complication, as seen with meningitis. Some partial complex seizures, which originate from a specific area, spread diffusely throughout the brain to the extent that they become full, general complex seizures.

As the name suggests, *general complex seizures* do not have a specific focus or point of origin; rather, neuronal instability occurs throughout the entire brain.

The underlying pathophysiology is the same for all seizures. Specifically, they result from a paroxysmal event in which massive electrical discharge is emitted from a group of abnormal neurons in the brain. These abnormal neurons are technically referred to as "*epileptogenic foci*," more commonly known as a seizure focus. A seizure focus is a cluster of neurons that are damaged by either structural or metabolic lesions. As a result of the damaged neurons, the permeability of the membranes increases. Subsequently, sodium and potassium ions diffuse more readily across the membranes of the damaged neurons, thereby increasing the ability of the neurons to emit an electrical charge. This increased ability to emit an electrical charge (stimulation) is known as excitability. Neurons within the seizure focus are said to be hyperexcitable. Therefore, seizures occur as a result of an overabundance of electrical discharge emitted from a cluster of hyperexcited neurons in the brain.

Assessment

Understanding the pathophysiology of seizures can help the paramedic anticipate their occurrence in various patients. In assessing the seizure patient, priority must be given to responsiveness, airway, breathing, and circulation. If the patient is postictal (period following a seizure), the paramedic needs to watch for a steady improvement in the mental status. In certain types of seizure, the patient experiences a period of unconsciousness and, therefore, is unable to protect the airway. Frequently, these patients vomit during the seizure. Also, they have a tendency to bite their tongue. Thus, particular attention and care should be given to clearing and maintaining the airway. After these measures are taken, a full, systematic head-to-toe survey should be performed.

Patient history is an important factor in the assessment of the seizure patient. It include information about past seizure disorders, frequency of the attacks, prescribed medications, and regularity in taking medications. The paramedic needs to become familiar with these types of medications. Common anticonvulsant home medications include Tegretol, phenobarbital, phenytoin (Dilantin), and Depakote. Further, history of head trauma is a significant finding. Other important aspects to explore include alcohol and drug abuse, recent fever, nuchal rigidity (stiff neck, as seen in meningitis), history of heart disease, diabetes, or stroke.

If the paramedic did not witness the attack, an attempt should be made to elicit characteristic behavior displayed during the attack, as seen by any family member or bystander. The paramedic should become familiar with the different types of seizures and the various kinds of behaviors that characterize them.

Within each of the two categories of seizures, the manifestation and types of seizure vary. Partial complex or focal seizures are usually precipitated by some type of prodrome, including certain smells or tastes, such as a metallic taste in the mouth, just before the onset of the attack. These patients repeat certain words or phrases and also display local, nonpurposeful movements, such as "lip smacking" and rolling their fingers as if moving a marble between them. Though these patients may be unable to communicate with the surroundings, they remain conscious.

A **Jacksonian seizure** is a partial complex seizure that progresses into a general complex attack. In this case, the specific site of origin gradually begins to spread until massive electrical discharge occurs throughout the entire brain. These seizures are characterized by twitching, which begins in only one part of the body, such as an arm, that eventually develops to the stage of full tonic–clonic activity. The term "*tonic*" means a simultaneous contraction of flexor and extensor muscles that leads to rigidity. The term "*clonic*," on the other hand, denotes alternate contraction of flexor and extensor muscles.

Several types of general complex seizures exist. Grand mal seizures are marked by loss of consciousness, tonic-clonic movements, tongue biting, incontinence (loss of control over bladder and bowel), mental confusion, and a postictal period. The postictal period is marked by a steady improvement in the patient's mental status. Focal motor seizures cause twitching in only one part of the body but may progress to grand mal seizures. Psychomotor seizures result in altered personality states, sometimes including unexplained attacks of rage. They are often preceded by dizziness or a metallic taste in the mouth. Petit mal seizures occur in children and are characterized by a brief loss of motor tone. They practically never require the services of a paramedic.

All of these seizures are pathologic in nature. Hysterical seizures, on the other hand, are not pathologic and do not respond to normal treatment modalities. In fact, a differential diagnosis can often be made through the use of *aromatic ammonia* (smelling salts). Pathologic seizures do not respond to this treatment. In most cases, patients who exhibit hysterical seizures respond readily and profoundly. Hysterical seizures often result in bizarre movements that frequently can be interrupted by sharp command. These patients rarely injure themselves.

Management

Care of the patient should always begin with opening and securing an airway. In maintaining the airway of the seizure patient, objects should never be forced between the patient's teeth. Padded tongue blades may cause further complications, such as broken teeth, vomiting, aspiration, and laryngeal spasm. Use of the jaw-thrust technique and of nasopharyngeal airways is often sufficient under these circumstances. In addition, all seizure patients should receive oxygen, especially since many times the patient becomes apneic during the actual attack.

After gaining control of the airway, perhaps the most important thing a paramedic can do for a patient who is having a seizure is to protect the patient from injury. The patient should almost never need to be restrained. All seizure patients should be monitored for cardiac arrhythmias. The paramedic should institute this monitoring early in management and continue it throughout transport to the hospital. During transport to the hospital, the paramedic may consider placing the patient in a lateral recumbent position. This position facilitates suctioning if vomiting has occurred or if blood and secretions are noted. Also, the paramedic should provide a quiet and reassuring atmosphere, especially if the patient is prone to seizure activity. Bright lights and loud noise often aggravate the situation.

Depending on the status of the patient, the paramedic may consider IV therapy. In an isolated event, the patient rarely needs pharmacologic support. Common medications administered in care of the seizure patient include diazepam (Valium 5–10 mg), 50% dextrose solution (25 g), and at times naloxone (Narcan 0.4–0.6 mg).

Status Epilepticus

Status epilepticus is defined as two or more seizures without an intervening period of consciousness. This condition is a major medical emergency that, if not urgently treated, can result in respiratory failure and death. Associated complications of status epilepticus include aspiration of blood and vomit, brain damage from the resultant hypoxia, long bone and spine fractures, and severe dehydration.

Pathophysiology

Status epilepticus can occur at any age. Causes include severe head trauma, brain tumors, stroke, meningitis and other CNS complications, and certain metabolic processes.

One of the most common causes of status epilepticus is failure to take prescribed medications by people who have a history of seizure disorders. Because they take prescribed medications, these patients often go for a period of time without experiencing a seizure. They begin to think that they have been cured, so they cease taking their medication on a regular basis. Subsequently, though these patients do not realize it, the blood level of the drug begins to decrease. Over a period of time, the blood level of the drug reaches a critically low level, and the person suffers an extremely severe attack. Often this attack is in the form of a status seizure.

Status epilepticus also occurs in patients who suffer from severe systemic or neurologic disease but who have no history of seizures. Though encountered less frequently in the field than seizures caused by patients who neglect to take their medication, this cause of seizure should be considered when managing the status seizure patient. In so doing, various underlying conditions that could possibly result in seizure activity should be considered, and correction of any positive findings should be initiated.

Assessment

Basic assessment of the status epileptic patient is the same as with any seizure patient. The paramedic should pay particularly close attention to the condition of the airway and should institute protective measures as early as possible, since these patients are often apneic during the course of the attack.

In addition, the duration of the attack should be determined and communicated to the base physician. An attempt should be made to determine an accurate history up to the onset of the seizure. This information may help elucidate various circumstances that precipitated the event.

The base physician needs to be alerted to the type of behavior the patient is displaying. When the paramedic communicates this information, care should be taken to use descriptive terms. Precise terms improve communication between the paramedic and physician and foster an accurate and detailed account of the event.

Management

Managing the status epileptic patient should be aimed at maintaining a patent airway. This maintenance is essential since these patients tend to become severely acidotic because of hypoxia. Though the paramedic should not attempt to force objects into the patient's mouth, the use of a nasopharyngeal airway is often ideal as an initial method of protecting the patient's airway. These patients frequently secrete large amounts of saliva. Further, many bite their tongues during the attack, causing blood to collect in the mouth. The lumen of the nasopharyngeal airway functions not only as a passage for air but also allows suction tips to be passed to suction the base of the pharynx where blood and saliva collect. Aggressive suctioning helps decrease the risk of aspiration. Oxygen in high concentrations and high-flow rates should be administered. If the need presents, the bag-valve-mask device should be used to assist ventilation.

An IV line is established in preparation for administration of anticonvulsant drugs. A universal medication used to treat status epilepticus is diazepam (Valium). It hinders the spread of the seizure focus throughout the brain. Diazepam's peak effects occur within 5 to 10 minutes. The recurrence of seizure activity should be anticipated shortly after the drug's administration. It may be necessary to repeat the drug if seizures recur.

One main side effect of diazepam is respiratory depression. After administration of this drug, closely monitor the patient's respiratory status. Supplemental oxygen should always be administered with diazepam. The drug should be given in 2 to 5 mg increments until the seizure stops or to a total of 10 mg. If the seizure activity ceases after the initial dose of diazepam, record the exact amount of the drug that had been administered when the activity stopped. If, on the other hand, after 10 mg the seizure is still persisting, contact the base physician for further instructions.

If the person is already taking seizure medications at home, such as phenytoin (Dilantin), the physician occasionally may order this drug to be given IV once the seizure activity has ceased. This action increases the blood level of the drug, perhaps preventing further attacks.

Another medication to consider is glucose (50% dextrose in water). Since a great deal of energy is lost during the status attack, the patient may become hypoglycemic. The administration of glucose (e.g., 25 g) helps to replace some of the energy lost during the attack. On the other hand, the paramedic has to consider that the patient may be hyperglycemic as a result of dehydration. Therefore, a blood sugar level should be obtained before the administration of glucose. Obtaining blood sugar levels may also help determine the origin of the status event.

Stroke

A **stroke** is a sudden interruption in blood flow to the brain with resultant neurologic deficits. Numerous factors can impede blood flow to the brain and result in a stroke. The technical name for stroke is **cerebrovascular accident**. Thus, it is a cardiovascular problem that affects the cerebral vessels. It is one of the most common medical emergencies encountered in the field.

Statistically, strokes are the third most common cause of death in the United States. They frequently leave the older population severely debilitated. Because of more advanced diagnostic tools, such as computerized tomography, improved medications, and progressive therapy after the stroke, the prognosis for partial or full recovery has greatly improved.

Diagnosis and management often begin with the paramedic. Signs and symptoms depend on the area of the brain damaged. Areas commonly affected are the motor, speech, and sensory centers. It is quite possible and common, therefore, for the patient to lose all means of appropriate expression, frequently leading to frustration in both the patient and the paramedic. Understanding this effect beforehand, however, will help the paramedic manage the problem. Predisposing factors to stroke include hypertension, diabetes, abnormal blood lipid levels, sickle cell disease, and some cardiac arrhythmias.

Pathophysiology

Strokes have various causes. The underlying pathophysiology for all strokes, however, is the same: blood flow in the cerebral vessels is impeded. Thrombosis and embolism are the most common causes of cerebrovascular accidents. A stroke can also result from a cerebrovascular hemorrhage, such as when a cerebral artery aneurysm ruptures. Emboli that result from atherosclerotic plaque, air, tumor, or fat often originate in the carotid arteries. They travel to the brain and eventually become lodged in one of the small cerebral vessels. Often the embolus lodges in and thus occludes the middle cerebral artery. In this circumstance, cardiac arrhythmias may be seen. The specific type of deficits seen in strokes that result from embolism depend on the location of the occlusion. Symptoms or deficits caused by embolism usually come on suddenly.

In other cases, an artery may gradually become occluded as a result of plaque build-up from atherosclerosis. Such atherosclerotic plaques are commonly the sites of clot formation and result in vessel occlusion by a blood clot. This condition is called thrombosis. Vascular occlusion by thrombosis causes necrosis (death) of cerebral tissue and produces cerebral infarction, which is analogous to myocardial infarction caused by thrombotic occlusion in a coronary artery. The onset of thrombotic stroke is usually much slower than that of embolic and hemorrhagic stroke. Signs and symptoms can develop at any time, even during rest, and are not associated with activity or trauma.

Strokes result also from intracerebral vessels that rupture because of chronic hypertension, head injury, aneurysm, or arteriovenous malformation. Strokes that occur as a result of hemorrhage many times are fatal. Blood from a ruptured vessel often leaks into the subarachnoid space, subsequently compressing the contents of the brain. A common manifestation of strokes that result from hemorrhage is hemiplegia. Coma rapidly progresses in these patients because of the increase in pressure exerted on the brain.

Assessment

In the stroke patient, the level of consciousness often fluctuates. Any changes in the mental status of the patient should be documented and the base physician notified immediately.

The history should include both medical conditions and a detailed account of the presenting event. Does the patient suffer from any cardiovascular complications, such as hypertension or coronary artery disease? Have strokes occurred previously? If the patient has a history of stroke and the paramedic notices specific neurologic deficits, the patient should be asked if these are new or if they were a result of an earlier stroke. This information is important to note in the run report. In addition, it should be determined if the onset of the stroke was rapid or gradual and if the signs and symptoms were precipitated by activity or if they occurred while at rest.

The paramedic should compile a detailed list of even the slightest sign of neurologic change. Is there weakness on one side? Does the patient have any apparent speech disturbances? Is there peculiar behavior, such as uncontrolled laughing or excessive crying? Is the patient confused or easily agitated? If able to walk, the patient should be checked for any gait disturbances. Is the patient experiencing unusual visual problems? The paramedic also should note any changes in these initial signs and if they progress in severity. Repeated and thorough head-to-toe surveys are often helpful.

Management

Management is largely aimed at supportive care. The paramedic should maintain a high level of suspicion that the condition is subject to rapid change. Preventive and supportive care should be instituted early in stroke patients. Since they are often confused and frightened, the paramedic should take care to explain procedures to them, even if they cannot speak.

The first priority for any patient is always to establish and maintain an adequate airway. These patients should receive oxygen until the underlying cause can be determined. If the patient is comatose, the paramedic may elect to intubate. It is necessary to constantly evaluate the adequacy of the airway. If IV therapy is indicated, blood should be drawn to determine the glucose level. If hypoglycemic, the base physician should be notified; an injection of 50% dextrose may be authorized. The use of pharmacologic support, however, varies among emergency services. Hyperglycemia can provoke cerebral acidosis during cerebral ischemia, necessitating documentation of hypoglycemia before glucose administration can even be considered.

Since cardiac arrhythmias are common with strokes, the patient should be monitored throughout transport. If ventricular ectopy is present, it should be treated accordingly. The paramedic should notify the hospital if any changes in the rhythm occur.

In the transport of stroke patients, position is an important factor. They should be transported in a position of comfort. If hemiparesis or hemiplegia is present, care should be exercised to assure that the extremities are protected. As stated above, these patients are often frightened and confused. The paramedic needs to convey a calm and reassuring attitude when caring for these patients.

SUMMARY

Medical or traumatic disruption of the nervous system is a frightening and potentially life-threatening condition that requires the knowledge, skill, and tact of the responding paramedic. Because many nervous system disorders are treatable, if not reversible, prompt, appropriate care by the paramedic can contribute to recovery and a reduction in morbidity and mortality.

SUGGESTED READING

Bates B: A Guide to Physical Examination and History Taking, 4th ed. Philadelphia, JB Lippincott, 1987

Callahan ML: Current Therapy in Emergency Medicine. Philadelphia, BC Decker, 1987

Caroline NL: Emergency Care in the Streets, 3rd ed. Boston, Little, Brown & Co, 1987

Rosdahl CB: Textbook of Basic Nursing, 4th ed. Philadelphia, JB Lippincott, 1985

Tortora GJ, Anagnostakos NP:Principles of Anatomy and Physiology, 6th ed. New York, Harper and Row, 1990

US Department of Transportation, National Highway Traffic Safety Administration: Emergency Medical Technician–Paramedic: National Standards Curriculum. Washington, DC, US Government Printing Office, 1985

CHAPTER 23

Gastrointestinal, Urinary, and Reproductive System Emergencies

Anatomy and Physiology of the Gastrointestinal System
   Primary Structures and Organs
   Accessory Structures and Organs
Anatomy and Physiology of the Abdomen
Anatomy and Physiology of the Urinary System
Anatomy and Physiology of the Reproductive Systems
   Male Reproductive System
   Female Reproductive System

The Acute Abdomen
   Pathophysiology
      Conditions That Result in Acute Abdominal Pain
         Intestinal Obstruction
         Duodenal Ulcer
         Cholecystitis
         Diverticulitis
         Appendicitis
         Aortic Aneurysm
      Conditions Responsible for Acute Gastrointestinal Bleeding
         Esophageal Bleeding
   Assessment
      History
   Physical Examination
      Primary Survey
      Secondary Survey
   Management of Acute Abdominal Disorders

Pathophysiology of the Urinary System
   Acute
   Chronic
   Kidney Stones
   Urinary Tract Infections
   Assessment
   Management
      Hemodialysis
         Management of the Dialysis Patient
Pathophysiology of Reproductive System Disorders
   Male Reproductive System
      Management
   Female Reproductive System
      Management
Summary

BEHAVIORAL OBJECTIVES

On successful completion of this chapter, the reader will be able to:

1. Identify the primary and secondary structures and organs of the gastrointestinal system
2. Locate organs of the abdomen using the four quadrant method
3. Identify the organs and structures of the urinary system
4. Identify the organs and structures of the male and female reproductive systems
5. Describe the pathophysiology of an acute abdomen
6. Define the conditions that result in acute abdominal pain
7. Define the conditions that result in acute gastrointestinal bleeding
8. Describe the assessment and management of a patient with an acute abdominal disorder
9. Describe the pathophysiology of the urinary system

(continued)

BEHAVIORAL OBJECTIVES (continued)

10. Explain the process of hemodialysis
11. Describe the pathophysiology of the male and female reproductive systems
12. Discuss management procedures for male and female reproductive system disorders
13. Define all of the key terms listed in this chapter

KEY TERMS

The following terms are defined in the chapter and glossary:

acute abdomen
anuria
appendicitis
appendix
cholecystitis
colic
diverticulitis
duodenal ulcers
dysuria
epididymitis
epiglottis
hematuria
melena
oliguria
peristalsis
peritoneum
retroperitoneal space

This chapter discusses the anatomy, physiology, and pathophysiology of the gastrointestinal, urinary, and reproductive systems. When a patient presents with an acute emergency that involves any of these systems, a detailed patient evaluation must be completed efficiently and quickly. Medical- or trauma-related problems can result in rapid deterioration of the patient's condition unless they are quickly identified and managed. The goal of prehospital care is to manage these life-threatening disorders and provide supportive care and transport to a medical facility at which definitive treatment can be provided.

ANATOMY AND PHYSIOLOGY OF THE GASTROINTESTINAL SYSTEM

The gastrointestinal structures and organs can be classified as either primary or accessory. The primary structures and organs include the mouth, pharynx, esophagus, stomach, small and large intestines, and the rectum. The accessory organs include the salivary glands, the teeth, liver, gallbladder, pancreas, and appendix. Figure 23-1 illustrates the gastrointestinal system.

Primary Structures and Organs

The *mouth*, or oral cavity, receives food, prepares it for digestion, and begins the digestion of starch. It is surrounded by the lips, cheeks, tongue, palate, and teeth.

The *pharynx*, or throat, is that portion of the airway between the nasal cavity and larynx. The function of the pharynx is to serve as a passageway for air into the lungs and food into the esophagus. As food is swallowed, the flaplike **epiglottis** closes off the opening to the larynx and prevents food from entering the lungs.

The *esophagus* is a straight collapsible tube. It begins at the base of the pharynx and extends downward behind the trachea, penetrating the diaphragm and opening into the stomach. Wavelike muscular movements (**peristalsis**) of the wall of the esophagus move solid food particles into the stomach.

The *stomach* is a hollow J-shaped organ that receives food from the esophagus. It lies under the diaphragm predominantly in the left upper quadrant and is the major organ of digestion.

The *small and large intestines* occupy a major portion of the space in the peritoneal cavity. The small intestine consists of the duodenum, the jejunum, and the ileum. Together, these three portions measure about 7 m in length. The duodenum is frequently a site for the development of ulcers.

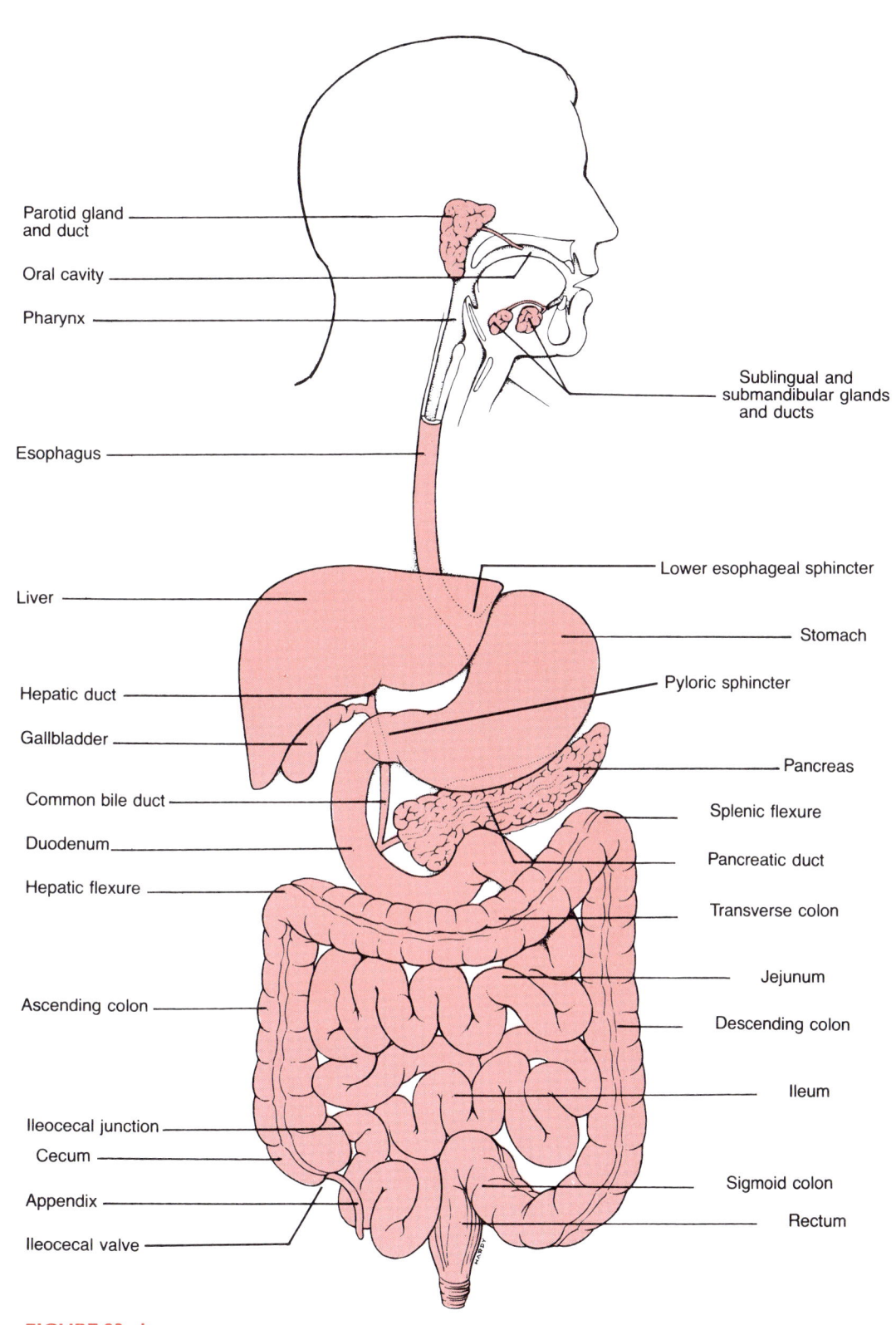

CHAPTER 23: Gastrointestinal, Urinary, and Reproductive System Emergencies 559

FIGURE 23-1.
Anatomy of the gastrointestinal system. (Brunner LS, Suddarth DS)

The large intestine extends from the ileum to the anus and consists of the colon and rectum. The colon is divided into the ascending, transverse, descending, and sigmoid portions. The rectum is the terminal end of the sigmoid colon. The large intestine averages 1.5 m in length and 6.25 cm in diameter.

Accessory Structures and Organs

The *salivary glands* connect to the mouth via small ducts, or tubes. They produce and secrete saliva and begin the digestion of carbohydrates.

The *teeth* break food into smaller particles and increase the surface area, making it possible for the digestive enzymes to react more effectively with the food particles.

The *liver* is the largest solid organ in the body and is located in the right upper quadrant just below the diaphragm. It is a highly vascular organ that secretes bile, produces many blood proteins, detoxifies drugs and harmful substances, and converts glucose to glycogen.

The *gallbladder* is a pear-shaped sac attached to the ventral surface of the liver. It stores, concentrates, and releases bile into the small intestine for the digestive process.

The *pancreas* is a soft oblong gland that lies behind the parietal peritoneum. It extends horizontally across the posterior abdominal wall, with one end in the C-shaped curve of the duodenum and the other against the spleen.

The functions of the pancreas are twofold: it secretes digestive enzymes, and it secretes the hormones glucagon and insulin, which help regulate blood glucose levels.

At the lower end of the colon, where it joins with the ileum, is a hollow narrow tube with a closed end that projects downward into the right lower quadrant. This structure, known as the **appendix,** has no known digestive function but is susceptible to inflammation, which may result in appendicitis.

ANATOMY AND PHYSIOLOGY OF THE ABDOMEN

The *abdominopelvic cavity* is subdivided anatomically into the abdominal cavity and the pelvic cavity. In common usage, the term abdomen refers to the entire region. For purposes of communication, the surface topography of the abdomen may be described by the four-quadrant method. In this method, the abdomen is divided into regions by two perpendicular lines that cross at the umbilicus (Fig. 23-2). The resulting four quadrants are the following:

Right upper quadrant (RUQ)
Left upper quadrant (LUQ)
Right lower quadrant (RLQ)
Left lower quadrant (LLQ)

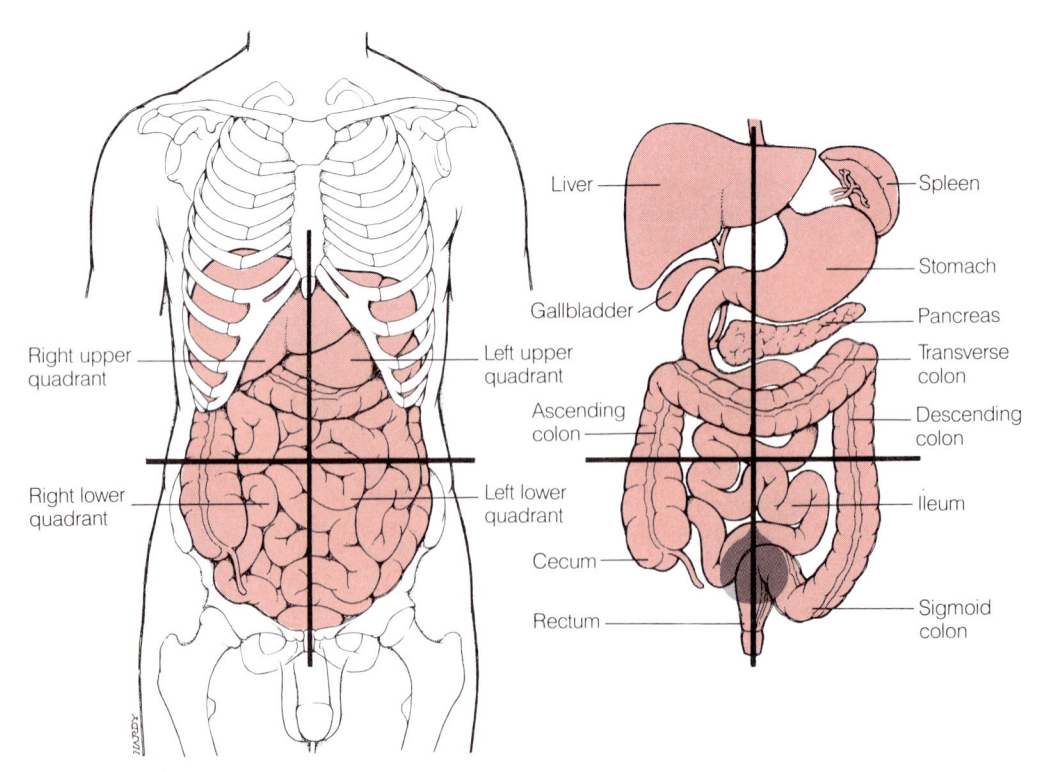

FIGURE 23–2.
Four quadrant divisions of the abdomen. (Brunner LS, Suddarth DS)

The intra-abdominal anatomy is framed by the abdominal cavity proper, which is bound superiorly by the diaphragm and extends downward to the pelvic bones, where its inferior boundary is demarcated by an imaginary plane between the pubic symphysis and the sacral promontory. Anteriorly and posteriorly, the cavity is bound by the muscular abdominal wall and its associated blood vessels, nerves, and cutaneous tissue. The major abdominal organs include the liver, gallbladder, stomach, spleen, small intestine, and large intestine. Together, these intra-abdominal organs are enclosed by a double layered membranous sac that lines the abdominal cavity; this is the **peritoneum.** The peritoneum is subdivided into two components; the *parietal* peritoneum lines the abdominal wall and is reflected back on itself to form the *visceral* peritoneum, which covers each of the abdominal organs. Outside and behind the confines of the peritoneum, lying between the peritoneal sac and the muscles of the back, is an area known as the **retroperitoneal space.** Several important structures are located within the retroperitoneum, including the kidneys, aorta, ureters, inferior vena cavae, pancreas, suprarenal glands, and duodenum (distal portion). Knowledge of the retroperitoneum and its associated structures is of practical importance, since major blood loss into this area can occur after abdominal trauma and produce life-threatening hypotension and shock.

Continuous with the abdominal cavity and extending below its inferior boundary is the pelvic cavity. This smaller portion of the abdominopelvic cavity contains the urinary bladder, rectum, and reproductive organs.

Organs of the abdominal cavity can be classified by their structure as either *solid* or *hollow*. The solid organs of the abdominal cavity include the liver, spleen, pancreas, and kidneys. The hollow organs are the stomach, intestines, gallbladder, urinary bladder, appendix, and, in the female, the uterus.

ANATOMY AND PHYSIOLOGY OF THE URINARY SYSTEM

The primary function of the urinary system is to maintain homeostasis by controlling the amount of water, solutes, and wastes. The organs that make up the urinary system include the kidneys, ureters, bladder, and urethra (Fig. 23-3).

The *kidneys* are located in the retroperitoneal space on either side of the vertebral column. In general, the upper and lower borders of these solid organs are at the level of the 12th thoracic and 3rd lumbar vertebrae respectively. The primary function of the kidneys is to maintain a normal composition and volume of the internal body fluids.

The *ureters* are tubular structures, about 25 cm long, that extend from the renal pelvis to the bladder. At the terminal end of the ureter is a flaplike fold of mucosal membrane. This flap acts as a one-way valve that allows

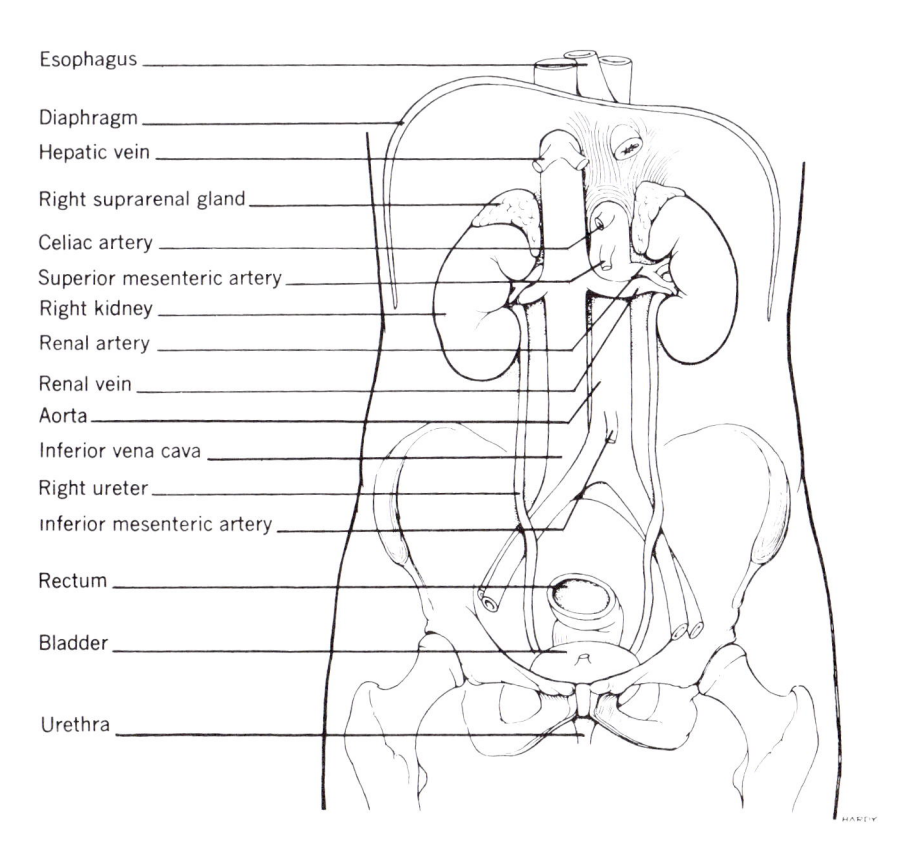

FIGURE 23-3.
Anatomy of the urinary system. (Rosdahl CB)

urine to enter the bladder and prevents it from refluxing into the kidneys.

The *urinary bladder* is a hollow muscular organ located in the pelvic cavity behind the pubic bone. It stores the urine that is produced by the kidneys. Damage to the urinary bladder can either result from blunt or penetrating trauma to the abdomen or from a pelvic fracture.

The *urethra* is a hollow tube that leads from the urinary bladder to the outside of the body. In the female, it is about 4 cm long. In the male, the urethra serves as a passageway for urine and secretions from various reproductive organs.

ANATOMY AND PHYSIOLOGY OF THE REPRODUCTIVE SYSTEMS

Male Reproductive System

The male reproductive system consists of the testes, epididymis, the vas deferens, penile urethra, and the prostate gland (Fig. 23-4). The testes are paired oval glands located outside the body and suspended in the saclike scrotum. The testes produce and secrete the male sex hormone, *testosterone*.

The *epididymis* is a tightly coiled, threadlike tube that emerges from the top of the testes and becomes the vas deferens. The epididymis houses the sperm cells for 18 hours to 10 days until they mature and are ready to fertilize a female egg.

The *vas deferens* is a small muscular tube that begins at the lower end of the epididymis and passes upward along the medial sides of the testes to become part of the spermatic cord. It conducts sperm from the epididymis to the urethra.

As discussed earlier, the penile urethra is the terminal duct of the male reproductive system and serves as a common passageway for semen and urine.

The *prostate gland* is an accessory organ of the male reproductive system. It is a doughnut-shaped gland that surrounds the beginning of the urethra, just below the urinary bladder. The prostate secretes an alkaline fluid. This fluid neutralizes seminal fluid and increases the motility of sperm cells.

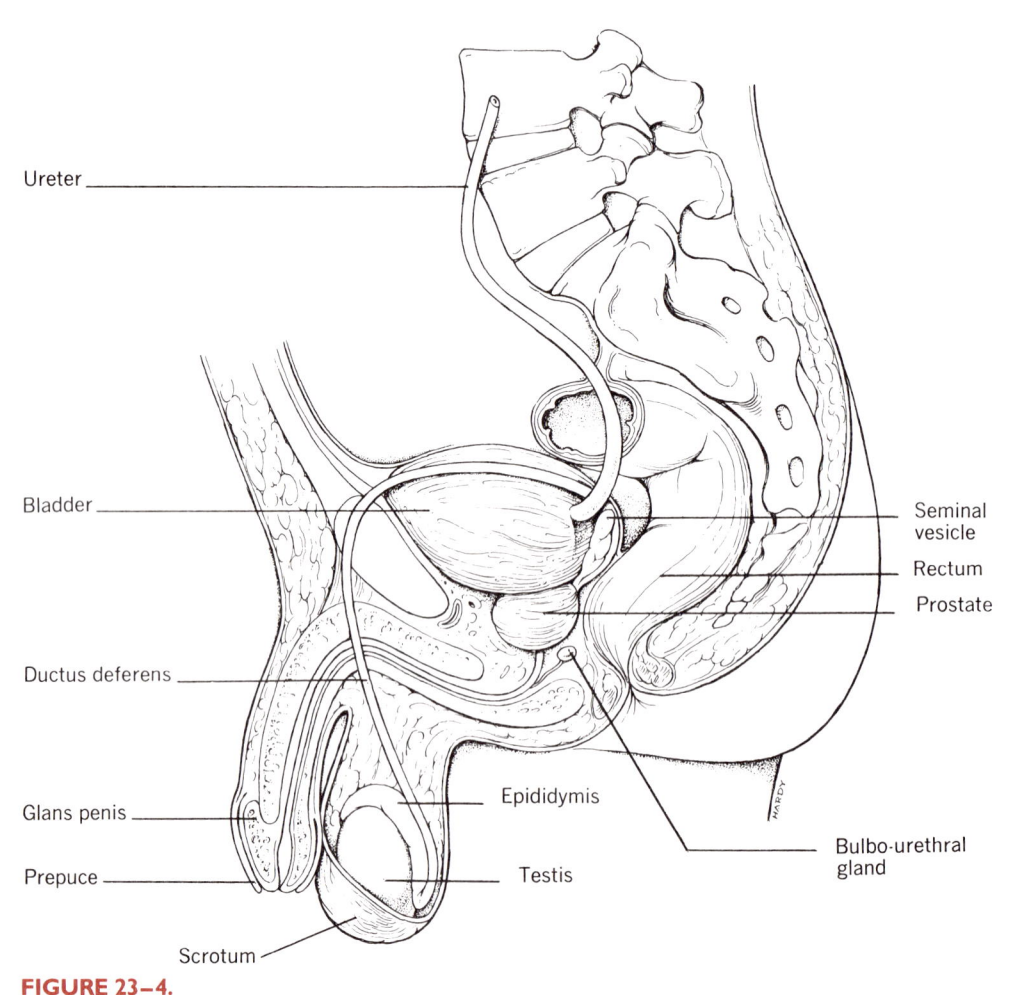

FIGURE 23-4.
Anatomy of the male reproductive system. (Brunner LS, Suddarth DS)

Female Reproductive System

The female reproductive system consists of the ovaries, fallopian tubes, uterus, vagina, and the external structures, the vulva. The ovaries are walnut-sized organs located on each side of the body that are attached to the pelvic cavity via ligaments. The ovaries produce and release eggs and secrete female sex hormones.

The *fallopian tubes* extend from the ovaries to the uterus. They serve as a passageway to convey egg cells to the uterus. Occasionally, a fertilized egg implants itself in the fallopian tube instead of the uterus. This condition is known as an *ectopic pregnancy* and can result in rupture of the tube. The *uterus* is situated between the urinary bladder and the rectum. This inverted pear-shaped organ receives the embryo that results from a fertilized egg cell and houses the developing fetus.

The *vagina* is a muscular tube that extends from the uterus to the vulva. It serves as a passageway for the menstrual flow and a receptacle for the penis during sexual intercourse and is the lower portion of the birth canal. Further discussion of the female reproductive system can be found in Chapter 30.

THE ACUTE ABDOMEN

The **acute abdomen,** by definition, means an abdominal disorder that develops quickly and is potentially severe in nature. Diagnosis of a specific abdominal disorder is difficult to do in the prehospital setting because so many disease states mimic one another. Pain may be referred to another area or overlap from quadrant to quadrant. Because of these facts, it is imperative to obtain an accurate clinical evaluation based on the history of the chief complaint and rapidly treat those disorders that may be life-threatening.

Pathophysiology

Gastrointestinal disorders have four general causes: inflammation, infection, obstruction, and hemorrhage. Injury to a solid organ is likely to result in hemorrhage, while injury to a hollow organ may lead to infection and inflammation. Obstruction results in the failure of the bowel to pass gas and intestinal contents normally through the tract.

When a hollow organ ruptures, its contents spill into the peritoneal cavity. The peritoneum is the smooth, thin lining of the abdominal cavity and is about the thickness of the lining of an egg shell. When gastrointestinal contents spill into the open peritoneal cavity, as with a perforated duodenal ulcer, this lining is immediately irritated and inflamed, causing pain. Peritonitis develops in 6 to 10 hours and can be fatal because of massive systemic infection.

Conditions That Result in Acute Abdominal Pain

Pain is the most frequent complaint of a patient who is experiencing an acute abdominal disorder. Pain can be caused by a variety of medical conditions, including intestinal obstruction, ulcers, inflammation of the gallbladder (*cholecystitis*), inflammation of the intestine (*diverticulitis*), appendicitis, or an abdominal aortic aneurysm.

INTESTINAL OBSTRUCTION. Intestinal obstruction is caused by a mechanical or neurogenic condition. Tumors and a twisting of the intestine are examples of mechanical disorders. In neurogenic obstruction, the peristaltic wave-like action of the intestinal wall is interfered with, causing gas, secretions, and intestinal contents to back up in the intestine.

The patient with an intestinal obstruction describes pain as being crampy (**colic**) and located in either the periumbilical or suprapubic area. Abdominal distention, nausea, and severe vomiting may also be present. As a result of the severe vomiting and fluid loss, hypovolemic shock may occur. Abdominal distention develops because the portion of the bowel proximal to the obstruction becomes filled with intestinal contents.

DUODENAL ULCER. **Duodenal ulcers** are a common disease among adults, particularly in a society of high stress and anxiety. The ulcer and its related signs and symptoms are caused by the digestive action of hydrochloric acid on the mucosa of the duodenum. Pain, which may be described as "gnawing" or "burning," occurs in the epigastric region. It develops suddenly, usually within 1 hour after meals and frequently awakens the patient from sleep.

When a duodenal ulcer perforates, the intestinal contents spill into the peritoneal cavity. This spillage results in sudden severe worsening of the pain, accompanied by abdominal rigidity, diaphoresis, tachycardia, and hypotension.

CHOLECYSTITIS. Acute **cholecystitis** is almost always due to the presence of gallstones that are obstructing the gallbladder ducts. Cholecystitis occurs more often in middle-aged women than in men. After a meal that contains fried, greasy, spicy, or fatty foods, the patient develops an acute onset of crampy pain in the right upper quadrant. This pain may also be referred to the right shoulder and may increase with deep inspiration. Nausea and vomiting can also occur. In addition to the pain, the patient may display symptoms similar to those of an acute myocardial infarction (see Chapter 20). Because of the similar symptoms, an accurate history is vitally important.

DIVERTICULITIS. *Diverticula* are sacs or pouches caused by a weakening in the muscular wall of the intestine.

The contents of the gastrointestinal tract often become trapped in these pouches, causing irritation, inflammation, infection, and, if severe enough, perforation of the intestinal wall. Acute **diverticulitis** results in a gradual onset of pain in the left lower quadrant, which is variable in nature but fairly constant. If perforation occurs, peritonitis and shock may result.

APPENDICITIS. *Appendicitis* is one of the most common abdominal emergencies that requires surgery. The appendix is located at the tip of the cecum. If obstruction occurs at the opening of the appendix, fecal material becomes impacted and bacterial infection and inflammation develop. Appendicitis can occur at any age. However, it is more common among adolescents and young adults. An attack of severe epigastric discomfort is the most common symptom. Classically, this symptom is followed hours later by localization of the pain to the right lower quadrant. *McBurney's point*, which is located about halfway between the umbilicus and the right iliac crest, is usually the site of the most severe pain. In addition to pain, the patient may have a low-grade fever, nausea, and vomiting. Pain and irritation cause the psoas muscles in the abdomen to contract. The patient feels more comfortable if the legs are flexed and pulled up. If perforation of the appendix occurs, the pain and discomfort may diminish; however, severe peritonitis and shock ensue.

AORTIC ANEURYSM. The walls of the arteries are inherently elastic. When the elasticity is weakened by disease or chronic hypertension, an outpouching may occur in the vessel wall. When this develops in the abdominal aorta, it is known as an *abdominal aortic aneurysm*. Patients with aortic aneurysm often have a history of lumbosacral pain. The pain may radiate into the groin or down the legs. Physical examination of the abdomen may reveal a pulsating mass.

As this condition worsens, the walls of the aorta may separate, with blood filling the newly created spaces. Nausea and vomiting can occur because of pressure on the intestines. Abrupt pain in the flanks or direct lumbar back pain, described as a "tearing" sensation, can also be experienced. As the pressure increases in the aneurysm, the pain worsens and the patient may become hypotensive with decreased or absent femoral and pedal pulses.

After rupture of the aneurysm, sudden deep cyanosis often develops and the patient rapidly becomes severely hypotensive and may proceed to cardiac arrest, most commonly in the form of electromechanical dissociation secondary to exsanguination.

Other conditions that can cause abdominal pain include chemical or food poisoning, medications (particularly aspirin or steroids), *gastroenteritis* (inflammation of the stomach and intestines), ectopic pregnancy, and hernias (umbilical or inguinal). Signs and symptoms of these conditions vary.

Conditions Responsible for Acute Gastrointestinal Bleeding

Acute bleeding in the gastrointestinal tract can be caused by mucosal bleeding of the esophagus, the stomach, duodenum, small intestine, or colon. Gastrointestinal bleeding manifests itself with the presence of bright-red blood or coffee-ground emesis, or bright-red or black tarry stools.

If a patient is vomiting blood or has coffee-ground emesis, possible causes include peptic ulcer, gastritis, inflammatory bowel disease, diverticulosis, hiatal hernia, esophageal varices, tumor, hemophilia, or drugs, especially aspirin, anticoagulants, and steroids. When bleeding occurs high in the gastrointestinal tract, such as in the stomach duodenum and small bowel, the stools appear black and tarry (**melena**). Bleeding from the lower gastrointestinal tract, such as that which can occur with hemorrhoids, produces bright- or dark-red bloody stools.

It should be understood, however, that many other causes for a change in stool color exist. Ingestion of iron supplements, beets, blueberries, or charcoal also cause the stool to darken in color. The paramedic must remember that obtaining an accurate history is especially important when caring for a patient who is experiencing gastrointestinal bleeding.

ESOPHAGEAL BLEEDING. Esophageal hemorrhage deserves special attention because of the often massive bleeding that occurs and the possibility of aspiration. Esophageal bleeding can occur when the esophagus tears or when the esophageal veins rupture. Esophageal varices are submucosal and may rupture, producing massive *hematemesis* (vomiting blood) and death. Rupture can be precipitated by prolonged vomiting or a history of liver disease and is more common in alcoholics. Signs and symptoms include severe vomiting, including bright-red blood, and hypovolemic shock. Management should be aimed at maintaining the airway, replacing fluids, and preventing or treating shock.

Regardless of the location of gastrointestinal bleeding, general signs and symptoms include diarrhea, vomiting, dizziness, tachycardia, and cold extremities. In severe cases, a decreased level of consciousness associated with hypotension may be seen.

Assessment

History

When obtaining a history of the present illness, the paramedic should identify the time of onset and surrounding circumstances. The patient should be asked when and what was last eaten. The onset of symptoms should be noted as either abrupt or gradual.

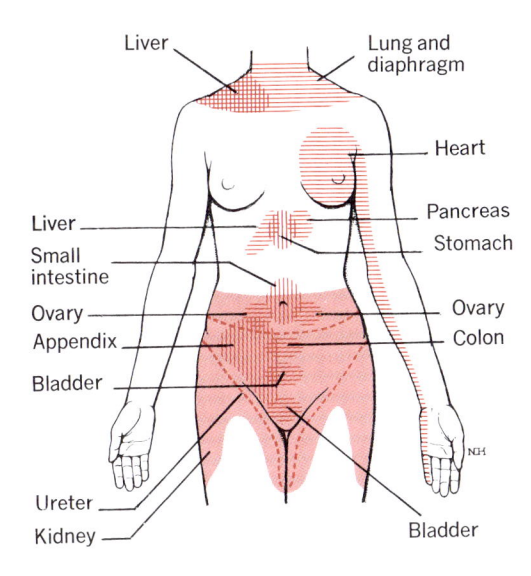

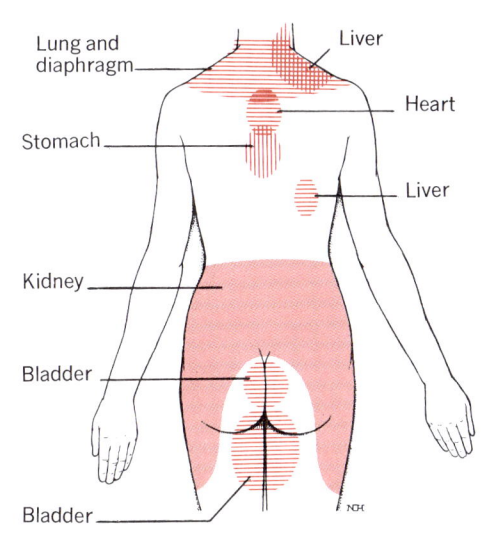

FIGURE 23-5.
(**A**) Referred pain, anterior view. The areas to which pain in the various organs is referred are indicated by colored lines and shading. (**B**) Referred pain areas, posterior view. (Chaffee EE, Lytle IM)

Pain is the most common complaint of a patient with an abdominal disorder. The following should be noted:

Location: The onset of the pain may be difficult to assess and may radiate from one location to another (Fig. 23-5). Asking the patient to specifically point to the area of pain may be helpful.

Character: The character of abdominal pain can be described as gnawing, burning, tearing, crampy, sharp, or dull. While it is important to remember not to be suggestive and "lead" the patient into describing the pain, it is also important to get as accurate a description as possible. Often the type of pain helps identify the abdominal disorder. Note whether the pain is constant or intermittent.

Aggravating or alleviating factors: Ask the patient if it feels more comfortable in one position or another. Patients may feel more comfortable lying supine with the legs flexed or lying on their side with legs flexed. Ask if eating or drinking makes the pain worse or better.

In addition to the above, the paramedic should ask the patient if any associated symptoms are present and the duration of these symptoms.

When eliciting a medical history, particular attention should be paid to a history of heart disease, as an acute myocardial infarction may present with substernal or upper abdominal pain. A history of diabetes should be noted, as ketoacidosis can also cause abdominal pain. Black patients should be asked about a history of sickle cell disease. Sickle cell crisis is also a cause of abdominal pain.

Respiratory diseases, particularly pneumonia in the right lower lobe, can mimic acute abdominal pain. Female patients should be questioned about their menstrual history and the possibility of pregnancy. Information about any recent operations or illnesses or similar pain in the past should be obtained.

Physical Examination

Primary Survey

As always, a primary survey should be conducted first and management instituted immediately for any life-threatening problems that are encountered. The primary survey must include a baseline of the patient's responsiveness, airway, breathing, and circulation.

Secondary Survey

During the secondary survey, vital signs should be recorded and repeated at frequent intervals. A pattern of increasing pulse rate and falling blood pressure may suggest internal hemorrhage. The respiratory rate may be normal or increased, reflecting anxiety, acidosis, hypoxia, or fever.

The general appearance of the patient should be noted with attention directed to the position adopted by the patient as well as any voluntary movements. Skin temperature, moisture, and turgor should all be assessed. Prolonged vomiting or diarrhea causes dehydration and hypovolemia. A low-grade temperature frequently is seen in acute appendicitis, while a higher temperature suggests an acute infection.

The abdomen should be inspected for any obvious bruises, scars, masses, or distention. The presence of a pulsating mass should suggest the possibility of an abdominal aortic aneurysm. If the patient also displays sign and symptoms of shock, management should be initiated immediately and rapid transport should be considered. The umbilicus may protrude when an over accumulation of fluid in the abdominal cavity or a hernia is present. Ecchymosis in the flanks or at the umbilicus may be due to retroperitoneal bleeding that can occur with acute hemorrhagic pancreatitis.

Palpation of the abdomen should be done with gentleness. It is unnecessary to elicit more pain in an already painful abdomen. Gently palpate, starting with the area farthest away from the area of tenderness. Note whether the abdomen is soft or rigid and if the pain radiates and to what area.

Auscultation, including all four quadrants, should be done for at least 1 minute to determine positively that bowel sounds are absent. Absence of bowel sounds indicates an inflammatory process. The presence of a high-pitched bowel sound may be due to an obstruction of the gastrointestinal tract.

Management of Acute Abdominal Disorders

Most abdominal disorders cannot be definitively managed in the field. Management should be supportive in nature, making the patient as comfortable as possible, replacing fluids as needed, and preventing or treating shock.

Management of the patient with an acute abdominal disorder or gastrointestinal bleeding includes the following:

1. Maintain the airway and administer high-flow oxygen.
2. Establish an intravenous (IV) line of lactated Ringer's or normal saline solution with a large-bore (14–16 gauge) catheter. Consider starting a second IV line if shock is present.
3. Closely monitor vital signs, electrocardiogram, and level of consciousness.
4. Apply the pneumatic anti-shock garment if indicated.
5. Transport rapidly but gently.

PATHOPHYSIOLOGY OF THE URINARY SYSTEM

As stated earlier, the function of the kidneys is to maintain homeostasis by controlling fluid volume, blood pH, and the composition of body fluids and by eliminating metabolic waste products. Normally, the kidneys filter about 150,000 mL of fluid each day. When renal failure occurs, metabolic waste products begin to accumulate. Over a period of days or weeks, this build-up of waste materials has a toxic effect on the body and produces a clinical picture of *uremia*.

Acute

Causes of acute renal failure include shock and dehydration, which result in decreased blood flow to the kidneys. Other causes include trauma, infection or obstruction of urine flow that results from tumors, prostate enlargement, kidney stones, or drugs.

When acute renal failure occurs, normal kidney function rapidly deteriorates. Urine output decreases (**oliguria**) or stops completely (**anuria**). The patient can exhibit signs and symptoms related to heart failure (*e.g.*, hypertension, generalized edema) or show signs of shock. In addition, nausea, vomiting, and deep rapid respirations (Kussmaul's respiration) may occur from metabolic acidosis. Arrhythmias may result because of the inability of the failing kidneys to regulate sodium and potassium.

Chronic

Chronic renal failure results in a slow, progressive, and irreversible decrease in kidney mass and ability to filter body fluids. It is caused by congenital disorders, decreased blood flow, or generalized infections. The problem may develop over such a long period of time that the patient may be unaware of the changes that occur in appearance and bodily function.

The skin gradually develops a brownish or yellowish tint. Because of protein loss and poor nutrition, the arms and legs appear thin. Edema around the eyes and pitting edema at the ankles may also be seen. In severe cases, urea crystals may form on the skin, resulting from waste products being excreted by the skin rather than the kidneys. This condition is known as "*uremic frost*."

With the availability of renal dialysis facilities, patients seldom die as a direct result of renal failure. However, the complications of renal failure are long term and can result in a dismal prognosis. Complications of renal failure include uremic pericarditis, pericardial tamponade, hyperkalemia, fluid overload, and pulmonary edema.

Kidney Stones

As a result of an inability to rid the body of waste products, calcium deposits may collect on the inner surface of the kidney. Eventually, these deposits, called renal calculi or kidney stones, break off and travel down the ureters. When this process occurs, excruciating pain develops in the flanks and may radiate to the groin. The pain may be so intense that the patient is unable to lie still.

Urinary Tract Infections

Acute infections of the urinary tract can result from any obstruction to the flow of urine. Signs and symptoms include painful urination, difficulty in starting urination, or a burning sensation. In addition, the patient may complain of lower abdominal pain.

Assessment

The history is the major source of information regarding disorders of the urinary system. As with the acute abdomen, the four major causes of urinary disorders are infection, inflammation, obstruction, and hemorrhage.

Typically, the chief complaint is pain on urination (*dysuria*) or blood in the urine (**hematuria**). If infection is the problem, the patient may complain of fever, chills, and pain or burning on urination. Obstruction of the urinary system can result in anuria, hesitancy in starting urination, or dribbling at the end of urination.

When obtaining a history of the chief complaint, the paramedic should ask the patient when and how the problem occurred. It should be determined if a similar incident has occurred in the past or if a recent illness has occurred. The patient should be questioned about any changes in the frequency, amount, or color of the urine.

As with any patient, the life-threatening injuries are managed immediately. During the secondary survey, the paramedic should inspect, auscultate, and palpate the abdomen and flanks appropriately.

Management

Prehospital management of urinary disorders is supportive in nature. In most cases, the airway is not compromised, and oxygen administration via nasal cannula or mask is adequate. If the patient is unconscious, intubation followed by 100% oxygen is indicated. An IV line of D_5W as a life-line drug route should be established. If the patient exhibits signs and symptoms of pulmonary edema, administration of diuretics, such as furosemide, should be requested. Monitor vital signs and cardiac rhythm as indicated, observing for arrhythmias.

Disorders of the urinary system can also be precipitated by trauma. The patient should be evaluated and treated for shock or other injuries as indicated by patient assessment.

Hemodialysis

Hemodialysis is performed for patients in renal failure in an effort to either prevent or treat uremia. The basic principle of dialysis is to bring the blood into contact with a semipermeable membrane and diffuse with water and solutes. This process results in an equilibrium of solute particles in the fluid compartments of the body. Through the use of ultrafiltration, the hydrostatic (fluid) pressure and osmotic (particle) pressure can be altered, and excess fluid and toxic substances can be removed from the body.

When a patient is going to be placed on a hemodialysis machine, cannulas are inserted into the blood vessels. Two types of vascular access are used: external arteriovenous shunts and internal fistulas. Shunts are comprised of two small tubes, one inserted into a superficial artery and one into a vein (Fig. 23-6). When the patient is not on dialysis, the tubes are connected to one another to form a shunt. In the event of trauma, the shunt could be severed. Since one limb of the shunt is connected to an artery, the patient can hemorrhage quickly. The exposed

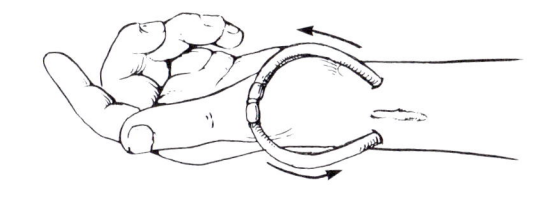

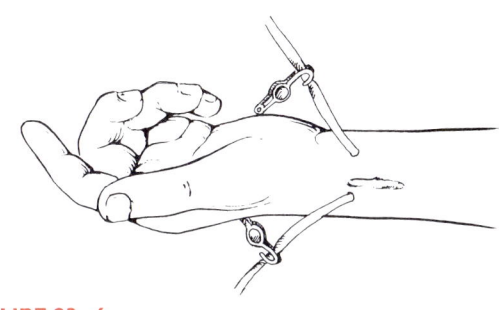

FIGURE 23-6.
An arteriovenous fistula allowing access to the circulation for hemodialysis.

ends need to be clamped rapidly to prevent extensive blood loss.

Other complications that can occur with a shunt are that the cannula tip can become dislodged from the vessel or that an aneurysm can develop at the shunt site and rupture. In either case, direct firm pressure must be applied as with any arterial bleeding.

Internal fistulas are surgically created, joining an artery and a vein. Together, they allow arterial blood to flow directly into the vein because of the lower blood pressure in the vein. Occasionally, a fistula develops an aneurysm and after repeated use could rupture. If bleeding in the area occurs, a large hematoma results or the patient quickly develops shock. As with the shunt, firm direct pressure must be applied and the patient must be treated for shock. Rapid transport is necessary so that the fistula can be surgically repaired.

Two additional complications related to the vascular access can occur. These complications are clotting at the shunt and infection. Both of these problems must be treated in-hospital, and only supportive care is indicated in the prehospital setting.

Patients may be on dialyzing machines in their homes. Three major complications can occur as a result of machine malfunction, including blood loss, thrombosis, and air embolism. If blood loss occurs while patients are on the dialysis machine, they may become hypotensive, dizzy, or have syncopal episodes. The machine should be turned off and an IV line of normal saline established, at a rate prescribed by the physician.

Thrombosis occurs when blood coagulates in the machine tubing and the clot is then pumped into the patient. The patient may exhibit seizures or decreased level of consciousness. If this problem occurs, the machine should be turned off, an IV line of normal saline started to replace the fluid lost in the machine, and the patient transported.

Most dialyzing machines have an air bubble detector that senses when blood is no longer present in the drip chamber and automatically stops the pump. If the sensor malfunctions, an air embolism can enter the bloodstream. The patient may exhibit severe dyspnea, cyanosis, and hypotension. If the patient displays these signs and symptoms, the machine should be turned off, the patient placed on the left side in the Trendelenburg position, and the airway, breathing, and circulation managed as with any patient in respiratory distress.

Patients who are undergoing hemodialysis can experience hypotension along with a lack of balance or stability during dialysis. Hypotension can result from a variety of causes, such as collapsed or kinked blood lines, blood leaks in the dialyzer, excessively rapid removal of fluid, or line separation. If hypotension occurs, the patient should be placed in the Trendelenburg position and an IV line of normal saline should be started and infused at a rate prescribed by the physician.

A lack of balance or stability is caused by excessive rapid fluid removal. The patient may complain of a headache or lethargy and develop seizures. In this instance, the symptoms should be treated as they present with oxygen therapy and fluid replacement. The need for diazepam should be anticipated if seizures occur.

MANAGEMENT OF THE DIALYSIS PATIENT. The following guidelines should be considered when managing a patient with a dialysis shunt or fistula:

1. No blood pressures should be obtained in the extremity with the shunt or fistula unless absolutely necessary. If another extremity is not available, do not leave the blood pressure cuff on afterward.
2. No venipuncture should be performed on that extremity.
3. If a fracture occurs in the extremity with the shunt or fistula, immobilization can be done, using caution so that the area is not wrapped too tightly.
4. If bleeding occurs at the sight, apply direct firm pressure for at least 10 minutes.
5. All patients who have been dialyzed that day have been given heparin. As a result, they bleed more readily and rapidly. Even a small laceration can cause a large blood loss. Head injuries can be more traumatic because of the increased risk of intracranial bleeding. These patients must be observed closely for the development of shock.

PATHOPHYSIOLOGY OF REPRODUCTIVE SYSTEM DISORDERS

In general, disorders of the male and female reproductive systems require little prehospital care. As with the other two systems discussed in this chapter, it is necessary to obtain an accurate history and provide supportive care. In rare instances, however, more aggressive therapy is indicated.

Male Reproductive System

Epididymitis is an inflammation or infection of the epididymis, which travels via the vas deferens. The symptoms include testicle pain, chills, and fever.

Torsion of the testes is a twisting or rotation of the spermatic cord. It is more common in preadolescent boys and can be precipitated by heavy exercise or something as simple as crossing the leg. The patient may have sudden testicular pain and may feel as though he received a traumatic injury to the testes. Unless the spermatic cord is untwisted soon, the testes can be quickly destroyed.

Management

Unless traumatic injury to the testes or penis has occurred, it is rare that aggressive therapy is needed. In general, management of the male patient with a disorder of the reproductive system should include managing the airway as indicated, monitoring vital signs, following shock protocols as indicated, and transporting in a position of comfort.

Female Reproductive System

The most common disorders of the female reproductive system result from infection, bleeding, or complications of pregnancy or trauma.

Pelvic inflammatory disease is the term used to describe an infection of the pelvic organs. The most frequent cause is the gonococcus organism, although other organisms such as streptococci or staphylococci can also be contributing factors. Typically, the patient complains of severe or aching abdominal or back pain, fever and chills, nausea, and vomiting. In addition, vaginal bleeding not consistent with the menstrual cycle may be present.

An ectopic pregnancy is one of the most serious emergencies that involve the female reproductive system. Almost all ectopic pregnancies occur in the fallopian tubes. Pain that is on one side of the abdomen is the most common symptom. This pain is intermittent but becomes sharper and more constant as the fallopian tube distends. After the tube ruptures, patients may also complain of referred shoulder pain as blood spills into the peritoneal cavity. Shock can develop quickly with a loss of 2000 to 3000 mL of blood into the peritoneal cavity. If vaginal bleeding is present, it is usually intermittent and slight. In some cases, the sudden onset of severe abdominal pain is associated with syncope and shock, and vital signs indicate hypovolemia.

Cysts commonly occur on the ovaries. Many times, they are symptomless and disappear. Occasionally, however, the cyst continues to grow and eventually ruptures.

When an ovarian cyst ruptures, the abdominal pain may have a gradual onset or develop rapidly. Guarding is also present. Syncope or shock may develop.

Management

Management of the female patient with a disorder of the reproductive system that does not involve trauma should include the following:

1. Manage airway as indicated.
2. Establish an IV life-line. If shock is present, start a lactated Ringer's or normal saline solution with a large-bore catheter. Consider use of the pneumatic anti-shock garment.
3. Monitor vital signs and cardiac rhythm.
4. Transport in a position of comfort.

SUMMARY

When a patient presents with signs and symptoms related to a disorder of the gastrointestinal, urinary, or reproductive system, it is vitally important to obtain an accurate and complete history. A detailed evaluation must be conveyed to the physician in an effort to provide a continuum of care once the patient reaches the hospital. Most conditions that involve these three body systems do not require aggressive prehospital management. However, the paramedic must keep in mind that, in some situations, the patient's condition may deteriorate rapidly unless the problem is quickly identified and appropriately managed.

SUGGESTED READING

Fontanarosa PB: Acute abdominal pain: Exploring the gut level causes. J Emerg Med Serv 14(11):28, 1989

Hunt D: Genitourinary problems: Case review. The Journal of Emergency Care and Transportation 19(3):62, 1990

Memmler RL, Wood DL: The Human Body in Health and Disease, 6th ed. Philadelphia, JB Lippincott, 1987

Rund DA: Gallbladder emergencies. The Journal of Emergency Care and Transportation 19(3):26, 1990

Stewart C: The liver: An overview. The Journal of Emergency Care and Transportation 19(3):22, 1990

US Department of Transportation, National Highway Traffic Administration: Emergency Medical Technician–Paramedic: National Standards Curriculum. Washington, DC, US Government Printing Office, 1985

CHAPTER 24

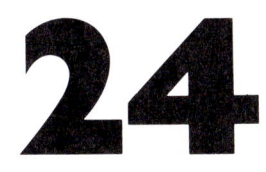

Allergic and Anaphylactic Reactions

Concepts and Terminology
Common Allergens
Pathophysiology
Assessment of the Anaphylactic Patient
Management of Allergic and Anaphylactic Reactions
Prevention and Patient Education
Summary

BEHAVIORAL OBJECTIVES
On successful completion of this chapter, the reader will be able to:

1. Discuss the terms antigen, antibody, allergy, allergic reaction, anaphylaxis, and immunity
2. List common allergens that cause allergies and anaphylaxis, including agents that are drugs, insects, and foods
3. Describe the pathophysiology of anaphylaxis to include the chemicals released, the general body system effects, and specific system effects
4. Describe the assessment of the patient in anaphylaxis
5. Discuss the management of the patient with a simple allergic reaction and the patient in anaphylaxis, including drug actions, precautions, and side effects
6. Discuss prevention and patient education for the victim of anaphylaxis
7. Define all of the key terms listed in this chapter

KEY TERMS

The following terms are found in the chapter and glossary:

allergy
allergic reaction
anaphylaxis
anaphylactic reaction
antibody
antigen
histamine
immunity
sensitization

Few situations encountered by paramedics can match the dramatic lifesaving intervention that is provided during a severe allergic or anaphylactic reaction. The patient frequently appears near death, and, yet, the astute paramedic, with the delivery of appropriate therapy, can often restore the patient's vital functions.

This chapter addresses allergic reactions, including the severe form, anaphylaxis. Anaphylaxis (or anaphylactic reaction) causes the most emergency runs related to allergies. Some people summon medical help, however, for simple allergic reactions without systemic signs and symptoms.

The exact incidence of anaphylactic reactions is difficult to pinpoint. Estimates of the incidence in the United States usually place a person's lifetime risk at 0.4%. One study of more than 20,000 healthy men revealed that 0.49% of that group had experienced anaphylaxis. Another study determined that 1% to 2% of all patients who receive penicillin have some form of allergy to the drug and that 1 in 50,000 injections of penicillin results in death. Estimates of anaphylactic death from insect stings number at least 50 per year.

CONCEPTS AND TERMINOLOGY

To understand what occurs in allergic reactions and in anaphylaxis, several concepts and terms need to be explained. The first concepts to clarify are the body's immune response and the allergic response. The body has a variety of protective mechanisms, such as the "fight or flight" response and metabolic responses, when injuries occur.

The immune response is a positive adaptive response. It is designed to guard the body against dangerous foreign substances, such as infection and antigens. In this normal immune response, the protective cells of the body recognize dangerous intruders, fight them, and destroy them. The ***allergic reaction*** or response, on the other hand, is an oversensitive and harmful response against foreign substances that may actually be harmless. The protective cells overestimate the danger of the harmless intruder and may produce needless damage to body tissue.

Immunity is the body's natural protective state of being resistant to poisons and foreign substances. This state requires that the body be able to distinguish between "self" and "nonself." Immunity can be natural, from birth, or acquired by inoculation. For example, the human body is naturally resistant to the distemper virus that kills 25% to 30% of all dogs that contract the disease. Also, most people in the United States have acquired immunity to small pox because of inoculation.

An ***antigen*** is a foreign substance that induces the formation of antibodies. Antigens are typically introduced into the body, such as bacteria or viruses. An ***antibody*** is a protective protein substance formed in the body as a result of contact with a foreign agent (antigen). Antibodies are also called immune bodies or immunoglobulins. The major function of antibodies is to defend the body from foreign antigen substances.

When antigens and antibodies interact in the body, an immune response develops, presenting protein against disease. However, this antigen-antibody reaction can also cause allergies and anaphylaxis, the oversensitive and severe allergic response. Therefore, an **allergy** is an abnormal and individual hypersensitivity to substances that are ordinarily harmless.

An important fact to note is that an allergic reaction cannot occur with the first contact with a potential antigen, because antibodies have not yet been produced by the body. This process of exposure to allergen and then production of antibodies is called **sensitization**. Sensitization may occur with repeated exposures to an allergen, such as a single bee sting, or from several bee stings over a period of time. It can also occur through more subtle exposures, such as inhalation of horse dander, which creates sensitization to horse serum, or sensitization to antibiotics by drinking milk from antibiotic-treated cows.

The term **anaphylaxis** is derived from "ana," which means without, and "phylaxis," which means protection. It is an acute generalized allergic reaction that occurs within minutes to hours after the body has been exposed to a foreign substance to which it is oversensitive. This **anaphylactic reaction** has systemic signs and symptoms that are exaggerated from a simple allergic reaction. It was first described in 1902 by two French physicians, Portier and Richet. Their investigations eventually won them a Nobel prize and are described as the most significant work in their field. They discovered that nonlethal injections of sea anemone poison into dogs were without effect; however, when subsequent injections of the same amounts were given to the dogs, they developed anaphylaxis.

COMMON ALLERGENS

An allergen is a substance that gives rise to hypersensitivity or allergy. The number of allergens that can elicit allergic reactions or anaphylaxis expands yearly, especially as new drugs are introduced. Allergen groups include drugs, insect venom, food, and pollen. The causative agent may be injected, ingested, absorbed through the skin or mucus membranes, or even inhaled. Injected drugs or foreign substances are the most common cause of anaphylaxis. Intravenous (IV), intramuscular (IM), or subcutaneous (SQ) injections usually cause rapid anaphylaxis. Ingested substances typically require a longer period for the development of allergic symptoms, as do absorbed substances. Inhaled substances rarely cause severe allergic reactions.

Any injected drug can cause anaphylaxis, but the most common one in the United States is penicillin and its derivatives. It has been estimated that 400 to 500 deaths per year occur in the United States from penicillin-related anaphylactic reactions. Patients allergic to penicillin are also at risk of having reactions to semisynthetic penicillins, such as methicillin and ampicillin. Other antibiotics can also be culprits.

Radiographic contrast material, such as IV pyelogram dye, is also a frequent allergen. Most exposure to this material, however, occurs inside the hospital. Aspirin is a common cause of allergic reactions, especially in patients with asthma. Horse serum used in some vaccines can cause anaphylaxis, as can the vaccines for tetanus, pertussis, diphtheria, measles, mumps, rubella, influenza, and yellow fever.

Paramedics encounter patients who describe an allergy to local anesthetics, such as the "caine" drugs. True anaphylactic reactions to local anesthetics are rare, and, in fact, no evidence of cross-sensitivity has been found among the ester-type local anesthetics, such as procaine (Novocaine), and the local anesthetic drugs with an amide structure, such as lidocaine.

Morphine and codeine are narcotics that can produce allergic reactions. Blood transfusions are an additional cause of allergic reactions, although usually they are limited to the hospital setting. Parenteral iron, muscle relaxants (Zomax especially), hormones, insulin, and vitamins have all been reported to cause anaphylaxis. Insect stings and bites are another important cause of anaphylaxis by injection. This physiologic reaction is different from toxic effects that some insects cause, even though the symptoms may be similar. The insect order Hymenoptera is the most common allergen. The four prominent members of the order include the bumblebee, honeybee, white-faced hornet, and the yellow jacket (Fig. 24-1). More annual deaths are reported in the United States from the venom of these insects than from snake bites. About 8 in 1000 people are allergic to stinging insects, and half of these are severely sensitive.

Most of the stinging insects are timid, although some may swarm. The insects in the order Hymenoptera have

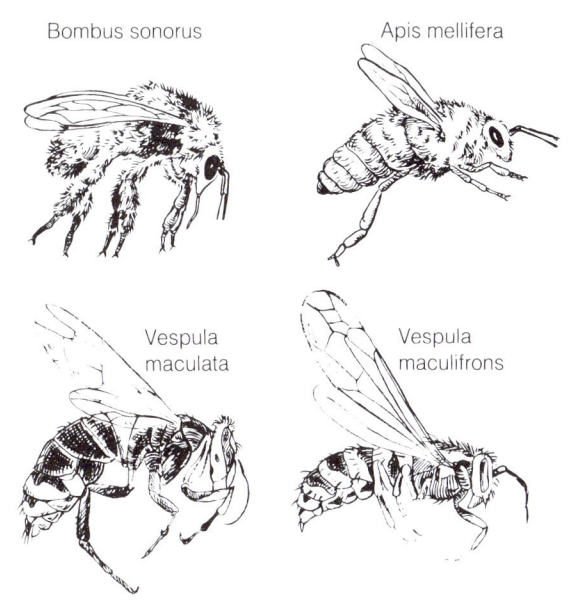

FIGURE 24-1.
Four prominent members of the order Hymenoptera that cause many anaphylactic reactions are the bumblebee (*Bombus sonorus*), honeybee (*Apis mellifera*), white-faced hornet (*Vespula maculata*), and yellow jacket (*Vespula maculifrons*).

an antigen cross-sensitivity, which means that an initial sting by any of the insects may lead to an allergic response from the sting of any of the others. Stings about the neck and head are more likely to cause a severe reaction.

In addition to the Hymenoptera order, ants (particularly some fire ant species) are becoming a major cause of both mild and severe allergic reactions. Fire ants can be found in many southern states and are spreading. They multiply rapidly, are temperamental, do not respond well to insecticides, and have well-developed abdominal stinging organs. Other insects that have been reported to cause allergic reactions include deer flies, ticks, and mosquitoes.

Various food and food additives can produce anaphylaxis. These are usually ingested, and the reaction occurs more slowly. Shellfish (shrimp, lobster), other fish (especially cod), nuts (especially peanuts), strawberries, and eggs are common culprits that cause allergic reaction. Food additives, such as tartrazine yellow (a coloring agent) and benzoic acid (an antimicrobial preservative), have been reported to cause anaphylactic reactions. Also, the substance sulfite, a preservative found in varying quantities in wines, jellies, carbonated beverages, salad bars, and other foods has been known to cause severe anaphylaxis and death.

Occasionally, highly sensitive people react to inhaled allergens. People have been reported to have had allergic reactions to the odor of fish, walnuts, and penicillin. Although unusual, cold, heat, exercise, sunlight, and human seminal fluid have also been reported to produce anaphylactic episodes.

PATHOPHYSIOLOGY

In a simple anaphylactic reaction, the antigen-antibody interaction causes mild allergic symptoms limited to usually one or two body systems and without systemic cardiovascular effects. In an anaphylactic reaction, the antigen-antibody reaction is severe. This antigen-antibody reaction occurs on the surface of specific types of white blood cells, called mast cells and basophils, and signals the release of several chemicals, primarily **histamine**. Other chemicals released that are less important include serotonin, bradykinin, and a substance called slow-reacting substance of anaphylaxis (SRS-A). These chemicals cause three primary responses: capillary dilatation, increased capillary permeability, and smooth muscle spasm. As these substances travel through the body, specific organs are affected, and the patient may exhibit any of a variety of signs and symptoms (Table 24-1).

The skin frequently is affected by the chemical mediators of the reaction, which cause urticaria (hives), itching, a red, flushed skin, a rash, and edema. This edema usually is noticed in the eyelids and lips. A sensation of warmth may accompany the signs and symptoms that affect the skin. The eyes may be itching and watery; the

TABLE 24-1.
EFFECTS OF HISTAMINE AND OTHER CHEMICALS DURING ANAPHYLAXIS

System	Signs and Symptoms
Skin	Flushing, itching, edema, hives, rash
Eyes	Itching, tearing, edema
Nose	Congestion, itching, sneezing, rhinorrhea
Upper airway	Pharyngeal or laryngeal edema or spasm, hoarseness, stridor, bronchospasm
Lower airway	Dyspnea, wheezing, use of accessory muscles to breathe, cyanosis, pulmonary edema
Cardiovascular	Tachycardia, irregular pulse, weak pulse, hypotension
Gastrointestinal	Nausea, vomiting, diarrhea, abdominal cramps
Neurologic	Anxiety, dizziness, syncope, weakness, seizure, headache

nose may be runny, congested, and itching; the patient may sneeze.

The airway may be affected with edema, including rapidly developing and severe laryngeal edema. Since the primary cause of death in anaphylaxis is airway obstruction, the paramedic must observe closely for signs of airway involvement. Stridor, choking, or tightness in the neck and throat may signal this danger. In addition to the upper airway, the entire respiratory system frequently is involved. The patient may exhibit wheezing, dyspnea, bronchospasm, coughing, hemoptysis, or pulmonary edema.

As gastrointestinal smooth muscle spasm develops, the patient may exhibit nausea, vomiting, cramping, and diarrhea. Anxiety, headache, dizziness, and a decrease in level of consciousness may ensue. These signs and symptoms may be a result of vascular collapse or central nervous system involvement. Seizures sometimes occur.

In the cardiovascular system, the increased capillary permeability displaces vascular fluid into the extravascular space. This process causes a form of hypovolemic shock, as a result of the decrease in intravascular volume. In addition, capillary dilation leads to a low resistance type of shock with peripheral pooling of blood, decreased venous return, and a fall in cardiac output. The vascular collapse and the hypotension stimulate the release of epinephrine from the adrenal medulla, the release of which is also stimulated by histamine. Tachycardia, pallor, dryness of the mouth, sweating, and other classic signs of shock are manifestations of compensatory epinephrine release and sympathetic nervous system stimulation. Cardiac arrhythmias may also occur. Supraventricular tachycardia, atrial fibrillation, premature ventricular contractions, ventricular tachycardia, and ventricular fibrillation have been reported. In addition, myocardial infarction may occur during anaphylaxis, usually secondary to shock.

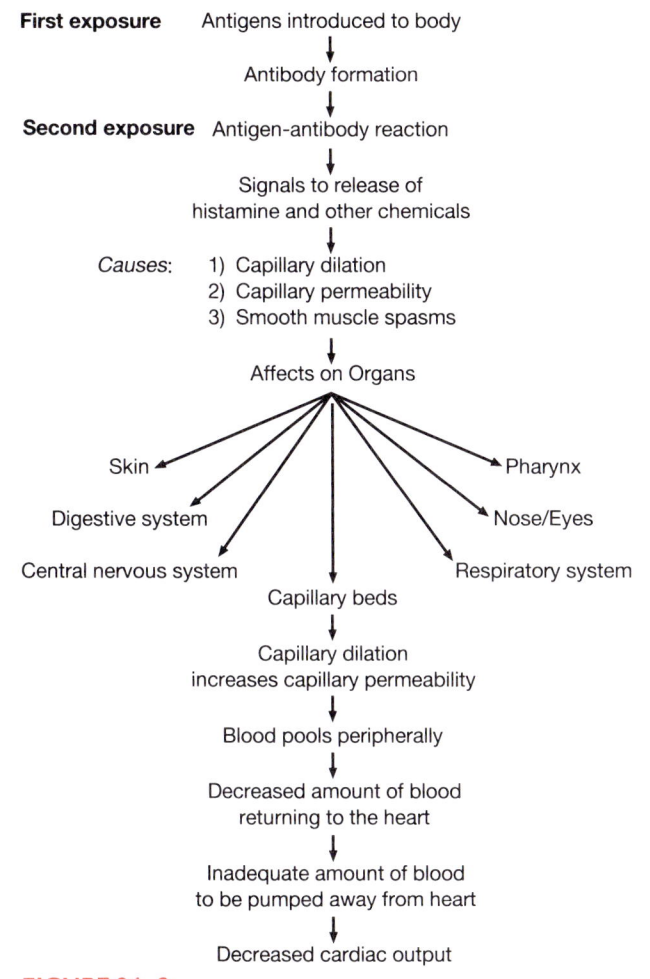

```
First exposure    Antigens introduced to body
                              ↓
                      Antibody formation
                              ↓
Second exposure   Antigen-antibody reaction
                              ↓
                      Signals to release of
                  histamine and other chemicals
                              ↓
       Causes:  1) Capillary dilation
                2) Capillary permeability
                3) Smooth muscle spasms
                              ↓
                      Affects on Organs
              ↙    ↙     ↓    ↘    ↘
        Skin                          Pharynx
     Digestive system                 Nose/Eyes
  Central nervous system          Respiratory system
                      Capillary beds
                              ↓
                     Capillary dilation
                increases capillary permeability
                              ↓
                   Blood pools peripherally
                              ↓
                 Decreased amount of blood
                     returning to the heart
                              ↓
                 Inadequate amount of blood
                to be pumped away from heart
                              ↓
                  Decreased cardiac output
```

FIGURE 24-2.
Pathophysiology of anaphylaxis.

A patient may experience symptoms within seconds after exposure to an allergen, or the reaction may be delayed for several hours. The initial signs and symptoms typically are manifest in the skin, although cardiovascular collapse and shock can occur without any skin changes. The severity of the initial signs does not correlate well with the eventual severity of the reaction.

The primary rule for any exposure is that, the earlier the onset of symptoms after exposure, the more severe the reaction is likely to be. Injected antigens can produce symptoms immediately, but they most commonly occur between 5 and 30 minutes after injection. An hour delay is unusual. Ingested antigens usually cause reactions within 2 hours. Figure 24-2 summarizes the effects of anaphylaxis.

ASSESSMENT OF THE ANAPHYLACTIC PATIENT

The patient who is suffering from anaphylaxis may seek help for a variety of reasons. If the patient has lost consciousness or is having respiratory difficulty, a family member or bystander may summon help. Severe itching, a feeling of warmth, tightness in the throat or chest, or a rash may be the first signs the patient notices. People who have experienced a prior severe anaphylactic reaction may call emergency medical services immediately after exposure, before the onset of symptoms, and may simply state that they are having an allergic reaction.

As in any situation to which paramedics respond, airway, breathing, and circulation must be immediately and quickly evaluated. Laryngeal edema may develop insidiously, as can pulmonary edema and shock. The primary survey, level of consciousness, and vital signs must be reevaluated constantly throughout management and during transportation to the hospital. The patient is likely to be anxious, and reassurance is an important part of the immediate intervention.

History should be elicited to determine when the exposure occurred, if known, and how quickly the first symptoms were noticed. This information is important to keep in mind, since as noted before the earlier the onset of symptoms, the more severe the reaction is likely to be. The cause of the reaction is known readily by some patients, such as those who were stung by a bee. Others may not be able to relate their symptoms easily to a specific cause, but questioning may reveal new medications or foods that may be the culprit. The medical history should seek information about previous reactions, with particular attention to the severity of the reaction relative to airway, breathing, and circulation. Whether or not the patient was seen in the emergency department or was hospitalized may give additional clues about the severity of past reactions. Other medical problems, especially heart disease and asthma, are important to note, as are any known allergies and any current medications. A history of heart disease or asthma should cause concern, as these patients have a higher mortality rate from anaphylaxis. Drugs such as β-blockers (e.g., propranolol) may impair the action of epinephrine and may necessitate additional therapy. The paramedic should look for medical alert tags.

The patient's environment should be assessed quickly for clues to an unknown allergen. A victim who was outside working in a garden or having a picnic when the symptoms began may be suffering from an insect bite. A victim who had recently finished a meal of shrimp might be having a reaction to that food. The specific cause is helpful, but management should not be delayed while searching for clues.

Another observation the paramedic should make about the patient's environment is to look for a self-administered epinephrine preparation. Several types are available by prescription, and physicians frequently prescribe this for their patients who are subject to anaphylaxis. Epi Pens are one type of injectable epinephrine. Inhalation products, such as Medihaler-Epi, do not achieve therapeutic systemic levels of epinephrine and may be effective only for bronchospasm. Information about the use of any medication for the allergic reaction is important, as a lower dose or temporary delay in administration of epinephrine may be indicated.

The physical examination should include a more thorough evaluation, including reassessment of the airway, breathing, and circulation. Dyspnea, stridor, coughing, and hoarseness may be related to upper airway involvement. Wheezing and dyspnea are common findings in the allergic patient, but coughing blood-tinged sputum, use of accessory muscles to breathe, and tracheal tugging signify more severe involvement of the lower respiratory tract.

Circulation should be thoroughly evaluated by the capillary refill test, evaluation of pulse rate, pulse quality, and regularity, and blood pressure measurement. As the capillaries become dilated and more permeable, the pulse quickens to compensate, and the blood pressure eventually falls.

Remember that, if the blood pressure has fallen, the patient's vascular system is no longer compensating, and the patient is in the latter stages of shock.

The patient's skin should be assessed for urticaria, flushed or ashen appearance, and for edema, either at a site of allergen injection or in the face. Continual reevaluation of these signs must be carried out. Respiratory and cardiac arrest should be appropriately treated with cardiopulmonary resuscitation as necessary.

MANAGEMENT OF ALLERGIC AND ANAPHYLACTIC REACTIONS

Some allergic reactions are mild, without respiratory problems or signs of shock. These simple reactions can be managed as follows:

1. Administer oxygen, 2 to 4 L/min.
2. Administer diphenhydramine, 25 to 100 mg IM or IV.
3. Frequently reassess airway, breathing, circulation, level of consciousness, and vital signs.
4. If respiratory involvement ensues without shock, 0.1 to 0.5 mg epinephrine 1:1000 subcutaneously may be given. Pediatric dose of epinephrine is 0.01 mg/kg. Diphenhydramine may be given IV in this case.

In the patient with severe anaphylactic reaction who is in shock, more aggressive therapy is indicated and treatment is as follows:

1. Manage airway with high-flow oxygen, intubation if necessary, and ventilation with a bag-valve-mask device if necessary.
2. Administer IV therapy of lactated Ringer's or normal saline solution; infusion rate depends on blood pressure.
3. Administer epinephrine 0.3 to 0.5 mg 1:10,000 IV, very slowly; if IV initiation is delayed for any reason, epinephrine 1:1,000, 0.3 to 0.5 mg dose may be given IM or subcutaneously; pediatric dose is 0.01 mg/kg.
4. Monitor cardiac rhythm.
5. Administer additional drug therapy as ordered: diphenhydramine, 25 to 100 mg IV. If symptoms of bronchospasm persist, administer theophylline ethylenediamine (aminophylline) at a loading dose of 6 mg/kg IV infusion, diluted in 100 mL D_5W or normal saline over a 20-minute period, if the patient has had no theophylline products in the last 36 hours. If patient has had theophylline products in the last 36 hours and symptoms of bronchospasm persist, use a loading dose of 1 mg/kg IV infusion diluted in 100 mL D_5W or normal saline over a 20-minute period. The pediatric dose for children older than 1 year is the same loading dose in D_5 0.9% NaCl.
6. Expedite transport to the hospital as soon as possible.
7. If the causative agent leaves a stinger, scrape the stinger away; do not pinch it.
8. Reevaluate airway, breathing, circulation, level of consciousness, and vital signs.
9. Inflate pneumatic antishock garment, if blood pressure remains low.

The primary goal of therapy in the patient with severe anaphylactic reaction is to restore respiratory and circulatory function. Epinephrine counteracts the effects of histamine and the other chemicals by vasoconstriction, bronchial dilation, and restoration of the tone and permeability of the vessels. Epinephrine's major side effect is the development of cardiac irritability. Intravenous administration or high doses of epinephrine may provoke serious or even fatal arrhythmias. The value of epinephrine should be weighed against the dangers in the patient with heart disease or hypertension; however, most experts agree that the drug is appropriate for the patient in anaphylactic shock or with respiratory difficulty. Very slow IV administration, subcutaneous administration (except when the patient is in profound shock or has lost consciousness), and close cardiac monitoring may help minimize problems related to epinephrine. Epinephrine is short acting and may need to be repeated every 10 to 15 minutes.

Diphenhydramine is an antihistamine that antagonizes the adverse effects of histamine and prevents further release of histamine. The usual dose is 25 to 100 mg IV for a severe anaphylactic reaction. A deep IM injection is appropriate if the reaction is not severe. The pediatric dose is 2 to 5 mg/kg. Bronchial asthma is a relative contraindication to diphenhydramine, and careful history should be taken to insure that the wheezing is not due to asthma. Pregnancy is also a contraindication. Diphenhydramine has sedative effects and may cause the patient to complain of a dry mouth.

Theophylline ethylenediamine may be used for bronchospasm that does not respond to epinephrine. Theophylline ethylenediamine is approaching toxic levels when nausea, vomiting, or other gastrointestinal symptoms occur; toxic levels or too rapid IV administration can cause cardiac arrhythmias.

PREVENTION AND PATIENT EDUCATION

When appropriate, victims of allergic and anaphylactic reactions should be encouraged to seek methods of prevention. All patients, even if their reaction is simple and self-limiting, need to seek medical care to evaluate their allergic status. This care frequently prevents misinformation about their experience and allows them to give a more accurate allergic history in the future. Some patients and prehospital personnel may understandably mistake a vasovagal reaction for an allergic reaction. This distinction is important. The patient's physician can also advise the victim about desensitization techniques and about carrying self-injectable epinephrine.

Medical alert tags can be lifesaving, particularly for patients who have severe anaphylactic reactions. The tags are available as a bracelet or necklace and usually have engraved medical information. The paramedic's encouragement of the use of these bracelets can often influence the patient and prevent or minimize future problems.

Several items can be discussed with patients to prevent insect stings. Avoiding bright colored clothing and floral perfumes can be helpful, as well as avoiding flower beds, clover fields, and picnic grounds. Shoes should be worn by sensitive people when outdoors.

SUMMARY

Allergic reactions and anaphylaxis can occur suddenly in sensitized people. A variety of allergens can cause a simple allergic reaction without systemic signs and symptoms or can cause a catastrophic anaphylactic event. Paramedics with keen observation, rapid assessment skills, and the ability to manage promptly can frequently reverse the potentially lethal effects of anaphylaxis.

SUGGESTED READING

Gupta S: Management of bee-sting anaphylaxis. Med J Aust 149:602, 1988

Kaplan AP: Allergy. New York, Churchill Livingstone, 1985

McNeil D: Exercise-induced anaphylaxis related to food intake. Ann Allergy 61:440, 1988

US Department of Transportation, National Highway Traffic Safety Administration: Emergency Medical Technician–Paramedic: National Standards Curriculum. Washington, DC, US Government Printing Office, 1985

CHAPTER 25

Toxicology and Drug and Alcohol Abuse

Poisoning and Overdose
  Poison Control Center
  **General Management of Toxico-
   logic Emergencies**
    Scene Survey
    Primary Survey
      Responsiveness
      Airway
      Breathing
      Circulation
    Secondary Survey
      History
      Level of Consciousness
      Physical Examination
    Decontamination
      Syrup of Ipecac
      Activated Charcoal
  **Specific Toxicologic Problems
   and Management**
    Caustics
      Alkalies
      Acids
      Hydrofluoric Acid

Petroleum Distillates
Alcohols
Smoke Inhalation
  Carbon Monoxide
  Cyanide
Other Toxic Inhalations
Pesticides
  Organophosphate and Carba-
   mate Insecticides
Food Poisoning
Poisonous Plants
  Mushrooms
Bites and Stings
  Arthropods
  Snake Bites
  Antivenins
  Marine Animals
Drug Overdose
  Prescription Narcotics
  Sedatives and Hypnotics
  Over-the-counter Analgesics
  Tricyclic Antidepressants
  Antipsychotics

Drug Abuse Emergencies
  Narcotics
  Stimulants
    Phencyclidine
    Amphetamine
    Phenylpropanolamine
    Cocaine
    Hallucinogens
  Solvent Abuse
  Abstinence Syndromes
Alcoholism
  Acute Intoxication
  Chronic Alcoholism
  Alcohol–Antabuse Reaction
  **Abstinence Syndromes and
   Delirium Tremens**
Summary

BEHAVIORAL OBJECTIVES
On successful completion of this chapter, the reader will be able to:

1. Explain the role of the regional poison control center in an emergency medical services (EMS) response and discuss how to access the center through existing local protocols
2. Describe the importance of the scene survey to assess the requirements for personal protection and potential patient care needs
3. Discuss the elements of the primary survey and specific management problems of toxicologic emergencies
4. Discuss the methods, limitations, and contraindications of decontamination and prevention of absorption from the skin and gastrointestinal tract
5. Describe the pathophysiology and management of specific toxicologic problems, such as caustics, hydrocarbons, smoke and toxic inhalation, pesticides, food poisoning, poisonous plants, and stings and bites

(continued)

BEHAVIORAL OBJECTIVES (continued)

6. Describe the pathophysiology and management of specific classes of drug overdose, such as narcotics, sedatives and hypnotics, salicylates and acetaminophen, tricyclic antidepressants, and antipsychotics
7. Describe the pathophysiology and management of acute drug abuse emergencies that involve narcotics, stimulants, solvents, and abstinence syndromes
8. Discuss the pathophysiology and management of acute ethanol intoxication
9. Define all of the key terms listed in this chapter

KEY TERMS
The following terms are defined in the chapter and glossary:

abstinence syndromes
acetaminophen
acid
activated charcoal
alcoholism
alkali
amphetamine
Antabuse
antipsychotic
carbon monoxide
caustic
cocaine
cyanide
decontamination
delirium tremens
ethanol
hallucinogens
hydrofluoric acid
hypnotics
narcotics
petroleum distillates
phencyclidine
phenylpropanolamine
poison control center
salicylates
sedatives
syrup of ipecac
tricyclic antidepressants

The likelihood that one will be exposed to toxins in the home or work place is increasing. Over-the-counter and prescription medications are common in the home. About two thirds of physician's visits result in a prescription. Household chemicals are a hazard, many times designed to have a pleasant odor and color. Industrial chemicals offer another dimension of potential toxic exposures. These chemicals may involve a single victim or may create a triage problem in a hazardous materials incident.

Overall, most toxic exposures occur in the home. About 47% of exposures reported occur in children between the ages of 1 and 3 years. About 90% of all reported poisonings are accidental. More than 65% are asymptomatic or produce only minor symptoms. The other reported toxic exposures involve newborns, adolescents, and adults. In adolescents and adults, intentional toxic exposures can occur. Although deaths from poisoning and drug overdose are not frequent, intentional toxic exposures tend to have a higher death rate and result in more serious symptoms than accidental exposures or adverse drug reactions. The most commonly encountered route of exposure is by ingestion of a toxic substance. A typical toxicologic emergency that results in an EMS response is a suicide attempt or gesture in the form of an oral drug overdose. Acute drug abuse emergencies may account for a significant number of urban EMS responses but are certainly not unique to urban EMS. The most common prehospital toxicologic problem, but the least likely to be thought of this way, is alcohol intoxication.

All three of these problems, attempted suicide, drug abuse, and alcoholism, represent medical and psychosocial problems that extend beyond the immediate prehospital-care emergency. Management of toxicologic emergencies is aimed at the specific symptoms and organ systems involved. At times, a specific treatment or antidote is available, but not usually. An additional step that follows the usual priorities of securing a patent airway and maintaining adequate ventilation and circulation is an effort at decontamination. This step may be as immediate as removing the victim from a toxic environment, or it may involve the removal of ingested substances from the patient's gastrointestinal tract.

POISONING AND OVERDOSE

Poison Control Center

When information about a poisoning or drug overdose is not readily available, the **poison control center** is a valuable resource. Poison control centers are designed to answer questions from health care professionals and the public. Many times, they can evaluate a nontoxic or mildly toxic exposure by telephone, instruct the caller in the use of syrup of ipecac to induce vomiting, and check on the progress by follow-up telephone calls. These abilities can make a hospital visit or EMS response unnecessary. In questionable or more potentially serious toxic exposures, the poison control center can be consulted from the hospital emergency department or from the emergency scene. Exactly how a poison control center is consulted from the scene depends on the design and protocol of local EMS communications. A poison control center may be called directly when a telephone is available, by cellular phone, or may be consulted through the base hospital medical control. The advantage of establishing contact through the base hospital is that the paramedics at the scene need only talk with one source, rather than juggle multiple communications. This system also allows better coordination between information obtained and management given to the patient.

The American Association of Poison Control Centers has established standards and recognizes regional poison control centers throughout the country. These centers are staffed by physicians, nurses, and pharmacists who are specifically trained or experienced in collecting information from a caller and retrieving information from many sources. In addition, records are kept on all calls made to a center. These records allow trends in toxicologic problems to be recognized. From this data collection, steps can be taken to identify solutions to changing toxic hazards to the public. Regional poison control centers are available to provide assistance 24 hours a day.

General Management of Toxicologic Emergencies

Few toxic substances have specific antidotes. As a result, management of the toxicologic emergency is aimed at the signs and symptoms present and organ systems involved. Decontamination and prevention of further absorption is done once the patient is relatively stable and the initial priorities have been addressed. The box "Routes of Exposure and Absorption" shows the various routes of entry of a poison into the body.

Scene Survey

As with any prehospital emergency, the first priority is to minimize hazards to the rescuers. Environmental hazards may be part of the toxicologic emergency. Gaining access and removing a victim from a hazardous environment requires protective gear. Structural fire fighting turnout gear and a self-contained breathing apparatus are basic to personal protection. Hazardous materials incidents require specialized protective gear.

ROUTES OF EXPOSURE AND ABSORPTION
Ingestion
- Most common
- Ingestion of drugs, household products, plants, contaminated food
- Absorption must occur across gastrointestinal mucosa before toxic effects occur
- Stomach can act as reservoir for continued absorption of large doses
- Most gastrointestinal absorption occurs in small intestine
- Early manifestations may be gastrointestinal or upper airway signs and symptoms
- Decontamination by dilution, emesis, activated charcoal

Inhalation
- Rapid absorption
- Noxious fumes from gases
- Upper and lower airway signs and symptoms may precede systemic toxicity; upper airway edema, laryngospasm, bronchospasm, pulmonary edema
- Hypoxia may be due to toxic effects or asphyxiation by displacement of air by gases, vapors, aerosols, or dusts
- Victim rescue may require full protective gear, including respiratory protection (*e.g.*, self-contained breathing apparatus)
- Move the patient to fresh air; use supplemental oxygen

Injection
- Immediate (intravenous) or rapid (intramuscular, subcutaneous) absorption
- Includes bites and stings; intravenous drug overdose
- Rapid onset of systemic symptoms, or causes intense local tissue destruction
- Immobilize extremity; provide basic life support

Cutaneous
- Slowest absorption, increased when skin is disrupted
- Contact with corrosives (*e.g.*, acids, alkalies)
- Local effects include cutaneous burns, blisters, erythema, contact dermatitis
- Remove clothing, dust off dry materials, flush with water

Primary Survey

RESPONSIVENESS. Rapid neurologic assessment can be accomplished by determining whether the patient is alert or unresponsive. This finding is important in the assessment of the toxicologic emergency. Many substances can cause impairment in the patient's overall level of responsiveness.

AIRWAY. Maintaining a patent airway is the highest medical priority. Patients who are sleepy but arousable or unconscious but responsive to stimulation of the posterior pharynx present a problem. In these situations, a nasopharyngeal airway may be tolerated when an oropharyngeal airway will not. A bag-valve-mask device and endotracheal tube should be on hand to assist ventilation if needed.

BREATHING. Many toxic substances depress ventilation. Inhalation of vapors or gases can cause physical injury to the oral pharynx and respiratory epithelium, resulting in edema and possibly airway obstruction. Aside from inadequate ventilation, other pulmonary problems may be part of a toxicologic emergency. Some drugs or chemicals, whether inhaled, injected, or ingested, can cause pulmonary edema. This form of pulmonary edema results from an increase in pulmonary capillary permeability so that fluid can enter the tissue between the alveoli and the alveoli themselves. Aspiration is another potential complication of toxic ingestions. Emesis may occur spontaneously without being induced. If emesis happens in a patient whose level of consciousness is declining and before rescuers arrive, the airway will be unprotected and aspiration is likely. Substances with a high volatility and low surface tension, as some hydrocarbons, can be aspirated even without emesis. A patient who has ingested a hydrocarbon and is coughing can be assumed to have aspirated.

CIRCULATION. The usual signs of circulatory insufficiency, such as pallor, diaphoresis, weakness, confusion, restlessness, and loss of consciousness, must be interpreted carefully when a toxic exposure is suspected. Toxic effects of drugs or chemicals can inhibit or enhance these signs. Hypotension in a toxicologic emergency can be due to arrhythmias, direct myocardial depression, vasodilation, or hypovolemia from trauma or loss of fluid into the lungs from acute pulmonary edema.

Secondary Survey

HISTORY. Many times the conclusion that a patient's problem is a toxicologic one is reached based on history alone. Establishing a toxicologic history is easy if the patient was seen ingesting or exposed to a toxin. Sometimes, however, suspicion may be the only guide. A few circumstances should trigger suspicion of a toxicologic problem: any patient with a psychiatric history; a trauma victim, especially a young one; coma of unknown cause; arrhythmias in a young person without a history; fire victims; children with unexplained lethargy or any unusual presentation; any patient with multiple, seemingly unrelated symptoms.

Once a toxicologic problem is suspected, an attempt can be made to identify the substance involved. Up to this point, management has been aimed at the presenting symptoms, and it may have to continue in this manner. If a container or sample of the suspected substance is available, it should be kept with the patient. An idea of the dose involved and the time since the ingestion or exposure should be obtained. Sometimes a patient intentionally ingests a drug, but not enough to be toxic. Although not necessarily a medical emergency, suicidal ideation or gesture is a behavioral emergency and becomes a different priority for the EMS responders.

LEVEL OF CONSCIOUSNESS. A common sign of a toxic exposure is a change in the level of consciousness. It is difficult or impossible to differentiate an altered level of consciousness in a victim with toxic exposure from that observed in a victim with head trauma. Since toxicologic problems and trauma may occur together, it is always wise to consider head and spinal trauma in any patient with altered consciousness. Toxic effects on the central nervous system (CNS) and alertness can range from delirium, such as confusion, hallucinations, delusions, disorientation, tremulousness, and aggressiveness, to unresponsiveness. These changes in consciousness also can be caused by problems other than those due to toxins or trauma. Metabolic derangements, such as ketoacidosis, uremia, and hypoglycemia, and nontraumatic CNS structural disorders like stroke can alter consciousness. Hypoxia can also alter the level of consciousness; however, establishing an airway and maintaining adequate ventilation and circulation are priorities that already should have been addressed by this stage of patient care.

Two causes of altered consciousness that can be reversed quickly are hypoglycemia and narcotic overdose. Therefore, early management steps are aimed at these problems. In any patient with an altered level of consciousness for which the cause is not evident, potential hypoglycemia is treated with 50% dextrose and potential narcotic overdose is treated with naloxone (Narcan). Naloxone also reverses respiratory depression due to narcotics. The 50% dextrose and naloxone should be given a minute or so apart to determine which was the effective drug if the patient's level of consciousness improves. The use of 50% dextrose in stroke victims has been controversial. It is argued that 50% dextrose can alter the viscosity of blood and worsen a stroke caused by an intracerebral bleed. There is also concern that elevated blood glucose levels can have an adverse effect on cerebral ischemic states by worsening cerebral intracellular acidosis.

Seizures may occur from hypoxia due to respiratory depression or from direct toxic effects. A single seizure may be self-limiting and require no specific treatment. Continued seizure activity may require control with diazepam (Valium), with the recognition of the potential need for subsequent ventilatory support. The Glasgow Coma Scale shown in Appendix C is used to report a patient's level of consciousness. The eye, motor, and verbal responses assessed by the Glasgow Coma Scale are useful to describe the level of consciousness in a toxicologic emergency. Unlike with a head injury, however, the Glasgow Coma Scale has no prognostic value in toxic or metabolic emergencies. A victim of a toxic exposure may have a low score on the Glasgow Coma Scale but still recover completely.

PHYSICAL EXAMINATION. A few observations during the secondary survey may be helpful in a toxicologic emergency. The odor of an ingested product may be detectable on the breath. Odor or presence of product on the victim's clothes or chemical burns of the skin or mouth may point to the degree or route of exposure. Needle tracks, bruises at injection sites, or burns related to drug paraphernalia also may be clues. Chronic abuse of some sedative and hypnotic drugs may cause cutaneous blisters. Specific physical findings associated with certain drugs or chemicals are discussed later in the chapter. In general, physical findings mostly help to support a history of suspected toxic exposure.

Decontamination

Corrosives can cause injury by direct contact with the eye, skin, or upper gastrointestinal and respiratory tracts. A substance that causes organ system toxicity, however, first has to be absorbed. For **decontamination,** skin and eyes with gross contamination should first be dusted off and then washed off with large amounts of water after removal of contaminated clothing. Because the eyelids have contours in which alkalies and other chemicals can be trapped and cause harm because of their extensive corrosive action, the eye should be flushed for 20 minutes or more. The most common skin and eye exposures are acids from exploding car batteries, alkalies such as lye, pesticides from both agricultural and commercial use, and mace.

SYRUP OF IPECAC. **Syrup of ipecac** is the most effective way to induce emesis. Poison control centers and pediatricians encourage parents to keep syrup of ipecac in the home but not to use it without the advice of their physician or poison control center. An informed and motivated parent may have already given syrup of ipecac before the paramedic arrives. Syrup of ipecac is derived from a plant; its components are absorbed in the small intestine and act on the region of the brain stem that triggers vomiting. The dose for syrup of ipecac is shown in the box "Syrup of Ipecac." Once the initial dose is administered, emesis usually is induced within about 20 minutes. If no emesis occurs, the dose can be repeated once. Inducing emesis is not recommended in children younger than 6 months of age without consulting a physician or poison control center. Before administering syrup of ipecac, however, a few considerations must be made.

By far the most important consideration is to protect the airway. The patient has to be awake and have an intact gag reflex and has to stay awake for as long as eme-

SYRUP OF IPECAC
Dose

Less than 6 months: do not give

6 months–1 year: 10 mL (2 teaspoons) with 2–4 oz clear fluid

1 year–5 years: 15 mL (3 teaspoons or 1 tablespoon) with 4–8 oz clear fluid

5 years–12 years: 15–30 mL (3–6 teaspoons or 1–2 tablespoons) with 8–16 oz clear fluid

12 years or older: 30 mL (6 teaspoons or 2 tablespoons) with 8–16 oz clear fluid

Repeat once if no emesis occurs within 30 minutes
Note: 5 mL = 1 teaspoon, 15 mL = 1 tablespoon, 1 tablespoon = 3 teaspoons

Contraindications

Coma

Absent gag reflex

Seizures

Caustic ingestion (acids, alkalies)

Sharp object ingestion

Strychnine, camphor ingestion (rapid onset of seizures)

Tricyclic antidepressant, narcotic ingestion (rapid loss of consciousness)

Hydrocarbon ingestion less than 1 mL/kg (unless it contains toxic solute)

Relative Contraindications

Myocardial infarction

Bleeding disorder (cirrhosis, thrombocytopenia)

---

sis can be expected (up to about an hour). If the patient is sleepy but easily arousable, the use of syrup of ipecac should be questioned. If the patient is slow to arouse or unarousable, syrup of ipecac should not be given. If syrup of ipecac has been given to the patient before the EMS arrival and the patient is now sleepy, the patient should be placed in a head-down left lateral position. If emesis occurs, aspiration is less likely in this position. Gastric lavage is the only way to remove a toxic substance from an unresponsive patient and is not a prehospital treatment. A patient who has ingested caustics such as strong acid or alkali should not be given syrup of ipecac because of the considerable injury that can occur to the esophagus. Also, patients who are having seizures or who are at risk for seizure are not given syrup of ipecac. Although the occurrence is rare, a patient who has ingested solid sharp objects, such as glass or nails, should not be made to vomit.

Some ingested drugs can cause a rapid change in the status of the patient. Ingested narcotics can cause a loss of consciousness, and tricyclic antidepressants can cause seizures, loss of consciousness, and arrhythmias. Strychnine (in some rodenticides) or camphor can cause seizures. All of these reactions can occur suddenly, so syrup of ipecac should not be used. Instead, these drug ingestions warrant gastric lavage.

Hydrocarbons are a special case. Because of their viscosity, they are easily aspirated, even in a conscious person; therefore, emesis usually is contraindicated. The exception to the no-emesis rule, however, is granted when the ingested hydrocarbon has another toxic substance dissolved in it, like a pesticide or heavy metal. Paramedics should be aware of their local poison control center guidelines regarding hydrocarbon ingestions and the use of syrup of ipecac.

ACTIVATED CHARCOAL. Neither emesis nor lavage can remove a drug or chemical that has made its way to the small intestine. Therefore, once the stomach has been decontaminated, further absorption in the small intestine must be prevented. In prehospital care, absorption is prevented by the administration of **activated charcoal.** Activated charcoal, with its large absorptive surface, can be given by the nasogastric tube after lavage or orally after emesis has stopped. Charcoal can absorb the components of syrup of ipecac, so the two should not be given together. Activated charcoal is available as a suspension of powder, which is mixed with water (one part activated charcoal to four parts water). The dose for children and adults is 1 to 2 g/kg body weight (see the box "Activated Charcoal"). One general exception to the routine use of activated charcoal is that it should not be administered when a specific oral antidote is to be given. Activated charcoal will absorb the antidote, diminishing its effectiveness. The most common situation in which an oral antidote may be administered is in an acetaminophen (*e.g.*, Tylenol) overdose. Acetaminophen blood levels and other metabolic monitoring determine the need for the antidote.

ACTIVATED CHARCOAL
Dose

Adult and child: 1–2 g/kg

If not in premixed slurry, mix one part charcoal with four parts water

Contraindications

Do not give until ipecac-induced emesis has stopped

If specific oral antidote is used (*e.g.*, acetaminophen ingestion)

Specific Toxicologic Problems and Management
Caustics

When a **caustic** substance has been ingested, treatment is cautious. An attempt to neutralize the acid or alkali should never be made. The *exothermic* (heat-generating) reactions can cause more damage. Syrup of ipecac should not be used. One sip of plain water should be offered and transport expedited. Back pain may indicate an esophageal perforation. Alkalies are more serious because they hydrolyze proteins and literally eat through tissue. Visible damage may be delayed for an hour or longer; therefore, it should not be assumed that everything is fine because no burns or pain are visible. In the worst case, the immediate emergency may be airway management. Sufficient injury to the posterior pharynx, epiglottis, and larynx may compromise the airway and make endotracheal intubation difficult or even hazardous. This patient may require a surgical airway.

ALKALIES. Accidental ingestion by children of a household **alkali** is the most common toxic exposure, although lye is frequently used in suicide attempts. If the product is gulped by the child, burns to the mouth may be minimal compared to those in the esophagus. A history of alkali ingestion with only mild injury to the mouth and oral cavity in a child who cannot swallow indicates potentially serious esophageal burns. Drain opener, oven cleaner, and electric dishwasher detergent are the strongest common household alkalies. Clinitest tablets used by diabetics to test their glucose concentration at home can cause alkali burns when ingested. Household bleach is not caustic, but household ammonia can produce significant oral and esophageal injury.

ACIDS. In contrast to alkalies, many **acid** exposures involve automotive or industrial accidents; ingestion may be seen occasionally in a suicide attempt. Many acid-based home cleaning chemicals also are available, such as Lime Away and nonscratch cleaners. Sulfuric acid from car or boat batteries and industrial exposure to hydrochloric, nitric, or phosphoric acids can cause skin or eye burns. Continuous irrigation is the most important management step. Acid fumes can cause upper airway burns and edema.

HYDROFLUORIC ACID. A special case of acid exposure is **hydrofluoric acid,** a strong acid like the others that causes the same kinds of injury. The additional danger with hydrofluoric acid, however, is the fluoride ion. Fluoride inhibits enzymes of cell metabolism and binds calcium. The fluoride ion can be absorbed through the skin or gastrointestinal tract if the acid or other fluoride salt is ingested. The fluoride ion can combine with calcium in the blood, causing hypocalcemia. This condition can cause seizures and cardiac arrhythmias, including ventricular fibrillation. In addition to the usual management of arrhythmias, calcium chloride can be given as a slow intravenous (IV) bolus (10 mL of 10% calcium chloride).

Hydrofluoric acid ingestion can cause gastric perforation and gastrointestinal bleeding, leading to hypovolemic shock. Industrial exposure to fluoride can occur through many fluoride salts. Commercial or household exposure is most common through rust removers, insecticides (roach powder), and rodenticides. Unlike other acids, hydrofluoric acid penetrates deep into tissues and causes intense pain at the site of exposure. However, if the patient is exposed to a relatively dilute solution, progressive pain may not be noticed until hours after the initial exposure.

Petroleum Distillates

Accidental ingestion of **petroleum distillates** accounts for a number of poisoning deaths in children younger than 5 years of age. The most commonly ingested petroleum distillates are kerosene, pine oil products, gasoline (from siphoning), and lighter fluids. Although kerosene may be colored for fuel in ornamental lamps and pine oil products can smell good, it seems that the reason these otherwise unpleasant products are ingested by children is because adults store them in beverage bottles and leave them in reach of children. These products have a low *viscosity* (resistance to flow) and high *volatility* (tendency to evaporate rapidly), making pulmonary toxicity the primary risk. Aspiration and subsequent hypoxia can be the immediate emergency. Sometimes ingestion of petroleum distillates can result in coma, seizures, and cardiac arrhythmias. Coughing is a sign of potential aspiration, and wheezing may result from bronchospasm. Epinephrine and theophylline ethylenediamine may be dangerous to use to treat bronchospasm because hydrocarbons can sensitize the myocardium to their actions and cause ventricular arrhythmias.

If drug therapy for bronchospasm is needed, it is better to use a β_2-stimulating drug, such as terbutaline (Brethine) or metaproterenol (Alupent), which has less effect on the myocardium. Inducing emesis is contraindicated unless the ingested amount is large (greater than 1 mL/kg) or the petroleum distillate contains a toxic substance dissolved in it. Inducing emesis is contraindicated whenever red furniture polish (mineral seal oil) is ingested because of its low viscosity and the likelihood of aspiration.

Alcohols

The challenge of poisoning by alcohols other than **ethanol** (ethyl alcohol) to prehospital care providers is recognition. Initial suspicion of ingestion of methanol, isopropanol, or ethylene glycol may be based on history alone. The toxicity of these alcohols is due to their metabolites.

Methanol (methyl alcohol) and ethylene glycol can cause a serious metabolic acidosis. Methanol and ethylene glycol are most commonly encountered in the home as automotive products; methanol is found in windshield washer fluid and gasoline antifreeze and ethylene glycol in radiator antifreeze. It has been reported that 5 mL of methanol caused blindness in one adult. Metabolism is slower than for ethanol, so symptoms can be delayed for hours. Ethylene glycol is metabolized more rapidly than methanol and may have a more rapid onset of symptoms.

Isopropanol (isopropyl alcohol) is found in rubbing alcohol and cosmetic and shaving products. Isopropanol produces effects of half the blood level of ethanol. Accidental ingestion can occur in the home, but these alcohols have been used in suicide attempts and by destitute alcoholics who cannot afford another drink. Children have been accidentally poisoned by well-intentioned but uninformed parents who use rubbing alcohol to sponge their febrile child.

Because ethanol absorption is so rapid, syrup of ipecac usually does not help prevent absorption. Milk may reduce ethanol-induced gastric irritation and temporarily delay absorption. The major problem with ethanol is hypoglycemia. This can be managed by offering the patient a sugar substitute.

Smoke Inhalation

Toxic inhalation can result in absorption virtually as fast as IV injection. Unlike ingestion, the toxic substance cannot be removed from the absorption site, the lungs, once inhalation has occurred. Industrial and commercial accidents can result in a toxicologic emergency by inhalation of a large number of chemicals; a common toxic emergency, however, is smoke inhalation.

By far, most fire deaths result from smoke inhalation rather than burns. In fact, the burns on a victim found during body recovery may have occurred postmortem. On the other hand, the management of a burn victim who was injured by a fire in a closed space should include consideration of smoke inhalation. Incomplete combustion of synthetic fabrics and plastics in furnishings and synthetic polymers in building materials can produce many toxic gases and particulates. Ironically, fire retardant fabrics and building materials resist combustion but promote *pyrolysis* (chemical change produced by heat), which generates toxic gases, such as hydrogen cyanide, carbon monoxide, aromatic hydrocarbons, phosgene, and hydrogen chloride. Smoke inhalation can be a medical emergency because of asphyxia from the displacement of air, direct pulmonary injury from heated or caustic gases, and organ system toxicity from toxic gases.

CARBON MONOXIDE. In addition to smoke inhalation, **carbon monoxide** poisoning can occur from gas or kerosene space heaters or any combustion engine that operates in an enclosed space. Carbon monoxide binds with hemoglobin, making it unavailable to transport oxygen. Because of this process, the organs affected by carbon monoxide first are those that use oxygen rapidly, the heart and brain. Early signs and symptoms of exposure include headache, nausea and vomiting, and visual disturbances followed by syncope, tachypnea, tachycardia, seizures, coma, and cardiopulmonary arrest. The definitive treatment for this exposure is the administration of 100% oxygen by a nonrebreathing face mask or tracheal intubation. Ventilation with 100% oxygen when ventilatory assistance is needed displaces carbon monoxide from hemoglobin. Ventricular arrhythmias that do not respond to oxygenation can be treated with lidocaine. Hyperbaric oxygen therapy may be considered for comatose patients with carbon monoxide poisoning; these patients may need to be transported to a hospital with a recompression chamber.

CYANIDE. *Cyanide* exposure may occur in several ways. Industrial exposures to hydrogen cyanide gas can be accidental, or ingestion of a cyanide salt may occur in a suicide attempt. Household exposure may occur by the accidental ingestion of silver polish or some rodenticides. The seeds of many fruits contain amygdalin, which, when metabolized, releases cyanide. Synthetic amygdalin (Laetrile) has been a controversial treatment for cancer. Inhaled or ingested cyanide can cause death within minutes to hours. The role of cyanide in fire deaths from smoke inhalation may be underestimated.

Carbon monoxide primarily prevents the transport of oxygen by hemoglobin. Cyanide allows oxygen transport but prevents the use of oxygen by the tissues. Together, carbon monoxide and cyanide can potentiate the effects of each other. Both can contribute to the mental confusion of fire victims during escape attempts. It has been suggested that unresponsive smoke inhalation victims should be treated empirically for cyanide inhalation. For cyanide ingestions, and inhalations if the patient is still alive, treatment is specific. A cyanide antidote kit (Eli Lilly and Company, Indianapolis, IN) is available and should be used according to local protocols. The kit contains amyl nitrite inhalants, 3% sodium nitrite injection, and 25% sodium thiosulfate injection. The nitrites are used to form *methemoglobin* from hemoglobin. Methemoglobin can then carry cyanide (as *cyanmethemoglobin*) and allow less cyanide to bind to the enzymes in cells that convert oxygen to energy. The sodium thiosulfate reacts with cyanide to form essentially nontoxic thiocyanate, which is then excreted in the urine. The sequence is to quickly give the amyl nitrite by inhalation, then establish an IV and give the sodium nitrite and sodium thiosulfate by injection. Intervention must be quick, as cyanide intoxication can be rapidly fatal.

Cyanide poisoning is treated as shown in the box "Management of Cyanide Poisoning." Two amyl nitrite inhalants crushed in a gauze pad and held about an inch

MANAGEMENT OF CYANIDE POISONING
Airway
Tracheal intubation as necessary

Breathing
100% O$_2$

Assist ventilation as necessary

Circulation
CPR as necessary

Cyanide Antidote Kit
Two amyl nitrite inhalants in gauze
    inhalation 15–30 seconds each minute

3% sodium nitrite (stop amyl nitrite)
    Adults: 10 mL slow IV push over 2–4 minutes
    Children: 0.2 mL/kg up to 10 mL over 5 minutes
    If hypotension occurs: Trendelenburg position, IV fluids, dopamine, stop nitrite

25% sodium thiosulfate
    Adults: 50 mL IV bolus
    Children: 5 mL sodium thiosulfate per 1 mL sodium nitrite given

---

from the victim's nose or under an oxygen mask for 15 to 30 seconds each minute form enough methemoglobin for immediate care. If the patient has to be ventilated, the gauze pad can be placed inside the face mask or held at the intake part of the bag-valve-mask device. Sodium nitrite is given as a 10 mL (300 mg) slow IV push over 2 to 4 minutes (to prevent sudden profound hypotension). This treatment is followed by a 50 mL (12.5 g) IV bolus of sodium thiosulfate.

Nitrites, which are potent vasodilators, may pose other potential problems. The sodium nitrite injection can result in significant hypotension, enough to warrant the use of dopamine. One way to treat the cyanide toxicity but avoid the hypotension in prehospital care is to use only the amyl nitrite and sodium thiosulfate. Inducing emesis or gastric lavage is only attempted after giving the antidote and is not done in the prehospital setting.

Other Toxic Inhalations

Even gases and vapors that have no organ system toxicity can cause asphyxia when they displace air in an enclosed space. For example, methane and carbon dioxide found in sewer gas and silos can cause asphyxia. Sewer gas also contains hydrogen sulfide, which reduces the oxygen-carrying capacity of hemoglobin. Flammable asphyxiant gases, such as methane, butane, and propane, also pose an explosion hazard. Silo gas contains nitrogen oxides formed by the degradation of fertilizers that can cause severe pulmonary edema. Anhydrous ammonia and chlorine can cause pulmonary injury and cutaneous chemical burns. Ammonia and chlorine may represent a hazardous materials transportation emergency. In addition, a leak in a chlorine storage tank at a swimming pool may be a triage problem. Mixing bleach with an acid can release chlorine and cause a household exposure to toxic fumes. In addition to airway control and oxygenation, dyspnea and wheezing from bronchospasm after a toxic inhalation may be treated with aminophylline.

Another potential triage problem is exposure to tear gas (CS, CN or CR gas). In general, once the victim is clear of the exposure, removal of contaminated clothing, irrigation of the eyes with water or saline, and washing of exposed skin relieve the discomfort. The effects of CS and CR gas are shorter than those of CN gas (mace). An inflammatory reaction in the eyes may last for days after exposure to CN gas, and direct eye contact with this agent from discharge of the canister can cause permanent damage to the cornea. Staying upwind and wearing gloves may limit personal discomfort during initial decontamination of a victim.

Pesticides

Pesticides (*i.e.*, insecticides, herbicides, and rodenticides) are a diverse group of chemicals. Of the insecticides, the majority of poisonings are due to the organophosphates. As expected, most poisonings occur in agricultural areas, but household versions of these insecticides are available, although they are also the least toxic. Carbamate insecticides have toxic effects similar to those of the organophosphates. The organochlorine insecticide lindane is important to mention because it is the active ingredient in Kwell, which is used to treat body lice. Household insect sprays may contain pyrethrins, which are plant derivatives of low toxicity. The diluted form of herbicides, such as paraquat and diquat, are considered potentially dangerous, and accidental or intentional ingestion of the concentrate can cause pulmonary toxicity or central nervous system disorders that may be fatal. Herbicides such as 2,4D and 2,4,5T (components of Agent Orange) may cause cancer and skin disorders, but rarely acute toxicity. Some fungicides are similar to the drug disulfiram (Antabuse) and can cause an alcohol-disulfiram reaction if alcohol is also involved in the poisoning (see the later discussion under Alcoholism). Rodenticides may contain strychnine, yellow phosphorous, or warfarin anticoagulants. Strychnine ingestion causes protracted seizures that may not respond to diazepam or phenobarbital.

ORGANOPHOSPHATE AND CARBAMATE INSECTICIDES. The most common insecticides involved in toxicologic problems are the organophosphate and carbamate insecticides. They are chemically unstable and are degraded once applied so that they do not accumulate in the environment. Toxicologic emergencies can result from accidental agricultural, industrial, or home exposure or from a hazardous materials transportation incident. Many reported organophosphate and carbamate insecticide exposures are from suicide attempts. Children are susceptible to accidental exposure anytime these products are improperly stored. These insecticides are absorbed well by all routes of exposure: inhalation, ingestion, and contact with skin and eyes.

The carbamates differ from the organophosphates in organ system toxicity because they do not penetrate the CNS and, therefore, do not cause CNS toxicity. Both act by inhibiting the enzyme acetylcholinesterase, which is involved in modulating nerve impulse transmission in the neuromuscular junction, where motor nerves stimulate skeletal muscle, and in the autonomic nervous system, in postganglionic parasympathetic nerves, and in both sympathetic and parasympathetic ganglia. The ganglia act as switching stations for these nerves before they go out to the organs they affect. Unlike the organophosphates, which irreversibly bind to acetylcholinesterase, the carbamates bind reversibly, and their effects are shorter and less severe. The symptoms of these insecticide poisonings all relate to the accumulation of acetylcholine in the central and peripheral nervous systems.

The easiest way to remember some of the signs of acetylcholinesterase inhibition is with the acronym *SLUD*: salivation, lacrimation, urination, and diarrhea. Central nervous system toxicity can cause anxiety, confusion, toxic psychosis, seizures, and unconsciousness. Peripheral and autonomic nervous system toxicity can cause pupillary constriction, blurred vision, wheezing from bronchoconstriction, muscle twitching and weakness, diaphoresis, and SLUD. Heart rate and blood pressure can go up or down. The most useful signs of serious toxicity are pupillary constriction, altered level of consciousness, muscle twitching (or paralysis), wheezing, diaphoresis, and SLUD.

The general principles of management take on new dimensions when organophosphate and carbamate insecticides are involved in the toxicologic emergency. Decontamination not only prevents further absorption by the patient but is a means of personal protection. If the patient vomits or emesis is induced for ingestion of the insecticide, contact with the vomitus should be avoided. In addition to the usual considerations of managing the airway, suction may be frequently necessary to keep up with the excessive salivation and pulmonary secretions. Respiratory distress from bronchospasm and obstruction due to bronchial secretions may require ventilatory assistance. If the patient is conscious and the airway protected, inducing emesis may be appropriate even when the ingested insecticide was dissolved in a hydrocarbon.

The definitive prehospital treatment of bronchospasm and hypersecretion is atropine. Inadequate ventilation due to bronchospasm and pulmonary secretions may represent the immediate emergency. Because of the potential for arrhythmias, theophylline ethylenediamine is contraindicated. In fact, adequate oxygenation may not be possible until atropine is given. Hypoxia may be contributing to the arrhythmias, so the electrocardiogram should be monitored as soon as is practical. The doses of atropine needed to control symptoms may be much greater than those used to treat bradyarrhythmias. The initial dose of atropine is 2 mg for an adult (0.05 mg/kg for children) repeated in 15 minutes if no effect is seen. Since the insecticide is inhibiting acetylcholinesterase, an excess of acetylcholine will be present. This effect is blocked by atropine. Atropine is continued in 2 mg increments every 15 to 60 minutes until the patient's skin appears flushed, the secretions in the mouth and lungs (clear to auscultation) regress, and the pupils dilate. Heart rate is not a reliable indicator of sufficient atropine doses. Tachycardia or bradycardia may be present before atropine is given. Atropine improves the respiratory status of the patient, which is the first priority, but does not stop the skeletal muscle twitching.

Food Poisoning

Food poisoning can occur when food or water is contaminated by certain bacteria or protozoa or by the presence of toxins produced by bacteria. Toxins that affect the gastrointestinal tract alone are called *enterotoxins*, but other toxins can be absorbed and cause organ system toxicity. The immediate vomiting and diarrhea may be the cause of prehospital problems when symptoms are severe. Syncope and weakness may be the chief complaints, and hypotension with electrolyte imbalance may be the immediate problem that requires treatment. The patient may present with pallor, diaphoresis, orthostatic vital sign changes or overt tachycardia, and hypotension. Cardiac arrhythmias and dyspnea may occur, particularly in the elderly or in patients with underlying cardiopulmonary disease. In general, the signs and symptoms of food poisoning include nausea, vomiting, abdominal pain or cramping, and diarrhea, although not all of these need occur simultaneously. Some types of food poisoning cause more upper gastrointestinal upset (nausea, vomiting) and others cause more lower gastrointestinal upset (abdominal pain, diarrhea). Treatment is aimed at managing hypovolemia with lactated Ringer's or normal saline infusion and the pneumatic anti-shock garment if necessary.

The most severe food poisoning is *botulism*, which may present as a respiratory emergency. The toxin of botulism is absorbed from the gastrointestinal tract. It then blocks the neurotransmitter acetylcholine at the neuromuscular junction, where motor nerves stimulate skeletal muscle. At this point, it can decrease skeletal muscle response to nerve stimulation. Initially, the reaction may be flulike weakness but can progress to respiratory paralysis several hours or days after ingestion. Botulism is rare; therefore, if it is not recognized when the patient seeks initial medical attention for the more mild and vague early symptoms, it may become a prehospital emergency in the form of unexplained respiratory arrest.

In general, food poisoning results from contamination of food stuffs during processing or from improper food preparation and storage. A typical patient history is the onset of symptoms several hours after eating foods left at warm temperatures during a picnic. Botulism, however, is more commonly associated with improperly prepared or stored home-canned low-acid foods, such as green beans. Infant botulism can occur from the ingestion of bacteria found in spores in dust or in honey. It has been implicated as one cause of sudden infant death syndrome (SIDS). In rare cases, direct infection of deep wounds by the bacterium, which is commonly found in soil, can cause wound botulism.

Poisonous Plants

The most commonly encountered problems with plants are the occasional ingestion of plant parts by curious children and skin rashes from contact or skin punctures by some plants. Hallucinogenic plants have an abuse poten-

---

COMMON TOXIC PLANTS
Oral, Pharyngeal Irritation: Airway obstruction (oxalate crystals)

Philodendron

Jack-in-the-pulpit

Dieffenbachia

Cardiac Glycosides: Bradycardia, Atrioventricular Block

Foxglove

Oleander

Lily of the valley

Central Nervous System Toxicity

Morning glory

Hemlock

Tobacco

Christmas rose

Jerusalem cherry

Nightshade

Autonomic Nervous System Toxicity: Cholinergic Effects

Jimson weed

Severe Vomiting, Diarrhea: Dehydration, Hypotension

Caster bean

Holly

Mistletoe

Daffodil

Nightshade

Jerusalem cherry

Rhubarb (leaf blade only)

tial. Foraging for plants as food can lead to serious toxicity; mushrooms are a potentially fatal example.

The poisonous quality of a plant depends on many factors:

- Type and amount of poison varies from plant to plant even among the same species
- The maturity of the plant or fruit
- Part of the plant (*e.g.*, rhubarb stalks are edible but leaves are poisonous)

Prehospital emergencies that involve plants are rare. Mechanical airway obstruction may be the primary concern in a child who ate plant parts. Some plants contain oxalate crystals that can cause intense irritation and edema of the mouth, pharynx, and possibly the larynx. Dieffenbachia and philodendrons are examples. Airway compromise may be the immediate emergency. Many plants can cause nausea, vomiting, or diarrhea if ingested.

Some plants, such as lily of the valley, contain alkaloids similar to the cardiac glycosides that can cause bradycardia and atrioventricular block. Treatment with atropine or external pacing may be necessary if the slow heart rate becomes symptomatic. Others can affect the CNS by causing arousal, sedation, or hallucinations. If enough of the plant is ingested, seizures may occur. Alkaloids similar to atropine in plants such as jimson weed can cause cholinergic toxicity, hallucinations, tachyarrhythmias, dilated pupils, and flushed and dry skin. Most plant ingestions are small and require no treatment except cleaning the mouth and contacting the poison control center for plant protocols.

The box "Common Toxic Plants" lists some of the more common poisonous plants.

MUSHROOMS. Mushrooms are a *fungus*. Most species are edible but a few are toxic, and recognizing the difference is not easy. Poisoning from mushrooms usually occurs when foragers mistake a toxic mushroom for an edible one. Sometimes this mistake is made when people are looking for hallucinogenic mushrooms. Mushroom poisoning results from toxins unique to a particular species. The initial signs and symptoms are nausea, vomiting, abdominal pain, and diarrhea. These reactions can be enough to cause hypovolemia and orthostatic vital sign changes and may be the immediate problem. Gastrointestinal manifestations begin within several hours of ingestion. Gastrointestinal symptoms that do not begin until more than 6 hours after ingestion may indicate serious toxicity. The problem is that toxicity may not stop here. If the patient is not treated for mushroom poisoning or if the diagnosis is missed, liver and kidney failure can occur days later and can be fatal. When poisonous mushroom ingestion is suspected, emesis should be induced, if it has not already occurred, with syrup of ipecac. When vomiting stops, activated charcoal should be administered. Recognizing the problem may be the real challenge, since serious complications may not occur until several days later. When available, a sample of the ingested mushrooms should be taken along with the patient for identification.

Figure 25-1 shows several types of poisonous and edible mushrooms.

FIGURE 25–1.
(**A**) *Amanita phalloides,* common name "death cap." The cap is fairly deep olive-green to olive-brown. It is deadly poisonous: as little as one cap can prove fatal to an adult. Symptoms do not occur for 10 to 12 hours (or longer). (**B**) *Amanita virosa,* common name "destroying angel." The white cap is never completely open. It is deadly poisonous and usually has an unpleasant, yeastlike odor. (**C**) *Morchella esculenta,* common name "morel." It has a yellow-brown cap with irregular depressions. It is excellent for eating and has a strong mushroomy odor and a sweetish flavor. (**D**) *Pleurotus ostreatus,* common name "oyster mushroom." The cap is violet-black to brownish gray, and it is excellent for eating. It can be found on stumps and trunks of various broad-leaf trees.

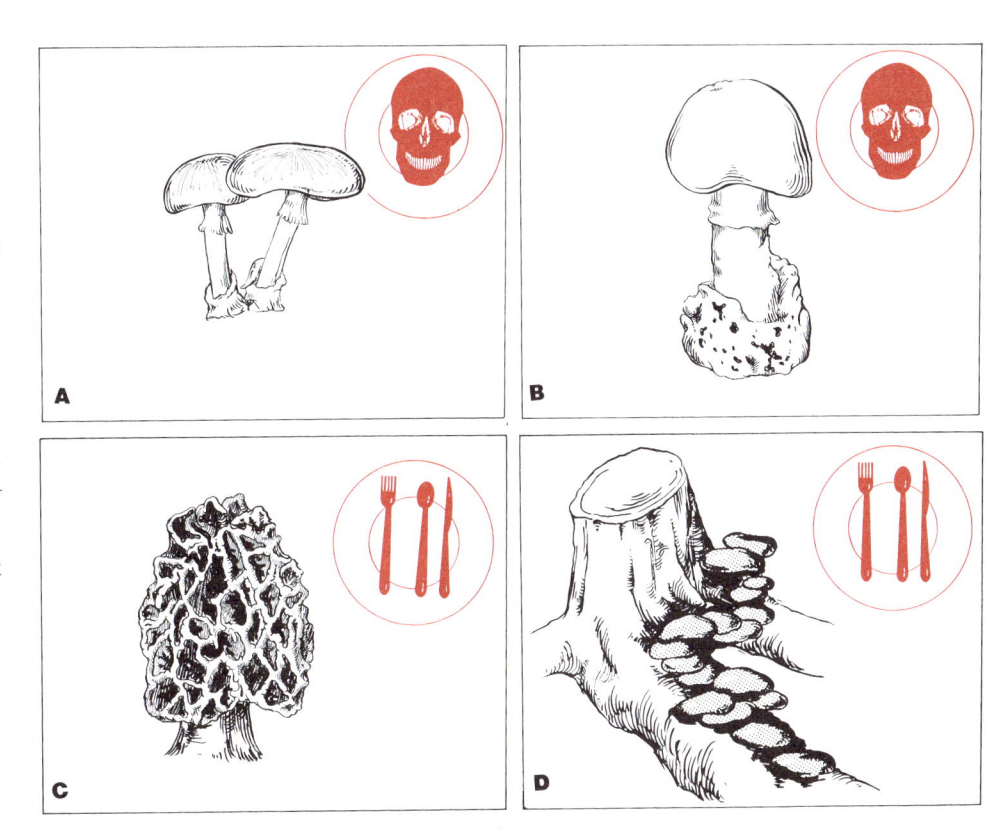

Bites and Stings

ARTHROPODS. The most common prehospital problem that results from biting and stinging insects is an allergic reaction. Allergy and anaphylaxis from bites and stings are treated as they are when they occur from any other cause. Insects of the *Hymenoptera* genus include bees, wasps, and ants. Honeybee stings leave behind the stinger, which should be scraped off with a sharp knife rather than squeezed or pulled out. This action prevents further envenomation. Almost all spiders use venom to kill their prey, but only two pose a threat to humans. However, allergic reactions to spider bites are also possible. The black widow spider (*Latrodectus* species) has a characteristic hourglass-shaped red mark on its abdomen, and its bite immediately produces burning pain. The neurotoxic venom can cause muscle spasm, rigidity, and paralysis initially in the anatomical region of the bite. If the reaction is severe enough, it can be treated with a slow IV bolus of 10 mL 10% calcium gluconate or 5 mg IV diazepam. The other dangerous spider bite is the brown recluse spider (*Loxosceles* species). It may be difficult to differentiate from other spiders but is generally brown or tan with a small *violin-shaped* mark on its head. Its bite can lead to a long-lasting, nonhealing ulcer often complicated by secondary infection. Occasionally, a hemolytic reaction can occur and progress to renal failure and intravascular coagulation. Scorpion stings are painful and locally irritating but rarely harmful. Some tick bites can cause a flaccid paralysis that is reversible when the tick is removed. In all these cases, the chances of more serious toxicity from the venoms are greater when children or the elderly are bitten or stung.

SNAKE BITES. The United States has four poisonous varieties of snakes: three pit vipers—rattlesnakes, water moccasins (cottonmouth), and copperheads (*Crotalidae* species)—and the coral snake (*Elapidae* species). The larger the snake, the greater the potential envenomation. The size can be judged from the distance between the two fang marks on the skin. If the fang marks are more than 12 mm apart, the snake was big, with greater potential envenomation than a small snake with fang marks less than 8 mm apart. Pit vipers get their name from the pit-like sensory organ in front of their eyes. Their heads tend to be triangular in shape. Coral snakes have an alternating red, yellow, and black coloration. Snake bites in infants and children and in elderly or debilitated victims can have more serious consequences than in healthy adults. Also, bites to the head and trunk tend to be more serious than bites to the extremities. Bites to the upper extremities tend to have a worse prognosis than bites to the lower extremities.

The symptoms and signs of envenomation vary, but immediate reactions at the site of envenomation include edema, ecchymosis, bleeding, and pain. Later, neurotoxins can cause difficulty in swallowing, weakness, muscle twitching, or seizures. Signs that the venom is being absorbed include nausea, vomiting, diarrhea, and restlessness. Arrhythmias may follow. The key to treatment is to start it early and limit absorption of the venom. If the bite has occurred within the last 30 to 45 minutes, the area should be immobilized and kept below heart level if possible. The patient should not be allowed to walk. A venous constricting band that maintains a distal arterial pulse on a limb should be placed proximal to the bite and reapplied ahead of advancing edema.

Ice or chemical cold packs should not be used because they may result in severe necrosis of the skin and deep frostbite injury at the bite and may make amputation necessary much later. Instead, treatment becomes symptomatic. In severe envenomation, hemorrhage, hypotension, seizures, and arrhythmias are possible.

ANTIVENINS. Specific antivenin therapy may be indicated in severe envenomation. Antivenin is of animal origin, so allergic reactions and anaphylaxis are possible adverse effects. Communication and transport to a facility with access to the necessary antivenin is the ultimate prehospital goal. Antivenin may be flown to the scene of a remote incident. Local protocols should specify the logistics. Zoos that exhibit poisonous exotic animals may keep a stock of specific antivenin available for emergencies.

MARINE ANIMALS. Ingestion of seafood can cause allergic reactions or anaphylaxis. Aside from direct trauma from some marine animals, other incidents can present a toxic problem. Occasionally, a toxic problem can result from eating seafood or fresh water fish from bacteria- or virus-contaminated water. Venomous marine animals can inflict injury by direct skin contact or by skin puncture. Stings from contact with jellyfish, stinging corals, and the Portuguese man-of-war result from specialized structures called *nematocysts*. Contact with the tentacles causes release of the nematocysts, which superficially adhere to the skin and release a venom that causes pain and redness. Signs and symptoms such as headache, nausea, vomiting, and muscle cramps may occur, but, aside from the painful discomfort, the primary concern is allergic reaction in susceptible people. The rare exception is the sea wasp of Australian or Philippine waters, the venom of which can cause progressive weakness, muscle spasms, pulmonary edema, dyspnea, shock, and even death. Nematocysts can also be released when dead jellyfish are stepped on in the sand.

Treatment of these stings begins by pulling off any adhering tentacles. Rubbing can fire more nematocysts and cause increased symptoms. Washing the area with rubbing alcohol (70% isopropyl alcohol) fixes the remaining nematocysts and prevents them from firing. Unless an allergic reaction occurs, the only other treatment necessary may be mild analgesics for pain and antihistamines for redness and itching.

Stingrays release their venom in a puncture wound or laceration. Since they tend to lie partially buried in sand under water, they can easily be stepped on, resulting in the sting. Usually, intense pain is the presenting problem, but the venom is a vasoconstrictor. Coronary vasospasm, with electrocardiographic changes, chest pain, and hypotension, is rare but can occur. The venom is easily destroyed by heat, so the foot or leg, where stings usually occur, should be immersed in water as hot as the patient can tolerate for about 1 hour. Since hot water can trigger nematocysts, a painful but unknown ocean sting should be treated with alcohol when no puncture wound or laceration is present.

Drug Overdose

PRESCRIPTION NARCOTICS. The effects of **narcotics** on the CNS include increased pain tolerance, sedation, anxiety reduction, drowsiness, and suppression of the cough reflex. Later, nausea, vomiting, and respiratory depression occur. In addition to CNS effects, narcotics are vasodilators that can result in orthostatic hypotension. They also reduce intestinal peristalsis and can cause cramps or reduce diarrhea. Narcotic overdose is most commonly a drug abuse problem, which is discussed later; however, other less expected circumstances can occur. Children can accidentally ingest such drugs as methadone, Darvon, or Lomotil that are prescribed for someone in the family. Darvon commonly is used in suicide attempts. Cancer patients on home care may be prescribed injectable narcotics, which can lead to accidental or intentional overdose. Narcotics are prescribed for pain relief but are also used in cough suppressants, antidiarrheal drugs (Lomotil), and some narcotic withdrawal programs (methadone) (see the box "Common Prescription Narcotics").

COMMON PRESCRIPTION NARCOTICS

Codeine
Morphine
Dilaudid (hydromorphone)
Percodan, Percocet, Tylox (oxycodone)
Stadol (butorphanol)
Cough suppressants (dextromethorphan)
Lomotil (diphenoxylate)
Sublimaze (fentanyl)
Demerol (meperidine)
Dolophine (methadone)
Nubain (nalbuphine)
Talwin (pentazocine)
Darvon, Darvocet (propoxyphene)

The classic presentation of narcotic overdose is pupillary constriction (pinpoint), decreased level of consciousness, and respiratory depression. The immediate priority is to restore adequate ventilation. Although respiratory depression occurs in time with a large dose of any narcotic, pupillary constriction may not be dramatic. In fact, if the patient has been hypoxic long enough, the pupils may begin to dilate. Because of this reaction, any unresponsive patient should be given a naloxone (Narcan) bolus, especially when a toxicologic problem cannot be ruled out. Naloxone is a narcotic antagonist that competes with the narcotic for its receptors. The only general management consideration that may need to be modified is the choice of airway management. Reversal of the effects of narcotics can be rapid when no other drugs or medical and trauma problems are involved. It is better to postpone endotracheal intubation and especially the esophageal obturator airway until after naloxone has been given. If the airway can be satisfactorily managed with an oropharyngeal airway and bag-valve-mask ventilation, the paramedic will be saved the problem of trying to deflate cuffs on an endotracheal tube or esophageal obturator airway in a gagging, fighting patient.

The immediate goal is to get the patient breathing again. Patients who are waking up may be agitated, delirious, or confused and occasionally overtly combative, especially when drugs are involved in the overdose. The paramedic should be prepared to restrain or withdraw from a patient given naloxone. The other side of this problem is that some narcotics are notoriously resistant to naloxone, necessitating higher doses. This fact is true of propoxyphene (Darvon), Talwin, and methadone, which have long durations of action. One way to handle this resistance is to give a 0.4-mg naloxone IV push and watch for an effect. If there is no response, repeat the dose. If there is still no response, give a 2-mg naloxone IV push. The dose in children is 0.01 mg/kg. Although all narcotics can cause hypotension if enough is taken, Darvon also can cause cardiac arrhythmias.

SEDATIVES AND HYPNOTICS. **Sedatives** and **hypnotics**, antianxiety drugs, minor tranquilizers, and anticonvulsants all affect the CNS. The two major drug classes involved are barbiturates and benzodiazepines.

Barbiturates: general CNS depressants; inhibit impulse conduction in the ascending reticular activating system, depress the cerebral cortex, alter cerebellar function, depress motor output, and can produce excitation, sedation, hypnosis, anesthesia, and deep coma
Benzodiazepines: exact mechanisms of action not understood; act mainly at subcortical levels of the CNS, leaving the cortex relatively unaffected; main sites of action may be the limbic system and reticular formation

The presenting problem usually is decreased level of consciousness. Hypotension can also occur. The prehos-

> **COMMON SEDATIVES AND HYPNOTICS, ANTIANXIETY DRUGS, MINOR TRANQUILIZERS, AND ANTICONVULSANTS**
>
> | Barbiturates | Anticonvulsants | Benzodiazepines |
> |---|---|---|
> | Phenobarbital | Dilantin (phenytoin) | Xanax (alprazolam) |
> | Butabarbital | Zarontin (ethosuximide) | Librium, Librax (chlordiazepoxide) |
> | Amobarbital | Tegretol (carbamazepine) | Clonopin (clonazepam) |
> | Secobarbital | Depakene (valproic acid) | Tranxene (clorazepate) |
> | Pentobarbital | | Valium (diazepam) |
> | Quaalude (methaqualone) | | Dalmane (flurazepam) |
> | Ethchlorvynol | | Ativan (lorazepam) |
> | Miltown, Equagesic (meprobamate) | | Serax (oxazepam) |
> | Glutethimide | | Centrax (prazepam) |
> | Ethinamate | | Restoril (temazepam) |
> | Noludar (methyprylon) | | |

pital management of overdose follows the general principles described earlier. Unfortunately, these drugs are manufactured under many trade names and as combination drugs (see the box "Common Sedatives and Hypnotics, Antianxiety Drugs, Minor Tranquilizers, and Anticonvulsants"). Consultation with the poison control center or base hospital can help identify the drugs involved and management priorities.

OVER-THE-COUNTER ANALGESICS. **Salicylates** and **acetaminophen** are in many nonprescription and prescription drugs. Overdoses with these drugs can cause serious metabolic derangements, liver failure, and death. Infants and children can become critically ill with acid-base and electrolyte imbalance. Common clinical features of salicylate toxicity are tinnitus (ringing in the ears), diaphoresis, hyperventilation, nausea, and vomiting. The problem with acetaminophen overdose is that, if it goes untreated or unappreciated, serious and even fatal liver failure can occur several days later. An oral antidote, acetylcysteine, is available but must be started within 24 hours. This medication is given orally, and activated charcoal should not be given when acetylcysteine will be used. The severity of the ingestion for both acetaminophen and salicylates is determined by measuring their concentrations in the blood. Even when nontoxic doses have been ingested, suicidal gestures may mandate medical evaluation. If the dose ingested cannot be determined or substantiated, the patient should be evaluated at a hospital for potential subsequent toxicity.

TRICYCLIC ANTIDEPRESSANTS. It is ironic that the drugs of choice for endogenous depression have significant toxicity. The **tricyclic antidepressants** are effective antidepressants and are prescribed to patients who may become or who already are suicidal. Imipramine (one type of tricyclic antidepressant) is used to treat nocturnal enuresis (bed wetting) in children, so it is commonly available for accidental or intentional overdose in the home. Antidepressants are some of the most commonly prescribed medications (see the box "Common Tricyclic Antidepressants"). In addition to their antidepressant effects, tricyclic antidepressants also cause sedation and have central and peripheral anticholinergic effects. Overdose can rapidly lead to coma and seizures. Usually, however, the immediate toxicologic problem is cardiac arrhythmias and hypotension, with sinus tachycardia progressing to ventricular fibrillation. The best indicator of severe toxicity is loss of consciousness.

Again, the principles of general poisoning management apply but with a few new considerations. First of all, the onset of seizures, ventricular arrhythmias, and loss of consciousness can occur rapidly; for this reason, some authorities maintain that a conscious patient should not be given syrup of ipecac to induce emesis. Supraventricular tachycardia, ventricular arrhythmias, and hypotension

> **COMMON TRICYCLIC ANTIDEPRESSANTS**
>
> Tofranil (imipramine)
> Elavil, Triavil, Limbitrol (amitriptyline)
> Norpramin (desipramine)
> Aventyl (nortriptyline)
> Sinequan (doxepin)
> Vivactil (protriptyline)
> Ludiomil (maprotiline)

occur in part from the anticholinergic effects of tricyclic antidepressants. However, these drugs also have a direct effect on ion flux across myocardial conduction fibers. The second consideration is early administration of sodium bicarbonate. The mechanism of action is alkalinization of blood to decrease the potential for cardiac arrhythmias. Sodium bicarbonate, in the same dose as used in refractory pulseless rhythms during cardiopulmonary resuscitation (1 mEq/kg), has been reported to stop seizures and arrhythmias and to increase blood pressure in tricyclic antidepressant overdose. Hyperventilation with a bag-valve-mask device can be used in place of sodium bicarbonate, but it is not as effective.

ANTIPSYCHOTICS. **Antipsychotic** drugs are from several different chemical groups, but the phenothiazines are a group commonly encountered (see the box "Common Antipsychotic Drugs"). Phenothiazines may cause CNS effects and an altered level of consciousness as well as effects on the cardiovascular system. They can block α-adrenergic receptors and histamine receptors and, therefore, cause vasodilation. They also exert an anticholinergic action. Together, these effects lead to tachycardia and hypotension. Myocardial conduction can be affected, causing a wide-complex tachycardia. Another unusual but characteristic adverse effect of this class of drugs is *dystonia*, which is known as an extrapyramidal effect. Dystonia refers to abnormal motor activity of skeletal muscle groups. Normally, skeletal muscle motor function is controlled by portions of the cerebral cortex on the opposite side of the body. These nerve tracts cross over in the brain stem and form two bundles of motor nerve fibers called the pyramids, which then descend in the spinal cord to eventually exit as spinal nerves to skeletal muscle. Other motor nerve tracts that are separate from the pyramids, the extrapyramidal tracts, descend in the spinal cord. They are controlled in part by the basal ganglia in the brain, which is where the antipsychotic drugs act to affect motor function. These dystonic reactions are striking and unforgettable. The eyes can deviate to one side (*oculogyric crisis*), the head and neck can turn to one side (*torticollis*), the tongue can become paralyzed, and the limbs can jerk and writhe (*choreoathetosis*). All of these actions are totally involuntary on the part of the patient. The reaction can be differentiated from a tonic seizure by the fact that the patient remains conscious during the episode, which can subside and recur. There is no postictal period. The situation is uncomfortable for the patient, and the patient can completely recall the event.

Dystonia can occur in overdose or after any dose of most antipsychotic drugs. Sometimes, dystonia is the reason for an EMS response and can demonstrate the problem many municipalities have in dealing with the indigent mentally ill. A common story is one in which an indigent patient with a mild to moderate psychiatric history is evaluated at a clinic and, without other resources,

COMMON ANTIPSYCHOTIC DRUGS

Mellaril (thioridazine)
Sparine (promazine)
Thorazine (chlorpromazine)
Vesprin (triflupromazine)
Stelazine (trifluoperazine)
Trilafon (perphenazine)
Prolixin (fluphenazine)
Haldol (haloperidol)
Taractan (chlorprothixene)
Loxitane (loxapine)

given "an injection and some pills" and sent back to the streets. The injection was an antipsychotic to control behavior, and the pills were probably diphenhydramine (Benadryl) to prevent a dystonic reaction. Either the dystonic reaction occurred before the patient took the Benadryl dose, or it was not taken as directed. An EMS unit is requested for a patient who is experiencing a "seizure." Prehospital treatment of dystonia is with IV diphenhydramine, 25 to 50 mg (2 mg/kg in children). Cardiovascular reactions from an overdose are treated with general management principles. Since the phenothiazines do have antiemetic properties, it has been argued that syrup of ipecac will not work. However, in general it is effective, so a conscious patient with protective airway reflexes can be given syrup of ipecac to induce vomiting. If no emesis occurs, the next alternative is gastric lavage.

DRUG ABUSE EMERGENCIES

Narcotics

Respiratory depression and coma from narcotic abuse can occur in nontolerant users or in addicts when a higher purity of narcotic hits the streets. The drugs usually involved are IV heroin, fentanyl (china white), or oral methadone. Street narcotics are invariably cut (diluted) with other substances, such as quinine, lidocaine, lactose, sucrose, starch, baking soda, or talc. As with other narcotic overdoses, the classic presentation is coma with respiratory depression and constricted or pinpoint pupils. Needle tracks may be evident on the skin from *mainlining* (IV injection) or *skin popping* (intradermal injection).

Initial management is to secure an airway and provide adequate ventilation and oxygenation. The definitive treatment is naloxone (Narcan) as described in the drug overdose section. It is not uncommon for patients who regain consciousness to refuse transport to a hospital. In this

TABLE 25-1.
CONTROLLED SUBSTANCES: USES AND EFFECTS

Drugs	Schedule	Trade or Other Name	Medical Uses	Physical Dependence	Psychological Dependence
NARCOTICS					
Opium	II, III, V	Dover's powder, paregoric, Parepectolin	Analgesic, antidiarrheal	High	High
Morphine	II, III	Morphine, Pectoral Syrup	Analgesic, antitussive		
Codeine	II, III, V	Codeine, Empirin compound with codeine, Robitussin A-C	Analgesic, antitussive	Moderate	Moderate
Heroin	I	Diacetylmorphine, horse, smack	Under investigation		
Hydromorphone		Dilaudid	Analgesic		
Meperidine (Pethidine)	II	Demerol, Pethadol	Analgesic	High	High
Methadone		Dolophine, methadone, Methadose	Analgesic, heroin substitute		
Other narcotics	I, II, III, IV, V	LAAM, Leritine, Levo-Dromoran, Percodan, Tussionex, Darvon*, Talwin*, Lomotil Fentanyl	Analgesic, antidiarrheal, antitussive	High-Low	High-Low
DEPRESSANTS					
Chloral hydrate	IV	Noctec, Somnos	Hypnotic	Moderate	Moderate
Barbiturates	II, III, IV	Amobarbital, Phenobarbital, Butisol, Phenoxbarbital, Secobarbital, Tuinal	Anesthetic, anticonvulsant, sedative, hypnotic	High-Moderate	High-Moderate
Glutethimide	III	Doriden	Sedative, hypnotic	High	High
Methaqualone	II	Optimil, Parest, Quaalude, Somnafac, Sopor			
Benzodiazepines	IV	Ativan, Azene, Clonopin, Dalmane, Diasepam, Librium, Serax, Tranxene, Valium, Verstran	Antianxiety, anticonvulsant, sedative, hypnotic	Low	Low
Other depressants	III, IV	Equanil, Miltown, Noludar, Placidyl, Valmid	Antianxiety, sedative	Moderate	Moderate
STIMULANTS					
Cocaine†	II	Coke, flake, snow	Local anesthetic		
Amphetamines	II, III	Biphetamine, Delcobese, Desoxyn, Dexedrine, Mediatric	Hyperkinesis, narcolepsy, weight control	Possible	High
Phenmetrazine	II	Preludin			
Methylphenidate		Ritalin			
Other stimulants	III, IV	Adipex, Bacarate, Cylert, Didrex, Ionamin, Plegine, PreSate, Sanorex, Tenuate, Tepanil, Voranil			
HALLUCINOGENS					
LSD		Acid, microdot		None	
Mescaline and peyote	I	Mesc, buttons, cactus	None		Degree unknown
Amphetamine variants		2,5-DMA, PMA, STP, MDA, MMDA, TMA, DOM, DOB		Unknown	
Phencyclidine	II	PCP, Angel dust, hog	Veterinary anesthetic	Degree unknown	High
Phencyclidine analogs	I	PCE, PCPy, TCP	None		Degree unknown
Other hallucinogens		Bufotenine, Ibogaine, DMT, DET, Psilocybin, Psilocyn		None	

Tol-erance	Duration of Effects (in hours)	Usual Methods of Administration	Possible Effects	Effects of Overdose	Withdrawal Syndrome
Yes	3–6	Oral, smoked	Euphoria, drowsiness, respiratory depression, constricted pupils, nausea	Slow and shallow breathing, clammy skin, convulsions, coma, possible death	Watery eyes, runny nose, yawning, loss of appetite, irritability, tremors, panic, chills, sweating, cramps, nausea
		Oral, injected, smoked			
		Oral, injected			
		Injected, sniffed, smoked			
	12–24	Oral, injected			
	Variable				
Possible	5–8	Oral	Slurred speech, disorientation, drunken behavior without odor of alcohol	Shallow respiration, cold and clammy skin, dilated pupils, weak and rapid pulse, coma, possible death	Anxiety, insomnia, tremors, delirium, convulsions, possible death
Yes	1–16				
		Oral, injected			
	4–8				
Possible	1–2	Sniffed, injected	Increased alertness, excitation, euphoria, increased pulse rate and blood pressure, insomnia, loss of appetite	Agitation, increase in body temperature, hallucinations, convulsions, possible death	Apathy, long periods of sleep, irritability, depression, disorientation
Yes	2–4	Oral, injected			
		Oral			
Yes	8–12	Oral	Illusions and hallucinations, poor perception of time and distance	Longer more intense "trip" episodes, psychosis, possible death	Withdrawal syndrome not reported
		Oral, injected			
	Up to days				
		Smoked, oral, injected			
Possible	Variable	Oral, injected, smoked, sniffed			

(continued)

TABLE 25–1. (continued)
CONTROLLED SUBSTANCES: USES AND EFFECTS

Drugs	Schedule	Trade or Other Name	Medical Uses	Physical Dependence	Psychological Dependence
CANNABIS					
Marijuana		Pot, Acapulco gold, grass, reefer, sinsemilla, Thai sticks	Under investigation		
Tetrahydrocannabinol	I	THC		Degree unknown	Moderate
Hashish		Hash			
Hashish oil		Hash oil	None		

(Drug Enforcement Administration, United States Department of Justice)
*Not designated a narcotic under the Controlled Substance Act
†Designated a narcotic under the Controlled Substance Act

situation, the IV naloxone can be followed with an intramuscular (IM) injection of another 0.4 to 1 mg. Since the duration of effect of the naloxone may be shorter than that of the injected narcotic, the IM injection of naloxone is slowly absorbed and reduces the risk of repeated respiratory depression. Naloxone given to a narcotic addict to treat respiratory depression can cause some symptoms of a withdrawal syndrome within the first hour after administration. The withdrawal signs and symptoms are usually mild and limited to perspiration, *piloerection* ("goose flesh"), flushing, twitching, restlessness, and irritability. Naloxone-induced narcotic withdrawal does not usually cause fever, nausea, vomiting, diarrhea, or involuntary muscle spasm, and it does not cause the seizures seen in acute withdrawal syndrome.

Occasionally, a pregnant narcotic addict gives birth to an infant who is lethargic and cyanotic. If the infant's APGAR (see Chapter 29) score is low and respiratory efforts weak or even absent, naloxone may be given after the airway is secured and bag–valve–mask ventilation started. The dose is 0.01 mg/kg given IV or IM. Neonatal naloxone is available in a lower concentration to facilitate administration of this small dose.

Another frequently encountered problem of narcotic abuse is acute pulmonary edema. The cause in most cases is an increase in pulmonary capillary permeability (increased capillary leak). The onset of pulmonary edema can be rapid and can cause death shortly after the narcotic is injected. Recommended treatment is positive-pressure ventilation. Since the cause is not pulmonary congestion, diuretics, such as furosemide, are not effective. Pulmonary edema is not reversible with naloxone.

Stimulants

Phencyclidine

The immediate emergency in **phencyclidine** (PCP, angel dust, crystal) abuse may be trauma. If trauma is not the problem, then the management priority amounts to hazard control. Usually, the presenting problem is psychotic agitation. Because phencyclidine can be easily synthesized, it is a commonly abused drug and sometimes sold on the street as THC, mescaline, LSD, or psilocybin. Usually, it is smoked in cigarettes or joints or snorted, but it can be taken orally. Most phencyclidine abuse occurs at doses that cause CNS stimulation, but at higher doses it can cause coma. Unlike the coma of narcotics or sedatives, these patients have good respiratory function, significant hypertension, and brisk reflexes. It is more common, though, for the patient to be awake with a catatonic blank stare or to be disoriented, agitated, combative, or excited.

The psychotic response can be highly variable. Sensory anesthesia to pain presents a problem for both the patient and EMS responders. The patient can sustain and inflict considerable trauma. Methods of passive and active restraint that are otherwise effective may be futile. In the extreme case, IV diazepam may be a final alternative. Tonic-clonic seizures or even status epilepticus can occur. Although not always present, a useful sign to differentiate phencyclidine from other stimulants is *nystagmus*. Rhythmic oscillations of the eyes can be up and down or side to side, vertical or horizontal nystagmus, and can occur in awake or comatose patients. Keep the patient in a quiet dark environment if possible.

Amphetamine

Amphetamine abuse is by ingestion or IV injection, and amphetamines may be mixed with other drugs. Abuse may substitute for a reduction in available heroin. Although the substance sold on the streets as speed, Black Beauties, bennies, dexies, or uppers is assumed to be amphetamines, it may be caffeine, phenylpropanolamine, or ephedrine. The presenting problem is usually a drug-induced psychosis. Unlike phencyclidine, the patient is less disoriented and, although agitated, generally is controllable. Higher

Tolerance	Duration of Effects (in hours)	Usual Methods of Administration	Possible Effects	Effects of Overdose	Withdrawal Syndrome
Yes	2–4	Smoked, oral	Euphoria, relaxed inhibitions, increased appetite, disoriented behavior	Fatigue, paranoia, possible psychosis	Insomnia, hyperactivity, and decreased appetite occasionally reported

doses of amphetamines can result in acute drug abuse emergencies. Dangerous hypertension can cause intracranial hemorrhage, and tachyarrhythmias can lead to ventricular fibrillation. Seizures can develop from excessive CNS stimulation. Amphetamines can also cause a significant and even dangerous rise in core body temperature, leading to a heatstroke-like syndrome. If the drug was ingested, syrup of ipecac and activated charcoal can be given to an awake patient.

Seizures are treated with diazepam, and ventricular arrhythmias are treated with lidocaine. Prehospital treatment of malignant hypertension is a problem to be resolved. The drugs of choice are usually arteriolar vasodilators or β-adrenergic blockers, which generally are not included in prehospital protocols. The best choice may be sublingual nitroglycerin. Its vasodilator properties can be fairly predictable dose to dose, and it has a relatively short duration of action.

Phenylpropanolamine

Phenylpropanolamine is available in over-the-counter diet pills, nasal decongestants, and cold preparations. It can be intentionally abused, but, even when used as directed, it occasionally can cause profound hypertension. The patient may present with neurologic signs and symptoms of an intracranial bleed or stroke.

Cocaine

Cocaine abuse can be found throughout all socioeconomic groups. It is usually snorted but can be injected IV. Free basing is done by dissolving the cocaine in an alkaline solution (in water) and then extracting it, usually with diethyl ether. The free base is recovered by evaporating the ether and is smoked in a cigarette or pipe. The extremely volatile and flammable diethyl ether can cause burns from flash fires. Cocaine produces an alert euphoria in the occasional user but can leave the chronic abuser in a paranoid psychosis. In addition to the behavioral crisis, prehospital medical emergencies that result from cocaine use are seizures and cardiac arrhythmias. Seizures are treated with diazepam, but status epilepticus may be resistant to this drug. Ventricular arrhythmias usually respond to lidocaine, but if not propranolol is the drug of choice.

Hallucinogens

Hallucinogens include marijuana. The prehospital problem that involves hallucinogens is usually a behavioral emergency. History is usually poor or unavailable. In fact, the user may not even know what was taken. Usually, these drugs are ingested, but syrup of ipecac and activated charcoal are generally not necessary. The discomfort may aggravate the behavioral crisis, and this treatment does not usually change the outcome. A complicating problem is that other drugs may also have been used.

Table 25-1 lists the uses and effects of some common controlled substances.

Solvent Abuse

Inhalation of solvent vapors from a plastic bag or a cloth causes an inebriated feeling with vivid hallucinations. Materials such as glues and adhesives, gasoline, aerosols (fluorocarbon propellants), paints, varnishes and lacquers, dyes, and nail polish remover typically are used. Solvents in general, but especially fluorocarbon propellants (Freon) from aerosol cans, sensitize the myocardium to the effects of hypoxia from the displacement of air by solvent vapors. The immediate emergency may be cardiac arrhythmias or cardiopulmonary arrest.

Abstinence Syndromes

In addition to acute drug abuse emergencies, the opposite problem of abstinence may be the reason for an EMS request. ***Abstinence syndromes*** result when a habitual drug user cannot get another dose or elects to stop the drug use. Tolerance can develop to drugs such as narcotics, amphetamines, and barbiturates. As abuse continues, larger doses are necessary for the same effect. Drug dependency, which can lead to tolerance, can be physical or psychologic. Psychologic drug dependency, as occurs early with cocaine, is compulsive, neurotic behavior aimed at acquiring another dose. A compulsive coffee-drinker is a common example. Physical dependency, however, is a poorly understood change in physiology with habitual drug abuse that literally requires another dose to prevent withdrawal symptoms. Narcotics cause a physical dependency. In the early stages of drug abuse, psychologic dependency may precede physical dependency. Drug dependency occurs for alcohol, barbiturates and other sedative-hypnotics, narcotics, amphetamines, marijuana, cocaine, and hallucinogens.

Abstinence symptoms begin about the time of the next dose, peak in 2 or 3 days, and decline over the next week or so. Early signs and symptoms include perspiration, *rhinorrhea* (runny nose), and yawning. These can progress to insomnia, anorexia, abnormal sleep patterns, twitching, tremor, restlessness, flushing, piloerection, and tachycardia. Peak signs of abstinence include delirium, nausea, vomiting, abdominal cramps, diarrhea, muscle spasm, and possibly progressive seizure activity. From the prehospital point of view, it is important to recognize an abstinence syndrome from other drug abuse symptoms based on history. Seizures may need to be controlled with diazepam.

ALCOHOLISM

The most common prehospital toxicologic problem and the largest drug abuse problem in the United States is **alcoholism.** Usually alcohol intoxication presents as a prehospital emergency that involves trauma or unconsciousness. When trauma is involved, the trauma assessment findings take priority over the toxicologic problem.

Acute Intoxication

When trauma is not the problem, a common reason for an EMS response that involves alcohol intoxication is an altered level of consciousness. Management of an unresponsive patient with suspected acute alcohol intoxication follows the general principles of airway management, ventilation, and oxygenation, IV D$_5$W TKO (to keep the vein open), 50% dextrose (D$_{50}$W), and naloxone. One other factor must be considered when the patient is believed to be an alcoholic: alcoholism is frequently accompanied by some degree of malnutrition, sometimes serious. Chronic alcoholism and malnutrition cause many chronic medical problems. However, one aspect of malnutrition, B-complex vitamin deficiency, has significance for emergency prehospital care. Thiamine, vitamin B$_1$, is necessary for the body to use carbohydrates.

Hypoglycemia can occur in alcoholics and, particularly, in children who accidentally ingest alcohol. Hypoglycemia needs to be ruled out in any patient with an altered level of consciousness. To prevent the dangerous effects of potential hypoglycemia on the brain, 50% dextrose, a carbohydrate, is routinely given to unresponsive patients. This load of carbohydrate in a thiamine-deficient alcoholic can cause a metabolic abnormality called *Wernicke's encephalopathy.* Wernicke's syndrome presents as mental confusion, vertical and horizontal nystagmus, disconjugate gaze, and *ataxia* (gait disturbances). If untreated, it can progress irreversibly to a syndrome called *Korsakoff's psychosis,* which is characterized by amnesia, gaps in memory, and inability to remember sequences of events. To prevent the onset of Wernicke's encephalopathy, an unresponsive suspected alcoholic should be given an IM injection of 100 mg thiamine before the IV 50% dextrose.

Chronic Alcoholism

A large number of chronic medical problems result from chronic alcoholism. Gastritis, pancreatitis, and liver disease can present as nausea, vomiting, weakness, and abdominal pain. These symptoms may be severe enough to be accompanied by tachycardia and orthostatic hypotension. The inebriating and vasodilative properties of ethanol make hypothermia a possibility in alcoholics. Aside from body temperature, hypothermia may present as cardiac arrhythmias. Destitute alcoholics may resort to other substances when they cannot afford ethanol. Windshield washer fluid (methanol), antifreeze (ethylene glycol), and rubbing alcohol (isopropanol) all have an inebriating effect but also have serious toxicity. Solvent abuse is suspected to be more common among destitute alcoholics. Because of liver disease, venous blood flow through the portal vein may be restricted. When this restriction occurs, veins that connect with the portal vein become enlarged under higher pressure than they normally handle. One place of particular importance where this enlargement occurs is the lower esophagus, in which dilated esophageal veins (*varices*) can rupture, causing severe, even exsanguinating, hemorrhage and hypovolemic shock. Upper gastrointestinal bleeding can also occur from other sites.

Alcohol–Antabuse Reaction

One method of rehabilitation for properly motivated alcoholics is the use of disulfiram (**Antabuse**) as a deterrent to ethanol. Antabuse works by inhibiting the metabolism of ethanol and, in part, allowing the accumulation of the metabolite acetaldehyde. Acetaldehyde produces symptoms through its effects on the gastrointestinal, cardiovascular, and autonomic nervous systems. For example, it is thought to be the cause of the discomfort of a hangover. If a patient who is voluntarily taking Antabuse drinks ethanol, the face and chest become flushed and a pounding headache begins. Dyspnea, nausea, vomiting, sweating, weakness, dizziness, blurred vision, and confusion may ensue. The severity of the symptoms parallels the amount of ethanol ingested and may last a few minutes to a few hours. If enough ethanol is consumed, hypotension and shock can occur even to the point of being life-threatening.

Because Antabuse is used only in association with other rehabilitation measures, the patient should be well aware of the dangers of drinking. Occasionally, a patient may test the drug's effects by drinking a little ethanol or may accidentally use over-the-counter elixirs like cough syrups, which contain ethanol. Treatment is aimed at oxygenation, IV fluid replacement, and correction of severe hypotension. This problem is not particularly common, so recognition is the key to management.

Abstinence Syndromes and Delirium Tremens

Alcohol abuse results in both psychologic and physical dependence. When an alcoholic stops drinking, a withdrawal period follows. The abstinence syndrome begins with agitation, anxiety, and insomnia. The longer and more severe the alcohol dependency was, the further these symptoms progress. Within about 6 to 8 hours after abstinence begins, symptoms appear and a tremor develops. Grand mal seizures may occur early in withdrawal, within about 12 hours. If the patient had been an alcoholic long enough for major medical complications to develop, then the abstinence syndrome can progress to hallucinations, total disorientation, and changes in vital signs.

The most severe phase of abstinence is **delirium tremens** (DT's), which occurs 2 to 3 days after the patient stops drinking. Tremulousness, visual hallucinations, agitation, confusion, and disorientation occur. Autonomic nervous system overactivity can cause cardiac arrhythmias, hypertension, and heatstroke. All of these reactions may have serious or even fatal consequences in alcoholics with underlying disease. It is important to remember that, if lidocaine is used to treat ventricular arrhythmias, the dose has to be reduced because of the underlying liver disease. Seizures are usually self-limiting, but repeated seizure activity may require diazepam. Oversedation, however, may then require airway management and bag-valve-mask ventilation.

SUMMARY

The number of prescription and over-the-counter drugs, drugs of abuse, and industrial and agricultural chemicals is ever increasing. A toxicologic emergency that requires an EMS response may involve a single victim, as an accidental or intentional ingestion, or may involve a multicasualty incident, in which transportation of hazardous materials are involved. Because of the vast diversity of toxicologic problems, management has to be systematic and focused on basic priorities: hazard control and personal protection, primary survey, secondary survey, and decontamination. Occasionally, specific antidotes are available, but usually treatment is aimed at protecting the airway, assisting ventilation when necessary, inducing emesis when appropriate, and treating arrhythmias and extremes in blood pressure.

Drug abuse, alcoholism, and abstinence syndromes may be the reason for an EMS response or may represent underlying problems during the management of a trauma emergency. In either case, the prehospital management of substance abuse represents one phase of a long treatment process, often with many remissions before recovery.

SUGGESTED READING

Carlton FB: General management of the poisoned patient. Emergency Care Quarterly 6(3):1, 1990

Harwood–Nuss A: The Clinical Practice of Emergency Medicine. Philadelphia, JB Lippincott, 1991

Lampe KF, McCann MA: AMA Handbook of Poisonous and Injurious Plants. Chicago, American Medical Association, 1985

Lincoff GH: Simon and Schuster's Guide to Mushrooms. New York, Simon and Schuster, 1981

Noll GG, Hildebrand MS, Yvorra JG: Hazardous Materials: Managing the Incident. Annapolis, Peake Productions, 1988

Parker F. The skin and the elements: Sun, plants, and stinging and biting organisms. Emergency Care Quarterly 4(3):21, 1988

US Department of Transportation, National Highway Traffic Safety Administration: Emergency Medical Technician–Paramedic: National Standards Curriculum. Washington, DC, US Government Printing Office, 1985

CHAPTER 26

Infectious Diseases

Immune System
 Immune Response
 Infectious and Communicable
Communicable Diseases of Adults and Children
 Tuberculosis
 Hepatitis Types A and B
 Hepatitis C
 Meningitis
 Herpes
  Herpes Simplex Types 1 and 2
  Herpetic Whitlow
  Varicella
  Herpes Zoster
  Cytomegalovirus
 Syphilis
 Gonorrhea
 Scabies and Lice
 Mumps
 Measles: Rubella and Rubeola
 Acquired Immunodeficiency Syndrome
Techniques of Management
 Universal Precautions
 Hand Washing
 Handling and Disposal of Needles
 Disposal of Contaminated Articles
 Gloving Technique
 Gowns
 Protective Eye Wear
 Face Mask
 Cleaning a Blood Spill
 Cleaning the Vehicle
 Blood Exposure Follow-up
Summary

BEHAVIORAL OBJECTIVES

On successful completion of this chapter, the reader will be able to:

1. Describe the immune system's role in the immune response
2. Explain the difference between infectious and communicable
3. Describe each of the following communicable diseases: tuberculosis, hepatitis A and B, hepatitis C, herpes viruses, syphilis, gonorrhea, scabies, lice, mumps, measles, acquired immunodeficiency syndrome
4. Explain the rationale for universal precautions
5. Describe the techniques for universal precautions
6. Discuss the handling and disposal of needles and contaminated articles
7. Describe the process of cleaning a blood spill
8. Describe the process of cleaning the vehicle after contamination
9. Explain blood exposure follow-up
10. Define all of the key terms listed in this chapter

KEY TERMS

The following terms are defined in the chapter and glossary:

airborne transmission
acquired immuno-
 deficiency syndrome
 (AIDS)
B lymphocytes
cellular immunity
communicable disease
congenital rubella
 syndrome
cytomegalovirus
gonorrhea
hepatitis
hepatitis A
hepatitis B
hepatitis C
herpes zoster
herpes simplex types
 1 and 2
herpetic whitlow
human immunodefi-
 ciency virus (HIV)
humoral immunity
IgA
IgE
IgG
IgM
immune system
immune response
immunoglobulins
incubation period
infectious disease
Kaposi's sarcoma
Koplik's spots
lice
lymphatic system
meningitis
mumps
percutaneous
permucosal
phagocytosis
rubella
rubeola
scabies
syphilis
T lymphocytes
tuberculosis
universal precautions
varicella
vehicle transmission

Many diseases, such as syphilis and herpes, have existed for thousands of years. It was not until people began to venture out of their environment and explore other areas that infectious disease became a factor in survival. Human contact with other humans has been the major factor in the spread of these diseases.

Until the early 1900s, infectious diseases were the leading cause of death for children and young adults. Since 1900, great achievements have been made in the identification, treatment, and prevention of infectious diseases. Some diseases, such as smallpox, have been totally eradicated; others have been brought under control by *immunization* (vaccination), medication, improved sanitary practices, and public education.

Paramedics come in direct contact with patients who have a wide range of illnesses. The paramedic must have a good working knowledge of infectious diseases with a basic understanding of the infectious process. This chapter includes a discussion of the methods by which each disease is transmitted, the signs and symptoms associated with each disease, and the measures by which the paramedic can prevent acquisition of the disease.

IMMUNE SYSTEM

To understand how the body responds to exposure to a specific organism or infection, the paramedic must have an understanding of the function of the body's protective mechanism, the **immune system**. The immune system is not made up of organs but of separate cells and molecules. Included among these are the white blood cells, connective tissue cells, and the protein molecules. The immune system's primary function is to prevent disease by searching for any foreign microscopic organisms found in the body and setting out to destroy them.

The **lymphatic system** is a vital component in the overall functioning of the immune system and is sometimes described as a "middle man" between the blood and the tissues of the body. The lymphatic system functions to move fluids and molecules from tissue spaces to the blood. The lymph fluid within the lymphatic system transports waste away from tissues and blood and carries nourishment from the blood to the tissues. At various points throughout the lymphatic network, nodes are found. These nodes function within the lymphatic system to produce lymphocytes (lymph cells) and antibodies. As the lymph fluid passes through the nodes, the lymphocytes and antibodies are added to the circulating fluid. The nodes also function as filters and serve as a defense against the spread of infection within the body.

Immune Response

The **immune response** is made up of two different but interrelated systems, the humoral and cellular systems. The actions of these systems are regulated by the B- and T-type lymphocytes. The working relationship between these two systems is formed by the action of the cells and antigen. **Humoral immunity** is the major system that defends against bacterial infection by circulating antibodies. **Cellular immunity** is the system that defends the body against infections caused by viruses, fungi, and some bacteria. Its action is regulated by T lymphocyte products.

During fetal development, lymphocyte precursors located in the thymus gland are transformed into the lymphocytes responsible for cellular immunity, the **T lymphocytes.** The **B lymphocytes** are transformed in the fetal liver and spleen. After transformation, these cells travel to the lymph nodes and bone marrow. The T lymphocytes are responsible for antibody production, and the B lymphocytes are responsible for the transformation of plasma cells that secrete antibodies into the circulatory system. These antibodies are termed **immunoglobulins.** Four primary immunoglobulins can be detected in the laboratory using immunofluorescent techniques. The primary immunoglobulins are: **IgG,** the presence of this antibody signifies past exposure to a disease; **IgA,** this antibody appears in the serum within a few days to a week after onset of certain viral illnesses; **IgM,** this antibody is the first to respond to the presence of a new antigen; and **IgE,** this antibody induces the cell to release a number of pharmacologically active agents, for example histamine; this release activates symptoms of an allergic reaction.

Humoral defenses play a major role in bacterial infection. Antibodies act to render bacteria ineffective. This body defense system activates and increases the production of *leukocytes* (white blood cells). White blood cells seek out, attack, and destroy certain *antigens* (invading bacteria). This process is known as **phagocytosis.**

Infectious and Communicable

Infectious and communicable are two terms that are not synonymous. An **infectious disease** is an illness caused by the invasion of an organism, be it a virus, bacterium, or a fungus. Examples of infectious diseases include pneumonia, meningitis, and hepatitis A. Each of these illnesses is caused by either bacteria or a virus and in some cases may be communicable, depending on the causative organism. A **communicable disease** is one that can be transmitted from one person to another. It is important to note that not all infections are communicable. For example, peritonitis caused by a specific bacteria is an infection, but it is not communicable directly from one person to another. Certain types of pneumonia and meningitis are communicable (*e.g.,* influenza, meningococcal), while other types are not (*e.g.,* pneumococcal pneumonia, viral meningitis).

Infectious diseases are transmitted by direct or indirect contact. For direct contact, a person physically touches the infected body area or fluid. For indirect contact, a person touches an object or surface that may have organisms on it and then introduces the organism into the body. Diseases are also transmitted by other means: they can be transmitted by infected droplets introduced into the air (*airborne transmission*) or by ingestion into the body (*vehicle transmission*). Drinking contaminated water is an example of vehicle transmission. Infectious diseases can also be spread by vectors; for example, malaria is spread by a certain type of mosquito.

Examples of communicable diseases, which are transmitted from one human being to another, include the common cold, the flu, measles, and mumps. Often, people are exposed to a disease and do not develop it; development of the disease depends on the response of the immune system. If a person is under physical or emotional stress, the immune system may not be normally responsive, resulting in increased susceptibility to infection.

COMMUNICABLE DISEASES OF ADULTS AND CHILDREN

Tuberculosis

Tuberculosis is a communicable disease caused by an organism known as *Mycobacterium tuberculosis*. This disease is spread by airborne transmission of droplets created by the coughing of an infected patient. The bacteria are introduced into the air in the form of droplets. The patient presents with symptoms of a productive cough, fever, and profuse night sweats. The patient also complains of weight loss, fatigue, and swollen glands. Often, the sputum contains blood (hemoptysis). The **incubation period** for tuberculosis is 4 to 12 weeks. Exposure is defined as prolonged contact with a patient who is actively coughing. Paramedics can protect themselves by using a face mask. The risk of acquiring tuberculosis while transporting a patient is low. Prolonged exposure is defined as working daily with or living in the same household as the infected person. Since this disease is spread by airborne droplets, the paramedic should place a face mask on the patient.

If a paramedic is exposed to a patient later found to have tuberculosis, the medical director should be notified to determine the need for any follow-up. If the paramedic is exposed to a coughing patient, follow-up should include administration of a tuberculin skin test (PPD). If the paramedic had a negative skin test when hired, a retest should be done 12 weeks after the exposure incident. If no skin test was performed before this exposure, testing should be done immediately after the exposure and again in 12 weeks. For paramedics with a previously positive tuberculin skin test, follow-up testing should be by chest film or observation of signs and symptoms. Should the paramedic test positive after an exposure, evaluation for drug therapy with isoniazid (INH) should be done.

Hepatitis Types A and B

The term **hepatitis** means inflammation of the liver. This condition can be the result of a virus, drug, or chemical reaction. It should be noted that not all types of hepatitis are communicable. For example, alcoholic and chemical hepatitis are not communicable. The most common type of communicable hepatitis is **hepatitis A,** caused by the hepatitis A virus. This disease is most common in children but does occur in adults.

The signs and symptoms for hepatitis A include low-grade fever, complaints of weakness and loss of appetite, nausea and vomiting, headache, and right upper-quadrant pain. As these signs and symptoms progress, the patient's stool takes on a clay-colored appearance, the urine becomes dark, and the patient's skin may take on a yellow appearance (*jaundice*). The incubation period for hepatitis A is 15 to 50 days after exposure, depending on dose; the average is 28 to 30 days.

Hepatitis A is transmitted through direct contact with the stool and urine of an infected patient. The paramedic can prevent acquisition of this disease by practicing good hand-washing techniques after contact with infected body excretions and by using disposable gloves. If exposed to the urine or stool of a patient with hepatitis A, the paramedic's medical director should be notified and *prophylaxis* (precautions taken to prevent a disease) with immune serum globulin may be recommended.

Hepatitis B is caused by the hepatitis B virus. This viral infection is transmitted through blood, urine, and other body fluids. In a nonmedical setting, people usually come in contact with hepatitis B through sexual exposure to carriers or through the use of dirty needles. This infection has a more insidious onset than hepatitis A. The incubation period can be 42 to 180 days after exposure; the average is 60 to 90 days. In many cases, the signs and symptoms are not always obvious. The signs and symptoms for hepatitis B include those that were described for hepatitis A; however, jaundice, clay-colored stools, and dark urine may never become evident. Patients may simply feel, from the presenting signs and symptoms, that they have a bad case of the flu. In other words, a large percent of infected people are not aware of their infection.

The paramedic can prevent acquisition of this disease by the practice of good hand-washing techniques and the use of disposable gloves when in contact with blood or body fluids. Since hepatitis B is a blood-borne disease, a contaminated needle stick injury requires immediate follow-up. The risk of acquiring hepatitis B as the result of an exposure to hepatitis B positive blood is estimated to be between 6% and 30%. Exposure can be defined as ***percutaneous*** (intravenous, intramuscular, subcutaneous, or intradermal) or ***permucosal*** contact with contaminated blood or body fluids, as can occur in needle stick accidents or blood splattered into eyes, mouth, or fresh wounds. Risk can be diminished by recurring hepatitis B vaccine.

Several studies list prehospital providers in the high-risk group for hepatitis B. One study demonstrated a three to five times greater risk for the prehospital provider than for that of the general public. The Centers for Disease Control and the Occupational Safety and Health

BLOOD EXPOSURE FOLLOW-UP

1. Document on the employer's accident report form any blood and body fluid exposure on the day the exposure occurs.
2. Follow state or department's procedure regarding hand delivery of that form to the patient's receiving health care facility and a copy to your department.
3. In some states, further testing of the patient for HBV, hepatitis C, and HIV may be initiated on receipt of documentation of a blood exposure. In other states, testing may not be initiated, but EMS departments are notified if patient has a known communicable disease.
4. Prophylaxis should be given within the first 24 hours in the following situations:

Patient Results	Prophylaxis
Hepatitis B surface antigen positive or known carrier	Hepatitis B immune globulin and hepatitis B vaccine
Hepatitis C or elevated alanine aminotransferase	Immune serum globulin
HIV Positive or AIDS	No prophylaxis currently recommended; baseline HIV test and 3-month, 6-month, and 1-year follow-up testing of exposed care giver

Administration recommend vaccine for all emergency care providers. This counsel is an important example of why vaccine programs are recommended. In the absence of vaccine, note the specific procedure to follow up a contaminated needle stick injury reflected in the box "Blood Exposure Follow-up."

Hepatitis C

Hepatitis C was formerly known as non-A, non-B hepatitis. Little is known about this form of hepatitis. Hepatitis C usually is associated with receipt of contaminated blood during transfusion. It is the most common post-transfusion hepatitis in the United States, accounting for approximately 90% of such disease. The incidence of this disease is growing in the intravenous drug user group. The incubation period ranges from 2 weeks to 6 months, but most fall within 6 to 9 weeks. Since it is transmitted by blood, it becomes an occupational health risk if a contaminated needle stick injury is sustained while working with an infected patient.

In February 1991, the Food and Drug Administration approved the first effective treatment for hepatitis C. Diagnosis is made on signs, symptoms, history, negative testing for hepatitis A and hepatitis B, positive hepatitis C antibody, and elevated liver enzymes.

The paramedic can protect against acquisition of this virus by handling needles and other blood-contaminated sharp objects carefully, by not recapping needles whenever possible, and by avoiding mucous membrane contact with blood and body fluids. If an injury occurs, it should be documented and medical follow-up should be sought. Prophylaxis may include receipt of immune serum globulin; dosage is based on body weight.

Meningitis

The term **meningitis** refers to the inflammation of the membranes that surround the brain and spinal cord. This inflammation is caused primarily by bacteria or viruses, more infrequently by fungi. The specific cause for each case is determined by the result of first a Gram's stain or direct antigen test and then a culture of the cerebrospinal fluid. Bacterial meningitis is a disease primarily seen in young children.

The symptoms and signs for meningitis whether caused by a bacteria or virus are much the same: fever, headache, nausea, and vomiting with a rash. The incubation period varies with the causative organism, depending on whether it is bacteria or virus. The average incubation period is between 2 to 10 days.

The mode of transmission for bacterial meningitis is direct contact with upper respiratory (e.g., nasopharyngeal, throat) secretions from an infected person. Viral meningitis is acquired by the inhalation of droplets from the respiratory tract of an infected person.

The primary difference between the two types of meningitis is their degree of communicability. Bacterial meningitis is often described as being highly communicable, particularly after prolonged direct contact with the patient's respiratory secretions. Viral meningitis, however, is not readily communicable.

The paramedic cannot determine, based on signs and symptoms, which type of meningitis the patient may have; therefore, prevention should include the use of an artificial resuscitation device, rather than direct mouth-to-mouth resuscitation. The paramedic should also wear a face mask, protective eye wear, and gloves when coming in close, direct contact with the patient's respiratory secretions (e.g., intubation, suctioning). A face mask should be placed on the patient whenever possible.

If prevention was not practiced by the paramedic or if there is risk of exposure, it should be reported to the medical director. Once the type of meningitis has been identified, the need for prophylactic medication can be evaluated.

Herpes

The herpesvirus family has many members, including herpes simplex virus 1 and 2, varicella-zoster virus, and cytomegalovirus. The herpesvirus generally enters the body through a mucous membrane, such as the lips or genital area. It may also enter through breaks in the skin and result in herpetic whitlow. Once the herpesvirus has invaded the body, it takes up residence in the ganglia of nerve and resides there until triggered to be active. This time is referred to as the latency period. This latent characteristic explains why the herpesvirus family is responsible for chronic infections with oftentimes multiple reactivations. Activation can be brought on by physical or emotional stress. Herpes lesions can appear anywhere on the body, depending on the nerve affected. The onset of lesions usually is signaled by itching, tingling, or a burning sensation. This reaction is referred to as the prodrome or warning phase. A person is considered communicable from the time of the prodrome until the lesions are crusted and dried. Recent studies have shown that the herpesvirus may continue to be present in secretions when obvious lesions are not present.

Herpes Simplex Types 1 and 2

Herpes simplex types 1 and 2 can only be differentiated by immunologic testing, not by location on the patient's body. The clinical presentation of herpes simplex is usually a fluid-filled vesicle, usually located near a mucous membrane, for example, on the lip, labia, or genitalia. Lesions located on the lip or oral area are commonly referred to as "*cold sores*" or "*fever blisters*." Usually, these herpetic vesicles are caused by the herpes simplex virus 1, but genital herpetic lesions or vesicles can transmit herpes simplex virus 2 to the oral area during oral intercourse and vice versa, type 1 oral lesions can be spread to the genital area. Therefore, no hard and fast guidelines place herpes simplex type 1 above the waist and type 2 below the waist. Herpes simplex is transmitted by direct contact with drainage from the lesion, mucous membranes of the mouth, saliva, or genital area, including the buttocks and thighs. The incubation period for developing herpes simplex vesicles or lesions is 1 to 12 days after contact exposure. Since many people shed this virus and are not aware of it, the paramedic can prevent acquisition of this disease by using a face mask when ventilating a patient in respiratory distress. When clearing an airway, disposable gloves should be worn. Since herpesvirus can infect the eye, protective eye wear should be worn if spray or splatter is anticipated.

Since genital herpes is a sexually transmitted disease and lesions may be present in the vaginal canal during the birth process, there is a significant risk of transmission to the infant. Any lesions noted during a field delivery should be reported immediately. This notation will assist in the proper identification and treatment of the newborn. Transmission of genital herpes is similar to oral herpes, that is, with direct contact of mucous membranes with fluid-filled vesicles or lesions; therefore, barrier precautions should be used.

If the paramedic comes into contact with lesions while performing a physical assessment of a patient, good hand washing is required and disposable gloves should be worn. This disease is not spread through contact with toilet seats, hot tubs, pools, or stretcher bedding. If the paramedic is exposed, the occurrence should be documented. No follow-up treatment is indicated.

Herpetic Whitlow

One form of herpesvirus infection listed as an occupational health risk for health care providers is herpetic whitlow. **Herpetic whitlow** is herpes simplex virus infection of the finger or fingers. It can be acquired if a cut, open sore, or torn hangnail comes in direct contact with secretions from a person who is shedding herpesvirus. Because many people shed herpesvirus in their oral secretions, the use of disposable gloves and good hand washing is strongly recommended when in contact with oral secretions.

Similar to other herpesvirus infections, the incubation period is between 2 to 12 days after the exposure. If acquired, there is no cure for this disease. Antiviral treatment with acyclovir (Zovirax) is available and may shorten the duration of the outbreak and minimize the symptoms. If herpetic whitlow develops, it should be clearly documented as a work-related disease.

Varicella

Varicella (chickenpox) is one of the most common childhood diseases and is the only childhood disease for which no routine preventative vaccine is available. The causative agent is varicella-zoster virus, a member of the herpesvirus family. This disease is usually a mild one that begins with sore throat, sudden onset of low-grade fever, and headache. This initial phase lasts about 2 days, then the rash appears. The rash usually begins on the face and back then spreads to the rest of the body (Fig. 26-1). The rash then progresses to become vesicles that rupture and scab during the recovery phase. A person with chickenpox is communicable until all the lesions are crusted and dried, usually within 5 to 7 days.

Chickenpox is transmitted by direct contact with the secretions from the lesions and also by airborne droplets from the respiratory tract. The incubation period is 10 to 21 days after exposure. This fact is particularly important to the paramedic who has not had chickenpox and is exposed.

The paramedic who is exposed to chickenpox and who is not immune has to be removed from duty from the 10th day after the exposure to the 21st day to see if chickenpox develops. However, the paramedic can prevent exposure by not caring for a child deemed to have chickenpox, by using a face mask and gloves when caring for a patient with symptoms suggestive of chickenpox, or by receiving Varicella Zoster Immune Globulin (VZIG) for prophylaxis. Gloves are also required for contact with drainage from the vesicles. Exposure should be promptly reported to the medical director. Blood testing for antibodies to varicella-zoster virus can determine whether the paramedic is immune or nonimmune. This testing must be done before the 10th day after exposure.

Herpes Zoster

Herpes zoster (shingles) is also caused by a member of the herpesvirus family. However, one important difference in the virus content of these lesions is that they contain live varicella-zoster virus. As previously discussed, the herpesvirus can remain dormant for long periods of time; herpes zoster is a good example of this phenomenon. Herpes zoster is a local manifestation of a reactivation with the virus that causes chickenpox.

Shingles usually presents as a unilateral rash that progresses to pustules (Fig. 26-2). The patient complains of itching and a constant burning pain. The risk with shin-

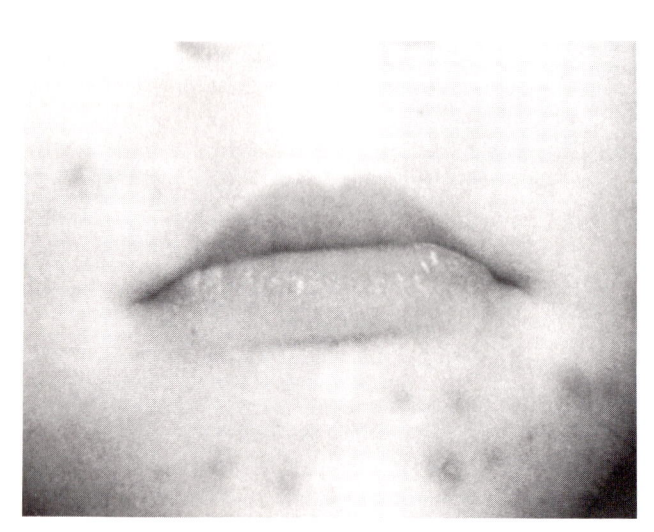

FIGURE 26-1.
Varicella.

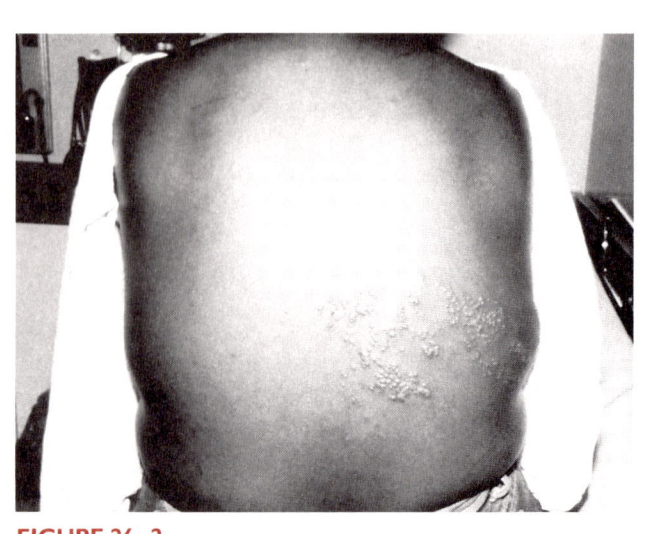

FIGURE 26-2.
Herpes zoster.

gles is that, if the care giver has not had chickenpox, direct contact with drainage from the lesions could cause the care giver to develop chickenpox. Shingles is not readily transmitted through droplets as is chickenpox.

The paramedic should wear disposable gloves when in contact with lesions. Good hand-washing technique also remains an important procedure. If gloves are not available and direct contact with drainage from lesions occurs, it should be determined from the medical record if the paramedic ever had chickenpox; if not, the exposure should be documented and the medical director notified.

Cytomegalovirus

Cytomegalovirus (CMV) is also a member of the herpesvirus family. As with the many other diseases discussed, most people infected with this virus do not exhibit any symptoms. This virus is common in immune-compromised people, such as those who are infected with human immunodeficiency virus, who have leukemia, and who have undergone transplant surgery. This virus is also the cause of congenital abnormalities as the result of transmission from mother to fetus.

Cytomegalovirus is transmitted by direct contact with infectious secretions or excretions. Cytomegalovirus is excreted in urine, saliva, breast milk, cervical secretions, and semen during primary or reactivated infection. *Viremia* (virus in the blood) may be present in asymptomatic people, and the virus may be transmitted by blood transfusion, probably associated with leukocytes. Infection from patient to care giver is not well documented in the literature. The paramedic should wear gloves and practice good hand washing when in direct contact with blood and body fluids.

Syphilis

Syphilis is a sexually transmitted disease that has been prevalent worldwide since the time of ancient Egypt. The incidence of syphilis in this country has been increasing since the late 1960s, apparently a result of the sexual revolution. Syphilis is a treatable disease, but, if not treated, long-term problems may result. The causative organism is a spirochete known as *Treponema pallidum*. The incubation period for this disease is 10 days to 10 weeks, usually 3 weeks after exposure. The disease has a course of three stages; the first is called the primary phase when the lesion or *chancre* is first noted. This lesion is painless and resolves without treatment in 4 to 6 weeks. The second stage begins about 6 weeks after the lesion first appeared. At this time, lymph nodes begin to enlarge and a reddish brown rash appears on the hands and feet. The person also presents with fever, headache, sore throat, and a loss of appetite. If not treated, the disease proceeds into the third or latent stage. During this phase, the blood serology test is positive but no other symptoms are present.

During the latent stage, syphilis can affect various organs, the central nervous system, and the heart and major vessels. Syphilis is a blood-borne disease and can be transmitted to a fetus in utero or through blood transfusion. The donor's blood is screened for syphilis before transfusion.

Syphilis should not pose a risk for the paramedic who is caring for a patient with syphilis. Since this disease can also be spread through blood transfusion, disposable gloves should be worn when handling blood. Risk of infection by blood exposure is negligible since the number of spirochetes that circulate in the bloodstream is small. Infection by indirect contact with contaminated articles is theoretically possible but rarely occurs. Health professionals have developed primary lesions on the hands after clinical examination of infectious lesions. When caring for people in the field, the paramedic does not always know what disease the patient may have; therefore, the use of gloves is required whenever handling blood or body fluids or whenever in direct contact with lesions or rashes. If genital lesions are noted when assisting in field deliveries, the attending physician at the hospital should be informed.

Gonorrhea

Gonorrhea is another common sexually transmitted diseases. It is caused by a bacterium called *Neisseria gonorrhoeae*. This disease is seen in both males and females but may differ in course, severity, and ease of recognition. In women, chronic infection can lead to infertility and pelvic inflammatory disease. As with syphilis, gonorrhea has been prevalent throughout the world for many years, with reported cases increasing since the onset of the sexual revolution of the late 1960s. This disease, for the most part, is treatable. Some new strains brought into the United States from southeast Asia and the Philippines are resistant to penicillin (penicillinase-producing *Neisseria gonorrhoeae* strains).

The incubation period for this disease is about 2 to 7 days after exposure. The presenting symptoms differ somewhat in men and women. In the male, a yellow discharge may be noted from the penis, and the patient may complain of pain on urination. In the female, symptoms may include a vaginal or urethral discharge, pain on urination, or simply lower abdominal pain. Some women show no symptoms at all. In both sexes, pharyngeal and anal infections are common. Septicemia may occur, with arthritis, skin lesions, endocarditis, and meningitis.

Because the disease is sexually transmitted, the newborn is at risk for exposure during the birth process. The disease should be identified early and treatment for the infant prescribed. All newborns are prophylactically treated with either 1% silver nitrate solution, erythromycin, or tetracycline ophthalmic ointments to prevent gonococcal conjunctivitis. If unusual discharge is noted in a field delivery, the attending physician at the hospital should be informed.

Mode of transmission is by direct contact with exudates from mucous membranes of infected people, almost always as a result of sexual activity. Good hand washing after contact with potential infectious secretions should adequately protect care givers.

Scabies and Lice

Both scabies and lice are occupational hazards for the paramedic. Since the paramedic has direct contact with a wide variety of people, the transfer of the scabies mite and lice is not uncommon.

Scabies is an eight-legged mite that burrows beneath the layers of the skin. The waste products deposited under the skin produce symptoms of intense itching, which may not begin until 2 to 6 weeks after exposure. Inflammation may accompany the itching. The areas that may be affected include the abdomen, lower buttocks, wrists, elbows, genital area, and the area between the fingers.

Lice have six legs and reproduce by laying eggs. They are divided into three types. Head lice, *Pediculus capitis*, are prevalent in young school children. Body lice are *Pediculus corporis*, and pubic lice (crab lice) are *Phthirus pubis*. Head and pubic lice attach their eggs to hair shafts with a cementlike substance. To survive, lice need a blood meal at least every 24 to 48 hours. Lice can live away from the human body on fomites, such as clothing or stuffed animals, for brief periods of time.

The paramedic can prevent exposure to both scabies and lice by using disposable gloves when handling a potentially infested patient. If the paramedic's clothing has been in direct contact with the patient, the clothing should be washed by normal laundering with soap and hot water. No special chemicals need to be used. If the paramedic develops symptoms of scabies or lice, the medical director should be notified and the paramedic examined and treated if infested. Kwell is the usual prescription drug of choice; however, some over-the-counter medications are also effective. Lotions or shampoos recommended for treatment should be used once and repeated in 10 to 14 days. This procedure kills any eggs that hatch within a week.

Mumps

Mumps is a viral disease caused by the mumps virus, a member of the genus *Paramyxovirus*. It is less common than other childhood diseases. It is estimated that about one third of exposed people develop an asymptomatic infection. This disease has been decreasing in incidence because of the availability of the MMR vaccine (measles, mumps, rubella vaccine), which is part of the routine immunization program for children. It is somewhat seasonal, appearing mostly in the winter and spring.

Mumps is transmitted by direct contact with the oral secretions of an infected person. The incubation period is 2 to 3 weeks, commonly 18 days after exposure. The presenting symptoms include fever, swelling, and tenderness in the area of the salivary glands. In adult men, *orchitis* (inflammation of the testes) may be the major manifestation of mumps. The central nervous system may be involved, either early or late in the disease, usually as an aseptic meningitis.

The paramedic can avoid acquisition of mumps by receiving recommended immunization if nonimmune. In lieu of immunization, the use of disposable gloves when in direct contact with secretions and good hand washing are recommended. A mask is also indicated, as this disease is transmissible by respiration.

Measles: Rubella and Rubeola

Rubella is caused by a virus that is a member of the genus *Rubivirus*. It occurs worldwide and is most prevalent in the winter and spring. This disease is also decreasing in incidence because preventative vaccine (MMR) is available and is part of the recommended childhood immunization program. This disease is transmitted by direct contact with nasopharyngeal secretions from an infected person. It is also transmitted by droplets and by direct contact with articles contaminated with blood, urine, and stool.

Children may begin their illness with few initial symptoms, including fever, headache, malaise, runny eyes, and generalized swollen lymph glands. The rash associated with this disease is difficult to distinguish from other rashes. It is usually a diffuse macular rash. As many as half of infections may occur without evident rash. The incubation period is 14 to 23 days after exposure, and the person is communicable 1 week before to 4 days after the rash appears.

The paramedic can protect against acquiring this disease first by receiving appropriate immunization if not immune. Immunity is essential for care providers because infection poses a risk to pregnant women. If a woman becomes infected during the first trimester of her pregnancy, her infant could develop **congenital rubella syndrome.** This disease is associated with multiple congenital anomalies and mental retardation. The Centers for Disease Control recommends that all health care providers be immune to reduce the risk of exposure to themselves and those they treat. In addition, prevention includes the use of a mask and gloves when caring for a person with symptoms suggestive of rubella.

Rubeola, also known as the red measles or hard measles, is caused by a virus that belongs to the genus *Morbillivirus*. This form of measles is also decreasing in incidence; although recent outbreaks have occurred in teenage children and young adults. Rubeola is also preventable by vaccine administration. In fact, measles, mumps, and rubella are given as a triple vaccine, the MMR vac-

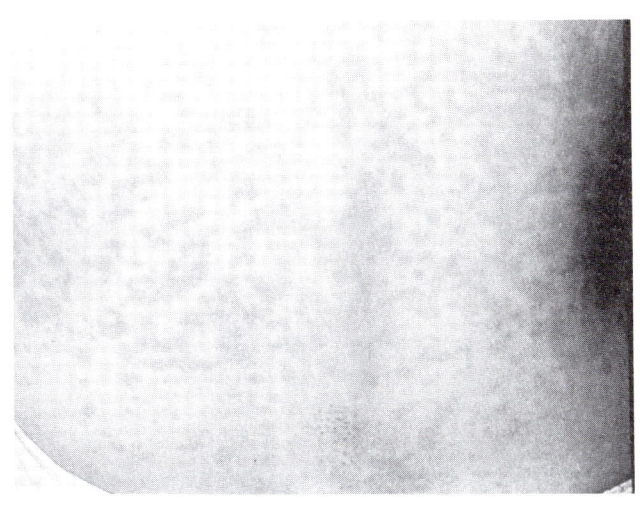

FIGURE 26–3.
Rubeola rash.

cine, to children older than 12 months of age. A second, booster shot is currently recommended to prevent outbreaks of vaccine-failure measles.

The person with rubeola presents with fever, conjunctivitis, cough, and white spots noted on the buccal mucosa known as **Koplik's spots.** The rash associated with rubeola is red, diffuse, and blotchy (Fig. 26-3). The incubation period varies from 8 to 13 days after exposure for development of fever and about 14 days until rash occurs. Transmission is by droplet spread and direct contact with nasal and throat secretions; it is less commonly spread by air or by articles freshly soiled with secretions of nose and throat.

As with rubella, the paramedic can prevent acquisition of rubeola by obtaining the recommended immunization if not immune. In lieu of immunity, the use of a mask and gloves are recommended when in direct contact with secretions. Good hand washing is also a routine procedure in patient care.

Acquired Immunodeficiency Syndrome

Acquired immunodeficiency syndrome (AIDS) was first identified in 1980, although the first cases occurred in the United States as early as 1978. At that time, the agent responsible for AIDS had not been identified, but the epidemiology of AIDS appeared to be similar to hepatitis B. Therefore, the first recommendations were modeled after previous Centers for Disease Control recommendations designed to prevent the transmission of hepatitis B. In 1984, scientific research discovered the viral agent responsible for AIDS and, subsequently, in 1985 developed serologic tests for antibodies directed against the virus. Initially, this virus was named human T-cell lymphotrophic virus, type III (HTLV-III). Later, the scientific community changed the name of this virus to **human immunodeficiency virus (HIV).** Because of these advances, it is possible to gain a clearer understanding of the risk for occupational and nosocomial transmission of HIV.

Infection with HIV occurs worldwide. Because of the effect this virus has on the immune system, opportunistic infections and malignancies can occur and allow the HIV infection to be classified as AIDS. Infection with HIV alone may not result in any symptoms of illness. For this reason, universal precautions when resuscitating or providing medical care in the field are necessary. Figure 26-4 shows reported and projected cases of AIDS in the United States.

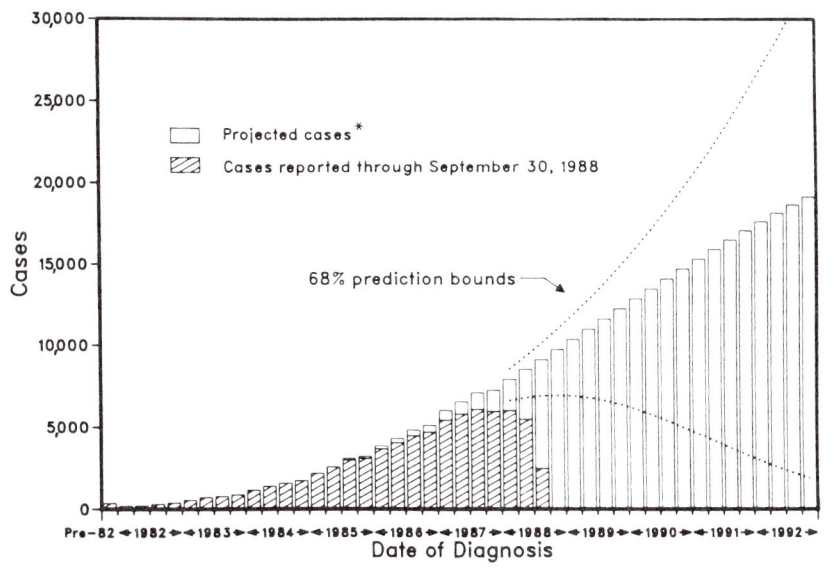

FIGURE 26–4.
Incidence of AIDS, by quarter and year of diagnosis, in the United States, pre-1982 to 1992. (Centers for Disease Control: AIDS and human immunodeficiency virus infection in the United States: 1988 update. MMWR 38 (No. S-4:36, 1989)

Infection with HIV is transmitted primarily by sexual intercourse with an infected person, sharing contaminated intravenous needles, infected mother to her baby, and multiple blood transfusions before March 1985. Antibody screening methods have been available and required of blood donors since that time. Infection with HIV is primarily a sexually transmitted disease. Even though the virus is present in most body fluids, no evidence has been documented that HIV infection, and subsequently AIDS, can be acquired by contact other than sexual or blood to blood. This assertion is supported by serologic antibody studies of nonsexual household contacts and health care workers, illustrating the intimate contact required for transmission of the virus.

The incubation period appears to be in the range of 2 months to 10 years or longer, with a mean of 2 years in transfusion-associated cases. The presenting symptoms of AIDS are weight loss unrelated to dieting (greater than 10% of total body weight), fever (greater than or equal to 104°F) and night sweats, pneumonia caused by an opportunistic organism, persistent diarrhea, swollen glands in the neck, groin, and axillary region that do not resolve, or the presence of "purplish" lesions on the skin or mucous membranes (***Kaposi's sarcoma***).

It is important to note that studies of health care personnel with documented blood exposure to HIV-infected blood have shown that health care personnel are at low risk for acquiring HIV infection. Information gathered from ten prospective studies that were designed to assess the magnitude of risk for HIV transmission in the health care setting reveal this risk to be 0.36%. This low risk of acquiring infection may be due to the low numbers of viruses per milliliter of blood and the need for efficient transmission of significant numbers of viruses into the appropriate mucous membranes of the exposed person. Many describe this need as the intimate nature of transmission of this virus. Many natural barriers, such as intact skin and gastric acids, may provide some initial protection. Additional first aid measures, such as cleaning the injury with soap, water, and then alcohol, also provide inhibitory measures to the establishment of the virus; health care workers also have an opportunity to clean up spills and disinfect reusable instruments, equipment, or linen used in providing medical care.

The paramedic and all health care personnel are required to use disposable gloves when in contact with blood or body fluids while caring for all patients. This universal precaution protects care givers from asymptomatic as well as symptomatic (or known) carriers of this virus. Good hand washing remains important even with the use of gloves. Care should be taken to avoid contaminated needle stick injuries. If ventilatory assistance is necessary as part of the care, an artificial resuscitator, such as a pocket mask or bag–valve–mask device, should be used.

Many studies involve health care workers who have had direct exposure to HIV; direct exposure is described as a contaminated needle stick injury, mucous membrane (e.g., eye, nose, mouth) contact with secretions, and contact with open lesions. Needle stick injury presents the primary risk. Disposal of used needles and syringes at the point of use into a puncture-proof impervious container without recapping is recommended to reduce needle stick injuries. If direct contact is made with the blood or body fluids of a person with HIV infection, the paramedic's medical director should be contacted. The procedure for

TABLE 26–1.
SUMMARY CHART

Disease	Method of Transmission	Prevention Measure
Chickenpox	Airborne	Mask
	Lesion contact	Gloves/hand washing
Measles	Airborne	Mask
	Contact with respiratory secretions	Gloves/hand washing
Mumps	Airborne	Mask
	Contact with saliva	Gloves/hand washing
Meningitis	Airborne	Mask
	Contact with respiratory secretions	Gloves/hand washing
Tuberculosis	Airborne	Mask
Hepatitis A	Urine, stool contact	Gloves/hand washing
Hepatitis B	Blood, saliva contact, semen, vaginal secretions	Gloves/hand washing
Hepatitis C	Blood contact	Gloves/hand washing
AIDS (or HIV infection)	Contact with blood, certain body fluids, cerebrospinal fluid, semen, vaginal secretions	Gloves/hand washing
Syphilis	Blood, lesion contact	Gloves/hand washing
Gonorrhea	Contact with genital secretions	Gloves/hand washing
Herpes	Contact with lesions, drainage, saliva	Gloves/hand washing

follow-up (see the box "Blood Exposure Follow-up") serves to continue collecting data that documents the low risk and to document types of occupational exposure.

Table 26-1 is a summary chart of disease transmission and prevention.

TECHNIQUES OF MANAGEMENT

Universal Precautions

In August of 1987, the Centers for Disease Control adopted the concept that the blood and body fluids of all persons should be considered potentially infectious for HIV, hepatitis B virus (HBV), and other blood-borne pathogens. This concept was termed **universal precautions.** This chapter has reviewed many diseases in which a person can be infected and not exhibit any signs or symptoms (*e.g.*, hepatitis B, hepatitis C, herpes). Thus, the concept of universal precautions offers a common sense approach to health care.

Universal precautions are intended to prevent parenteral, mucous membrane, and nonintact skin exposure of health care workers to blood-borne pathogens. Appropriate barriers should be used to protect the mucous membranes and skin of health care workers from direct contact with the blood and other body fluids that contain blood of all patients. Universal precautions also apply to semen and vaginal secretions. The risk of transmission from these sources to the care giver in the health care setting is limited, since gloves are routinely worn for vaginal examinations.

Universal precautions also apply to tissues and to the following fluids: cerebrospinal fluid, synovial (joint) fluid, pleural fluid, peritoneal fluid, pericardial fluid, and amniotic fluid. The risk of transmission of HIV and HBV from these fluids is unknown, since epidemiologic studies of health care exposures are limited. Appropriate barrier precautions, such as gloves, during the aseptic procedure and masks and eye wear to protect against splatter should be applied. Extreme caution should be used to guard against penetrating injuries due to contaminated needles or other sharp instruments.

Protective barriers are used in the application of universal precautions to reduce the risk of exposure to blood, body fluids that contain visible blood, and other fluids. Examples of protective barriers include gloves, gowns, masks, and protective eye wear (Fig. 26-5). Gloves should reduce the incidence of contamination of hands, but they cannot prevent penetrating injuries due to needles or other sharp instruments. Gowns protect general exposed body parts. Masks and protective eye wear or face shields should reduce the incidence of contamination of mucous membranes of the mouth, nose, and eyes (Figs. 26-6 and 26-7). Gloves, gowns, masks, and protective eyewear are required by law to be present on all emergency vehicles that respond or potentially respond to medical emergencies or victim rescues.

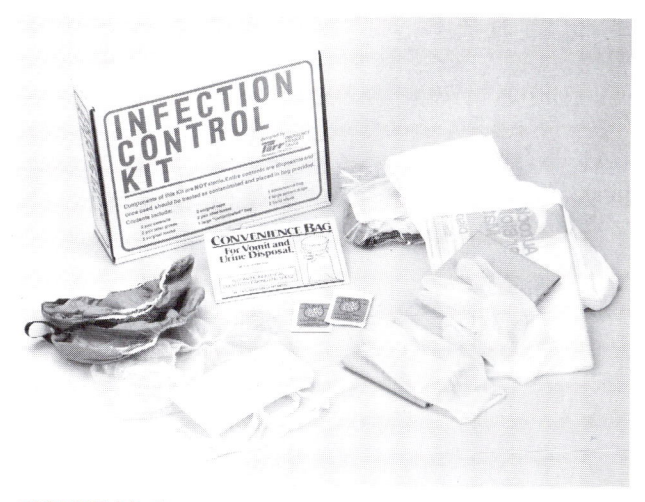

FIGURE 26–5.
Infection control kit. (Courtesy of Parr Emergency Product Sales, Inc., Galloway, Ohio.)

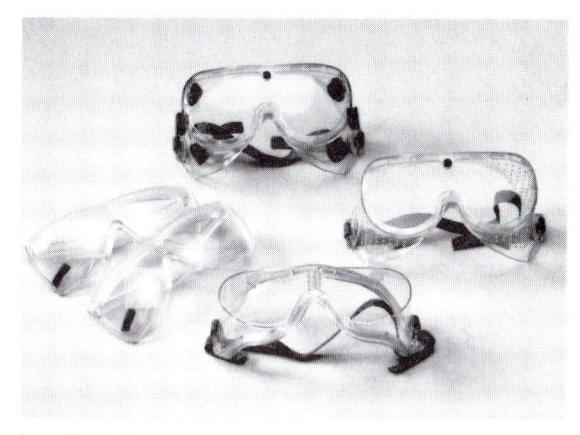

FIGURE 26–6.
Types of protective eye wear. (Courtesy of Parr Emergency Product Sales, Inc., Galloway, Ohio.)

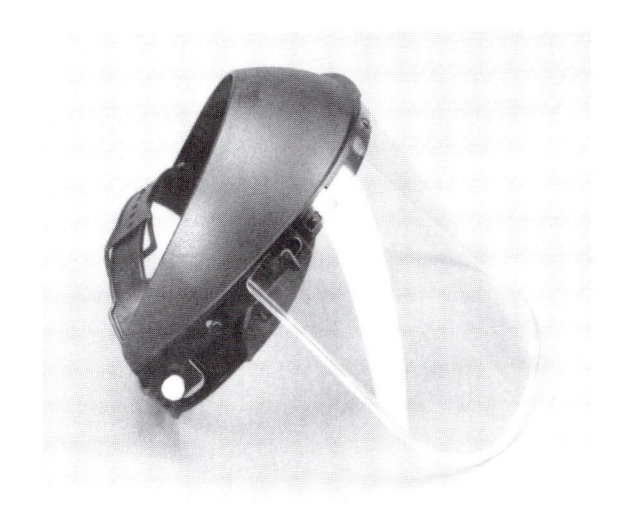

FIGURE 26–7.
Face shield. (Courtesy of Parr Emergency Product Sales, Inc., Galloway, Ohio.)

Universal precautions are intended to supplement rather than replace recommendations for routine infection control, such as hand washing and using gloves to prevent gross microbial contamination of hands. Because specifying the types of barriers needed for every possible clinical situation is impractical, some judgment must be exercised.

The risk of transmission of HIV, HBV, and other blood-borne pathogens can be minimized if health care workers use the following general guidelines:

1. Take care to prevent injuries when using needles, scalpels, lancets, and other sharp instruments or devices, when handling sharp instruments after procedures, when cleaning used instruments, and when disposing of used needles. Do not recap used needles; do not remove used needles from disposable syringes; and do not bend, break, or otherwise manipulate used needles. Place used disposable syringes and needles, scalpel blades, lancets, and other sharp items in puncture-resistant containers for disposal. Place the puncture-resistant containers as close to the use area as is practical.
2. Use protective barriers to prevent exposure to blood, body fluids that contain visible blood, and other fluids to which universal precautions apply. The type of protective barriers should be appropriate for the procedure being performed and the type of exposure anticipated (Table 26-2).
3. Immediately and thoroughly wash hands and other skin surfaces that are contaminated with blood, body fluids that contain visible blood, or other body fluids to which universal precautions apply.

Hand Washing

Throughout this chapter, the importance of good hand washing has been addressed. This technique is the single and most effective way to be protected when rendering care. Hand washing should be practiced before and after each patient contact and before performing any invasive

TABLE 26–2.
SUGGESTED INFECTION CONTROL PROCEDURES FOR SELECTED PARAMEDIC SKILLS

Skill	Precautions	Rationale
Establishing peripheral IV access Administering medications by the intradermal, subcutaneous, intramuscular, rectal, or sublingual routes Controlling hemorrhage in dressing wounds that do not exhibit spurting blood	Gloves	To prevent blood and body fluid contact with nonintact skin
Assessing and managing a patient who exhibits productive coughing or sneezing Assessing and managing a patient when the paramedic is experiencing productive coughing or sneezing	Mask, gloves	To prevent exposure to respiratory droplets, to prevent blood and body fluid contact with nonintact skin
Situations in which managing a patient's airway requires suctioning Endotracheal suctioning; inserting nasogastric or orogastric tubes Endotracheal intubation Esophageal intubation Establishing central intravenous access Controlling arterial bleeding Field delivery	Gloves, mask, protective eye wear	To prevent blood and body fluid contact with nonintact skin or with mucous membranes
Field delivery Controlling hemorrhage in dressing wounds that exhibit spurting blood	Gloves, mask, protective eye wear, gown	To prevent blood and body fluid splashes with nonintact skin or mucous membranes

procedure, such as starting an intravenous line or passing an endotracheal tube. Hand washing should also be performed after removing gloves, since gloves may not be a 100% effective barrier.

In the field, the use of alcohol-based hand wash products is recommended. For alcohol to be effective in degerming, the *proteinaceous* (gross) matter must first be removed. Alcohol cannot penetrate through protein to kill bacteria or viruses. In the hospital setting, the following steps are involved in a proper hand-washing procedure:

1. Use the soap that is recommended in the hospital. It is the mechanical action and friction used, not the specific soap, that is important.
2. Using friction, create a lather and wash for at least 15 seconds.
3. Rinse hands and dry with a paper towel.
4. Use the paper towel to turn off the water.

Handling and Disposal of Needles

The Centers for Disease Control recommend that needles not be recapped after use. The recapping procedure often results in needle stick injuries. Needles should not be cut or bent for disposal. Instead, the needle and syringe should be disposed of as one intact unit into a puncture-resistant container right after their use. Needles and syringes need to be disposed of as infectious waste, rather than as regular trash.

Disposal of Contaminated Articles

Articles that have been in direct contact with blood or body fluids should be handled as infectious waste. The Environmental Protection Agency recommends the following procedures for disposal:

1. Dressings should be placed in plastic bags to contain the secretions for disposal. Incineration is recommended.
2. Suction secretion containers should be sealed and then bagged. If disposable units are not available, contents should be carefully poured down the drain (sewer) and the container cleaned with a disinfectant solution. Appropriate protective barriers should be worn to protect mucous membranes from splatter.
3. Soiled linens should be bagged in a heavy-gauge plastic bag, which should be available in the emergency department. The outer bag, if required by the hospital, is color coded and shows the universal symbol for infectious waste. Check the hospital's procedure.

Gloving Technique

Sterile gloves are not required for routine care and self-protection in the field. Vinyl and latex nonsterile gloves are adequate and protective. Gloves should be worn for all procedures in which the paramedic anticipates contact with blood or other body fluids. Sterile gloves are indicated for sterile procedures; sterility, however, is difficult to maintain in the field. Vinyl and latex gloves do not require any special procedure to apply.

1. Apply disposable gloves and conduct procedures.
2. To remove, grasp disposable glove cuff. Pull the glove down over the hand to remove so that the glove is turned inside out after removal. This procedure reduces contact with the outer contaminated surface of the glove.
3. Remove gloves immediately after the procedure, taking care not to contaminate articles with patient's secretions.
4. Wash hands after removing gloves.

Gowns

Gowns or aprons should be worn to protect clothing from splashes with blood. If large splashes or quantities of blood are present or anticipated, impervious gowns or aprons should be worn. An extra change of work clothing should be available at all times.

Protective Eye Wear

The use of protective eye wear is recommended for situations in which blood splatter is anticipated. If prescription glasses are worn, these offer protection. If not, safety glasses are recommended. The type of face shields and goggles used depends on the EMS system. In the selection of eye wear, the time to apply, ease of application, cost, and the visual effect to the patient should be considered.

Face Mask

The use of a face mask is recommended for procedures that produce coughing and splatter of respiratory secretions (*e.g.*, intubation of patient). As with the use of protective eye wear, the purpose of the mask is to protect the care giver's mucous membranes from direct contact with the patient's potentially infectious secretions.

Cleaning a Blood Spill

Blood presents the greatest risk for carrying infection caused by HBV or HIV. Therefore, it is important to clean all blood-contaminated areas after completion of a call. The following procedure is recommended:

1. Put on gloves (heavy duty rubber).
2. Clean area with soap and water.
3. Soak area with a hospital-approved disinfectant agent or a bleach and water solution. Bleach and water

mixed at approximately 1½ cup bleach per gallon of water (1-to-10 solution) is effective and nontoxic.
4. Do not apply a bleach-water solution at a 1-to-10 ratio to delicate stainless steel items (*e.g.*, surgical instruments); this strength results in pitting of the surface and permanent damage to the item.

Cleaning the Vehicle

Infection control is for the benefit of the patient as well as the paramedic. To achieve a clean working environment that reduces the chance for cross infection, vehicle surfaces need to be cleaned on a routine basis. Cleaning routines should be conducted after each run and on a weekly basis.

To clean after the run, the following procedures should be conducted:

1. Put on gloves (heavy-duty rubber).
2. Using the proper cleaning agent, wipe down visibly soiled areas. These include the areas that the patient or the patient's blood or body fluids covered. It also includes areas that were touched while caring for the patient.
3. The cleaning solution should be a hospital-approved disinfectant that is effective against *Mycobacterium tuberculosis*. *M. tuberculosis* is not an organism that is spread by contact; however, this organism is one of the most difficult to kill by chemical means. Therefore, an effective cleaning agent must be used. If a commercial disinfectant is not available, bleach and water (1-to-10) is an acceptable cleaning solution.

Areas to include in weekly cleaning are doors, floors, walls, and windows. All cleaning routines should be documented.

Blood Exposure Follow-up

Criteria for a blood exposure include the following:

- Percutaneous puncture or cut with a contaminated needle or sharp instrument
- Splashing blood or body fluid contaminated with blood into the eyes, mouth, or nose (*e.g.*, mucous membranes)
- Contamination of open cut or abrasion with blood
- Human bites that break the skin

The exposure should be documented within 24 hours of the occurrence. The appropriate form should be filled out according to the department's policy. This procedure serves two purposes. It provides the necessary patient identification information for medical follow-up and vaccine prophylaxis, if necessary, for HBV exposure, and it also provides information about inappropriate use or nonprotective application of barriers for further safety evaluation.

Patient follow-up occurs according to department and hospital policy or State Board of Health requirements. As a general overview, the following may be involved:

1. The patient involved may be tested for hepatitis B surface antigen. If negative, no prophylaxis for HBV is necessary for the exposed health care worker. If the patient is positive for hepatitis B surface antigen, the exposed health care worker should be given hepatitis B immune globulin and a hepatitis B vaccine within 3 to 5 days of the exposure. For those health care workers who have previously been vaccinated with hepatitis vaccine, postexposure prophylaxis may include a blood test of the health care worker to determine the level of hepatitis B surface antibody and need for one dose of hepatitis B immune globulin or an additional dose of vaccine.
2. Hepatitis C follow-up of the patient is performed by testing for elevated liver enzymes (*e.g.*, with alanine aminotransferase). If elevated in the patient, the exposed health care worker should receive a dose of immune serum globulin.
3. HIV follow-up of patients may require the informed consent of the patient in many states. Baseline HIV antibody testing and counseling should be offered to the exposed health care worker with a repeat follow-up antibody test again at 3 months, 6 months, and 1 year.

SUMMARY

In this chapter, the most common diseases that pose a potential risk to the paramedic have been discussed. Particular attention was given to the measures for self-protection for each disease. These protective measures illustrate the proper use of universal precautions in the field situation. It is the responsibility of the paramedic to know the proper measures for self-protection and to practice these on a routine basis. Health care does not offer a 100% risk-free environment, but use of these simple measures greatly reduces the incidence of exposure in the field care environment.

SUGGESTED READING

Brookmeyer R, Gail MH: Methods for projecting course of acquired immunodeficiency syndrome epidemic. JNCI 80:900, 1988

Brunner LS, Suddarth DS: The Lippincott Manual of Nursing Practice, 5th ed. Philadelphia, JB Lippincott, 1991

Centers for Disease Control: Recommendations for prevention of HIV transmission in health-care settings. MMWR 36:25, 1987

Centers for Disease Control: Update: Universal precautions for prevention of transmission of human immunodeficiency virus, hepatitis B virus,, and other blood borne pathogens in health-care settings. MMWR 37:377, 1988

Centers for Disease Control: AIDS and human immunodeficiency virus infection in the United States: 1988 update. MMWR 38 (No.S-4), 1989

Cezus VP, Sawyer WM: Prehospital perspective on non-blood-borne contagious infectious diseases. Emergency Care Quarterly 5(4):8, 1990

Corey L, Spear PG: Infections with herpes simplex viruses. N Engl J Med 314:686, 1986

Dondero TJ Jr, Pappaioanou M, Curran JW: Monitoring the levels and trends of HIV infection: The Public Health Service's HIV surveillance program. Public Health Rep 103:213, 1988

Fineberg HV: Education to prevent AIDS: Prospects and obstacles. Science 239:592, 1988

Hafen BQ: Answers About AIDS for EMS Personnel. Englewood, NJ, Morton, 1988

Hart G: Syphilis tests in diagnostic and therapeutic decision making. Ann Intern Med 104:368, 1986

Hoffmann SA: Infection and the emergency care provider. Emergency Care Quarterly 5:43, 1989

Lipsky BA, Boyko EJ, Inui TS et al: Risk factors for acquiring pneumococcal infections. Arch Intern Med 146:2179, 1986

Sachs GM: OSHA mandates infection control for EMS and Fire services. J Emerg Med Serv 15(8):36, 1990

US Department of Transportation, National Highway Traffic Safety Administration: Emergency Medical Technician–Paramedic: National Standards Curriculum. Washington, DC, US Government Printing Office, 1985

West KH: Infectious Disease Handbook for Emergency Care Personnel. Philadelphia, JB Lippincott, 1987

CHAPTER 27

Environmental Emergencies and Hazardous Materials

Thermoregulation
  The Hypothalamus and Thermostasis
  Physical Principles of Heat Transfer
    Radiation
    Conduction
    Convection
    Evaporation
  Organ Mediation of Heat Transfer
Disruptions of Thermoregulation
  Hyperthermia
    Heat Cramps
      Management
    Heat Exhaustion
      Management
    Heat Stroke
      Management
    Febrile Illness
      Management
  Hypothermia
    Rate of Onset
    High-risk Groups
    Intoxicants
    Medical Conditions
    Trauma
    Pathophysiology
      Moderate Hypothermia
      Severe Hypothermia
    Management

Frostbite
  Superficial
  Deep
  Management
Water Emergencies
  Drowning
    Near Drowning
    Salt vs. Fresh Water Drowning
    Cold Water Drowning
    Management of Drowning
    Management of Cold Water Drowning
  Pressure-related Injury
    Nitrogen and Decompression Sickness
      Management of Decompression Sickness
        Recompression
        Fluid and Drug Therapy
    Gas Expansion and Air Embolism
      Management of Air Embolism
Hazardous Materials
  Recognition of Hazardous Materials
    Occupancy and Location
    Container Shapes
    Markings and Colors
      Fixed Facility
      Bulk Transportation Containers
      Nonbulk Packages and Containers
    Placards and Labels
    Shipping Papers
    Senses

Planning and Preparedness
  Vehicle Equipment
  Communications
  Rescue Considerations
  Responding to a Call
Exposure to Hazardous Materials
  Routes of Entry
    Absorption
    Inhalation
    Ingestion
    Injection
  Ionizing Radiation
  Acute vs. Chronic Exposures
Protection from Hazardous Materials
  Forms of Chemical Intrusion
  Self-care Precautions
  Levels of Protection
  Ambulance Protection
Decontamination
Management
Triage
Transport
Postevent Considerations
Summary

BEHAVIORAL OBJECTIVES
On successful completion of this chapter, the reader will be able to:

1. Describe the physical principles of heat transfer
2. Identify emergencies that may occur with a disruption of thermoregulation
3. Identify the different types of environmental emergencies
4. List special considerations when dealing with environmental emergencies
5. Differentiate among specific water emergencies and the treatment of each
6. List the locations in the community where hazardous materials might be found
7. Identify the various definitions of hazardous materials
8. List and describe the six clues for detecting hazardous materials
9. List the nine hazard classes and list some common hazardous materials in each
10. List in order the six steps of the D.E.C.I.D.E. process
11. Describe the information and assistance available from various emergency resources
12. Describe the relevant planning and preparedness procedures
13. List the primary function of emergency personnel in hazardous materials emergencies
14. Explain the types of harm that a person may experience when exposed to toxic materials
15. Describe the three types of ionizing radiation
16. Describe the various levels of protection available for emergency personnel
17. Describe how to protect the ambulance from contamination
18. Demonstrate how to decontaminate a contaminated victim
19. Describe decontamination procedures for emergency responders
20. Describe management, triage, and transport considerations in a hazardous materials incident
21. Define all of the key terms listed in this chapter

KEY TERMS
The following terms are defined in the chapter and glossary:

absorption
air embolism
α particles
barotrauma
β particles
bottom time
Boyle's law
chokes
cold zone
conduction
convection
decompression sickness
degradation
dose
drowning
evaporation
febrile illness
frostbite
frostbite—superficial, deep
τ rays
hazardous material
hazardous materials incident
heat cramps
heat stroke
heat exhaustion
Henry's law
homeostasis
hot zone
hydrostatic pressure
hyperthermia
hypothalamus
hypothermia
inhalation
ingestion
injection
immersion hypothermia
mammalian diving reflex
near drowning
nitrogen narcosis
normothermic
Osborne wave (J wave)
penetration
permeation
radiation
radioactive substances
roentgen
sweat glands
thermostasis
warm zone

Environmental emergencies include a broad range of loosely related conditions, several of which result from exposure to extreme temperature. Many of these thermal disorders can arise from the body's internal imbalances. In either case, understanding the mechanisms of homeostasis is central to patient assessment and management. The other environmental conditions—drowning, near drowning, pressure-related injuries, and hazardous materials incidents and exposure—are more specialized cases. Because they tend to cause problems that the body is not as prepared to resist, their management requires special care and easy reference to technical information.

THERMOREGULATION

Temperature is one of the many variables to which the body adjusts in the process of maintaining homeostasis. **Homeostasis** is defined as a state of physiologic equilibrium. As warm blooded animals, human beings depend on the ability to limit core body temperature within a range of several degrees. This range centers around a normal core temperature, measured rectally, of 37.6°C (99.6°F). Peripheral temperature is usually lower, as seen by a normal value of 37°C (98.6°F) for oral readings. The definition of normal thus varies with location. Temperature also fluctuates over a range of several degrees under entirely healthy circumstances. To take advantage of the patient's body temperature as an assessment tool, both rectal and oral thermometers should be available.

The Hypothalamus and Thermostasis

Because it is a component of homeostasis, the body's control of temperature is known as **thermostasis**. The **hypothalamus**, the prime organ of temperature control, can be thought of as a mechanical thermostat. The hypothalamus senses body temperature and activates mechanisms for heat gain or loss to offset changes from normal. This constant sensing of environmental feedback, coupled with the ability to reverse or negate changes from the desired setting, is shown in Figure 27-1.

The hypothalamus also detects the return to normal temperature when compensation efforts begin and shuts down the compensatory mechanisms accordingly, much like the thermostat in a heating system.

Physical Principles of Heat Transfer

The total amount of heat in the human body is a fluctuating balance between heat produced and heat lost. The body generates heat as a by-product of its metabolism. Heat production also increases in response to skeletal muscle contraction or exercise, but metabolic rate is the dominant factor in heat production at rest.

Heat loss results from four physical mechanisms: radiation, conduction, convection, and evaporation. All of these mechanisms can operate either passively or under the direction of the hypothalamus when it senses increased core heat. Radiation, conduction, and convection all operate in a similar way: heat migrates from warmer substances to relatively cooler substances in an attempt to equalize temperatures.

Evaporation follows different rules. Because it requires conditions that promote the transformation of water from fluid to vapor, evaporation actually works best at high temperatures. Low relative humidity also strongly favors evaporation. These traits explain evaporation's importance as the body's only means of heat loss when environmental temperature exceeds that of the skin. They also emphasize the potential dangers of weather that is both humid and hot. Although evaporation works best at high temperatures, a high relative humidity impedes the action of evaporation.

Understanding the four heat transfer methods is important to further understand problems with thermoregulation; each is summarized in Figure 27-2.

Radiation

Radiation (or *radiant heat*), the type that is felt when the sun shines, is a form of electromagnetic wave. It is a law of nature that warmer materials tend to radiate heat to cooler ones, in keeping with the thermal gradient principle. No physical contact between surfaces occurs in the transfer of radiant heat. Whether the body emits this heat or absorbs it depends on the relation of skin temperature to that of other temperatures in the environment.

Conduction

Conduction, direct physical contact between materials of different temperature, is another method of heat exchange. Unlike radiant transfer, which is an energy wave form, conduction depends on the direct passage of heat from molecule to molecule or on movement of the molecules. Heat loss by conduction requires contact with a cold substance, such as the ground, snow, or water.

Convection

Convection is the transport of heat away from the skin by air movement. A particularly important combination of heat loss mechanisms involves wet skin. Fluid greatly enhances conduction and evaporation, which in turn promotes convective loss if a breeze is present.

Evaporation

Physical laws dictate that water absorbs considerable heat in the process of vaporizing. **Evaporation** is the process by which the body sweats to draw heat out of the core; the heat then leaves the skin surface with the water vapor (when external conditions favor evaporation). The process also takes place in the mucous membrane linings of the respiratory system, resulting in further heat and water loss during exhalation. As external temperature rises to that of the skin, the other three heat transfer methods begin to be liabilities. When outside temperature actually exceeds skin temperature, heat gain is promoted, rather than the loss that the body needs. Evaporation remains the only working compensatory mechanism.

When associated with evaporation, the processes of radiation, conduction, and convection can harm the body if ignored. Heat loss when a person is sweating in a cool breeze can lead to hypothermia, and exposure of bare skin to the radiant, evaporative, and convective forces of a

620 UNIT FOUR: MEDICAL EMERGENCIES

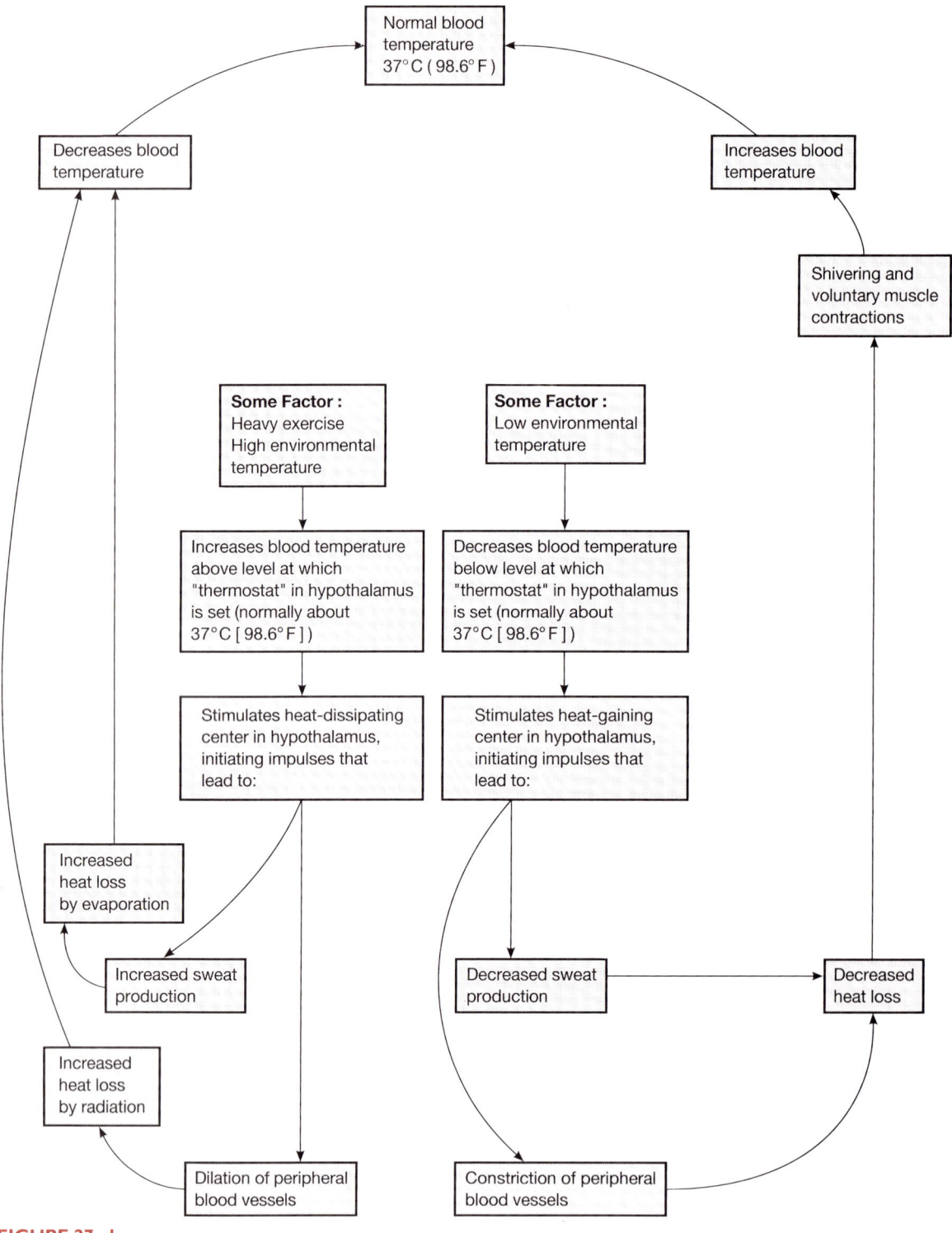

FIGURE 27-1.
Homeostasis of body temperature.

desert climate risks dangerous dehydration and hyperthermia. If a person is sweating and touches a cold metal object, the skin surface may adhere to the metal. The body's complete thermal stability in extreme temperature conditions demands use of conscious areas of the brain, in addition to the autonomic work of the hypothalamus.

Organ Mediation of Heat Transfer

Hypothalamic control of heat gain and loss takes place through manipulation of several organ systems. By varying the degree of skeletal muscle tone and stimulating involuntary muscle activity (*shivering*), the hypothalamus

PROCESS	DEFINITION	EXAMPLE	ILLUSTRATION
Radiation	The diffusion or dissemination of heat by electromagnetic waves	The body gives off waves of heat from uncovered surfaces.	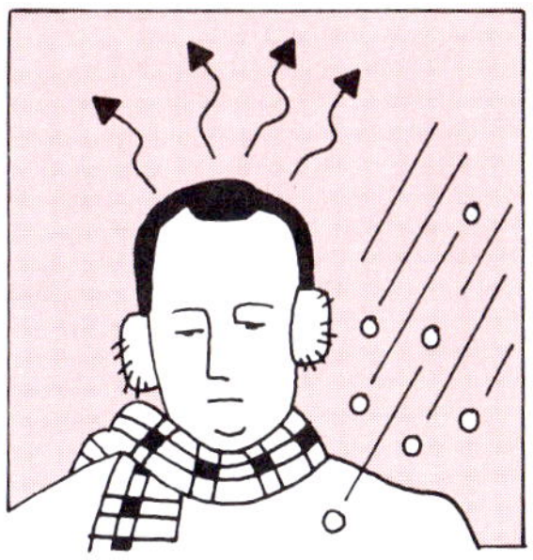
Convection	The dissemination of heat by motion between areas of unequal density	An oscillating fan blows currents of cool air across the surface of a warm body.	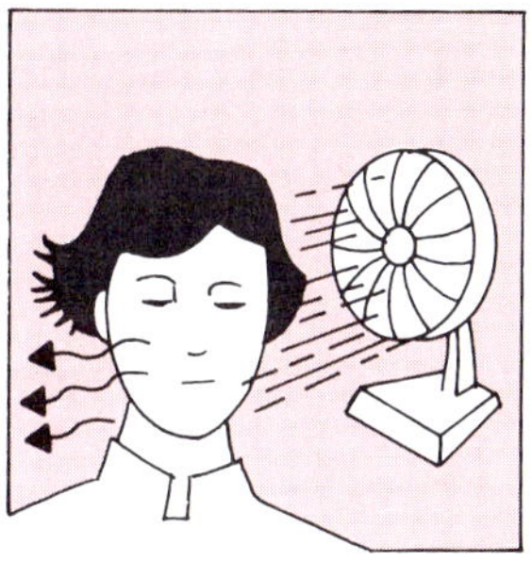
Evaporation	The conversion of a liquid to a vapor	Body fluid in the form of perspiration and insensible loss is vaporized from the skin.	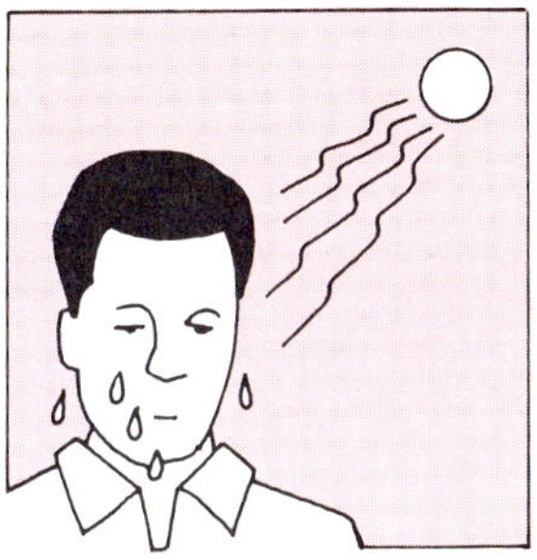
Conduction	The transfer of heat to another object during direct contact	The body transfers heat to an ice pack, causing the ice to melt.	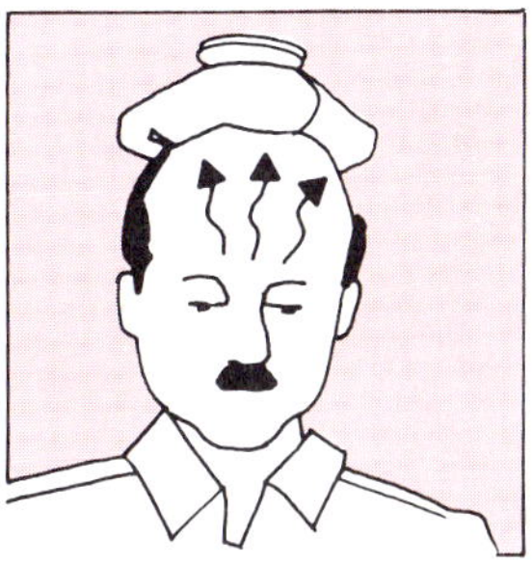

FIGURE 27–2.
Mechanisms of heat transfer. (Taylor C, Lillis C, Le Mone P)

modifies the amount of heat produced both metabolically and by friction between contracting muscle fibers. Shivering can increase heat production by 500%. A person's conscious tendency to step up physical activity when cold and rest when too hot adds a voluntary component to heat regulation. Together, voluntary and involuntary responses make heat production in muscle the most important defense against excessive heat loss in cold weather.

The **sweat glands** provide an effective route for evaporative heat loss. The hypothalamus regulates the sweat glands through the sympathetic nervous system, as it does the arterioles in the skin. Dilation and constriction of peripheral arterioles can cause dramatic changes in the skin's capacity to radiate and conduct heat. These vascular changes aid in both rapid cooling and efficient heat conservation.

When the hypothalamus senses a need for more heat production, it stimulates two endocrine glands, the adrenal medulla and the thyroid, which secrete epinephrine and thyroxine, respectively. Both hormones increase heat production by stimulating metabolism. The sympathetic response mediated by epinephrine also increases cardiac output. This increased cardiac output acts to distribute heat throughout the body, which may enhance heat loss if it serves to deliver more blood to dilated peripheral vessels.

Since blood plays a central role as a vehicle for heat transport, dehydration becomes an enemy of compensatory systems in both hot and cold conditions. Ironically, these thermal extremes actively produce dehydration. Sweating in hot weather is the obvious example, but heat conservation carries a similar danger. *Peripheral vasoconstriction*, which shunts blood to the body's core in response to cold, gives central blood pressure sensors the mistaken impression that blood volume is rising. As a result, a *reflex diuresis* (increased amounts of urine) depletes the blood volume. Once again, the conscious mind can assist homeostatic function, in this case by assuring adequate fluid intake.

DISRUPTIONS OF THERMOREGULATION

Several conditions disrupt the normal heat regulating mechanisms of the body. They are divided into two main categories, hyperthermia and hypothermia.

Hyperthermia

Hyperthermia refers to the general condition of excess body heat. Correct management depends on assessment of underlying causes. Heat cramps, heat exhaustion, and heat stroke result from imbalances between heat production and heat loss, while febrile illness results from interference with the hypothalamic thermostat setting.

Heat Cramps

Heat cramps are actually a chemical rather than thermal disruption that results from profuse sweating. Most often, the cramping follows a period of physical exertion in a hot environment. Heavy sweating leads to high sodium losses, and at some point the sodium deficit compromises muscle function.

Replacement of fluid without sodium does not help heat cramps and may aggravate them by further diluting the remaining sodium in the blood. The cramps are a consequence of sweating, a healthy compensatory mechanism, and usually present without evidence of more severe thermal problems.

The patient complains of cramps most commonly in the calves of the legs and in the abdomen. Cramps may also occur in the hands, arms, and feet. The patient's skin is cool and usually wet. Mental status and blood pressure should be normal, though tachycardia is common.

MANAGEMENT. Heat cramps signal the need for cooling and rest. In uncomplicated cases, the patient is often able to take fluid by mouth, but nausea may make intravenous (IV) infusion of 0.9% NaCl the desired management. Infuse 0.9% NaCl rapidly, 150 to 200 mL or more per hour, to maintain the patient's vital signs. If the patient is able to take fluid by mouth, add ½ to 1 teaspoon of salt per pint of water or fruit juice or give one of the commercial electrolyte solutions, such as Gatorade. Cramps can sometimes be prevented entirely with similar oral intake before physical exertion. Salt tablets are not recommended, as they may precipitate nausea.

Heat Exhaustion

Heat exhaustion indicates a more advanced stage of the homeostatic imbalance that sometimes begins with heat cramps. Heat exhaustion results most often from physical exertion in the heat without adequate fluid replacement; in this case, however, the fluid loss itself takes on greater importance. Heat exhaustion is primarily a circulatory rather than chemical problem. The combination of sweat loss and peripheral blood pooling, as the hypothalamus attempts to maximize evaporation, radiation, and convection of heat into the environment, threatens core perfusion.

Heat exhaustion is not a total thermal imbalance. Temperature usually remains normal or only slightly above, and active compensation continues. Patients often present with central nervous system symptoms, such as headache, fatigue, dizziness, or syncope. Skin is typically damp, and the pulse rate is high. Skin color, blood pressure, and respiratory rate are all variable, depending on the degree to which compensatory efforts are succeeding in holding off circulatory distress. Patients with later stages of heat exhaustion have pale skin, low blood pressure, and an increased respiratory rate.

MANAGEMENT. The primary management concern in heat exhaustion is breaking the cycle of lower circulating blood volume and loss of cooling ability that could lead to heat stroke. Management used for heat cramps may suffice in the early stages, but any hint of decreased mental status or unstable vital signs demands closer attention.

The patient should be removed from the heat and fluid replaced with an IV infusion of 0.9% NaCl or lactated Ringer's solution. Infuse fluid rapidly, 150 to 200 mL or more per hour, to maintain vital signs. Use aggressive cooling measures, as described for heat stroke, if rectal temperature is above 39°C (102°F).

Heat Stroke

Heat stroke is a true emergency. As the body's compensatory mechanisms such as vasodilation and sweating are exhausted, or actually cause further trouble through shock and dehydration, hypothalamic control weakens, then collapses. Core temperature threatens brain damage as it rises rapidly past 41°C (105°F). During this final phase, only immediate and aggressive intervention can prevent death.

Heat stroke patients can deteriorate quickly to coma. They often have seizures, and the skin is classically hot, flushed, and dry, though gradual onset, age, and other factors can alter this sign. Vital signs rise initially, then drop later, culminating in cardiorespiratory arrest.

MANAGEMENT. Heat stroke demands rapid cooling. The patient should be moved quickly to a cool area, clothing removed, and cold water, ice, or wet sheets placed on the patient's body. Concentrate on the "*core surface*" areas where the ability to cool central blood is greatest: the scalp, neck, axillae, and groins. Cool to 39°C (102°F), monitoring the patient's rectal temperature. Scene time should be minimal, and transport to the hospital with continued cooling en route is required. Remember that overcooling is also dangerous since the hypothalamus is not functioning.

The patient should be given oxygen and placed on a cardiac monitor. Administer an IV infusion of 0.9% NaCl or lactated Ringer's solution to replace lost fluid and sodium and to counteract vasodilation. Infusion rate should be monitored to maintain the patient's blood pressure. Monitor vital signs and breath sounds. Not all heat stroke patients are profoundly hypovolemic; hypotension may partially reflect cardiac function. Overhydration is a special concern in congestive heart failure patients and the elderly. Cooling is the top priority in the management of patients who are suffering from heat stroke.

Febrile Illness

In **febrile illness,** toxic by-products of infection called *pyrogens* reset the hypothalamic thermostat to a higher temperature by producing substances called *prostaglandins,* which act directly on the hypothalamus. Aspirin and acetaminophen fight fever by inhibiting the production of prostaglandins.

The chills and shivering common to febrile illness represent the body's perception that it is cold, relative to the new thermostat setting. The hypothalamus activates vasoconstriction and increases metabolic rate in an attempt to warm up to the new level. When pyrogen activity wanes and the hypothalamic setting drops, flushed skin and sweating signify the compensatory effort to lose what is now recognized as excess heat.

MANAGEMENT. Management usually centers on the cause, that is, the underlying infection. Adults do not commonly need emergency therapy for the increased temperature itself.

Children are particularly sensitive to rapid rises in temperature and may experience febrile seizures. Pediatric seizures merit contact with the child's physician, if not immediate transport. Febrile seizures are discussed in detail in Chapter 29. Rapid cooling procedures described for heat stroke should be instituted for temperatures of 41°C (105°F) or higher.

Table 27-1 summarizes the signs and symptoms of hyperthermic-related emergencies.

Hypothermia

The body's core temperature can drop several degrees in the normal course of body function. Even when the heat

TABLE 27-1.
SIGNS AND SYMPTOMS OF HYPERTHERMIC-RELATED EMERGENCIES

Signs and Symptoms	Heat Cramps	Heat Exhaustion	Heat Stroke	Febrile Illness
Respiration	Normal	Increased	Increased	Normal
Pulse	Normal	Increased	Increased	Normal
Blood pressure	Normal	Low	High then low	Normal
Temperature	Normal	Normal or high	Very high	High
Skin	Cool, pale, moist	Cool, pale, moist	Hot, flushed, dry	Warm, flushed, moist
Consciousness	Normal	Stuporous	Decreased	Normal
Nausea	Present	Present	Absent	Absent
Cramps	Present	May be present	Absent	Absent
Underlying illness	None	None	Possibly	Yes

loss is not routine, the body usually tolerates a 3° to 4° drop without symptoms. Rectal readings below 35°C (95°F) constitute **hypothermia.** Internal metabolic factors and heat loss to the external environment can both lead to hypothermia. Exploration of origins is crucial to management and patient outcome.

Rate of Onset

The rate of onset of hypothermia is variable. Very cold air and immersion in cold water can cause rapid drops in core temperature. Gradual onset is also common, indoors or outdoors, and is easy to miss because of its subtle early signs and the absence of extreme environmental hints. Prolonged exposure to air temperatures of 10°C (50°F) or even warmer, especially when wind and rain or humidity accelerate convective and evaporative heat losses, can lead to hypothermia just as more obvious conditions do. Wet clothing and bare wet skin both greatly speed heat loss by convection and evaporation.

High-Risk Groups

Heat loss can be more serious in groups at high risk for hypothermia. Children, particularly newborns and infants, have thermoregulation systems that are not completely developed, and their ratio of skin surface to body mass is higher than that of adults. Both of these factors predispose them to rapid heat loss. The elderly tend to lose heat gradually. Their thermal balancing mechanisms and other defense systems that would otherwise protect them from excessive heat loss lose sensitivity with age. Additional risks for the elderly may include poor circulation, physical immobility, the tendency of friends and family to dismiss early mental changes as senility, and other factors such as malnutrition and poorly heated homes. Hypothermia in the elderly can develop over a period of days in indoor surroundings that feel comfortable to the young healthy adult.

Intoxicants

Many intoxicants also increase the risk of heat loss. They dull the conscious perception of cold that would encourage exercise and extra clothing. Alcohol and other substances directly counteract compensatory mechanisms by inhibiting shivering, dilating peripheral vessels, and promoting diuresis.

Medical Conditions

A number of medical conditions can also contribute to the development of hypothermia. Hypothyroidism reduces metabolic heat production secondary to thyroxine action, and brain tumors, strokes, and head injuries alter hypothalamic function. Sepsis, congestive heart failure, and other conditions that affect metabolism and circulation can also contribute to hypothermia. Diabetic ketoacidosis results in lowered heat production, dehydration, and tissue glucose starvation, all risk factors even in warm environments. At the other extreme, insulin shock, with its combined mental changes and heavy sweating, typical of insulin reactions leads to profound heat loss if the patient is not discovered quickly.

Trauma

Finally, trauma also increases the risk of hypothermia. Patients with head injuries, pain, shock, and fractures all deteriorate more rapidly in cold surroundings.

Pathophysiology

Core temperature drops when mechanisms for producing and conserving heat are out-paced by heat loss. Metabolic rate then decreases, lowering metabolic heat production. As is true in hyperthermic disorders, these changes are initially opposed by the body's compensatory measures but can decay into a cycle reversible only by external intervention. Prevention includes sensible safety and clothing precautions and steady fluid consumption to maintain circulatory volume during long exposures to cold.

For the purposes of assessment and management, hypothermia can be divided into two broad categories of severity. Rectal temperature is useful in distinguishing between moderate and severe hypothermia, though state of consciousness, vital signs, and other findings make the distinction in most cases. The box, "Levels of Hypothermia," lists the signs and symptoms of hypothermia with regard to changes in the body's core temperature. Low reading thermometers should be available since regular thermometers only measure to 34°C (94°F). A thermometer cannot be used, however, with combative patients and should not take priority over maintaining the patient's airway, breathing, and circulation.

MODERATE HYPOTHERMIA. *Moderate hypothermia* refers to the early stage where the patient is alert and physically coordinated. The body is still attempting compensation by shivering. Core temperature remains above 32°C (90°F).

SEVERE HYPOTHERMIA. *Severe hypothermia* exists in any cold patient with depressed vital signs, altered level of consciousness, absent shivering, core temperature of 32°C (90°F) or lower, or any serious complicating illness or injury. Remember that alcohol may retard shivering, regardless of heat loss.

The brain and the heart are the organs most sensitive to cold. Changes in the patient's level of consciousness and cardiac rhythm signal not only temperature drop but also the need for rewarming measures to augment physiologic compensation. The classic **Osborne wave (J wave)** may be seen after the QRS complex (Fig. 27-3). Oxygen dissociates less readily from hemoglobin when the blood cools, so sensitive organs face the threat of hypoxia in addition to changes in cellular function due to the cold.

LEVELS OF HYPOTHERMIA

°F	°C	Signs and Symptoms of Hypothermia
99.6	37.6	"Normal" rectal temperature
98.6	37	"Normal" oral temperature
96.8	36	Increased metabolic rate in an attempt to balance temperature
95.0	35	Shivering maximum at this temperature
93.2	34	Patients usually responsive with normal blood pressure
91.4	33	**Severe hypothermia below this temperature**
89.6	32	Consciousness clouded; pupils dilated; shivering ceases
87.8	31	Blood pressure difficult to obtain
86.0	30	Progressive loss of consciousness; increased muscular rigidity
85.2	29	Slow pulse and respiration; cardiac arrhythmia develops
82.4	28	Ventricular fibrillation may develop if heart is irritated
80.6	27	Voluntary motion lost along with pupillary light reflex; deep tendon and skin reflexes; appearance of death
78.8	26	Victim seldom conscious
77.0	25	Ventricular fibrillation may appear spontaneously
75.2	24	Pulmonary edema develops
73.4	23	
71.6	22	Maximum risk of fibrillation
69.8	21	
68.0	20	Heart standstill
66.2	19	
64.4	18	Lowest accidental hypothermic patient with recovery
62.6	17	Isoelectric electrocardiogram
48.2	9	Lowest artificially cooled hypothermic patient with recovery

(Moderate: 99.6–91.4°F; Severe: 89.6–48.2°F)

At 29°C to 32°C (85°F–90°F), the heart becomes "*irritable*." Rough physical handling and the "*afterdrop*" in core temperature that is thought to accompany recirculation of cold acidotic blood from the periphery can precipitate ventricular fibrillation. This effect is particularly relevant in the rapidly developing hypothermia of cold water immersion. Water conducts heat 25 to 30 times more efficiently than air. Brief immersion can cool peripheral blood without a major fall in core temperature, but the latter begins to drop after about 20 minutes. Rest and gentle handling are critical for the cold water immersion patient.

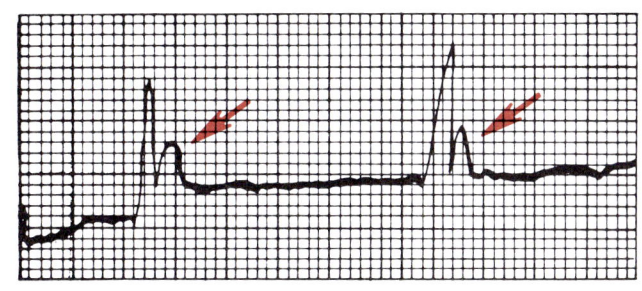

FIGURE 27–3.
Classic Osborne wave ("J" wave) may be seen following the QRS complex in a person with severe hypothermia.

Management

Basic management of hypothermia includes handling the patient gently, removing wet clothing, and covering the patient to prevent further cooling. Give warm oral fluids only if evidence of active rewarming is seen. The patient should be alert and able to swallow easily and control shivering. Avoid drinks that contain caffeine (coffee and tea), which constricts peripheral blood vessels, and alcohol, which dilates them. Warm beverages with sugar, such as hot chocolate, can be given to begin replacement of the metabolic fuel the body needs to restore normal heat production. No oral fluids should be administered to patients with changing levels of consciousness.

When transport time is short, active rewarming therapy probably does not accomplish much. Rapid rewarming and numerous other therapies encourage peripheral recirculation and may trigger circulatory, metabolic, and thermal disruptions. In any severely hypothermic patient, avoid showers or baths, cold IV fluids, and massaging or warming of extremities.

Longer transport may call for active rewarming of severely hypothermic patients. If active rewarming is necessary, use central rather than peripheral methods and carry out gradually. Give heated humidified oxygen. Apply warm packs, carefully wrapped to avoid burning poorly perfused skin, to "*core surface*" areas: the head, neck, axillae, and groins.

More specific field therapy is limited. Most medications work poorly and are abnormally metabolized in cold blood. Defibrillation often is not successful unless rewarming is in progress, possibly until core temperature reaches about 29°C (85°F). Indications for pneumatic anti-shock garments and airway control adjuncts are similar to those for **normothermic** (normal body temperature) patients, although the vagal stimulation associated with tracheal and esophageal airways (and Foley catheters) increases the chance of provoking ventricular fibrillation.

The probability of hypovolemia in the severely hypothermic patient indicates a need for volume replacement using 0.9% NaCl or lactated Ringer's solution. An initial challenge of 250 to 500 mL may improve perfusion, with further infusion based on monitoring of vital signs and breath sounds. Intravenous fluids should be warmed before being administered to the patient, for example, by keeping the fluids in the back of a warm ambulance or by holding the IV container next to the paramedic's body under the coat.

Intravenous infusions are often difficult to start in the hypothermic patient and should not receive priority over more critical management. The cardiac rhythm should be monitored, though arrhythmias may be difficult to treat. Atrial fibrillation and bradycardic rhythms are common. Remember that muscle artifact in shivering can mimic fibrillation. Extreme bradycardia can be mistaken for cardiac arrest if an adequate interval is not taken for monitoring the pulse rate and electrocardiogram. The respiratory rate may also be extremely slow. Muscular rigidity typical of severe hypothermia has been mistaken for rigor mortis. Rigidity is not a reliable sign of death in the cold patient, even when a careful check reveals no vital signs. Hypothermic patients have proven viable after long periods of this deathly appearance, giving rise to the saying that cold patients are *"not dead until they are warm and dead."*

When extended pulselessness and a rhythm on the cardiac monitor indicates certain cardiac arrest, cardiopulmonary resuscitation is indicated. Although drug and electrical therapies may not prove as successful as in the normothermic patient, they should be followed according to the cardiac management procedures outlined in Chapter 20.

Frostbite

Windy subfreezing weather creates the greatest risk to frostbite. **Frostbite** occurs when small body parts with a high ratio of surface area to tissue mass (fingers, toes, ears, and the nose) are exposed to extreme cold. Larger areas of the extremities are vulnerable in more profound cooling. This cold exposure causes an initial spasm in the small blood vessels and slows or blocks circulation. Tissues freeze, and ice crystals form and grow between cells. The cells are deprived of water, and dehydration results. The fluid in the cells becomes more concentrated and the cells eventually die.

The *type* and *duration* of contact are the two most important factors in determining the extent of frostbite injury. Touching cold fabric is not nearly as dangerous as coming into direct contact with cold metal, particularly if one's hands are wet or even damp. In the latter case, the skin usually is cemented instantly to the cold metal and is torn off when the hand is removed. Air itself is a poor thermal conductor. Cold air alone is not nearly as dangerous a freezing factor as a combination of wind and cold. It is astounding but true that the chilly effect of a temperature of −6°C (20°F) combined with a 45 mile/hour wind is identical to that of a −26°C (−15°F) temperature coupled with a 3 mile/hour wind. The box, "Wind Chill Chart," shows temperature effects of wind and cold.

All frostbite victims should be assessed for signs of hypothermia as well. Clothing offers good protection against weather only if it is loose enough to avoid restricting circulation. Tight gloves, cuffs, boots, and straps add to the danger. As is true of other heat and cold maladies, dehydration intensifies frostbite problems. It further compromises heat distribution that has already been reduced by vasoconstriction in response to the cold.

Superficial

Like burns, frostbite is a thermal emergency that can affect superficial or deeper tissue. **Superficial frostbite** appears as firm and waxy gray or yellow skin in an area that loses sensation after hurting or tingling. Warming with another body surface immediately after onset of numbness should prevent damage beyond later skin peeling.

Deep

Prolonged exposure can lead to blistering and eventually **deep frostbite,** which most often afflicts hands and feet. No warning symptoms appear after the initial loss of feeling. Freezing progresses painlessly once the nerve endings are numb. Skin becomes inelastic and the entire area feels hard to the touch. In anything beyond superficial frostbite, the true depth and functional effect of freezing is impossible to assess immediately. Figure 27-4 shows the effects of frostbite after a 24-hour period.

Management

Management for more than superficial frostbite is rapid rewarming after any system-wide hypothermia has been corrected. Deep frostbite should only be managed in the field if necessary to prevent further damage. Immerse the frozen tissue in 41°C (105°F) water until tissue pliability, color, and sensation return. Since this effect may take at least 20 minutes in most cases, transport to the hospital should not be delayed. Discontinue warming after 20 to 30 minutes. Dry heat, cold therapy, massaging, and any handling that breaks blisters are harmful actions.

Several aspects of the rewarming process make rewarming difficult in the field. Pain can be extremely intense without analgesia, and exact control of water temperature is nearly impossible. Maintaining it in the range of 38°C to 43°C (100°F–110°F) suffices, but even this

WIND CHILL CHART

Wind Speed		Cooling Power of Wind Expressed as "Equivalent Chill Temperature"																			
Knots	MPH	Temperature (°F)																			
Calm	Calm	40	35	30	25	20	15	10	5	0	−5	−10	−15	−20	−25	−30	−35	−40	−45	−50	−55	−60
		Equivalent Chill Temperature																			
3–6	5	35	30	25	20	15	10	5	0	−5	−10	−15	−20	−25	−30	−35	−40	−45	−50	−55	−65	−70
7–10	10	30	20	15	10	5	0	−10	−15	−20	−25	−35	−40	−45	−50	−60	−65	−70	−75	−80	−90	−95
11–15	15	25	15	10	0	−5	−10	−20	−25	−30	−40	−45	−50	−60	−65	−70	−80	−85	−90	−100	−105	−110
16–19	20	20	10	5	0	−10	−15	−25	−30	−35	−45	−50	−60	−65	−75	−80	−85	−95	−100	−110	−115	−120
20–23	25	15	10	0	−5	−15	−20	−30	−35	−45	−50	−60	−65	−75	−80	−90	−95	−105	−110	−120	−125	−135
24–28	30	10	5	0	−10	−20	−25	−30	−40	−50	−55	−65	−70	−80	−85	−95	−100	−110	−115	−125	−130	−140
29–32	35	10	5	−5	−10	−20	−30	−35	−40	−50	−60	−65	−75	−80	−90	−100	−105	−115	−120	−130	−135	−145
33–36	40	10	0	−5	−15	−20	−30	−35	−45	−55	−60	−70	−75	−85	−95	−100	−110	−115	−125	−130	−140	−150
Winds above 40 have little additional effect		Little danger					Increasing danger (Flesh may freeze within 1 min)							Great danger (Flesh may freeze within 30 seconds)								

DANGER OF FREEZING EXPOSED FLESH FOR PROPERLY CLOTHED PERSONS

U.S. Government Printing Office, 1973.

---

regulation proves a real challenge. The largest possible basin slows cooling of the water, but its temperature must still be boosted periodically by removing the frostbitten part and pouring in new water.

Apply dry sterile dressings and handle gently after thawing. If rewarming is not attempted, the frostbitten part should be bandaged with dry sterile dressings and the patient transported to the hospital. Frostbitten flesh also shares burned tissue's vulnerability to infection, so care should be taken to keep the affected part as clean as possible.

WATER EMERGENCIES

Every year millions of people take to the nation's lakes, oceans, and streams. Swimming, sailing, rowing, water skiing, and scuba diving are just some of the activities enjoyed on and about the water that require careful consideration as to water safety. Ironically, of all the equipment used by boaters, they are least knowledgeable about flotation gear.

Not only does a personal flotation device aid in keeping the victim afloat, but it also provides protection against hypothermia.

Drowning

Drowning accounts for about 8000 deaths annually in the United States; 4700 of the victims never intended to get wet. Fifty percent of these deaths occur in children younger than 5 years of age. More than two thirds of drowning victims are nonswimmers and die less than 10 ft from safety. In 85% of the cases, personal flotation devices were not used. Five factors influence a drowning victim's chances for survival: age, ability to swim,

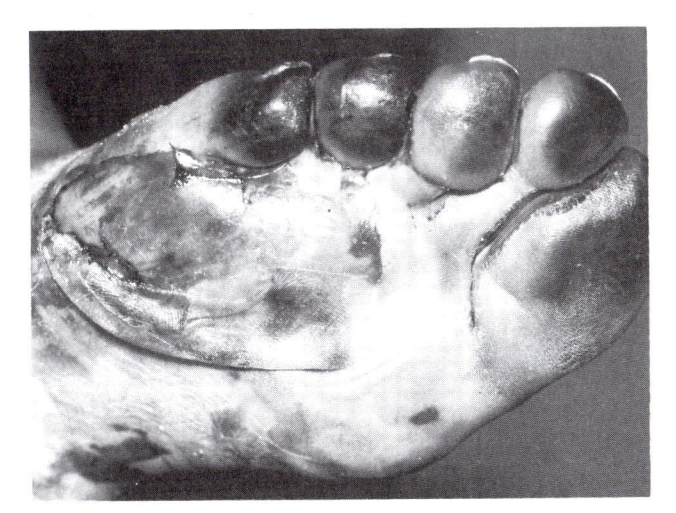

FIGURE 27–4.
Effects of frostbite on a patient 24 hours after exposure. Note the blisters and necrotic tissue around the toes.

medical history, water temperature, and length of time immersed.

Drowning is defined as death from asphyxia during an immersion episode with or without inhalation of the surrounding medium. Two types of drowning are characterized, wet and dry. A *wet drowning* occurs when fluid is inhaled or aspirated into the lungs. This drowning usually happens after the vocal cords relax and the lungs become partially flooded with water. This type typically represents 85% of all drownings. A *dry drowning* occurs when no fluid has been inhaled or aspirated into the lungs. An estimated 15% of all victims drown without aspiration of water because of prolonged laryngospasm. Because no water enters the tracheal airway, dry drowning responds readily to artificial ventilation, and victims of this type of drowning account for 90% of those successfully resuscitated.

Most drownings follow a common pattern. Cold water can stimulate involuntary gasping soon after it contacts the face, often distracting from or disabling the victim's attempts to resurface. After a period of breath holding, a reflex swallowing mechanism forces the intake of some water. Laryngospasm usually minimizes water aspiration during the early stages of consciousness and struggling, so the lungs remain relatively dry. Swallowing frequently takes place, however, making aspirations of vomitus a risk after even brief uncontrolled submersions. Laryngospasm relaxes after the victim loses consciousness, opening the trachea to free water flow. Figure 27-5 diagrams the stages of wet and dry drowning.

Near Drowning

Near drowning can be wet or dry. The term implies that recovery has occurred after initial submersion. Dry near drowning victims usually fully recover. Victims of wet near drownings usually die because of pulmonary edema hours or days later and are referred to as secondary drownings. Near drowning episodes may involve, either as cause or effect, numerous complicating problems: drug and alcohol use, spinal injuries or other trauma, especially in shallow diving accidents, suicidal depression, hypothermia, and cardiac problems. As usual, astute scene survey and history taking can yield vital information.

Salt vs. Fresh Water Drowning

In salt water drowning, the high concentration of salt contained in the water that has collected in the lungs draws fluid from the bloodstream into the lungs to equalize the concentration of salt. Salt water aspiration has been shown to be twice as lethal as fresh water aspiration. Victims drown in their own fluids as much as in the salt water itself.

Fresh water in the lungs can chemically alter the alveolar-capillary interface and alter the normal pulmonary surfactant. Recall that *surfactant* is a chemical in the alveoli of the lungs that is responsible for the stability of the alveoli. The fresh water also passes through the lungs into the bloodstream, diluting all the electrolytes except potassium. Red blood cells rupture from the water that is diffusing into the cells. Potassium is released from the lysis of the cells and is therefore at a higher extracellular level than normal.

Water components other than salt complicate patient survival. Silt, organic matter, pollutants, and pool chlorine all promote either physical obstruction of alveoli, body chemistry alterations, or later pulmonary infection.

The management of fresh water and salt water drowning is the same. Immediate therapy focuses on basic resus-

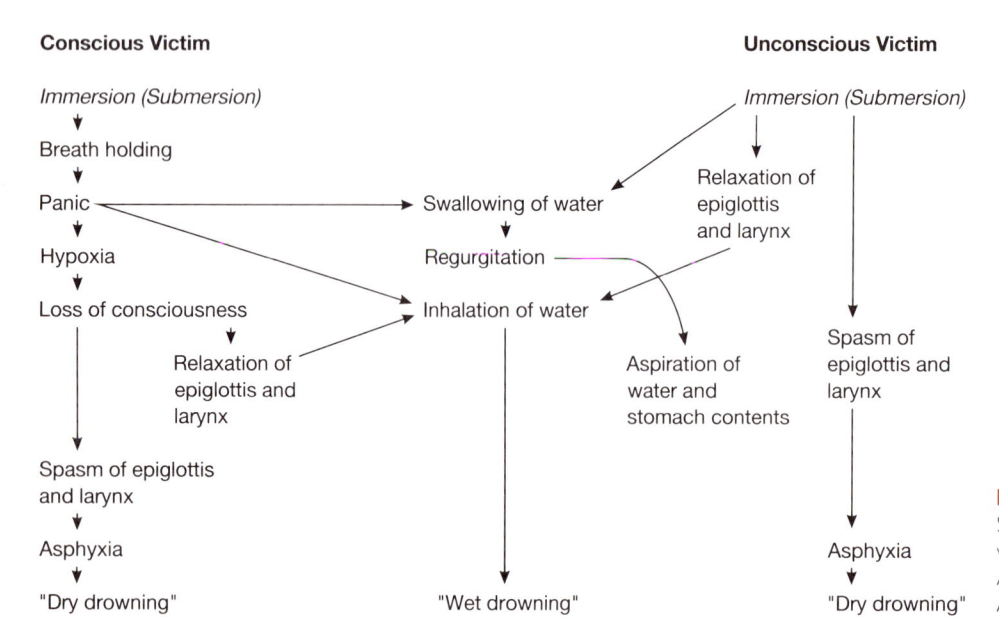

FIGURE 27–5.
Sequence of events in a drowning victim. (From Spoor JE: Drowning: An overview. Emerg Med Serv Mar/Apr 1980)

citation. The differences between salt water and fresh water drowning are primarily shown to affect the pulmonary system.

Cold Water Drowning

Cold water drowning, in addition to the prior effects given for drowning victims, involve immersion hypothermia. **Immersion hypothermia** is the chain of events associated with prolonged exposure, shivering, and loss of body temperature caused by immersion in cold water (less than 21°C (70°F)) and is a major cause of deaths in boating accidents. Victims who have succumbed to hypothermia lose consciousness and then drown.

Survival time is affected by body type, body size, mental attitude, physical condition, amount of subcutaneous fat, and the will to survive. As with children, small body size is associated with faster cooling rates.

Although victims of cold water drowning may give the physical appearances of being dead, they are ideal candidates for resuscitation because of the **mammalian diving reflex.** This reflex is triggered by immersing the face in cold water. Blood is diverted from the arms and legs and circulates at a heart rate as low as 5 to 6 beats per minute. A small sufficient supply of oxygen is very slowly circulated among the lungs, heart, and brain. This diving response has been observed in air-breathing aquatic mammals, such as the whale, porpoise, and seal.

Aggressive resuscitative attempts should be used on victims of cold water drowning where submersion time has been an hour or less.

Management of Drowning

The patient should be raised to the surface and removed from the water as rapidly as concern for spinal injuries and rescuer safety allows. Ensure particularly that rescuers do not become hypothermic or drowning patients themselves. The use of safety lines, wet and dry suits, and so on must be organized and practiced in advance, especially for rescue in fast moving or cold water. Paramedics not formally trained in water rescue should not attempt any type of rescue.

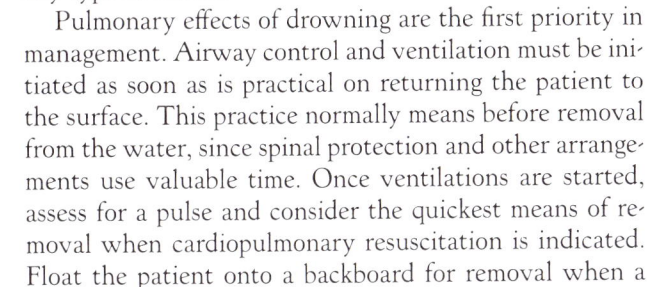

Pulmonary effects of drowning are the first priority in management. Airway control and ventilation must be initiated as soon as is practical on returning the patient to the surface. This practice normally means before removal from the water, since spinal protection and other arrangements use valuable time. Once ventilations are started, assess for a pulse and consider the quickest means of removal when cardiopulmonary resuscitation is indicated. Float the patient onto a backboard for removal when a fall or dive is suspected and add further spinal protection.

Avoid initial attempts to drain fluid from the lungs or stomach, including abdominal compression, in favor of beginning ventilation. Later, gastric emptying may be considered if distension obstructs ventilation, but aspiration risks make gastric emptying undesirable in the absence of endotracheal intubation.

Establish direct airway control as early as possible after initial ventilations. Endotracheal intubation provides the best protection. If this procedure cannot be accomplished, other devices, such as the esophageal obturator airway, esophageal gastric tube airway, or pharyngeotracheal lumen airway, can be used. Ready access to suction equipment is mandatory. Ventilate with 100% oxygen. If hypothermia is suspected, oxygen should be warmed and humidified before administration.

Most patients submerged long enough to stop breathing have become acidotic and may develop ventricular ectopy as well as hypoxemia as a result. Hyperventilation is the first-line method of treating acidosis. Administration of 1 mEq/kg IV sodium bicarbonate may be authorized, along with hyperventilation. The IV may be difficult to start in a cold patient, since peripheral veins tend to be constricted. Attempt a 0.9% NaCl or lactated Ringer's IV infusion en route rather than delay transport. If oxygenation, hyperventilation, and possibly sodium bicarbonate injection do not suppress ventricular ectopy, a bolus of lidocaine, 1 mg/kg, followed by additional 0.5 mg/kg bolus injections to 3 mg/kg, or a 2 to 4 mg/min IV infusion can be used to suppress the ectopy. Further medications are generally not called for, particularly when hypothermia reduces the likelihood that the drugs will exert expected actions.

Management of Cold Water Drowning

Management of cold water drowning or immersion hypothermia should be aimed at rewarming the body's core temperature. Wet clothing should be removed as quickly as possible because it is up to 24 times more conductive than the surrounding still air. Further management is aimed at aggressive sustained resuscitation, since cold water survival times can be extended much further than previously thought.

Victims of short submersion episodes sometimes revive on the spot and appear healthy and unaffected. Nevertheless, the incidence of serious pulmonary complications within 24 hours is high in this group. Hospital examination is extremely important for anyone submerged long enough to ingest water, stop breathing, or lose consciousness. A significant number of deaths after near drownings occur in the following several days as a result of progressive deterioration in pulmonary function that might have been corrected if promptly diagnosed.

Pressure-related Injury

Barotrauma, or *pressure-related injury*, arises most frequently among self-contained underwater breathing apparatus (SCUBA) divers as an effect of underwater pressure on the process of respiration. It also appears in caisson workers, those who work in pressurized environments underground or underwater building tunnels, for example. Decompression sickness, one type of barotrauma, was first known as *caisson disease*.

The gases breathed underwater are essentially breathed at the pressure of the water at that level. At 33 ft below the salt water surface (34 ft for fresh water), pressure is twice that of sea level atmosphere, and it continues to increase by one "*atmosphere*" for each succeeding 33 ft (34 ft in fresh water) in depth.

A physical principle expressed in **Henry's law** states that the amount of a gas that dissolves in a fluid is directly proportional to the pressure of that gas as it contacts the fluid. The pressure of a gas forces it into solution; in other words, a higher pressure means more dissolved gas (Fig. 27-6). In barotrauma, the pressure is the surrounding atmospheric or **hydrostatic** (water) **pressure,** and the fluid is the body's total water content. Gas content in the blood responds directly to pressure in the lungs, and the resulting changes spread throughout the body as the dissolved gases diffuse out of the blood vessels. The gases are the same as those breathed in room air, normally 0.03% carbon dioxide, 21% oxygen, and 78.97% nitrogen, unless a diver uses a special mixture.

Nitrogen and Decompression Sickness

The gas of concern in the most common pressure disorders is nitrogen. It accounts for most of our inspired air and can only travel in the blood in dissolved form. Nitrogen has no substance to bind and transport it as hemoglobin does for oxygen.

At 99 ft, water pressure forces four times the normal quantity of nitrogen into solution in the blood. The tissues absorb dissolved nitrogen at varying rates depending on their water content and other factors. This nitrogen saturation process goes on constantly during both descent and **bottom time** (amount of time the diver is at a certain depth).

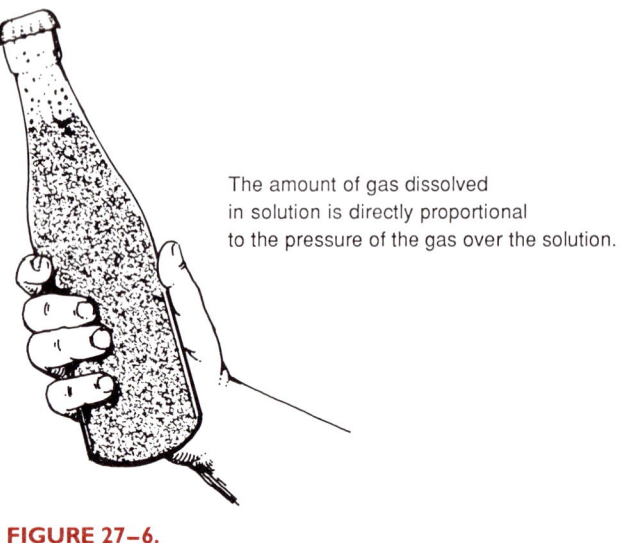

Since nitrogen physiologically is partially an *inert gas* (inactive) at normal pressures, it does not directly affect metabolism. Most tissues feel little change even as its pressure rises; the brain, however, displays a special sensitivity. A syndrome of disorientation and other mental changes called **nitrogen narcosis** has led divers to use completely inert gases (inactive at all pressures), especially helium, on prolonged dives and at great depths.

The real problem with nitrogen has to do with ascending. As a diver returns to the surface, water pressure drops and Henry's law dictates that gradually less nitrogen remains in solution. If the ascent is slow enough, the gas diffuses smoothly from the tissues back into the blood for transport to the lungs and excretion. The diffusion and transport have distinct rate limits, however, and ascent time is likely to be much shorter than the total nitrogen "*loading*" time (descent plus bottom interval). Too rapid an ascent encourages nitrogen to bubble out of solution in the tissues and the blood, according to Henry's law.

This process in the body, known as **decompression sickness,** or "*the bends,*" is painful and sometimes dangerous. Flying in a plane after diving, unless done in a cabin maintained at sea level pressure, adds greatly to the chance of developing decompression sickness, a critical point when transporting barotrauma patients. Most symptoms develop within 1 hour after diving, and almost all within 6 hours, though delayed symptoms are possible. Complete excretion of excess nitrogen can take more than 24 hours.

Nitrogen bubble formation causes both intravascular and extravascular derangements. *Bubbles* in sufficient quantity in the blood obstruct its flow, leading to hypoxia. The bubbles also promote *platelet aggregation* (clumping) and consequent clotting disorders. Extreme intravascular bubble formation can lead to tissue infarct. Bubbles outside of the vessels apply pressure to tissues, commonly causing pain.

The threat is much more serious in the central nervous system, as this tissue's fragility makes it vulnerable to damage from bubble pressure, particularly in the spinal cord where low space tolerances leave little room for expansion or shifting. Changes in neurologic function possibly due to decompression sickness call for immediate recompression chamber therapy to prevent permanent damage. Recompression forces the bubbles back into solution (again, via Henry's law) and then controls the speed of elimination.

Musculoskeletal pain, especially in the joints, and skin color changes, such as mottling, redness, and cyanosis, are other common signs and symptoms of decompression sickness. Another type of bends, called **chokes,** originates with bubbles in the pulmonary vasculature. Chokes pre-

FIGURE 27-6.
Henry's law.

The amount of gas dissolved in solution is directly proportional to the pressure of the gas over the solution.

sent with chest pain, dyspnea, and coughing and possibly hemoptysis. Decompression sickness has many other possible presentations. Any significant symptoms after diving should be evaluated for possible pressure-related origins.

MANAGEMENT OF DECOMPRESSION SICKNESS. Management of decompression sickness focuses on fundamental resuscitative measures when necessary and pain control in less severe cases. Chamber recompression is desirable with any serious symptoms and crucial in the presence of neurologic, pulmonary, and more than minor peripheral circulatory deficits (Figs. 27-7 and 27-8). Any patient with serious symptoms should be transported in the left lateral Trendelenburg's position to prevent any emboli in the ventricles from migrating to the arterial system. This position tends to trap air in the right ventricle and prevent its passage to the left side of the circulation.

Recompression. Recompression by returning to depth in the water is more dangerous than beneficial. Both the environment and the patient's airway are uncontrollable, and further nitrogen loading simply prolongs the problem.

The gas mixture in a chamber can be controlled to optimize nitrogen excretion. Administering 100% oxygen on the way to the chamber helps do the same by preventing intake of any new nitrogen while the excess is being excreted. It also improves tissue perfusion that may be compromised by nitrogen bubbles in the blood. The use of 100% oxygen is one of two direct treatments for decompression sickness before chamber recompression.

Fluid and Drug Therapy. Fluid therapy is the second management available for decompression sickness before chamber recompression. An IV infusion of 0.9% NaCl or lactated Ringer's solution is indicated for any patient ill enough to

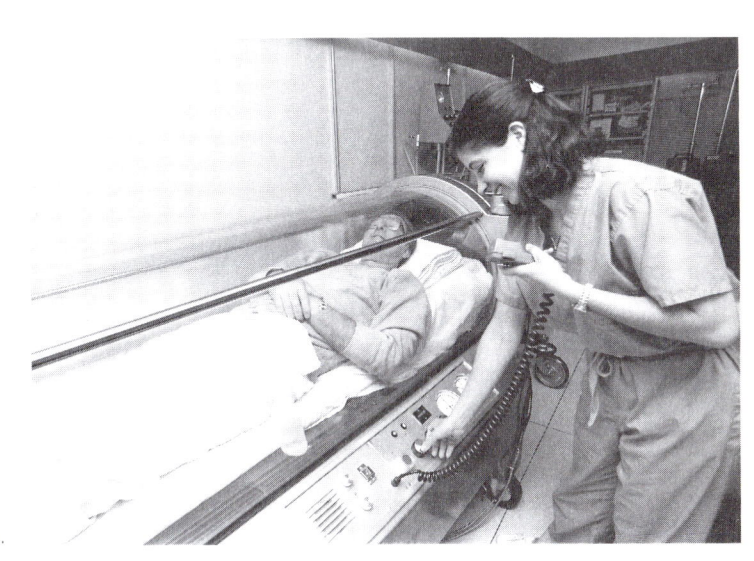

FIGURE 27-7.
Monoplace chamber for recompression.

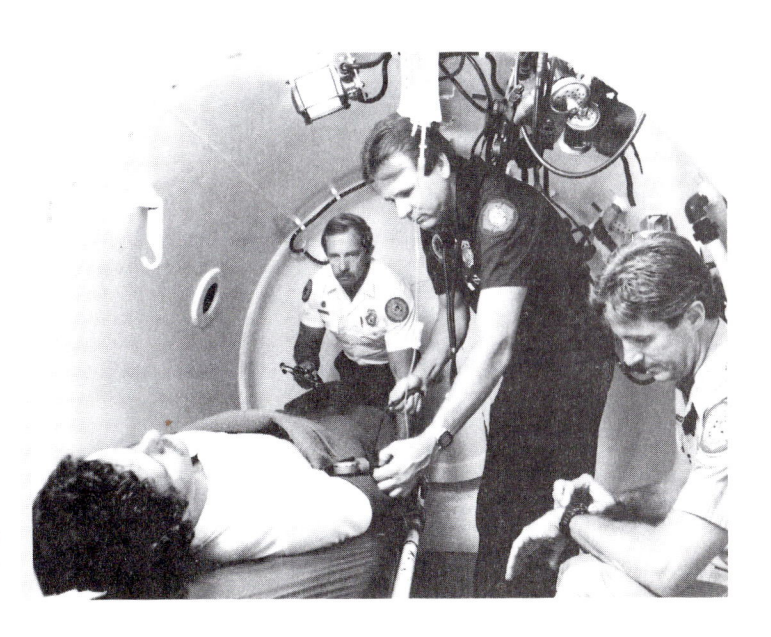

FIGURE 27-8.
Recompression chamber that allows medical personnel to be *in* the chamber with the patient. (Courtesy of Hyperbarics International)

be transported. Maintaining blood volume assists in the circulation (and thus excretion) of nitrogen and also enhances tissue oxygenation. Infuse at a rate to maintain blood pressure, and monitor frequently for early signs of overhydration, such as increased respiratory effort and pulmonary rales.

Aspirin relieves minor pain and reduces the potential for clotting problems. A physician may order steroids, often dexamethasone, when a neurologic involvement is found, or an anticoagulant such as heparin.

Gas Expansion and Air Embolism

The second major category of barotrauma originates with *gas expansion* rather than bubble formation. Another principle of physics, **Boyle's law,** says that the volume of a gas varies inversely with the external pressure applied to it. Increasing pressure compresses gas into a smaller volume, and lowering pressure allows the gas to expand and occupy more space, possibly rupturing the tympanic membrane.

The physiologic principles stated in Boyle's law also function in combination with those expressed in Henry's law to the patient's detriment. Once nitrogen bubbles evolve, they grow larger during ascent, compounding the effects of decompression sickness.

Boyle's law poses problems on descent primarily in the sinuses and inner ears. Normally, air being compressed can escape these soft-walled open spaces through connecting tubes or passages, but membrane inflammation and mucus congestion can obstruct the passages and prevent pressure equalization. Respiratory infections are thus important considerations for divers and aviators. Many regularly use decongestants to prevent pain and the chance of structural damage, such as tympanic membrane rupture.

Ascent, with its accompanying expansion of gas in closed compartments, presents the potential for similar problems. Air expansion, like compression, can injure sinuses and eardrums. Breath holding while ascending, however, poses much more serious threats, some of which can be fatal (Fig. 27-9). Turning the lungs into an enclosed space can cause several kinds of pulmonary "*overpressure*" injuries: air embolism, pneumothorax, and mediastinal and subcutaneous emphysema.

Air embolism is the most serious of the pulmonary overpressure accidents, and it can occur without breath holding if the lungs are diseased or some other mechanism encourages air entrapment. When pressure in the lungs reaches a critical point, it forces air bubbles across the alveolar membrane and into the pulmonary capillaries. The small bubbles may collect into larger ones as they flow through the pulmonary veins toward the left atrium.

Air embolism presents suddenly, during or immediately after the dive, with severe pain, paralysis or other neurologic signs, cardiac or respiratory collapse, or loss of consciousness. The formation of emboli at depth has devastating consequences. Symptoms make drowning likely, and the volume of trapped air and the emboli themselves expand with ascent to the surface.

MANAGEMENT OF AIR EMBOLISM. Management of embolism and the other pulmonary overpressure accidents is difficult without recompression therapy, but basic sup-

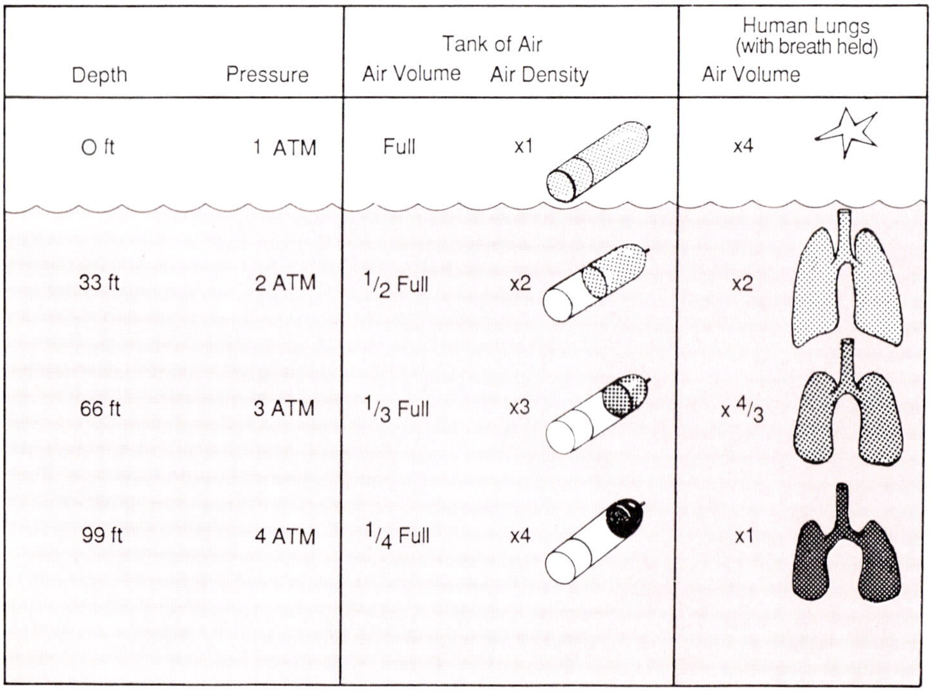

Depth	Pressure	Tank of Air Air Volume	Air Density	Human Lungs (with breath held) Air Volume
0 ft	1 ATM	Full	x1	x4
33 ft	2 ATM	1/2 Full	x2	x2
66 ft	3 ATM	1/3 Full	x3	x 4/3
99 ft	4 ATM	1/4 Full	x4	x1

FIGURE 27-9.
Gas expansion with altitude.

portive care can help. Support cardiopulmonary function as needed, give high concentration supplemental oxygen, and transport in the left lateral Trendelenburg's position to minimize migration of air into the arterial circulation. Positive-pressure ventilation can further complicate all of these conditions; if it is required, avoid gas-powered adjuncts and instead use a bag-valve-mask device. Skillful ventilatory support in this manner can keep inspiratory airway pressures to an absolute minimum.

Time is extremely important to overpressure patients. Begin transport to a recompression chamber absolutely as soon as possible and finish stabilizing treatment on the way. Specialized medical advice or safety information and the location of the nearest hyperbaric chamber are available Monday through Friday, 9 am to 5 pm Eastern Standard Time by calling the Diver's Alert Network: (919) 684-2948. For 24 hour information on diving emergencies, call (919) 684-8111 and ask for a diving physician.

Air evacuation of divers must be kept close to sea level. Even flight in pressurized cabins exposes patients to decreased atmospheric pressure and therefore further gas expansion, unless the aircraft holds to a low-altitude flight plan. Actual cabin pressure must remain below 1000 ft (above sea level). Below 500 ft is preferable.

Subtle temperature changes may complicate diving injuries. Heat loss through an insulated suit can be so gradual that it builds to significant levels without activating the normal compensatory mechanisms with their classic signs and symptoms. Suspect hypothermia in these patients and manage accordingly.

HAZARDOUS MATERIALS

The variety of scenarios of hazardous materials incidents is nearly endless: an industrial chemical spill, toxic gas release from a railroad tanker, the potential radiation danger of a collision between a truck that radiographs construction welding and a car, a family driven from the house by fumes from the attached garage, and many others.

Large or small, hazardous materials incidents are specialized problems, the correct handling of which requires advanced planning and training. Interagency cooperation is important to successful outcomes, as is a comprehensive regional view of likely exposure risks and response configurations.

Individual states have designed a series of courses that comply with the Occupational Safety and Health Administration's (OSHA) standard for hazardous waste operations and emergency response. The rule 29 CFR 1910.120 was signed into law March 6, 1989 and regulates the safety and health of employees during initial assessment and emergency medical response. This series of training courses is based on the duties and functions to be performed by each responder of an emergency response organization. Response personnel who participate, or who are expected to participate, will be given training according to the following course descriptions:

First Responder Awareness Level: Individuals who are likely to witness or discover a hazardous substance release and who have been trained to initiate an emergency response sequence by notifying the proper authorities (*i.e.*, police officers, industrial workers) of the release. They take no further action beyond notifying the authorities of the release. First responders at the awareness level will demonstrate competency in behavioral objectives 6 through 13 (at the beginning of this chapter). This course has no time requirement. An annual refresher requires training of sufficient content and duration to maintain competency, or demonstration of competency.

First Responder Operations Level: Individuals who respond to releases or potential releases of hazardous substances as part of the initial response to the site for the purpose of protecting nearby persons, property, or the environment from the effects of the release. They are trained to respond in a defensive fashion without actually trying to stop the release. Their function is to contain the release from a safe distance, keep it from spreading, and prevent exposures. First responders at the operations level shall have received at least 8 hours of training or have had significant experience to objectively demonstrate competency in behavioral objectives 6 through 20 (at the beginning of this chapter). This knowledge includes the objectives listed for the awareness level. An annual refresher requires training of sufficient content and duration to maintain competency, or demonstration of competency.

This section on hazardous materials meets the OSHA training requirements for both the First Responder Awareness and Operations Level courses. The term "*first responder*" should not be confused with the same term used by the U.S. Department of Transportation to designate a person with basic first aid skills. A first responder according to OSHA signifies a person with basic hazardous materials skills.

Recognition of Hazardous Materials

Hazardous materials can be defined in a number of ways, as shown in the box "Hazardous Materials Definitions." Each term in the box has its own applications. For example, the U.S Department of Transportation's definition only concerns itself with hazardous materials being transported. The OSHA definition applies only to those chemicals found in the workplace. Since a variety of definitions for hazardous materials exists, a broad definition developed by Ludwig Benner, Jr., a former hazardous materials specialist with the National Transportation Safety Board

HAZARDOUS MATERIALS DEFINITIONS

Hazardous materials—Any substance or material in a quantity or form that poses an unreasonable risk to health, safety, and property when transported in commerce.
 —U.S. Department of Transportation

Hazardous substance—Any substance designated under the Clean Water Act and the Comprehensive Environmental Response Compensation and Liability Act (CERCLA) as posing a threat to waterways and the environment when released.
 —U.S. Environmental Protection Agency

Hazardous materials—Any substance that causes or may cause adverse effects on the health or safety of employees, and general public, or the environment; any biologic agent and other disease-causing agent, or a waste or combination of wastes.
 —National Fire Protection Association

Hazardous waste—Any waste or compilation of wastes that pose a substantial presence or potential hazard to human health or living organisms because such wastes are nondegradable or persistent in nature or because they can biologically magnify or because they can be lethal or because they may otherwise cause or tend to cause detrimental cumulative effects.
 —U.S. Environmental Protection Agency

---

in Washington, D.C., states: A *hazardous material* is any substance that jumps out of its container when something goes wrong and hurts or harms the things it touches. A *hazardous materials incident* can then be defined as the release, or potential release, of a hazardous material from its container into the environment.

Proper recognition and identification of hazardous materials are accomplished by occupancy and location, container shapes, markings and color, placards and labels, shipping papers, and senses.

Occupancy and Location

Paramedics should be familiar with various *occupancies* and *locations* in their communities where hazardous materials are produced, transported, used, or stored. Since chemical exposures are no longer limited to industrial or transportation emergencies, the potential of being exposed is present at any emergency.

Container Shapes

The general classifications of containers for hazardous materials are individual containers, bulk transport containers, and bulk storage containers. Some hazardous materials require specialized containment that has a specific *shape*, which can give a clue to the identity of the contents. Some samples of characteristic shapes are shown in Figure 27-10.

CONTAINER SHAPE	DESCRIPTION	CONTENTS
Underground Storage Tank	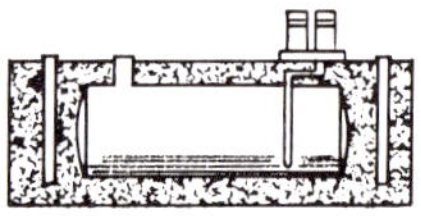 Low pressure storage tank. Horizontal tank constructed of steel or fiberglass	Stores primarily petroleum products
Corrosive Cargo Tank Trucks	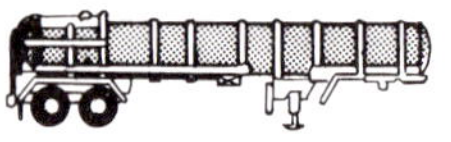 Circular cross section with external reinforcing ribs. Generally 5,000 to 6,000 gallons capacity	Transports strong corrosives
Pressurized Tank Cars	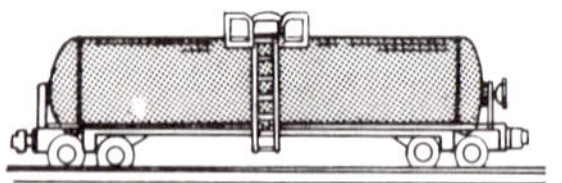 Horizontal tank with rounded ends. Fittings and valves enclosed in dome	Transports flammable and nonflammable compressed gases and Class A poisons
Multicell Packages	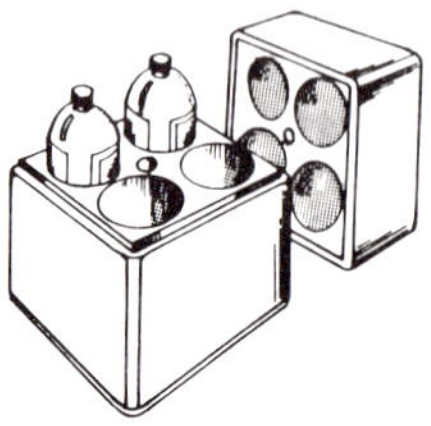 Fiberboard boxes with compartments for containers	Used to ship various solvents and corrosives such as sulfuric and hydrochloric acid

FIGURE 27-10.
The size, shape, and construction features of a container can provide a clue to the identification of hazardous materials.

Markings and Colors

Many unique general *markings* and *colors* are associated with hazardous materials containers and packages. Markings and colors are evaluated based on fixed facility, bulk transportation containers, and nonbulk packages and containers.

FIXED FACILITY. Many state and fire codes mandate the use of the National Fire Protection Association (NFPA) 704 marking system at all fixed facilities in their jurisdiction, including tanks and storage areas. The NFPA 704 system, which is shown in Figure 27-11, is not used on transport vehicles. The diamond-shaped hazardous identification symbol indicates what level of health, fire, reac-

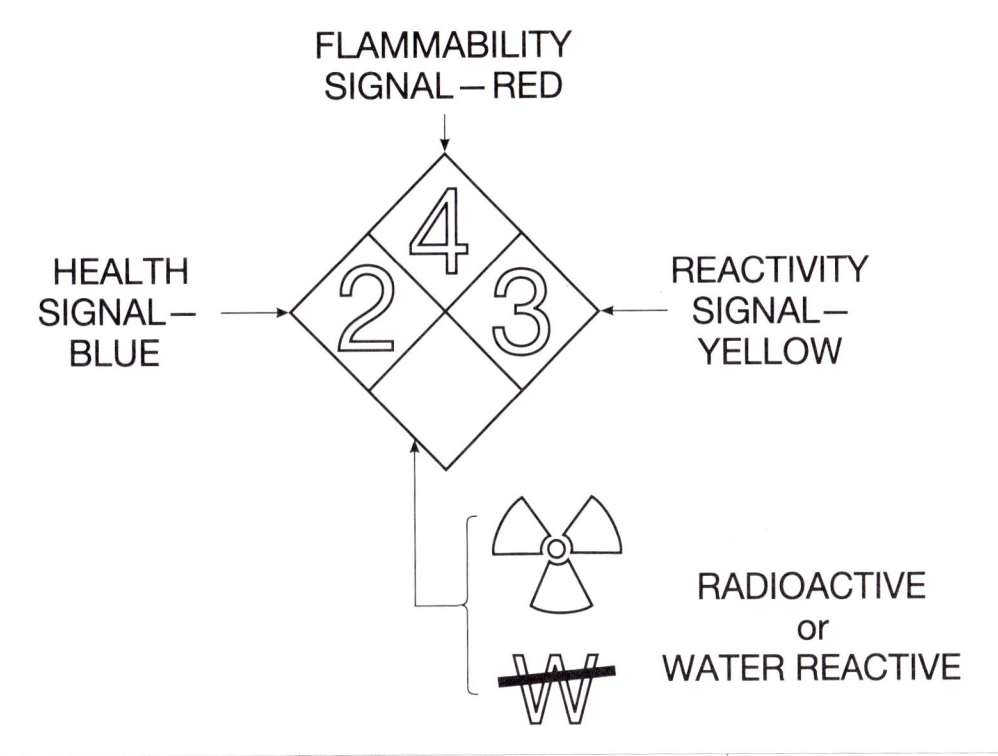

Identification of Health Hazard Color Code: BLUE		Identification of Flammability Color Code: RED		Identification of Reactivity (Stability) Color Code: YELLOW	
Signal	Type of Possible Injury	Signal	Susceptibility of Materials to Burning	Signal	Susceptibility to Release of Energy
4	Materials that on very short exposure could cause death or major residual injury even though prompt medical treatment were given.	4	Materials that will rapidly or completely vaporize at atmospheric pressure and normal ambient temperature, or that are readily dispersed in air and that will burn readily.	4	Materials that in themselves are readily capable of detonation or of explosive decomposition or reaction at normal temperatures and pressures.
3	Materials that on short exposure could cause serious temporary or residual injury even though prompt medical treatment were given.	3	Liquids and solids that can be ignited under almost all ambient temperature conditions.	3	Materials that in themselves are capable of detonation or explosive reaction but require a strong initiating source or that must be heated under confinement before initiation or that react explosively with water.
2	Materials that on intense or continued exposure could cause temporary incapacitation or possible residual injury unless prompt medical treatment is given.	2	Materials that must be moderately heated or exposed to relatively high ambient temperatures before ignition can occur.	2	Materials that in themselves are normally unstable and readily undergo violent chemical change but do not detonate. Also materials that may react violently with water or that may form potentially explosive mixtures with water.
1	Materials that on exposure would cause irritation but only minor residual injury even if no treatment is given.	1	Materials that must be preheated before ignition can occur.	1	Materials that in themselves are normally stable, but that can become unstable at elevated temperatures and pressures or that may react with water with some release of energy but not violently.
0	Materials that on exposure under fire conditions would offer no hazard beyond that of ordinary combustible material.	0	Materials that will not burn.	0	Materials that in themselves are normally stable, even under fire exposure conditions, and that are not reactive with water.

FIGURE 27-11.
National Fire Protection Association 704 marking system.

tivity, and specific hazards the material may have. Health hazard levels are located in the left quadrant in a blue color. The upper quadrant is red and indicates the level of fire hazard involved. The yellow right quadrant indicates the level of reactivity hazard, and specific hazards are indicated in the bottom white quadrant.

BULK TRANSPORTATION CONTAINERS. The U.S. Department of Transportation requires the commodity name of about 44 hazardous materials to be stenciled on both sides of railroad tank cars. In addition, other markings include the company name, telephone number, tank registration or serial number, and U.S. Department of Transportation container specification number. Cargo tank trucks, like tank cars, also have similar markings.

As of November 1, 1981, identification numbers were required on portable tanks, cargo tanks, and tank cars. Identification numbers may also be displayed on the containers. Any tank, vehicle, or rail car that carries hazardous materials of any kind is required by law to display a four-digit identification number on the end of the vehicle. In case of an accident, this number can be matched against a list of toxic substances so that the material can be quickly identified.

Pipelines are considered a hazardous materials transportation mode and often cross under or over roads, railroads, and waterways. At each of these crossovers, a marker should provide the pipeline contents and an emergency telephone number.

NONBULK PACKAGES AND CONTAINERS. Individual nonbulk packages and containers display useful information for identification and hazard assessment. Those containing pesticides and agricultural chemicals may include such markings as product name, ingredient list, environmental information, and physical or chemical hazard statement.

Placards and Labels

Hazardous materials that are being used, stored, or transported display a diamond-shaped *placard* with a symbol that identifies what properties are possessed by the material, such as flammable, corrosive, or explosive. This placarding system enables the initial responders to take any immediate action to contain the material and also to help advise the communications operator about additional vehicles or agencies that are needed. Placards are diamond shaped, 10¾ inch square. The placard provides recognition information in a number of ways: the colored background, the hazard symbol on top, the United Nations (UN) hazard class number at the bottom, and the hazard class or the four-digit identification number found in the center (Fig. 27-12). The nine hazard classes are shown in Table 27-2.

The *four-digit identification system* was adopted by the U.S. Department of Transportation to allow first responders to immediately access hazard information pro-

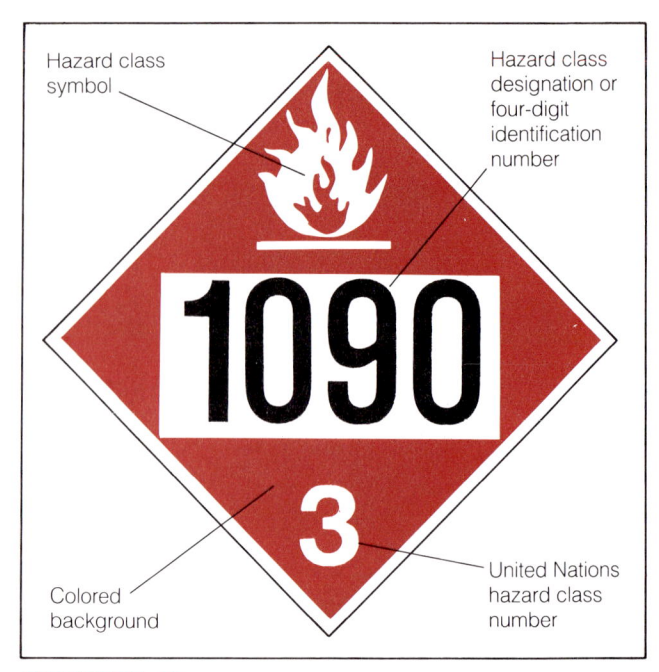

FIGURE 27-12.
Placards provide general hazard recognition in several ways.

vided in the U.S. Department of Transportation's *Emergency Response Guidebook*. Identification numbers are required on shipping papers and on or near bulk transport container placards. This number may be displayed on bulk containers in one of three ways (Fig. 27-13).

Labels are mostly small versions of placards. They are 4 inch by 4 inch markings applied to individual hazardous materials packages. Labels may be found not only on metal containers but also on those made of wood, plastic, cardboard, and even paper bags. Since federal laws require only one label on the outside of shipping containers, labels may not be visible because of the way they are loaded. Labels are used on individual packages of hazardous materials but do not use the four-digit identification number, instead they name the class of material.

A color chart of hazardous materials placards and labels appears on the inside front cover of this text.

Shipping Papers

All *shipping papers* have the following information: proper shipping name, hazard classification (such as flammable or explosive), four-digit identification number, type of packages, and correct weight. When required, shipping papers are kept in the cab of the motor vehicle, in the possession of a train crew member, in a holder on the bridge of a vessel, or in an aircraft pilot's possession.

Senses

Senses include any physiologic reaction to incident proximity, such as smell, taste, or feel. Senses should not be intentionally used to detect hazardous materials. Senses

TABLE 27–2.
PLACARD RECOGNITION INFORMATION

United Nations Hazard Class	Symbol	Background Color	Examples
CLASS 1			
Explosives	Bursting ball	Orange	Fireworks Ammunition Dynamite
CLASS 2			
Gases (compressed, liquified, or dissolved under pressure)	*Flammable* Flame	Red	Flammable: Butane Propane
	Nonflammable Cylinder	Green	Nonflammable: Ammonia Chlorine
CLASS 3			
Flammable liquids	Flame	Red	Brake fluid Camphor oil Glycol ethers Gasoline
CLASS 4			
Flammable solids or substances	*Flammable Solid* Flame	Red and white vertical stripes	Lithium Magnesium Phosphorus Titanium
	Water Reactive Materials Slashed W	Red and white vertical stripes with blue top quadrant	
CLASS 5			
Division 5.1: Oxidizing substances Division 5.2: Organic peroxides	Circle with flame	Yellow	Ammonium nitrate Benzoyl peroxide Calcium chlorite
CLASS 6			
Poisonous and infectious substances	Skull with crossbones	White	Chemical mace Pesticides Cyanide AIDS specimens
CLASS 7			
Radioactive materials	Propeller	Yellow over white	Cobalt 14 Plutonium Radioactive waste Uranium 235
CLASS 8			
Corrosives	Test tube over hand Test tube over metal	White over black	Caustic potash Caustic soda Hydrochloric acid Sulfuric acid
CLASS 9			
Miscellaneous dangerous substances	ORM-A ORM-B ORM-C ORM-D ORM-E	White	ORM-A: Dry ice ORM-B: Quick lime ORM-C: Sawdust ORM-D: Hair spray ORM-E: Hazardous waste

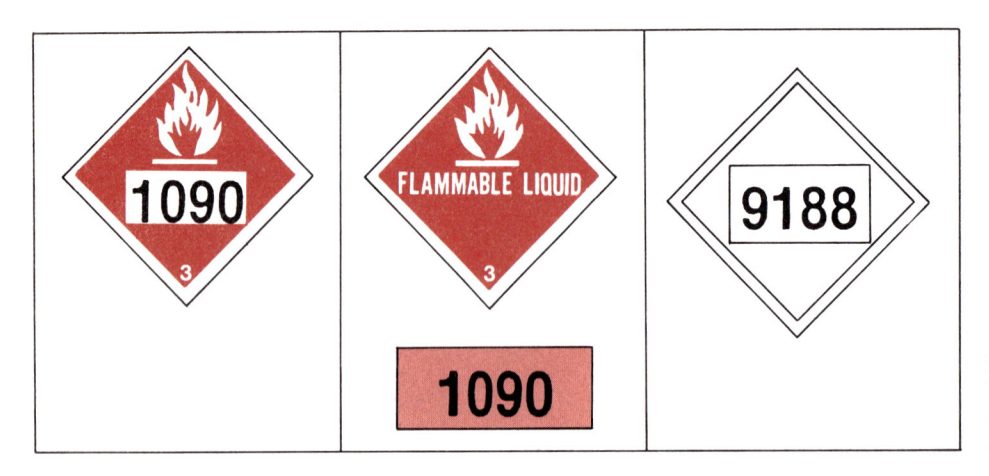

FIGURE 27–13.
The four-digit identification number may be displayed on bulk containers in one of three ways.

can, however, alert the first responder to the presence of hazardous materials. If a product does have a distinctive odor or other characteristic and it is inadvertently encountered, it serves as a signal that the product is close, and responders should go to an uncontaminated area.

Once a hazardous material is encountered, the following steps provide a guide for making decisions. The acronym *D.E.C.I.D.E.* is used to help remember these steps:

D Detect presence of hazardous materials
E Estimate likely harm
C Choose response objectives
I Identify action options
D Do the best option
E Evaluate the process

By following this six step process, favorable outcomes can be achieved during a hazardous materials incident. When identifying the action option, the responder must consider the dangers that exist before instinctively trying to get to the victims. Choosing the best option most likely means waiting until properly trained and protected responders arrive on the scene to remove the hazards or the patients.

Hazardous materials data and information can be obtained through various emergency response telephone centers. In the United States, the most recognized telephone information service is CHEMTREC (Chemical Transportation Emergency Center). Established in 1971, it is a public service of the Chemical Manufacturers Association (formerly Manufacturing Chemists Association) in Washington, D.C. CHEMTREC's purpose is twofold. First, it provides immediate advice on the nature of the product and steps to be taken in handling the early stages of a problem. Second, it promptly contacts the shipper of the material for more detailed information and appropriate follow-up. CHEMTREC operates 24 hours a day, 7 days a week and can be contacted at 800-424-9300. Other emergency response numbers that may be useful for both planning and response purposes are shown in the box, "Hazardous Materials Emergency Numbers."

HAZARDOUS MATERIALS EMERGENCY NUMBERS

Association of American Railroads,
Hazardous Materials System
  (formerly the Bureau of Explosives)
202-639-2222   24-hour service

- Assistance in handling railroad-related hazardous materials emergencies

CANUTEC
  (Canadian Transportation Emergency Center)
613-966-6666   24-hour service

- Canadian counterpart of CHEMTREC
- Assistance in identification and establishing contact with shippers and manufacturers of hazardous materials that originate in Canada

Centers for Disease Control
404-633-5313   24-hour service

- Assistance in handling infectious disease–related incidents

CHEMTREC
  (Chemical Transportation Emergency Center)
800-424-9300   24-hour service

- Identification of unknown chemicals
- Advice on response methods
- Assistance in contacting shippers, carriers, response teams

Texas Tech University Pesticide Hotline
800-858-7378   24-hour service

- Information on toxicity, handling, and cleanup

U.S. Coast Guard and the Department of Transportation National Response Center
800-424-8802   24-hour service

- Reporting of hazardous materials incidents that cause death, serious injury, property damage in excess of $50,000, or a continuing threat to life and property
- Assistance in identification, technical information, and initial response actions

Planning and Preparedness

To become familiar with the needs of their communities, responders should complete the following pre-emergency planning and inspection activities:

1. Know what major businesses and industries in the community use, store, or transport hazardous materials. If possible, meet with them to discuss their emergency plan in case of an accident. Get a list of contacts, including names and phone numbers. Ask if their plants have internal hazardous materials teams. Find out the location of decontamination showers in the plants.
2. Know who is available to provide a Hazardous Materials Emergency Response Team to the community and an alternate if they are not available. If possible, meet with them to discuss how to best work together in an emergency.
3. Provide means for having the necessary equipment available for personal protection of the emergency medical services (EMS) workers; consider disposable items to minimize unnecessary decontamination.

Vehicle Equipment

The items in the response vehicle must accommodate incidents that involve a variety of hazardous materials. The following is a partial list that should be refined and altered to suit the conditions of the most common incidents:

- Binoculars to assess scene from a safe distance
- Plastic sheeting and clear trash bags (3 or 4 mL) to protect equipment and dispose of contaminated articles
- Disposable blankets (plastic coated to contain liquids on the patient)
- Inexpensive stethoscopes, blood pressure cuffs, and other gear that can be discarded if contaminated
- Rubber or neoprene boots and gloves (not surgical rubber gloves or latex types)
- Skin-covering outerwear (long sleeve shirts, coveralls, disposable gowns)
- A generous supply of fresh water to flush away contaminates
- Goggles or face shields to protect EMS personnel from splashes
- A large supply of oxygen to treat breathing problems caused by exposure to hazardous materials
- Disposable gowns and slippers for patients who must remove contaminated clothes at the scene
- Copy of the current U.S. Department of Transportation's *Emergency Response Guidebook*

Communications

Communications from the initial call to 911 and to the actual on-scene dialogue is always a challenge. The following communication information is important in a hazardous materials incident:

1. Establish or review communication procedures for information collection and dissemination, as well as for operations. Will the necessary information be collected (Fig. 27-14)?
2. Establish or review communication procedures for operations. Do they follow the Incident Command System format (see Chapter 6)? Use of the Incident Command System at the scene of all hazardous materials incidents that are beyond the scope of the First Responder Awareness Level is now mandated by OSHA.
3. Maintain a list of radio frequencies used by local fire, police, EMS, and hazardous materials units. Is there a common frequency that all agencies are capable of using?
4. Record information transmitted about a hazardous materials incident.
5. Communications should be in plain language. They should be simple and concise.

Rescue Considerations

Request clear information while en route to the incident. Often the EMS unit is not the first on the scene. Fire or police units may be the first arriving emergency personnel. In some ways, a hazardous materials incident has more in common with a fire than with a standard medical run because rescuers are at risk every second they remain in the environment. The victims must be removed to a safe area quickly. Hazardous Materials Teams and some fire departments have equipment designed for hostile environments and generally have far more experience at rapid and safe removal of victims from hazardous environments than medical units have. The incident commander should direct those nonmedical rescue personnel to bring victims to the triage area.

On arrival at the incident scene, the responder should do the following:

1. Report to the incident commander. EMS personnel must follow the directions of the incident commander as to which areas they may not enter. These regulations are for the protection of all medical personnel.
2. Assess the situation. Determine the escape route, if necessary, and from which direction potential patients will likely arrive.
3. Get information to assess the risk to the EMS responders.
4. Medical personnel who monitor entry personnel should learn what chemicals are involved, the signs and symptoms of exposure, and any special personal safety, decontamination, or first aid considerations required.
5. When medical personnel arrive on the scene before qualified hazardous materials personnel, care must be

HAZARDOUS MATERIAL INCIDENT LOGG

Date ______________ Dispatch Time ________ AM/PM

Product Name ______________ U.N./N.A. No. ______________

E.P.A. No. ______________ S.T.C.C. No. ______________

Chemical Name ______________ Guide No. ______________

Manufacturer ______________ Tel. No. ______________

Address ______________ Contact ______________

Principal Uses ______________

Hazard Class ______________ Flash Point ______________

Flammable Range-Lower ______________ Upper ______________

Ignition Temp. ______________ Boiling Point ______________

Specific Gravity (Water = 1) ________ Vapor Density (Air = 1) ________

Routes of Entry ______________ Toxicity ______________

Water Solubility ______________ Reactivity ______________

HAZARD I.D.

CHEMTREC 1-800-424-9300 Poison Center # ______________

Narrative ______________

Diagram Area

WEATHERLOGG® USE PENCIL ONLY • ERASEABLE • CLEAN WITH CLEANSER

© 1985 Jones Research, P.O. Box 22008, Indianapolis, IN 46222

FIGURE 27–14. Types of information that should be gathered at a hazardous materials incident.

> taken to assess the situation, use appropriate personal protection measures, and make decisions with caution, regarding fire, explosion, and toxicity potential.

Emergency medical personnel should take and record the vital signs of hazardous materials entry personnel before they initially go into the ***hot zone*** (area that surrounds a hazardous materials incident that is dangerous to life and health) and on their exit into the ***warm zone*** (outside the hot zone, personal protection not required) or during self-contained breathing apparatus (SCBA) bottle changes at the edge of the warm zone. The ***cold zone*** is a safe area for agencies directly involved in the incident. See Figure 27-15 for hazard zone areas. This information must be promptly given to the safety officer, who is responsible for the safety of the personnel who are working at the incident.

Everyone who goes through decontamination procedures should be screened for signs and symptoms of exposure. If it appears that a worker has been exposed, the

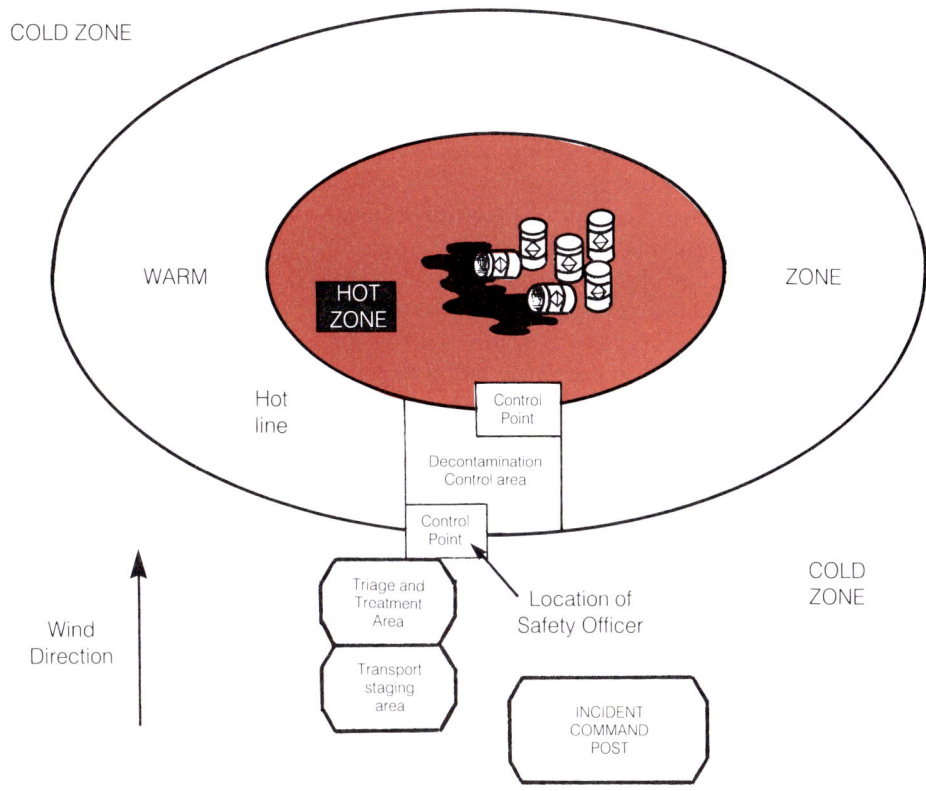

FIGURE 27–15.
Incident control and hazard zones.

safety officer should be notified immediately. Victims brought out of the hot zone should be assumed to be contaminated. As deemed appropriate, based on the extent of the injuries and risk to the medical personnel, emergency care may be initiated either simultaneously with or immediately once decontamination has progressed to the point to allow safe access to the patient.

Responding to a Call

Every piece of information acquired about an incident before arrival at the scene adds to effectiveness and safety. The communications operator plays a vital role in getting the needed information to perform the job safely. The communications operator should also be familiar with the current U.S. Department of Transportation's *Emergency Response Guidebook* to immediately identify the nature of the hazardous material. Incident control and hazard zones should be established for safety and incident operations (see Fig. 27-15).

Exposure to Hazardous Materials
Routes of Entry

Substances can enter the body by four pathways: absorption, inhalation, ingestion, and injection.

ABSORPTION. The skin acts as a barrier against the entry of foreign materials into the body. If this protective barrier is weakened or compromised, toxic chemicals can enter, resulting in **absorption.** The barrier is greatly diminished by lacerations and abrasions. Also, many organic solvents increase the permeability of the skin to materials that would otherwise not pass through it. The skin provides a large surface area for contact with toxic agents.

INHALATION. **Inhalation** is the most rapid route, immediately introducing chemical vapors or toxic products of combustion into respiratory tissues and the bloodstream. Once admitted into the blood through the lungs, these toxins are quickly transported throughout the body to contact all organs. In many cases, chemicals accumulate in a target organ.

INGESTION. Materials get into the mouth (**ingestion**) through hand-to-mouth contact and through coughing when inhaled particulate material is removed from the lungs to the throat and then swallowed. Since the gastrointestinal tract has acids, alkalies, and enzymes, the toxic nature of the compound may be enhanced or diminished.

INJECTION. The **injection** of hazardous materials into the body, however unlikely it sounds at first, can occur by stepping on or bumping against a sharp object while working at an incident site. The best precaution for the injection of a hazardous material is to wear protective clothing and observe safe work habits.

Ionizing Radiation

In its broadest sense, radiation is the method by which certain forms of energy, composed either of particles or waves, emanate from a central source. Light, heat, noise, and radio signals are all examples of radiant energy.

The type of energy emitted by **radioactive substances** is *ionizing radiation*, so named for its ability to damage organic matter by breaking loose the ions, electrically charged particles, that make up atoms. This process alters or destroys cellular structure. Cellular genetic materials are particularly prone to damage; long-term problems include sterility and birth defects, as well as immune system impairment, bone deterioration, and cancer.

Radioactive sources emit three principle types of ionizing radiation: *α particles, β particles, and τ rays* (see the box, "Types of Ionizing Radiation"). Understanding how they differ is important to patient care and personal safety.

The amount of radiation absorbed by the body is thought of as the **dose,** which is measured by calculating both the level of radiation present in the immediate area and the duration of exposure to that level. The common unit of measurement is the **roentgen,** abbreviated R. The Geiger counter provides a convenient portable measuring tool. Other units of measurement, the REM (roentgen equivalent in man) and the RAD (radiation absorbed dose), can be thought of as equivalent to the roentgen.

Several factors influence the total radiation dose that one receives from an emitting source, including density of shielding materials, time of exposure, the amount of body surface exposed, and distance from the source. Distance is particularly important because radiation intensity drops with the square of the distance, rather than in direct proportion. Doubling distance reduces exposure to one-quarter, tripling distance drops it to one-ninth, and so on.

Acute vs. Chronic Exposures

Important factors to consider when determining the toxicity of a material are the relationships between concentration, exposure time, and the threshold sensitivity of the person exposed. In general, an acute exposure refers to a large single dose received over a short period of time, and an immediate response occurs. Effects from acute exposures may not be evident for 24 to 72 hours after the initial exposure.

Chronic exposure is the result of repeated exposures to smaller doses of toxins over a period of time. This exposure may result in a delayed effect. The longer the exposure, the greater the likelihood of harm. Exposure time should be limited for all personnel. Ensure that unnecessary personnel remain out of range.

Protection from Hazardous Materials
Forms of Chemical Intrusion

Degradation is the loss in beneficial physical properties caused by exposed gloves, protective clothing, and other material to various liquid chemicals. Materials may get harder, stiffer, and brittle, or they may get softer, weaker, and swell to several times their original dimensions. The traditional method of testing rubber and plastic for chemical resistance has been a degradation test.

Penetration is the flow of a hazardous chemical through zippers, stitched seams and pores, or other imperfections in clothing material. Gloves that can be penetrated are generally only intended to prevent cuts, abrasions, thermal burns, and other similar physical (rather than chemical) hazards.

Permeation is the process by which hazardous chemicals move through protective clothing. No pinholes or other flaws are involved in allowing the chemical to reach the other side of the material. The process consists of the absorption of molecules of the liquid into the contacted (outside) surface of a material, the diffusion of the absorbed molecules through the material, and the desorption of the molecules from the opposite (inside) surface of the material.

Self-care Precautions

The rescuer must take self-care precautions to keep from becoming another victim and thereby part of the problem rather than part of the solution. All EMS personnel need training in the general principles of hazardous materials safety. Early recognition is the top priority. Maintaining a high index of suspicion when approaching home, indus-

---

TYPES OF IONIZING RADIATION

α particles are relatively large, heavy, and slow-moving particles that cannot travel more than a few inches from their source unless borne by smoke or other matter. Light materials such as clothing, even paper, prevent penetration of the particles and their ionizing force. Direct contact damages the skin surface a few cells deep. Internal organs are not at risk unless particles gain access by way of contaminated food, open wounds, or inhalation.

β particles are lighter and faster than α particles and have slightly more penetrating capacity. Light metal and possibly heavy clothing stop them. Their primary threat lies in internal access as mentioned with α particles, but they do cause internal damage, a few centimeters deep, from the surface. Rinsing the body thoroughly after exposure removes both α and β particles.

γ rays are electromagnetic waves similar to x-rays, rather than particles. They penetrate the air much farther from their source (hundreds of yards) than α or β particles do, although their concentration drops rapidly over distance. They penetrate clothing, body tissues, and all but the densest materials, damaging them as they pass through. Only thick layers of substances such as concrete and lead can shield against γ rays completely.

trial, laboratory, and transportation accidents helps alert initial responders before they become victims themselves.

First responders to a hazardous materials incident must take several important factors into consideration before making a decision to attempt an immediate rescue of victims. First, and most importantly, will anything be gained by rescuing the victim? If the victim is obviously dead or conditions point to a high probability of death from injury or the exposure already suffered, a rescue should not be undertaken. If severe injury to rescuers is likely, a rescue should not be attempted. In a case in which removing the victim will be a life-saving action, which can be accomplished with minimal adverse effect to the rescuers, initiation of a rescue may be a reasonable option.

Levels of Protection

When response activities are conducted where atmospheric contamination is known or suspected to exist, personal protective equipment is designed to prevent and reduce skin and eye contact as well as inhalation or ingestion of the chemical substance. Proper training is required to assess the need for the appropriate level to be used. The Environmental Protection Agency has a system for classifying protective clothing into levels A, B, C, and D. Selection of appropriate materials and the use of Level A, B, and C personal protective equipment require specific training.

Level A protection should be worn when the highest level of respiratory, skin, eye, and mucous membrane protection is needed (*e.g.*, vapors, gases, mists, and dusts). Level A personal protective equipment is called a totally encapsulating suit. This term means that the suit envelops the wearer totally, including the SCBA. If the SCBA is placed on the outside, it is called a partially encapsulating suit. This term means that the SCBA is not protected against the environment, but the wearer of the suit is.

Level B protection provides protection against liquid splashes and should be worn when the highest level of respiratory protection but a lesser level of skin and eye protection than level A is needed. Level B protection is the minimum level recommended on initial site entries until the hazards have been further identified and defined by monitoring, sampling, and other reliable methods of analysis and when personal protective equipment corresponding with those findings is used. The level B garment is nonencapsulating with the SCBA worn on the outside. It is usually a two-piece suit, typical of heavy rain gear.

Level C protection should be selected when the type of airborne substance is known, concentration measured, criteria for using air-purifying respirators met, and skin and eye exposure unlikely. Periodic monitoring of the air must be performed. The same level of chemical resistant clothing is used for skin protection as level B, but level C allows for the use of nonfire service respirators. Though level C is commonly found at work sites as the routine protection worn, it is rarely appropriate during hazardous materials emergency operations.

Level D protection is primarily a work uniform. It should only be worn when no possibility of respiratory or skin exposure exists. Level D protection includes surgical rubber gloves, protective eye wear, splash apron, and coveralls.

Ambulance Protection

When a contaminated patient is transported in an ambulance, the ambulance and its contents are considered contaminated. Actions to limit the spread of the contamination are possible and should be taken. For example, the patient may be clothed in a disposable gown or placed on disposable (plastic coated) blankets. In addition, supplies or equipment that come in contact with contaminated areas of the patient should be inexpensive and disposable.

The primary method of limiting the spread of contamination is to cover all exposed surfaces in the interior of the ambulance transport compartment with plastic sheeting. A heavy gauge (3–4 mm thickness) plastic should be used to minimize the possibility of ripping or tearing. Equipment and supplies likely to be needed should be stored in compartments that can be easily accessed through flaps in the plastic. All other items should be removed or stored where they cannot be contaminated.

Decontamination

Decontamination is the process by which a hazardous substance is removed from individuals and equipment. The protocols for decontamination of victims should be used to prevent further exposure to the victims, to limit the spread of contamination, and to prevent contamination of emergency personnel.

The presence of contamination is what makes responding to a hazardous materials incident different from a normal medical emergency run. The extent of decontamination necessary varies substantially, depending on the nature of the incident, the specific hazardous materials involved, and the quantity. The extent of appropriate decontamination necessary may need to be determined from CHEMTREC and the local or regional poison control center.

Normally, decontamination is handled by qualified personnel, such as Hazardous Materials Teams or in industrial settings by the company's health or safety officer. Medical personnel, even in proper personal protective equipment, should not attempt to initiate treatment of a contaminated victim unless the nature of the injuries is life-threatening and significant benefit may be achieved. In most hazardous materials incidents, medical personnel should not attempt to approach victims unless they are decontaminated. Emergency medical services personnel should never enter a designated hot zone unless they have been trained and equipped to do so.

The following basic points should be considered in assessing decontamination needs when, because of the nature and quantity of the hazardous material involved, medical personnel must decontaminate the patient:

1. Solid or particle contaminants should be brushed off as completely as possible before washing to reduce the chance of reaction with water. Heavy liquid contaminants should also be blotted from the body before washing.
2. Rinse patient with water and remove contaminated clothing, jewelry, shoes, and so on. Everything that is removed must be saved in separate plastic bags marked with the patient's name. The level of exposure can sometimes be estimated from the amount of contaminant on the patient's clothes.
3. Wash patient, if possible, with Tincture of Green soap or other mild soap. Pay special attention to hair, nail beds, and skin folds. Be careful not to abrade the skin, and use extra caution over bruised or broken areas. Rinse with large quantities of water.
4. Control all runoff. Small children's wading pools or draft tanks may be useful. If no containers are available, channel runoff to a containment area.
5. If possible, use warm water because more extensive washing can be accomplished. If cold water must be used, watch for signs and symptoms of hypothermia.

Management

Medically trained personnel are often tempted to begin treatment within the hazardous area, before the victim has been removed to triage. Treatment should begin only after the patient is in the triage area. Treatment for victims of hazardous materials exposure is not like conventional emergency medical treatment. Although broken bones, bleeding, and other conventional injuries may be evident, respiratory distress, skin burns, and exposure should be detected and treated first.

Heavy gloves and other protective garments must be worn continuously during treatment even though many health professionals would prefer fewer restrictions to their actions. Since more than basic life support treatment is necessary for victims of hazardous materials incidents the following serves as a guideline:

1. Check with the safety officer for special emergency medical considerations.
2. Remove patient's clothes, shoes, and personal articles (*e.g.*, rings, contact lenses) that may trap toxic dust.
3. Unless the hazardous material reacts with water, flush exposed skin with large amounts of lukewarm water.
4. Flush exposed eyes with isotonic saline for at least 15 minutes before transport (and during transport, if possible). Use potable water if saline solution is not available or is in short supply.
5. Provide oxygen, the antidote for most inhalation exposures. Do not use mouth-to-mouth or pocket face mask resuscitation.
6. In case of ingestion, do not induce vomiting without consulting a physician or poison control center.

Triage

The victims removed from the hot zone must be brought to a safe place where preparation for treatment can begin. A triage area should be established away from (and upwind of) the site. In medical triage, the most critical injuries are identified and the priorities for treatment are established. When hazardous materials are involved, however, all personnel must remain on guard to avoid being contaminated by the victims. Techniques similar to those of isolation wards in hospitals should be used to protect personnel. In addition to normal triage assessment (see Chapter 6), the following information must be determined:

To what degree is each injury related to the hazardous materials involved?
Which injuries are most severe (and should be treated first)?
What is the route of entry to the body?
Are the materials still acting on the patient? A patient who has not been fully decontaminated may be delivered to the EMS personnel if the patient's condition is such that complete decontamination cannot be performed or the chemical involved cannot be removed from the patient in the field.

Transport

Transporting patients to the hospital involves knowing which hospital's are best prepared to receive the victims of hazardous materials exposure. While medical professionals in the transport vehicle require protection from contamination, it is unsafe to drive wearing heavy boots, breathing apparatus, and goggles. A driver not wearing protective gear must avoid contact with the victim or contaminated medical professionals in the vehicle. A separate driver's compartment usually provides adequate protection.

The vehicle must be considered contaminated as soon as it has been used to transport victims. After arrival at a treatment facility, the vehicle must not be left unattended because of the possibility that unauthorized people will come in contact with contamination on the vehicle. All emergency personnel who were in the ambulance with the patient must also be considered to be contaminated and go through proper decontamination procedures for their protection.

Whether air or ground transport, make sure the admitting hospital is properly informed in advance and is prepared to treat victims of the specific hazardous materials involved in the incident.

Postevent Considerations

Experienced professionals never assume that they are clean of contamination after an incident. Medical personnel must be decontaminated according to the established policies of the environmental agencies and industry experts. The response vehicle and equipment must also be decontaminated according to the established policies of environmental agencies and industry experts. Some equipment is discarded rather than decontaminated.

Once the hazardous materials incident is over, a review session should be held to cover the following topics:

- Assess need for a critical incident stress debriefing
- Areas of strongest performance
- Areas that need additional work
- Additional personnel and equipment needed next time
- Items transported that were unnecessary
- Restocking requirements

Hospital personnel should also have a postevent evaluation, considering most of the list above. In addition, hospitals must be concerned with the effect of the hazard (if any) on the public, staff, and other patients in the hospital, the security of the contaminated vehicles that must be parked in public places, the efficiency of specialized lab services, and the adequacy of equipment, staff, and facility.

SUMMARY

If time affords only a quick look at specialized topics such as near drowning, barotrauma, and hazardous materials during initial paramedic education, the paramedic should follow up with extensive specialized training later.

Each area covered in this chapter can provide the paramedic with many hours of additional study and would allow specialization within the field of EMS. Although incidents such as drowning, barotrauma, and hazardous materials happen less frequently than other types of emergencies, they may be far more devastating, both physically and mentally, to the paramedic as well as to the patients involved. For this reason, the paramedic should be prepared to handle the initial aspects of scene management and direct attention, once qualified personnel have arrived, toward patient care and crew safety.

SUGGESTED READING

Bibb J: Environmental emergencies. Emergency Care Quarterly 4(3):61, 1988

Currance PL: EMS crosses hazmat lines. J Emerg Med Serv 14(2):58, 1989

Currance PL: Personal hazmat protection. Rescue 3(2):33, 1990

Dunford R: Decompression sickness and arterial gas embolism. Emergency Care Quarterly 4(3):39, 1988

Kurzeja W: Hazwoper and you. J Emerg Med Serv 22(9):35, 1990

Noll GG, Hildebrand MS, Yvorra JG: Hazardous Materials: Managing the Incident. Annapolis, Peake Productions, 1988

Persons D: Profound hypothermia. J Emerg Med Serv 13(1):60, 1988

Roberts SW: Spinal injuries in water. J Emerg Med Serv 13(5):34, 1988

Staten C: Hazardous materials: The EMS response. Journal of Emergency Care and Transportation 18(10):34, 1989

Steinman AM: Prehospital management of immersion hypothermia. Emergency Care Quarterly 4(3):33, 1988

Steinman AM: Prehospital management of hypothermia. Response 6(2):18, 1987

Title 29 of the Code of Federal Regulations. Hazardous Waste Operations and Emergency Response; Final Rule, Part 1910.120, March 1990

US Department of Transportation: 1990 Emergency Response Guidebook for Hazardous Materials Incidents. Washington, DC, US Government Printing Office, 1990

US Department of Transportation, National Highway Traffic Safety Administration: Emergency Medical Technician–Paramedic: National Standards Curriculum. Washington, DC, US Government Printing Office, 1985

Weinberg AD, Hamlet MP, Paturas JL et al: Cold Weather Emergencies: Principles of Patient Management. Branfort, CT, American Medical Publishing Company, 1990.

Wilkerson JA (ed), Bangs C, Hayward JS: Hypothermia, frostbite and other cold injuries: Prevention, recognition, and prehospital treatment. Seattle, The Mountaineers, 1986

UNIT FIVE

Caring for Patients With Special Needs

CHAPTER 28

Geriatric Emergencies

Anatomy and Physiology of the Aging Process
  Respiratory System
  Cardiovascular System
  Renal System
  Nervous System
  Musculoskeletal System
  Gastrointestinal System
Assessment of the Geriatric Patient
  General Communication
    Principles
  Conducting the Patient History
  Conducting the Physical
    Examination
Respiratory Emergencies
  Chronic Obstructive Pulmonary
    Disease
  Pulmonary Embolism
  Pulmonary Edema
  Pneumonia
  Management of Respiratory
    Emergencies
Cardiovascular Emergencies
  Myocardial Infarction
  Congestive Heart Failure
  Syncope
  Arrhythmias
  Management of Cardiovascular
    Emergencies

Neurologic Emergencies
  Coma
  Seizures
  Cerebrovascular Accident
  Transient Ischemic Attacks
  Dizziness
  Dementia
  Management of Neurologic
    Emergencies
Psychiatric Disorders in the Elderly
  Affective Disorders
  Paranoid Disorders
  Other Functional Disorders
  Management of Psychiatric
    Disorders
Musculoskeletal Problems
  Osteoarthritis
  Osteoporosis
  Management of Musculoskeletal
    Problems
Gastrointestinal Emergencies
  Upper Gastrointestinal Bleeding
    Peptic Ulcers
    Esophageal Varices
    Mallory–Weiss Syndrome
  Lower Gastrointestinal Bleeding
    Diverticula
    Ischemic Colitis
    Cancer of the Large Intestine

  Bowel Obstruction
  Management of Gastrointestinal
    Emergencies
Trauma in the Elderly
  Pathophysiology of Trauma
  Contributing Factors
  Management of Trauma
Pharmacology in Geriatrics
  Drug-induced Illness
  Drugs that Cause Toxicity
Environmental Emergencies
  Hypothermia
  Hyperthermia
    Heat Exhaustion
    Heatstroke
Geriatric Abuse
Summary

BEHAVIORAL OBJECTIVES
On successful completion of this chapter, the reader will be able to:

1. Discuss the impact of the growing elderly population on the emergency medical services (EMS) system
2. List four factors that complicate the clinical evaluation of an elderly patient
3. Explain the age-related changes that occur in the respiratory system
4. List six causes of respiratory distress in the elderly
5. Describe the complicating effects of chronic obstructive pulmonary disease in the elderly patient
6. Discuss the effects of aging on the cardiovascular system
7. Describe the management of acute pulmonary edema in the elderly patient
8. Describe the effects of aging on drug distribution and clearance

(continued)

649

BEHAVIORAL OBJECTIVES (continued)

9. List five conditions that may cause seizures in the elderly
10. Explain cerebrovascular accident and transient ischemic attacks and distinguish between their signs and symptoms
11. Review the management of coma in an elderly patient
12. Discuss the effects of aging on the musculoskeletal system
13. List three causes of gastrointestinal bleeding and discuss the significance of blood loss in the elderly patient
14. Explain polypharmacy and its significance to the elderly patient
15. Describe two contributing factors for the development of hypothermia in the elderly population
16. Explain the significance of heat-related illnesses in the elderly
17. Define all of the key terms listed in this chapter

KEY TERMS

The following terms are defined in the chapter and glossary:

Alzheimer's disease
chronic obstructive pulmonary disease (COPD)
collateral circulation
dementia
geriatric
hemoptysis
ischemic colitis
kyphosis
Mallory–Weiss syndrome
nocturia
osteoarthritis
osteoporosis
transient ischemic attacks
vial of life

The dramatic expansion of the average life span during this century has caused the **geriatric** (elderly) population, those over the age of 65 years, to grow steadily in proportion to the total population of the United States. This over-65 age group has become the fastest growing group in America. It is estimated that by the year 2030, the elderly population will be nearly 18% of the total population of the United States. The reasons for this increase are many, varied, and complex and include the following:

- An increase in the mean survival age, which implies better housing, sanitation, and nutrition
- A declining birth rate
- Improved medical care and better drugs
- Improved access to care

In general, the elderly describe their health as good; fewer than 20% are confined to their homes. However, the elderly have a higher per capita percent usage of our nation's health care facilities. The population older than 65 years of age tends to develop acute medical problems more frequently and, thus, uses the EMS system more frequently than any other age group. In the prehospital setting, there is often a biased generalization that the majority of the elderly population is prone to sickness. It is important that paramedics and all health care providers be aware of their attitudes toward aging. These attitudes may have an effect on the care that is provided to their patients. Figure 28-1 lists important rights of the older adult that are sometimes taken for granted.

The three leading causes of death in the elderly population are heart disease, cancer, and cerebrovascular accident. Elderly people may be more susceptible to disease and injury than younger people, and the course of their illnesses may be more severe. Many elderly people may be poorly nourished; for example, laboratory tests have shown deficient levels of serum albumin, protein, vitamins, and hemoglobin in the elderly. Nutritional habits may be affected by the medications they take, their poverty, physical disabilities, chronic illnesses, and dental problems. Years of exposure to air pollutants and smoking may have accelerated the normal age-related changes that occur in the lungs. Cardiovascular efficiency may have decreased, and, as a result, the elderly may be more vulnerable to sudden death and heart failure.

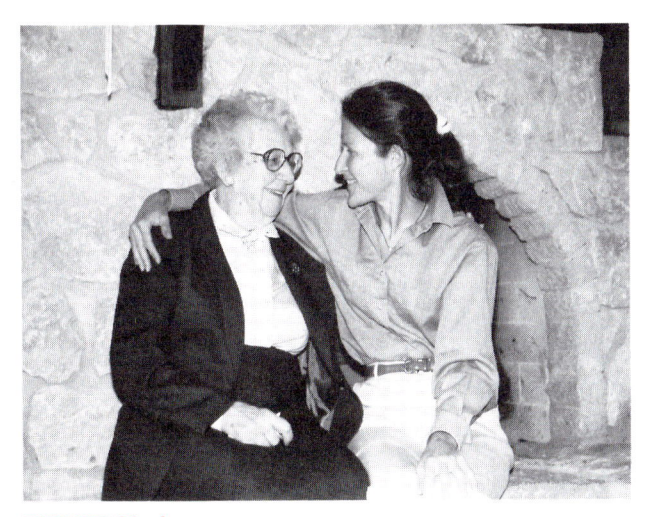

FIGURE 28–1.
Rights of the older adult.
- To share their wisdom and experience
- To be recognized as individuals
- To strive for self-esteem and self-actualization
- To be independent and make their own decisions
- To be creative
- To be recognized for their strengths
- To have control over their own destiny
- To follow their own lifestyles and goals
- To follow their own ethnic and cultural beliefs
- To be loved and have respect
- To be productive
- To have dignity

ANATOMY AND PHYSIOLOGY OF THE AGING PROCESS

During the aging process, normal age-related changes occur in the body that affect various body systems. The body systems that are discussed in this section are the respiratory, cardiovascular, renal, nervous, musculoskeletal, and gastrointestinal systems.

Respiratory System

The normal, age-related changes that occur within the lungs are extensive. The structural changes may cause ventilation to become less efficient. The chest muscles may gradually become weakened. The increased stiffness in the chest wall and the calcification of the costochondral junctions along with other structural changes may result in a less pliable chest wall. **Kyphosis,** the posterior angulation of the spine due to changes in the cartilage in the spinal column, may cause asymmetry of the chest, resulting in an inadequate use of the respiratory muscles. These structural changes affect ventilation by limiting the tidal volumes during each breath.

The lungs begin to lose elasticity in the aging process and they distend more easily. The smaller airways that rely on the elasticity of the surrounding tissues to keep them open during exhalation may begin to collapse prematurely. This premature collapse eventually causes some of the smaller airways to remain closed during normal breathing. In addition, the alveolar walls rupture and then fuse with neighboring walls, causing emphysemalike structures and symptoms. Loss in the vital capacity of the lungs is as high as 50% when a person reaches the age of 80. The capillary beds may also change with age, and this change can contribute to a decrease in gas exchange at the alveolar-capillary membrane.

As a result of these anatomical and physiologic changes in the respiratory system, elderly people can suffer significantly from inadequate ventilations and chronic states of hypoxia. With aging, a reduction in the sensitivity to carbon dioxide levels may also be found. Patients may lose the ability to increase their respiratory rate in response to blood gas levels; this mechanism is an important protective one that deteriorates in the aging process.

Other factors, such as obesity, years of exposure to air pollutants, smoking, and recurring respiratory diseases in the elderly, may cause even greater reductions in respiratory function and result in severe respiratory distress. Therefore, the paramedic must be constantly alert to the respiratory condition of elderly patients.

Cardiovascular System

The aging process affects the cardiovascular system in a number of ways. Reduction in cardiac output is as high as 50% by age 80; this reduction is caused by a decrease in stroke volume, decrease in heart rate, degeneration of the conduction system, and left ventricular hypertrophy. Peripheral vascular resistance may increase because of arteriosclerosis and, thus, often results in systemic hypertension. There may be a decrease in cardiac reserve or the ability of the myocardium to respond to increased demands for cardiac output. Also, the lack of physical fitness may cause atrophy of the myocardial fibers. Exercise is an important factor in the health of the elderly. When people do not exercise regularly, fat and connective tissue replace myocardial fibers and valve calcification occurs.

Overall, the aging of the cardiovascular system may tend to result in a decrease in the system's ability to compensate for stress and a decrease in its ability to maintain a normal cardiac output. In addition, the recovery time for the cardiovascular system to return to normal after a stressful incident may increase as a person ages, and, as a result, syncope, falls, and heart failure can occur while the system is trying to compensate for a sudden drop in cardiac output.

The cardiovascular system is responsible for the delivery of oxygen and nutrients to the tissues throughout the body. When the body's needs for oxygen, nutrients, and the removal of wastes increase, because of exercise or stress, the cardiovascular system responds to these needs. The long-term effects of cardiovascular disease cause a reduction in the elderly patient's ability to respond effectively to and withstand the stresses of hypoxia and hypovolemia.

The baroreceptors, or stretch receptors, located in the aortic arch and carotid sinuses, are instrumental in the regulation of arterial blood pressure; however, they become less sensitive to changes in blood pressure because of atherosclerotic changes in the arteries. As a person ages, it becomes increasingly difficult for the body to adjust to changes in systolic blood pressure that result from changes in body position, exercise, or other causes of the minute adjustments necessary to maintain a constant blood pressure. Even the otherwise healthy older person may experience periodic orthostatic hypotension due to changes in body position. Hypertension is of particular significance in the elderly trauma patient because a systolic blood pressure of 100 mm Hg may not provide adequate tissue perfusion if the elderly patient is normally hypertensive.

Aging may affect the venous system by causing a rupture in the valves of the leg veins, which facilitate the movement of blood from the lower extremities back to the heart. Varicose veins, which result from the damaged valves, lead to the diminished ability of an older person to walk or move about well.

Aging also tends to cause a decrease in the automaticity of the heart and a decrease in the heart rate. These decreases are partially due to the fact that the myocardial fibers found along the conduction pathways and surrounding the sinoatrial node in the atria are replaced over time with fibrous tissue. Arrhythmias may occur, and the frequency of atrial arrhythmias, which is common in the elderly population, is thought to be the result of the heart's response to the stress of exercise.

The valves of the aging heart have a tendency to develop an increase in thickness and rigidity of their walls. Atherosclerosis causes narrowing of the coronary arteries, resulting in decreased blood flow to the myocardium. However, the aging heart has the unique ability to develop collateral circulation between coronary arteries. This **collateral circulation** allows the blood from occluded areas to be diverted to distal myocardial tissues. A myocardial infarction may be relatively pain-free because of this phenomenon.

Respiratory infections, which are seen frequently in the elderly population, can cause both congestive heart failure and fast irregular heart rates because the myocardium is not as capable of withstanding stress as well as it was in earlier years. The congestive heart failure commonly is transient, subsiding when the stress is reduced, and the body systems return to normal. Overall, the aging of the cardiovascular system results in its inability to compensate as quickly and as effectively in stressful situations.

Renal System

The kidneys are primarily responsible for the excretion of waste products from the blood; they also participate in fluid balance, acid-base balance, and in the regulation of blood pressure. As a person ages, accumulations of fat deposits develop between nephron cells, and renal blood flow is reduced, as high as 50% in some cases. The decrease in blood flow is partly related to the decrease in cardiac output associated with aging. When the circulating blood volume decreases significantly, the filtration rate through the kidneys decreases, at a rate of about 6% every 10 years, and the rate of reabsorption decreases. Aging also causes a reduction in the overall size of the kidneys, from 250 g at age 40 to about 200 g at age 80. The smaller size of the kidneys causes a significant reduction in the size of the vascular bed.

Arteriosclerosis affects the renal arterioles, and, as a result, less circulating blood volume is filtered through the kidneys.

As a person ages, a reduction in the number and effectiveness of the nephrons, the functional units of the kidneys, results in a decrease in the kidney's ability to concentrate urine. In younger people, urine production decreases at night. In the elderly, urine is produced at the same rate day and night. The bladder becomes distended with urine at night, and the elderly suffer from a condition called nocturia. **Nocturia** is excessive urination at night. Also, bacteria accumulate asymptomatically in the kidneys, urine, and bladder. It is thought that this accumulation is one cause of the weakening in the normal functioning of the nephrons.

The kidneys are adversely affected by chronic hypertension and diabetes. The age-related disorders in fluid and electrolyte balance cause recovery time after illness to become extended. In situations of stress, the kidneys are normally able to keep up and adjust to the needs of the body. However, recovery time for the kidneys after periods of stress in the elderly is often longer.

Nervous System

The nervous system, responsible for the integration and coordination of all body systems, can be significantly affected by multisystem diseases and the drugs ingested by elderly patients. Within the nervous system, the loss of neurons begins as early as age 25; this loss marks the beginning of the reduction in the nervous system's ability to adapt quickly to the needs of the body.

As the number of central nervous system cells decreases, the transmission rate, or the nerve conduction velocity, also decreases. Reaction time tends to be slower because of slower conduction velocities along the nerve.

Although decrease in velocity is only about 15%, more time may be needed to perform complex tasks. Slower reaction time in the elderly is also related to increased caution and decreased willingness to take risks. The patient needs to be given time to answer the questions and perform the requested motor skills.

Intelligence is not affected by aging, nor is the ability to verbalize. Long-term memory is intact and short-term memory may decrease. Therefore, learning new tasks that are not based on long-term experiences is sometimes difficult for the elderly.

Musculoskeletal System

Muscle strength is at its peak in the midtwenties and may decline with each advancing year. Muscle weakness is common among elderly people. This weakness may be due to medications taken for diseases, or it may be due to atrophy of the muscles from decreased use. Although muscle strength decreases, the musculoskeletal system retains its ability to maintain an adequate amount of strength necessary for daily living. Kyphosis may be responsible for the loss of up to 2 inches in height, and it may have damaging effects on the respiratory system, as described earlier. The joint capsules become calcified and bone spurs may begin to develop around the joints, particularly in the fingers. Some muscle fibers are replaced by fat and connective tissue.

A direct relationship is seen between mobility and health status in the elderly population. Decreased mobility may cause fear and even withdrawal from daily activities. Some elderly people may move and respond more slowly, not because of their inability to respond, but because of the limitations of their muscular ability. A degree of loss of flexibility may affect the elderly's balance and range of motion in the neck and extremities. Even with a lack of mobility, elderly people can still adapt to their changing environment.

Gastrointestinal System

The gastrointestinal tract, which is responsible for the absorption of nutrients from food, is the most common site of chronic distress in the elderly. About 56% of complaints are related to poor eating and bowel habits and are caused by an intense preoccupation with stomach and bowel function.

The effects of aging on the gastrointestinal system are numerous. The loss of teeth is partly due to the fundamental changes of aging as well as the result of gum disease. The grinding surfaces of teeth are worn down, and, as a result, chewing effectiveness is diminished. A reduction in the secretions from the salivary glands may occur and result in a decrease in the chemical breakdown of starches and a decrease in the moistening of food. The total number of taste buds decreases with age, and the muscles of the mouth, cheeks, and tongue atrophy, resulting in a significant decrease in taste sensation and food appeal.

Many elderly people experience heartburn after meals, which is due to the relaxation of the muscles in the walls of the esophagus. These muscle walls also thin out and become more sensitive. Peristalsis may slow, and the production of stomach acids and enzymes decreases. A reduction in blood flow to the intestines is another cause of some intestinal problems.

Complicating the organic changes in the gastrointestinal system are the stress and psychological pressures of aging, which manifest themselves most frequently as gastrointestinal problems. Many elderly people complain of weight loss. The factors that have been identified as the cause of these symptoms are emotional tension, fear of illness, fear of death, fear of being old, and depression.

ASSESSMENT OF THE GERIATRIC PATIENT

Because the elderly population has a higher per capita use of the EMS system than any other identifiable group in society, prehospital care is commonly related to the care of the elderly patient. Elderly people call for the assistance because they feel something is wrong, and paramedics must take into consideration all of the physiologic, social and psychological concerns of elderly patients when caring for them.

General Communication Principles

The paramedic should use a proper introduction and approach the elderly patient with an attitude of respect and kind concern. The patient's surname should be used unless the patient requests otherwise. The use of first names is too personal, and elderly patients are often offended by this. Addressing the patient by Mr., Mrs., or Ms. makes data gathering easier by putting the patient at ease. Gentleness in manner, voice, and touch throughout the patient assessment is genuinely appreciated by the elderly (Fig. 28-2).

It is important to remember that being "old" does not mean a person is out of touch with reality. Often, an elderly patient thinks that getting sick means that they will have to be admitted to a nursing home or, if there is psychiatric history, a state hospital.

Conducting the Patient History

Conducting the patient history for an elderly patient may take longer than for a younger patient because of visual and hearing problems, patient fatigue, and poor concentration. Response time for answers to questions may also

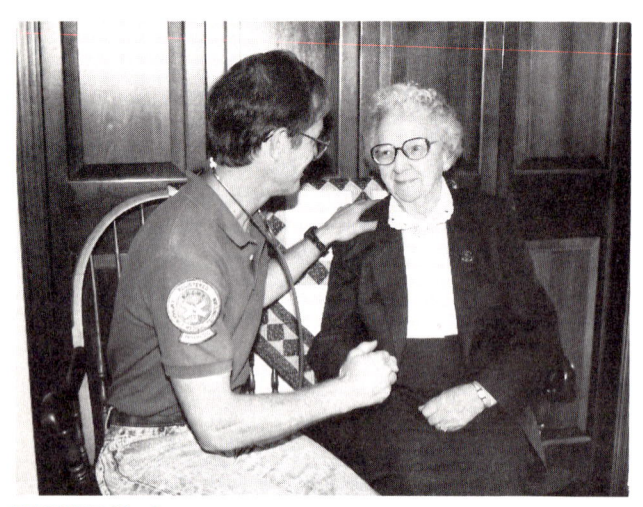

FIGURE 28-2.
The elderly should be treated with gentleness and respect.

be quite lengthy. Points to remember when developing rapport with an elderly patient include the following:

- Establish an appropriate environment for communication
- Encourage and facilitate accuracy in response to questions
- Validate the information received with a family member
- Incorporate information received from the patient history in the overall evaluation of the patient

Other points to consider when conducting the patient history of an elderly patient include the following:

- Keep background noise to a minimum
- Speak slowly and clearly
- Face the patient at eye level when conducting an interview
- Be patient
- Give the patient adequate time to answer the questions

It is also important to gather information from other sources as well as from the patient. The assistance of a family member may increase the patient's compliance with the history and physical exam. However, if the patient's history is described by a person other than the patient, that information should never take the place of a direct interview with the patient.

Acquiring an accurate medical history from an elderly patient requires an awareness of the diseases of the elderly, the complicating factors of aging, and the various manifestations of the diseases. When an altered mental status is the chief complaint, it is difficult for the paramedic to acquire an accurate medical history from the patient. Also, many elderly patients have been taking long-term medication for chronic diseases since youth, and the dosages have never been changed. This patient may be overmedicated for that illness, a fact that may be causing the altered mental status.

It is helpful to interview the patient in an environment that is familiar to the patient. The familiar surroundings make the patient more at ease and provide the paramedic with a more complete and accurate medical history. The paramedic should always remember to ask, "Are there any other things you would like to tell me about your medical history?" before completing this segment of the assessment process. Gentleness and patience are important. Information about recent hospitalizations and surgical procedures may help identify a present condition. However, lengthy discussions are inappropriate. The physician in the emergency department completes the information when the patient is interviewed about the medical history.

The paramedic must ask to see all of the patient's medications. If it cannot be quickly determined which medications belong to the patient, it is appropriate for the paramedic to bring all medications found to the hospital.

The paramedic should evaluate the patient as a whole, considering each piece of positive data in relationship to the total picture. Diseases in the elderly may not present with the classic signs and symptoms. The manifestations can be subtle. The paramedic should concentrate on collecting and documenting the important historical data and provide this information to the physicians for their use in the evaluation of the patient in the emergency department.

Conducting the Physical Examination

When conducting the physical examination on an elderly patient, the paramedic will find the following considerations useful:

1. Elderly people may be sensitive to modesty. Their modesty should be respected fully unless it interferes with patient care. A complete head-to-toe examination must be performed.
2. The elderly may be sensitive to cold and may be wearing many layers of clothing.
3. Elderly patients may tend to forget parts of their medical conditions, or they may not be aware of evidence of trauma, necrotic toes, or decubitus ulcers.
4. Patients may have a high pain threshold and may minimize small discomforts.

It is helpful to the emergency department physician if the paramedic takes the time to observe the patient's room for evidence of alcohol, medications, and so on. When examining the refrigerator for the *vial of life*, which is a container that lists the patient's medical history and medications, the paramedic should note if any food is in the refrigerator. This information provides clues to the patient's nutritional status. Many elderly people have limited resources. It is important to remember, however, that all patients have Medicare and are not medically indigent. Often their housing facilities have no access to social services, and neighbors provide no support. It is helpful to the physician if the paramedic can provide clues to the psychological health of the patient in addition to observing and reporting the physical surroundings of the scene.

Overall, it is important to approach the elderly patient with gentleness, reassurance, and an understanding of the types of problems and difficulties unique to this age group. The manifestations of disease may be subtle or even disguised, and determining the nature of the illness often requires the assistance of other family members or friends as well as the patient.

RESPIRATORY EMERGENCIES

The four respiratory diseases common to the elderly are chronic obstructive pulmonary disease, pulmonary embolism, pulmonary edema, and pneumonia.

Chronic Obstructive Pulmonary Disease

Chronic obstructive pulmonary disease (COPD) is the term used to describe patients with combined chronic bronchitis, emphysema, and asthma. The disease is ranked sixth as the cause of death in the United States, although it is on a decline because of decreased smoking habits. It is most frequently seen in elderly men who are or have been smokers. The incidence of moderate to severe COPD in men older than the age of 70 is about 40%. The incidence of COPD in women has been increasing dramatically during the past few years and was approaching about 20% in 1986. One of the most debilitating results of COPD is decreased exercise tolerance, which has a limiting effect on the lifestyle of the elderly person.

Paramedics see COPD patients at the acute phases of the disease. The acute phase usually is precipitated by a viral infection, dehydration, hot and humid weather, heart failure, or exposure to noxious fumes or air pollutants. The acidosis that is associated with an acute phase of COPD seriously affects the patient. It reduces the responsiveness of β-adrenergic stimulating drugs used in the bronchodilators and contributes to the arterial vasoconstriction that commonly occurs with hypoxemia. Therefore, the administration of oxygen to COPD patients as soon as possible is extremely important.

Patients with COPD and acute decompensation are almost always observed to be tachycardic. Electrocardiographic monitoring reveals an irregular narrow complex tachycardia usually diagnosed as atrial fibrillation. Closer inspection often reveals this to be multifocal atrial tachycardia (MAT). If the ventricular rate is very rapid, verapamil 5 mg IV can slow the ventricular rate (and often the atrial rate), or sometimes restore sinus rhythm.

Patients with chronic bronchitis have a cough with significant secretions, central cyanosis, and inspiratory rales and use accessory muscles to breathe. **Hemoptysis,** the coughing up of blood, is most commonly seen as streaking of sputum. This condition is an important diagnostic indication in the elderly patient; it also produces a degree of anxiety in the patient. The most common cause of blood streaking is chronic bronchitis associated with cigarette smoking. It occurs as a result of the rupture of small vessels in the bronchial mucosa.

Hemoptysis of several hundred milliliters of blood is a significantly different problem. This volume of blood loss is usually the result of one of the following:

- Chronic use of anticoagulants
- Heavy use of aspirin
- Bleeding from the nose (*epistaxis*)

Massive hemoptysis of more than 200 mL of blood per day, caused by lung disease or a vascular aneurysm, should be considered life-threatening.

Patients with emphysema exhibit a high level of anxiety. They usually are found seated, leaning forward, and using accessory muscles to breathe. They may be breathing through pursed lips. Breath sounds are distant and an expiratory wheeze is heard.

Acute bronchial asthma in the elderly usually is precipitated by exercise, anxiety, viral infections, or exposure to cold air, toxic fumes, or air pollutants. A high percentage of the elderly population have bronchial asthma. The symptoms of coughing, wheezing, and nocturnal episodes of asthma increase with age. The frequency of bronchial asthma attacks after meals and after ingesting cold food and drink, especially red wine, increases as well.

Pulmonary Embolism

The leading cause of death in hospitalized patients is pulmonary embolism. About 80% of the pulmonary emboli originate in the deep veins of the leg. Advancing age is just one of the predisposing factors that contribute to the development of emboli. Patients with heart disease, particularly those with atrial fibrillation and congestive heart failure, are at higher risk of developing a pulmonary embolism. Other contributing factors include the following:

- Trauma
- Major surgery
- COPD
- Prolonged bed rest
- Cancer
- Obesity

A pulmonary embolism that occludes greater than 50% of the pulmonary circulation is likely to cause acute right heart failure and cardiovascular collapse. If a clot fragments and moves to smaller branches of the pulmonary circulation, the signs and symptoms are less severe, and the patient responds well to treatment. When a pulmonary vessel becomes blocked by an embolus, the body releases substances that immediately constrict the airways, leading to 1 to 2 minutes of relatively little air movement at all throughout the lungs. This condition improves quickly and usually is not witnessed by the paramedic.

Elderly people with preexisting cardiopulmonary disease are at extremely high risk of profound hypoxia and, therefore, must be given high concentrations of oxygen as soon as possible at the scene and throughout transport to the hospital. Elderly patients with poor response to the oxygen therapy usually are candidates for lethal arrhythmias and sudden death.

Pulmonary Edema

Acute pulmonary edema is a life-threatening condition that is commonly seen in the elderly patient with acute left-sided heart failure. The two ventricles of the heart normally eject the same volume of blood with each contraction. When the left ventricle fails, blood begins to accumulate within the pulmonary system, resulting in acute pulmonary edema within a few minutes. The paramedic must recognize this emergency quickly and initiate care and transportation immediately if the patient is to survive.

The use of oxygen is of particular importance in the elderly patient because of the probable presence of coexisting coronary artery disease. High concentrations of inspired oxygen are necessary to increase the alveolar–blood oxygen pressure difference and thus increase arterial partial pressure of oxygen. The administration of both furosemide and morphine can produce marked relief of respiratory distress as well as beneficial cardiovascular actions.

Pneumonia

After age 75, pneumonia becomes the fourth leading cause of death in men and women. About 10% of all hospitalizations are due to pneumonia. Several factors are responsible for the elderly population's susceptibility to pneumonia. These include the following:

- Reduced salivation
- An abnormal cough reflex
- Residence in extended care facilities
- Altered mental status
- Metabolic acidosis
- Impairment of the normal defenses in the upper and lower respiratory tracts
- An increased aspiration of oral pharyngeal organisms
- Chronic disease

Bacterial and viral pneumonias are more common in the elderly population than in young adults, and they have an especially high mortality rate when secondary to the influenza virus.

Pleuritic pain is difficult to evaluate thoroughly in the prehospital setting. Patients who complain of pleuritic pain must always be evaluated at a medical facility because the causes of this pain can be life-threatening.

A pulmonary embolism causes pleuritic pain. The pain is dull and is gradual in onset. However, over time the quality of the pain changes to sharp. If the pain is abrupt in onset, the pain increases with deep breathing or coughing and may also increase with postural changes. The pain is commonly located in the posterior lung bases.

Management of Respiratory Emergencies

Oxygen by nasal cannula or mask is always indicated for the patient in acute respiratory distress. The patient should be asked to cough. If the cough is weak, ventilatory support may also be needed. The administration of a bronchodilator by aerosol is indicated if bronchospasm is present.

Epinephrine is not recommended for elderly patients because of the possibility of *tachyphylaxis* (rapid production of immune tolerance), particularly if the patient is acidotic. The administration of intravenous (IV) aminophylline is acceptable in elderly patients if the patient has not recently received theophylline. However the safety, efficacy, and relative ease of administration of aerosolized bronchodilators such as metaproterenol and albuterol make them the drugs of choice. Theophylline ethylenediamine (Aminophylline) administered intravenously has considerable potential for toxicity. It has rapidly been replaced by aerosolized bronchodilators as the drugs of choice in this circumstance. The administration of a sedative is never appropriate, even if the patient is agitated and restless.

CARDIOVASCULAR EMERGENCIES

More than 50% of all Americans will die of heart disease, and more than 70% of these are people older than age 60. Specific age-related changes occur within the cardiovascular system. The valves of the heart become stiffer (sclerotic) as a result of fibrous and calcific changes. Aortic valve sclerosis can contribute to development of left ventricular hypertrophy (muscle thickening). Decreased compliance in the arterial vasculature with aging is accompanied by increases in systolic arterial pressure (systolic hypertension). The time required for the cardiovascular system to return to normal after a stressful incident increases as a person ages. Also, the stress of emotional and physical strains, infections, and so on may cause acute congestive heart failure, myocardial infarction, arrhythmias, syncope, and falls with injury.

Myocardial Infarction

An acute myocardial infarction in an elderly person may present quite differently from the signs and symptoms the paramedic is accustomed to seeing. The pain may be mild. Shortness of breath may be significant, and signs and symptoms of acute congestive heart failure and anginal pain, substernal pressure, or a feeling of indigestion may be present. Therefore, it is important for the paramedic to have a high degree of suspicion of a myocardial infarction and to manage the patient accordingly when observing these kinds of signs and symptoms.

Acute myocardial infarction also may be the first sign of heart failure in the elderly person. A careful, individualized examination by a physician is required to determine the type of acute heart event that the patient is developing.

Extreme caution must be exercised in the use of pain medications for the elderly because of the possibility of respiratory depression.

Congestive Heart Failure

As noted earlier, congestive heart failure is commonly found in the elderly patient. The causes include the following:

- Hypertensive heart disease
- Cor pulmonale
- Mitral stenosis
- Pulmonary embolism
- Pneumonia
- Calcific aortic stenosis

The clinical features of congestive heart failure include wheezing, cough, dyspnea (also related to pulmonary disease), orthopnea, nocturia (associated with diuretics), pulmonary rales, nausea (also associated with digitalis excess), and weakness (also associated with malnutrition). Ankle edema is associated with malnutrition, varicose veins, anemia, lymphedema, neurologic conditions, and intra-abdominal disease as well as with chronic congestive heart failure and, therefore, cannot be relied on as a sign.

Syncope

In a myocardial infarction without pain, syncope is commonly the first sign. Arrhythmias can also produce syncope, as discussed in Chapter 20. Ventricular tachycardia, however, is rarely a cause of syncope in the elderly patient, unless it is related to an acute myocardial infarction. Other causes of syncope include the following:

- Stokes–Adams syndrome
- Sick sinus syndrome
- Hyperventilation
- Sudden decrease in blood pressure
- Carotid sinus syndrome
- Urination

Hyperextension of the neck in patients with atherosclerotic carotid arteries can temporarily occlude the arteries in the cervical spine. This state is thought to be the cause of syncope and falls when elderly people reach up to change a ceiling light bulb or reach for objects on high shelves.

Syncope also results from hypoglycemia, and, if not treated in the elderly patient, hypoglycemia can result in a myocardial infarction or a cerebrovascular accident.

Failure of the baroreceptors in the neck and changes in the flow of blood throughout the body with pooling of venous blood also cause syncope in the elderly patient.

Arrhythmias

The degenerative process of aging may cause calcification and fibrosis of the structures within the heart. Resulting from this condition are the following:

- Sinus node dysfunction (sinus arrest or exit block)
- Sinus bradycardia
- Atrial fibrillation
- Atrioventricular block
- Left or right bundle branch block

The symptoms of this degenerative process include fatigue, syncope, angina, palpitations, and congestive heart failure.

Coronary artery disease can cause the following types of arrhythmias in the elderly: sinus bradycardia, sinus arrest, atrial escape rhythms, and varying degrees of heart block. Other causes of cardiac arrhythmias are digitalis, which causes arrhythmias through direct effects and vagal effects, previous rheumatic fever, and metastases from lung carcinoma. The types of cardiac arrhythmias most frequently seen in elderly patients are atrial arrhythmias, ventricular premature beats, bundle-branch blocks, and second and third degree heart block. These types of arrhythmias can cause death in the elderly patient if untreated.

Management of Cardiovascular Emergencies

The management of cardiovascular emergencies for the elderly is generally the same as for younger patients (see Chapter 20). The patient's airway and respiratory status are of primary concern. Supplemental oxygen is of critical importance to elderly patients. The patient's pulse and cardiac rhythm must be monitored and any life-threatening arrhythmias treated according to management guidelines in Chapter 20. Pain management for acute myocardial infarction is also given in Chapter 20.

NEUROLOGIC EMERGENCIES

As aging occurs, some areas of the brain may lose a significant number of brain cells with subsequent compromises in the functioning of brain tissue. Patients with neurologic problems present an interesting challenge to the paramedic because these patients may also have other chronic medical problems and may take medications that affect their neurologic status.

Coma

Coma in the elderly patient poses a challenge to both prehospital and emergency department personnel. Coma is defined as a state of profound unconsciousness from which one cannot be aroused. In the elderly, it is frequently a result of a combination of disorders that affect the functioning of the central nervous system, as opposed to coma in the young patient, which usually is caused by only one factor. The elderly have aging neurons and atherosclerotic vessels that compound the problem. Also, they frequently are taking medications that can cause changes in the level of consciousness.

When evaluating the pupils of an elderly patient in coma, it is necessary to remember that chronic diseases, like glaucoma and cataracts, as well as previous eye surgery and some medications may cause pupillary changes not directly related to the present problem.

Seizures

The effects of the aging process on vessels and neurons make the elderly more vulnerable to seizure activity. One of the most common causes of seizures in the elderly is cerebral vascular accident. However, the following conditions can also cause seizures in the elderly population:

- Renal and hepatic failure
- Diabetes mellitus
- Hypoglycemia
- Cardiac arrhythmias
- Stokes–Adams syndrome
- Infections
- Tumors
- Head trauma

Drugs, such as tranquilizers, tricyclic antidepressants, amphetamines, β-adrenergic agonists, theophylline, and alcohol, can precipitate seizures. It is possible for Alzheimer's disease, transient ischemic attacks, and vertigo to mimic seizure activity also, so it is important for the paramedic to get an accurate description of the seizure and the events immediately preceding the seizure from family members or bystanders.

Cerebrovascular Accident

Cerebrovascular accidents (strokes) result from hemorrhage within the brain itself, caused by rupture of a blood vessel; hemorrhage outside the brain in the subarachnoid space (subarachnoid hemorrhage) caused by a ruptured aneurysm; and ischemia as a result of an occluded vessel in the brain. Mortality in the elderly from cerebrovascular accidents caused by hemorrhage is about 80%, particularly those caused by hypertensive bleeds. Most cerebrovascular accidents are sudden in onset, within several minutes to hours. If a patient's symptoms developed over a period of more than 24 hours, the condition probably is not a cerebrovascular accident.

Transient Ischemic Attacks

Transient ischemic attacks are most commonly caused by plaque from atherosclerotic arteries that breaks off and occludes distant cranial arteries. Transient ischemic attacks are a common cause of syncope in the elderly; the neurologic symptoms of hemiparesis, motor or sensory loss, *aphasia* (language disorder due to brain dysfunction), *diplopia* (double vision), *vertigo* (dizziness), *tinnitus* (ringing in the ear), or *ataxia* (lack of muscular coordination) are transient, lasting less than 24 hours. It is important to rule out cardiac arrhythmias, orthostatic hypotension, and hypoglycemia as the cause of the syncope when assessing these patients.

Dizziness

Dizziness in the elderly patient is frequently the result of the aging process, which may cause the degeneration of the nerve cells in the inner ear. By quickly moving the head in any direction, the patient can become unsteady and lose balance. Simple acts like getting up from a chair, bending over, and changing directions while walking can cause dizziness.

Atherosclerosis of the arteries of the spine may also cause dizziness. This condition can occur when an elderly person flexes the neck backwards to reach a high shelf, for example. This movement of the head partially occludes the arteries of the cervical spine and, therefore, diminishes the amount of blood that flows to the brain through the vertebral arteries. The results of this condition are falls and injuries in the home. Atherosclerosis of the carotid arteries may cause similar results when the patient turns the head to one side. Motor vehicle accidents may occur when an elderly patient turns to look into the side mirror for traffic and becomes dizzy.

Postural hypotension may also cause dizziness. One out of ten elderly patients has this problem, and it indicates cerebrovascular disease. Some patients also have deficient baroreceptor reflexes, venous pooling, and uncompensated decreased cardiac output, and many elderly patients have low serum sodium levels, all of which can cause dizziness.

Dementia

The etiology of **dementia** (**Alzheimer's disease**) is not clearly understood. The changes in brain function may be caused by aging, or dementia or may be a disease process itself. Age, however, is a significant risk factor in the development of dementia. Millions of elderly Americans suffer from this problem and are confined to extended care facilities as a result. The onset of dementia is more common with advancing age.

A certain subset of patients with dementia may have a genetic predisposition. This predisposition affects the neurons of the cerebral cortex in all six layers in every lobe. The degeneration of these neurons affects their normal function and may accelerate functional decline.

Dementia is not a natural condition of aging, but it may occur commonly in the elderly. Dementia is demonstrated by knowledge and memory loss in any or all of the following ways:

- Disorientation to person, place, time
- Impaired memory of recent events
- Impaired ability to recall numbers or perform simple mathematical problems
- Decreased general memory and creative thought

Dementia has no specific treatment. Patients who are moderately to severely disoriented or confused may receive psychotherapy. The underlying causes of the problem are treated with pharmacologic therapy, and many of these patients are hospitalized for treatment.

Management of Neurologic Emergencies

An IV infusion, usually normal saline or lactated Ringer's solution, should be started. Dextrose-containing solutions should not be administered to any patient with the potential for underlying acute cerebral ischemia, such as a cerebrovascular accident, because dextrose may worsen cerebral intracellular acidosis. Only if hypoglycemia is confirmed to be present, as with a glucometer, should dextrose be administered. In consideration of the fact that malnutrition and alcoholism are common in the elderly population, 100 mg thiamine can be administered, followed by 0.8 mg naloxone. Because dehydration is a common cause of coma in the elderly, IV fluid therapy should be directed toward correcting hypovolemic hypotension. The paramedic should always be aware of potential pulmonary edema. Blood pressure and pulse should be the guide for fluid therapy in the comatose patient.

PSYCHIATRIC DISORDERS IN THE ELDERLY

Most psychiatric disorders of the elderly are initially diagnosed by the primary care physician and not by emergency medical personnel. Heredity may play an important role in the dementias, and many of these patients may have been hospitalized for such conditions. The functional disorders, such as depression, neurotic disorders, paranoid states, and hypochondriasis, are found in the elderly population, but they are generally more difficult to diagnose because they do not conform to the usual pattern of symptoms, they frequently appear as various physical ailments or complaints, and because the high incidence of physical illnesses in the elderly masks the psychological problems.

Affective Disorders

Depression is common in elderly people. Studies have shown that about 25% of elderly people who live independently are depressed. The symptoms vary from mild to severe and suicidal. Elderly people who are depressed exhibit some of the following symptoms and signs:

- Withdrawal
- Apathy
- Insomnia
- Weight loss
- Reluctance to talk
- Solitude

These signs and symptoms, although frequently seen in elderly patients, are not a natural part of aging. When these signs and symptoms are observed, a careful history should be obtained, and the paramedic should be aware that a depressive illness may be present. Successful attempts at suicide do occur in the elderly population.

Mania also occurs in the elderly population, although less frequently than depression. It is often overlooked as just an individual's exaggerated expression of moods and behaviors of earlier years. The patient may appear agitated, hostile, hyperactive, or paranoid and may even exhibit dementia. Manic states frequently follow periods of depression.

Paranoid Disorders

Symptoms of paranoid disorders frequently are found in patients with dementia and multi-infarct dementia. In addition to the elderly mental patients with schizophrenia who have been hospitalized for many years, some elderly patients develop schizophreniclike symptoms later in life. This type of illness is called paraphrenia. The clinical signs can range from mild paranoid reactions to severe psychotic reactions that require hospitalization. These disorders affect older women more frequently than men. The illness may begin as exaggerated personality traits of earlier years, such as irritability, suspiciousness, hostility, fatigue, insomnia, and nervousness, and may progress to include hallucinations, euphoria, or depression. In some cases, it may be difficult to distinguish these disorders from dementia or depression disorders.

Other Functional Disorders

Functional disorders, also called psychogenic disorders, comprise a broad list of conditions, including neurotic reactions, alcoholism, drug dependence, and personality disorders. Many elderly patients are also hypochondriacal. Their physical complaints include a wide range of symptoms, including those of cardiovascular disease, gastrointestinal disease, or intracranial disease. It is often difficult to determine whether the pain is physical or psychological in origin. Unfortunately, the risk of suicide in patients who do not find relief is an ongoing problem.

Management of Psychiatric Disorders

The management of elderly patients who exhibit signs and symptoms of psychiatric disorders is the same as for any other age group (see Chapter 31). It is not necessary for the paramedic to identify the specific disorder. It is important, however, for the paramedic to provide reassurance to the patient and to remain in the presence of the patient at all times. By observing and recording the behavior of these patients, the paramedic can provide vital information to the emergency department physician.

MUSCULOSKELETAL PROBLEMS

Decreased physical activity, the effects of medications, changes in acid-base balance, menopause, decreased bone formation, increased bone reabsorption, cancer, and other diseases affect the musculoskeletal system of elderly adults. Osteoarthritis and osteoporosis are two of the problems that most commonly affect the musculoskeletal system. No known dietary plan can prevent the loss of bone with aging. Fractures secondary to osteoporosis are the leading cause of death from accidents in patients older than age 75. Femur fractures are five times more common after age 70, and the incidence doubles in women every 5 years thereafter.

Osteoarthritis

Osteoarthritis, seen more commonly in women than men, causes degeneration of the joints, particularly the weight-bearing joints of the hip, knee, and spine. About 85% of people older than age 70 suffer from osteoarthritis. Maintaining a program of mild physical exercise relieves the stiffness associated with this disease and also helps to maintain muscle tone.

Osteoporosis

Osteoporosis is seen most often in postmenopausal women, and it affects about 33% of all women older than age 60. The disease causes a decrease in actual bone mass, which causes the bones to become more fragile. Hundreds of thousands of serious bone fractures every year are attributed to osteoporosis. At the cellular level, an increase in the rate of bone reabsorption occurs. When bone mass is lost, the calcium in the bone is actually lost. As a result, the incidence of fractures in the elderly significantly increases. The addition of calcium to the diet can help delay the development of this disease. Vegetarian diets can actually maintain calcium levels and maintain greater bone mass in elderly people.

Management of Musculoskeletal Problems

The management of fractures and other musculoskeletal injuries in the elderly should include all of the priorities and management plans of younger patients (see Chapter 18). Positioning, immobilization, and packaging of the elderly patient may have to be modified to accommodate the physical abnormalities present, and padding of splints is important because of the decreased fat stores in elderly people. Reassurance and communication are also important.

The extreme pain of the injury, however, is also complicated by the patient's fear of being permanently disabled and confined to a nursing home, thus losing all independence.

GASTROINTESTINAL EMERGENCIES

Aging produces many changes within the gastrointestinal system, as noted earlier in this chapter. The gastrointestinal symptoms experienced by all people during life increase with aging. In addition, the elderly complain of dry mouth, soreness in the mouth, belching or burping, heartburn, diarrhea, intestinal gas pains, and abdominal discomfort and dysphagia. Many of these complaints are due to a decrease in the secretion of hydrochloric acid and digestive enzymes and an altered motility through the system. Gastrointestinal bleeding is a common problem in emergency medicine.

Upper Gastrointestinal Bleeding

Gastrointestinal bleeding is a common problem in elderly adults. The blood loss is manifested in many ways: by hematemesis (vomiting bright red material or material like coffee grounds), melena (black, tarry, malodorous stool with 500 mL of blood or more), and rectal bleeding.

Peptic Ulcers

Peptic ulcer disease is the most common cause of upper gastrointestinal bleeding in nonalcoholic elderly patients. The areas of ulceration usually are in the esophagus, stomach, and duodenum. Also, changes in the mucosal barrier with aging make the gastric mucosa more vulnerable to irritation or frank ulceration, for example, from drugs. This gastritis or gastric ulceration can result in bleeding, and, if the patient is a smoker, the time required for recovery can be greatly extended.

Esophageal Varices

Esophageal varices, as a complication of portal hypertension, are a potential cause of severe or recurrent bleeding. The patient has a history of liver disease, and the clinical presentation includes massive hematemesis. The bleeding may be life-threatening and may also cause serious airway management problems for the paramedic. Intravenous fluid therapy and blood replacement are necessary. However, fluid overload is of constant concern to emergency personnel when managing elderly patients.

Mallory–Weiss Syndrome

Mallory–Weiss syndrome is a condition that usually heals itself. With this syndrome, tears occur in the mucosa just below the gastroesophageal junction secondary to vomiting. The patient history reveals that the patient vomited gastric contents, then bright red blood. These tears usually heal spontaneously.

Lower Gastrointestinal Bleeding

Bright red blood in the stool is an important sign of bleeding from the large bowel. Dark blood is also possible if movement through the bowel is slow or if the bleeding is not massive. A good patient history is important, such as recent weight loss, change in bowel habits, and previous rectal bleeding. Bleeding from the large bowel in the elderly is frequently the result of diverticula, polyps, cancers, or ischemic colitis. Lesions of the colon are a part of the degenerative process of aging and are one of the most common causes of lower gastrointestinal bleeding in the elderly population.

Diverticula

In the lower gastrointestinal tract, diverticula are found in about 50% of the population older than age 60. The bleeding source is in the arterioles in the mesenteric walls, and, therefore, bright red blood is found in rectal bleeding. Bleeding may be massive without much complaint of pain or minimal with moderate abdominal pain on physical examination.

Ischemic Colitis

Ischemic colitis is seen in patients older than age 50. This disease should be suspected in elderly patients who are experiencing the signs and symptoms of ulcerative colitis for the first time. The patient may not appear to be sick but may experience sudden cramping pain in the abdomen, usually the left side, followed by bright red or dark red bloody diarrhea. The patient may also have a low-grade fever. Blood loss amounts vary and are usually not so severe that hypovolemia is a problem. Ischemic colitis usually resolves itself. The bleeding stops and the symptoms subside within 1 to 2 days, and a complete recovery occurs within 10 to 14 days.

Cancer of the Large Intestine

The incidence of colon cancer increases with age after a person reaches age 40, and, after age 50, the incidence doubles every 10 years. Tumors of the small intestine are rare, but the incidence of tumors of the large intestine doubles every 10 years after the age of 50. These tumors are second only to lung cancer as a cause of cancer deaths in the United States. Women suffer from cancer of the colon more frequently than men, and the reverse is true for cancer of the rectum. Risk factors appear to include the following:

- High beef diets
- High fat diets
- History of ulcerative colitis
- Family history of cancers

The signs and symptoms of bowel cancer include weight loss, change in bowel habits, and the signs and symptoms of a bowel obstruction.

Tumors of the colon and rectum have a good prognosis. They are generally noninvasive and have a high rate of cure when detected early. The history of the present illness, the medical history, and the physical examination may provide information to lead to the suspicion of bowel cancer.

Bowel Obstruction

Bowel obstruction may be caused by tumors, depending on the location of the obstruction. The tumors have a tendency to ulcerate and bleed. Because of the variable nature of the development of cancer, the clinical evaluation may be nonspecific except for the presence of blood in the stool.

Management of Gastrointestinal Emergencies

Assessment priorities include a good medical history that addresses previous episodes, use of alcohol, aspirin, and prescription and nonprescription drugs, previous abdominal operations, and anticoagulant therapy. Any information that can be acquired from the patient, family, or friends about previous episodes of gastrointestinal problems may help to identify the source of the bleeding.

Airway, breathing, and circulation are obviously of primary importance. An IV infusion should be initiated, and fluid therapy should be administered depending on the signs and symptoms. The pneumatic anti-shock garment may help manage hypovolemia in elderly patients. Constant monitoring of vital signs is paramount when administering fluid therapy to the elderly.

TRAUMA IN THE ELDERLY

Trauma is the fifth leading cause of death in the elderly population. The primary types of trauma suffered by the elderly are blunt trauma from auto accidents, pedestrians struck by automobiles, falls, and burns.

The aging process and the various diseases of the elderly may make these patients more vulnerable to the serious effects of trauma (*e.g.*, hypotension, hypoxemia, and shock) than younger patients. A greater sense of urgency in both extrication and transportation is needed with these patients. Elderly trauma patients usually do not compensate as effectively, and they begin to deteriorate much earlier. The effects of years of cardiovascular disease, respiratory disease, hypertension, cerebrovascular accident, and atherosclerosis may cause these patients to have a diminished ability to handle the stress of trauma.

Pathophysiology of Trauma

Rib fractures can be seen in elderly trauma patients because their chest wall is not as elastic. After blunt trauma to the chest from an automobile accident or cardiopulmonary resuscitation, multiple rib fractures and even lung contusions result. The risk of pneumonia is so great after rib fractures in the elderly that these injuries should be considered significant. Rib fractures also can lacerate the pleura, causing pneumothorax and possibly tension pneumothorax, both of which are life-threatening in the elderly because of the decrease in cardiac output. Also, an elderly patient's level of fatigue contributes to hypoventilation and hypoxia in chest trauma.

The normal physiologic response to traumatic blood loss is to increase heart rate in an effort to maintain cardiac output. Tachycardia and increased respiratory rate with delayed capillary refill, anxiety, and restlessness are signs of significant blood loss in elderly people.

As blood loss continues, the release of the catecholamines, epinephrine and norepinephrine causes peripheral vasoconstriction and an increase in blood pressure. However, the cardiac and respiratory response to the increased catecholamine release is not as effective in the elderly patient. The cardiac response may not maintain the cardiac output in the elderly patient in early stages of hypotension and hypovolemia. The presence of coronary atherosclerosis makes the heart susceptible to ischemia and infarction with hypotension from blood loss. A decreasing pulse pressure, less than 35 mm Hg, is a sign of significant blood loss in elderly patients. Shock is lethal in elderly patients, and it must be recognized early and managed quickly

Contributing Factors

Many physical and psychological factors may contribute to the significant number of traumatic injuries in the elderly adult population. The elderly tend to refuse to accept the physical limitations of aging related to operating motor vehicles, the work environment, and misjudging their capabilities of walking. Dementias cause confusion, disorientation, and wandering. Reflexes tend to be slower, and hearing and eyesight are diminished. For an object to be seen, the illumination of the object must be doubled every 13 years after the age of 20. Glare and a decreasing field of vision and decreased night acuity contribute to motor vehicle accidents by elderly drivers.

Dizziness plays an important role in falls down stairs. An elderly person may get dizzy when looking down the stairs and then may fall. Elderly people who are climbing the stairs may also become dizzy and fall backward down the stairs, because of the compression of vertebral and carotid arteries when looking up, to the side, or over their shoulder, as described earlier in this chapter. Much more serious injuries occur when the elderly fall backward down the stairs. Head and spinal injuries are particularly serious in the elderly.

The loss of acuity of smell causes the elderly to be at greater risk of accidental gas poisoning from unignited jets on gas stoves or open jets that were extinguished when a pot boiled over.

Management of Trauma

A patent airway is of immediate concern in the elderly patient. The airway must be carefully inspected for dentures, partial plates, loose teeth, vomitus, and blood. Partial plates can cause significant trauma and bleeding in the oral cavity if not found. The tongue is the most common cause of upper airway obstruction, and this is often found in the unconscious elderly patient. Aging causes the pharyngeal muscle and the tongue to lose tone; therefore, the oropharyngeal or nasopharyngeal airway can effectively maintain an open airway. The elderly also have a less sensitive gag reflex, and weakened muscle tone results in an ineffective cough. Active intervention by the paramedic is essential in this case.

PHARMACOLOGY IN GERIATRICS

Elderly people have a wide range of differences in drug sensitivity and metabolism. Many of the disease processes that affect the elderly population require patients to take medications. As the aging process affects most body systems, it is not difficult to understand how the older adult can fall victim to drug-induced illness. Specific drugs commonly used to treat disease processes in the elderly are usually the culprits in causing drug toxicity.

Drug-Induced Illness

Drug-induced illness is common in elderly people. Elderly patients may take more medications, have more illnesses, and have more adverse effects from drugs than younger patients. About 10% of hospital admissions are due to patients 60 years of age or older with drug-induced illnesses.

The most common situations that cause drug-induced problems are the following:

- Forgetting to take a medication
- Taking an incorrect dosage
- Taking over-the-counter medications in addition to prescriptions
- Continuing to take old prescription medications for prior medical events along with new medications
- Changing dietary, smoking, exercise, and alcohol habits
- Running out of medications
- Abusing drugs

Because of the potential contribution of polypharmacy to the clinical situation, an accurate history of specific drug use is essential and must be collected from patients, family, friends, pharmacy, and doctors.

The absorption of a drug is affected by gastric pH, motility, and ingestion of a fatty meal. The distribution of a drug is affected significantly by changes in percent body fat. As people age, a change in body composition results in an increase in percent body fat, a decrease in lean body mass, and a decrease in total body water. Drugs like acetaminophen, morphine, and meperidine, which are adjusted according to body weight, appear in significantly higher concentrations in a 70-year-old patient than in a 30-year-old patient. This concentration can be important if the drug has a narrow therapeutic range.

Most drugs are eliminated through the kidneys or metabolized by the liver. As a person ages, both of these systems experience changes, and these changes ultimately affect drug clearance. Drugs like digoxin and lithium, which have a narrow therapeutic index, must be administered in decreased dosages as the patient ages, because renal function and renal blood flow both decrease with age. Blood flow through the liver also declines with age, particularly in the presence of congestive heart failure. The liver also decreases in size. Therefore, several important factors of drug metabolism and clearance in the elderly patient should be considered:

- Drug disposal in the elderly patient may be impaired
- Diet affects the metabolism and the disposal of certain drugs
- Aging causes the exaggeration of the effects of drugs
- Elderly patients lack an understanding of their drug therapy
- Elderly patients in the emergency setting present a variety of signs and symptoms of toxic reactions to drugs

Drugs That Cause Toxicity

The most common drugs that cause toxicity in the elderly are the following:

- Digitalis
- Anti-Parkinson's drugs
- Diuretics
- Anticoagulants
- Lidocaine
- Propranolol
- Theophylline
- Narcotic analgesics
- Acetaminophen
- Phenothiazine
- Tricyclic antidepressants

ENVIRONMENTAL EMERGENCIES

The ability of an elderly person to maintain a normal body temperature in excessive heat or excessive cold temperatures depends on many factors: the person's overall state of health, the ability to move about, diet, and the ability to control the ambient temperature with heat or air conditioning. As people age, the body loses some of its natural ability to protect itself from extreme changes in ambient temperature, and, therefore, the elderly suffer the ill effects.

The elderly may be on multiple medications, some of which facilitate heat loss, their cardiovascular and respiratory systems are not as efficient, their central nervous system functions are altered, and their electrolyte balances are altered. Any unusual situation, such as a fall or motor vehicle accident, place the elderly at greater risk of morbidity and mortality from a cold or hot environment.

Hypothermia

The increasing interest in hypothermia in the last 25 years has resulted in a better awareness of this condition by prehospital and emergency department personnel. This increased awareness has been life-saving to many patients, particularly the elderly, who have suffered from this condition. Hypothermia is defined as a body temperature of less than 35°C (95°F). Accidental hypothermia occurs when the body is not able to maintain its normal body temperature in a cool environment. The elderly population is one of several high-risk groups that are extremely susceptible to hypothermia. The mortality rate from hypothermia in the elderly population is about 80%.

The human body's ability to adapt to environmental temperature changes declines with advancing age; in the past, hypothermia was frequently not diagnosed because it was not suspected. It has finally become standard protocol for hospital emergency departments to take a rectal temperature reading of any patient with an oral temperature of 35°C (95°F) to assure an accurate temperature reading.

Contributing factors for hypothermia in the elderly population are many. The elderly frequently live alone and may be less active because of chronic, debilitating diseases or lack of family. On average, they have increased proportion of fat stores and have a decreased metabolic rate. They are also less responsive to the cold and, therefore, do not protect themselves from it. Alcohol use and abuse, mental confusion, and the use of certain medications can also result in hypothermia. Several of the medications commonly used by elderly patients actually induce hypothermia. Hypothermia may be observed in patients in the early stages of pneumonia, pulmonary embolism, myocardial infarction, and stroke.

Many of the signs and symptoms of hypothermia can also be associated with stroke, a diabetic emergency, or a cardiac event; therefore, hypothermia should always be suspected in the elderly patient who is living alone and who has a history of chronic diseases.

Hyperthermia

The elderly population may be susceptible to heat-related illnesses. The body's adaptability to increases in temperatures in the environment may be diminished by the process of aging. Abnormalities within the body that result from chronic disease, use or abuse of alcohol, and the use of medications like propranolol, antihistamines, anticholinergics, and phenothiazines may further predispose the person to hyperthermia. Obesity, fatigue, and lack of protection from the sun and heat are also contributing factors. Whenever the environmental temperature remains above 32°C (90°F) for more than 2 days, the paramedic should expect to receive emergency calls from elderly people who are suffering from the effects of the heat.

Heat Exhaustion

Heat exhaustion is generally a result of a lack of adequate fluid intake during periods of hot weather and high humidity. The elderly patient may suffer from mental confusion. The patient has a weak and rapid pulse, decreased blood pressure, nausea, diarrhea, visual problems, fatigue, and weakness.

Heatstroke

Heatstroke is another environmentally induced disorder. However, when the elderly person experiences heatstroke, it is a life-threatening situation that must be quickly recognized and correctly managed by the paramedic. When the environmental temperature is above 38°C (100°F) for several days, especially with high humidity, the elderly become at risk for heatstroke. The following predisposing conditions commonly are seen in the elderly person and should be recognized: infection with fever, potassium depletion from use of diuretics, heat exhaustion, heat cramps, dehydration, recent immunizations, alcohol, and certain medications.

GERIATRIC ABUSE

Geriatric abuse may be as widespread as child abuse in the United States. The abuse may be physical, psychological, or financial, or it may involve neglect of the needs of an elderly person. Geriatric abuse occurs in the home, in nursing homes, and in hospitals.

The risk factors for abuse may include the following:

- Multiple chronic diseases
- Dementia
- Incontinence
- Disturbances of sleep and nocturnal wandering
- Dependency on family members for daily activities and physical needs

These risk factors are reflective of the stress on the family members, friends, or health care workers who have become the caretakers of the elderly. Because of the close relationship between the patient and the caretaker, the elderly generally does not admit to the abuse or neglect. The paramedic must be aware of any clues in the environment or in the patient's history or physical condition that indicate that abuse may be occurring.

Signs of physical abuse include the following:

- Closed wounds of the scalp from severe hair pulling
- Various stages of healing of wounds from bites, cigarettes, and cutting instruments
- Burns from ropes
- Wounds or bruises on the chest, back, or extremities

Most states have adult protective services agencies that handle geriatric abuse cases. The paramedic should carefully document all evidence of suspected geriatric abuse or neglect and report it to the emergency department staff or appropriate agency according to local protocol.

SUMMARY

In general, the elderly have the same needs as younger people regarding health, safety, love, belonging, and the need for a certain level of self-esteem. However, elderly people frequently have fewer resources (financial, social, psychological, and physiologic) to meet their specific needs. Many of these needs are health related; however, since they are not specifically defined as such, insurance policies do not provide the necessary resources.

A normal state of health in the elderly person requires that each body system function adequately and that there be a balance among all body systems. The normal age-related changes that occur in the body are extensive and affect every body system. If any one system becomes adversely affected by trauma, disease, stress, or environmental changes, then the entire body's health is adversely affected.

In the prehospital care setting, a general bias that elderly people are sick and of deteriorated vitality is found. To some extent, paramedics share this negative stereotype of the elderly population. Therefore, it is important that paramedics and all health care providers be aware of their attitudes about aging and the effects that these attitudes may have on the care provided to geriatric patients.

SUGGESTED READING

Bosker G, Schwartz GR, Jones JS et al:Geriatric Emergency Medicine. St. Louis, Mosby Year Book, 1990

Gallo JJ, Reichel W, Anderson L: Handbook of Geriatric Assessment. Rockville, MD, Aspen Publishers, 1988

Gilmore GC, Whitehouse PJ, Wykle ML: Memory, Aging, and Dementia. Springhouse, PA, Springhouse Publishing, 1989

Judd RL, Warner CG, Shaffer MA: Geriatric Emergencies. Rockville, MD, Aspen Publishers, 1986

Kozier B, Erb G, Olivieri R: Fundamentals of Nursing, 4th ed. Redwood City, CA, Addison-Wesley, 1991

Lewis CB: Aging: The Health Care Challenge, 2nd ed. Philadelphia, FA Davis 1990

McSwain NE, Butman AM, McConnell WK et al: Prehospital Trauma Life Support, 2nd ed. Akron, Emergency Training, 1990

Spaite DW, Criss EA, Valenzuela TD:Geriatric injury: An analysis of prehospital demographics, mechanisms, and patterns. Ann Emerg Med 19: 1418, 1989

US Department of Transportation, National Highway Traffic Safety Administration: Emergency Medical Technician–Paramedic: National Standards Curriculum. Washington, DC, US Government Printing Office, 1985

CHAPTER 29

Pediatric Emergencies

Approach to the Pediatric Patient
    General Considerations
    General Approach
    Physical Examination
Developmental Stages
Common Pediatric Problems
Problems Specific to the Pediatric Patient
    Sudden Infant Death Syndrome
        Diagnosis
        Management
    Seizures
        Febrile Seizures
        Assessment
        Management
    Dehydration
    Infectious Processes
        Meningitis
        Septicemia
        Reye's Syndrome

Respiratory Emergencies
    Obstructed Airway
        Foreign Body
        Injuries to the Face and Neck
        Anaphylaxis
    Croup
    Epiglottitis
    Bronchiolitis
    Asthma
Cardiopulmonary Arrest
Shock
Trauma
Child Abuse
    Characteristics of the Abused Child
    Characteristics of Child Abusers
    Assessment of Child Abuse
    Management of the Abused Child

Techniques of Management
    Airway Management
        Oropharyngeal Airway
        Nasopharyngeal Airway
        Resuscitation Mask
        Resuscitation Bags
        Endotracheal Intubation
        Cricothyroidotomy
    Intravenous Insertion
        Selection of Needles and Cannulas
        Intravenous Fluids
        Selection of Vein
        Intraosseous Infusion
Summary

BEHAVIORAL OBJECTIVES

On successful completion of this chapter, the reader will be able to:

1. Describe therapeutic approaches to use when interacting with family members in a pediatric emergency
2. Identify significant information to be included when obtaining a pediatric history
3. Suggest three approaches to improve the child's cooperation during the physical assessment
4. Explain the five developmental stages of the child
5. Identify common anatomic and physiologic differences between children and adults in the following areas: airway, respiratory, neurologic, thermoregulation, and cardiovascular
6. Describe signs and symptoms and unique aspects of field management of sudden infant death syndrome, seizures, dehydration, meningitis, septicemia, Reye's syndrome, and shock
7. Describe signs and symptoms of the pediatric respiratory emergencies of obstructed airway, croup, epiglottitis, bronchiolitis, and asthma
8. Describe aspects of management of cardiac arrest unique to the pediatric patient
9. Recognize physical and behavioral signs of child abuse and neglect
10. Describe techniques of vascular access in the child
11. Describe techniques of airway management and ventilatory support in the child
12. Define all of the key terms listed in this chapter

KEY TERMS

The following terms are defined in the chapter and glossary:

asthma
adolescence
bronchiolitis
child abuse
child neglect
croup
dehydration
developmental stages
emotional abuse
epiglottitis
febrile seizures
fontanelle
infant
intraosseous infusion
meningitis
pediatrics
preschool
Reye's syndrome
school age
septicemia
sexual abuse
status asthmaticus
status epilepticus
sudden infant death syndrome (SIDS)
toddler

Few situations produce as much anxiety for paramedics as the management of the acutely ill or injured child. The severity of the presenting problem may appear out of proportion to the true extent of injury or illness, not only to the parents and bystanders, but to the paramedics as well. Somehow, it is hard to feel adequately prepared to care for the very young.

Pediatrics is the branch of medicine concerned with the care and development of children and the treatment of their diseases. As has often been pointed out, children are not just small adults; they present problems specific to their age group. Those processes that especially affect field care are discussed in this chapter. This discussion of pediatrics is intended not to review all pediatric emergencies but rather to cover the more common problems encountered by paramedics in the field. As with other areas of emergency care, it is often less important to accurately diagnose the specific problem than to recognize the need for expedient transport for definitive care.

It is crucial in the management of the pediatric patient that paramedics must recognize when not to delay treatment. They should not avoid an attempt at definitive airway management, such as endotracheal intubation, because they lack confidence in the ability to perform the procedure. These management decisions become even more difficult in the emotionally charged atmosphere that is encountered with the seriously ill or injured child. The paramedic must become familiar with assessing these young patients and practicing the techniques of management discussed in this chapter.

APPROACH TO THE PEDIATRIC PATIENT

General Considerations

Evaluation of the ill or injured child is frequently complicated by several factors. Any anxiety by the paramedic may interfere with the normal orderly and thorough approach to the evaluation and examination of the patient. After the precipitating event, the child may be frightened and become a poor historian, unable to relate pertinent facts. Fear also makes the child difficult to examine; it may even make it difficult to elicit accurate physical findings. Sometimes, when one thing hurts a child, everything hurts. A parent or caretaker's anxiety and at times guilt (often unjustified) may also make obtaining historical information more difficult.

The child's fear of strangers may complicate the usual paramedic-patient relationship and may further interfere with patient management. The very young child, who is unable to communicate, presents special problems in evaluation. As a general rule, the younger the child, the greater the anxiety produced in both the parent and paramedic.

General Approach

Establishing a relationship with both the patient and the parent or other caretaker is especially important when caring for pediatric patients. Both sources should be used to obtain information about the presenting problem. Depending on age, the child should not be dismissed as a source of history. School age children can be accurate in their descriptions and a valuable source of information. It is particularly important in the evaluation to observe the child's behavior and physical responses, since these may reflect data more accurately than the information the child gives or the parent or caretaker infers. Depending on the child's age and the urgency of the situation, the paramedic may wish to interview the child first and then the parent or caretaker. This approach is especially important for patients in adolescence; in addition to clarifying the clinical picture, it demonstrates concern for and trust in the patient. It may be wise to interview the adolescent alone, since important information may be withheld when parents are present.

It is important to remember that the general considerations in approach to the pediatric patient are operative when life-threatening problems are not present. Priorities of patient management are based on threat to life and the gathering of historical information and the method of physical examination may be altered depending on the urgency of the presenting problem.

The initial approach to the pediatric patient should be aimed at fostering cooperation and gaining the child's confidence. Approach the child slowly, begin by stating your name, and, depending on the child's age, ask permission to conduct the physical examination. Always call the child by name. Be as gentle as possible in handling the child; be aware that a firm touch indicates confidence and control of the situation. Avoid touching injured or painful areas first. Talking to the child, regardless of age and ability to understand, frequently provides a calming effect. If the child is old enough to understand, explaining what you are doing and what to expect in simple understandable terms helps to achieve cooperation and reduce fear. A calm, quiet, assured voice is soothing to both the pediatric patient and the parent and helps develop rapport. Tell the child what you want done, instead of asking if it can be done, to avoid giving the child the opportunity to say "no."

It is essential to be honest with the pediatric patient. Telling the child that a procedure does not hurt when it does or minimizing the pain involved destroys not only trust in the paramedic but in other health care professionals as well. Contrary to popular opinion, most children are cooperative if they know what is happening to them and what to expect. Give the child permission to cry (or express fear and pain) if something is painful. Let the child know when the procedure is finished, and, if appropriate, praise should be given for bravery and help. Children should never be threatened with punishment if they are uncooperative.

When possible, the child should not be separated from the parent. Separation anxiety only heightens the child's fear and causes unnecessary distress. Parental anxiety, however, is contagious, and every effort should be made to provide reassurance to the parents and to gain their cooperation. Procedures that benefit the patient may be perceived as harmful or uncomfortable by the parent and must be explained. Allow the child to keep a favorite toy, doll, blanket, or other object. Young children may be most easily examined while held by a parent.

While children may provide an important source of historical information, it must be recognized that they may not be honest if they were injured while involved in an activity that was forbidden to them. Guilt may also cause them to distort facts about an illness or injury. Children may confuse fantasy with reality, making an accurate history difficult to obtain.

Children may be extremely modest depending on their developmental stage. Undress children slowly, or have a parent do so, to maintain their modesty and warmth. Do not remove underwear unless necessary for the exam. If children are reluctant to permit a physical examination, ask them to point on a doll or a parent or yourself to where it hurts. Proceeding slowly and with a friendly manner more likely results in cooperation. When possible, reach the same physical level as the child to reduce fear and the feeling of being overpowered.

Enlist the child's cooperation in holding a dressing or stethoscope, for example, if possible. Children are easily distressed by unpleasant sights such as injuries; these should be covered from view as quickly as possible. If an accident has occurred, others, particularly parents and siblings, may also be injured.

The ill or injured child needs emotional and psychological support (Fig. 29-1). The use of *touch*, such as holding a hand, may be reassuring, especially if a parent is not present. It is usually advisable, however, to ask the child for permission first.

During patient hand-off, or transfer of care at any point, explain to the child what is happening and introduce the person who is assuming the care. Explain, when appropriate, the whereabouts and condition of parents and caretakers.

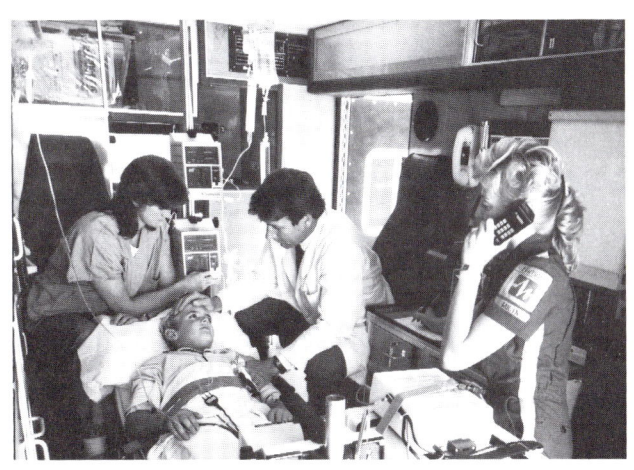

FIGURE 29-1.
Providing emotional support (e.g., the use of touch) is extremely important for this ill child, since he has been placed in an unknown environment with strange equipment and unfamiliar faces. (Courtesy of Hartson Medical Services, San Diego, CA.)

Finally, because the presentation of ill or injured children provokes tension in both caretaker and paramedic, each situation must be approached calmly and nonjudgmentally. Pediatric illness often develops precipitously. Parental guilt, demonstrated by statements like "I should have called for help sooner" or "I shouldn't have let him ride his bike in the street," is common. Do not impart to care givers an evaluation of their competency. Evaluate and report facts. For situations in which suspicion of abuse or neglect exists, follow appropriate reporting procedures. However, avoid compounding the conscientious parent's misplaced feelings of guilt.

Physical Examination

Establishing rapport with the child and parents before beginning an examination facilitates the child's cooperation. Begin the evaluation by a visual assessment. Observe skin color, respiratory rate and effort, and general appearance. Make eye contact with the child and let the child see what is happening. The physical examination should begin with the areas that are not injured or painful. This procedure gains the child's trust and confidence. Beginning the examination without instruments reduces fear. It allows the paramedic to obtain information that might be denied if the child becomes uncooperative. In children younger than age 2, it may be preferable to begin the examination in reverse, from *toe to head*. This procedure permits completion of most of the secondary survey before the fear response is elicited by approaching the young child's face. By age 4, children usually are cooperative with the standard patient head-to-toe survey.

Vital signs should be evaluated in all pediatric patients. Obtaining accurate measurements, particularly in the uncooperative patient, can be challenging. Respiratory rate should be obtained before beginning the physical examination and, in the young child, while held in a parent's arms. Because a young infant's respiratory rate is normally somewhat irregular, respirations should be counted for a full minute, if time permits, to obtain a more accurate rate. Note the respiratory effort and use of accessory muscles of respiration. The apical or brachial pulse may be most readily obtainable in the patient in infancy. It is important to remember that infants and young children have proportionately less myocardial mass and, therefore, depend more on heart rate to maintain adequate cardiac output. Partially because of an immature sympathetic nervous system, bradycardia often results from hypoxia and can rapidly progress to complete cardiac arrest.

For accurate blood pressure determination, the appropriate size cuff for the patient must be used (see Chapter 9). Normal values for vital signs vary with age and size. Approximate values for weight and vital sign parameters are shown in Table 29-1. Baseline determinations and serial measurements of vital signs help most to evaluate the child's clinical condition and significant changes. The pediatric patient should be reassessed frequently, since signs of shock can develop rapidly.

Many pediatric illnesses are accompanied by a change in body temperature. Temperature variations are wider in children than adults, and a child may develop a temperature above 39°C (103°F) during a mild illness. Infants and young children are especially susceptible to both rapid and substantial elevations in temperature and to hypothermia. If a thermometer is available, a rectal temperature may be obtained in 3 to 5 minutes in the preschool child. Oral temperatures are suitable for the older cooperative child. Axillary readings may be inaccurate and are normally lower than the true body temperature. Cooling with tepid water may be indicated for the patient with a significantly elevated temperature (over 39°C [103°F]). However, transport should not be delayed for these measures.

The **fontanelle** is any of the membrane-covered spaces between the incompletely ossified cranial bones of an in-

TABLE 29-1.
NORMAL WEIGHTS AND VITAL SIGNS IN THE PEDIATRIC AGE GROUP

Age	Weight (kg)	Pulse per minute	Respirations per minute	Blood Pressure systolic (±20)
Premature	<3	145	24–40	N/A*
Newborn	3–4	125	24–30	N/A
6 months	5–7	130	20–30	80 mm Hg
1 year	10	130	20–24	90 mm Hg
3 years	15	100	20–24	95 mm Hg
5 years	20	100	20–24	95 mm Hg
8 years	25	90	12–20	100 mm Hg
12 years	32–42	75	12–20	110 mm Hg
16 years	>50	70	12–18	120 mm Hg

*N/A = Not available

fant; commonly called the soft spot. The anterior fontanelle provides a window for evaluation of intracranial pressure in the infant. The normal fontanelle in the non-crying infant appears flat or level with the skull and may pulsate slightly. The fontanelle is best evaluated when the infant is in a sitting position. When intracranial pressure increases because of infection or other processes, the fontanelle begins to feel tense, may bulge slightly, and the normal pulsations may decrease or disappear. If dehydration is present, the fontanelle takes on a sunken appearance and falls below the level of the skull. The fontanelle is difficult to evaluate, however, when the child is crying, restless, or uncooperative.

As with adults, level of consciousness is an important clinical indicator. However, evaluation of level of consciousness in the pediatric patient may be more difficult because of fear and reluctance to communicate. The parent may be able to provide helpful information about the child's response to this illness or injury in relation to past experiences and to normal behavior. Evaluation of the mental status includes the child's ability to relate to others, level of activity, mood, attention span, ability or willingness to cooperate with the examination, and the appropriateness of responses. Assessment of motor strength may be tested by the ability to stand up from a supine position, when not contraindicated. Hand grip strength and leg strength should be evaluated in the cooperative child. Muscle tone is estimated by the resistance to passive movement of the extremities. Sensory evaluation can be tested by observing the response to pain from a pin prick, including withdrawal and emotional reaction (see Appendix C for the Pediatric Glasgow Coma Scale). However, this step should be omitted, when possible, to avoid causing further distress.

Respiratory compromise is a major cause of pediatric cardiopulmonary arrest. Adequate assessment, early recognition, and appropriate management of respiratory impairment is essential in the pediatric patient. Important *anatomical* and *physiologic* differences in the airway include the following: the larynx is relatively cephalad in position; the epiglottis is "U" shaped and protrudes into the pharynx; the vocal cords are short and concave; and, in the child younger than age 8, the most narrow portion of the airway is at the cricoid cartilage. These differences have significance in visualization and tube selection in endotracheal intubation. The lower airway is particularly vulnerable to obstruction in the infant and young child because of the smaller size of the structures. Obstruction may result rapidly from a variety of causes, including edema, blood, mucus, pus, and bronchoconstriction, because a child's airway contains proportionally more smooth muscle, which is highly reactive to irritation. An equal amount of obstruction in the adult and small child, for example, produces a much larger decrease in the size of the pediatric airway. The rib cage is more pliable in the young child than in the adult. Sternal retractions may occur during inspiration, limiting lung expansion. The tidal volume also depends more on adequate excursion of the diaphragm.

Hypoxemia in the pediatric patient may be aggravated by a high metabolic rate that is about twice that of an adult. Injury or disease that increases respiratory effort, therefore, increases an already high oxygen demand. When assessing a child with respiratory distress, attempt to gather as much information as possible before touching the child. It is normal for young children to be anxious when approached by a stranger, and agitation can adversely affect a child who already has breathing problems.

Several unique factors indicate increased respiratory effort in the child. Use of accessory muscles, as in the adult, reveals that the older child is working at breathing. In the infant or younger child, retractions may be noted in the suprasternal, intercostal, or substernal areas. As noted above, severe retractions can decrease intrathoracic volume and further inhibit breathing. The presence of stridor indicates upper airway obstruction, which can be caused by edema, foreign bodies, or an infectious process such as croup or epiglottitis. Expiratory grunting or gasping is a physiologic mechanism to increase airway pressure and correct hypoxia. *Paradoxical* (seesaw) breathing in the infant, in which the abdomen expands on inspiration but the chest lags behind or actually "pulls in," also indicates impending fatigue. Nasal flaring, an attempt to expand the air passages, is also a sign of increased respiratory effort.

In assessing breath sounds in the child, it is helpful to have a pediatric size stethoscope. Because of the thin chest wall, normal breath sounds can be transmitted to an area of atelectasis or otherwise decreased breath sounds; this effect is more pronounced with a large stethoscope and can lead to inaccurate assessment of air exchange.

DEVELOPMENTAL STAGES

Appropriate assessment of the child requires some understanding of growth and **developmental stages.** Since children change continually and rapidly, the task of assessment may be a difficult one, especially for the paramedic who deals with pediatric patients infrequently. To complicate matters further, numerous descriptions that use varying age groups and categories are available. Children may not fall into any usual category or behavioral pattern. However, attempts to structure developmental stages help the paramedic to recognize specific needs by age group and to determine how to respond to those needs. It must also be remembered that the stress of illness or injury can cause the child to regress to a lower level of behavior.

Growth refers to an increase in body size. *Development* denotes improvement or maturation in organs and systems as well as skills and functions. Both occur in an

TABLE 29-2.
DEVELOPMENTAL APPROACH TO PEDIATRIC EMERGENCY CARE PATIENTS

Age	Developmental Characteristics	Important Concerns of the Child	Helpful Techniques
Infant (younger than 1 year) Rolls over Crawls	Limited language Requires physical contact with parents for security No independent sense of self No control over physical environment	Separation anxiety	Examine in parent's lap if possible Maintain warm environment Warm hands and stethoscope before patient contact Allow child to suck pacifier if possible
Toddler (1–3 years) Walking, running Climbing	Limited language, understands but may be unable to express thoughts Tests reality Short memory and attention span Beginning to see self as separate from parents and environment	Separation anxiety Fears pain	Examine in parent's lap if possible Communicate with child on his or her level Allow choices when possible Allow child to hold security blanket or favorite toy
Preschool (3–5 years) Very active Growth spurts	Imaginative, displays magical thinking and fantasy life Verbal skills improving, but comprehension may remain limited Strong self-concept May display regression during stressful periods	Separation anxiety Fears pain, blood, disfigurement	Allow choices when possible Maintain communication on child's level Allow play and participation in care with simple tasks (e.g., holding stethoscope) Cover wounds Use adhesive bandage as "badges of courage"
School age (5–12 years) Frequent growth spurts "Daredevil" Peer pressure	Language skills well developed Tends toward modesty Begins to use logic, reason, and self-control Improved understanding of body functions	Fears pain, disfigurement, and loss of function Often fears death	Explain procedures, including reasons why Be honest but stress expectation of positive outcome Respect modesty Stress child's strength and courage
Adolescence (12–19 years) Peer pressure Emerging sexual identity	Developing independence but may regress when stressed Peer group may be more important than family May be hysterical or overreact in emergencies Realistic view of death but may not relate mortality with dangerous actions	Fears loss of control, disfigurement, death Needs peer acceptance	Allow choices when possible Respect independence and modesty Allow peer contact when possible Maintain honest communication

orderly sequential fashion, allowing for individual variations. An interrelationship exists between the child's intellectual growth, social environment, and emotional experiences. These factors may serve to enhance or retard a child's development. Knowledge of the psychosocial development presented in Table 29-2 helps the paramedic understand the appropriate approach to a child and anticipate the child's response.

COMMON PEDIATRIC PROBLEMS

Common causes of disease and disability in children are predictable by age group. Less than 1 year of age, major causes of infant death are infection, specifically those of respiratory and gastrointestinal origin, and sudden infant death syndrome. Between ages 1 and 15, accidents of all types are the leading cause of death. Preschoolers are more susceptible to accidents of all types because they begin to investigate their surroundings. Because of lack of muscular coordination, lack of previous experience and therefore judgment, and lack of the ability to relate cause and effect, they are prone to injuries, including falls, other musculoskeletal trauma, and burns. The tendency to investigate the world with their mouths leads to ingestion of harmful substances, including household products, medications, and foreign objects. Failure to use vehicular restraints also results in increased morbidity and mortality in this age group. Common illnesses of the preschooler include croup, asthma, seizures, epiglottitis, and meningitis.

Accidents in the school age group are the major cause of morbidity and mortality. Accidents occur more often outside the home and include vehicular accidents, injuries from sports activities, bicycle accidents, falls, and drownings. Injuries from child abuse may occur in any age group. The incidence of toxic ingestion due to abuse or suicide gesture increases in the adolescent age group.

PROBLEMS SPECIFIC TO THE PEDIATRIC PATIENT

Sudden Infant Death Syndrome

Sudden infant death syndrome (SIDS) is traditionally described as the sudden death of an infant or young child that is unexpected and for which the postmortem examination fails to reveal an adequate cause for death. This devastating event is the leading cause of death in infants between 1 week and 1 year of age. Two deaths from SIDS occur per 1000 live births, and about 7500 infant deaths each year in the United States are attributed to SIDS. The peak incidence occurs between 2 and 4 months of age. Nine out of ten deaths occur in the first 6 months of life. Death is unexpected and typically occurs between midnight and 6:00 AM; there are no warning signs. At present, no known cause has been discovered for SIDS. While some risk factors have been identified, it is not possible to predict which infants will be affected. Several theories about the etiology of the syndrome have been advanced and include sleep apnea, chronic hypoxia, cardiac electrical conduction abnormalities, immaturity of the nervous system, metabolic imbalances, and abnormal upper airway function.

As research into the cause continues, it is perhaps easier to identify what SIDS is not. The syndrome is not caused by external suffocation, for example from a blanket or pillow. It is not caused by vomiting and aspiration of vomitus. It is not the result of child abuse. It is important to recognize these facts and not make premature judgments about the circumstances surrounding an infant death while on the scene or immediately thereafter. Inappropriate responses by the paramedic increase the guilt and self-reproach of the parents. Though SIDS is not hereditary, children in the same family do have a somewhat higher incidence of occurrence.

The greatest incidence of SIDS occurs during the winter and early spring months. Male infants are slightly more at risk (60%). Also included in the at-risk group are premature infants, infants of young mothers, and low birth weight babies. Though SIDS occurs in all social strata, infants from lower socioeconomic groups have a higher incidence of occurrence.

Typically, the infant is discovered during the early morning hours. Frothy or blood-tinged fluids may be around the mouth, and vomitus may be in the mouth and trachea. The vomitus and aspiration represent a terminal event rather than a cause of death. The infant may appear in an unusual position because of muscle spasm at the time of death. Incontinence of bowel and bladder is common. Dependent lividity may be present depending on time of death. Death occurs quietly, and the parents or caretakers usually recall no sound of distress or struggle. The infant is most often described as healthy, although some have had symptoms of mild upper respiratory infection.

Diagnosis

The diagnosis of SIDS is made by ruling out specific causes of death at autopsy, by typical postmortem examination findings, and by excluding other disease processes. It is also confirmed by excluding pneumonia by chest radiograph, central nervous system hemorrhage by lumbar puncture, and septicemia by blood culture. Common findings at autopsy include intrathoracic petechiae, pulmonary congestion and edema, microscopic inflammatory changes in the trachea, and aspiration of gastric contents.

Management

Management of SIDS includes assisting the other victims of the syndrome, the parents. A resuscitation effort may reassure the parents that every attempt was made to save the infant. Despite physical evidence to the contrary, the parents often have difficulty believing that the child is dead. Do not falsely encourage parents, however; regardless of time down, resuscitation efforts are rarely, if ever, successful in true cases of SIDS. Each EMS system should have a protocol that addresses pediatric resuscitation. The decision to initiate or continue resuscitation may be made in conjunction with the medical control physician. Paramedics must be familiar with normal grief reactions and be prepared to deal with them. Reactions include shock, disbelief, denial, anger, rage, hostility, blame, guilt, self-reproach, feelings of inadequacy as a parent, helplessness, confusion, and fear. These reactions may normally continue for 1 to 2 years.

Parents need unconditional support from the paramedics who arrive on the scene. They should be provided with accurate information about what was done, both by the paramedics and hospital personnel. Closure is important to the grief process, and, after resuscitation efforts, the parents should be permitted to see and hold the infant if they desire to do so. An autopsy should be performed whenever possible to further confirm the diagnosis of SIDS. While obtaining history and background information about the child, the paramedic should not imply neglect on the part of the parents or give advice about what they should have done. Perceived accusations of failure to act as a responsible parent remain with the person and compound the guilt already present. At the hospital, information about SIDS should be given to the parents. Printed information from a SIDS resource center can be given to them to take home and review. Local and national organizations are available to provide support for grieving families of SIDS victims.

Seizures

Seizures are, of course, not specific to the pediatric age group. They are relatively common in childhood and cause frequent pediatric emergency calls. Seizures are frightening to observers at any time, and they are particularly distressing when the patient is a young child. Most grand mal types of seizures are self-limiting and require no direct intervention.

As with the adult patient, seizures may be caused by hypoxia, hypoglycemia, meningitis, head trauma, idiopathic epilepsy, toxic ingestion and exposure, tumors, drug toxicity, and failure to take anticonvulsant medications as prescribed. In addition, children are susceptible to febrile seizures caused by a high temperature.

Febrile Seizures

Febrile seizures occur most commonly between the ages of 6 months and 6 years. If the body temperature is elevated, fever should be considered as a possible predisposing factor for the seizure. Febrile seizures account for about 40% of all first seizures in children. Pharyngitis, tonsillitis, and otitis media (infection of the middle ear) are the most common illnesses associated with febrile seizures. Meningitis must always be considered as a possible associated infection. Irrespective of the suspected etiology, all pediatric patients who have suffered a seizure should be transported for evaluation. Febrile seizures are usually self-limiting and do not result in a serious condition.

Not all seizure activity resolves without serious consequence. Seizures may result in death from anoxia, hypoxic encephalopathy, or aspiration. ***Status epilepticus*** may produce any of these disastrous consequences. Status epilepticus is defined as continuous seizure activity for 20 to 30 minutes or more than two seizures without a lucid interval. Status epilepticus requires rapid intervention.

Seizures in children are not always manifested by grand mal and clonic-tonic types of activity. Children demonstrate all types of seizures, including grand mal, petit mal, focal or Jacksonian seizures, and psychomotor seizures. See Chapter 22 for a discussion of seizures.

Assessment

Assessment of the pediatric patient who has had a seizure requires a careful history. Try to determine the following information:

1. Is there a history of previous seizures? Has there been a diagnosis of idiopathic epilepsy?
2. Have there been previous seizures that have been associated with an elevated temperature?
3. Does the child have a fever at the present time?
4. How many seizures has the child had at this time?
5. How does the child act at this time?
6. Is there any history of head trauma, headache, stiff neck, endocrine disorder (*e.g.*, diabetes), or recent illness?
7. Is there a possibility of toxic ingestion?
8. Does the child take any medication?
9. Is there a history of lethargy or irritability before the seizure? (May indicate central nervous system infection or disorder.)
10. What is the description of the seizure activity?

During the physical examination, evaluate level of consciousness, adequacy of respirations, evidence of injury or head trauma on secondary survey, and signs of dehydration. Note if the body temperature appears to be elevated.

Management

The first priority of management is attention to the airway, breathing, and circulation. Assure airway patency and assist respiratory effort if needed. Do not attempt to use a bite block if the patient is in active seizure. Potential hypoxia due to seizures requires particular attention to airway management. Supplemental oxygen at 4 to 6 L/min is indicated. Suction as needed. Vital signs must be evaluated and monitored on a serial basis. Position the patient on the side and protect from further injury. If status epilepticus is present, initiate an intravenous (IV) line of $D_5 0.9\% NaCl$ or $D_5 LR$ at a keep-open rate en route to the hospital. Strip test for blood glucose; if the reading is less than 45, administer 2 to 4 mL/kg of 25% dextrose. If hypoglycemia is suspected for any reason (*e.g.*, newborn or child less than 1 year of age with first-time seizure), do not wait for the results of a strip test for blood glucose. Administer 25% dextrose immediately. If the seizure persists, diazepam 0.2 to 0.3 mg/kg IV push, slowly (over 3 minutes or until seizure activity subsides) may be indicated. The maximum dose of diazepam is 10 mg.

If fever is suspected as a cause of the seizure, cooling measures may be indicated. However, do not delay transport for cooling. Remove excess clothing (a natural tendency is for the parent to overdress or wrap the ill child). Apply cool wet towels en route.

In some locales, pediatric specialists prefer to use IV or intramuscular phenobarbital in the field setting to control prolonged seizures rather than IV diazepam. Pediatric seizure activity responds well to phenobarbital with less respiratory depression than may accompany diazepam use. Phenobarbital may also prevent recurring seizures.

Phenobarbital is administered at 3 to 5 mg/kg IV push, slowly (over 5–10 minutes).

Dehydration

Dehydration can develop rapidly in infants because of their small fluid reserves and results in serious consequences. Of key importance is to recognize the potential for dehydration and to transport for further evaluation and management. Contributing causes include fever, vomiting, and diarrhea.

The history should determine the presence of any of the contributing causes mentioned and the length of time they have persisted. Determine the frequency of vomiting and diarrhea. Dehydration may be classified as mild, moderate, or severe. The following signs and symptoms appear in varying degrees: dry mucous membranes, absence of tears, reduced skin turgor, depressed anterior fontanelle, sunken eyeballs, orthostatic hypotension, tachycardia, and hyperpnea. The severely dehydrated child may present in shock.

Management of dehydration in the field is minimal unless shock is present. Assure adequacy of airway, breathing, and circulation. Monitor vital signs and remain alert to changes suggestive of decreased circulatory status. If shock is present, initiate an IV line of normal saline or lactated Ringer's solution and transport rapidly. A fluid bolus of 20 mL/kg of either solution should be infused in less than 20 minutes. Reassess the patient and repeat the fluid bolus as necessary. Intravenous placement may be complicated by compromised vascular status. Do not spend excessive time trying to establish an IV line prior to transport.

Infectious Processes

The paramedic is generally not expected to diagnose and differentiate the various infectious processes. However, three of the more significant infections are briefly discussed here along with special considerations for each. The reader is referred to Chapter 26 for further discussion, including appropriate procedures for self-protection and infection control.

Meningitis

Meningitis is an infection of the tissues that cover the brain and spinal cord and is most commonly caused by either bacterial or viral organisms. Various bacteria may cause meningitis. *Haemophilus influenzae B* is a bacteria that causes meningitis and two-thirds of the cases are found in children under the age of 5. Bacterial and viral meningitis appears in all age groups. In the young patient, the clinical picture is often nonspecific with signs and symptoms that include fever, dehydration, lethargy, bulging fontanelle, irritability, loss of appetite, vomiting, seizures, respiratory distress, and cyanosis. Older children may exhibit the same symptoms as well as stiffness of the neck, *Kernig's sign* (pain on extension of the legs), and headaches. Ear infections are common. The child may have been ill for one to several days. Complications include cerebral edema with increased intracranial pressure and brain stem herniation, septic shock, and disseminated intravascular coagulation. When paramedics are summoned, the child usually appears acutely ill.

Management of the child with suspected meningitis involves maintaining the airway, breathing, and circulation, making the child comfortable, monitoring vital signs, and transport. Once the diagnosis has been confirmed, all emergency personnel who were in close contact with the patient should be notified and appropriate therapy instituted if bacterial meningitis is diagnosed.

Septicemia

Septicemia is a generalized infection of the bloodstream in which the patient appears seriously ill. It may be associated with a localized or focal infection, such as pneumonia or meningitis, or it may occur without an apparent source of infection in infants and susceptible children. Shock and disseminated intravascular coagulation are serious sequelae. History reveals that the child may have become ill suddenly, or the illness may have developed over several days. On physical examination, signs and symptoms include vomiting, lethargy, and irritability. The fontanelle in infants is usually normal. Fever is present initially; however, hypothermia develops and is a clinical sign suggestive of sepsis. Signs of shock include hypotension, cold clammy skin, mottling, cyanosis of the extremities, and a rapid thready pulse.

Management includes monitoring the airway, breathing, circulation, vital signs, positioning the child for comfort, and rapid transport. If shock is present, initiate an IV line of normal saline or lactated Ringer's solution and transport rapidly. A fluid bolus of 20 mL/kg of either solution should be infused in less than 20 minutes. Reassess the patient and repeat the fluid bolus as necessary. Do not spend excessive time trying to establish an IV line prior to transport.

Reye's Syndrome

Reye's syndrome was first recognized as a disease entity in 1963. As the name implies, Reye's is a syndrome or a collection of signs and symptoms associated with a disease process. The signs and symptoms constitute the clinical picture of the disease. Reye's syndrome is a disease process that affects multiple body systems. Damage to liver cells results in changes in protein metabolism and increased serum ammonia levels. Fatty acid levels also increase, leading to fatty infiltration of vital organs, including the brain. The final result is organ dysfunction and cerebral edema. No single etiologic factor has been identified; however, possible toxic, drug, viral, and metabolic causes have been implicated. Outbreaks tend to cluster during influenza B epidemics. In some cases, Reye's syndrome appears to be related to resolving chicken pox. Salicylate ingestion may be a predisposing factor. Often a history of gastroenteritis (especially in infants) is present, and a history of mild upper respiratory infection is common.

Reye's syndrome is a rare, acute, life-threatening condition. It affects all age groups, but the peak incidence is

6 years of age, with most cases occurring between 4 and 12 years. Incidence increases in fall and winter seasons and is higher in suburban and rural populations.

Early symptoms include nonspecific irritability, lethargy, confusion, and personality changes. A history of minor upper respiratory infection for 2 to 3 days is common. The spectrum of symptoms may begin with sudden onset of vomiting. Irrational behavior and hyperexcitability lead to progressive stupor and restlessness. Seizures and coma follow. Signs and symptoms encountered by the paramedic vary depending on the progression of the disease process.

On physical examination, the patient may have rapid and deep or irregular respirations and a subnormal temperature. Pupils are dilated and react sluggishly. Other signs and symptoms of increased intracranial pressure occur. Reye's syndrome can be rapidly fatal. Complications include respiratory failure, cerebral edema with herniation, cardiac arrhythmias, and acute pancreatitis. Most patients die of cerebral complications, such as herniation of the brain stem.

The diagnosis of Reye's syndrome is not made in the field. It is based on clinical and laboratory findings as well as signs and symptoms. Clinical staging of Reye's syndrome is shown in Table 29-3. Assessment in the field reveals a delirious child of unknown etiology. It is important to consider and rule out other causes, such as alcohol or drug ingestion.

Airway management is important, especially in the comatose patient. Oxygen should be administered at moderate to high flow, depending on patient status. Support ventilation and suction as necessary. Transport rapidly for further evaluation and treatment.

Respiratory Emergencies

Obstructed Airway

Respiratory emergencies represent one of the most common calls for emergency medical care for children. Respiratory distress may develop rapidly or over a period of time and usually requires immediate attention and intervention. The clinical picture and physical findings vary depending on the cause and type of obstruction. Upper airway problems interfere primarily with ventilation, while lower airway disorders can cause disturbances in both ventilation and perfusion. Normal respiration is not noisy. Breath sounds that indicate airway obstruction include wheezing, snoring, and stridor.

FOREIGN BODY. Children's natural curiosity and tendency to explore the environment by placing objects in their mouths frequently lead to the aspiration of foreign bodies. The onset of sudden respiratory distress and stridor should alert the paramedic to the possibility of airway obstruction by a foreign body. History may be helpful, but usually the aspiration was not observed. Foreign body aspiration occurs most commonly in the child between 6 months and 4 years of age. Common objects include coins, candy, buttons, beads, nuts, and pins. The symptoms presented depend on the location of the lodged object, its size, and the patency of the remaining airway. Classic findings include an acute episode of choking, gagging, coughing, and wheezing. Laryngotracheal obstruction results in acute life-threatening respiratory distress. Cyanosis and apnea may be present. Facial petechiae may occur as a result of increased intrathoracic pressure. Bronchial foreign bodies produce subacute obstruction.

Appropriate management depends on accurate assessment of respiratory status. The patient who has a partial upper airway obstruction and who is exchanging air adequately should be transported to definitive care for removal of the foreign body. Attempts to remove the obstruction in the field may cause complete obstruction. Likewise, attempts to remove a bronchial foreign body may result in a totally obstructed airway.

If inadequate air exchange is present, however, vigorous attempts must be made to clear the airway following the American Heart Association obstructed airway pro-

TABLE 29-3.
CLINICAL STAGING OF REYE'S SYNDROME

Effects	Stages				
	I	II	III	IV	V
Level of consciousness	Lethargy; follows verbal commands Behavioral changes	Combative/stupor; verbalizes inappropriately	Coma	Coma	Coma
Response to pain	Purposeful	Purposeful/nonpurposeful	Decorticate	Decerebrate	None
Pupillary reaction	Quick	Slow	Slow	Slow	None
Oculocephalic reflex (doll's eyes)	Normal	Conjugate deviation	Conjugate deviation	Inconsistent or absent	None
Posture	Normal	Normal	Decorticate	Decerebrate	Flaccid

tocols (see Appendix B). If these procedures are not rapidly successful, an attempt should be made to remove the obstruction with a laryngoscope and Magill forceps. After removal of the foreign body, apply moderate flow oxygen, monitor closely, and transport for evaluation. If attempts at removal are unsuccessful, translaryngeal jet ventilation (needle cricothyroidotomy) may be considered. This procedure is described in Chapter 10. Surgical cricothyroidotomy is generally contraindicated in children in the field because of the difficulty in performing the procedure in children and the high complication rate.

Complications of airway obstruction include respiratory arrest, cardiac arrhythmias, and cardiac arrest. Sinus bradycardia in an infant or child is a sign of hypoxia and is an indication for cardiac monitoring.

INJURIES TO THE FACE AND NECK. Injuries to the face and neck should alert the paramedic to potential obstruction of the upper airway and to possible aspiration of blood, teeth, or other material. Laryngeal fracture results when an unrestrained child is thrown against the dashboard of a car during sudden deceleration. If this injury is suspected, careful observation of the airway is required. Patient survey includes evaluation for subcutaneous crepitus (air in the interstitial space). Injuries also include chemical or thermal burns. The small upper airways in children can be rapidly compromised by minimal swelling.

Management of the traumatized airway includes careful suctioning, maneuvers to maintain an open airway, oxygen administration, and endotracheal intubation. If complete obstruction occurs with laryngeal fracture, a needle cricothyroidotomy may be indicated. If burns are suspected, respiratory status should be monitored carefully.

ANAPHYLAXIS. A third cause of upper airway obstruction or lower airway bronchospasm in children, though less common, is a systemic allergic reaction. Antigens that produce anaphylaxis may be ingested, inhaled, or injected. Common causative agents include antigen extracts used for desensitization, antibiotics (particularly penicillin), insect stings, foods (especially nuts, shellfish, eggs, and milk), aspirin, and inhaled allergens.

Upper airway symptoms include stridor, laryngeal and epiglottic edema, and obstruction. Lower airway bronchospasm causes coughing, wheezing, and severe distress. Complications include circulatory collapse and arrhythmias. Other systemic reactions are urticaria (hives), itching, nausea, vomiting, abdominal cramping, and diarrhea.

Management is directed at oxygenation and intubation if airway obstruction is present. Bronchospasm may be relieved with a subcutaneous injection of epinephrine 0.01 mg/kg of 1:1000 solution (maximum of 0.35 mg/dose). If shock is present, epinephrine should be administered IV or via endotracheal tube, using the 1:10,000 solution, 0.01 mg/kg repeated every 5 minutes. If shock is not present, initiate a maintenance IV fluid of $D_5 0.9\%NaCl$ or D_5LR at 4 mL/kg/hour for infants less than 10 kg or infuse 40 mL/hour for children more than 10 kg.

Croup

Croup, or *laryngotracheobronchitis*, is a viral infection that usually occurs during late fall or early winter months in children between the ages of 3 months and 3 years. Croup is a pediatric obstructive disease commonly encountered in the field. Symptoms occur primarily because of inflammation and edema in the subglottic area and may cause significant narrowing of the airway at the level of the cricoid cartilage (Fig. 29-2).

The onset of signs and symptoms is usually gradual, over a period of several days. Early symptoms include those of upper respiratory tract infection with mild temperature elevation. A characteristic barking cough or "*seal bark*" develops, followed by inspiratory stridor. The acute episode typically occurs at night or early in the morning. The patient usually is found sitting upright and refuses to lie down. Crying aggravates the signs and symptoms. Inflammation of the mucosa of the conducting airways may be present, and wheezing may occur. If respiratory obstruction progresses, nasal flaring and suprasternal and intercostal retractions occur, and breath sounds are decreased. Hypoxia causes the patient to be restless and anxious, and tachycardia develops. Cyanosis develops as a late sign. A mild attack may subside in a few hours but may recur for 2 or 3 nights in succession.

Management includes maintenance of a patent airway and supplemental oxygen. The child should be allowed to assume a position of comfort. Mild attacks frequently subside or improve after exposure to cool night air or cool mist from running a shower with the bathroom door closed. If respiratory distress is severe, racemic epineph-

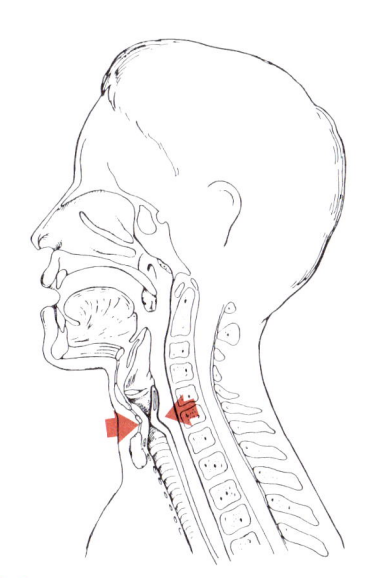

FIGURE 29-2.
Croup is a viral infection of the trachea.

rine should be administered in a solution of 0.3 to 0.5 mL in 4 mL of normal saline by updraft nebulizer. The patient should inhale the mist until all of the medication is gone. Rebound obstruction can occur after 15 to 30 minutes, and the need for racemic epinephrine frequently means the patient must be hospitalized.

Epiglottitis

Epiglottitis is one of the most frightening respiratory emergencies encountered by the paramedic. It is a potentially lethal disease that most commonly affects children between the ages of 3 and 7 years. Epiglottitis is a bacterial disease that has a sudden onset, usually over a few hours, and progresses rapidly. The hallmark of epiglottitis is a swollen *cherry-red* epiglottis that may rapidly obstruct the airway (Fig. 29-3). Symptoms include a high fever, difficulty and pain on swallowing, a muffled voice, a sore throat, and hypersecretion with subsequent drooling. The child may appear extremely ill, may be tachycardic, is usually found sitting upright, and is drooling. Breathing may be shallow, and, if respiratory distress is severe, nasal flaring and suprasternal, supraclavicular, and intercostal retractions may be present. Anxiety progresses to agitation and disorientation. Visualization of the oral cavity and pharynx may precipitate laryngospasm and complete airway obstruction; therefore, visualization of the airway must be avoided in any patient with potential epiglottitis.

Management priorities include rapid transport to an appropriate facility. Oxygen should be administered by mask, and the patient should be permitted to assume a position of comfort. Reassurance should be provided, and increased agitation should be avoided. The use of oropharyngeal airways and endotracheal intubation is contraindicated unless total airway obstruction occurs. In this situation, intubation is difficult if not impossible. Do not waste time with multiple attempts, but ventilate with a bag-valve-mask device and transport rapidly. Translaryngeal jet ventilation (needle cricothyrotomy) may be a beneficial technique in the rare event of complete obstruction. This procedure is described in Chapter 10.

Bronchiolitis

Bronchiolitis is a respiratory infection of young children that is characterized by wheezing. It is most commonly caused by a virus and occurs with the highest frequency in the winter months in children younger than 2 years of age. The highest incidence occurs in the 2- to 8-month age group. Some authorities restrict the diagnosis of bronchiolitis to children younger than 1 year of age. In this condition, the bronchioles become inflamed, and the resulting narrowing of the airway produces expiratory obstruction and air trapping (Fig. 29-4). Mucus plugging may lead to atelectasis. Bronchiolitis may also be caused by an allergy or a combination of allergy and infection.

The clinical picture includes low-grade fever, tachypnea, tachycardia, cough, expiratory wheezing, and prolonged expiration. Signs of respiratory distress, such as intercostal and subcostal retractions, nasal flaring, and cyanosis, develop. Other evidence of viral infection, such as otitis media, may be seen. The patient frequently has a history of a mild upper respiratory infection with nasal discharge and sneezing. If hypoxia becomes marked, the child may become restless and apprehensive. Complications include dehydration, pneumonia, pneumothorax, apnea, and respiratory failure.

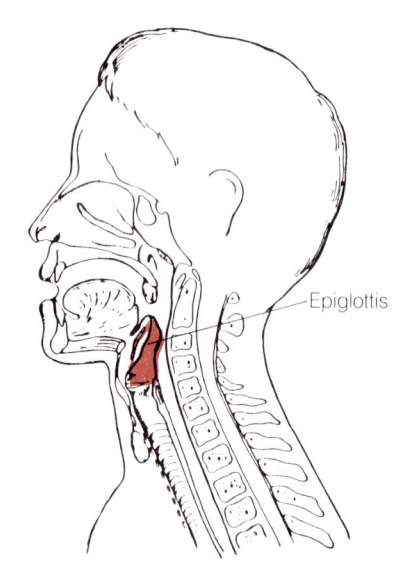

FIGURE 29-3.
Epiglottitis is a bacterial infection of the epiglottis.

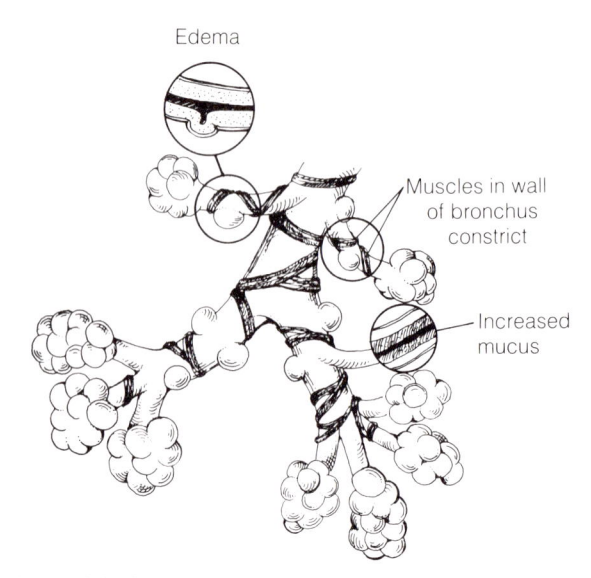

FIGURE 29-4.
Air trapping in bronchiolitis and asthma.

Assessment of the child should include determination of previously identified allergies, family history of allergies, and a description of the onset of symptoms. Bronchiolitis produces similar symptoms to bronchial asthma. Asthma, however, rarely occurs in children younger than 1 year of age.

It is important not to confuse lower airway obstruction with upper airway obstruction. Adequate history and assessment reveals two different clinical pictures, including onset, signs of infection, and unilateral vs. bilateral air trapping.

Management of bronchiolitis is directed at reducing hypoxia. Humidified oxygen should be delivered by mask if possible. If fatigue develops, ventilatory assistance may be required. The child should be allowed to assume a position of comfort. Although bronchiolitis is not a bronchospastic disease, occasionally children with bronchiolitis also have accompanying bronchospasm. If bronchospasm is severe, subcutaneous injection of epinephrine 0.01 mg/kg of 1:1000 solution (maximum dose of 0.35 mg/dose) may be given, although response to epinephrine is often poor. Albuterol 0.05 to 0.1 mg/kg in 2 mL of normal saline by updraft nebulizer may be indicated in the child older than 6 months of age. The patient should inhale the mist until all of the medication is gone. Racemic epinephrine, 0.3 to 0.5 mL in 4 mL of normal saline by updraft nebulizer, is used less commonly. Vital signs, particularly respiratory rate and function, and cardiac rhythm should be monitored while the patient is being transported.

Asthma

Asthma is a reactive airway disease characterized by bronchoconstriction that results from autonomic dysfunction or sensitizing agents (see Fig. 29-4). Precipitating factors include allergens (*e.g.*, foods, medications, environmental agents), exercise, irritants, viral infection, weather changes, and emotional stress. **Status asthmaticus** is the failure to respond to an appropriate therapeutic regimen initially. An asthmatic attack may result in hypoxia, hypercapnia, acidosis, dehydration, and electrolyte imbalance. Asthma is relatively common in children and is the most common chronic disease in the pediatric age group.

On physical examination, the patient demonstrates labored respirations, retractions, nasal flaring, tachypnea, and tachycardia. Diffuse inspiratory and expiratory wheezing can be heard in all fields. Localized wheezing suggests obstruction by a foreign body. The chest is hyperinflated and hyperresonant. The expiratory phase is prolonged. As the attack progresses, inspiratory wheezes develop. Hypoxia and hypercapnia may produce agitation, confusion, or drowsiness. Cyanosis and falling blood pressure are late findings. As fatigue increases, the child becomes more lethargic and eventually comatose. If complete closure of the small airways occurs, wheezing becomes diminished or absent.

Peak flow readings are usually not taken on children, since they are frequently inaccurate because of the child's lack of cooperation. If a peak flow reading is taken (see Chapter 19), the outcome is used as an assessment tool to test the effectiveness of bronchodilation. If the peak flow is higher after bronchodilation therapy, therapy generally is not repeated.

History should include previous episodes of this nature, routine medications, any treatment or medication administered for this attack, and previous hospitalization for asthma. It should also be determined when the attack began, the amount of fluid intake, and if there is any history of recent respiratory infection. The attack may have begun with nasal and conjunctival itching, sneezing, and nasal discharge. Mild cough and tightening of the chest precede increased coughing and wheezing. Fever is absent or minimal. Complications include pneumonia, atelectasis, respiratory failure, dehydration, cardiac arrhythmias, and cardiac arrest.

Management includes humidified oxygen at 4 to 6 L/min and position of comfort. If the attack is severe, albuterol may be administered by updraft nebulizer. Mix 0.05 to 0.1 mg/kg of solution for inhalation in 2 mL of normal saline in the nebulizer. The child should inhale as much of the mist as possible. Children less than 5 years of age may be given a treatment for half the time, about 3 minutes. If the child is uncooperative, epinephrine may be administered subcutaneously, 0.01 mg/kg of 1:1000 preparation (maximum of 0.35 mg/dose). Careful consideration must be given to onboard medications before administration of epinephrine. Epinephrine should not be given if the heart rate is greater than 180 beats per minute.

Theophylline ethylenediamine (Aminophylline) may also be considered for status asthmaticus in the child older than 1 year of age. It should first be determined if the patient has taken any theophylline-containing compounds, including the amount and time of last dose and duration of therapy. Theophylline products include Marax, Primatene, Quibron, Slo-Phyllin, Slo-bid, Somophyllin, Tedral, and Theo-Dur. If the patient has not received theophylline products in the last 36 hours, the loading dose of theophylline ethylenediamine is 6 mg/kg diluted in 100 ml of $D_5 0.9\%NaCl$ placed in a calibrated volume set, given IV over a 20-minute period. The dose is 1 mg/kg IV over 20 minutes if the patient has taken theophylline products in the last 36 hours.

If respiratory distress is marked, ventilatory assistance may be required. Monitor cardiac rhythm and vital signs with particular attention to respiratory status and level of consciousness. The previously agitated child who becomes calm and drowsy may be developing increasing hypoxia, respiratory failure, and impending arrest.

Cardiopulmonary Arrest

Cardiopulmonary arrest in infants and children is primarily related to shock or respiratory events and is rarely caused by primary cardiac disorders. It is usually secondary to hypoxia and respiratory arrest. Therefore, management targets airway control and appropriate ventilatory technique. Cardiopulmonary arrest may be the end point of any of the respiratory emergencies discussed in this chapter. Other contributing causes include near drowning, poisoning, shock, and central nervous system depression or injury.

Since cardiopulmonary arrest in children typically follows a prolonged period of hypoxemia, chances of a successful outcome are poor. Infants and children demonstrate a greater ability to survive and recover from respiratory arrest. In any event, resuscitation measures should be instituted if there is any question about down time or viability of the pediatric patient. Even if chances of survival appear poor, such as in a suspected SIDS death, transportation with life support measures may provide support for the parents and demonstrates that all possible attempts were made to save the child.

If the arrest is secondary to trauma, rapid transport to the appropriate facility with maintenance of an open airway, oxygenation and respiratory support, IV insertion, and pneumatic anti-shock garment application en route are indicated.

A complete discussion of cardiopulmonary resuscitation techniques is not included in this text. The reader is referred to the current American Heart Association Standards and Guidelines for Cardiopulmonary Resuscitation and Emergency Cardiac Care for recommended procedures and techniques. A summary of these guidelines is shown in Appendix B.

Shock

Shock has been defined as a state of inadequate tissue perfusion that results in the inability of the cells to maintain function. The pediatric patient may present in hypovolemic shock that results from blunt or penetrating trauma, burns, and dehydration due to vomiting and diarrhea. Distributive or vasogenic shock is associated with an abnormality in the distribution of blood flow and may be caused by spinal cord injury, anaphylaxis, or sepsis. Cardiogenic shock that results from myocardial insufficiency or cardiac obstruction may occur but is uncommon.

Relatively small amounts of fluid loss may be critical in the pediatric patient. The amount of body fluid and the circulating blood volume are larger per kilogram in the child than the adult. While the circulating volume in the average adult is 5000 mL, a 13-kg child has an average volume of about 1000 mL. If the volume of blood lost from an injury is equal in both the adult and child, the adult may suffer no or minimal effects, while the child has lost a significantly larger proportion of blood volume and may be in hemorrhagic shock.

Clinical signs of shock develop as the total circulating volume is reduced by 10% to 20%. In acute blood loss, supine blood pressure may remain normal with a 20% to 25% loss. Evaluation of early signs, including altered level of consciousness, agitation, and delayed capillary refill, should be repeated frequently. If no contraindication exists (e.g., spinal injury) orthostatic vital signs should be obtained. This is performed by placing the child in a sitting or semisitting position. Supine blood pressure tends to be maintained in the previously healthy child because of excellent vascular tone. Consequently, by the time supine blood pressure changes appear, a significant amount of volume may already have been lost. As the shock state continues, the heart rate increases, and the pulse becomes weak and thready. The skin becomes cool and moist, and peripheral vascular collapse occurs. The patient becomes less responsive, and coma ensues.

Management of the child in shock, or the child in whom shock is anticipated, begins with 100% oxygen. Establish an IV line with the largest needle or catheter possible. Since hypovolemia is the most common cause of shock in children, initiate an IV line of normal saline or lactated Ringer's solution and transport rapidly. A fluid bolus of 20 mL/kg of either solution is infused in less than 20 minutes. Reassess the patient and repeat the fluid bolus as necessary. Do not spend excessive time trying to establish an IV line on the scene. Intravenous placement may be complicated by compromised vascular status. Apply an appropriate size pneumatic anti-shock garment and monitor vital signs carefully. Support respirations as necessary. Keep the patient warm to prevent hypothermia, which significantly increases oxygen demands and contributes to acidosis.

Trauma

Injuries are the leading cause of death in the pediatric patient. They account for about 44% of the deaths between the ages of 1 and 4 years. In decreasing order of frequency, categories include motor vehicle accidents, drowning, burns, firearms, and poisoning. For those younger than 1 year of age, leading causes of death involve poisons, suffocation, and motor vehicles.

The approach to managing the injured child includes the same priorities that it does for the adult patient:

1. Maintain airway and establish cervical spine precautions.
2. Evaluate respiratory status and support ventilation as necessary.
3. Evaluate circulatory status and support as necessary. Control hemorrhage. Anticipate potential life-threatening internal hemorrhage.
4. Manage shock.
5. Assess level of consciousness.
6. Perform a secondary survey and immobilization if the patient is not in a critical condition. Do not focus on obvious injuries, perform a thorough evaluation.

7. Transport with continuous monitoring and reassessment.

If the child is conscious, proceed as usual with the examination, introducing yourself and explaining what you are about to do. A calm, firm approach helps allay the child's fears and gain cooperation. If possible, do not separate the child from the parents or care givers. Separation increases both the child's and parent's anxiety and sense of fear. Pediatric injuries are particularly stressful for the parent, and the paramedic can provide support and reassurance.

Special considerations for the traumatized pediatric patient include the following:

Head injuries: Children experience better neurologic recovery from head injury than adults do. Diffuse cerebral edema may occur. Increased intracranial pressure should be managed by aggressive hyperventilation when altered mental status appears.

Chest injuries: Pulmonary contusions are common because of the mechanism of many childhood accidents. Flail chest occurs less frequently than in adults, since the child's ribs are more flexible. Trauma to the heart and intrathoracic vessels is uncommon.

Abdominal injuries: Liver injuries are common in children because of the relatively larger size of the organ, as well as the relative lack of protection offered by immature abdominal muscles. Injury to the spleen is also common. Cases of blunt trauma should be evaluated carefully for possible injury to the liver or spleen.

Burns: Infants are at higher risk for complications from burn injury. Inhalation injuries may rapidly compromise airway patency.

Child Abuse

Child abuse is a form of domestic violence in which a child or adolescent is maltreated by a parent, guardian, or other caretaker. Child abuse is not new. However, the recognition and reporting of the problem have dramatically increased over the past 20 to 25 years. It is difficult to establish with accuracy the frequency of child abuse. Reports estimate that 10% of the injures seen in the hospital emergency department to children younger than 5 years of age are due to abuse. Child abuse causes about 2000 deaths per year in the United States.

While abuse can occur in any age group, the majority of cases occur in children younger than age 6. Complications include death, permanent physical damage, neurologic sequelae, and psychological and emotional damage.

The four types of abuse are physical abuse or nonaccidental trauma, emotional or psychological abuse, sexual abuse, and neglect. Physical abuse involves physical injury, such as fractures, hematomas, lacerations, and burns. The abuse was inflicted by a relative in 90% of the cases. Other potential abusers include the mother's boyfriend, a baby-sitter, and, rarely, a sibling. Child discipline that leads to bruises or other injuries is considered abuse. Other injuries that result from abuse include central nervous system trauma (especially subdural hematomas), internal injuries from visceral trauma, sensory organ injury, dental trauma, poisoning, and intentional starvation.

Emotional abuse results from withholding or depriving the child of normal emotional and psychological nurturing. The child consistently feels unwanted, unloved, and rejected. The child is usually told directly or indirectly that he or she is worthless and a bad child.

Sexual abuse is being recognized as a problem of previously unrevealed proportions. It may be in the form of molestation, touching, or fondling of a child's genitals or asking the child to do so to the adult. This category also includes pornography. Sexual intercourse is a second type of abuse and includes vaginal, rectal, or oral penetration. In this situation, the child is enticed into sexual activity with a family member or other person. In the third type of sexual abuse, the child is forced into sexual intercourse by threats of physical violence (family-related rape). This type is least common. Without intervention, molestation eventually leads to sexual intercourse.

Some cases of sexual abuse occur over a long period of time, for example years, but the majority happen over a shorter time span. It occurs equally in all socioeconomic groups, is somewhat more common with stepfathers than fathers, and occurs with similar frequency in all pediatric age groups. Most sexual abusers are males.

Child neglect includes failure to thrive in infants and young children. Excluding organic disorders, the main cause of failure to thrive is lack of enough food. The mother may pay inadequate attention to the child's nutritional needs or may dislike the baby and withhold food. These children are usually emotionally deprived as well.

Child neglect may also include failure to provide medical attention for specific illness or injury or on a routine preventative basis. Hygiene is neglected, the child appears unwashed, and clothing may be inappropriate for the environment. Untreated skin infections and severe diaper rash in infants are common. The child's education may also be neglected, and the parent leaves the child unattended for long periods of time without regard to safety or physical needs.

Characteristics of the Abused Child

Children who are abused are often seen as special for a variety of reasons. The child may require additional care because of chronic illness, physical handicap, or retardation. They may be seen as more demanding of time and attention, such as a premature baby or the "difficult" or exceptionally "gifted" child. The infant or child who cries frequently and is not easily comforted is seen as demanding as well. Physical abuse is somewhat more common in boys, perhaps because of their active nature and tendency to appear more trying. Sexual abuse is more common among girls. The quiet child who is not openly expressive is also at greater risk, as is the child who is not what the parents wanted or expected, for example the wrong sex (a girl instead of a boy). The illegitimate child may also be more likely to be abused when sacrifices in career or schooling have been made for an unplanned and often unwanted child.

Characteristics of Child Abusers

Although any person has the potential to abuse a child in particular circumstances, certain characteristics increase the likelihood of realizing that potential. Child abuse is not restricted to particular socioeconomic, religious, ethnic, educational, or occupational groups. It is more common in lower socioeconomic classes because of the number of stress factors that occur, such as unemployment, poverty, and poor living conditions. Episodes of abuse often begin as discipline but are escalated by anger. The child abuser has frequently been a victim of abuse and repeats learned behavior patterns.

Abusers may have unrealistic expectations of the child and may be perfectionists. The concept of strict discipline, including a military or law enforcement background or strict religious beliefs, can lead to abusive situations. Abusers see themselves as unworthy, isolated, and without a support network and feel helpless yet unwilling to seek assistance. Dissatisfaction with a marriage or relationship may be present. The parent who feels the child will provide a source of love may find disappointment and frustration. Coping mechanisms to deal with financial difficulties, relationship problems, and unemployment are poorly developed. Substance abuse is a complicating factor.

Child abuse does not equal a lack of love. The majority of abusing parents care for the child they mistreat. However, in the stress of recurring family crises, the abuser is unable to cope with the situation and acts out against the child.

Assessment of Child Abuse

Paramedics may be called to treat a child because of injuries or problems that resulted from abuse or neglect directly, or they may become suspicious of abuse while called to a home for other reasons. During assessment, the following indicators of abuse and neglect may be detected and should alert the paramedic:

- Evidence of bruises in various stages of healing, especially old and new bruises
- Bruises, burns, or welts in the shape of an object used to inflict injury (Figs. 29-5 and 29-6)
- Injuries not compatible with the child's ability at that age
- Immersion burns on ankles, buttocks, and so on (Fig. 29-7)

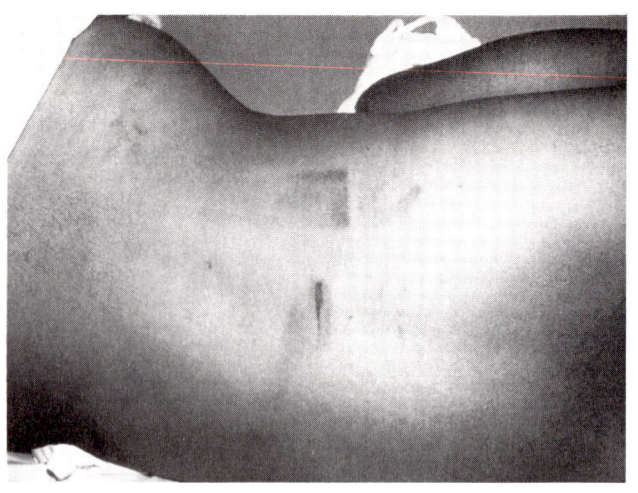

FIGURE 29–5.
Bruises in the shape of a belt buckle are shown across the back of this child. (Schmitt BD: Child Abuse/Neglect: The Visual Diagnosis of Non-Accidental Trauma and Failure to Thrive. Elk Grove Village, IL, American Academy of Pediatrics, 1979)

- Injuries that do not match with the reported mechanism of injury
- Bald patches where the hair has been pulled from the scalp
- Bruises to the face, neck, back, chest, buttocks, and thighs
- Evidence or history of old fractures and the presence of spiral-type fractures from twisting of an extremity

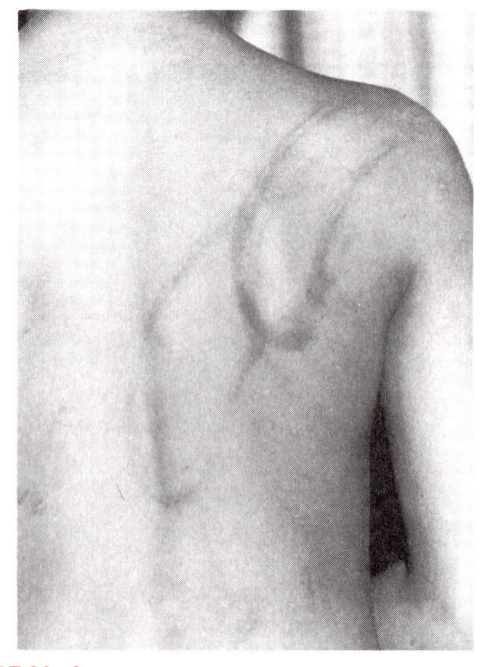

FIGURE 29–6.
Welts on the back of this child were caused by a whipping with an electrical cord. (Schmitt BD: Child Abuse/Neglect: The Visual Diagnosis of Non-Accidental Trauma and Failure to Thrive. Elk Grove Village, IL, American Academy of Pediatrics, 1979)

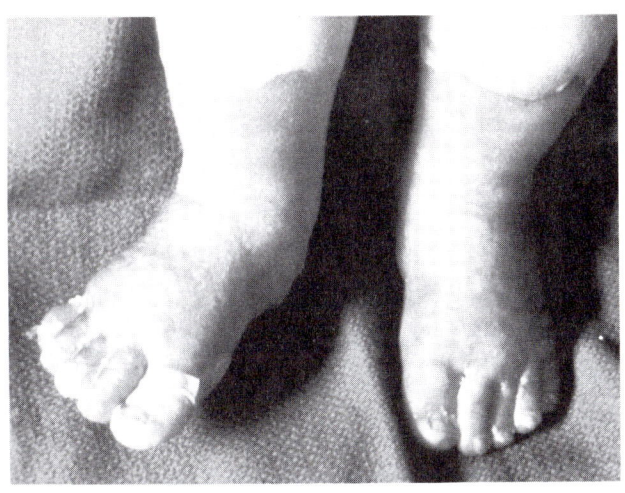

FIGURE 29–7.
"Sock burns" are immersion burns caused by the child being held down in scalding water (e.g., a bathtub). (Schmitt BD: Child Abuse/Neglect: The Visual Diagnosis of Non-Accidental Trauma and Failure to Thrive. Elk Grove Village, IL, American Academy of Pediatrics, 1979)

- Injuries that appear in patterns, such as from cigarette burns (Fig. 29-8) or teeth marks, that suggest nonaccidental infliction; rope marks or burns may be present
- Injuries to the mouth in infants that may result from force during feedings
- Undernourished and uncared for appearance
- Signs of abdominal distention in infants
- Poor hygiene, inappropriate dress
- Withdrawn, apathetic behavior
- The child appears fearful but submits to treatment and does not cry

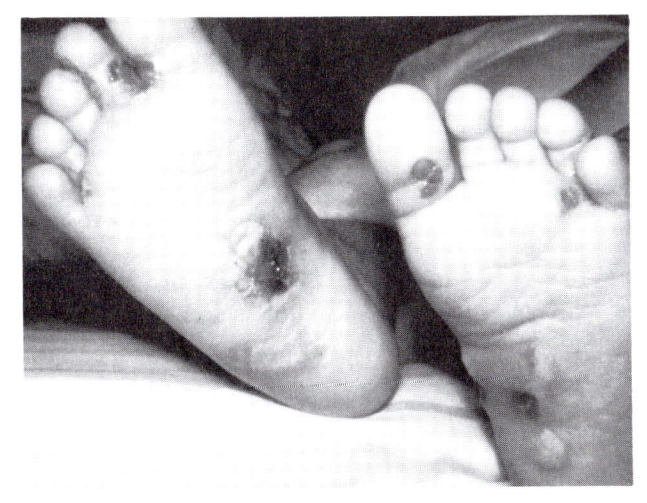

FIGURE 29–8.
Cigarette burns inflict painful second- and third-degree burns. (Schmitt BD: Child Abuse/Neglect: The Visual Diagnosis of Non-Accidental Trauma and Failure to Thrive. Elk Grove Village, IL, American Academy of Pediatrics, 1979)

- The child has been abandoned or left unattended for long periods

In addition, there may have been a delay in seeking treatment for the injury. The parent's story may be inconsistent over time, and the parent is evasive regarding details of the accident. They may label the child as careless, accident prone, with frequent injuries. The spectrum of parental reactions is broad and may include anger and hostility at the child, each other, or emergency care workers. They may appear quiet and withdrawn or aggressive. They may overreact to the situation and display great concern or underreact and minimize the injuries and events.

Assessment of the potential child abuse victim includes the normal trauma evaluation. Observations of the environment, affect and behavior of both the caretaker and the child, and the caretaker-child interactions are especially important. The child should be carefully observed for signs of injury, especially evidence of bruises or other injuries in various stages of healing. An abused child usually protects the abusing parent and does not truthfully relate how the injury occurred. This response may be out of love (abused children still love the abusing parent), protection of the parent, or fear of further injury.

Victims of sexual abuse should receive limited physical evaluation. As with any sexual abuse victim, limited intervention is indicated in the absence of threat to life. A detailed history is obtained in the emergency department and need not be repeated in the field. Provide reassurance and a safe environment.

Establish rapport with both the child and parents. Talk to the child on the child's level, for example kneel or sit down. Be alert to verbal clues from the child and to inconsistencies in the parent's description of events.

Management of the Abused Child

Management of the abused child begins with attention to current injuries. When abuse is suspected, it is not the paramedic's responsibility to confront the parent or suspected abuser. The paramedic should ensure, however, that the child receives a medical evaluation. This requirement generally involves transportation to the emergency department. Do not restrict the parents from accompanying the child to the hospital, but do not permit them to transport the child by private auto.

The paramedic must report the findings and observations to the emergency department staff. In addition, a written report should be completed as mandated by state statute. All states have laws that require professionals who deal with children in their work to report suspected child abuse. It is the paramedic's responsibility to be familiar with state requirements and local procedures for verbal and written reports. Paramedics should not assume that another agency, for example law enforcement or the hospital, will report the case and therefore relieve them of the responsibility. It is important for paramedics to record their own observations.

Management of the abusive situation, especially when severe physical injuries or sexual abuse has occurred, can be especially difficult for emergency workers. The natural tendency is to protect the child, and the anger produced when faced with such abusive situations is difficult not to express. It is important, however, to maintain a nonjudgmental attitude to enlist cooperation in providing appropriate care. Also, the suspected abuser may not be the one who has inflicted the injuries. The dynamics of the situations that produce the abusive outbursts are usually complex and not apparent during initial evaluation of the child. The long-term goal of management is to treat both the child and the abuser, to break the cycle that produces abuse, and to improve the functioning of the family unit. Long-term effects of abuse on the child can be minimized by successful treatment in the family setting.

TECHNIQUES OF MANAGEMENT

Airway Management

Airway adjuncts must be selected by appropriate size for the pediatric patient. Tables that estimate appropriate equipment size may be useful, but the most accurate determinations result from evaluation of the size of the child's airway. Types of adjuncts do not vary from adult to pediatric, only their sizes and considerations in use vary. Therefore, this chapter does describe the basic methods of use detailed in Chapter 10. However, some helpful hints in selecting the most appropriate adjuncts and maintaining the airway are included.

Small pediatric airways may become easily plugged by mucus, blood, and vomitus. Careful attention to clearing the airway is mandatory. Pediatric suction catheters are also proportionately smaller and increase the difficulty of removing secretions. Remember that, when suctioning, oxygen is removed as well as secretions. Therefore, adult suction catheters should not be used on pediatric patients.

The pediatric airway varies anatomically somewhat from the adult. The tongue is relatively larger, and the airway is smaller and more flexible. The glottis is higher in the neck. These differences are relevant when positioning the head to maintain an open airway and when performing endotracheal intubation.

Basic life support may be effectively administered without the use of airway adjuncts. Mouth-to-mouth ventilation is an acceptable method of ventilation and should be initiated without delay for the selection of adjunctive equipment.

The pediatric patient with upper airway obstruction from severe croup, epiglottitis, or laryngeal edema related to anaphylaxis may be difficult or impossible to intubate. Adequate air exchange may be possible using mouth-to-mask ventilation or a bag–valve–mask device.

Oropharyngeal Airway

The selection of the appropriate size oropharyngeal airway is especially important for the child. An airway that is too large may obstruct the airway or displace the tongue into the pharynx, producing obstruction.

Nasopharyngeal Airway

Nasopharyngeal airways offer the advantage of being better tolerated in the patient who is not comatose. However, the smaller pediatric sizes may become easily occluded.

Resuscitation Mask

To provide an adequate seal, the resuscitation mask must be an appropriate size for the child's face. Masks with soft air-filled cuffs are usually preferable for forming an effective seal. If the only mask available is larger than required, a better seal usually is obtained by turning it upside down or putting the narrow end toward the chin.

Resuscitation Bags

All resuscitation bags should be equipped with a reservoir to allow for delivery of 100% oxygen. The paramedic unit should stock both infant and child bags and masks. Bags used for resuscitation should not be equipped with a pressure-relief or "pop-off" valve, or the valve should be easily occluded, since the pressures required for ventilation during cardiopulmonary resuscitation may exceed the pop-off limit. Resuscitation bags deliver considerably less volume than mouth-to-mouth ventilation. Lung compliance is more easily monitored using mouth-to-mouth or mouth-to-mask technique. Exercise caution using either technique.

Endotracheal Intubation

Pediatric intubation is relatively uncommon in most response areas. If the paramedic does not feel confident in the procedure, an attempt should be made to maintain the airway by more basic measures. When intubation is attempted, select the appropriate size endotracheal tube and laryngoscope blade. Since children's sizes at the same age may vary considerably, choose equipment based on patient size. Uncuffed tubes are generally used in children younger than 8 years of age, and cuffed tubes are used in older children. Guidelines for selection of endotracheal tubes and suction catheters are shown in Table 29-4.

Do not hyperflex the child's neck backward during the intubation. The head should be in the "*sniffing*" position with the neck slightly flexed backward. Intubation attempts should occur after preoxygenating the patient and should not last more than 30 seconds. Monitor the heart rate continuously. If bradycardia develops, discontinue attempts and ventilate with a bag-valve-mask device. Brady-

TABLE 29-4.
GUIDELINES FOR SELECTION OF ENDOTRACHEAL TUBES AND SUCTION CATHETERS*

Age	Endotracheal Tube (mm)	Suction Catheter (French)
Premature	2.5	5
Newborn	3.0	6
6 months	3.5	8
1 year	4.0	8
3 years	4.5	8
5 years	5.0	10
8 years	6.0	10
12 years	6.5	10
16 years	7.0	10

*One size larger and one size smaller should be allowed for individual variations.

cardia is a heart rate of less than 80 beats per minute in infants and less than 60 beats per minute in a child.

A straight laryngoscope blade may be preferred for infant intubation. The tip of the blade is positioned under the epiglottis, allowing it to be lifted up and the vocal cords visualized. A straight or curved blade may be used for children. The tip of the curved blade is placed into the vallecula and lifted, allowing for visualization of the glottic opening. Guidelines for laryngoscope blades are shown in Table 29-5. Visualization may be enhanced by slight elevation or padding under the head and by gentle pressure over the larynx. After intubation, evaluate tube placement thoroughly in the upper and lower lung fields and over the epigastrium. Observe for rise and fall of the chest, condensation in the tube, and improvement in skin color. Confirmation of correct tube placement is imperative. Secure the tube adequately and avoid movement of the head and neck, which causes the endotracheal tube to move. Remember that, in the infant, even a small amount of movement may displace the tube.

Cricothyroidotomy

Surgical cricothyroidotomy is not recommended in children because of anatomical differences from the adult and the risk of incising highly vascular tissue. The technique of translaryngeal jet ventilation (needle cricothyroidotomy) may be considered with a 14 gauge over-the-needle catheter. The procedure is performed the same as in the adult patient (see Chapter 10). A high-pressure source of oxygen and a mechanism to control delivery are required for effective ventilation.

Intravenous Insertion

The basic technique of establishing an IV infusion is the same for both the adult and pediatric patient. Attention to technique in performing the venipuncture, aseptic precautions, and securing the IV are the same. Site selection may vary with the size of the pediatric patient. Other variables include choice of fluids and, to some extent, selection of equipment.

Volume overload, especially in the small child, is a serious potential problem. The rate of fluid administration must be carefully monitored. Adjuncts to assist in limiting fluid administration in the younger patient include the microdrip or minidrip IV tubing, which delivers 60 drops per milliliter. Regular or macrodrip sets (which delivers 10 drops per minute) may be used for the older child when large volumes are required. In addition, a calibrated volume set is a device placed in-line between the IV bag and the tubing (Fig. 29-9) that allows a controlled volume of fluid, for example 100 or 150 mL, to be administered to the patient. The chamber may be filled with a lesser amount of fluid as well. While this device does not prevent rapid infusion of the fluid in the chamber, it prevents administration of the entire contents of the IV bag. The disadvantage of the volume set in the field is the lowering of the fluid chamber in relation to the patient. The ambulance roof does not typically allow for the additional height sometimes required to permit the IV fluid to infuse by gravity.

Selection of Needles and Cannulas

In the pediatric patient, IVs may be started using an over-the-needle catheter or a scalp vein or butterfly needle. Though easier to use and gain access to a vein than a traditional needle, the scalp vein needle has the disadvantage of potentially puncturing the vein once in place and infiltrating. Both catheters and scalp vein needles must be securely taped and the extremity immobilized to an arm board, or other means of restraint must be applied. Intravenous lines become easily dislodged in the active or restless child.

Intravenous Fluids

Intravenous solutions in the field are primarily used for venous access but also serve to maintain fluid balance. The maintenance IV fluid of choice for children contains both electrolytes and dextrose. Dextrose is indicated since the nutritional reserves of the child are limited and may be

TABLE 29-5.
GUIDELINES FOR LARYNGOSCOPE BLADES

Age	Blade Size
Newborn to 3 years	No. 1 straight Miller
3 years to adolescence	No. 2 straight Miller or curved Macintosh
Adolescence	No. 3 curved Macintosh

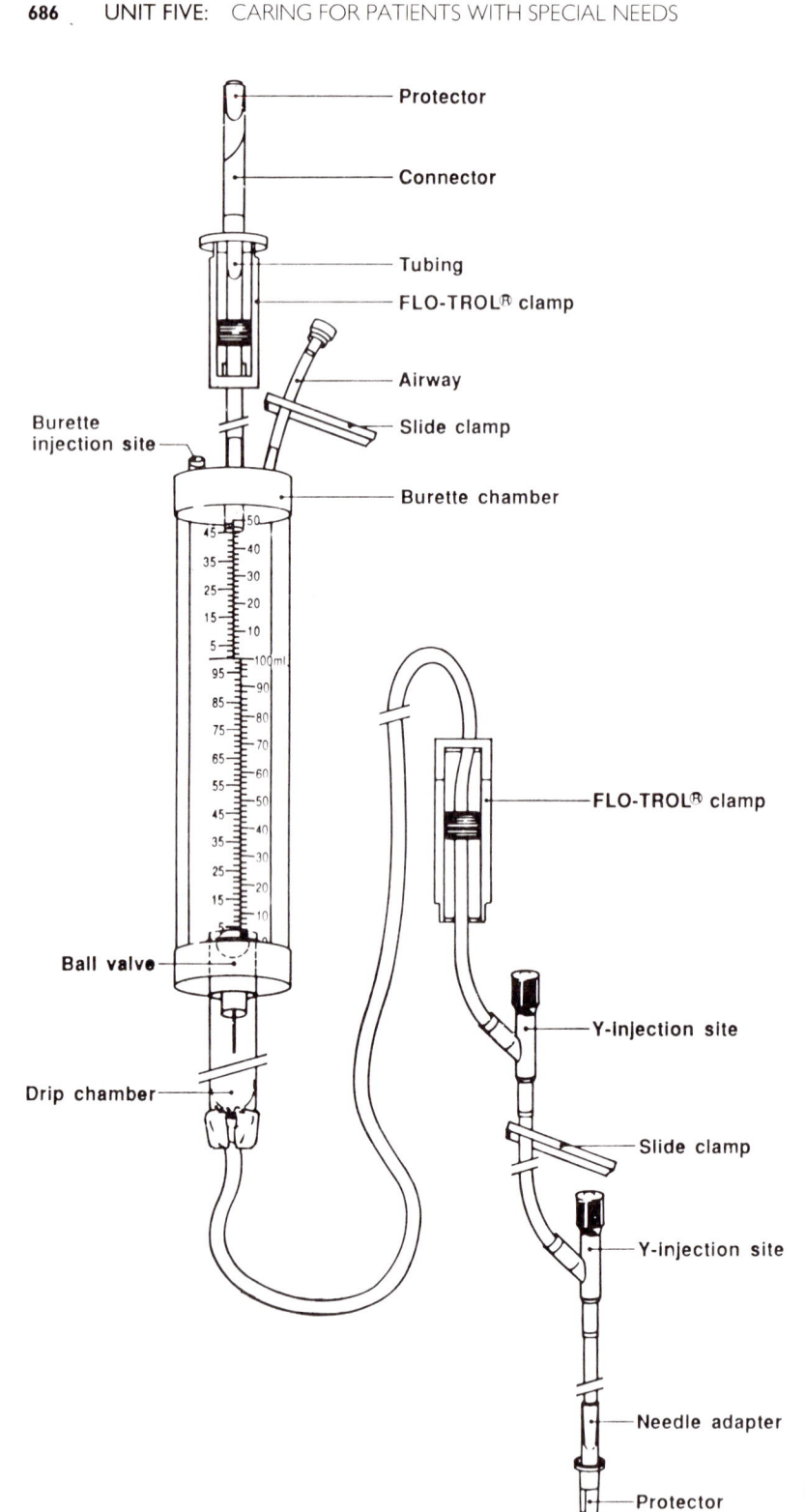

686 UNIT FIVE: CARING FOR PATIENTS WITH SPECIAL NEEDS

FIGURE 29–9.
A calibrated volume set allows for a controlled volume of fluid.

taxed during illness or injury. For routine pediatric IV therapy, $D_5 0.9\%NaCl$ or D_5LR should be available. Both solutions are hypertonic, providing fluid and glucose and maintaining electrolyte balance. To prevent the possibility of fluid overload and to maintain fluid balance during transport, the following rates are recommended: infants less than 10 kg, infuse 4 mL/kg per hour; children more than 10 kg, infuse 40 mL per hour. Stock should include 250- or 500-mL bags. D_5W is not appropriate for the pediatric patient. D_5W is an isotonic solution but becomes hypotonic once it enters the bloodstream and, therefore, can contribute to overhydration and electrolyte shifts. Children need the electrolytes available in $D_5 0.9\%NaCl$ and D_5LR, as well as glucose, because they have greater glucose needs and fewer glucose stores.

However, when volume expansion is necessary, IV fluids should not include glucose because of the possibility of inducing hyperglycemia and subsequent osmotic diuresis. Therefore, normal saline or lactated Ringer's solution are the fluids of choice for fluid resuscitation. In the patient with suspected hypovolemic shock (*e.g.*, from dehydration or trauma), an initial fluid bolus of 20 mL/kg should be infused in less than 20 minutes. The patient should then be reassessed. If the signs and symptoms of shock persist, the fluid bolus should be repeated as long as the child's breath sounds remain clear and the liver does not become enlarged and firm. As much as 60 to 80 mL/kg of fluids may be required for stabilization in the first hour.

As discussed previously, glucose administration may worsen intracellular cerebral acidosis if cerebral ischemia is present, as in cardiorespiratory arrest. Unless hypoglycemia is confirmed to be present, or strongly suspected, non-glucose-containing fluids should be used in this circumstance.

Selection of Vein

Selection of an appropriate vein is usually more difficult in the child, whose veins are deeper in the subcutaneous tissues and are smaller. Veins are often not easily visualized and must be palpated. When fluid replacement is required, select the largest accessible vein. Veins of the hands, arms, and feet and the external jugular veins may be used. Scalp veins may also be used in young infants, but this technique is infrequently performed in the field. A rubber band substitutes for a tourniquet in this procedure (Fig. 29-10). Select a vein in the forehead or temporal area and point the 21- or 23-gauge scalp vein needle toward the infant's face or neck. Cut the rubber band before infusing fluids to prevent rupture of the thin vein wall.

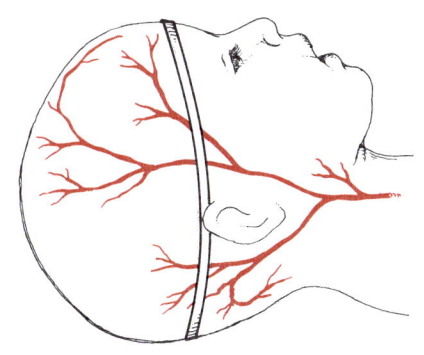

Intraosseous Infusion

Intraosseous infusion refers to the placement of a rigid needle into a bone and infusing fluid and medications directly into the bone marrow. Since bone marrow is highly vascular and has direct communication to the peripheral circulation, both fluids and medications may be administered effectively in this way.

The technique of intraosseous infusion has been known for many years but has only recently been emphasized as a relatively fast and safe means of fluid and drug administration. While it is effective in adults, the intraosseous technique is of particular value to critically ill or injured children when no other peripheral venous access can be established. See Chapter 12 for a discussion of intraosseous infusion and the skill procedure.

SUMMARY

Management of the pediatric patient is most challenging and yet rewarding. Few field or general emergency department personnel see enough acute pediatric patients in their practice to establish a relative comfort level in this area of medicine. Frequent review of the pathophysiology, assessment, and management of pediatric emergencies, careful observation of normal and abnormal behaviors, and periodic clinical experiences with this patient population reinforce the paramedic's knowledge base and confidence in managing the pediatric patient.

SUGGESTED READING

Behrman RE, Vaughan VS: Nelson Textbook of Pediatrics, 13th ed. Philadelphia, WB Saunders, 1987

Chameides L: Textbook of Pediatric Advanced Life Support. Dallas, TX, American Heart Association and American Academy of Pediatrics, 1988

Dierking BH, Everidge JM, Ramenofsky ML: Initial prehospital assessment of the pediatric patient. J Emerg Med Serv 13(4):59, 1988

Dierking BH, Ramenofsky ML, Reynolds EA: Hypovolemic shock in pediatric trauma. J Emerg Med Serv 13(6):68, 1988

Hadley MN, Zambramski JM, Browner CM, Rekate H, Sonntag VK: Pediatric spinal trauma: Review of 122 cases of spinal cord and vertebral column injuries. J Neurosurg 68:18, 1988

Harris BH, Latchaw LA, Murphy RE, Schwaitzberg SB: The critical hour. Pediatr Ann 16(4):301, 1987

Harte FA, Chalmers PC, Walsh RF, Danker PR, Sheikh FM: Intraosseous fluid administration: A parenteral alternative in pediatric resuscitation. Anesth Analg 66:687, 1987

Hensinger RN, Herzenberh JE, Dedrick DK, Phillips WA: Po-

FIGURE 29-10.
A rubber band around an infant's scalp serves as a tourniquet in vein selection.

tential hazards of backboards in emergency transport of children with neck injuries. Pediatr Emerg Care 4:146, 1988

Jacobs LM: Results of aggressive roadside treatment of pediatric trauma patients. Pediatr Emerg Care 4:63, 1988

Kempe CH, Silver HK, O'Brien DO: Current Pediatric Diagnosis and Treatment, 9th ed. Los Altos, Lange Medical Publications, 1987

Lynch FP, Rodarte A, Wotherspoon L: Impact of prehospital treatment on pediatric trauma outcome. Pediatr Emerg Care 4:162, 1988

McNamara RM, Spivey WH, Unger HD, Malone DR: Emergency applications of intraosseous infusion. J Emerg Med 5:97, 1987

Manley LK: Pediatric trauma: Initial assessment and management. Journal of Emergency Nursing 13(2):77, 1987

Manley LK, Haley K, Dick M: Intraosseous infusion: Rapid vascular access for critically ill or injured infants and children. Journal of Emergency Nursing 14(2):63, 1988

Perkin RM, von Stralen D: Putting the brakes on pediatric shock. J Emerg Med Serv 15(9):58, 1990

Schmitt BD: Child Abuse/Neglect: The Visual Diagnosis of Non-Accidental Trauma and Failure to Thrive. Elk Grove Village, IL, American Academy of Pediatrics, 1979

Seidel JS, Hornbein M, Uoshiyama K: Emergency medical services and the pediatric patient: Are the needs being met? Pediatrics 73:769, 1987

Simon JE, Goldberg AT: Prehospital Pediatric Life Support. St. Louis, CV Mosby, 1989

Smith JP, Keseg DP, Manley LK, Standeford TS: Intraosseous infusions by prehospital personnel in critically ill pediatric patients. Ann Emerg Med 17:491, 1988

Templeton JM, Delgado-Paredes C, Templeton JJ, Fleisher G: Experimental prehospital resuscitation for hemorrhagic shock in the young. Pediatr Emerg Care 4:157, 1988

US Department of Transportation, National Highway Traffic Safety Administration: Emergency Medical Technician-Paramedic: National Standards Curriculum. Washington, DC, US Government Printing Office, 1985

CHAPTER 30

Gynecologic, Obstetric, and Newborn Emergencies

Anatomy and Physiology of the Female Reproductive System
   Ovaries and Ovulation
   Fallopian Tubes
   Uterus
   Vagina
   External Genitalia
Ovulation and the Menstrual Cycle
   Proliferative Phase
   Secretory Phase
   Premenstrual Phase
   Menstrual Phase
Pregnancy and Fetal Growth
   Fertilization
   Fetal Growth
   Maternal Changes During Pregnancy
Assessment of the Gynecologic and Obstetric Patient
   Patient History
      History of Present Illness
      Medical History
      Obstetric and Menstrual History
      Vaginal Discharge
   Physical Examination
   Fetal Assessment

Gynecologic Emergencies
   Abdominal Pain
   Vaginal Bleeding: Traumatic
   Vaginal Bleeding: Nontraumatic
   Sexual Assault
Complications of Pregnancy
   Trauma in Pregnancy
   Medical Conditions in Pregnancy
   Complications of Early Pregnancy
      Ectopic Pregnancy
      Abortion
   Complications of Late Pregnancy
      Preeclampsia and Eclampsia
      Third Trimester Bleeding
         Placenta Previa
         Abruptio Placentae

Labor and Delivery
   Labor
   Delivery
   Abnormal Presentations
      Breech Presentation
      Other Abnormal Presentations
   Multiple Births
   Abnormal Deliveries
      Prolapsed Umbilical Cord
      Precipitous Delivery
   Complications of Delivery
      Postpartum Hemorrhage
      Uterine Rupture
      Uterine Inversion
Care of the Newborn
   Airway
   Breathing and Circulation
   Initial Evaluation
   Maintaining Warmth
   Premature Infant
   Management of the Distressed Infant
Summary

BEHAVIORAL OBJECTIVES
On successful completion of this chapter, the reader will be able to:

1. Describe the anatomy and physiology of the reproductive system, including the ovaries and ovulation, fallopian tubes, uterus, vagina, and external genitalia
2. Explain the menstrual cycle
3. Describe the process of pregnancy and fetal growth

(continued)

BEHAVIORAL OBJECTIVES (continued)

4. Describe the assessment scheme for gynecologic and obstetric patients
5. Give a brief description of the assessment and management of abdominal pain, traumatic and nontraumatic vaginal bleeding, and sexual assault
6. List the complications of early and late pregnancy
7. Describe the management of complications of early and late pregnancy
8. Describe the stages of labor
9. List the sequence of a normal delivery
10. Explain the problems in abnormal presentations and deliveries
11. List and describe three complications of delivery
12. Explain the process for care of the newborn
13. Define all of the key terms listed in this chapter

KEY TERMS
The following terms are defined in the chapter and glossary:

abortion
abruptio placentae
amniotic sac
amniotic fluid
Apgar score
attitude
Bartholin's glands
breech
cephalic
clitoris
complete breech
crowning
eclampsia
ectopic pregnancy
endometrium
engagement
fallopian tubes
footling breech
frank breech
fraternal twins
gravida
identical twins
labia minora
labia majora
labor
meconium
menopause

menstrual cycle
myometrium
ovaries
ovulation
para
parity
pelvic inflammatory disease (PID)
perimetrium
placenta
placenta previa
postpartum hemorrhage
precipitous delivery
preeclampsia
presentation
prolapsed umbilical cord
shoulder lie
station
umbilical cord
uterine inversion
uterine rupture
uterus
vagina
vaginal show
vulva

Gynecologic and obstetric problems make up a small percentage of paramedic practice in the field. Intervention usually is required for potential life-threatening hypovolemia or to assist in delivery. Pregnancy and its complications should always be considered in the woman in the child-bearing age range who presents with abdominal pain. While management of the patient with impending hypovolemia is the same regardless of the cause, it is useful to understand the underlying etiology and pathophysiology of gynecologic and obstetric problems. Causes of abdominal pain and vaginal bleeding are discussed in this chapter.

The out-of-hospital delivery generally is uncomplicated and requires the paramedic to assist in a natural process and provide appropriate care for the newborn. The paramedic must be alert, however, to complications and expedite transport for obstetrical care to reduce maternal and fetal morbidity and mortality.

ANATOMY AND PHYSIOLOGY OF THE FEMALE REPRODUCTIVE SYSTEM

Ovaries and Ovulation

The functions of the **ovaries** include the production, maturation, and release of *ova* (eggs). The ovaries, one on each side of the uterus, are held to the posterior pelvic wall by the uterine broad ligament. The ovaries are small, about 4 cm long, 2 cm wide, and 8 mm thick. Each ovary is connected to the uterus by the ovarian ligament. The ovary is suspended by ligaments in the pelvis and is close to the fimbriated projections of the ends of each fallopian tube. The ovarian (or primary) follicles are vesicles (containers) on the cortex (surface) of each ovary. The lining of the primary follicles produces the two ovarian hormones, *estrogen* and *progesterone*. The position of the ovaries is shown in Figures 30-1 and 30-2.

Fallopian Tubes

The ***fallopian tubes***, one on either side of the uterus, extend laterally from the superior margin of the uterus. The three sections of the fallopian tube are the *isthmus* (portion adjacent to the uterus), the *ampulla* (middle section), and the *infundibulum* (most distal section).

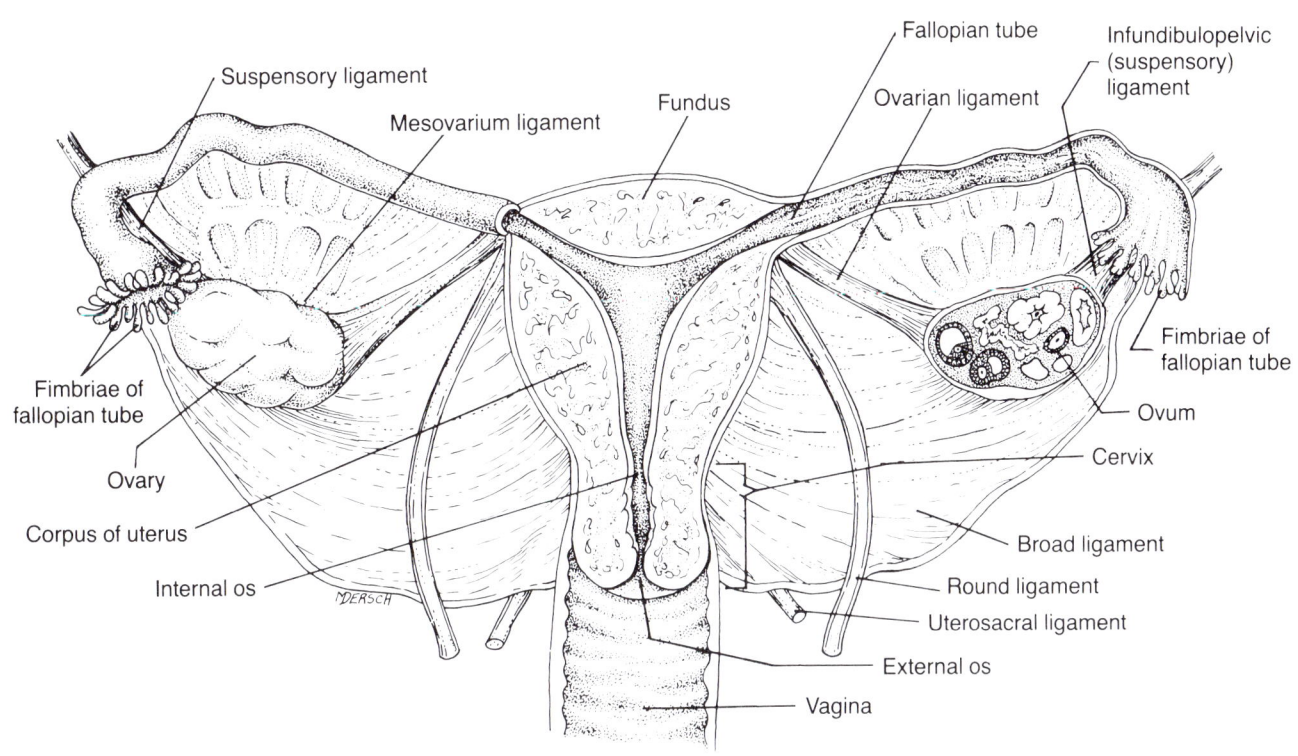

CHAPTER 30: Gynecologic, Obstetric, and Newborn Emergencies 691

FIGURE 30-1.
Anterior view of the uterus and related structures. (Reeder S, Martin L)

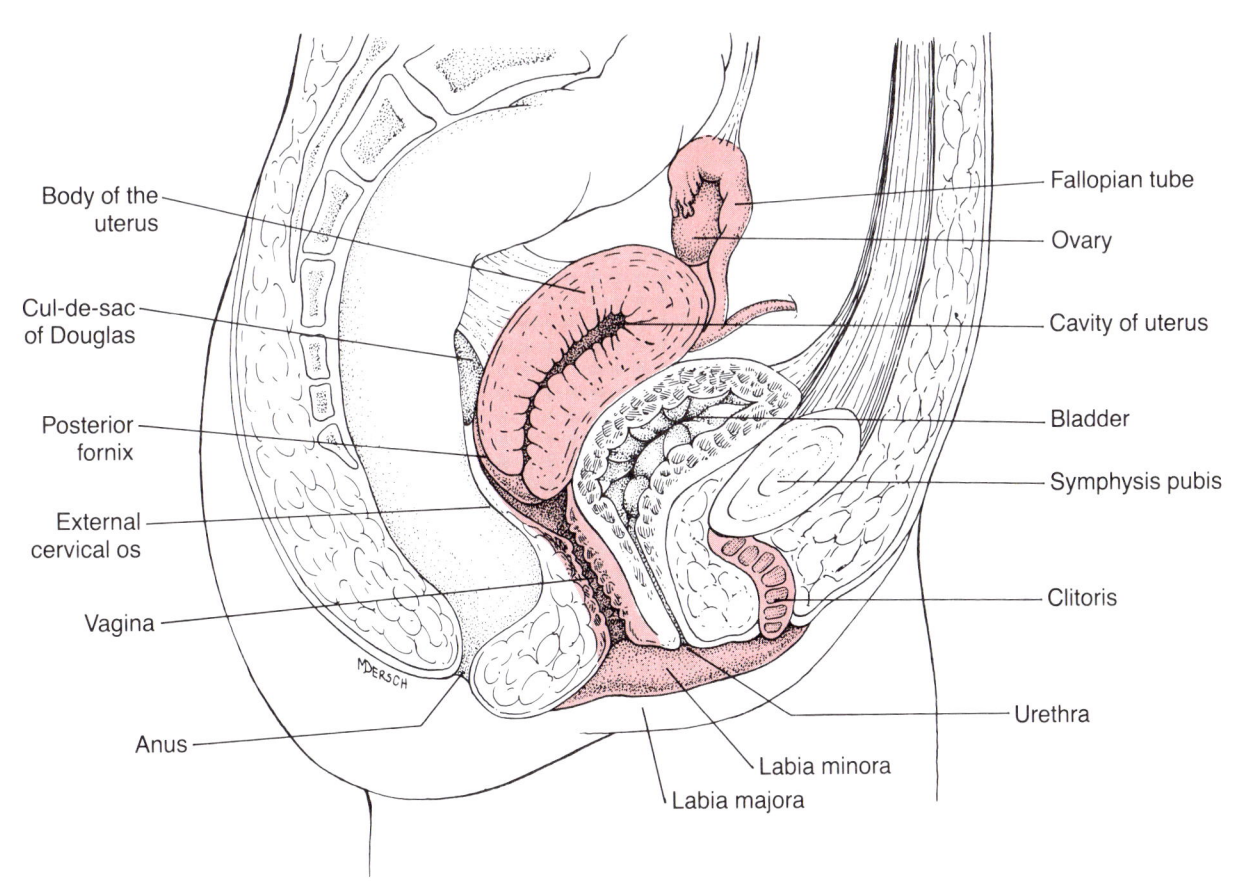

FIGURE 30-2.
Female reproductive organs as seen in the sagittal plane. (Reeder S, Martin L)

Each fallopian tube is 10 cm in length. The ampulla is where fertilization of the ovum usually takes place. The inside of the fallopian tube is lined with a mucous membrane. Between the underlying layer of circular muscles and this mucous membrane is a layer of connective tissue. The ovarian fimbria of the fallopian tubes attach to each ovary. *Fimbria* are the fingerlike projections at the distal end of the tube and are collections of hair-covered cells. They help propel the ovum from the ovary into the tube. The fallopian tube functions as the conduit for transporting the fertilized ovum into the uterus. The muscle layer causes peristaltic movement and both ciliated and mucous-secreting cells aid in the migration of the ovum to the uterus. The position of the fallopian tubes is shown in Figures 30-1 and 30-2.

Uterus

The **uterus** is located in the pelvis. The bladder is anterior to the uterus, and the rectum is situated posteriorly. The uterus changes in size and position as pregnancy progresses. The nonpregnant uterus is a hollow, muscular, pear-shaped organ that weighs between 35 and 60 g. The fallopian tubes communicate with the uterus at its superior-lateral border. The upper portion of the uterus is the body, and the elongated lower part is the cervix. The cervix or neck of the uterus is about 2 to 5 cm long. The opening into the cervix at the vaginal end is the external os. The fundus is the upper rounded portion of the uterus. The body of the organ enlarges during pregnancy as the fetus grows and matures. The uterus is not a fixed organ but is suspended in the pelvis by the cardinal, broad, and uterosacral ligaments. The *levator ani*, a thin muscle that forms the floor of the pelvis, also helps to support the uterus and maintain its position. The peritoneum covers the uterus. The position of the uterus is shown in Figures 30-1 and 30-2.

The three layers of the uterus are the perimetrium, myometrium, and the endometrium. The **perimetrium** is the outer layer. The middle layer, the **myometrium**, is composed of muscle fibers, blood vessels, nerves, and lymphatic vessels. The muscles of the myometrium are interwoven layers of smooth muscle arranged in transverse, oblique, and longitudinal directions. The muscle fibers of this layer enlarge as the uterus grows with advancing gestation of the fetus. The inner layer, the **endometrium**, is the mucous membrane. This membrane extends through the opening of the fallopian tubes into the peritoneum and extends within the uterus through the cervix to the vaginal lining. The endometrium contains uterine glands that enlarge under hormonal influence to support an implanted fertilized ovum. If implantation does not occur, this layer is expelled during the menstrual phase of the cycle.

Vagina

The vaginal opening is visible on direct examination and lies posterior to the urethral opening. The hollow **vagina** extends to the cervix and is 8 to 12 cm long. The position of the vagina is shown in Figures 30-1 and 30-2. The vagina is the passageway for sperm, the excretory duct for menstrual flow, and part of the birth canal. The mucous membranous lining of the vagina is continuous and also lines the uterus. The second layer of the vagina is muscular. This layer is subdivided into an external layer, with muscle fibers that run longitudinally, and an internal layer, with muscle fibers in a circular configuration. A connective tissue layer contains large veins. The pH of the vagina is acidic to protect against bacterial infections.

External Genitalia

A number of external structures of the female genitalia collectively form the **vulva.** Pubic hair in the postpubescent female covers the skin over the mons pubis, the rounded protuberant collection of adipose tissue over the bony symphysis pubis. The larger longitudinal outer lips over the vaginal and urethral orifices are the **labia majora.** The outer labial surface is covered with pubic hair. The inner labial surface is smoother and has sebaceous glands.

The smaller inner lips that cover the vaginal and urethral openings are the **labia minora.** They extend from the clitoris posteriorly to where the labia majora end. The *clitoris* is composed of erectile tissue and is situated between the anterior ends of the labia minora. The rounded portion of the clitoris that can be seen on direct visualization is the glans clitoris and is composed of erectile corpus cavernosa (analogous to the male penis). **Bartholin's glands** lie on either side of the vaginal opening. They secrete an alkaline lubricant that supports sperm survival. Blockage of these glands can cause painful infected Bartholin's cysts. Structures of the external genitalia are shown in Figure 30-3.

OVULATION AND THE MENSTRUAL CYCLE

Ovulation occurs when the mature graafian follicle ruptures onto the surface of the ovary. The ovum, once it leaves the ovary, is swept into the fallopian tube opening. The now-empty follicle fills with a yellow substance called *lutein* and becomes the corpus luteum. If the ovum is fertilized at this point, the corpus luteum continues to grow. If not fertilized, the corpus luteum degenerates.

The **menstrual cycle** describes the changes that occur in the ovaries and uterus between puberty (12 to 14 years of age) and the end of child-bearing potential. The phases of the usual 28-day cycle are described below and shown in Figure 30-4.

Proliferative Phase

After the menstrual phase, follicle-stimulating hormone (FSH) is secreted from the anterior lobe of the pituitary gland in the *proliferative phase*. The stimulus for the release of FSH is gonadotropin-releasing hormone from the hypothalamus. The FSH is the stimulus for the ovary to develop ovarian follicles, hence its label as a gonadotropin hormone. Trophic refers to growth, and gonad refers to the ovary. An additional hormone, *estrogen*, is produced by growing follicles. The endometrium of the uterus is stimulated and a proliferation ensues, enlarging the glands of the uterus to produce thickening of the endometrium.

Secretory Phase

The ovarian follicle grows and eventually the graafian follicle ruptures in the *secretory phase*. As the ovum is released, luteinizing hormone (LH) is secreted, stimulat-

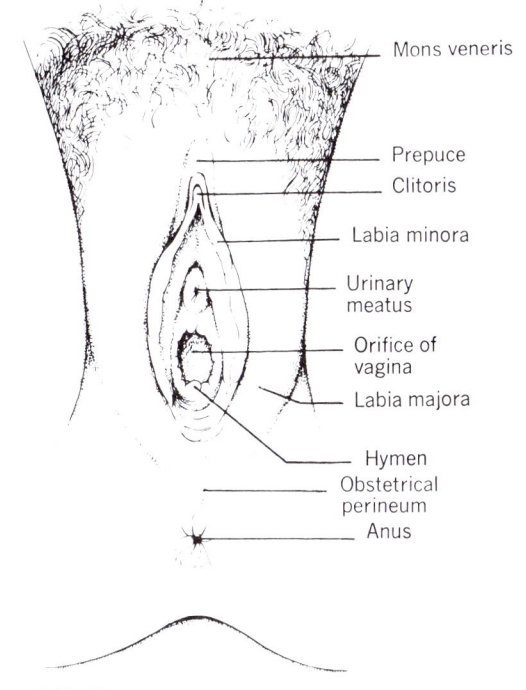

FIGURE 30–3.
External female genitalia. (Reeder S, Martin L)

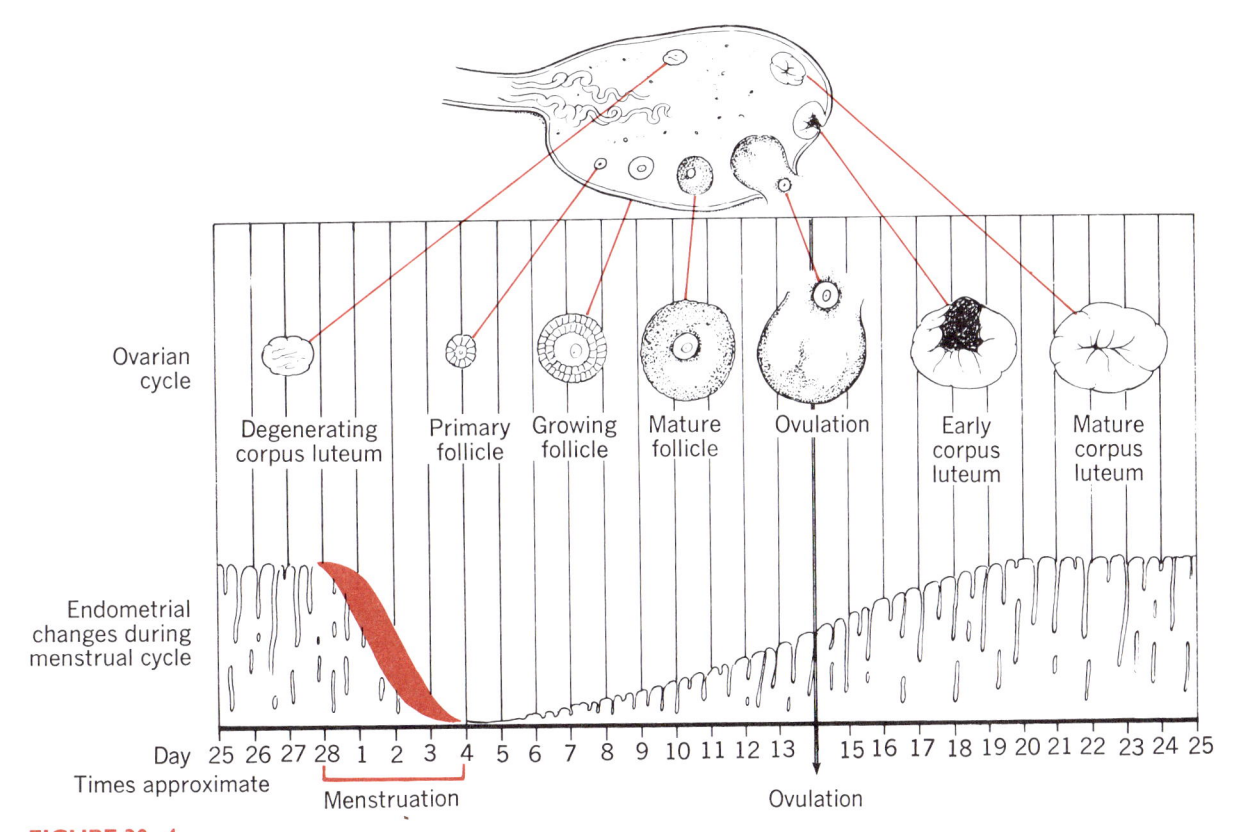

FIGURE 30–4.
Schematic representation of one ovarian cycle and the corresponding changes in thickness of the endometrium. It is thickest just before the onset of menstruation and thinnest just as it ceases. (Reeder S, Martin L)

ing the development of the corpus luteum. Further enlargement of the uterine glands of the endometrium is stimulated by release of another hormone, *progesterone*, from the corpus luteum. This phase prepares the uterus for the fertilized ovum. The number of endometrial capillaries increases during this phase.

Premenstrual Phase

The direction of the cycle at this point depends on the presence or absence of a fertilized ovum. If fertilization takes place, the fertilized ovum continues to mature within the uterus. If fertilization of the ovum does not occur, hormonal secretion ceases, and the corpus luteum, still in the ovary, degenerates. During this phase, the uterus and the enlarged endometrium undergo significant changes that lead to deterioration of the endometrial tissue.

Menstrual Phase

If fertilization of the ovum has not occurred, the premenstrual phase continues to the menstrual phase. The endometrium sloughs the portion formed by the enlarged glands and augmented capillary supply. This sloughing and bleeding from the ruptured capillaries produces the menstrual flow and discharge. **Menopause** is permanent cessation of ovulation and menstrual activity. The average age for menopause is between age 45 and 50.

PREGNANCY AND FETAL GROWTH

Fertilization of the ovum produces physiologic changes in the maternal system. The development of the fetus and maternal physiology are interrelated and interconnected.

Fertilization

Although only one egg usually is released during ovulation for every menstrual cycle, each male ejaculation contains an average of more than 200 million sperm. If a spermatozoa fertilizes the ovum, the resulting fusion results in the formation of a *zygote*, which contains 46 chromosomes. It is the sex chromosome from the sperm that determines the gender of the fetus. If the sperm has an X chromosome, the embryo will be female (XX). If the sperm has a Y chromosome, the embryo will be male (XY). The male, therefore, determines the sex of the child.

Cell division begins before the zygote travels to the uterus. The zygote changes as it grows into a *blastocyst*. The blastocyst attaches to the endometrium and implants high in the uterus on the posterior wall. The outer structure of the blastocyte contains a layer of cells called a *trophoblast*.

These cells produce the placenta. The **placenta** is the structure that provides nutrition, excretion, and circulation to the fetus. Fingerlike projections termed chorionic villi are formed from the trophoblastic cells and eventually produce the **umbilical cord** that grows to about 21 inches. The cord has one vein that carries oxygen and nutrients from the mother through the placenta's villi to the fetus. The cord has two arteries. Both carry blood with waste products from the fetus back to the villi of the placenta. A gelatinous substance (*Wharton's jelly*) forms the cord and protects the three vessels from pressure. The umbilical cord is a vital structure. Blood flow is so rapid that twisting or kinking is prevented. The cord is not innervated and, therefore, does not cause pain to the infant when it is cut after delivery.

Chorionic villi are also involved in the development of the **amniotic sac.** The medial villi surface that does not invaginate the endometrium forms the outermost chorionic membrane, which gives the amniotic sac its support. The inner membrane of the sac is the amniotic membrane. Both membranes cover the fetal surface of the placenta. The fetus drinks and excretes the **amniotic fluid.** It is absorbed from the intestine into fetal blood circulation and transported via arteries back to the placenta. About 500 to 1000 mL of amniotic fluid is found at birth. The functions of amniotic fluid are to protect the fetus from pressure or blows to the mother's abdomen, to permit fetal movement within the amniotic sac, and to regulate temperature. No pain is associated with the rupture of the amniotic membranes before delivery, since the membranes are not innervated.

Fetal Growth

Fetal development begins immediately on fusion of the ovum and the sperm and progresses over the 36 to 40 weeks of pregnancy. The stages are summarized in Table 30-1. The early development of the heart and vascular system is of particular importance. The fetal circulation is different from *postnatal* circulation. It is helpful to understand the fetal circulation when assessing a newborn in the event that one of the fetal structures persists after birth. The heart chambers and the valves develop from the fourth to the seventh week. Fetal circulation does not rely on the lungs for oxygenation. The necessary oxygen and nutrients are received from the mother and the chorionic villi and placenta. Circulation within the fetus takes the path identified in Figure 30-5.

The development of the respiratory system is important, since infants born prematurely may be in significant respiratory distress because of immaturity of the lungs. By the fourth gestational week, the digestive and respiratory systems, which were previously united, separate. However, it is not until the 24th to 28th week that alveoli and corresponding capillaries form. Formation continues until the 40th week. *Premature birth* (before 28 weeks) is seri-

TABLE 30-1.
EMBRYO AND FETAL DEVELOPMENT *IN UTERO*

Gestational Weeks	Development Events
Four	Formation of placenta
	Heartbeats
	Buds form for limbs, esophagus, stomach, pancreas, liver, and lungs
	Brain and neural tube begin to form
Eight	Ventricular septum forms and heart has form
	Limbs growing, fingers and toes separating
	Distinct facial features
	Further lung development to bronchiolar level
Twelve	Kidneys make urine
	Brain and spinal cord developed
	Lungs develop definite shape
	Fetus growing in length
	May recognize gender
Twenty	Fetal heartbeat auscultated
	Lanugo (hair on shoulders and back)
	Hair on head
	Mother may sense movement
Twenty-eight	Fetus more rounded in appearance
	Eyelids open, eyebrows and eyelashes
	Alveoli developing after 24th week
Thirty-six	Completion of fissure development in brain (furrows of cerebral hemispheres)
Forty	Bronchioles and alveoli developing at final stages
	Rest of body systems fully developed (e.g., skull)
	Bones firmer, kidneys in position lateral to second lumbar vertebra

ous, since the lungs are too immature to support ventilation, diffusion, and perfusion. The formation of surfactant is a necessary component of respiratory system development. Surfactant lines the alveoli and reduces the surface tension. If the surface tension is not controlled, the alveoli remain collapsed after expiration. It is not until the 35th gestational week that the main component of surfactant, lecithin, is produced at high levels.

Maternal Changes During Pregnancy

The systemic changes that occur during pregnancy are important to understand, since values may vary from normal. The total blood volume increases as pregnancy progresses, with the largest increase occurring around the 24th week. The reason for the change is the maternal demand to support the fetal circulation.

In addition to changes in blood volume, the heart rate, stroke volume, and cardiac output increase. Arterial blood pressure and vascular resistance decrease. Heart rate may increase by 15 beats per minute over the nonpregnant rate. Stroke volume increases 25% to 30%, and cardiac output increases 40%. Other cardiovascular changes are more obvious during the last trimester. The greatly enlarged uterus may cause pressure on veins from the lower extremities and torso. Interference with venous return may cause lower extremity edema and venous congestion that result in varicosities of the legs and rectum (hemorrhoids).

Supine-induced hypotension may also occur. As the patient rests in the supine position, the pressure of the uterus on the inferior vena cava may cause a decrease in venous return with a drop in cardiac output and subsequent hypotension. Therefore, it is important to avoid the supine position during transport, since *supine hypotensive syndrome* compromises both fetal and maternal perfusion. The patient should be positioned on the left side.

The maternal respiratory system undergoes alterations. Pregnant women may complain that shortness of breath, nasopharyngeal congestion, and an increased respiratory rate limit their activity. As the diaphragm rises with the growing uterus, the anterior-to-posterior diameter of the thoracic cage is increased during inspiration to compensate for the decreased superior-to-inferior dimension. Tidal volume also increases. The arterial partial pressure of carbon dioxide ($PaCO_2$) is lower than in the nonpregnant female because carbon dioxide from the fetal circulation crosses the placenta to the mother's circulation where the carbon dioxide level is lower. The maternal $PaCO_2$ remains lower in spite of the additional carbon dioxide because of the mother's increased ventilation and resultant elimination of carbon dioxide. The metabolic buffering system compensates for the respiratory alkalosis by eliminating bicarbonate. The box "Normal Signs of Preg-

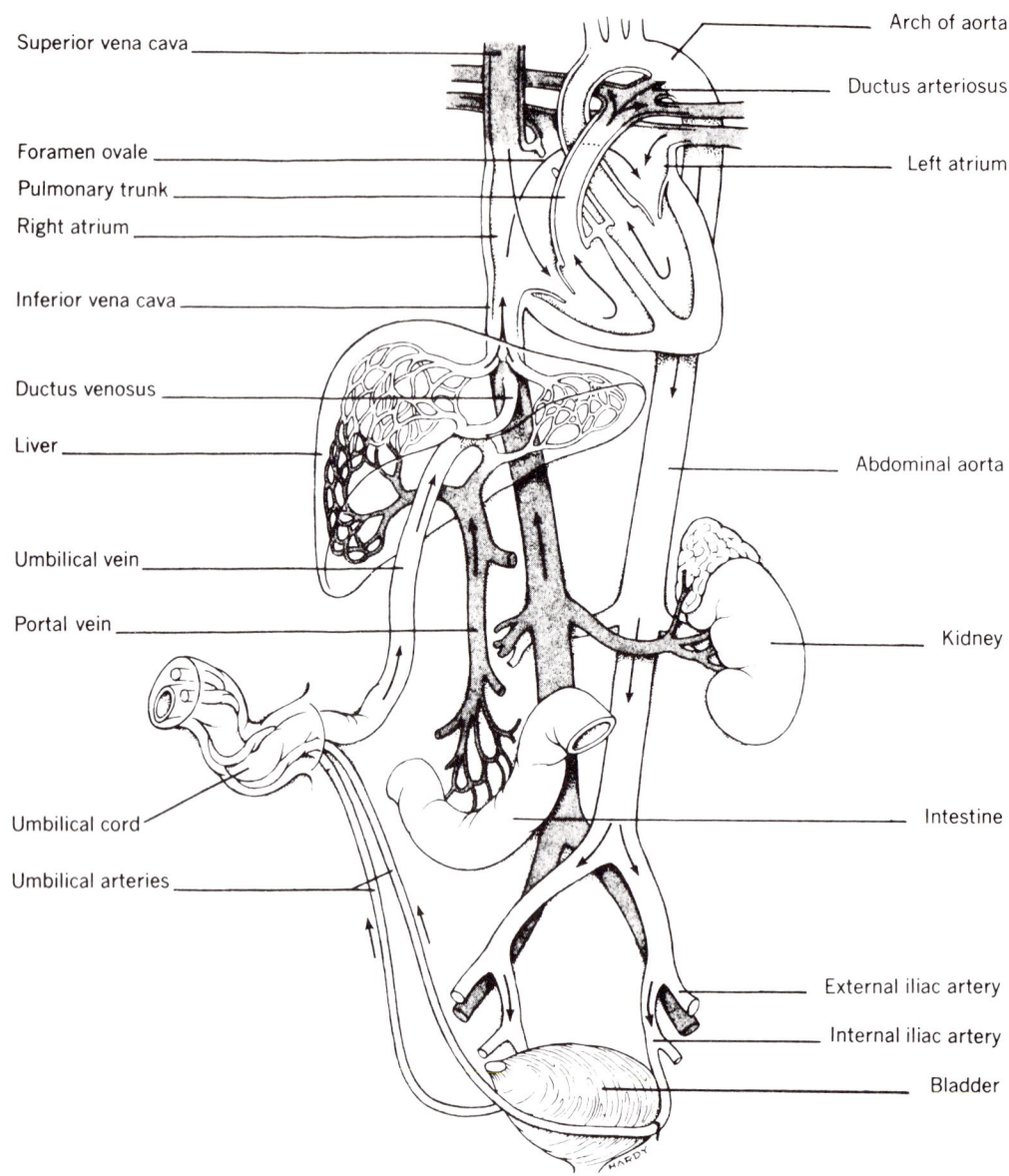

FIGURE 30–5.
Diagram of fetal circulation shortly before birth; the course of blood is indicated by arrows. The baby's blood travels through the blood vessels in the umbilical cord to and from the placenta, where exchanges of gases (oxygen and carbon dioxide) and digestive products (nutrients and wastes) take place. Here is an exception to the rule of veins and arteries: the fetal umbilical arteries carry deoxygenated blood and the umbilical vein carries oxygenated blood. (Rosdahl CB)

nancy" lists other common changes during pregnancy that may be noted on examination.

ASSESSMENT OF THE GYNECOLOGIC AND OBSTETRIC PATIENT

Although a significant number of problems can constitute an obstetric or gynecologic emergency, few require access to prehospital emergency medical services. Those that do, however, may be life-threatening to the obstetric patient and her unborn infant. Emergencies due to problems with the female genitalia that are not related to pregnancy are less common but require comprehensive and sensitive management. General principles of assessment are related to physical examination and history taking. The severity of the patient's condition, the possibility of an imminent at home or on-scene delivery, complications of delivery, and the proximity of the patient to an appropriate obstetric service hospital determine the rapidity of obstetric assessment and transport decisions.

NORMAL SIGNS OF PREGNANCY

Early Signs

Missed menstrual period

Nausea and vomiting

Frequent urination

Breast fullness and tenderness

Dark blue coloration of vaginal tissues

Darkening of pigmentation around nipples and between the umbilicus and the pubic symphysis

Striae gravidarum (red or pink streaks on abdomen)

Probable Signs

Increase in uterine size, abdomen size

Positive pregnancy test

Weight gain (20–30 lb during pregnancy)

Fetal outline

Braxton–Hicks contractions

Positive Signs

Fetal movement

Fetal heart sounds

The physical examination in the field should be conducted with clear objectives in mind. Because the patient is female and the problem is gynecologic or obstetric in nature, additional psychologic support and sensitivity during the interview and examination are required. Any examination that does not lend information about the patient's condition, help determine the severity of the problem, or influence management should be avoided. The examination includes a primary and secondary survey as found in Chapter 9. The patient history is different and is discussed in the next section. The severity of the problem usually can be rapidly determined and guides the extent of the survey and the need for prompt intervention.

Patient History

The paramedic must first ascertain what prompted the call for help. The patient may be reluctant to describe her problem in detail if it is related to menstrual or sexual activities or events. Collection of the history must be done in conjunction with the physical examination for those women who present with an urgent or life-threatening problem. Important historical information is described below.

History of Present Illness

Information about the history of the present illness includes the following:

- Patient's age
- Present problem, including time of onset and, if pain is present, its location, distribution, character (dull, ache, crampy, sharp, intermittent, or constant), what aggravates or alleviates it, and whether it had a gradual or sudden onset
- If bleeding is present, the amount (often measured by the number of tampons or perineal pads used or saturated in a given time frame), time of onset, character (clots, tissue-containing, dark or bright red)
- Unprovoked onset or related trauma
- Associated symptoms (fever, chills, urinary symptoms, including frequency, urgency, and burning)

Medical History

Information about the medical history includes the following:

- Occurrence of the same problem in the past
- Major cardiovascular disorders (hypertension); endocrine (diabetes); genitourinary diseases (infections)
- Previous vaginal infections, vaginal bleeding, or other gynecologic difficulties
- Use of birth control adjuncts (birth control pills, intrauterine devices, diaphragms, foams or jellies)
- Current medications and allergies; inquire specifically about blood thinners and hormones

Obstetric and Menstrual History

If pregnancy is obvious or a possibility (*i.e.*, woman is in child-bearing years), the following information should be ascertained:

- Previous pregnancies (**gravida**)
- Previous live births (**para**)
- Anticipated date of delivery, if known
- Type of previous deliveries (vaginal or cesarean section), length of labor, and any complications
- Date of last menstrual period (regularity, character)
- Early signs of pregnancy (changes in breast tenderness, nausea, vomiting, frequent urination, missed period)
- Prenatal care, single or multiple birth anticipated, and any complications of pregnancy that have occurred
- Any problems with pregnancy before the current event
- Recent history of ruptured membranes or vaginal bleeding or bloody show

Vaginal Discharge

Information about vaginal discharge includes the following:

- If discharge is present: time of onset, length of occurrence, color, character, associated factors (postmenses or premenses, odor, amount)
- If discharge is associated with pregnancy: time of onset, duration, presence of blood
- If bleeding: amount, time of onset, duration, similarities to normal menstrual flow
- If evidence of products of conception: time of expulsion, associated symptoms (contractions)

Physical Examination

Speaking to the patient alerts the paramedic to the patient's level of consciousness and orientation. The patient who is not obviously alert is evaluated for responsiveness to verbal and painful stimuli and orientation to person, place, and time.

The alert patient with a gynecologic problem who does not demonstrate compromised cardiovascular and respiratory status is unlikely to have airway difficulties. However, the severity of the illness or complications of pregnancy may result in airway compromise if the problem is left untreated. Look, listen, and feel for air exchange via the nose and mouth. Check for the presence of foreign material in the oropharynx. Check for facial trauma. Assess respiratory rate, depth, and exertion, symmetrical chest movements, skin and lip color, and breath sounds.

Assess the pulse rate and rhythm, blood pressure, presence or absence of cyanosis, skin temperature, diaphoresis, and EKG rhythm. A patient who appears to be in shock should not be evaluated for orthostatic vital sign changes.

The presenting complaint determines the extent of the secondary survey. The objective is to determine the severity of the patient's problem to initiate the appropriate intervention. The secondary survey includes observations of the general appearance of the patient (e.g., ill, frightened, anxious, obviously pregnant). Note skin color (e.g., pale or ashen). Vital signs should be evaluated serially. The gynecologic or obstetric patient may require examination of the abdomen. Inspection should be carried out with notation of distention and signs of trauma, such as ecchymosis, lacerations, or abrasions.

For the obviously pregnant female, note the height of the uterus. When the patient complains of abdominal pain, palpation should be performed with care to avoid provoking undue distress. Asking the patient to locate the pain helps the paramedic avoid that area during the initial examination. Do not palpate the area that is painful until the last step of the abdominal examination. Tenderness, rigidity, and guarding should be noted. Vaginal or digital examination is not indicated in the field.

If bleeding is present, a visual inspection of the external vaginal orifice may be necessary. Estimate the amount of blood loss. If the patient is in labor, inspect the perineum for presence of bloody show, crowning, or evidence of ruptured membranes. Evaluation of orthostatic vital signs is indicated when supine hypotension is not present to assess for concealed blood loss.

Fetal Assessment

If the patient appears to be in active labor, it is important to check the cardiac status of the fetus. Risk to fetal circulation is increased by possible compression of the umbilical cord during strong uterine contractions. A specially designed stethoscope facilitates auscultation of the heart beat. However, this equipment is generally not available in the field. Evaluating the position of the fetus determines the most appropriate area to auscultate. In the normal vertex presentation, sounds are best heard by placing the stethoscope over the back of the fetus, since sounds are better heard when the fetus' upper body is convex. Begin listening low in the abdomen in the right and left lower quadrants. If sounds are not present in either area, move the stethoscope to the lateral areas of the uterus and above the umbilicus. Auscultate between contractions. Normal fetal heart rates are as follows:

Between contractions: 120 to 160 beats per minute
During contractions: May drop to 100 beats per minute but returns to 120 to 160 beats per minute
Baseline variability: Normal to fluctuate 5 to 15 beats per minute
Tachycardia: More than 160 beats per minute
Bradycardia: Less than 120 beats per minute

GYNECOLOGIC EMERGENCIES

The majority of the patients with gynecologic problems seek medical attention without the need for prehospital intervention. The most common gynecologic emergencies seen in the field are abdominal pain, vaginal bleeding, sexual assault, and sepsis secondary to toxic shock syndrome or pelvic inflammatory disease.

Abdominal Pain

Abdominal pain may be due to a number of causes. Determining whether the problem is of gynecologic, urinary, infectious, or gastrointestinal origin is not always possible or appropriate in the prehospital setting. The general assessment of abdominal pain in the field includes establishing priorities of care and managing airway, breathing, and circulatory compromise. Determine the history of the pain, including type, length, severity, time of onset, character, location, radiation, and what increases or decreases the pain. Identify accompanying symptoms (e.g., nausea, vomiting, diarrhea, rectal pressure), previous episodes of similar pain, previous abdominal surgery, and date of last menstrual period. Determine the possibility of pregnancy and examine the abdomen.

Pelvic inflammatory disease (PID) is a gynecologic problem that causes acute abdominal pain. It is an infectious process that leads to inflammation of the pelvic organs, the uterus, ovaries, and fallopian tubes. If the infection is untreated, it may spread to supporting structures and involve the peritoneum and abdominal viscera. The disease is sexually transmitted in most cases, and the history provides more information than the physical examination. Extensive abdominal examination is unnecessary and provokes needless additional pain.

Management of the patient with abdominal pain includes positioning the patient for comfort. If shock is impending, the patient should be supine with the legs elevated. Initiate intravenous (IV) fluid replacement with normal saline or lactated Ringer's solution. Withhold oral fluids and save vomitus, perineal pads, clots, and so on. Monitor blood pressure, pulse, and respirations. Transport for further evaluation and management.

Vaginal Bleeding: Traumatic

Direct injury to the external genitalia may cause vaginal bleeding if the soft tissues are injured either by direct force, insertion of foreign bodies into the vagina, attempts at aborting an unwanted pregnancy, or sexual assault. In addition to the general assessment and management of the patient, it may be necessary to inspect the perineum. Direct pressure over any obvious lacerations or punctures may be needed to control bleeding. Perineal pads are useful. Never pack the vagina with dressings or perform a manual examination. If bleeding is significant, interventions include administration of oxygen, placement in shock position, initiation of a large-bore IV catheter, and infusion of normal saline or lactated Ringer's solution. The pneumatic anti-shock garment (PASG) may be indicated for systolic blood pressure lower than 90 mm Hg.

Vaginal Bleeding: Nontraumatic

Most nontraumatic uterine bleeding is caused by the following three conditions:

Hormonal disturbances: no ovulation cycle, estrogen therapy
Tumors: lesions of the cervix, ovaries, tubes, or endometrial polyps
Complications of pregnancy: first trimester bleeding from an abortion or ectopic pregnancy and third trimester bleeding due to disorders such as abruptio placentae or placenta previa (discussed later in the chapter)

The bleeding varies in quantity and may or may not indicate the seriousness of the problem. General assessment and management for possible hypovolemia should be instituted.

Sexual Assault

Sexual assault refers to sexual contact without permission. It is one of the fastest growing crimes in the United States. It has been estimated that less than 40% of cases are reported. There is no typical victim; sexual assault occurs in all age, economic, and cultural groups.

While both males and females may be subject to sexual assault, discussion in this section is limited to the female victim. Sexual assault (referred to in legal terms as rape) is a crime of violence. It is not motivated by passion or sexual attraction. The rapist seeks to inflict humiliation and pain on his victim through this act of aggression. Forced submission of the victim allows him to feel a sense of power and control.

When the paramedic encounters the patient who has been sexually assaulted, varying degrees of injury may be present. If the patient has significant physical injuries, she should be assessed and managed as any other multiple trauma patient. Genital trauma may include lacerations, abrasions, and contusions. More severe injury can result from objects placed inside the vagina, possibly leading to perforation of the uterus or other pelvic or abdominal viscera. Cases have been reported of objects inserted into the vagina that have perforated the uterine wall and the diaphragm, causing hemopneumothorax and serious multiple trauma. These occurrences are rare, but the paramedic should suspect this type of injury if the patient presents with signs of serious breathing or circulatory compromise.

Sexual assault may cause profound emotional and psychological effects. Phases of psychological reaction include the following:

Impact or acute reaction: Anxiety, fear, feelings of guilt, shame, and humiliation; the patient may cope expressively (e.g., with tears, anger, confusion) or in a controlled way (e.g., by being calm, logical, composed).
Recoil or outward adjustment: The patient denies the impact and resumes normal activities.
Resolution or integration: Depression and feelings of helplessness are felt, and the patient becomes preoccupied with the event and attempts to resolve the conflict.

The paramedic usually encounters the patient in the acute reaction phase. Reactions vary depending on the patient's personality, previous experience with crisis, and coping mechanisms.

General assessment and management of the sexual assault victim is similar to that of any trauma patient. However, some special considerations exist. Do not question the patient about details of the event. Do not ask if penetration occurred. Do not inquire about the patient's sex-practices. Avoid questions that may lead [to] guilt, such as "why were you out so late[?]" [Be fle]xible in your approach. Adopt a nonjudg[mental styl]e and expect a wide range of emotional expression. Do not assume that the patient who is calm and composed is little affected by the event.

Examine the genitalia only if injury is present. Question the patient about other physical injuries and perform a secondary survey only if it appears appropriate. Avoid touching the patient without her permission. Explain all procedures before proceeding with them. Allow the patient to regain a sense of control over her environment by involving her in her care and allowing choices when possible. If a female paramedic is available, it may be appropriate for her to assess and treat the patient. However, the gender of the care giver is less important than an empathetic, gentle, and caring approach.

Aside from airway, breathing, and circulation in life-threatening situations, the most important component in management of the sexual assault victim is psychological support. Respond appropriately to the feelings the patient expresses. Respect her need for privacy, confidentiality, and modesty. Provide a safe environment to help reduce her anxiety and fear.

Follow local protocols for handling evidence and preservation of the crime scene. Instruct the patient not to change or discard clothes or to bathe (usually an initial reaction). Do not clean wounds. Handle clothing that was removed as little as possible. Bag each item separately and transport with the patient to the hospital as evidence. Disturb the potential crime scene as little as possible. Take the patient to the ambulance for evaluation, if possible, to remove the victim from the scene and provide her with additional privacy.

Sexual assault can produce devastating psychological and emotional consequences. Psychological support from emergency care givers is important in both short-term and long-term management of the victims.

COMPLICATIONS OF PREGNANCY

Both trauma and various preexisting medical conditions can complicate the course of pregnancy.

Trauma in Pregnancy

Trauma during pregnancy presents obvious risks to both the mother and fetus. The key to preserving the fetus is appropriate treatment of the mother. The paramedic should have a high index of suspicion for concealed injury when evaluating the traumatized pregnant patient.

Injuries from trauma increase during pregnancy. Motor vehicle accidents and falls are the leading causes of blunt trauma. Fatigue, syncope, clumsiness due to weight gain and altered center of gravity, and an unsteady gait contribute to an increased incidence of falls. Domestic violence and assaults may increase with the family stress of the pregnancy.

Physiologic changes during pregnancy have been previously identified. These changes are important to consider when evaluating the traumatized pregnant patient.

Pregnancy places the mother and fetus at increased risk for several types of injuries. The uterine size and prominence make it the most frequently injured abdominal organ by gunshot and stab wounds. Penetrating uterine wounds rarely produce maternal death but are likely to cause fetal death. Blunt injuries may produce trauma to the bladder, liver, or spleen. Uterine rupture and abruptio placentae are discussed later. Increased vascularity of the pelvic vessels may result in increased hemorrhage after pelvic fracture.

Motor vehicle accidents are the leading cause of maternal and fetal injury. Combination shoulder and lap belts, properly applied, decrease the risk of injury from ejection. The lap belt portion should be applied below the abdomen and made snug. The shoulder restraint strap should be worn across the shoulder and abdomen in the normal position.

Most fetal complications related to trauma are caused by maternal hypotension, hypoxia, acidosis, or placental injuries. Injuries to the fetus itself occur rarely.

Trauma assessment and management should be conducted consistent with any trauma survey. If a significant mechanism of injury has occurred, consider the patient as potentially seriously injured. Blunt trauma can produce serious life-threatening injuries to both mother and child. Determine whether a complication of pregnancy exists or could have caused the accident or injury (*e.g.*, eclampsia). Oxygen should be administered when any potential for serious injury exists.

Since hypotension may be a late finding in concealed blood loss, establish large-bore IV lines of normal saline or lactated Ringer's solution. Shock should be treated with aggressive fluid replacement. Volume replacement may be higher than anticipated since the mother has a greater reserve. Remember that blood volume increases during pregnancy. Clinical signs of shock may not appear until 30% to 35% of the total volume has been lost. The PASG may be used with inflated leg sections. The abdominal compartment should not be inflated on a patient in her third trimester. If not contraindicated by mechanism of injury, place the patient beyond 20 weeks gestation on her left side. When spinal immobilization is required, elevate the head of the long spine board 10 to 15° to reduce compression of the vena cava.

Any pregnant patient who has received trauma to the abdomen, no matter how minor, should be transported for medical evaluation. When a significant mechanism of injury has occurred, transport should be rapid.

Medical Conditions in Pregnancy

Medical conditions that complicate pregnancy include acute appendicitis, acute cholecystitis, and infectious diseases. Preexisting disease processes may also aggravate the pregnancy. Diabetes becomes unstable, and hypoglycemia or hyperglycemic coma can occur with greater frequency. The patient with essential hypertension is at greater risk to develop preeclampsia and eclampsia. Neuromuscular disorders may also be aggravated by pregnancy. Pregnancy places an additional strain on the heart if cardiac function is previously compromised.

Complications of Early Pregnancy

Several complications of early pregnancy are relatively common. Early recognition and appropriate management are required to assure a satisfactory outcome.

Ectopic Pregnancy

An ectopic pregnancy is an emergency, since the patient may rapidly develop hypovolemic shock. The appropriate history and presenting complaints should raise a high index of suspicion for the paramedic.

A fertilized ovum that implants outside the uterus results in an *ectopic pregnancy* (Fig. 30-6). Although a fertilized ovum may implant anywhere along the path from the surface of the ovary to the cervix, 95% of ectopic pregnancies are located in the fallopian tubes. The reasons why a fertilized ovum may implant in a tube instead of progressing toward the uterus include the following:

- Changes in tube size from previous endosalpingitis caused by an episode of PID or infection that has left the lumen of the tube constricted or obstructed
- Abnormalities of the tube from birth (congenital)
- Adhesions around the tube, which may develop after a peritoneal or pelvic infection or surgery
- Tubal compression, for example from a uterine or pelvic tumor

Other factors that may contribute to the risk of ectopic pregnancy include the use of an intrauterine device, previous tubal sterilization, and the use of low-dose progesterone oral contraceptives.

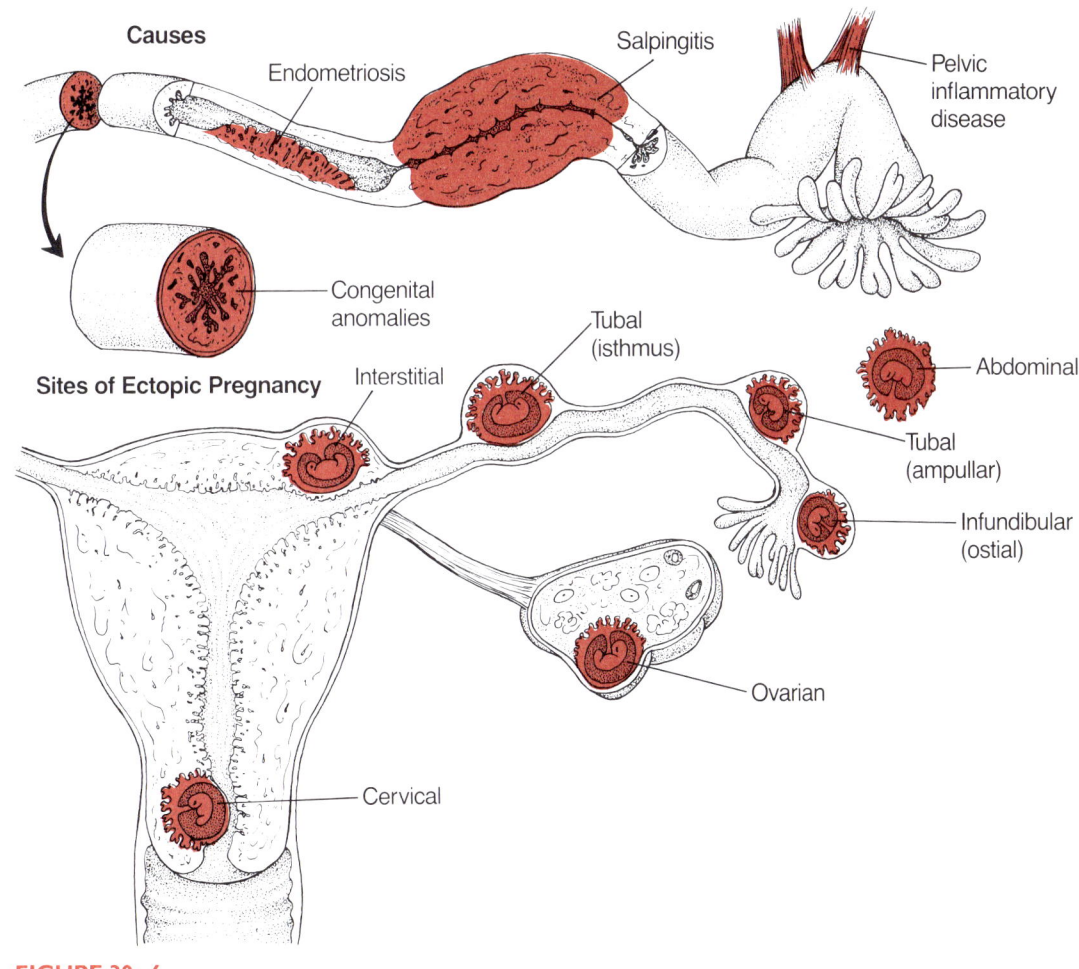

FIGURE 30-6.
Causes and sites of ectopic pregnancy. (Reeder S, Martin L)

In about 1 in every 200 pregnancies, the fertilized ovum implants in the wall of the fallopian tube rather than the uterine cavity. Since the fallopian tube is incapable of expanding sufficiently for the developing ovum, rupture of the tube occurs. The site of implantation determines the length of time the *conceptus* (products of conception) develops before the tube ruptures. For example, an implantation in the most narrow part of the tube (*isthmus*) ruptures sooner than one in the distal ampulla. Once the event occurs, the conceptus and blood from torn vessels pass into the peritoneal cavity. The time from fertilization to rupture varies. Rupture may occur from 2 to 12 weeks after fertilization. Most commonly, it develops between 5 and 9 weeks. Since fertilization has occurred, progesterone and estrogen are produced, causing symptoms of early pregnancy. After death of the conceptus, the endometrium breaks down, causing vaginal bleeding, which may appear as spotting or as a normal menstrual period. In ruptured ectopic pregnancy, external bleeding is minimal. The life-threatening hemorrhage occurs intra-abdominally from torn vessels as the tube ruptures.

The presenting signs and symptoms vary, depending on the gestational age of the fetus and the location of implantation and rupture. The patient may exhibit mild intermittent symptoms over several weeks or may develop acute severe manifestations. The paramedic may encounter a patient with minimal symptoms or may respond to a patient in profound life-threatening shock. Important historical and clinical data include the following:

- History of a missed or delayed menstrual period that may be abnormal
- Red or brown vaginal discharge in small amounts
- Repeated episodes of pain
- Early signs and symptoms of pregnancy
- Acute severe lower abdominal pain
- Syncope
- Signs and symptoms of vascular collapse, such as tachycardia, diaphoresis, thready pulse, decreased sensorium, hypotension, cool clammy skin, pallor, and tachypnea

The hallmark signs of ectopic pregnancy are abdominal pain accompanied by vaginal bleeding. The paramedic must rely on an accurate history and a high index of suspicion based on presenting signs and symptoms. Any female patient of child-bearing age with abdominal pain and vaginal bleeding should be managed as if shock is imminent. Transport to a hospital for definitive diagnosis and operative intervention must be expeditiously achieved. Assessment includes an appropriate history and a brief examination of the abdomen, locating areas of pain, tenderness, rigidity, and distention. Obtain orthostatic vital signs if the patient is not hypotensive in the supine position. Estimate amount of external vaginal blood loss by history and direct inspection.

Management includes placing the patient in the supine position with legs elevated if shock is pending or obvious. Administer 100% oxygen. Initiate a large-bore IV line. A second IV line is appropriate if marked hypotension exists. Infuse normal saline or lactated Ringer's solution at a rate in accordance with blood pressure response. Apply and inflate the PASG for hypotension (systolic below 90 mm Hg). Monitor and record vital signs, including blood pressure, pulse, and respirations, every 5 minutes. Transport to the hospital for definitive care.

Abortion

The two most common reasons for abnormal bleeding during the first trimester are **abortion** and ectopic pregnancy. An abortion is the termination of pregnancy before the fetus is viable. Viability is usually defined as 24 to 26 weeks gestation or a weight of 400 to 600 g. The terms for various types of abortion are given in the box "Types of Abortions."

Most abortions occur during the first trimester, usually before the 12th week. Bleeding may be minimal to exces-

---

TYPES OF ABORTIONS

Spontaneous: Loss of a fetus that results from natural causes and begins of its own accord. Vaginal spotting is the primary symptom; 10% of all pregnancies end in a spontaneous abortion.

Threatened: Vaginal bleeding occurs early in pregnancy, but the fetus has not yet aborted. The cervix is not dilated. The symptoms may subside and the pregnancy may proceed to term.

Inevitable: Uterine contractions and cervical dilatation accompany the vaginal bleeding, and the abortion is imminent.

Complete: Expulsion of the entire conceptus (fetus, placenta, and membranes) occurs.

Incomplete: Expulsion of a portion of the conceptus, usually the fetus, occurs. May cause significant bleeding, and the patient requires hospitalization for operative care.

Missed: Death of the fetus occurs *in utero* without expulsion for more than 4 weeks.

Induced (therapeutic): An elective abortion procedure is used to terminate the pregnancy. This procedure is performed by a physician for an unwanted pregnancy or if the pregnancy threatens the mother's life. Abortions up to 12 weeks' gestation are allowed in all states. In certain states and circumstances, abortions beyond 12 weeks' gestation may be permitted.

Criminal: An abortion procedure that is performed illegally by someone not licensed to practice medicine.

sive. The common causes of abortion are abnormalities in fetal development, structure, and implantation. Other causes include a hormonal imbalance of progesterone and infection.

Determine if the patient has passed tissue that could represent conceptus. Evaluate the amount of bleeding by history, number of pads used, and presence of current bleeding. Ask about the onset and duration of pain and cramping. Save and transport tissue for evaluation. Evaluate for volume depletion. Orthostatic vital signs are appropriate if the patient is not hypotensive in the supine position. Therapeutic intervention depends on the clinical status. Oxygen and IV volume replacement are indicated if circulatory status is marginal or if bleeding is excessive. The PASG can be used if volume depletion is severe. Transport for further evaluation and treatment. Loss of a fetus is usually a traumatic event for the patient. Provide empathy and psychological support.

Complications of Late Pregnancy

Complications of late pregnancy include preeclampsia, eclampsia, placenta previa, and abruptio placentae.

Preeclampsia and Eclampsia

Preeclampsia and **eclampsia** are hypertensive disorders specific to pregnancy. They occur late in pregnancy (after the 20th week) or soon after delivery. Preeclampsia is characterized by an elevation in blood pressure, protein in the urine, hyperreflexia, and edema in a person who has previously been normal. The rise in blood pressure may be sudden or develop over time. The significance of the rise in blood pressure depends on the baseline nonpregnant level. The blood pressure does not need to be high by normal standards to be significant. Elevation of blood pressure above 140/90 in the pregnant patient should alert the paramedic to preeclampsia. However, a 30 mm Hg rise in systolic pressure or a 15 mm Hg rise in diastolic pressure over prepregnancy levels may be diagnostic.

Edema is usually most pronounced in the hands and face. Excessive weight gain may occur and results from accumulation of fluid in the tissues. Other signs and symptoms include severe continuous headaches, dizziness, blurring of vision, persistent vomiting, and epigastric pain. The exact cause of preeclampsia or eclampsia is unknown. However, it occurs most frequently with the first pregnancy, age extremes (younger than age 20 or older than age 35), multiple gestation, diabetes mellitus, preexisting hypertensive, vascular, or renal disease, a family history of hypertension or vascular disease, and dietary deficiencies. Preeclampsia can progress to the convulsive state or eclampsia. Seizures are grand mal in nature. Eclamptic seizures can occur with relatively moderate increases in blood pressure.

The pregnant patient who has had a seizure must be evaluated for eclampsia. History of a previous seizure disorder must be determined. Eclampsia is a life-threatening event and may produce cerebral hemorrhage, renal failure, pulmonary edema, and death. The only definitive management of preeclampsia or eclampsia is delivery of the fetus. Assessment may reveal any or all of the physical findings described. The blood pressure is elevated to some degree from prepregnancy levels. The face and hands appear edematous. The patient may appear pale and quite ill. She should be kept calm and quiet. Darken the environment if possible, or dim the lights. Circumstances such as loud noises, bright lights, and sudden jarring may precipitate a seizure. Position the patient on her left side. Administer oxygen by nasal cannula. Initiate an IV line of D_5W TKO (to keep vein open). If a seizure has occurred, maintain the airway. The drug of choice for eclamptic seizures is magnesium sulfate 4 g IV not to exceed 1 g/min. The initial dose usually is followed by a continuous infusion of 1 to 2 g/hour. Diazepam 5 to 10 mg slow IV push (5 mg/min) may also be considered. Transport to a facility that can provide the appropriate level of obstetric care.

Third Trimester Bleeding

Vaginal bleeding in the third trimester should always be regarded as a serious complication. Both the survival of the fetus and the health of the mother may be jeopardized. Two primary causes are placenta previa and abruptio placentae.

PLACENTA PREVIA. **Placenta previa** is the implantation and development of the placenta in the lower uterine segment so that the placenta partially or completely covers the internal cervical os (Fig. 30-7). The placenta normally develops higher in the uterus. Three types of previa are identified. The total placenta previa covers the internal os completely. Partial placenta previa occurs when the placenta partially covers the internal os. Low implantation or marginal placenta previa occurs when the placenta is adjacent to but does not extend beyond the margin of the os. Total placenta previa is rare, and partial or marginal placental previa occurs in about 1 of every 200 deliveries. Predisposing factors include multiparity, advancing maternal age (greater than 35 years), multiple gestation, uterine scars (e.g., from previous cesarean section or uterine surgery), and repeated pregnancies with short intervals between them. Bleeding usually starts in the third trimester as the cervix begins to withdraw. Painless vaginal bleeding is the cardinal sign of placenta previa. It may begin as spotting or appear as profuse hemorrhage. It is unusual, however, for hemorrhage to appear without a previous episode of some degree of bleeding. Sexual intercourse may precipitate heavy bleeding in the patient with placenta previa.

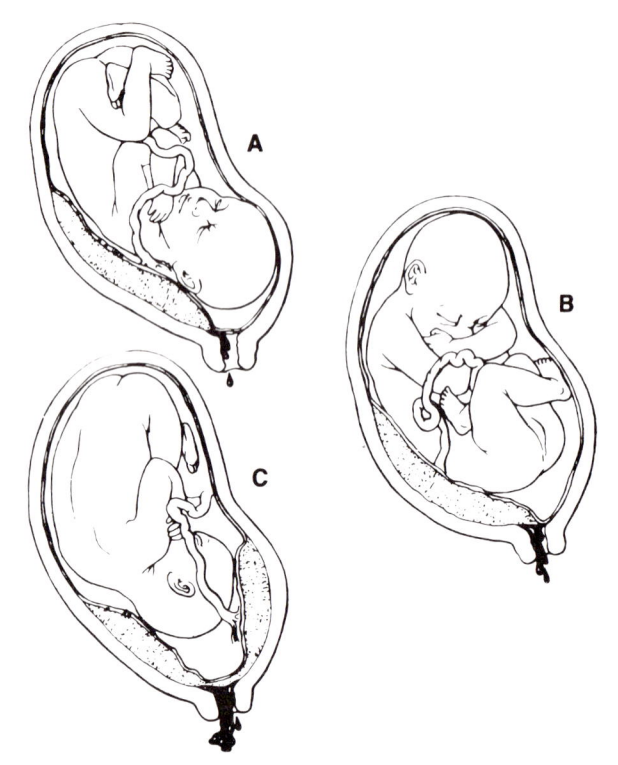

FIGURE 30–7.
Placenta previa. Low implantation (**A**), partial placenta previa (**B**), and central (complete) placenta previa (**C**). (Rosdahl CB)

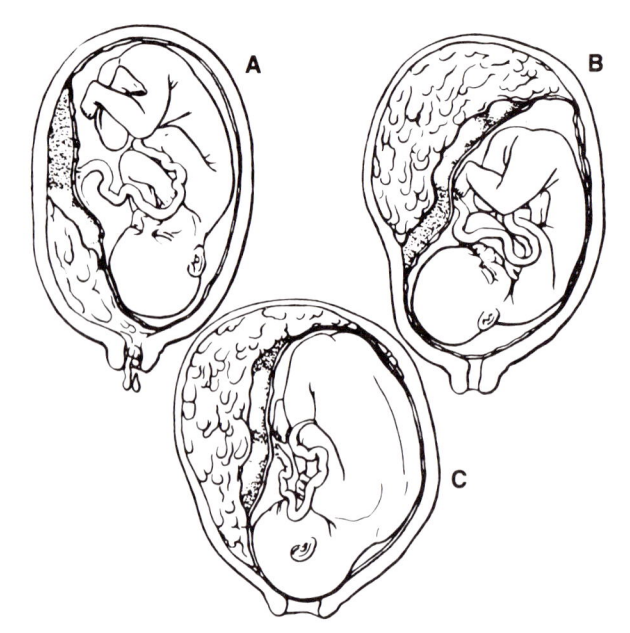

FIGURE 30–8.
Abruptio placentae at various separation sites. (**A**) The separation is low and not complete; vaginal hemorrhage is evident. (**B**) Separation is high in the uterine segment and there is internal or concealed hemorrhage. (**C**) Complete separation. External hemorrhage is prevented by the presence of the fetal head in the cervical os. This fetus is in grave danger, and an immediate cesarian section probably is needed to save the baby's and the mother's lives. (Rosdahl CB)

In addition to the usual assessment, other clues may alert the paramedic to the presence of placenta previa. History may reveal one or more episodes of vaginal bleeding during the first trimester, occurrence of placenta previa with an earlier pregnancy, five or more previous pregnancies, and bleeding immediately after intercourse. Bleeding is usually bright red and painless.

Third trimester bleeding should be treated aggressively, regardless of the amount of suspected blood loss. Apply oxygen and initiate a large-bore IV infusion of normal saline or lactated Ringer's solution for volume replacement. Transport should be initiated early for definitive therapy. The PASG may be used if shock is present. Inflate the leg compartments only.

ABRUPTIO PLACENTAE. *Abruptio placentae* is the premature separation of the placenta from its uterine attachment (Fig. 30-8). The separation may occur at the center of the placenta or at the margins or as a combination of both. The amount and location of the separation determine the amount and location of blood loss. Abruptio placentae occurs in about 1 of every 250 pregnancies. Several factors appear to predispose to premature separation of the placenta. Hypertension of any cause, whether preeclampsia or essential hypertension, may contribute to abruptio placentae. This complication also increases with **parity** (the number of pregnancies) and with a short umbilical cord. Trauma may also produce premature separation. If separation occurs in the central portion of the placenta, blood loss may be trapped between the uterine wall and the placenta. Hemorrhage is concealed, possibly masking the seriousness of the situation. When separation occurs at the margin of the placenta, blood loss is external. Complete separation is associated with massive hemorrhage, which may not be readily apparent, depending on the position of the fetus.

The patient may or may not present with a history and evidence of dark vaginal bleeding. If bleeding occurs behind the placenta, external bleeding may be absent. Pain may also be present or absent, depending on the degree of separation. When pain is present, onset may have occurred with physical activity or trauma. Localized uterine tenderness may be present on palpation. The finding of abdominal tenderness also varies with degree and location of the separation. In severe abruption, fetal heart tones may be absent, and shock is frequently out of proportion to the amount of external bleeding. Aggressive management is indicated and is the same as for placenta previa.

LABOR AND DELIVERY

Labor is the process of expelling the fetus and placenta from the uterus and the vagina. Labor has been described as the three "P"s. The "*passage*" refers to the birth canal and the contour of the mother's pelvis to accommodate the "*passenger*" or fetus. "*Power*" refers to the ability of the uterus to contract in a manner that facilitates the birth.

Labor

The fetus must pass through the ring formed by the pelvic bones. The ring is composed of the two hips, the sacrum, and the coccyx. The hip is composed of the ilium, ischium, and the pubis; it forms the anterior and lateral portions of the ring. The sacrum forms the posterior portion of the ring, and the coccyx is below the sacrum and also forms the posterior ring. The coccyx has some flexibility and can be pushed backward during the birthing process. The normal position of the fetus is head first (cephalic). *Vertex* is the term used to denote the portion of the fetal cranium between the anterior and posterior fontanelles. The anterior-to-posterior dimension of the cranium is the widest, and the transverse dimension is the smallest. Therefore, the fetus usually presents with the transverse diameter first. The following obstetric terms describe the position of the fetus at delivery:

Station: the presenting part of the fetus and its relationship to the mother's ischial spines
Engagement: occurs when the fetus is at the midpoint of the pelvis at the ischial tuberosities
Attitude: the degree of flexion of the fetus
Presentation: the presenting part of the fetus
Cephalic: vertex, brow, face, or chin
Frank Breech: buttocks
Complete Breech: thighs flexed on abdomen and legs on thighs
Footling Breech (incomplete): one foot or both feet
Shoulder Lie: position (*e.g.*, transverse, oblique, vertical)

The power of labor is due to uterine contractions that result from the coordinated activity of the uterine muscle fibers. These fibers have important properties. First, they can elongate to permit growth of the uterus during the advancing pregnancy. Second, they have elasticity, which prevents the fibers from remaining stretched after delivery. Third, and most important for effective labor, is the property of contractility to expel the fetus during labor and delivery. As the fetus passes into and through the birth canal, the uterine muscle fibers become shorter and thicker to remain in close contact with the fetus.

The mother may have experienced relatively painless contractions at intervals throughout the pregnancy after the 12th week. These are *Braxton–Hicks* contractions and are of little consequence clinically. Pathophysiologically, they aid nutrient exchange by maintaining pressure in spaces between the villi.

During the first stage of labor, contractions are short and mild and occur 10 to 15 minutes or more apart. The contractions of true labor gradually increase in frequency, intensity, and duration. Labor sometimes is experienced initially as discomfort in the back and abdomen. Some women may continue to feel contractions primarily in the back. During the second stage, the contractions last from 50 to 70 seconds and occur at intervals of 2 to 3 minutes. Toward the end of the second stage, the urge to push or bear down becomes strong.

Vaginal show is a discharge composed of blood and mucus that is a sign of impending labor. The presenting fetal part ruptures capillaries, and a small amount of blood mixes with cervical mucus. The show is pinkish in color and is related to dilatation of the cervix.

Rupture of the amniotic sac usually occurs early in the second stage of labor. At times, however, the membranes may rupture before the onset of active labor. A large or scant amount of amniotic fluid may drain from the vagina. When rupture occurs before labor, the risk of prolapsed cord increases if the presenting part is not adequately engaged.

Cervical effacement is the shortening and thinning of the cervical canal. Cervical dilatation is the widening of the cervical canal. Complete dilatation is about 10 cm.

The stages of labor are the following:

Stage one: Begins with the onset of labor and concludes with full cervical dilatation
Stage two: Begins with full cervical dilatation and concludes with delivery of the fetus
Stage three: Begins with delivery of the fetus and concludes with delivery of the placenta

Wide variations occur in the duration of labor. However, the average length of first labor is 14 hours. Subsequent labors are about 6 hours shorter than the first.

During active labor, the mother experiences an increase in blood pressure, pulse rate, cardiac output, and respiratory rate. The mother may lose between 300 to 500 mL of blood during delivery. However, blood volume is increased during pregnancy; therefore, the loss is somewhat compensated.

Uterine contractions are a key component of the labor process that the paramedic evaluates to determine imminent delivery. Labor is an individual experience, and, although averages in time can be estimated, each labor is different, depending on parity, the size and attitudinal position of the fetus, the ability of the uterine contractions to propel the passenger along the passage, the mother's pelvic contour, cervical changes, and overall psychological attitude. Because evaluation of cervical dilatation is not field practice, uterine contractions, presence of show, and crowning determine the decision to transport. Emergent normal deliveries may be encountered in the multiparous patient with a rapidly progressing labor and the adolescent who does not recognize or who denies active labor. The premature infant may also present a precipitous delivery.

TABLE 30-2.
STATISTICS OF CONDITIONS OF PREGNANCY AND DELIVERY

Condition	Statistics
Early abortion (first 12 weeks)	10%–15% of all pregnancies
Placenta previa	1 in 200 deliveries
Abruptio placentae	
Mild	1 in 250 deliveries
Severe	1 in 500 deliveries
Preeclampsia and eclampsia	4.3%–23.5% of all pregnancies, reports vary
Transverse lie	0.25% of all deliveries
Face presentation	1 in 600 deliveries
Brow presentation	1 in 2000 deliveries
Twins	1 in 85 births
Identical twins	⅓ of all twin pregnancies
Fraternal twins	⅔ of all twin pregnancies
Triplets	1 in 7629 births
Quadruplets	1 in 670,734 births
Quintuplets	1 in 41,600,000 births
After taking ovulation-inducing drugs*	
Triplets	1 in 1696 births
Quadruplets	1 in 5370
Breech presentation	3.5% of all deliveries
Prolapsed cord	1 in 300 deliveries
Vertex presentation	95% of births

Seventy-two percent of triplets and quadruplets are born to those who take ovulation-inducing drugs.

Delivery

While the majority of pregnancies and deliveries are uneventful, a significant number are considered of high risk, in which the mother or the fetus has an increased risk of death or disability (Table 30-2). Imminent delivery occurs late in the second stage of labor and is characterized by intense contractions with a short duration between contractions, uncontrollable pushing by the mother, pressure on the rectum that produces the sensation of impending bowel movement, perineal bulging, rectal bulging, and crowning of the fetal head. The head may appear and disappear, but birth is usually near when it remains visible between contractions, and this is called ***crowning.***

The goal of field delivery is to assist delivery with minimal trauma to the mother and without injury to the infant. Priorities include anticipating and recognizing problems during birth and protecting the child from cold stress after birth.

If delivery is imminent, the following procedure is followed:

1. Explain to the mother and bystanders (*i.e.*, husband or family members) the reason for the decision not to transport. Provide reassurance that this process is normal. Focus on the mother's role in the birth and emphasize that you are there to assist.
2. Prepare a comfortable location and position for the mother.
3. One crew member should monitor the mother's condition and stay close to her head and upper torso. The paramedic should assume the responsibility for delivering the infant. Communicate with the mother throughout the delivery, offering support and encouragement. Allay anxiety. After delivery, one care giver must manage the newborn (see newborn section) while the other attends to the mother.
4. During the delivery, the care giver at the head of the patient should instruct the mother to push only when a contraction occurs and to try to relax between contractions. Before delivery of the head, panting-type breathing may be beneficial with contractions to prevent a precipitous delivery. During this stage, a semi-Fowler's position with knees flexed is suggested. Encourage the mother to push to assist in the delivery. Repeat instructions and encouragement frequently and provide reassurance.
5. Wash hands thoroughly, open the obstetric kit, put on gloves, and arrange drapes and instruments in an organized easy-to-reach pattern near the delivery area.
6. The need for oxygen and the initiation of an IV infusion is determined by the immediacy of delivery and the mother's vital signs. If complications exist or are anticipated, apply oxygen. The IV fluid to use is normal saline or lactated Ringer's solution at about 100 mL/hour.
7. The mother may be supine with knees flexed and

hips externally rotated for delivery; elevation of the hips facilitates delivery.
8. Cleanse the perineum beginning at the vaginal opening and extending outward to include the entire perineum and upper medial thighs, if time permits.
9. Drape the mother to preserve modesty and to provide a clean area for delivery of the infant. As the delivery progresses, support the perineum with a sterile 4-by-4 inch dressing over the anus. This dressing can protect the infant from contamination and ease tension on the perineum.
10. During preparation and delivery, the primary concern is to prevent any uncontrolled delivery that results in trauma to the mother and infant. Place one hand on the fetal head and apply gentle pressure with the palm of the hand to the crowning head and perineum to prevent rapid expulsion of the head. Precipitous delivery can cause intracranial hemorrhage. Never try to hold the head back or delay delivery.
11. Fetal position changes automatically during the delivery. The infant makes these cardinal movements to maintain the narrowest diameter of the body to travel the birth canal (Fig. 30-9).
12. As the mother experiences the almost involuntary need to push, the fetal head passes the cervix and presses on the vagina (Fig. 30-10). The infant's head is then flexed forward onto the chest (flexion). Next, the head internally rotates so that the occiput is in the superior rotation below the symphysis pubis (internal rotation). Extension of the head causes the head, chin, and face to exit the birth canal (extension). This process usually takes 1 to 3 contractions. At this point, the paramedic should use both hands to guide the birth. With one hand on the infant's chin and the other hand on the occiput, guide the extension maneuver. Do not turn the infant yourself. Never put any pressure on the uterus to speed the delivery. This pressure is extremely dangerous and may cause uterine rupture. Instructing the mother to pant between contractions facilitates delivery of the head. It is preferable to deliver the head between contractions. Use a bulb syringe to aspirate secretions from first the infant's mouth and then the nose. If meconium (fecal material) is present, suction thoroughly. Aspiration of meconium can result in damage to the lungs and can be fatal. On rare occasions, the amniotic sac does not rupture. If it doesn't, nip the membranes at the back of the neck to prevent aspiration of fluid as the infant takes its first breath. After delivery of the head, inspect the neck for a looped umbilical cord. If the cord is looped, it usually can be easily loosened and slipped down over the infant's head. If the cord cannot be loosened, it must be cut between two clamps. Next, the head externally rotates back to the transverse position from the anterior–posterior of extension (restitution). The shoulders present in an anterior–posterior position, with the anterior shoulder usually delivering first. Gentle downward traction may be applied using both hands on the head to assist delivery of the anterior shoulder. The rest of the infant is born (expulsion) without any additional fetal maneuvers.
13. Note the gender of the infant and time of birth. Perform Apgar scoring at 1 and 5 minutes (see section on newborn).
14. After delivery, blood-tinged amniotic fluid usually flows from the birth canal.
15. Hold the infant with the head slightly down to facilitate drainage of secretions. Maintain a firm grip on the infant. Do not hold the infant upside down by the feet. Suctioning and vigorous drying should initiate crying. Position the infant on the mother's abdomen or close to the birthing area. Never place the infant below the level of the birth canal.
16. Repeat suction of the mouth and nose.
17. After birth, the cord continues to pulsate. Do not hurry to cut it. Waiting until pulsation stops and keeping the infant at the level of the birth canal give the infant additional blood from the umbilical cord.
18. Cut the cord about 8 to 10 inches from the infant's umbilicus, between 2 secure clamps placed 2 inches apart. Keep the clamp on the portion of the infant's cord that remains attached to the infant.
19. Dry the infant and wrap in a dry clean or sterile blanket and give to the mother to hold.
20. After the infant is born, the uterus can be palpated just below the umbilicus. It should feel firm and round.
21. After an interval of uterine resting, contractions begin to separate the placenta from the uterine wall. Placental separation may occur from 1 to 20 minutes after delivery of the baby. Indications that the placenta has separated include further delivery of more of the umbilical cord and sudden release of blood from the vagina; the uterus also becomes more firm and globular in shape, while rising higher in the abdomen. Transport should not be delayed for delivery of the placenta. No attempt should be made to manually deliver the placenta. Pulling on the cord or placenta can cause serious consequences, such as uterine inversion. If the placenta is spontaneously delivered, save it and the attached cord in a plastic bag. Take it to the hospital to be inspected for completeness.

The first hour after delivery of the placenta is sometimes called the fourth stage of labor. The mother requires continued monitoring to assess for signs of postpar-

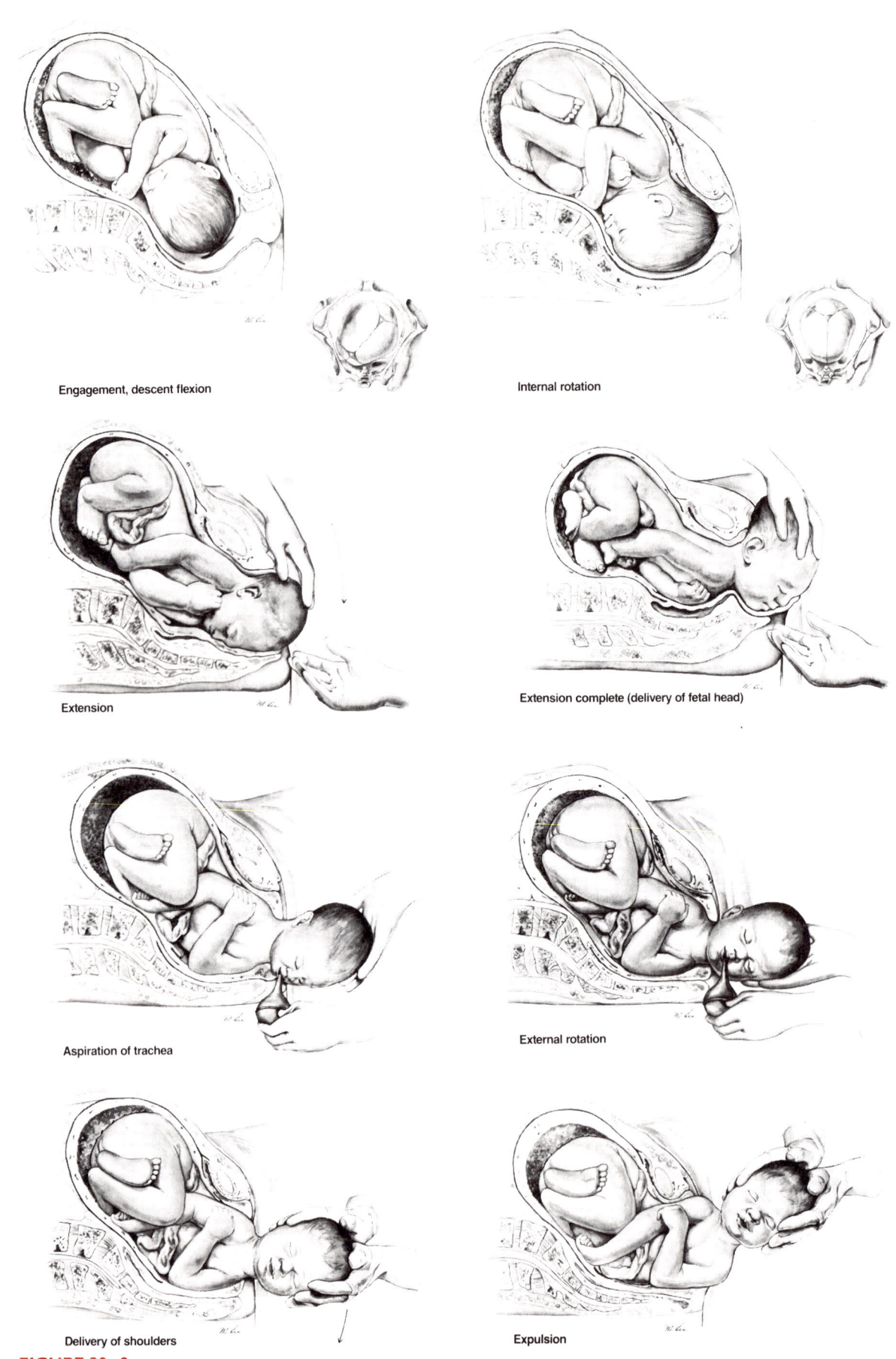

FIGURE 30–9.

Mechanism of delivery for a vertex presentation. (Reeder S, Martin L)

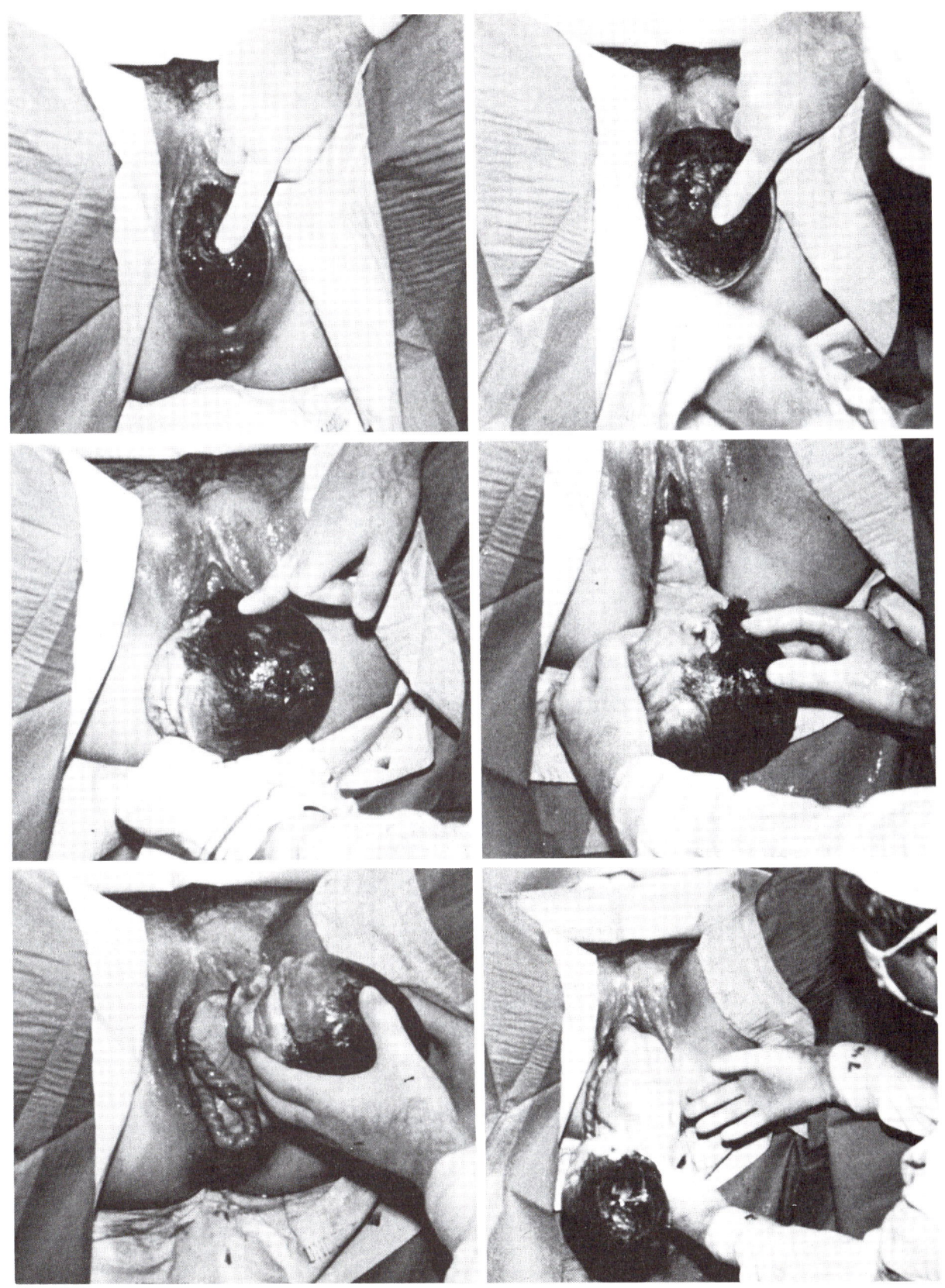

CHAPTER 30: Gynecologic, Obstetric, and Newborn Emergencies   709

FIGURE 30-10.
Assisting an emergency birth. Apply gentle, even pressure with the flat of your hand or fingers on the emerging head to slow the baby's progress and protect the mother's perineum. Gently support the head during restitution and external rotation. Placing palms over baby's ears, apply gentle traction downward until the anterior shoulder appears fully, then upward to lift out the other shoulder. As the body emerges, slide your hand down the baby's back, cradling the buttocks in one hand, the head and the upper back in the other. Hold the head lower than the trunk. (Reeder S, Martin L)

(continued)

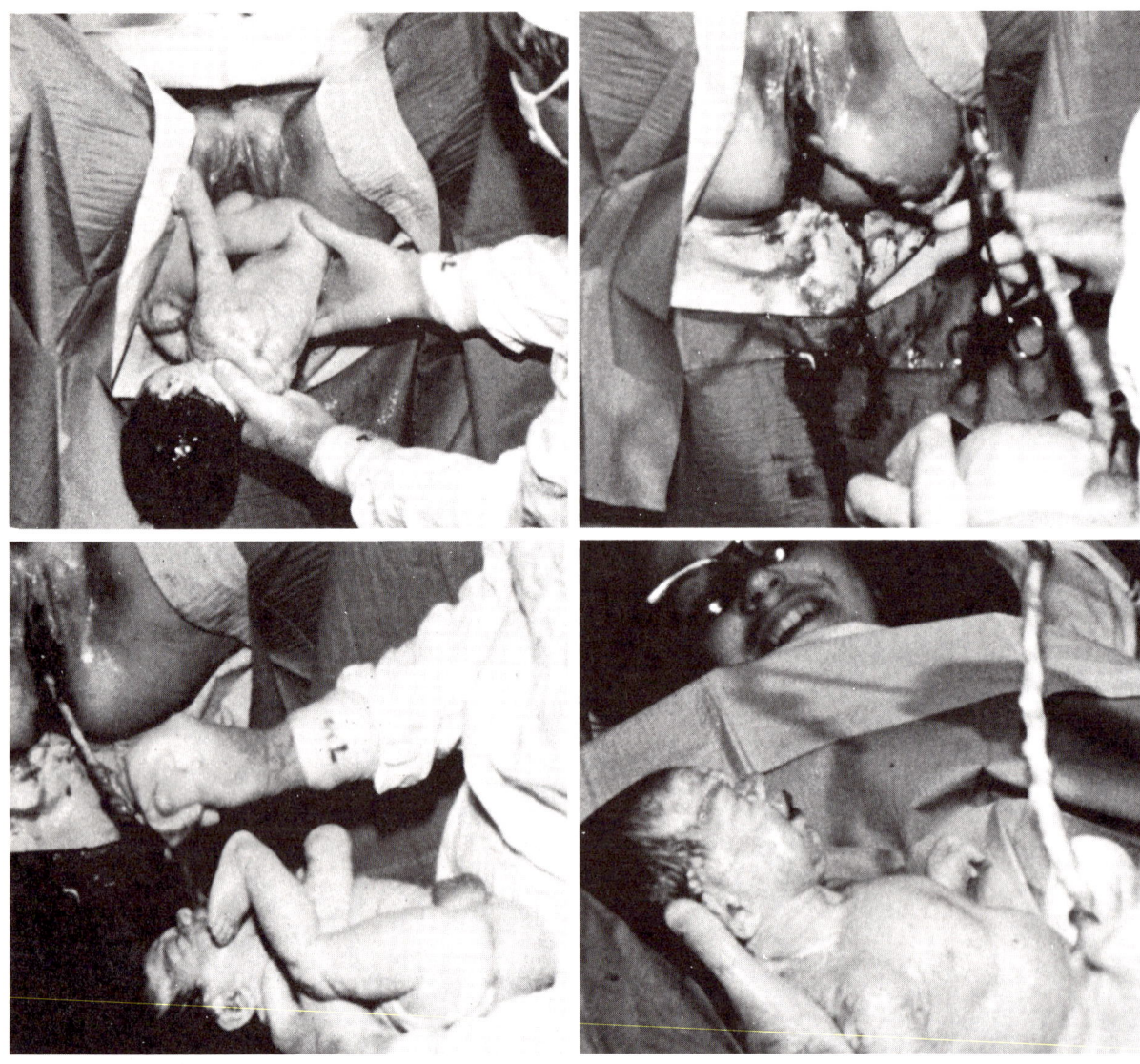

FIGURE 30–10.
(Continued)

tum hemorrhage. Continued uterine contractions of the myometrium produce vasoconstriction. If the uterus is permitted to relax, this hemostatic mechanism fails, and hemorrhage can ensue. To care for the mother during this stage, monitor the pulse, blood pressure, and respirations. Assess the amount of vaginal bleeding. A 300 to 500 mL blood loss is normal. Initiate IV therapy as necessary. Check the fundus of the uterus frequently to be sure it is contracted or firm (Fig. 30-11). If the uterus relaxes, massage the fundus to promote contraction (see postpartum hemorrhage). If perineal tears have occurred, apply direct pressure using a perineal pad or large dressing. Dry the blood and fluid and provide a clean drape or blanket. Allow the mother to hold the baby. Keep both patients warm and transport without lights and siren if both are stable.

Abnormal Presentations

In 95% of all labors, the fetus is in the occiput or vertex presentation. Delivery of an infant in other than an occiput or vertex presentation may cause *dystocia* (difficult delivery). If an abnormal presentation is expected, attempt to avoid an at-home delivery. Definitive obstetrical care is needed, and an emergency cesarean section may be required. Most abnormal presentations require intervention beyond the scope of paramedic practice. Delay in transportation may jeopardize the infant's need for adequate oxygenation and perfusion. If a foot, arm, or shoulder is presenting, the mother and child should be immediately transported.

Breech Presentation

A **breech** presentation occurs when the buttocks, lower extremity, or extremities are the presenting part (Fig. 30-12). The most common type is the *frank breech*. The buttocks present with the hips flexed and the legs extended against the chest and abdomen. In the *incomplete breech* position, one or both feet or the knees extend below the buttocks (footling breech). Rarely, the hand may present

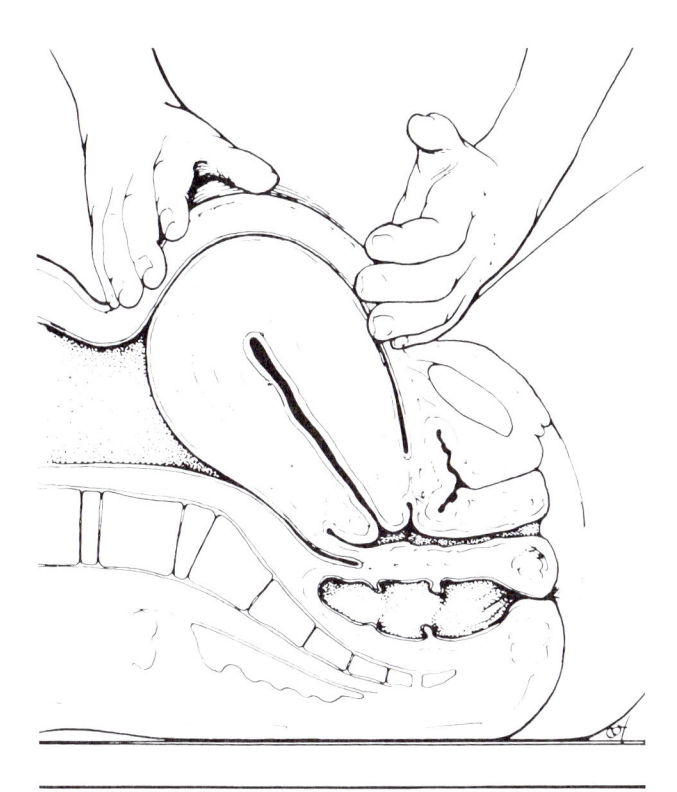

FIGURE 30–11.
Method for palpating the fundus. (Reeder S, Martin L)

with the buttocks. Breech presentation is more common in the premature infant and with multiple births. The infant is at greater risk for delivery trauma and anoxia from compression of the umbilical cord. The incidence of prolapsed cord is also increased. The mother should be transported to the hospital for delivery if at all possible. Consider use of a helicopter if available, as transport time is significant.

If delivery is imminent or in progress, position the mother with her buttocks on the edge of the bed. Have someone help her hold her legs in a flexed position. Never pull on the infant's legs to hasten delivery. Encourage the mother to push, and allow the baby to be delivered with the contractions. Do not touch the breech until after the umbilicus has been delivered so that the temptation to exert traction or "assist" the delivery is eliminated. After delivery of the umbilicus, support the baby as the arms are delivered. When the head is past the pelvis, gentle traction may be applied until the mouth appears over the perineum. The head should be delivered slowly to reduce cranial trauma and intracranial hemorrhage. Once the head is delivered, suction the mouth and nose. Continue routine management of the newborn. Monitor closely for signs of distress.

Other Abnormal Presentations

The shoulder presentation, or the transverse lie, occurs when the infant lies crosswise in the uterus instead of longitudinally. The shoulder is the usual presenting part at the inlet, and the infant cannot enter the pelvic outlet for vaginal delivery. The arm may prolapse into the vagina. If the membranes rupture, the umbilical cord may prolapse. Complications include rupture of the uterus and death of the mother and fetus. The transverse position is apparent on observation and palpation of the abdomen. The mother should be rapidly transported for possible cesarean section.

Face presentations occur less commonly. The face presents at the vulva with the chin anterior. Due to the usual edema of the presenting part, the face may not be immediately recognizable and may be mistaken for a breech. Delivery may be spontaneous. If delivery does not progress, however, transport rapidly for possible cesarean section.

In the brow presentation, which occurs rarely, the brow rather than the vertex is the presenting part. Vaginal delivery is not possible in this position since the largest diameter of the head is presenting. Rapid transport is indicated.

Compound presentations occur when an extremity enters the pelvis at the same time as the presenting part. The most common is an arm that prolapses along the

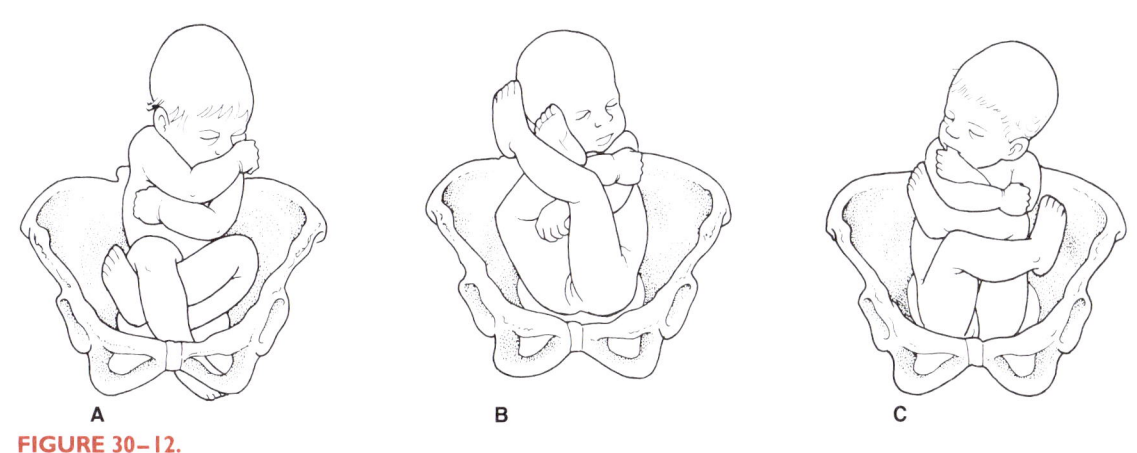

FIGURE 30–12.
Breech presentation may be incomplete or footling breech (**A**), frank breech (**B**), or complete breech (**C**). (Martin L, Reeder S)

head. The incidence of prolapse of the umbilical cord is increased in this presentation. Management includes alleviating pressure from the cord.

Successful management of abnormal presentations includes early recognition of the complication. Provide reassurance to the mother. Transport as soon as possible for definitive management.

Multiple Births

Fraternal twins result from the fertilization of two ova by two spermatozoa. Fraternal twins each have their own placenta, usually do not look alike, may be of different genders, and are separated by individual amniotic membranes. **Identical twins** are less common (one out of three twin conceptions) and result from fertilization of a single ovum. Identical twins are the same gender and look alike. Identical twins may share a common placenta and amniotic sac or may have separate structures.

The mother usually has been informed about the multiple birth by her physician. If she has not received prenatal care and is unaware of the presence of twins, be prepared to deliver a second infant after delivering a smaller than average infant or if the uterus still seems unusually large after the first delivery. The first infant should be handled as a normal delivery as previously described. The cord should be clamped and cut. Be sure that the clamps are secure, especially if the other infant is sharing the same placenta. The position or lie of the second infant may change after delivery of the first. The delivery has a more favorable outcome if the second twin is born 5 to 10 minutes after the first. In general, twin or other multiple births should be delivered in the hospital and transport should be expedited. If twins are delivered, additional assistance is needed since three patients need to be monitored and transported.

Multiple births may result in premature delivery. The infants may be smaller than normal and have special needs for warming. The second infant is at increased risk for hypoxia and prolapse of the cord. Be prepared for resuscitative measures. Postpartum hemorrhage is not uncommon because of a large placental site and hypotonic uterus.

Abnormal Deliveries

Cephalopelvic disproportion is a complication of labor and delivery. The term implies a relationship between the size of the fetal head and the pelvis. The problem may originate with either the passenger (fetus) or the passageway (pelvis). Causes are a contracted pelvis, an oversized baby, or fetal abnormalities. Excessive size of the infant (4000 g or more) may be due to maternal diabetes, large size of one or both parents, multiparity, and possibly postmaturity. Hydrocephalus, cojoined twins, and fetal tumors are congenital abnormalities that can cause difficult childbirth.

Extended labor can produce fetal distress and demise and uterine rupture. The mother is frequently in her first pregnancy and reports the experience of frequent strong contractions for a prolonged period of time. Labor does not progress normally. Management includes administration of oxygen to help prevent fetal anoxia. Initiate an IV line of normal saline or lactated Ringer's solution for volume expansion as needed and transport for possible cesarean section.

Prolapsed Umbilical Cord

During the course of labor, the umbilical cord may prolapse through the pelvic outlet into the birth canal ahead of the presenting part (Fig. 30-13). A **prolapsed umbilical cord** is a grave complication for the fetus, since the cord is then compressed between the presenting part and the bony pelvis. Fetal circulation is impaired or obstructed completely. Any factor that prevents proper adaptation of the presenting part to the maternal pelvis predisposes to prolapse of the cord, including abnormal presentations, multiple births, premature delivery, and premature rupture of the membranes when the presenting part is not sufficiently engaged. The prolapse may or may not be visible at the vaginal opening.

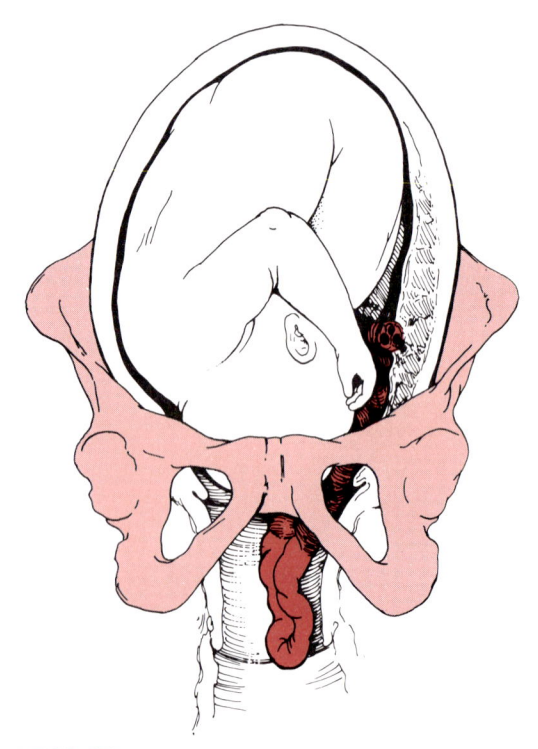

FIGURE 30-13.
Prolapse of the cord. As the head comes down, the compression of the cord between the fetal skull and the pelvic brim shuts off the fetus' circulation completely. (Reeder S, Martin L)

Immediate management of a prolapsed cord is to minimize the pressure of the presenting part on the cord. Check for pulsations of the cord. Positioning the mother may help alleviate pressure by gravity. Depending on the situation and point in the delivery process, the Trendelenburg position with the hips elevated on a pillow or the knee–chest position may be used. In the knee–chest position, the hips are raised above the level of the shoulders. The mother assumes the face-down position with the shoulders and upper chest and knees on the bed or stretcher and the hips elevated. The thighs are perpendicular to the surface. This position may be difficult to achieve and maintain in a moving ambulance and can present safety considerations.

The paramedic may insert two fingers into the vagina to elevate the presenting part off the cord. Apply pressure evenly over the occiput or other presentation. Do not attempt to push the cord back into the birth canal. Apply a towel moistened with normal saline solution to the cord to prevent drying. Administer 100% oxygen to the mother. Transport rapidly. Cesarean section may be required. The mother most likely is aware that the delivery is not normal. Provide reassurance and psychological support.

Precipitous Delivery

A *precipitous delivery* is a rapid spontaneous delivery of less than 3 hours from the onset of labor to birth. It occurs most frequently in the woman who has completed two or more pregnancies. The primary danger is cerebral trauma to the infant or tearing of the umbilical cord. The mother may sustain lacerations of the perineum, which bleed profusely. Precipitous delivery should be anticipated when labor is progressing rapidly. Attention should be focused on the mother. Be prepared for rapid delivery. Handle the infant securely as delivery progresses to minimize further injury from being dropped if delivery is explosive. Monitor the newborn closely and provide adequate warming measures, since the newborn may have difficulty with temperature regulation after rapid delivery.

Complications of Delivery

Postpartum Hemorrhage

Hemorrhage during the postpartum period is the most common cause of serious blood loss in pregnancy. *Postpartum hemorrhage* is the loss of more than 500 mL of blood in the 24-hour period after birth. Estimation of blood loss is always difficult, and the clinical condition of the patient must be evaluated. Excessive postpartum bleeding occurs in about one fourth of all deliveries. The most common causes of postpartum hemorrhage include loss of uterine tone or poor uterine tone, lacerations of the birth canal, and retained fragments of the placenta. The patient with a clotting disorder is also at risk. Infection and uterine inversion are less common causes.

A number of predisposing factors should alert the paramedic to the possibility of postpartum hemorrhage. These include any situation that overdistends the uterus, such as a large infant or multiple births. Past births and previous postpartum hemorrhage increase the risk for excessive bleeding. Abruptio placentae, placenta previa, prolonged labor, and precipitous delivery are also predisposing factors.

The paramedic may encounter postpartum hemorrhage after a field delivery. The emergency medical services system may also be called after delivery at home or at an independent birthing center when excessive blood loss occurs. Assessment and management are similar to third trimester bleeding as described previously. In addition, the uterus should be palpated for firmness or loss of tone. Ascertain the date and time of delivery if the paramedic was not in attendance. If the uterus does not feel firm, apply fundal massage (see Fig. 30-11). Support the lower uterine segment with the edge of one hand just above the symphysis. Massage the fundus gently but firmly with the other hand. The uterus is cupped between the hands and supported while it is massaged. Continue massage until the uterus feels very firm. Do not overmassage once it is well contracted. Overstimulation can cause fatigue of the muscle with subsequent relaxation and further hemorrhage. If possible, keep one hand lightly on the fundus. If this is not possible, recheck frequently and reapply massage as necessary.

Placing the newborn at the mother's breast to nurse may also help cause the uterus to contract. If the mother's condition is unstable, however, this action is not recommended. If bleeding is excessive, oxytocin may be administered. Oxytocin is a hormone that increases electrical and contractile activity in uterine smooth muscle. The uterus is sensitive to the actions of oxytocin near full term. It should be used in postpartum hemorrhage only when it is certain that a second fetus is not present in the uterus. Administration should follow delivery of the placenta whenever possible. Oxytocin is supplied in 10 *United States Pharmacopeia* (*USP*) units (20 mg) per mL. The IV dose is 10 to 20 *USP* units in 1000 mL normal saline or lactated Ringer's solution. Administer at 1 to 4 mL/min titrated to the severity of hemorrhage and uterine response. Side effects may include a transient but marked vasodilative effect, tachycardia, cardiac arrhythmias, uterine spasm, and uterine rupture.

Uterine Rupture

Uterine rupture is a rare but serious complication of pregnancy. Mortality rate for both mother and infant is extremely high. The wall of the uterus ruptures when it is unable to withstand the strain placed on it. Uterine rupture may occur during the pregnancy but is more common after the onset of labor. Occasionally, it may result from direct trauma. Predisposing factors include previous cesarean section, previous operative scar (noncesarean), prolonged or obstructed labor, certain faulty positions or fetal abnormalities, past births, and excessive fetal size.

When rupture occurs during labor, the patient complains of severe, shearing, sudden pain during a strong contraction. Fetal movements and heart tones are lost. If the rupture is complete, the pain ceases. Abdominal tenderness is present in both complete and incomplete rupture. After complete rupture, the uterus may be palpated as a hard mass beside the fetus. Fetal parts are more readily palpable. Profound shock develops rapidly. External blood loss may be minimal because of concealed hemorrhage. Fetal heart tones are usually absent. If rupture is incomplete, pain continues and shock may develop more slowly. Management includes aggressive therapy for shock and rapid transport for cesarean section.

Uterine Inversion

Uterine inversion is a rare event in which the uterus turns inside out after birth. It is most frequently caused by applying pressure to the umbilical cord in an attempt to hasten delivery of the placenta and by applying pressure to the uterus when it is relaxed. Profound shock ensues and should be managed appropriately. The patient should be transported rapidly to the hospital.

CARE OF THE NEWBORN

Initial evaluation of the newborn determines if the airway is clear, respirations are adequate, and the circulation is effective.

Airway

The newborn's airway must be cleared before the first breath to prevent aspiration. Suction the mouth and then the nose as soon as the newborn's head is delivered, before delivery of the chest. The nose should not be suctioned first, since the infant could take a breath as the nose is being irritated and swallow or aspirate fluid and mucus in the oropharynx. The head should be kept dependent to help drain mucus. Do not oversuction and deprive the newborn of needed oxygen.

Breathing and Circulation

The cardiac and respiratory systems are interrelated, and the use of the lungs alters the circulation after birth. Breathing status is evaluated for synchronized inspirations, absence of intercostal retraction, xiphoid retraction, dilatation of the nares, and expiratory grunt (Fig. 30-14). During the first 30 minutes of life, a period of transition from intrauterine to extrauterine life, the newborn is likely to have irregular respirations, with some retraction and

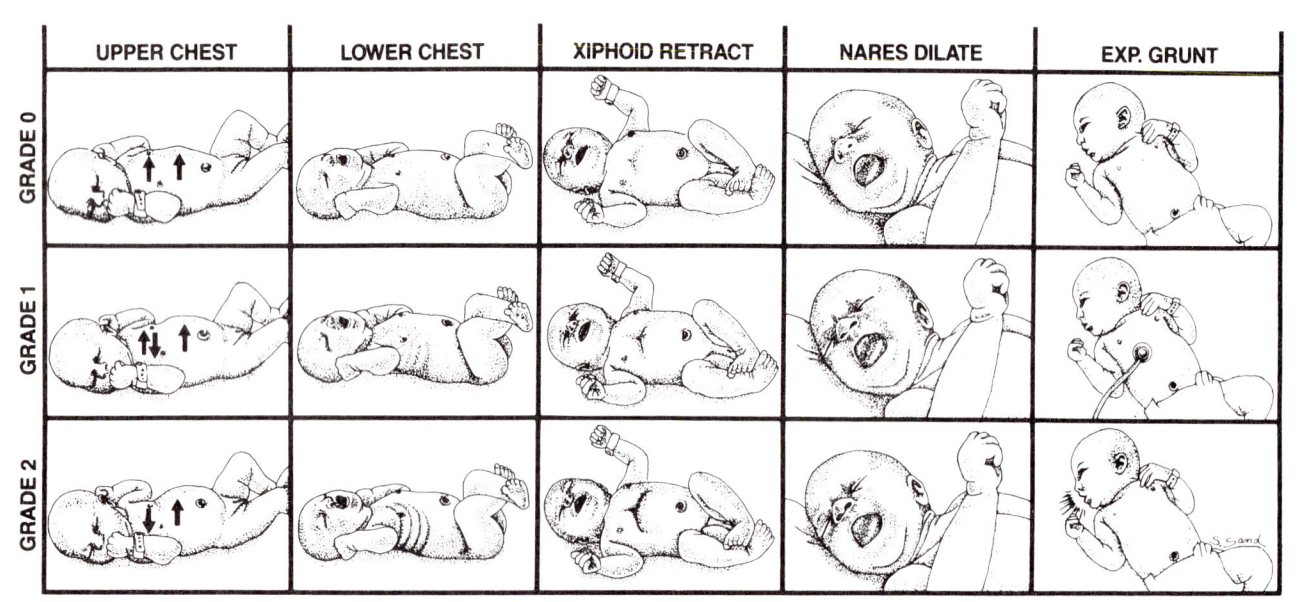

FIGURE 30–14.
Observation of respirations. An index of respiratory distress is determined by grading each of five arbitrary criteria; grade 0 indicates no difficulty, grade 1, moderate difficulty, and grade 2, maximum respiratory difficulty. The retraction score is the sum of these values. A total score of 0 indicates no dyspnea; a total score of 10 denotes maximal respiratory distress. (Rosdahl CB)

nasal flaring, and breathe at a rate in the range of 30 to 90 breaths per minute. Watch the diaphragm and the abdominal muscles.

Crying should be spontaneous and is a signal that the newborn is breathing. Short episodes of crying allow the infant to inflate and expand the lungs. However, too much crying may be exhausting for the newborn. The newborn should cry within the first 30 seconds of life. If the newborn does not cry, gently rub the back to elicit a response. Avoid vigorous spanking or rubbing. The first breath is a result of a drop of the newborn's PaO_2 from 80 mm Hg to below 50 mm Hg, a rise in $PaCO_2$, and stimulation of cold receptors. The fluid in the lungs actually makes the alveoli expand with less difficulty than if the alveoli were dry. After the first breath, the lungs are inflated and the pulmonary artery pressure decreases and the PaO_2 rises. These changes lead to closure of the ductus venosus, since the umbilical arteries and vein no longer have blood flow (obliteration is complete in 2–3 months); closure of the foramen ovale, since pressure is greater in the left heart than the right because of the increase in blood volume (obliteration is complete in 12 months); and closure of the ductus arteriosus (obliteration is complete in 1 month).

As breathing is initiated, the newborn's heart rate increases from an intrauterine rate of 120 to 160 beats per minute to 180 beats per minute. After about an hour, the rate drops to 120 to 140 beats per minute. Activities such as crying increase the rate. Apical rates should be counted for 1 minute. The femoral pulse is the most easily palpable to assess circulation. Blood pressure readings usually are not auscultated in the newborn. However, normal blood pressure is about 80/50 mm Hg. In general, skin color in the newborn is a ruddy hue because of a higher concentration of red blood cells. Because the peripheral circulation takes about 24 hours to normalize, the hands, feet, and the lips appear cyanotic and feel cold. These findings are considered normal for the first day of life. The newborn may also appear mottled.

Initial Evaluation

Characteristics of the newborn are shown in Tables 30-3 and 30-4. These criteria are important in determining the newborn's status.

The **Apgar score** is an index for determining the newborn's physiologic status (Table 30-5). The five-element score is done at 1 and 5 minutes after birth. The score serves to standardize the evaluation of the status of the newborn physiologically. The purpose of the Apgar score is to identify infants who require routine care and those who need further assistance. Each element is given a 0, 1, or 2, and the five scores are added to obtain a total score of 0 to 10.

In general, the Apgar score reflects the following:

Less than 4 = serious condition that requires some degree of resuscitation
4 to 6 = condition is guarded
7 to 10 = normal stable infant

The newborn should respond to airway support with a subsequent rise in the Apgar score. Heart rate, respiratory effort, and color have been described. When assessing muscle tone, the extremities remain flexed, and the newborn resists attempts to extend them. The newborn moves the extremities and attempts to control head movement. Flaccid and limp extremities are abnormal. Reflex irritability is elicited by either a slap to the sole of the foot or irritation of the nose with a suction catheter.

TABLE 30–3.
CHARACTERISTICS OF THE NEWBORN

Characteristic	Measurement
Weight	Average 7.5 lb (3.4 kg) female
	Average 7.7 lb (3.5 kg) male
	Low birth weight is less than 5.5 lb (2.5 kg)
Height	Average 20.9 inches (53 cm) female
	Average 21.3 inches (54 cm) male
	Low birth length is less than 18 inches (46 cm)
Head circumference	13.5–14 inches (34–35 cm)
Temperature	99°F
	98.6°F after first 24 hours of stabilization
Pulse	160–180 beats per minute initially
	120–140 beats per minute within 1 hour of stabilization
Respiration	30–50/min once stabilized at rest
Blood pressure	80/50 mm Hg
Blood volume	80–110 mL/kg, average of 300 mL

TABLE 30-4.
REFLEXES AND OTHER CHARACTERISTICS OF THE NEWBORN

Reflex	Function
Blink	To protect the eye
Rooting	To locate food, the infant moves his or her mouth toward stimulus, e.g., a stroke on the cheek (lasts for 6 weeks)
Sucking	To take in food
Extrusion	To prevent swallowing, the infant sticks out tongue if something is placed on it (lasts for 4 months)
Palmar grasp	Closes fingers around something placed in the palm of the hand (lasts for 6–12 weeks)
Plantar grasp	Toes grasp something that touches the sole of the foot (lasts for 8–9 months)
Moro	For protection, the newborn abducts and extends the arms and legs when startled and then brings the arms to the chest and pulls up the legs onto the abdomen
Hearing	Present within hours after birth
Sight	Present immediately after birth: the irises are gray or blue until the infant develops true eye color in 3 months
Lanugo	Fine hair on shoulders, back, and arms (disappears in 2 weeks)
Head	¼ of total length, forehead prominent
Fontanelles	Anterior: junction of two parietal bones and frontal bone; diamond-shaped; closes in 2–18 months
	Posterior: junction of two parietal bones and occipital bone; triangular-shaped
	Fontanelles may bulge if intracranial pressure is high or if the infant cries; fontanelle may pulsate; may be indented if the infant is dehydrated
Molding	Shaping of that portion of the head that engaged the cervix

Maintaining Warmth

Assessment and management of the newborn are performed simultaneously. After the airway, breathing, and circulation are evaluated and resuscitative intervention has begun if indicated, the newborn must be kept warm. Airway support and maintenance of temperature are the keystones in the care of the newborn. The newborn's temperature may drop because of general heat loss and a poorly functioning temperature regulating system. The four mechanisms of heat loss are the following:

Evaporation: The newborn is covered with fluid from the amniotic sac, and the liquid converts to a vapor. This form of heat loss is the most extensive.

Radiation: The newborn may lose body heat as it is transferred to a nearby cold surface or object.

Convection: Body heat is lost if the surrounding air is cooler. Convection causes more heat loss if the room has a draft, thereby increasing air velocity and increasing heat loss.

Conduction: Conduction is heat loss to a cooler object that is in contact with the newborn.

After delivery, the newborn should be dried with a clean or sterile towel. Wrap the infant in a dry blanket and keep warm. Do not wrap in the towel used to dry the amniotic fluid. The damp towel causes additional heat loss and cooling. The environmental temperature should be kept at 23 to 24°C (74–76°F). Prevent air drafts and do not place the newborn on a cold surface. Position on one side with the head in a slightly dependent position to facilitate drainage of secretions. A stockinet cap reduces heat loss from the head, which represents a large vascular surface of the body. An isolette is ideal for transport, if available. Well-insulated hot water bottles or rubber gloves filled with warm water may be used with great care. They must be well insulated and should not touch the newborn, since burns may result. Never use chemical hot packs.

Premature Infant

The preterm or premature infant is born before the 38th week of gestation. The infant's weight is usually less than 2500 g (5.5 lb). After premature birth, the newborn is at increased risk for hypothermia because of lack of subcutaneous fat, high surface-mass ratio, and insensible loss

TABLE 30-5.
APGAR SCORE

Category	0 Points	1 Point	2 Points
A Appearance	Blue, pale	Body pink, extremities blue	Completely pink
P Pulse rate	Absent	Below 100	Above 100
G Grimace	No response	Grimaces	Cries
A Activity	Limp	Some flexion of extremities	Active motion
R Respiratory	Absent	Slow, irregular	Good strong cry

from respiratory distress. Respiratory problems are common, since the alveoli are not mature until 34 to 36 weeks. Cardiovascular problems can occur because of immaturity of the cardiovascular system and failure of fetal circulatory structures to close.

The premature infant requires special attention and observation. Perform routine care for the newborn with emphasis on warming and clearing the airway. The umbilical clamp must be secure to prevent bleeding from the umbilical cord.

Management of the Distressed Infant

Resuscitation of the distressed infant is primarily concerned with ventilation and oxygenation. Advanced life support procedures, including IV therapy, pharmacologic intervention, and other cardiac care, are not generally indicated. Adequate suctioning is required. The infant should be dried rapidly, wrapped, and kept warm. Hypoxic infants have greater difficulty with thermoregulation and may easily become hypothermic. Foil blankets may be useful as an outer wrap to conserve body heat. If stimulation is required, it includes gentle rubbing along the back and gentle slapping of the soles of the feet.

Oxygen should be administered at 4 to 5 L/min from tubing or a mask held near the face. Avoid using oxygen from a tank stored in an outside compartment when the weather is cold. Do not aim the oxygen stream directly at the infant's face. If the infant is pale or cyanotic, administer oxygen until the color improves and becomes pink. Oxygen toxicity is unlikely since time of administration in the field is short. If ventilatory assistance is required, use an infant bag–valve–mask device to avoid excessive volumes that might inadvertently be delivered with an adult bag. Monitor chest expansion closely. Use a clear mask that is an appropriate size to minimize dead space. Maintain the head in a neutral position. Overextension or underextension may occlude the airway. Avoid hyperinflating the lungs. Mechanical resuscitators should not be used for this reason. Endotracheal intubation may be required if bag–valve–mask ventilation is ineffective. Ventilation rate is 40 to 60 breaths per minute. If chest compression is required, two fingers are placed in the middle of the sternum and compressed ½ to 1 inch at a rate of 100 times per minute. A 5:1 ratio of chest compression to ventilation with 100% oxygen should be used (see Appendix B).

Before or during delivery, the paramedic should be alert for the presence of meconium in the amniotic fluid. **Meconium** is the dark green or black substance found in the large intestine of the fetus. Hypoxia in the distressed infant stimulates reflex relaxation of the anal sphincter and accelerated intestinal peristalsis. Therefore, meconium in the amniotic fluid signals fetal distress. Meconium causes severe lung inflammation if inhaled. Vigorous suctioning should be performed before the first breath. Repeated suctioning may be required and should be applied judiciously. Do not continue to suction for longer than 10 seconds to avoid inducing further hypoxia. The lungs should be ventilated, either spontaneously or assisted, and 100% oxygen should be supplied between suctioning procedures. If meconium is noted in the field, it should be reported to the physician.

SUMMARY

Care of the patient with a gynecologic emergency requires knowledge and skills in the areas of physical assessment, history taking, and the management of the patient in hypovolemic shock. Paramedics need the skills of IV cannulation, use of the PASG, and general shock management. Caring for the obstetric patient can take one of two paths. The uncomplicated on-scene delivery can be a heart-warming and sensitive experience for all of those involved. The complicated delivery can pose difficult decisions for the paramedic. The two leading causes of maternal mortality are hemorrhage and infection. Understanding the pathophysiologic consequences of hypovolemia, the compensatory mechanisms, and the appropriate management enhances the paramedic's ability to reduce mortality from hemorrhage. In general, the patient in labor should be transported to a hospital setting, where the delivery can be performed in a controlled environment with the resources of an operating room for a possible cesarean section. Paramedics, with sensitivity and experience, can be of great assistance to those women who require prehospital intervention.

SUGGESTED READING

American Heart Association: Standards and Guidelines for Cardiopulmonary Resuscitation and Emergency Cardiac Care. Dallas, American Heart Association 1986

Bocka JJ: OB trauma: Prehospital care of the pregnant trauma patient. J Emerg Med Serv 13(10):51, 1988

Bocka JJ, Courtney J, Pearlman M et al: Trauma in pregnancy. Ann Emerg Med 17(8):829, 1988

Dierking BH: Neonatal resuscitation. J Emerg Med Serv 21(8):19, 1989

Dickinson ET: Life-threatening gynecological emergencies: When pain calls for action. J Emerg Med Serv 15(3)20, 1990

Henzler H, Martin ML, Young J: Delayed diagnosis of traumatic diaphragmatic hernia during pregnancy. Ann Emerg Med 17(4):350, 1988

Reeder S, Martin L: Maternity Nursing, 16th ed. Philadelphia, JB Lippincott, 1987

Tortora GJ, Anagnostakos NP: Principles of Anatomy and Physiology, 6th ed. New York, Harper & Row, 1990

US Department of Transportation, National Highway Traffic Safety Administration: Emergency Medical Technician–Paramedic: National Standards Curriculum. Washington, DC, US Government Printing Office, 1985

CHAPTER 31

Behavioral and Psychiatric Emergencies

Misconceptions
Forms of Emotional Disorders
Characteristics of Emotional Disorders
   Psychiatric Emergency vs. Emotional Crisis
Assessment of Behavioral Emergencies
   Sources of Information in Emergency Assessment
   The Emergency Interview
   The Mental Status Examination
   Transportation to Emergency Departments
   Factors That Affect Emotional States

Other Factors Associated With Behavioral Emergencies
   Substance Abuse
   Factors Associated With Reactions to Substances
   Domestic Violence
   Child, Spouse, or Elder Abuse
   Sexual Assault
   Suicide

Principles of Crisis Intervention
   Crisis Intervention Outline
   Emotional Reactions to Crisis
   General Crisis Intervention Strategies
   Managing Severe Mental Disturbances
   Controlling the Violent Situation
      Methods of Restraint
      Procedures for Restraining a Patient
   Legal Ramifications of Crisis Care
Summary

BEHAVIORAL OBJECTIVES
On successful completion of this chapter, the reader will be able to:

1. Identify two misconceptions a paramedic may encounter when caring for behavioral emergency patients
2. Identify the three main types of emotional disorders
3. List the common causes of transient disorders, anxiety states, and psychoses
4. Distinguish between a psychiatric emergency and an emotional crisis
5. Recognize three characteristics and behaviors exhibited by the behavioral emergency patient that the paramedic can use to assess patient status
6. Discuss six other factors associated with behavioral emergencies
7. Explain three ways to control a violent situation
8. Discuss emotional reactions that people exhibit during crisis situations
9. Identify several methods of restraint in crisis intervention
10. Identify legal ramifications of crisis care
11. Define all of the key terms listed in this chapter

KEY TERMS

The following terms are defined in the chapter and glossary:

crisis
crisis intervention
delusions
domestic violence
emotional crisis
hallucinations
illusions
mental status examination
psychiatric emergency
psychosis
restraints
sexual assault
suicide

Paramedics have been accused of "turning off" or "tuning out" the "human elements" of their care. Some people see the high degree of technical proficiency and rapid decision making in paramedics as a sign that they are insensitive or uncaring. People may also misinterpret the paramedics' sense of urgency on a call as well as their professional mannerisms and concise and rapid speech.

A more careful evaluation of paramedics, however, shows them to be sensitive, action-oriented, dedicated people who pride themselves on quick but accurate decisions to rapidly resolve problem situations on the behalf of ill and injured people. Frequently, a lack of training in the "human elements" is the cause of the misinterpretation of the paramedic's image. Because words like psychiatric, psychological, or behavioral are commonly related to images of "crazy" people out of control, paramedics avoid training programs in behavioral emergencies and crisis intervention. When given the choice between reading an article on cardiac arrest or one on a behavioral issue, paramedics usually pick the one on cardiac arrest, even though they encounter many more emotionally distressed people than people in cardiac arrest. In fact, every ambulance call involves emotional elements that occur in the victims, their families, the community, and even in the paramedics.

New materials and courses have been developed for training emergency personnel to manage behavioral emergencies, but few paramedics have taken advantage of these materials and courses. Dr. Calvin Frederick has stated, with a degree of certainty, that those "... who provide ambulance, fire, or police service are almost totally unprepared to render psychological first aid in the management of acute mental problems."

This chapter will stir interest in paramedics who wish to add the human element to patient care. The addition of the human element makes the paramedic's job safer and more personally satisfying.

MISCONCEPTIONS

Rumors and misconceptions are found in virtually every form of human experience. These rumors and misconceptions are also present in emergency medical services. Some of the more common rumors and misconceptions that paramedics encounter are that behavioral emergencies always involve "crazy" people and that people who are experiencing an emotional disturbance are likely to hurt themselves or others and should be considered dangerous. An even more ludicrous misconception is that a person can become crazy simply by coming in contact with a disturbed person. Another myth is that behavioral emergency patients are always problem cases for the paramedic.

The truth is that psychological distress and disturbance can apply to a range of human behaviors that stretch from the perfectly normal person to the severely disturbed psychotic. It is also impossible to become crazy simply by being in contact with someone who is.

One of the first steps in helping others is to examine personal misconceptions and prejudices related to behavioral emergencies. On becoming aware of the obstacles that block improved management of patients, the paramedic must develop an open mind to a new way of thinking, that is, to see emotionally disturbed people as people with a problem instead of "problem people."

FORMS OF EMOTIONAL DISORDERS

The range of human behavior from the normal person to the severe psychotic is so complex that it is difficult to discuss without some form of categorization. Table 31-1 is provided to help paramedics understand the various forms of emotional distress. It is important to remember that psychological distress may be mild, moderate, or severe in nature. The degree of intensity tempers the type and amount of intervention necessary.

Organically caused disturbances, which are behavioral disturbances caused by ingestion of some type of toxic substance (e.g., drugs), are most likely transient or progressive and permanent. In addition, anxiety states occasionally may be apparent with organic involvement. In all cases of behavioral emergencies, organic causes must always be initially ruled out. A thorough history and a mental status examination (described later) are extremely important. If any indication in the patient's medical history supports the possibility of organic involvement, other factors, such as the degree of disturbance or disability and family or other support, should be determined.

Transient states, or short duration personality disorders, can be successfully managed in the field, depending on the circumstances of the incident that triggered the response and the amount and type of help that is available during the crisis. Specific guidelines for intervention in a variety of situations are given later in this chapter.

Many anxiety states and psychotic reactions can be temporarily managed under crisis conditions; however, anxiety states and psychotic reactions are not finally resolved until adequate long-term professional mental health services are made available to the patient. Some anxiety states and psychotic conditions are permanent lifelong situations that cause repeat episodes over the years.

TABLE 31-1.
GENERAL CATEGORIES OF EMOTIONAL DISTURBANCE

Types	Causes	General Symptoms
ORGANIC		
Physiological cause (must always be ruled out first)		
Transient disorders	Toxicity	Mental confusion
	Infections	
	Substance abuse	Impaired thinking
Anxiety states	Advanced alcoholism	Poor attention span
	Brain injury	Impaired memory
	Fevers	Changes in level of consciousness
Psychosis	Dementia	Impaired emotions
	Delirium	
	Presenile	Disorientation
	Senile	
FUNCTIONAL		
No physiological cause (consider after organic is ruled out)		
Transient disorders	Stress	Anxiety
	Injury	Confusion
	Illness	Poor decision making
	Marital problems	Overcontrol
	Sudden death in family	Feelings of frustration
		Anger
		Grief
		Guilt
Anxiety states	Developmental problems	Anxiety
		Fear
	Threat	Phobias
		Depression
Psychosis	Stress development	Hallucinations
		Delusions and illusions
		Thought disorders
		Significant behavioral disorders

CHARACTERISTICS OF EMOTIONAL DISORDERS

To present a simple classification of emotional disorders is difficult because the disorders overlap, and time elements, such as transient vs. permanent, add to the complexity. The International Classification of Diseases places emotional disorders in the following categories:

I. Organic psychotic conditions with four subgroups, such as senile, alcohol, drugs, and others
II. Other psychoses with breakdown into schizophrenia, affective psychoses, and paranoid states
III. Neurotic and personality disorders
IV. Mental retardation

This section focuses on three types of emotional disorders: transient or situational disorders, anxiety states, and psychoses. The transient emotional disorders are the least severe and the psychoses are the most severe. This breakdown pertains more to the paramedic in the field than the International Classification, since it focuses on the behavioral elements and common causes. Summary material is presented in Table 31-2.

Psychiatric Emergency vs. Emotional Crisis

One of the difficulties faced by paramedics in behavioral emergencies is that at least 250 psychiatric conditions have been identified. It would be a monumental task for the paramedic to become completely familiar with each of the psychiatric disturbances, taking years of training. Trimming the broad spectrum of material down to a useful summary is of greater benefit to facilitate quick decisions under stressful circumstances.

When working with a behavioral problem in a patient, the paramedic must know what constitutes a psychiatric emergency and what is better classified as an emotional crisis. A *psychiatric emergency* is any situation in which patients' moods, thoughts, or actions are so disordered or disturbed that they have the potential to produce danger,

TABLE 31–2.
CHARACTERISTICS OF THE THREE MAIN EMOTIONAL DISTURBANCES

Disturbance	Common Causes	Characteristics
TRANSIENT DISORDERS (A temporary mental derangement that usually occurs after severe stress)	Overwhelming stress Physical injury Drugs Severe threat Sudden loss	Sudden onset is usual Resolves when the situation that is causing the condition is resolved Total recovery usually expected May become a permanent condition without proper help to resolve the problem
ANXIETY STATES (A form of emotional disturbance that disrupts one or two main areas of life but allows normal function in others; usually a long-term or even life-long problem)	Problems in early development Previous emotional trauma Loss Threat Fear Severe stress	Anxiety Apprehension Nervousness Doubts Tension Guilt Fear Phobias Depression Loss of self-confidence Lasts longer than current situation Person is able to function in most important areas of life Might need psychotherapy Repeats itself May need psychiatric hospitalization
PSYCHOSIS (Severe mental derangement sufficient to impair reality in most areas; usually a long-term or life-long problem with occasional acute episodes)	Genetic factors Severe emotional trauma at critical stages of development Problems in parenting, e.g., absence of love Biochemical malfunctioning in the brain	Disturbed motor behavior Disruption in emotions Disruption in orientation Hallucinations Delusions and illusions Often life-long condition Frequently causes a disruption in normal life functions May need frequent hospitalizations

harm, or death to themselves or to others if the situation is not quickly controlled.

An *emotional crisis,* on the other hand, is a situation with much less intensity. It is distressing but in most cases is not likely to end in danger, harm, or death if not responded to immediately. However, if neglected entirely, an emotional crisis may escalate to a full psychiatric emergency.

ASSESSMENT OF BEHAVIORAL EMERGENCIES

Paramedics who work with behavioral emergencies need to triage the patients quickly into one of three categories: emergency, urgent, and nonemergency.

A true behavioral emergency, like a medical emergency, has an element of serious threat attached to it. Without immediate intervention, true behavioral emergencies can end in injury or death to the patient or to someone else near the patient. True behavioral emergencies include the following:

- Suicidal activity
- Mental derangement, which produces an inability to care for one's basic needs
- Violent behavior, especially when a history of violence is found
- Medical problems that complicate or cause behavioral symptoms
- Severe psychoses
- Severe depression

Urgent behavioral situations are those that must be attended to as soon as possible after the more severe emergencies have been managed. Urgent behavioral situations generally require less intense expenditures of energy on the part of the paramedic. Overall, urgent behavioral situations have less potential for serious harm but may escalate to dangerous conditions if ignored. Because urgent conditions usually require some form of professional intervention, the patient should be transported to a hospital for evaluation. A typical list of urgent behavioral situations includes the following:

- Acute agitated state
- Panic attacks
- Drunkenness from alcohol (usually associated with behavioral problems)
- Bizarre behaviors
- General suicidal or homicidal thinking without a specific plan of action
- Serious but not extreme state of depression
- Those in a state of grief due to the sudden death of a loved one

The nonemergency cases have a far less degree of urgency attached to them. Nonemergency situations are less likely to result in potentially dangerous behaviors. Kindness, reassurance, and general support are usually sufficient until specialized services are available. Nonemergency situations include the following:

- Situational problems such as job, family, or marriage (depends on individual and degree of stress)
- A person needing emotional support and a listening ear
- Those who might need information to resolve some of their anxiety
- Mild generalized anxiety cases
- Known chronic cases who are involved in on-going treatment programs in the community

Sources of Information in Emergency Assessment

To determine in which behavioral emergency category to place a distressed person, the paramedic must rely on a variety of sources of information. Unfortunately, many disturbed or distressed people are not able to present a complete, coherent, and accurate history. The paramedic must be prepared to obtain information from alternate sources, including the following:

- Observations
- Conversation with the distressed person
- The person's family
- Friends of the distressed person
- Employers or coworkers
- Clergy
- The police
- Other medical personnel involved with the case
- Neighbors
- Bystanders
- A mental health professional who knows the person
- Written notes
- The physical environment
- Medication containers

The Emergency Interview

When a patient is able to communicate appropriately, significant insight can be gained into that patient's problems, and a plan of action can be developed to manage the situation.

The interview should start with the presenting problem. The patient should be asked what the major problem is at that time. Once it has been established what may be causing the problem, the patient should be asked why it has now become an emergency. It should be determined, during the interview process, what circumstances triggered the present problem and whether or not this problem has occurred before. In developing a plan of action, it frequently helps to know what served to resolve the problem in the past.

The paramedic should be careful to keep most of the conversation related to the current problem. Some distressed people like to get off on a tangent and discuss their entire life's problems. This tendency causes a distraction to properly managing the current problem. The paramedic should be comfortable and proficient in conducting the emergency interview so that the patient receives quick and appropriate care.

The emergency interview can be divided up into several distinct parts. Questions should cover the following:

- Personal information
- Presenting problems
- Brief history
- Physical findings
- Mental status examination

No fixed amount of information needs to be obtained, but the box "Emergency Interview Information" outlines some of the information that helps complete a behavioral assessment. Because it is of great importance, the mental status examination is presented separately.

The Mental Status Examination

A short organized format for emergency interviewing has been developed by psychiatrists and has been used by paramedics for many years. Called the **mental status examination,** it is used to help gather information about the patient's behavioral, psychological, and intellectual functions.

The mental status examination begins with observation of the appearance and general behavior of the patient. The following physical characteristics and behaviors can tell the paramedic a great deal about the patient being assessed:

- Dress and grooming
- Eye contact (appropriate)
- Posture (depressed people do not stand and sit with an air of self-confidence, they look beaten)
- Slowed body movements (depression)
- Wringing of hands (agitation)
- Violence
- Facial grimaces
- Actions
- Mannerisms

Speech is the second part of the mental status examination. It should be observed whether or not the person's speech has the following characteristics:

- Spontaneous or pressured
- Slow or fast
- Soft or loud
- Clear or slurred
- Understandable or not
- Appropriate or inappropriate

Seriously distorted or unusual speech patterns are indicative of problems. The more disturbance in speech, the more likelihood of serious internal disturbance.

EMERGENCY INTERVIEW INFORMATION

Personal

Name
Age
Gender
Occupation
Years employed
Marital status
Lives with whom
Address
Phone number
Closest relative
Address of closest relative
Living conditions
Family supports

History

Previous similar problems
Psychiatric hospitalizations
Physical illnesses
Significant distressing events
Past use of drugs or alcohol
Family history of problems
Coping strategies
Military history
Criminal record (be cautious)
Involvement in psychotherapy

Major Problem

Chief complaint or problem
When problem started
What has made it an emergency
What help is person seeking
Is this a first-time problem
Expectations of those involved

Physical Findings

Allergies
Current use of drugs or alcohol
Blood pressure
Medications
Pulse
Respirations
Temperature
Pupil size
Pupil reactivity
Nystagmus
Signs of head injury
Stiff neck
Skin color and texture
Tremors

The next concern is the patient's mood. It is important to note whether the person is any of the following:

- Depressed
- Euphoric
- Manic
- Anxious
- Angry
- Agitated
- Fearful
- Guilty

The patient's mood should be assessed as to its appropriateness or inappropriateness according to the current circumstances.

The mental status examination then moves into the area of thought. Note if the distressed person is having any of the following thoughts:

- Racing thoughts
- Hallucinations that are auditory (e.g., hearing voices), visual, or somatic (e.g., strange bodily sensations)
- Obsessive thoughts
- Delusions (false beliefs)
- Suicidal thoughts
- Unconnected thoughts
- Disturbed or distorted thoughts

A natural subdivision of the thought segment of the mental status examination is perception. Consistently misinterpreting actual stimuli or perceiving things that do not exist are indications of serious mental derangement and are key signs of **psychosis.** The most common distortions in perception are the following.

Hallucinations: sensing (seeing, smelling, tasting, feeling, hearing) things that do not exist
Illusions: misinterpreting actual stimuli
Delusions: maintaining a false belief in spite of having facts presented to the contrary

The final step in the mental status examination is to evaluate the cognitive abilities of the person. It must be determined if the patient is oriented to person, place, time, and situation. In addition, it should be observed if the patient is having problems paying attention or concentrating on the information provided by the paramedic. Problems in cognitive ability also include difficulties with memory, thinking clearly, insight, and judgment. Again, the more serious the disruption in cognitive abilities, the more significant the mental derangement.

One way to quickly remember the mental status examination under emergency conditions is to remember "*SEA-3,*" which means the following:

S: speech
E: emotions
A-3: alertness, awareness, actions (or behaviors)

Transportation to Emergency Departments

Paramedics are often faced with an uncomfortable dilemma when making a decision to transport an emotionally distressed patient to an emergency department. The decision is relatively easy when obvious physical injuries are present but not in the absence of injuries.

When injuries are present, the primary duty of a paramedic is to care for the life and safety of the patient. All other considerations are secondary. If a serious illness or injury is present, the patient should be transported to an emergency department in accordance with the medical protocols of the jurisdiction.

In cases without serious physical injuries, the paramedic should consider what might be in the best interest of the patient. If patients are so disturbed that danger to themselves or others is possible, they should be brought to an emergency department. Other circumstances that usually require hospitalization include the need for medications and behavior that is so bizarre that the person will become involved in serious conflict with society if left without care. If the patient's family refuses to assist in the patient's care or if the environment intensifies the symptoms, it is best to transport the patient to a hospital. Finally, when crisis intervention strategies fail, an emergency department evaluation is indicated.

The pressure to hospitalize is less if the symptoms are not severe and if the environment is one that can support and assist the distressed person through the crisis period. If the paramedic has any doubt about whether or not an emergency department visit is required, the patient should be transported for evaluation. It is always better to make an error that is in the best interest of the patient.

Factors That Affect Emotional States

Emotional states change frequently. As events change, emotions are generated and people react. Many factors make the impact of an event more or less powerful. The following are some of the key factors that influence the impact of events on people:

- History of psychosis
- The type of event
- Intensity or magnitude of the event
- The speed of onset of the event
- Duration of the event
- The simultaneous occurrence of multiple distressing events
- Amount of warning (if any)
- Amount of time to prepare
- Previous traumatic events
- Existence of a support network including family and friends
- The existence of well-developed and practiced coping strategies

- Manner in which the threat or event is perceived (whether it is looked at as the most tragic event or one that can be managed)
- Self-image of the person who encounters the problem
- Attitude of others toward the victim
- The possibility of escape from the distressing event
- Age of the victim
- Existence of resources to manage the situation
- Amount and type of outside help available
- The speed at which help becomes available

OTHER FACTORS ASSOCIATED WITH BEHAVIORAL EMERGENCIES

Many times the paramedic encounters behavioral emergencies that are precipitated or influenced by factors other than emotional states. The paramedic should be alert for these additional factors and alter patient care as is appropriate to the situation.

Substance Abuse

Some of the most frequently encountered behavioral emergencies in the United States involve patients who are intoxicated from one or more substances, ranging from alcohol to glue to a variety of controlled dangerous substances. Substances of any kind intensify the potential for uncontrolled erratic activity and threat of injury to others. Poor attitudes and inappropriate behavior on the part of the paramedic can easily turn a bad situation into an explosive one. In addition to the potential for dangerous activity, substance abuse cases are associated with medical, legal, law enforcement, and behavioral complications that usually are not found in other forms of crises.

This segment does not intend to provide a thorough coverage of the various types of substances and their effects on people. Instead, it offers practical general information that can be useful for paramedics under field conditions.

Factors Associated With Reactions to Substances

Chemicals and personalities mixed together produce highly unpredictable reactions. Extreme caution and a state of alertness are essential for paramedics who wish to remain both safe and effective. Reactions to chemical substances from alcohol to cocaine depend on the following factors:

- Type and dosage of the chemical
- The size, weight, and metabolism of the person who is using the substance
- The situation; where, when, and under what circumstances the substance has been used
- The mental attitudes, expectancies, and motivations of the user
- The personality of the user; how mature the person is, whether or not the person has experienced drug abuse before, and if psychological conditions exist previously
- Tolerance; how much of the substance the person needs to gain the same effect as earlier uses
- Contaminants; foreign substances in the chemical of abuse or other drugs used in combination may change the entire drug reaction and produce unusual or dangerous reactions

Domestic Violence

Domestic violence is a particularly dangerous variety of violence for emergency personnel. When violence breaks out in a family, the participants are even less rational than in other forms of violence. Their emotions are extraordinarily high, and anyone from the outside (*i.e.*, police, paramedics, or other emergency workers) is likely to stir enormous resentment and negative reactions from the involved family members.

To stay out of harm while attempting to intervene in a family situation in which violence has broken out and a person has been injured, the following suggestions should be kept in mind:

1. Never take sides.
2. Separate the combatants into different rooms.
3. Make sure the police are called in immediately.
4. Do not work alone.
5. Keep your voice under control; that is, use a calm steady voice.
6. Do not take unnecessary risks.
7. Jealousy runs rampant in disturbed families. Be careful not to pay too much attention to one particular family member unless the medical condition requires such attention.
8. Do not lie to the family.
9. Attempt to gain the cooperation of at least one family member.
10. Separate young children out of the "combat zone" and assign the calmest and most responsible adult to care for them.

Child, Spouse, or Elder Abuse

A disturbed family system may turn its violence on one or more family members. Younger, old, weak, defenseless, quiet, or needy members of a family system frequently become the targets of people who have uncontrolled rage reactions. Paramedics may get involved in these situations when called by family members or neighbors. The scene is either chaotic or calm, but the emotions are intense under either circumstance. Immediate action is necessary, but it must be applied with caution.

The first step is to calmly but effectively protect the child or elderly person, separate them from the potentially dangerous situation, and treat their medical emergencies. Reduce stress in the environment, and ask the family members to stay outside the room while the patient is being assessed and treated.

Select words carefully. The conversation with young children needs to be simple and brief. Elderly people, on the other hand, should be addressed as adults with respect for their dignity.

It is difficult for children to place blame for their injuries on their parents. It is equally difficult for spouses to blame each other or for elders to point accusing fingers at the family, which they perceive to be their primary caretaker.

The paramedic cannot solve all the problems of the family. Intervention should be done carefully in the current situation, making appropriate referrals for family counseling and reporting child abuse to the police. The emergency room staff should be informed of any suspicions of family member abuse. Punitive action against the perpetrators of family member abuse never solves the problem and usually compounds the situation.

People who are in an abusing environment are terrified for their safety and need accurate information, reassurance, and encouragement. Tell them in advance what care and treatment will be given to them. Keep surprises to a minimum.

Never provoke the abuser in the family. Nothing protects the paramedic from his or her rage; they can easily throw the paramedic out of the house. They may deprive the children of protection and may set up a need for revenge on the family member when the paramedic is no longer present.

Sexual Assault

Sexual assault is a crime of violence, not of sex. It causes not only the physical injuries that usually bring the paramedic to the scene but also a broad spectrum of short- and long-term psychological after-shocks. Victims most often feel terrorized, out of control, violated, and intruded on. They have a great need for protection and security as well as reassurance, emotional support, and respect.

Steps to assist the sexual assault victim include the following:

1. Listen to the victim carefully.
2. Advise the victim not to do anything that might destroy evidence.
3. Reassure the victim of safety.
4. Do not question the victim about the details of the situation; this type of questioning is best left to the investigating team from the police department. It is best for the victim to go through the story only one time.
5. Believe the victim's story.
6. Avoid unnecessary touching of the victim.
7. Ask for permission before proceeding to treat the victim.
8. Let the victim know what the plan of action is.
9. Do not examine the genital area unless the wounds are severe enough to require some inspection before treatment.
10. Stay with the victim unless the victim specifically requests a private time.
11. Talk to the victim about the victim's fear and pain.
12. Allow the victim to cry or otherwise express emotions.
13. Protect the victim's privacy.
14. Provide for immediate needs if that is possible.
15. Do not offer false hopes to the victim.
16. Document all evidence encountered.
17. Provide accurate information to the victim.
18. Treat victim with respect, kindness, and gentleness.

The paramedic should keep in mind that sexual assault victims are not always female. Anyone can be a sexual assault victim and should be treated with equal respect, dignity, and reassurance.

Suicide

The incidence of **suicide** has increased alarmingly over the last several decades. Therefore, paramedics are exposed to this ultimate form of personal violence more frequently.

Most suicidal people are experiencing profound feelings of hopelessness, helplessness, and worthlessness after a precipitating event, such as the following:

- Diagnosis of serious illness
- Loss of a loved one by death
- Breakup of a close relationship
- Economic loss
- Arrest or imprisonment
- Failure
- Retirement
- Other emotional and exhausting events

The profile of the typical suicide victim is shown in the emergency assessment scheme (Table 31-3). The crucial factors that suggest immediate and serious danger are part of that profile.

The following steps should help reduce the potential for suicide in most situations:

1. Reduce stress in the immediate environment.
2. Build the person's trust: Introduce yourself and offer assistance; let the person know you are taking the threat seriously; listen to the person as he or she discusses the situation; do not argue with the person's feelings; talk openly about the suicide threat and the plan of action; offer food and other items that suggest support.

TABLE 31-3.
EMERGENCY ASSESSMENT SCHEME FOR THE SUICIDE VICTIM

Factor	High-Risk Group
Age	Males older than age 35
	Elderly
Method	Immediately available
	Highly lethal
Location of the attempt	Isolated area
Person's present state	Distorted and disorganized
	Contemplative
	Depressed
	Hostile
Onset of self-destructive behavior	Previous attempt
Alcohol	Chronic abuse
	Present intoxication
Precipitating events	Loss of a loved one
	Loss of a job
	Threat of arrest, prosecution
	Chronic or serious illness
	Anticipated surgery
Resources: personal (family and friends), other (social, community, financial)	Limited or absent
Social integration vs. isolation	Isolation
Emotional background	Chronic emotional disturbance
	Chronic emotional instability

3. Evaluate the potential for suicide by asking questions that pertain to the emergency assessment scheme in Table 31-3.
4. Continuously offer emotional support and understanding of the person's particular problems.
5. Focus on the main problem.
6. Offer alternatives to suicide that the person may not have considered.
7. Suggest specific short-term actions to reduce the current suicide potential.
8. Take the person to a hospital when it becomes possible.
9. Take care of the family members and close friends if the suicide has already occurred when you arrive. They are now the victims.
10. Never dismiss a threat of suicide or moralize about it.
11. Never move too quickly unless a life-threatening medical emergency (e.g., slashed wrists) is present.
12. Avoid unnecessary risks. Suicidal potential can easily turn into homicidal threat under certain circumstances.

PRINCIPLES OF CRISIS INTERVENTION

Crisis intervention is a set of action-oriented, but temporary, strategies designed to reduce the negative impact of a distressing event (or state of mental distress) on a person or group and to restore those affected to as normal a level of function as possible.

A *crisis* occurs when a person or group of people enter a sudden state of emotional turmoil regardless of the cause. People in a state of crisis are unable to resolve the situation with their own resources and usually need outside assistance. Crisis situations need to be resolved quickly because the situations have the potential to degenerate into dangerous, self-destructive, or socially unacceptable conditions. Unattended crises can turn into genuine emergencies with a serious threat to life, safety, or the overall well-being of the people involved.

Three main objectives should be considered when working with people in a crisis: protect the people from any additional stress, help the distressed people mobilize their resources, and restore them to as much function as possible.

A number of basic elements help during a crisis. Paramedics will find crisis intervention an easier task when they become accustomed to working within a framework that contains the following elements:

- Taking charge
- Careful assessment of the problem
- Setting limited goals
- Immediate action to solve the problem
- Problem-solving activities focused on the immediate situation
- Encouraging the distressed person or group to take some action on their own behalf

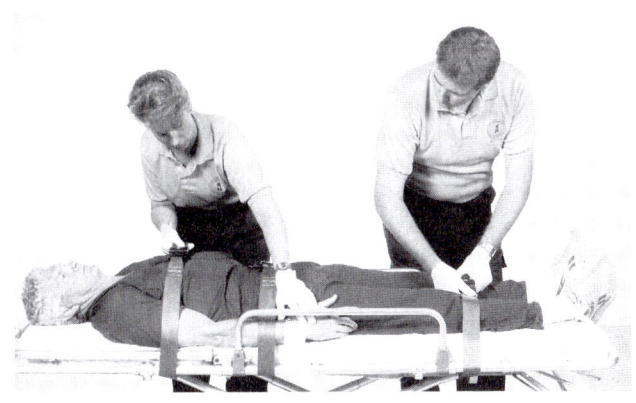

CHAPTER 31: Behavioral and Psychiatric Emergencies   731

FIGURE 31–3.
Awareness of the patient's range of motion can save injury to others. This patient has been secured by straps around the torso and legs. The wrists and ankles have been secured by soft roller bandages.

may be injured. It may set up a confrontation and aggravate the situation, and continuous physical restraint requires more than one paramedic or person per patient. In addition, physical restraint prevents the paramedic from dealing with other matters. Mechanical restraints should be applied as soon as possible after the initial period of restraint.

The paramedic should be familiar with different types of restraining devices and their operation before having to use them. Commercially manufactured restraints are shown in Figure 31-5. If commercially manufactured restraints are not available, the paramedic may improvise with materials stocked in the ambulance. Small towels or face cloths can be wrapped securely around the wrists and ankles. Tape is then used to cover the cloth and secure the restraints to the stretcher. Cravats and roller bandages or simple blanket rolls may also be used. Regardless of which types of restraints are used, they should be secure enough to produce the desired effect but should not be limiting to circulatory or respiratory status.

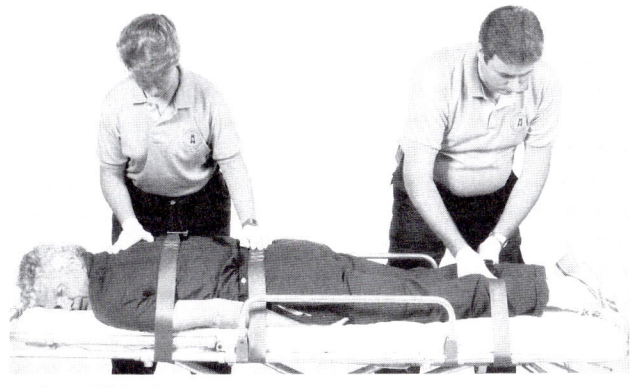

FIGURE 31–4.
Placed in a prone position on the stretcher, the patient's range of motion is decreased.

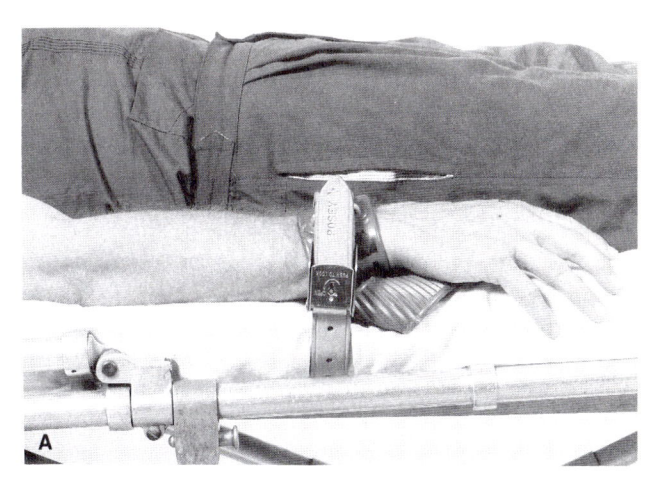

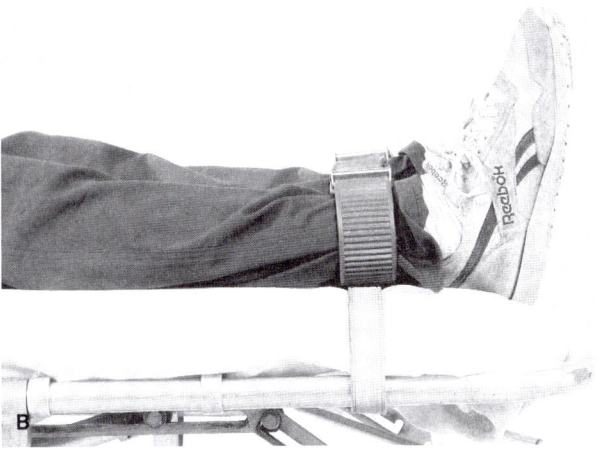

FIGURE 31–5.
Leather wrist (**A**) and ankle (**B**) restraints.

Procedures for Restraining a Patient

An attempt should be made to de-escalate any potentially violent situation as soon as possible. Once the situation has escalated to a point at which restraint techniques are necessary and adequate assistance is available, a plan of action should be taken. In general, once the decision has been made to restrain a patient, it must be accomplished swiftly. If two people move toward the patient together, the patient cannot focus on both. This lack of focus coupled with the swift motion of the emergency personnel reduces the accuracy of a kick or blow. During this time, one person should still continue to talk with the patient. Both personnel should attempt to position themselves close to but slightly behind the patient. The patient may calm down, and restraints may not be necessary. The patient needs continual reassurance and should be laid down on the stretcher. Once in the ambulance, personnel should position themselves between the patient and the doors to avoid a rapid exit attempt while the vehicle is in motion. If at any time the patient becomes dangerous, restraints should be applied.

Rarely is the paramedic in a position to attempt negotiations for extended periods of time. This job is better left to people trained specifically in the skills of negotiation. Occasionally, the paramedic may be exposed to a situation that requires some negotiation with the patient. A thorough understanding of the events that occur during a violent outburst and a general knowledge of the human body and how to use it to the best advantage are imperative. Since paramedics are not frequently exposed to violent outbursts from patients that result in restraint techniques, they should understand the principles of restraint so that they can be applied effectively when needed.

Legal Ramifications of Crisis Care

Each state has specific laws that govern emergency medical practices in relation to disturbed patients. Each paramedic has an obligation to gain a thorough understanding of the laws of patient care as they apply to the paramedic in the field. The comments in this segment are broad and generalized and may not have equal force in all jurisdictions and under all circumstances.

In general, the same rules that apply to the management of medical emergencies also apply to emotionally distressed cases. Paramedics must maintain the same professional standards with the uninjured emotionally distressed case as with the serious trauma or medical case. The paramedic must follow the appropriate written protocols and medical direction. Care should be taken that the paramedic does not say or do anything that could be interpreted as abandonment or negligence. Whenever possible, paramedics should obtain actual consent before treatment. However, the paramedic must also remember that when people are unable to care for themselves because of intoxication or other serious mental impairment, it is necessary for the paramedic to provide more than the ordinary care that would be provided in such cases.

Paramedics must be more acutely aware of the special needs of emotionally distressed patients. The paramedic needs to maintain the absolute highest level of patient confidentiality. This confidentiality is necessary in all emergency cases but takes on a special significance with the mentally disturbed patient, since the circumstances are so sensitive to violations of the right to privacy.

At times it is necessary to force an unwilling person, who is a danger to himself or herself or others, to obtain emergency care for a severe mental disturbance. Police assistance is necessary to assure the safety of the paramedic and to insure that the distressed patient's rights are not violated. The regulations that govern such cases vary from state to state, and the paramedic needs to know what is required by local statutes.

SUMMARY

A thorough presentation of every form of crisis situation that may be encountered by paramedics in the field cannot be covered in a few pages of a textbook. However, the key elements presented here can do much to restore the "human elements" to emergency work. They certainly go far to reverse Dr. Calvin Frederick's comments. It will no longer be possible to say with honesty that those who provide ambulance service, at least, are not prepared to render psychological first aid. A beginning has been made. The human element is being incorporated into emergency medical services.

SUGGESTED READING

Baehren D, Werman HA: Altered mental states: Grappling with the unknown. J Emerg Med Serv 14(3):67, 1989

Brizer DA, Convit A, Krakowski M: A rating scale for the assessment of aggressive behaviors. Hosp Community Psychiatry 38:769, 1987

Butler JP: Safe transportation of the psychiatric patient. J Emerg Med Serv 13(3):40, 1988

Dubin WR, Weiss KJ: Handbook of Psychiatric Emergencies. Springhouse, PA, Springhouse Corporation, 1991

Mitchell JT: Assessing and managing the psychologic impact of terrorism, civil disorder, disasters and mass casualties. Emergency Care Quarterly 2:51, 1986

Parrillo JE: Current Therapy in Critical Care Medicine. Philadelphia, BC Decker, 1987

US Department of Transportation, National Highway Traffic Safety Administration: Emergency Medical Technician–Paramedic: National Standards Curriculum. Washington, DC, US Government Printing Office, 1985

APPENDIX A.
NATIONAL REGISTRY OF EMERGENCY MEDICAL TECHNICIANS ADVANCED LEVEL PRACTICAL EXAMINATIONS*

**Paramedic Practical Examination
(for the Emergency Medical Technician-Paramedic)**

All candidates must complete the following skill stations and subskills:

Patient Assessment/Management
    Primary Survey/Resuscitation
    Secondary Survey

Respiratory Management

Cardiac Arrest Skills
    Dynamic Cardiology
    Static Cardiology

Intravenous and Medication Skills
    Intravenous Therapy
    Intravenous Bolus
    Intravenous Piggyback

Spinal Immobilization (Seated Patient)

In addition, each candidate must complete two of the following six skills in the Random Basic Skills station. The skills are paired and have been balanced for performance and time.

Supplemental Oxygen Administration

Bleeding–Wounds–Shock

Splinting (Joint)

Splinting (Long Bone)

Splinting (Traction Splint)

Spinal Immobilization (Lying Patient)

**Intermediate Practical Examination
(for the Emergency Medical Technician-Intermediate)**

All candidates must complete the following skill stations and subskills:

Patient Assessment/Management
    Primary Survey/Resuscitation
    Secondary Survey

Respiratory Management (not included)

Intravenous Therapy

Spinal Immobilization (Seated Patient)

In addition, each candidate must complete two of the above listed random basic skills.

*This was a draft on publication and some areas may be subject to change. Confirm any changes with the National Registry of Emergency Medical Technicians, 6610 Busch Blvd., Columbus, OH 43229

(continued)

APPENDIX A.
NATIONAL REGISTRY OF EMERGENCY MEDICAL TECHNICIANS
ADVANCED LEVEL PRACTICAL EXAMINATION (*continued*)

PATIENT ASSESSMENT/MANAGEMENT

Candidate: _____ Examiner: _____

Date: _____ Signature: _____

Scenario # _____ Time Start: _____ Time End: _____

PRIMARY SURVEY/RESUSCITATION		Possible Points	Points Awarded
Takes or verbalizes infection control precautions		1	
AIRWAY with C-spine control	Assesses airway (1 pt) Opens airway with manual cervical spine precautions (1 pt) Inserts adjunct (1 pt)	3	
BREATHING	Assesses breathing (1 pt) Initiates appropriate oxygen therapy (1 pt) Assures adequate ventilation of patient (1 pt) Manages any injury which may compromise breathing (1 pt)	4	

CIRCULATION	Checks pulse (1 pt)
	Assesses peripheral perfusion (1 pt)
	  [checks either skin color, temperature, or capillary refill]
	Assesses for and controls major bleeding if present (1 pt)
	Takes vital signs (1 pt)
	Applies PASG if needed (1 pt)
	  [candidate must assess body parts to be enclosed prior to application]
		5	

	Volume Replacement [usually deferred until patient loaded] • Initiates first IV line (1 pt) • Initiates second IV line (1 pt) • Selects appropriate catheter (1 pt) • Selects appropriate IV solution and administration set (1 pt) • Infuses at appropriate rate (1 pt)	5	
DISABILITY	Performs mini neuro assessment: AVPU (1 pt) Applies cervical collar (1 pt)	2	
EXPOSE	Removes clothing	1	
STATUS	Calls for immediate transport of the patient	1	
	SUB-TOTAL	22	

APPENDIX A.
NATIONAL REGISTRY OF EMERGENCY MEDICAL TECHNICIANS
ADVANCED LEVEL PRACTICAL EXAMINATION (continued)

SECONDARY SURVEY NOTE: Areas denoted by ''**'' may be integrated within sequence of Primary Survey

HEAD	Inspects mouth** and nose** and assesses facial area (1 pt) Inspects and palpates scalp and ears (1 pt) Checks eyes: PEARRL** (1 pt)	3
NECK**	Checks position of trachea (1 pt) Checks jugular veins (1 pt) Palpates cervical spine (1 pt)	3
CHEST**	Inspects chest (1 pt) Palpates chest (1 pt) Auscultates chest (1 pt)	3
ABDOMEN/PELVIS**	Inspects and palpates abdomen (1 pt) Assesses pelvis (1 pt)	2
LOWER EXTREMITIES**	Inspects and palpates left leg (1 pt) Inspects and palpates right leg (1 pt) Checks motor, sensory, and distal circulation (1 pt/leg)	4
UPPER EXTREMITIES	Inspects and palpates left arm (1 pt) Inspects and palpates right arm (1 pt) Checks motor, sensory, and distal circulation (1 pt/arm)	4
POSTERIOR THORAX/ LUMBAR** AND BUTTOCKS	Inspects and palpates posterior thorax (1 pt) Inspects and palpates lumbar and buttocks area (1 pt)	2
Manages fractures and wounds appropriately (1 pt. per each correctly managed fracture or wound)		4

SUB-TOTAL 25

TOTAL 47

CRITERIA FOR MANDATING FAILURE

_____ Failure to initiate or call for transport of patient within ten (10) minute time limit
_____ Failure to immediately establish and maintain spinal protection
_____ Failure to provide high concentration of oxygen
_____ Failure to evaluate and find all presented conditions of airway, breathing, and circulation (shock)
_____ Failure to appropriately manage/provide airway, breathing, hemorrhage control, or treatment for shock
_____ Failure to differentiate patient's needing transportation versus continued on-scene survey
_____ Does other detailed physical examination before assessing & treating threats to airway, breathing & circulation

(continued)

APPENDIX A.
NATIONAL REGISTRY OF EMERGENCY MEDICAL TECHNICIANS
ADVANCED LEVEL PRACTICAL EXAMINATION (continued)

RESPIRATORY MANAGEMENT

Candidate: _____   Examiner: _____

Date: _____   Signature: _____

NOTE: If candidate elects to initially ventilate with BVM attached to reservoir and oxygen, full credit must be awarded for areas denoted by "**" so long as first ventilation is delivered within initial 30 seconds

	Possible Points	Points Awarded
Takes or verbalizes infection control precautions	1	
Opens the airway manually	1	
Elevates tongue, inserts simple adjunct [either oropharyngeal or nasopharyngeal airway]	1	
NOTE: Examiner now informs candidate no gag reflex is present and patient accepts adjunct.		
**Ventilates patient immediately with bag-valve-mask device unattached to oxygen	1	
**Hyperventilates patient with room air	1	
NOTE: Examiner now informs candidate that ventilation is being performed without difficulty.		
Attaches oxygen reservoir to bag-valve-mask device and connects to high flow oxygen regulator [12-15 liters/minute]	1	
Ventilates patient at a rate of 12-20 minute and volumes of at least 800 ml	1	
NOTE: After 30 seconds, examiner auscultates and reports breath sounds are present and equal bilaterally and medical control has ordered intubation. The examiner must now take over ventilation.		
Directs assistant to hyperventilate patient	1	
Identifies/selects proper equipment for intubation	1	

Checks equipment for:
  -Cuff leaks (1 pt)
  -Laryngoscope operational and bulb tight (1 pt)
	2	

NOTE: Examiner to remove OPA and move out of way when candidate is prepared to intubate.		
Positions head properly	1	
Inserts blade while displacing tongue	1	
Elevates mandible with laryngoscope	1	
Introduces ET tube and advances to proper depth	1	
Removes laryngoscope blade from mouth	1	
Inflates cuff to proper pressure and disconnects syringe	1	
Directs ventilation of patient	1	
Confirms proper placement by auscultation bilaterally and over epigastrium	1	
NOTE: Examiner to ask "If you had proper placement, what would you expect to hear?"		
Secures ET tube [may be verbalized]	1	
TOTAL	**20**	

CRITERIA FOR MANDATING FAILURE

_____ Failure to initiate ventilations within 30 seconds or interrupts ventiliations for greater than 30 seconds at any time
_____ Failure to take or verbalize infection control precautions
_____ Failure to voice and ultimately provide high oxygen concentrations [at least 85%]
_____ Failure to ventilate patient at rate of at least 12/minute
_____ Failure to provide adequate volumes per breath [maximum 2 errors/minute permissable]
_____ Failure to hyperventilate patient prior to intubation
_____ Failure to successfully intubate within 3 attempts
_____ Using teeth as a fulcrum
_____ Failure to assure proper tube placement by auscultation bilaterally and over the epigastrium
_____ If used, stylette extends beyond end of ET tube

(continued)

APPENDIX A.
NATIONAL REGISTRY OF EMERGENCY MEDICAL TECHNICIANS
ADVANCED LEVEL PRACTICAL EXAMINATION (*continued*)

CARDIAC ARREST SKILLS STATION
DYNAMIC CARDIOLOGY

Candidate: _____ Examiner: _____

Date: _____ Signature: _____

Set # ____ Time Start: _____ Time End: _____

	Possible Points	Points Awarded
Checks level of responsiveness	1	
Checks ABC's	1	
Initiates CPR if appropriate [verbally]	1	
Performs "Quick Look" with paddles	1	
Interprets initial rhythm as:	1	
Manages initial rhythm by: _____	2	
Notes change in rhythm	1	
Checks patient condition to include pulse and, if appropriate, BP	1	
Interprets second rhythm as:	1	
Manages second rhythm by: _____	2	
Notes change in rhythm	1	
Checks patient condition to include pulse and, if appropriate, BP	1	
Interprets third rhythm as:	1	
Manages third rhythm by: _____	2	
Notes change in rhythm	1	
Checks patient condition to include pulse and, if appropriate, BP	1	
Interprets fourth rhythm as:	1	
Manages fourth rhythm by: _____	2	
Orders high percentages of supplemental oxygen at proper times	1	
TOTAL	**23**	

SHOCK SEQUENCE TO INCLUDE:
1. Verbalizes use of conductive medium [gel, pads, etc.]
2. Proper paddle placement
3. Charges appropriately, verbalizing correct energy level
4. Re-verifies rhythm and absence of pulse
5. Clears self and others [verbally and visually]
6. Appropriately delivers shock

CRITERIA FOR MANDATING FAILURE

____ Failure to deliver first shock in a timely manner due to operator delay in machine use or treatments other than CPR with simple adjuncts
____ Failure to deliver second or third shocks without delay other than the time required to reassess and recharge paddles
____ Failure to order or perform pulse checks before and after shocks
____ Failure to ensure the safety of self and others [verbalizes "All clear" and observes]
____ Inability to deliver DC shock [doesn't use machine properly]
____ Failure to verify pulse after rhythm change or treatment
____ Failure to order initiation or resumption of CPR when appropriate
____ Failure to order correct management of airway [ET when appropriate]
____ Failure to order administration of appropriate oxygen at proper time
____ Failure to treat 2 or more rhythms correctly
____ Failure to correctly diagnose or adequately treat v-fib, v-tach, or asystole

(*continued*)

APPENDIX A.
NATIONAL REGISTRY OF EMERGENCY MEDICAL TECHNICIANS
ADVANCED LEVEL PRACTICAL EXAMINATION (*continued*)

CARDIAC ARREST SKILLS STATION
STATIC CARDIOLOGY

Candidate:_____   Examiner:_____

Date:_____   Signature:_____

Set #____

NOTE: No points for treatment may be awarded if the diagnosis is incorrect. Concisely document all responses in spaces provided.

	Possible Points	Points Awarded
STRIP #1 Diagnosis:	1	
Treatment: _____	2	
STRIP #2 Diagnosis:	1	
Treatment: _____	2	
STRIP #3 Diagnosis:	1	
Treatment: _____	2	
STRIP #4 Diagnosis:	1	
Treatment: _____	2	
TOTAL	12	

(*continued*)

APPENDIX A.
NATIONAL REGISTRY OF EMERGENCY MEDICAL TECHNICIANS
ADVANCED LEVEL PRACTICAL EXAMINATION (*continued*)

INTRAVENOUS THERAPY

Candidate: _____   Examiner: _____

Date: _____   Signature: _____

Time Start: _____   Time End: _____

	Possible Points	Points Awarded

Checks selected IV fluid for:
  -Proper fluid (1 pt)
  -Clarity (1 pt)
  -Expiration date (1 pt)
	3	

Selects appropriate catheter	1	
Selects proper administration set	1	
Connects IV tubing to the IV bag	1	
Prepares administration set [fills drip chamber and flushes tubing]	1	
Cuts or tears tape [at any time before venipuncture]	1	
Takes/verbalizes infection control precautions [prior to venipuncture]	1	
Applies tourniquet	1	
Palpates suitable vein	1	
Cleanses site appropriately	1	

Performs venipuncture
  -Inserts stylette (1 pt)
  -Notes or verbalizes flashback (1 pt)
  -Occludes vein proximal to catheter (1 pt)
  -Removes stylette (1 pt)
  -Connects IV tubing to catheter (1 pt)
	5	

Releases tourniquet	1	
Flushes IV for a brief period	1	
Secures catheter [tapes securely]	1	
Adjusts flow rate as appropriate	1	
Disposes/verbalizes disposal of needle in proper container	1	
TOTAL	22	

CRITERIA FOR MANDATING FAILURE

_____ Failure to take or verbalize infection control precautions prior to performing venipuncture

_____ Contaminates equipment or site without appropriately correcting situation

_____ Any improper technique resulting in the potential for catheter shear or air embolism

_____ Failure to successfully establish IV within 3 attempts during 6 minute time limit

_____ Failure to dispose/verbalize disposal of needle in proper container

(*continued*)

APPENDIX A.
NATIONAL REGISTRY OF EMERGENCY MEDICAL TECHNICIANS
ADVANCED LEVEL PRACTICAL EXAMINATION (*continued*)

INTRAVENOUS BOLUS

Candidate: _____ Examiner: _____

Date: _____ Signature: _____

Time Start: _____ Time End: _____

NOTE: Check here (__) if candidate did not establish a patent IV and do not evaluate these skills.

	Possible Points	Points Awarded
Asks patient for known allergies	1	
Selects correct medication	1	
Checks expiration date	1	
Assures correct concentration of drug	1	
Assembles prefilled syringe correctly and dispels air	1	
Continues infection control precautions	1	
Cleanses injection site [Y-port or hub]	1	
Reaffirms medication	1	
Stops IV flow [pinches tubing]	1	
Administers correct dose at proper push rate	1	
Flushes tubing [runs wide open for a brief period]	1	
Adjusts drip rate to TKO [KVO]	1	
Voices proper disposal of syringe and needle	1	
Verbalizes need to observe patient for desired effect/adverse side effects	1	
TOTAL	**14**	

CRITERIA FOR MANDATING FAILURE

____ Contaminates equipment or site without appropriately correcting situation
____ Failure to adequately dispel air resulting in potential for air embolism
____ Injects improper drug or dosage [wrong drug, incorrect amount, or pushes at inappropriate rate]
____ Failure to flush IV tubing after injecting medication
____ Recaps needle or failure to dispose/verbalize disposal of syringe and needle in proper container
____ Failure to take infection control precautions

INTRAVENOUS PIGGYBACK

Time Start: _____ Time End: _____

	Possible Points	Points Awarded
Has confirmed allergies by now [award point if previously confirmed]	1	
Checks selected IV fluid for: -Proper fluid (1 pt) -Clarity (1 pt) -Expiration date (1 pt)	3	
Checks selected medication for: -Clarity (1 pt) -Expiration date (1 pt) -Concentration of medication (1 pt)	3	
Injects correct amount medication into IV solution given scenario	1	
Connects appropriate administration set to medication solution	1	
Prepares administration set [fills drip chamber and flushes tubing]	1	
Attaches appropriate needle to administration set	1	
Continues infection control precautions	1	
Cleanses port of primary line	1	
Inserts needle into port without contamination	1	
Adjusts flow rate of secondary line as required	1	
Stops flow of primary line	1	
Securely tapes needle	1	
Verbalizes need to observe patient for desired effect/adverse side effects	1	
Labels medication/fluid bag	1	
TOTAL	**19**	

CRITERIA FOR MANDATING FAILURE

____ Contaminates equipment or site without appropriately correcting situation
____ Administers improper drug or dosage [mixes wrong drug, incorrect amount, or infuses at inappropriate rate]
____ Failure to flush IV tubing of secondary line resulting in potential for air embolism
____ Failure to shut-off flow of primary line

(*continued*)

APPENDIX A.
NATIONAL REGISTRY OF EMERGENCY MEDICAL TECHNICIANS
ADVANCED LEVEL PRACTICAL EXAMINATION (continued)

SPINAL IMMOBILIZATION
(SEATED PATIENT)

Candidate: _____   Examiner: _____

Date: _____   Signature: _____

Time Start: _____   Time End: _____

	Possible Points	Points Awarded
Assures patient's head in neutral, in-line position	1	
Directs assistant to maintain cervical immobilization	1	
Applies appropriately sized extrication collar	1	
Positions the immobilization device behind the patient	1	
Secures device to the patient's torso and adjusts as necessary	1	
Evaluates torso fixation and adjusts as necessary	1	
Evaluates and pads behind the patient's head as necessary	1	
Secures patient's head to the device	1	
Evaluates motor function in extremities	1	
Evaluates sensory function in extremities	1	
Evaluates peripheral circulation in extremities	1	
Verbalizes moving the patient to a long board properly	1	
TOTAL	12	

CRITERIA FOR MANDATING FAILURE
____ Did not immediately direct or take manual immobilization
____ Releases or orders release of manual immobilization before it was maintained mechanically
____ Patient manipulated or moved excessively causing potential spinal compromise
____ Did not complete immobilization of the torso prior to immobilizing the head
____ Device moves excessively up, down, left, or right on patient's torso
____ Torso fixation inhibits chest rise resulting in respiratory compromise
____ Head immobilization allows for excessive movement
____ Upon completion of immobilization, head is not in neutral, in-line position

(continued)

APPENDIX A.
NATIONAL REGISTRY OF EMERGENCY MEDICAL TECHNICIANS
ADVANCED LEVEL PRACTICAL EXAMINATION (continued)

RANDOM BASIC SKILLS

Candidate: _____   Examiner: _____
Date: _____   Signature: _____
                                        Time Start: _____ Time End: _____

AIRWAY-OXYGEN-VENTILATION
SUPPLEMENTAL OXYGEN ADMINISTRATION

	Possible Points	Points Awarded
Assembles regulator to tank	1	
Opens tank	1	
Checks for leaks	1	
Checks tank pressure	1	
Attaches nasal cannula to oxygen	1	
Adjusts liter flow to 6 liters/minute or less	1	
Applies nasal cannula to patient	1	
The examiner must advise the candidate to change to a non-rebreather mask		
Attaches non-rebreather mask to oxygen	1	
Prefills reservoir	1	
Adjusts liter flow to 6 liters/minute or greater	1	
Applies and adjusts mask to face	1	
The examiner must advise the candidate to discontinue oxygen therapy.		
Removes non-rebreather mask from patient	1	
Shuts off regulator	1	
Relieves regulator pressure	1	
TOTAL	**14**	

CRITICAL CRITERIA
_____ Did not adjust device to a correct liter flow for nasal cannula (2-6L)
_____ Did not adjust device to a correct liter flow for a non-rebreather mask (6L or greater)
_____ Did not assemble tank & regulator without leaks
_____ Did not prefill reservoir

(continued)

APPENDIX A.
NATIONAL REGISTRY OF EMERGENCY MEDICAL TECHNICIANS
ADVANCED LEVEL PRACTICAL EXAMINATION (continued)

RANDOM BASIC SKILLS

Candidate: _____ Examiner: _____
Date: _____ Signature: _____
                                    Time Start: _____ Time End: _____

BLEEDING-WOUNDS-SHOCK

	Possible Points	Points Awarded
Takes or verbalizes infection control precautions	1	
Applies direct pressure to the wound	1	
Elevates the extremity	1	
Applies pressure dressing to the wound	1	
Bandages wound	1	
NOTE: The examiner must now inform the candidate that the wound is still continuing to bleed. The second dressing does not control the bleeding.		
Locates and applies pressure to appropriate pressure point	1	
NOTE: The examiner must indicate that the victim is in compensatory shock		
Applies high concentration oxygen	1	
Properly positions patient (supine with legs elevated)	1	
Prevents heat loss (covers patient as appropriate)	1	
NOTE: The examiner must indicate that the victim is in profound shock		
Removes clothing or checks for sharp objects	1	
Quickly assesses areas that will be under the PASG	1	
Positions PASG with top of abdominal section at or below last set of ribs	1	
Secures PASG around patient	1	
Attaches hoses	1	
Begins inflation sequence (examiner to stop inflation at 15 mm Hg)	1	
Checks blood pressure	1	
Verbalizes when to stop inflation sequence	1	
Operates PASG to maintain air pressure in device	1	
Reassess vital signs	1	
	TOTAL 19	

CRITICAL CRITERIA

____ Did not apply high concentration of oxygen
____ Applies tourniquet before attempting other methods of hemorrhage control
____ Did not control hemorrhage
____ Did not use PASG
____ Inflates abdominal section of PASG before the legs or to a higher pressure than the legs
____ Did not reassess patient's vital signs
____ Places PASG on inside-out
____ Allows deflation of PASG after inflation
____ Positions PASG above level of lowest rib

(continued)

APPENDIX A.
NATIONAL REGISTRY OF EMERGENCY MEDICAL TECHNICIANS
ADVANCED LEVEL PRACTICAL EXAMINATION (*continued*)

RANDOM BASIC SKILLS

Candidate: _____   Examiner: _____

Date: _____   Signature: _____

Time Start: _____   Time End: _____

SPLINTING
(JOINT)

	Possible Points	Points Awarded
Directs manual stabilization of injury	1	
Assesses distal neurological function	1	
Assesses distal circulation (Note: Present and normal)	1	
Selects proper splinting materials	1	
Immobilizes site of injury	1	
Immobilizes bones above injured joint	1	
Immobilizes bones below injured joint	1	
Reassesses distal neurological function	1	
Reassesses distal circulation (Note: Present and normal)	1	
TOTAL:	9	

CRITICAL CRITERIA

____ Did not immobilize bone above/below injured joint

____ Did not support joint so that it doesn't bear distal weight

____ Did not assess neurological function/circulation after splinting

(*continued*)

APPENDIX A.
NATIONAL REGISTRY OF EMERGENCY MEDICAL TECHNICIANS ADVANCED LEVEL PRACTICAL EXAMINATION (*continued*)

RANDOM BASIC SKILLS

Candidate: _____ Examiner: _____
Date: _____ Signature: _____
                                Time Start: _____ Time End: _____

**SPLINTING
(LONG BONE)**

	Possible Points	Points Awarded
Directs application of manual stabilization	1	
Assesses distal neurological function	1	
Assesses distal circulation (Note: Present and normal)	1	
Measures splint	1	
Applies splint	1	
Immobilizes joint above fracture	1	
Immobilizes joint below fracture	1	
Secures entire injured extremity	1	
Immobilizes hand/foot in position of function	1	
Reassesses distal neurological function	1	
Reassesses distal circulation (Note: Present and normal)	1	
	TOTAL: 11	

CRITICAL CRITERIA

____ Grossly moves injured extremity
____ Did not immobilize adjacent joints
____ Did not assess neurological function/circulation after splinting

(*continued*)

APPENDIX A.
NATIONAL REGISTRY OF EMERGENCY MEDICAL TECHNICIANS
ADVANCED LEVEL PRACTICAL EXAMINATION (*continued*)

RANDOM BASIC SKILLS

Candidate: _____ Examiner: _____
Date: _____ Signature: _____
                                     Time Start: _____ Time End: _____

SPLINTING (TRACTION SPLINT)

	Possible Points	Points Awarded
Directs manual stabilization of injured leg	1	
Directs application of manual traction	1	
Assesses distal neurological function/circulation (Note: Present and normal)	1	
Prepares/adjusts splint to proper length	1	
Positions splint at injured leg	1	
Applies proximal securing device (eg. groin strap)	1	
Applies distal securing device (eg. ankle hitch)	1	
Applies mechanical traction	1	
Positions/secures support straps	1	
Re-evaluates proximal/distal securing devices	1	
Reassesses distal neurological function/circulation (Note: Present and normal)	1	
NOTE: Examiner must ask candidate how he/she would prepare for transport.		
Verbalizes securing on long board to immobilize hip	1	
Verbalizes securing splint to long board to prevent movement of splint	1	
TOTAL	13	

CRITICAL CRITERIA
_____ Loss of traction at any point after it is assumed
_____ Did not reassess neurological function/circulation after splinting
_____ The foot is excessively rotated or extended after splinting
_____ Did not secure ischeal strap before taking traction

NOTE: If sager is used without elevating the leg, application of manual traction is not necessary. Candidate will be awarded 1 point as if manual traction were applied.

NOTE: If the leg is elevated manual traction must be applied before elevating the leg; however, manual traction may be applied after application of the ankle hitch.

(*continued*)

APPENDIX A.
NATIONAL REGISTRY OF EMERGENCY MEDICAL TECHNICIANS
ADVANCED LEVEL PRACTICAL EXAMINATION (*continued*)

RANDOM BASIC SKILLS

Candidate: _____ Examiner: _____

Date: _____ Signature: _____

Time Start: _____ Time End: _____

SPINAL IMMOBILIZATION SKILLS
(Lying Patient)

	Possible Points	Points Awarded
Directs assistant to move patient's head to the neutral in-line position	1	
Directs assistant to maintain cervical immobilization	1	
Applies cervical collar	1	
Gathers appropriate immobilization device/equipment	1	
Positions immobilization device appropriately	1	
Moves victim onto device without compromising the integrity of the spine	1	
Applies padding to all voids between the torso and the board as necessary	1	
Immobilizes torso to the device	1	
Evaluates and pads under the patients head as necessary	1	
Immobilizes the patient's head to the device	1	
Secures legs to the device	1	
Secures victims arms to the board	1	
Evaluates motor function	1	
Evaluates sensory function	1	
Evaluates peripheral circulation	1	
Total:	15	

CRITICAL CRITERIA

_____ Did not immediately direct manual immobilization

_____ Orders release of manual immobilization before it was maintained mechanically

_____ Did not complete immobilization of the torso prior to immobilizing the head

_____ Device excessively moves up, down, left or right on patient's torso

_____ Head immobilization allows for excessive movement

_____ Head is not immobilized in the neutral in-line position

_____ Patient moved excessively causing potential spinal compromise

APPENDIX B.
PERFORMANCE SHEETS FOR CARDIOPULMONARY RESUSCITATION AND FOREIGN BODY AIRWAY OBSTRUCTION MANAGEMENT

Adult One-Rescuer CPR

Adult Foreign Body Airway Obstruction Management — Conscious and Conscious Becomes Unconscious

Adult Foreign Body Airway Obstruction Management — Unconscious

Child One-Rescuer CPR

Child Foreign Body Airway Obstruction Management — Conscious and Conscious Becomes Unconscious

Child Foreign Body Airway Obstruction Management — Unconscious

Infant CPR

Infant Foreign Body Airway Obstruction Management — Conscious and Conscious Becomes Unconscious

Infant Foreign Body Airway Obstruction Management — Unconscious

Adult Two-Rescuer CPR

Child Two-Rescuer CPR

Summary Performance Sheets: Adult, Child, and Infant Combined

   Cardiopulmonary Resuscitation (CPR)

   Foreign Body Airway Obstruction (FBAO) Management

© American Heart Association: Healthcare Provider's Manual for Basic Life Support, pp. 95–108. Dallas, American Heart Association, 1988.

(continued)

APPENDIX B.
PERFORMANCE SHEETS FOR CARDIOPULMONARY RESUSCITATION AND FOREIGN BODY AIRWAY OBSTRUCTION MANAGEMENT (*continued*)

BLS Performance Sheet
Adult One-Rescuer CPR

Name _____ Date _____

Step	Objective	Critical Performance	S	U
1. **A**IRWAY	Assessment: Determine unresponsiveness.	Tap or gently shake shoulder.		
		Shout "Are you OK?"		
	Call for help.	Call out "Help!"		
	Position the victim.	Turn on back as unit, if necessary, supporting head and neck (4–10 sec).		
	Open the airway.	Use head-tilt/chin-lift maneuver.		
2. **B**REATHING	Assessment: Determine breathlessness.	Maintain open airway.		
		Ear over mouth, observe chest: look, listen, feel for breathing (3–5 sec).		
	Ventilate twice.	Maintain open airway.		
		Seal mouth and nose properly.		
		Ventilate 2 times at 1–1.5 sec/inspiration.		
		Observe chest rise (adequate ventilation volume.)		
		Allow deflation between breaths.		
3. **C**IRCULATION	Assessment: Determine pulselessness.	Feel for carotid pulse on near side of victim (5–10 sec).		
		Maintain head-tilt with other hand.		
	Activate EMS system.	If someone responded to call for help, send him/her to activate EMS system.		
		Total time, Step 1—Activate EMS system: 15–35 sec.		
	Begin chest compressions.	Rescuer kneels by victim's shoulders.		
		Landmark check prior to hand placement.		
		Proper hand position throughout.		
		Rescuer's shoulders over victim's sternum.		
		Equal compression–relaxation.		
		Compress 1½ to 2 inches.		
		Keep hands on sternum during upstroke.		
		Complete chest relaxation on upstroke.		
		Say any helpful mnemonic.		
		Compression rate: 80–100/min (15 per 9–11 sec).		
4. Compression/Ventilation Cycles	Do 4 cycles of 15 compressions and 2 ventilations.	Proper compression/ventilation ratio: 15 compressions to 2 ventilations per cycle.		
		Observe chest rise: 1–1.5 sec/inspiration; 4 cycles/52–73 sec.		
5. Reassessment*	Determine pulselessness.	Feel for carotid pulse (5 sec).† If there is no pulse, go to Step 6.		
6. Continue CPR	Ventilate twice.	Ventilate 2 times.		
		Observe chest rise: 1–1.5 sec/inspiration.		
	Resume compression/ventilation cycles.	Feel for carotid pulse every few minutes.		

* If 2nd rescuer arrives to replace 1st rescuer: (a) 2nd rescuer identifies self by saying "I know CPR. Can I help?" (b) 2nd rescuer then does pulse check in Step 5 and continues with Step 6. (During practice and testing only one rescuer actually ventilates the manikin. The 2nd rescuer simulates ventilation.) (c) 1st rescuer assesses the adequacy of 2nd rescuer's CPR by observing chest rise during ventilations and by checking the pulse during chest compressions.

† If pulse is present, open airway and check for spontaneous breathing: (a) If breathing is present, maintain open airway and monitor pulse and breathing. (b) If breathing is absent, perform rescue breathing at 12 times/min and monitor pulse.

Instructor _____ Check: Satisfactory _____ Unsatisfactory _____

(*continued*)

APPENDIX B.
PERFORMANCE SHEETS FOR CARDIOPULMONARY RESUSCITATION
AND FOREIGN BODY AIRWAY OBSTRUCTION MANAGEMENT (continued)

BLS Performance Sheet
Adult FBAO Management: Conscious

Name _____ Date _____

Step	Objective	Critical Performance	S	U
1. Assessment	Determine airway obstruction.	Ask "Are you choking?"		
		Determine if victim can cough or speak.		
2. Heimlich Maneuver	Perform abdominal thrusts.	Stand behind the victim.		
		Wrap arms around victim's waist.		
		Make a fist with one hand and place the thumb side against victim's abdomen in the midline slightly above the navel and well below the tip of the xiphoid.		
		Grasp fist with the other hand.		
		Press into the victim's abdomen with quick upward thrusts.		
		Each thrust should be distinct and delivered with the intent of relieving the airway obstruction.		
		Repeat thrusts until either the foreign body is expelled or the victim becomes unconscious (see below).		

Victim with Obstructed Airway Becomes Unconscious (Optional Testing Sequence)

Step	Objective	Critical Performance	S	U
3. Positioning	Position the victim.	Turn on back as unit.		
		Place face up, arms by side.		
	Call for help.	Call out "Help!" or, if others respond, activate EMS system.		
4. Foreign Body Check	Perform finger sweep.*	Keep victim's face up.		
		Use tongue–jaw lift to open mouth.		
		Sweep deeply into mouth to remove foreign body.		
5. Breathing Attempt	Ventilate.	Open airway with head-tilt/chin-lift.		
		Seal mouth and nose properly.		
		Attempt to ventilate.		
6. Heimlich Maneuver	(Airway is obstructed.) Perform abdominal thrusts.	Straddle victim's thighs.		
		Place heel of one hand against victim's abdomen, in the midline slightly above the navel and well below the tip of the xiphoid.		
		Place second hand directly on top of first hand.		
		Press into the abdomen with quick upward thrusts.		
		Perform 6–10 abdominal thrusts.		
7. Foreign Body Check	(Airway remains obstructed.) Perform finger sweep.*	Keep victim's face up.		
		Use tongue–jaw lift to open mouth.		
		Sweep deeply into mouth to remove foreign body.		
8. Breathing Attempt	Ventilate.	Open airway with head-tilt/chin-lift.		
		Seal mouth and nose properly.		
		Attempt to ventilate.		
9. Sequencing	(Airway remains obstructed.) Repeat sequence.	Repeat Steps 6–8 until successful.†		

* During practice and testing, simulate finger sweeps.

† After airway obstruction is cleared, ventilate twice and proceed with CPR as indicated.

Instructor _____ Check: Satisfactory _____ Unsatisfactory _____

(continued)

APPENDIX B.
PERFORMANCE SHEETS FOR CARDIOPULMONARY RESUSCITATION AND FOREIGN BODY AIRWAY OBSTRUCTION MANAGEMENT (*continued*)

BLS Performance Sheet
Adult FBAO Management: Unconscious

Name _____ Date _____

Step	Objective	Critical Performance	S	U
1. Assessment	Determine unresponsiveness.	Tap or gently shake shoulder. Shout "Are you OK?"		
	Call for help.	Call out "Help!"		
	Position the victim.	Turn on back as unit, if necessary, supporting head and neck (4–10 sec).		
	Open the airway.	Use head-tilt/chin-lift maneuver.		
	Determine breathlessness.	Maintain open airway.		
		Ear over mouth, observe chest: look, listen, feel for breathing (3–5 sec).		
2. Breathing Attempt	Ventilate.	Maintain open airway.		
		Seal mouth and nose properly.		
		Attempt to ventilate.		
	(Airway is obstructed.) Ventilate.	Reposition victim's head.		
		Seal mouth and nose properly.		
		Reattempt to ventilate.		
	(Airway remains obstructed.) Activate EMS system.	If someone responded to call for help, send him/her to activate EMS system.		
3. Heimlich Maneuver	Perform abdominal thrusts.	Straddle victim's thighs.		
		Place heel of one hand against victim's abdomen in the midline slightly above the navel and well below the tip of the xiphoid.		
		Place second hand directly on top of first hand.		
		Press into the abdomen with quick upward thrusts.		
		Each thrust should be distinct and delivered with the intent of relieving the airway obstruction.		
		Perform 6–10 abdominal thrusts.		
4. Foreign Body Check	Perform finger sweep.*	Keep victim's face up.		
		Use tongue–jaw lift to open mouth.		
		Sweep deeply into mouth to remove foreign body.		
5. Breathing Attempt	Ventilate.	Open airway with head-tilt/chin-lift maneuver.		
		Seal mouth and nose properly.		
		Reattempt to ventilate.		
6. Sequencing	Repeat sequence.	Repeat Steps 3–5 until successful.†		

* During practice and testing simulate finger sweeps.

† After airway obstruction is cleared, ventilate twice and proceed with CPR as indicated.

Instructor _____ Check: Satisfactory _____ Unsatisfactory _____

(*continued*)

APPENDIX B.
PERFORMANCE SHEETS FOR CARDIOPULMONARY RESUSCITATION AND FOREIGN BODY AIRWAY OBSTRUCTION MANAGEMENT (continued)

BLS Performance Sheet
Child One-Rescuer CPR*

Name _____ Date _____

Step	Objective	Critical Performance	S	U
1. **A**IRWAY	Assessment: Determine unresponsiveness.	Tap or gently shake shoulder.		
		Shout "Are you OK?"		
	Call for help.	Call out "Help!"		
	Position the victim.	Turn on back as unit, if necessary, supporting head and neck (4–10 sec).		
	Open the airway.	Use head-tilt/chin-lift maneuver.		
2. **B**REATHING	Assessment: Determine breathlessness.	Maintain open airway.		
		Ear over mouth, observe chest: look, listen, feel for breathing (3–5 sec).		
	Ventilate twice.	Maintain open airway.		
		Seal mouth and nose properly.		
		Ventilate 2 times at 1–1.5 sec/inspiration.		
		Observe chest rise.		
		Allow deflation between breaths.		
3. **C**IRCULATION	Assessment: Determine pulselessness.	Feel for carotid pulse on near side of victim (5–10 sec).		
		Maintain head-tilt with other hand.		
	Activate EMS system.	If someone responded to call for help, send him/her to activate EMS system.		
		Total time, Step 1—Activate EMS system: 15–35 sec.		
	Begin chest compressions.	Rescuer kneels by victim's shoulders.		
		Landmark check prior to initial hand placement.§		
		Proper hand position throughout.		
		Rescuer's shoulders over victim's sternum.		
		Equal compression–relaxation.		
		Compress 1 to 1½ inches.		
		Keep hand on sternum during upstroke.		
		Complete chest relaxation on upstroke.		
		Say any helpful mnemonic.		
		Compression rate: 80–100/min (5 per 3–4 sec).		
4. Compression/Ventilation Cycles	Do 10 cycles of 5 compressions and 1 ventilation.	Proper compression/ventilation ratio: 5 compressions to 1 slow ventilation per cycle.		
		Observe chest rise: 1–1.5 sec/inspiration (10 cycles/60–87 sec).		
5. Reassessment†	Determine pulselessness.	Feel for carotid pulse (5 sec).‡ If there is no pulse, go to Step 6.		
6. Continue CPR	Ventilate once.	Ventilate one time.		
		Observe chest rise: 1–1.5 sec/inspiration.		
	Resume compression/ventilation cycles	Feel for carotid pulse every few minutes.		

* If child is above age of approximately 8 years, the method for adults should be used.

† 2nd rescuer arrives to replace 1st rescuer: (a) 2nd rescuer identifies self by saying "I know CPR. Can I help?" (b) 2nd rescuer then does pulse check in Step 5 and continues with Step 6. (During practice and testing only one rescuer actually ventilates the manikin. The 2nd rescuer simulates ventilation.) (c) 1st rescuer assesses the adequacy of 2nd rescuer's CPR by observing chest rise during ventilations and by checking the pulse during chest compressions.

‡ If pulse is present, open airway and check for spontaneous breathing. (a) If breathing is present, maintain open airway and monitor breathing and pulse. (b) If breathing is absent, perform rescue breathing at 15 times/min and monitor pulse.

§ Thereafter, check hand position visually.

Instructor _____ Check: Satisfactory _____ Unsatisfactory _____

(continued)

APPENDIX B.
PERFORMANCE SHEETS FOR CARDIOPULMONARY RESUSCITATION AND FOREIGN BODY AIRWAY OBSTRUCTION MANAGEMENT (continued)

BLS Performance Sheet
Child FBAO Management: Conscious*

Name _____ Date _____

Step	Objective	Critical Performance	S	U
1. Assessment	Determine airway obstruction.*	Ask "Are you choking?"		
		Determine if victim can cough or speak.		
2. Heimlich Maneuver	Perform abdominal thrusts (only if victim's cough is ineffective and there is increasing respiratory difficulty).	Stand behind the victim.		
		Wrap arms around victim's waist.		
		Make a fist with one hand and place the thumb side against victim's abdomen, in the midline slightly above the navel and well below the tip of the xiphoid.		
		Grasp fist with the other hand.		
		Press into the victim's abdomen with quick upward thrusts.		
		Each thrust should be distinct and delivered with the intent of relieving the airway obstruction.		
		Repeat thrusts until either the foreign body is expelled or the victim becomes unconscious (see below).		

Victim with Obstructed Airway Becomes Unconscious (Optional Testing Sequence)

Step	Objective	Critical Performance	S	U
3. Positioning	Position the victim.	Turn on back as unit.		
		Place face up, arms by side.		
	Call for help.	Call out "Help!" or if others respond, activate EMS system.		
4. Foreign Body Check	Manual removal of foreign body if one is found. DO NOT perform blind finger sweep.	Keep victim's face up.		
		Use tongue–jaw lift to open mouth.		
		Look into mouth; remove foreign body ONLY IF VISUALIZED.		
5. Breathing Attempt	Ventilate.	Open airway with head-tilt/chin-lift.		
		Seal mouth and nose properly.		
		Attempt to ventilate.		
6. Heimlich Maneuver	(Airway is obstructed.) Perform abdominal thrusts.	Kneel at victim's feet if on the floor, or stand at victim's feet if on a table.		
		Place heel of one hand against victim's abdomen, in the midline slightly above navel and well below tip of xiphoid.		
		Place second hand directly on top of first hand.		
		Press into the abdomen with quick upward thrusts.		
		Perform 6–10 abdominal thrusts.		
7. Foreign Body Check	(Airway remains obstructed.) Manual removal of foreign body if one is found. DO NOT perform blind finger sweep.	Keep victim's face up.		
		Use tongue–jaw lift to open mouth.		
		Look into mouth; remove foreign body ONLY IF VISUALIZED.		
8. Breathing Attempt	Ventilate.	Open airway with head-tilt/chin-lift.		
		Seal mouth and nose properly.		
		Reattempt to ventilate.		
9. Sequencing	(Airway remains obstructed.) Repeat sequence.	Repeat Steps 6–8 until successful.†		

* This procedure should be initiated in a conscious child only if the airway obstruction is due to a witnessed or strongly suspected aspiration and if respiratory difficulty is increasing and the cough is ineffective. If obstruction is caused by airway swelling due to infection such as epiglottitis or croup, these procedures may be harmful; the child should be rushed to the nearest ALS facility, allowing the child to maintain the position of maximum comfort.

† After airway obstruction is cleared, ventilate twice and proceed with CPR as indicated.

Instructor _____ Check: Satisfactory _____ Unsatisfactory _____

(continued)

APPENDIX B.
PERFORMANCE SHEETS FOR CARDIOPULMONARY RESUSCITATION AND FOREIGN BODY AIRWAY OBSTRUCTION MANAGEMENT (continued)

BLS Performance Sheet
Child FBAO Management: Unconscious

Name _____ Date _____

Step	Objective	Critical Performance	S	U
1. Assessment	Determine unresponsiveness.	Tap or gently shake shoulder.		
		Shout "Are you OK?"		
	Call for help.	Call out "Help!"		
	Position the victim.	Turn on back as unit, if necessary, supporting head and neck (4–10 sec).		
	Open the airway.	Use head-tilt/chin-lift maneuver.		
	Determine breathlessness.	Maintain open airway.		
		Ear over mouth, observe chest: look, listen, feel for breathing (3–5 sec).		
2. Breathing Attempt	Ventilate.	Maintain open airway.		
		Seal mouth and nose properly.		
		Attempt to ventilate.		
	(Airway is obstructed.) Ventilate.	Reposition victim's head.		
		Seal mouth and nose properly.		
		Reattempt to ventilate.		
	(Airway remains obstructed.) Activate EMS system.	If someone responded to call for help, send him/her to activate EMS system.		
3. Heimlich Maneuver	Perform abdominal thrusts.	Kneel at victim's feet if on the floor, or stand at victim's feet if on a table.		
		Place heel of one hand against victim's abdomen in the midline slightly above navel and well below tip of xiphoid.		
		Place second hand directly on top of first hand.		
		Press into the abdomen with quick upward thrusts.		
		Each thrust should be distinct and delivered with the intent of relieving the airway.		
		Perform 6–10 abdominal thrusts.		
4. Foreign Body Check	(Airway remains obstructed.) Manual removal of foreign body if one is found. DO NOT perform blind finger sweep.	Keep victim's face up.		
		Use tongue–jaw lift to open mouth.		
		Look into mouth; remove foreign body ONLY IF VISUALIZED.		
5. Breathing Attempt	Ventilate.	Open airway with head-tilt/chin-lift maneuver.		
		Seal mouth and nose properly.		
		Reattempt to ventilate.		
6. Sequencing	Repeat sequence.	Repeat Steps 3–5 until successful.*		

* After airway obstruction is cleared, ventilate twice and proceed with CPR as indicated.

Instructor _____ Check: Satisfactory _____ Unsatisfactory _____

(continued)

APPENDIX B.
PERFORMANCE SHEETS FOR CARDIOPULMONARY RESUSCITATION AND FOREIGN BODY AIRWAY OBSTRUCTION MANAGEMENT (*continued*)

BLS Performance Sheet
Infant CPR

Name _____ Date _____

Step	Objective	Critical Performance	S	U
1. **A**IRWAY	Assessment: Determine unresponsiveness.	Tap or gently shake shoulder.		
	Call for help.	Call out "Help!"		
	Position the infant.	Turn on back as unit, supporting head and neck.		
		Place on firm, hard surface.		
	Open the airway.	Use head-tilt/chin-lift maneuver to sniffing or neutral position.		
		Do not overextend the head.		
2. **B**REATHING	Assessment: Determine breathlessness.	Maintain open airway.		
		Ear over mouth, observe chest: look, listen, feel for breathing (3–5 sec).		
	Ventilate twice.	Maintain open airway.		
		Make tight seal on infant's mouth and nose with rescuer's mouth.		
		Ventilate 2 times at 1–1.5 sec/inspiration.		
		Observe chest rise.		
		Allow deflation between breaths.		
3. **C**IRCULATION	Assessment: Determine pulselessness.	Feel for brachial pulse (5–10 sec).		
		Maintain head-tilt with other hand.		
	Activate EMS system.	If someone responded to call for help, send him/her to activate EMS system.		
		Total time, Step 1—Activate EMS system: 15–35 sec.		
	Begin chest compressions.	Imagine line between nipples (intermammary line).		
		Place 2–3 fingers on sternum, 1 finger's width below intermammary line.		
		Equal compression–relaxation.		
		Compress vertically, ½ to 1 inches.		
		Keep fingers on sternum during upstroke.		
		Complete chest relaxation on upstroke.		
		Say any helpful mnemonic.		
		Compression rate: at least 100/min (5 in 3 sec or less).		
4. Compression/Ventilation Cycles	Do 10 cycles of 5 compressions and 1 ventilation.	Proper compression/ventilation ratio: 5 compressions to 1 slow ventilation per cycle.		
		Pause for ventilation.		
		Observe chest rise: 1–1.5 sec/inspiration; 10 cycles/45 sec or less.		
5. Reassessment	Determine pulselessness.	Feel for brachial pulse (5 sec).* If there is no pulse, go to Step 6.		
6. Continue CPR	Ventilate once.	Ventilate 1 time.		
		Observe chest rise: 1–1.5 sec/inspiration.		
	Resume compression/ventilation cycles.	Feel for brachial pulse every few minutes.		

* If pulse is present, open airway and check for spontaneous breathing. (a) If breathing is present, maintain open airway and monitor breathing and pulse. (b) If breathing is absent, perform rescue breathing at 20 times/min and monitor pulse.

Instructor _____ Check: Satisfactory _____ Unsatisfactory _____

(*continued*)

APPENDIX B.
PERFORMANCE SHEETS FOR CARDIOPULMONARY RESUSCITATION AND FOREIGN BODY AIRWAY OBSTRUCTION MANAGEMENT (continued)

BLS Performance Sheet
Infant FBAO Management: Conscious*

Name _____ Date _____

Step	Objective	Critical Performance	S	U
1. Assessment	Determine airway obstruction.*	Observe breathing difficulties.*		
2. Back Blows	Deliver 4 back blows.	Supporting head and neck with one hand, straddle infant face down, head lower than trunk, over your forearm supported on your thigh.		
		Deliver 4 back blows, forcefully, between the shoulder blades with the heel of the hand (3–5 sec).		
3. Chest Thrusts	Deliver 4 chest thrusts.	While supporting the head, sandwich infant between your hands and turn on back, with head lower than trunk.		
		Deliver 4 thrusts in the midsternal region in the same manner as external chest compressions, but at a slower rate (3–5 sec).		
4. Sequencing	Repeat sequence.	Repeat Steps 2 and 3 until either the foreign body is expelled or the infant becomes unconscious (see below).		

Infant with Obstructed Airway Becomes Unconscious (Optional Testing Sequence)

Step	Objective	Critical Performance	S	U
5. Call for Help.	Call for help.	Call out "Help!" or, if others respond, activate EMS system.		
6. Foreign Body Check	Manual removal of foreign body if one is found (tongue–jaw lift, NOT blind finger sweep).	Keep victim's face up.		
		Place thumb in infant's mouth, over tongue. Lift tongue and jaw forward with fingers wrapped around lower jaw.		
		Look into mouth; remove foreign body ONLY IF VISUALIZED.		
7. Breathing Attempt	Ventilate.	Open airway with head-tilt/chin-lift.		
		Seal mouth and nose properly.		
		Attempt to ventilate.		
8. Back Blows	(Airway is obstructed.) Deliver 4 back blows.	Supporting head and neck with one hand, straddle infant face down, head lower than trunk, over your forearm supported on your thigh.		
		Deliver 4 back blows, forcefully, between the shoulder blades with the heel of the hand (3–5 sec).		
9. Chest Thrusts	Deliver 4 chest thrusts.	While supporting the head and neck, sandwich infant between your hands and turn on back, with head lower than trunk.		
		Deliver 4 thrusts in the midsternal region in the same manner as external chest compressions, but at a slower rate (3–5 sec).		
10. Foreign Body Check	(Airway remains obstructed.) Manual removal of foreign body if one is found.	Keep victim's face up.		
		Do tongue–jaw lift, but NOT blind finger sweep.		
		Look into mouth, remove foreign body ONLY IF VISUALIZED.		
11. Breathing Attempt	Ventilate.	Open airway with head-tilt/chin-lift.		
		Seal mouth and nose properly.		
		Reattempt to ventilate.		
12. Sequencing	(Airway remains obstructed.) Repeat sequence.	Repeat Steps 8–11 until successful.†		

* This procedure should be initiated in a conscious infant only if the airway obstruction is due to a witnessed or strongly suspected aspiration and if respiratory difficulty is increasing and the cough is ineffective. If the obstruction is caused by airway swelling due to infections, such as epiglottitis or croup, these procedures may be harmful; the infant should be rushed to the nearest ALS facility, allowing the infant to maintain the position of maximum comfort.

† After airway obstruction is cleared, ventilate twice and proceed with CPR as indicated.

Instructor _____ Check: Satisfactory _____ Unsatisfactory _____

(continued)

APPENDIX B.
PERFORMANCE SHEETS FOR CARDIOPULMONARY RESUSCITATION
AND FOREIGN BODY AIRWAY OBSTRUCTION MANAGEMENT (continued)

BLS Performance Sheet
Infant FBAO Management: Unconscious

Name _____ Date _____

Step	Objective	Critical Performance	S	U
1. Assessment	Determine unresponsiveness.	Tap or gently shake shoulder.		
	Call for help.	Call out "Help!"		
	Position the infant.	Turn on back as unit, if necessary, supporting head and neck.		
		Place on firm, hard surface.		
	Open the airway.	Use head-tilt/chin-lift maneuver to sniffing or neutral position.		
		Do not overextend the head.		
	Determine breathlessness.	Maintain open airway.		
		Ear over mouth, observe chest: look, listen, feel for breathing (3–5 sec).		
2. Breathing Attempt	Ventilate.	Maintain open airway.		
		Make tight seal on mouth and nose of infant with rescuer's mouth.		
		Attempt to ventilate.		
	(Airway is obstructed.) Ventilate.	Reposition infant's head.		
		Seal mouth and nose properly.		
		Reattempt to ventilate.		
	(Airway remains obstructed.) Activate EMS system	If someone responded to call for help, send him/her to activate EMS system.		
3. Back Blows	Deliver 4 back blows.	Supporting head and neck with one hand, straddle infant face down, head lower than trunk, over your forearm supported on your thigh.		
		Deliver 4 back blows, forcefully, between the shoulder blades with the heel of the hand (3–5 sec).		
4. Chest Thrusts	Deliver 4 chest thrusts.	While supporting the head and neck, sandwich infant between your hands and turn on back, with head lower than trunk.		
		Deliver 4 thrusts in the midsternal region in the same manner as external chest compressions, but at a slower rate (3–5 sec).		
5. Foreign Body Check	(Airway remains obstructed.) Manual removal of foreign body if one is found (tongue–jaw lift, NOT blind finger sweep).	Keep victim's face up.		
		Place thumb in infant's mouth, over tongue. Lift tongue and jaw forward with fingers wrapped around lower jaw.		
		Look into mouth; remove foreign body ONLY IF VISUALIZED.		
6. Breathing Attempt	Ventilate.	Open airway with head-tilt/chin-lift.		
		Seal mouth and nose properly.		
		Reattempt to ventilate.		
7. Sequencing	Repeat sequence.	Repeat Steps 3–6 until successful.*		

* After airway obstruction is cleared, ventilate twice and proceed with CPR as indicated.

Instructor _____ Check: Satisfactory _____ Unsatisfactory _____

(continued)

APPENDIX B.
PERFORMANCE SHEETS FOR CARDIOPULMONARY RESUSCITATION AND FOREIGN BODY AIRWAY OBSTRUCTION MANAGEMENT (continued)

BLS Performance Sheet
Adult Two-Rescuer CPR*

Name _____ Date _____

Step	Objective	Critical Performance	S	U
1. AIRWAY	**One rescuer (ventilator):** Assessment: Determine unresponsiveness.	Tap or gently shake shoulder.		
		Shout "Are you OK?"		
	Position the victim.	Turn on back if necessary (4–10 sec).		
	Open the airway.	Use a proper technique to open airway.		
2. BREATHING	Assessment: Determine breathlessness.	Look, listen, and feel (3–5 sec).		
	Ventilate twice.	Observe chest rise: 1–1.5 sec/inspiration.		
3. CIRCULATION	Assessment: Determine pulselessness.	Feel for carotid pulse (5–10 sec).		
	State assessment results.	Say "No pulse."		
	Other rescuer (compressor): Get into position for compressions.	Hands, shoulders in correct position.		
	Locate landmark notch.	Landmark check.		
4. Compression/Ventilation Cycles	**Compressor:** Begin chest compressions.	Correct ratio compressions/ventilations: 5/1.		
		Compression rate: 80–100/min (5 compressions/3–4 sec).		
		Say any helpful mnemonic.		
		Stop compressing for each ventilation.		
	Ventilator: Ventilate after every 5th compression and check compression effectiveness.	Ventilate 1 time (1–1.5 sec/inspiration).		
		Check pulse occasionally to assess compressions.		
	(Minimum of 10 cycles.)	Time for 10 cycles: 40–53 sec.		
5. Call for Switch	**Compressor:** Call for switch when fatigued.	Give clear signal to change.		
		Compressor completes 5th compression.		
		Ventilator completes ventilation after 5th compression.		
6. Switch	Simultaneously switch:			
	Ventilator: Move to chest.	Move to chest.		
		Become compressor.		
		Get into position for compressions.		
		Locate landmark notch.		
	Compressor: Move to head.	Move to head.		
		Become ventilator.		
		Check carotid pulse (5 sec).		
		Say "No pulse."		
		Ventilate once (1–1.5 sec/inspiration).†		
7. Continue CPR	Resume compression/ventilation cycles.	Resume Step 4.		

* (a) If CPR is in progress with one rescuer (lay person), the entrance of the two rescuers occurs after the completion of one rescuer's cycle of 15 compressions and 2 ventilations. The EMS should be activated first. The two new rescuers start with Step 6. (b) If CPR is in progress with one healthcare provider, the entrance of a second healthcare provider is at the end of a cycle after check for pulse by first rescuer. The new cycle starts with one ventilation by the first rescuer, and the second rescuer becomes the compressor.

† During practice and testing only one rescuer actually ventilates the manikin. The other rescuer simulates ventilation.

Instructor _____ Check: Satisfactory _____ Unsatisfactory _____

(continued)

APPENDIX B.
PERFORMANCE SHEETS FOR CARDIOPULMONARY RESUSCITATION AND FOREIGN BODY AIRWAY OBSTRUCTION MANAGEMENT (continued)

BLS Performance Sheet
Child Two-Rescuer CPR*

Name _____ Date _____

Step	Objective	Critical Performance	S	U
1. AIRWAY	**One rescuer (ventilator):** Assessment: Determine unresponsiveness.	Tap or gently shake shoulder.		
		Shout "Are you OK?"		
	Position the victim.	Turn on back if necessary (4–10 sec).		
	Open the airway.	Use a proper technique to open airway.		
2. BREATHING	Assessment: Determine breathlessness.	Look, listen, and feel (3–5 sec).		
	Ventilate twice.	Observe chest rise: 1–1.5 sec/inspiration.		
3. CIRCULATION	Assessment: Determine pulselessness.	Feel for carotid pulse (5–10 sec).		
	State assessment results.	Say "No pulse."		
	Other rescuer (compressor): Get into position for compressions.	Hand, shoulders in correct position.		
	Locate landmark notch.	Landmark check.		
4. Compression/Ventilation Cycles	**Compressor:** Begin chest compressions.	Correct ratio compressions/ventilations: 5/1.		
		Compression rate: 80–100/min (5 compressions/3–4 sec).		
		Say any helpful mnemonic.		
		Stop compressing for each ventilation.		
	Ventilator: Ventilate after every 5th compression and check compression effectiveness.	Ventilate 1 time (1–1.5 sec/inspiration).		
		Check pulse occasionally to assess compressions.		
	(Minimum of 10 cycles.)	Time for 10 cycles: 40–53 sec.		
5. Call for Switch	**Compressor:** Call for switch when fatigued.	Give clear signal to change.		
		Compressor completes 5th compression.		
		Ventilator completes ventilation after 5th compression.		
6. Switch	Simultaneously switch:			
	Ventilator: Move to chest.	Move to chest.		
		Become compressor.		
		Get into position for compressions.		
		Locate landmark notch.		
	Compressor: Move to head.	Move to head.		
		Become ventilator.		
		Check carotid pulse (5 sec).		
		Say "No pulse."		
		Ventilate once (1–1.5 sec/inspiration).†		
7. Continue CPR	Resume compression/ventilation cycles.	Resume Step 4.		

* (a) If CPR is in progress with one rescuer (layperson), the entrance of the two rescuers occurs after the completion of one rescuer's cycle of 5 compressions and 1 ventilation. The EMS should be activated first. The two new rescuers start with Step 6. (b) If CPR is in progress with one healthcare provider, the entrance of a second healthcare provider is at the end of a cycle after check for pulse by first rescuer. The new cycle starts with one ventilation by the first rescuer, and the second rescuer becomes the compressor.

† During practice and testing only one rescuer actually ventilates the manikin. The other rescuer simulates ventilation.

Instructor _____ Check: Satisfactory _____ Unsatisfactory _____

(continued)

APPENDIX B.
PERFORMANCE SHEETS FOR CARDIOPULMONARY RESUSCITATION AND FOREIGN BODY AIRWAY OBSTRUCTION MANAGEMENT (continued)

BLS Summary Performance Sheet
Cardiopulmonary Resuscitation (CPR)

	Objectives	Actions Adult (over 8 yrs.)	Child (1 to 8 yrs.)	Infant (under 1 yr.)
A. Airway	1. Assessment: Determine unresponsiveness.	Tap or gently shake shoulder.		
		Say, "Are you okay?"		Observe
	2. Get help.	Call out "Help!"		
	3. Position the victim.	Turn on back as a unit, supporting head and neck if necessary. (4–10 seconds)		
	4. Open the airway.	Head-tilt/chin-lift		
B. Breathing	5. Assessment: Determine breathlessness.	Maintain open airway. Place ear over mouth, observing chest. Look, listen, feel for breathing. (3–5 seconds)		
	6. Give 2 rescue breaths.	Maintain open airway.		
		Seal mouth to mouth		mouth to nose/mouth
		Give 2 rescue breaths, 1 to 1½ seconds each. Observe chest rise. Allow lung deflation between breaths.		
	7. Option for obstructed airway	a. Reposition victim's head. Try again to give rescue breaths.		
		b. Activate the EMS system.		
		c. Give 6–10 subdiaphragmatic abdominal thrusts (the Heimlich maneuver).		Give 4 back blows.
				Give 4 chest thrusts.
		d. Tongue–jaw lift and finger sweep	Tongue–jaw lift, but finger sweep only if you see a foreign object.	
		If unsuccessful, repeat a, c, and d until successful.		
C. Circulation	8. Assessment: Determine pulselessness.	Feel for carotid pulse with one hand; maintain head-tilt with the other. (5–10 seconds)		Feel for brachial pulse; keep head-tilt.
	9. Activate EMS system.	If someone responded to call for help, send them to activate the EMS system.		
	Begin chest compressions: 10. Landmark check	Run middle finger along bottom edge of rib cage to notch at center (tip of sternum).		Imagine a line drawn between the nipples.
	11. Hand position	Place index finger next to finger on notch:		Place 2–3 fingers on sternum, 1 finger's width below line. Depress ½–1 in.
		Two hands next to index finger. Depress 1½–2 in.	Heel of one hand next to index finger. Depress 1–1½ in.	
	12. Compression rate	80–100 per minute		At least 100 per minute
CPR Cycles	13. Compressions to breaths.	2 breaths to every 15 compressions.	1 breath to every 5 compressions.	
	14. Number of cycles.	4 (52–73 seconds)	10 (60–87 seconds)	10 (45 seconds or less)
	15. Reassessment.	Feel for carotid pulse. (5 seconds)		Feel for brachial pulse.
		If no pulse, resume CPR, starting with 2 breaths.	If no pulse, resume CPR, starting with 1 breath.	
Option for entrance of 2nd rescuer: "I know CPR. Can I help?"	1st rescuer ends CPR.	End cycle with 2 rescue breaths.	End cycle with 1 rescue breath.	
	2nd rescuer checks pulse (5 seconds).	Feel for carotid pulse.		Feel for brachial pulse.
	If no pulse, 2nd rescuer begins CPR.	Begin one-rescuer CPR, starting with 2 breaths.	Begin one-rescuer CPR, starting with 1 breath.	
	1st rescuer monitors 2nd rescuer.	Watch for chest rise and fall during rescue breathing; check pulse during chest compressions.		
Option for pulse return	If no breathing, give rescue breaths.	1 breath every 5 seconds	1 breath every 4 seconds	1 breath every 3 seconds

(continued)

APPENDIX B.
PERFORMANCE SHEETS FOR CARDIOPULMONARY RESUSCITATION AND FOREIGN BODY AIRWAY OBSTRUCTION MANAGEMENT *(continued)*

BLS Summary Performance Sheet
Foreign Body Airway Obstruction Management

	Objectives	Actions		
		Adult (over 8 yrs.)	**Child** (1 to 8 yrs.)	**Infant** (under 1 yr.)
Conscious Victim	1. Assessment: Determine airway obstruction.	Ask, "Are you choking?" Determine if victim can cough or speak.		Observe breathing difficulty.
	2. Act to relieve obstruction.	Perform subdiaphragmatic abdominal thrusts (Heimlich maneuver).		Give 4 back blows.
				Give 4 chest thrusts.
	Be persistent.	Repeat Step 2 until obstruction is relieved or victim becomes unconscious.		
Victim Who Becomes Unconscious	3. Position the victim; call for help.	Turn on back as a unit, supporting head and neck, face up, arms by sides. Call out, "Help!" If others come, activate EMS.		
	4. Check for foreign body.	Perform tongue–jaw lift and finger sweep.	Perform tongue–jaw lift. Remove foreign object only if you actually see it.	
	5. Give rescue breaths.	Open the airway with head-tilt/chin-lift. Try to give rescue breaths.		
	6. Act to relieve obstruction.	Perform subdiaphragmatic abdominal thrusts (Heimlich maneuver).		Give 4 back blows.
				Give 4 chest thrusts.
	7. Check for foreign body.	Perform tongue–jaw lift and finger sweep.	Perform tongue–jaw lift. Remove foreign object only if you actually see it.	
	8. Try again to give rescue breaths.	Open the airway with head-tilt/chin-lift. Try to give rescue breaths.		
	9. Be persistent.	Repeat Steps 6–8 until obstruction is relieved.		
Unconscious Victim	1. Assessment: Determine unresponsiveness.	Tap or gently shake shoulder. Shout, "Are you okay?"		Tap or gently shake shoulder.
	2. Call for help; position the victim.	Turn on back as a unit, supporting head and neck, face up, arms by sides. Call out, "Help!" If others come, activate EMS.		
	3. Open the airway.	Head-tilt/chin-lift.		Head-tilt/chin-lift, but do not tilt too far.
	4. Assessment: Determine breathlessness	Maintain an open airway. Ear over mouth; observe chest. Look, listen, feel for breathing. (3–5 seconds)		
	5. Give rescue breaths.	Make mouth-to-mouth seal.		Make mouth-to-nose-and-mouth seal.
		Try to give rescue breaths.		
	6. Try again to give rescue breaths.	Reposition head. Try rescue breaths again.		
	7. Activate the EMS system.	If someone responded to the call for help, that person should activate the EMS system.		
	8. Act to relieve obstruction.	Perform subdiaphragmatic abdominal thrusts (Heimlich maneuver).		Give 4 back blows.
				Give 4 chest thrusts.
	9. Check for foreign body.	Perform tongue–jaw lift and finger sweep.	Perform tongue–jaw lift. Remove foreign object only if you actually see it.	
	10. Rescue breaths.	Open the airway with head-tilt/chin-lift. Try again to give rescue breaths.		
	11. Be persistent.	Repeat Steps 8–10 until obstruction is relieved.		

APPENDIX C.
TRAUMA SCORES

Adult Glasgow Coma Scale

EYES OPENING

Spontaneous	4
To voice	3
To pain	2
None	1

VERBAL RESPONSE

Oriented	5
Confused	4
Inappropriate words	3
Incomprehensible words	2
None	1

MOTOR RESPONSE

Obeys command	6
Localizes pain	5
Withdraws (pain)	4
Flexion (decorticate)	3
Extension (decerebrate)	2
None	1

TOTAL 3 to 15

Crams Score

CIRCULATION

Normal capillary refill and blood pressure more than 100	2
Delayed capillary refill or blood pressure equals 85–99	1
No capillary refill or blood pressure less than 85	0

RESPIRATION

Normal rate and effort	2
Abnormal: labored, shallow, or rate more than 35	1
Absent	0

ABDOMEN/THORAX

Abdomen and thorax not tender	2
Abdomen or thorax tender	1
Abdomen rigid, thorax flail, or deep penetrating injury	0

MOTOR

Normal in obeying commands	2
Responds only to pain, no posturing	1
Postures or no response	0

SPEECH

Normal and oriented	2
Confused or inappropriate	1
None or unintelligible sounds	0

Total

(continued)

APPENDIX C.
TRAUMA SCORES (continued)

Adult Trauma Score

RESPIRATORY RATE	10–24/min	4
	25–35/min	3
	36/min or greater	2
	1–9/min	1
	None	0
RESPIRATORY EXPANSION	Normal	1
	Retractive	0
SYSTOLIC BLOOD PRESSURE	90 mm Hg or greater	4
	70–89 mm Hg	3
	50–69 mm Hg	2
	0–49 mm Hg	1
	No Pulse	0
CAPILLARY REFILL	Normal	2
	Delayed	1
	None	0

Adult Glasgow Coma Scale

EYES OPENING	Spontaneous	4	*Total Adult Glasgow Coma Scale Points*
	To voice	3	
	To pain	2	14–15 = 5
	None	1	11–13 = 4
VERBAL RESPONSE	Oriented	5	8–10 = 3
	Confused	4	5– 7 = 2
	Inappropriate words	3	3– 4 = 1
	Incomprehensible words	2	
	None	1	
MOTOR RESPONSE	Obeys command	6	
	Localizes pain	5	
	Withdraws (pain)	4	
	Flexion (decorticate)	3	
	Extension (decerebrate)	2	
	None	1	

Total Adult Trauma Score 1–15

(continued)

APPENDIX C.
TRAUMA SCORES (continued)

Pediatric Glasgow Coma Scale

	Score	Older Than 1 Year	Younger Than 1 Year
EYES OPENING	4	Spontaneously	Spontaneously
	3	To verbal command	To shout
	2	To pain	To pain
	1	No response	No response
BEST MOTOR RESPONSE	6	Obeys	
	5	Localizes pain	Localizes pain
	4	Flexion: withdrawal	Flexion: normal
	3	Flexion: abnormal (decorticate rigidity)	Flexion: abnormal (decorticate rigidity)
	2	Extension (decerebrate rigidity)	Extension (decerebrate rigidity)
	1	No response	No response

	Score	Older Than 5 Years	2–5 Years	0–23 Months
BEST VERBAL RESPONSE	5	Oriented and converses	Appropriate words and phrases	Smiles, coos, cries appropriately
	4	Disoriented and converses	Inappropriate words	Cries
	3	Inappropriate words	Cries and/or screams	Inappropriate crying and/or screaming
	2	Incomprehensible sounds	Grunts	Grunts
	1	No response	No response	No response

Pediatric Trauma Score

	Score		
Component	+2	+1	−1
Weight	>44 lb (>20 kg)	22–44 lb (10–20 kg)	<22 lb (<10 kg)
Airway	Normal	Maintainable without invasive procedures	Requires invasive procedures
Level of consciousness	Completely awake	Obtunded or any decreased level of consciousness	Comatose
Systolic blood pressure	Pulse at wrist >90 mm Hg	Carotid or femoral pulse palpable 50–90 mm Hg	No palpable pulse, <50 mm Hg
Open wounds	None	Minor	Major/penetrating
Fractures	None	Closed fracture	Open or multiple fractures

APPENDIX D.
EMERGENCY DRUGS

activated charcoal (Charcola)*
adenosine (Adenocard)
albuterol (Proventil, Ventolin)
amyl nitrite (See Cyanide Antidote Package)*
atropine sulfate*
bretylium tosylate (Bretylol)*
calcium chloride*
calcium gluconate*
codeine phosphate
Cyanide Antidote Package*
dexamethasone sodium phosphate (Decadron, Hexadrol)*
dextrose 50%*
diazepam (Valium)*
diazoxide (Hyperstat)
digoxin (Lanoxin)
diphenhydramine (Benadryl)*
dobutamine (Dobutrex)
dopamine (Intropin)*
epinephrine (Adrenalin)*
furosemide (Lasix)*
glucagon*
glucose (oral) (Glucola, Insta-glucose)*
haloperidol (Haldol)
heparin sodium
hydralazine (Apresoline)
hydrocortisone sodium succinate (Solu-Cortef)
insulin (Regular Insulin, Humulin R, others)
isoetharine (Bronkosol, Bronkometer)*
isoproterenol (Isuprel)*
lidocaine HCL (2%) (Xylocaine)*
mannitol 20% (Osmitrol)
meperidine (Demerol, Pethadol)
metaproterenol sulfate (Alupent, Metaprel)
metaraminol bitartrate (Aramine)
methylprednisolone sodium succinate (Solu-Medrol)
morphine sulfate*
nalbuphine HCL (Nubain)
naloxone (Narcan)*
nifedipine (Procardia)
nitroglycerine (Nitrostat)*
nitrous oxide, N_2O, dinitrous monoxide*
norepinephrine (Levophed, Levarterenol)*
oxygen*
oxytocin (Pitocin, Syntocin)*
phenobarbital sodium (Luminal Sodium)
phenytoin sodium (Dilantin)
physostigmine salicylate (Antilirium)
potassium chloride (KCL)
procainamide (Pronestyl)
propranolol (Inderal)
quinidine gluconate (Quinaglute, Quinidex)
racemic epinephrine*
sodium bicarbonate*
sodium nitoprusside (Nipride)
sodium nitrite (See Cyanide Antidote Package)*
sodium thiosulfate (See Cyanide Antidote Package)*
streptokinase, r-TPA (Kabikinase, Activase)
succinylcholine chloride (Anectine)
syrup of ipecac*
terbutaline sulfate (Brethine, Bricanyl)
theophylline ethylenediamine (Aminophylline)*
thiamine (Betalin)*
verapamil HCL (Calan, Isoptin, Verelan)*

* required by U.S. Department of Transportation Emergency Medical Technician-Paramedic: National Standard Curriculum

It is advisable to obtain up-to-date information from package inserts for use and dosage approved by the FDA before administering drugs.

(continued)

APPENDIX D.
EMERGENCY DRUGS (continued)

Generic Name: activated charcoal
Brand Name: Charcola
Class: adsorbent

Mechanism of Action:
Adsorbs toxic substances from GI tract (can adsorb up to 90% of another substance to render it inert)
Forms a barrier between toxic substances and gastric mucosa

Indications and Field Use:
Oral poisonings and overdoses
Used after evacuation of gastric contents

Contraindications:
Oral administration to comatose patient
Simultaneous administration of other oral drugs

Adverse Reactions:
Black stools

NOTES ON ADMINISTRATION
Incompatibilities/Drug Interactions:
Bonds with whatever it is mixed with

Adult Dosage:
1–2 g/kg; if not in pre-mixed slurry, mix one part charcoal with four parts water

Pediatric Dosage:
1–2 g/kg; if not in pre-mixed slurry, mix one part charcoal with four parts water

Routes of Administration:
Oral or nasogastric tube

Onset of Action:
Immediate

Peak Effects:
Not applicable

Duration of Action:
Dependent upon GI function; acts until excreted

Dosage Forms/Packaging:
Powder; pre-mixed slurry

Special Notes:
Often used in conjunction with magnesium citrate

Generic Name: adenosine
Brand Name: Adenocard
Class: antiarrhythmic

Mechanism of Action:
Slows conduction time through AV node; can interrupt re-entrant pathways through the AV node
Slows sinus rate
Has a direct effect upon supraventricular tissue

(continued)

APPENDIX D.
EMERGENCY DRUGS (continued)

Indications and Field Use:
Conversion of supraventricular tachycardias, including those caused by Wolff–Parkinson–White syndrome

Not effective in conversion of atrial fibrillation or flutter or ventricular tachycardia

Contraindications:
Sick sinus syndrome (except in patients with a functioning ventricular pacemaker)
Second- or third-degree AV block

Adverse Reactions:
Facial flushing, shortness of breath, chest pain (these occur in roughly 20% of patients; are very short-lived and well-tolerated if the patient is informed of the possibility of their occurrence)

NOTES ON ADMINISTRATION

Incompatibilities/Drug Interactions:
Methylxanthines (theophylline-type drugs) prevent binding of adenosine at receptor sites; larger doses may be needed

Dipyridamole (Persantine) causes potentiation of adenosine's effects; smaller doses may be effective

Carbamazepine (Tegretol) may result in development of high-degree blocks

May cause bronchoconstriction in asthmatic patients

Adult Dosage:
6 mg IV bolus as rapidly as possible, followed by flushing the IV line; if rhythm does not convert within 2 minutes, repeat using 12 mg bolus

Pediatric Dosage:
Not used

Routes of Administration:
Rapid IV push

Onset of Action:
Seconds

Peak Effects:
Seconds

Duration of Action:
10–12 seconds

Dosage Forms/Packaging:
6 mg in 2 ml vials (3 mg/ml)

Special Notes:
Short half-life (<10 seconds) limits side effects, but may permit arrhythmia to recur in some patients

---

Generic Name: albuterol
Brand Name: Proventil, Ventolin
Class: sympathomimetic

Mechanism of Action:
β agonist (primarily β_2)—relaxes bronchial smooth muscle, resulting in bronchodilation
Also relaxes vascular and uterine smooth muscle

(continued)

APPENDIX D.
EMERGENCY DRUGS (continued)

Indications and Field Use:
Treatment of bronchospasm from emphysema or asthma
Prevention of exercise-induced bronchospasm

Contraindications:
Synergistic with other sympathomimetics
Use caution in patients with diabetes, hyperthyroidism, and cerebrovascular disease

Adverse Reactions:
Excessive use may cause paradoxical bronchospasm and arrhythmias, tachycardia, tremors, nervousness, peripheral vasodilation, nausea, vomiting, hyperglycemia

NOTES ON ADMINISTRATION

Incompatibilities/Drug Interactions:
Tricyclic antidepressants (TCA's) and monoamine oxidase (MAO) inhibitors; other sympathomimetics

Adult Dosage:
Give 2.5 mg; dilute 0.5 ml of the 0.5% solution for inhalation with 2.5 ml normal saline in nebulizer over 10–15 minutes
2 inhalations with metered-dose inhaler every 4–6 hours

Pediatric Dosage:
Not recommended in children younger than 12 years

Routes of Administration:
Nebulized
Inhaler; also available in syrup

Onset of Action:
5–15 minutes

Peak Effects:
30 minutes–2 hours

Duration of Action:
3–4 hours

Dosage Forms/Packaging:
Metered-dose inhaler

Special Notes:
Antagonized by β-blockers (i.e., Inderal, Lopressor)

Generic Name: amyl nitrite, sodium nitrite, sodium thiosulfate
Brand Name: Cyanide Antidote Package
Class: antidote

Mechanism of Action:
Amyl nitrite—has affinity for cyanide ions; reacts with hemoglobin to form methemoglobin (low toxicity)
Sodium nitrite—same as amyl nitrite
Sodium thiosulfate—produces thiocyanate, which is then excreted

Indications and Field Use:
Cyanide or hydrocyanic acid poisoning

(continued)

APPENDIX D.
EMERGENCY DRUGS (continued)

Contraindications:
Not applicable

Adverse Reactions:
Excessive doses of sodium nitrite and amyl nitrite can induce severe life-threatening methemoglobinemia. Use only recommended doses

NOTES ON ADMINISTRATION

Incompatibilities/Drug Interactions:
Not applicable

Adult Dosage:
Amyl nitrite—breathe 30 seconds out of every minute
Sodium thiosulfate and sodium nitrite—dose dependent on hemoglobin level

Pediatric Dosage:
Same as adult

Routes of Administration:
Amyl nitrite—sniffed, or placed inside mask of bag–valve–mask device
Sodium thiosulfate and sodium nitrite—IV

Onset of Action:
Immediate

Peak Effects:
2 hours

Duration of Action:
Variable

Dosage Forms/Packaging:
Amyl nitrite—in pledgettes similar to ammonia capsules

Special Notes:
In cyanide poisoning, cyanide binds onto enzymes and interrupts the mitochondrial system; this blocks aerobic metabolism and the energy production system. Anaerobic metabolism continues briefly, contributing to acidosis.
Cyanide poisoning must be quickly recognized and treated; if pulse persists, even though patient is apneic, prognosis is good with treatment
Must be used in conjunction with oxygen

Generic Name: atropine sulfate
Brand Name: None
Class: parasympatholytic

Mechanism of Action:
Competitive inhibitor of acetylcholine in smooth muscle and glands, blocking parasympathetic response and allowing sympathetic response to take over
CNS effects:
Low doses—sedation
High doses—stimulation
Systemic effects:
Depresses salivary and GI secretions
Bronchodilation

(continued)

APPENDIX D.
EMERGENCY DRUGS (continued)

Cardiac effects:
Increases heart rate by increasing rate of SA discharge
Increases AV conduction

Indications and Field Use:
Sinus bradycardia with significant hypotension or ventricular ectopy
AV block
Asystole
Organophosphate insecticide poisoning
Counteracts physostigmine (Antilirium), neostigmine, edrophonium (Tensilon)

Contraindications:
Glaucoma
Bronchial asthma (may thicken secretions)
Mitral stenosis
Use with caution, if at all, in second degree AV block, Mobitz type II, because of risk of slowing ventricular rate

Adverse Reactions:
Increased cardiac workload
Pupil dilation
Dry mouth

NOTES ON ADMINISTRATION

Incompatibilities/Drug Interactions:
Sodium bicarbonate, norepinephrine, isoproterenol

Adult Dosage:
Bradycardia: 0.5–1.0 mg rapid IV push or ET
Asystole: 1.0 mg rapid IV push or ET
(For either) — may be repeated at 5 minute intervals; maximum of 2 mg except in insecticide poisoning

Pediatric Dosage:
0.01 mg/kg (minimum of 0.2 mg) rapid IV push

Routes of Administration:
IV, ET

Onset of Action:
1 minute

Peak Effects:
2–5 minutes

Duration of Action:
2 hours

Dosage Forms/Packaging:
0.1 mg/ml, 5 ml and 10 ml prefilled syringes

Special Notes:
Administering too small doses or administering too slowly may result in paradoxical bradycardia
Signs and symptoms of poisoning/overdose of atropine-like drugs: dry mouth; thirst; hot, dry, flushed skin; fever; palpitations; restlessness; excitement; delirium

(continued)

APPENDIX D.
EMERGENCY DRUGS (continued)

Generic Name: bretylium tosylate
Brand Name: Bretylol
Class: antiarrhythmic

Mechanism of Action:

Elevates ventricular fibrillation threshold

Biphasic autonomic (sympathetic) response—transient, slight adrenergic (sympathetic) response (increased heart rate, blood pressure, cardiac output, and possibly ventricular ectopy) due to norepinephrine release from nerve terminals, followed by a decrease in arterial pressure from vasodilation (due to norepinephrine depletion)

Does not suppress phase 4 depolarization

Does not affect conduction time or prolong P–R, Q–T, or QRS segments

Decreases re-entry by decreasing refractory time imbalance between normal and infarcted tissue
Prolongs action potential and refractory period

Indications and Field Use:
Intractable ventricular fibrillation and ventricular tachycardia as a second-line drug

Contraindications:
None, when used to treat life-threatening arrhythmias

Adverse Reactions:
Hypotension 15–20 minutes after administration (can usually be controlled with fluids and/or pressors)
Increased sensitivity to catecholamines
Nausea/vomiting after rapid IV administration

NOTES ON ADMINISTRATION

Incompatibilities/Drug Interactions:
None known

Adult Dosage:
5 mg/kg (350–500 mg) initially, over 1 minute
10 mg/kg (700–1000 mg) second dose, if needed, 10 minutes later (second dose is twice the first dose); total dose generally 30 mg/kg followed by infusion of 2 mg/min

Pediatric Dosage:
Same as adult (rarely given)

Routes of Administration:
IV bolus, followed by IV infusion

Onset of Action:
5 minutes to 2 hours

Peak Effects:
6–9 hours

Duration of Action:
5–10 hours

Dosage Forms/Packaging:
10 ml ampule, 50 mg/ml

Special Notes:
Not applicable

(continued)

APPENDIX D.
EMERGENCY DRUGS (continued)

Generic Name: calcium chloride, calcium gluconate
Brand Name: None
Class: electrolyte

Mechanism of Action:
Increases cardiac contractile state (positive inotropic effect)
May enhance ventricular automaticity

Indications and Field Use:
Used as antidote for adverse hemodynamic effects of calcium channel blockers;
Acute hyperkalemia
Acute hypocalcemia

Contraindications:
Hypercalcemia

Adverse Reactions:
May slow heart rate
Use cautiously in patients on digitalis

NOTES ON ADMINISTRATION

Incompatibilities/Drug Interactions:
All drugs—flush line before and after administration

Adult Dosage:
5–10 ml of a 10% solution IV push every 5–10 minutes

Pediatric Dosage:
Calcium gluconate is used in children

0.6 mg/ml of a 10% solution infused in 5–10 minutes (Calcium gluconate is one third the strength of $CaCl_2$; if calcium gluconate is unavailable, $CaCl_2$ may be substituted at one third the calculated dose of calcium gluconate)

Routes of Administration:
IV bolus

Onset of Action:
Immediate

Peak Effects:
3–5 minutes

Duration of Action:
15–30 minutes

Dosage Forms/Packaging:
10 ml prefilled syringe

Special Notes:
For pediatrics, if calcium gluconate is unavailable, 1–2 ml of 10% calcium chloride solution, diluted with IV fluid, may be substituted

(continued)

APPENDIX D.
EMERGENCY DRUGS (continued)

Generic Name: codeine phosphate
Brand Name: None
Class: narcotic analgesic

Mechanism of Action:
Acts on sensory cortex of the frontal lobes and diencephalon to interfere with the perception of pain

Indications and Field Use:
Mild to severe pain

Contraindications:
Elderly patients
Hypothyroidism
Head injury, elevated intracranial pressure
Narcotic dependence
Tachyarrhythmias
Myocardial infarction
Renal or hepatic disease

Adverse Reactions:
Sedation
Nausea
Dizziness
Agitation
Hallucinations
Cramping
Tachycardia, bradycardia
Blood pressure fluctuations
Respiratory depression

NOTES ON ADMINISTRATION

Incompatibilities/Drug Interactions:
Thiazides
Sulfonamides
Phenothiazines
MAO inhibitors

Adult Dosage:
30 mg SQ every 4 hours

Pediatric Dosage:
0.5 mg/kg SQ

Routes of Administration:
SQ

Onset of Action:
15–30 minutes

Peak Effects:
1 hour

Duration of Action:
4–6 hours

(continued)

APPENDIX D.
EMERGENCY DRUGS (continued)

Dosage Forms/Packaging:
15 mg/ml, 30 mg/ml, 60 mg/ml Tubex cartridges

Special Notes:
Schedule III narcotic

Often used in-hospital for minor head injuries because it has considerably less sedative effect than other narcotics

Generic Name: dexamethasone sodium phosphate
Brand Name: Decadron, Hexadrol
Class: corticosteroid

Mechanism of Action:
Enters target cells and binds to cytoplasmic receptors, thereby initiating many complex reactions that are resspsonsible for its anti-inflammatory and immunosuppressive effects.

Indications and Field Use:
Elevated intracranial pressure (prevention and treatment)

Shock (as an adjunct to other treatment)

Anaphylaxis

Status asthmaticus

Croup

Contraindications:
None for single dose

Adverse Reactions:
None from single dose

NOTES ON ADMINISTRATION

Incompatibilities/Drug Interactions:
Calcium

Metaraminol

Adult Dosage:
1 mg/kg slow IV bolus

Pediatric Dosage:
40–60 mcg/kg slow IV bolus

Routes of Administration:
IV push

Onset of Action:
Hours

Peak Effects:
8–12 hours

Duration of Action:
Not applicable

Dosage Forms/Packaging:
100 mg/5 ml vials
or 20 mg/1 ml vials

Special Notes:
Toxicity and side effects may result from long-term use

(continued)

APPENDIX D.
EMERGENCY DRUGS (continued)

Generic Name: Dextrose 50%
Brand Name: None
Class: hyperglycemic

Mechanism of Action:
Rapidly increases serum glucose levels
Provides short-term osmotic diuresis

Indications and Field Use:
Coma of unknown origin
Hypoglycemia
Status epilepticus

Contraindications:
Intracranial hemorrhage

Delirium tremens

Use with caution in acute alcoholism—ineffective without thiamine; may make thiamine deficiency more severe

Severe pain (paradoxical excitement may occur)

Do not administer to patients with known or suspected cerebrovascular accidents unless hypoglycemia is documented

Adverse Reactions:
Extravasation leads to tissue necrosis

NOTES ON ADMINISTRATION

Incompatibilities/Drug Interactions:
Sodium bicarbonate, coumadin

Adult Dosage:
25–50 g IV bolus

Pediatric Dosage:
Gives 25% dextrose 2–4 ml/kg IV bolus

Routes of Administration:
IV bolus (rapid)

Onset of Action:
Immediate

Peak Effects:
Variable

Duration of Action:
Variable

Dosage Forms/Packaging:
Prefilled syringe—20 g in 50 ml

Special Notes:
Draw blood sugar before administering

(continued)

APPENDIX D.
EMERGENCY DRUGS (continued)

Generic Name: diazepam
Brand Name: Valium
Class: benzodiazepine

Mechanism of Action:
Affects multiple levels of CNS to decrease seizures by increasing the seizure threshold
Transient analgesia
Amnesic
Sedative

Indications and Field Use:
Grand mal seizures, especially status epilepticus
Agitation secondary to head injury or hypoxia (treat the cause first)
Transient analgesia/amnesia for medical procedures (e.g., fracture reduction, cardioversion)
Delirium tremens

Contraindications:
Hypersensitivity
Glaucoma

Adverse Reactions:
Thrombosis and phlebitis
Bradycardia, hypotension, cardiovascular collapse
Respiratory arrest, especially with elevated blood alcohol levels
Burning proximal to IV injection site

NOTES ON ADMINISTRATION

Incompatibilities/Drug Interactions:
Incompatible with most drugs
Must be given close to hub of needle—can precipitate or bind with tubing

Adult Dosage:
5–10 mg slow IV push; can repeat at 10–15 minute intervals; administer no faster than 5 mg/minute

Pediatric Dosage:
0.2–0.3 mg/kg every 15–30 minutes (max. of 10 mg/kg); administer IV over at least 3 minutes or until seizure activity subsides

Routes of Administration:
Slow IV push
May be taken orally for anxiety

Onset of Action:
Minutes

Peak Effects:
Minutes

Duration of Action:
20 minutes to 50 minutes

Dosage Forms/Packaging:
10 mg/5 ml prefilled syringes

(continued)

APPENDIX D.
EMERGENCY DRUGS (continued)

Special Notes:
Schedule IV controlled drug

Use caution in renal patients

Be prepared to assist ventilation

Diazepam is a narcotic agonist

Diluent is propylene glycol (cardiotoxic and caustic to tissue/veins)

Metabolism of drug impaired in patients with congestive heart failure, liver disease, and the elderly; Cannot by dialyzed

Generic Name: diazoxide
Brand Name: Hyperstat
Class: vasodilator

Mechanism of Action:
Non-diuretic antihypertensive—acts directly on arterioles resulting in dilation, probably by antagonizing calcium

Decreases afterload by causing arteriolar dilation

Indications and Field Use:
Hypertensive crisis, especially in pre-eclampsia

Contraindications:
Hypotension

Labor

Adverse Reactions:
Reflex tachycardia

Myocardial or cerebral ischemia (leading to angina, arrhythmias, or stroke)

Causes sodium and water retention, leading to volume expansion; usually needs to be followed up with a diuretic

Can cause hyperglycemia by stimulating catecholamine release, which decreases insulin secretion and increases glycogenolysis; may need to be followed up with insulin

Can also cause flushing, dizziness, fever, orthostatic hypotension

NOTES ON ADMINISTRATION
Incompatibilities/Drug Interactions:
Heat, light, or acid solutions

Adult Dosage:
5 mg/kg or 300 mg, undiluted; give rapid IV push over 10–30 seconds

Pediatric Dosage:
5 mg/kg

Routes of Administration:
Rapid IV push

Onset of Action:
Immediate

Peak Effects:
5 minutes

(continued)

APPENDIX D.
EMERGENCY DRUGS (continued)

Duration of Action:
3–12 hours

Dosage Forms/Packaging:
5 mg/ml 20 ml ampules

Special Notes:
Administer only while patient is supine

Generic Name: **digoxin**
Brand Name: **Lanoxin**
Class: **digitalis preparation**

Mechanism of Action:
Positive inotropic without catecholamine release

Slows heart rate at the cellular level by augmenting calcium influx to contractile mechanism
Augments sodium–potassium pump by inhibiting breakdown of ATP

Enhances potassium efflux and sodium influx in myocardial cells (all of the above contribute to a positive inotropic effect)

Increases automaticity

Slows conduction through AV node (prolonging P–R interval)

Indications and Field Use:
Rarely used in the field

Patients may be on digitalis orally for congestive heart failure, atrial fibrillation, or paroxysmal atrial tachycardia

Contraindications:
Hypokalemia
Hypercalcemia
Heart block
Ventricular tachycardia

Adverse Reactions:
Many adverse reactions—toxic levels and therapeutic levels are very close

May include complete heart block, hypotension, bradycardia, nausea, vomiting, headache, malaise, drowsiness, disorientation, visual disturbances (yellow–green haze), hallucinations

NOTES ON ADMINISTRATION

Incompatibilities/Drug Interactions:
Calcium, phenytoin, nitroprusside

Adult Dosage:
6–12 mcg/kg to "digitalize" (reach therapeutic blood levels)
Oral—125 mcg tablet

Pediatric Dosage:
6–12 mcg/kg loading dose
125 mcg elixir orally

Routes of Administration:
Oral
May be given IV, but rarely used in the field

(continued)

APPENDIX D.
EMERGENCY DRUGS (continued)

Onset of Action:
IV—minutes
Oral—30 minutes–2 hours

Peak Effects:
2–6 hours oral

Duration of Action:
1–2 days

Dosage Forms/Packaging:
Tablets, elixir

Special Notes:
If a patient is on digitalis and presents with any arrhythmia, suspect digitalis toxicity
If administered with overdose of tricyclic antidepressants, may result in cardiac arrest
Toxicity much more likely in patients with renal disease, hypokalemia, hypercalcemia

Generic Name: diphenhydramine
Brand Name: Benadryl
Class: antihistamine; anticholinergic

Mechanism of Action:
Blocks cellular histamine receptors, but does not prevent histamine release; results in decreased capillary permeability and decreased vasodilation, as well as prevention of bronchospasm
Has some anticholinergic effects
Antiemetic—decreases motion sickness
Sedation

Indications and Field Use:
Anaphylaxis
Phenothiazine reactions
Blood administration reactions
Over-the-counter drug used for motion sickness, hay fever, and as a hypnotic
May also be used to treat side effects of some antipsychotic drugs

Contraindications:
Asthma
Glaucoma
Prostatic hypertrophy
Pregnancy
Hypertension
Hyperthyroidism
Cardiac disease
Elderly patients and infants

Adverse Reactions:
Sedation, hypotension, palpitation, anaphylaxis, arrhythmias
Seizures, visual disturbances, vomiting, hemolytic anemia
Urinary frequency or retention, thickening of bronchial secretions
In children, may cause paradoxical CNS excitation, palpitations, seizures

(continued)

APPENDIX D.
EMERGENCY DRUGS (continued)

NOTES ON ADMINISTRATION
Incompatibilities/Drug Interactions:
Decadron
Prednisone
Cephalosporins
Potentiates atropine, other anticholinergics, alcohol
Inhibits anticoagulants, some steroids

Adult Dosage:
25–100 mg IV push over 1–4 minutes
May also be given deep IM

Pediatric Dosage:
2–5 mg/kg IV push over 1–4 minutes
May also be given deep IM

Routes of Administration:
IV, IM, PO

Onset of Action:
Oral—15–30 minutes

Peak Effects:
Oral—1 hour

Duration of Action:
3–6 hours

Dosage Forms/Packaging:
50 or 100 mg prefilled syringes or vials

Special Notes:
Not used in infants or in pregnancy
In anaphylaxis, used in conjunction with epinephrine and steroids

Generic Name: **dobutamine**
Brand Name: **Dobutrex**
Class: **sympathomimetic**

Mechanism of Action:
Increased myocardial contractility and stroke volume, increasing cardiac output (positive inotropy)
Minimally enhanced chronotropy
No effect on dopaminergic receptors, but renal blood flow may increase due to increased cardiac output
Enhanced SA node automaticity, AV node conduction

Indications and Field Use:
Second-line drug for cardiogenic shock, often used in conjunction with other drugs
Rarely used in the prehospital setting

Contraindications:
Atrial fibrillation

(continued)

APPENDIX D.
EMERGENCY DRUGS (continued)

Adverse Reactions:
Use in myocardial infarction may increase infarct size
Arrhythmias may occur, but less commonly than with other pressors

NOTES ON ADMINISTRATION

Incompatibilities/Drug Interactions:
Alkaline solutions

Adult Dosage:
2–10 mcg/kg/minute IV infusion

Pediatric Dosage:
Same as adult

Routes of Administration:
IV infusion

Onset of Action:
2 minutes

Peak Effects:
10 minutes

Duration of Action:
1–2 minutes after infusion discontinued

Dosage Forms/Packaging:
250 mg vial

Special Notes:
Not applicable

Generic Name: dopamine
Brand Name: Intropin
Class: sympathomimetic

Mechanism of Action:
Immediate metabolic precursor to norepinephrine

Effects are dose-dependent:
    1–2 mcg/kg/minute—acts on dopaminergic receptors to dilate vessels in kidneys and mesentery; no change in HR or BP; may increase urine output
    2–10 mcg/kg/minute—primarily β_1 stimulant action; increased chronotropy and inotropy
    10–20 mcg/kg/minute—primarily α stimulant; peripheral vasoconstriction
    20 mcg/kg/minute—reversal of renal effects by overriding alpha effects

Indications and Field Use:
Cardiogenic, septic, or spinal shock
Electromechanical dissociation

Contraindications:
Hypovolemic shock
Pheochromocytoma

(continued)

APPENDIX D.
EMERGENCY DRUGS (continued)

Adverse Reactions:
Cardiac arrhythmias may occur due to increased myocardial oxygen demand
Tachycardia, hypertension
Renal shutdown (at higher doses)
Extravasation may cause tissue necrosis

NOTES ON ADMINISTRATION

Incompatibilities/Drug Interactions:
Incompatible in any alkaline solution
On-board MAO inhibitors will cause enhanced effects of dopamine and other catecholamines

Adult Dosage:
2–20 mcg/kg/minute IV infusion

Pediatric Dosage:
Same as adult

Routes of Administration:
IV infusion

Onset of Action:
Almost immediate

Peak Effects:
5–10 minutes

Duration of Action:
Effects cease almost immediately when infusion is shut off

Dosage Forms/Packaging:
40 mg/ml or 80 mg/ml 5 ml prefilled syringes
400 mg in 250 ml D_5W premixed solutions

Special Notes:
Always monitor drip rate—never run "wide open"

Generic Name: epinephrine
Brand Name: Adrenalin
Class: sympathomimetic

Mechanism of Action:
Direct acting α and β agonist
Effects include:
  α—bronchial, cutaneous, renal, and visceral arteriolar constriction (increased systemic vascular resistance)
  β_1—positive inotropic and chronotropic actions (increases myocardial workload and oxygen requirements), increases automaticity
  β_2—bronchial smooth muscle relaxation and dilation of skeletal vasculature
  Blocks histamine release

Indications and Field Use:
Cardiac arrest—increases cerebral and myocardial perfusion pressure; can stimulate spontaneous contractions in asystole
Occasionally used as infusion for profound hypotension or in cardiac arrest, in combination with other pressors

(continued)

APPENDIX D.
EMERGENCY DRUGS (continued)

Severe bronchospasm, i.e., bronchiolitis, asthma
Anaphylaxis

Contraindications:
Hypertension
Hypothermia
Pulmonary edema

Adverse Reactions:
Hypertension
Ventricular arrhythmias
Pulmonary edema
Tachycardia
Palpitations
Anxiety
Psychomotor agitation

NOTES ON ADMINISTRATION

Incompatibilities/Drug Interactions:
Potentiates other sympathomimetics
Patients on MAO inhibitors, antihistamines, and tricyclic antidepressants may have heightened effects
Sodium bicarbonate
Nitrates
Lidocaine
Aminophylline

Adult Dosage:
Cardiac dosage: Use 1:10,000 solution; give 0.5–1.0 mg every 5 minutes, IV or ET
Anaphylaxis and asthma: Use 1:1000 solution, give 0.1–0.5 mg SQ or IM; or use 1:10,000 solution; give 0.3–0.5 mg ET or IV if cardiovascular collapse occurs

Pediatric Dosage:
Cardiac: Use 1:10,000 solution; give 0.01 mg/kg every 5 minutes, IV or ET.
Asthma/anaphylaxis/bronchiolitis: Use 1:1000 solution; give 0.01 mg/kg SQ (maximum of 0.35 mg/dose)

Routes of Administration:
Cardiac: IV push, IV infusion, ET, intracardiac (if no other routes are available)
Asthma/anaphylaxis/bronchiolitis: SQ, IM, IV, ET

Onset of Action:
Immediate

Peak Effects:
Minutes

Duration of Action:
Several minutes

Dosage Forms/Packaging:
Cardiac: 0.1 mg/ml, 10 ml, 1:10,000 solution
Asthma/anaphylaxis/bronchiolitis: 1 mg/ml ampules, 1:1000 solution

(continued)

APPENDIX D.
EMERGENCY DRUGS (continued)

Special Notes:
If given ET, may dilute with sterile normal saline (10 ml in adults) to ensure that the drug reaches lung tissue rather than remaining in the tube

Generic Name: furosemide
Brand Name: Lasix
Class: loop diuretic

Mechanism of Action:
Potent diuretic—inhibits electrolyte reabsorption in the ascending Loop of Henle, and promotes excretion of sodium, potassium, chloride

Vasodilation, which increases venous capacitance and decreases afterload

Indications and Field Use:
Pulmonary edema; congestive heart failure

Contraindications:
Anuria
Hypovolemia
Hypotension (relative contraindication)

Adverse Reactions:
May exacerbate hypovolemia
Hyperglycemia (due to hemoconcentration)
Hypokalemia
May decrease the response to pressors

NOTES ON ADMINISTRATION

Incompatibilities/Drug Interactions:
Acidic drugs
Epinephrine, norepinephrine, isoproterenol, dopamine, dobutamine

Adult Dosage:
0.5–1 mg/kg (usually 20–80 mg) IV, no faster than 20 mg/minute (if dose is > 40 mg, give at 4 mg/minute)

Pediatric Dosage:
1 mg/kg IV

Routes of Administration:
Slow IV push

Onset of Action:
5 minutes

Peak Effects:
20–60 minutes

Duration of Action:
Variable

Dosage Forms/Packaging:
100 mg/5 ml, 20 mg/2 ml, 40 mg/4 ml vials

Special Notes:
Ototoxicity and resulting deafness can occur with rapid administration

(continued)

APPENDIX D.
EMERGENCY DRUGS (continued)

Generic Name: glucagon
Brand Name: None
Class: hyperglycemic

Mechanism of Action:
Naturally-occurring substance produced by α cells of Islets of Langerhans in pancreas

Fuel mobilization—increases blood glucose by stimulating glycogenesis; intensity of response is dependent on glycogen stores

Unknown mechanism of stabilizing cardiac rhythm in beta-blocker overdose

Positive inotropic and chronotropic (but minimal)

Decreases GI motility and secretions, pancreatic secretions, and blood pressure

Indications and Field Use:
Not commonly used in the field

May be used in-hospital in hypoglycemia and beta-blocker overdose

Contraindications:
Hyperglycemia
Known hypersensitivity

Adverse Reactions:
Hypersensitivity (glucagon is a protein-based drug)
Nausea/vomiting

NOTES ON ADMINISTRATION

Incompatibilities/Drug Interactions:
Incompatible in solution with most other substances

Adult Dosage:
0.5–1.0 mg IV
Repeat 1–2 times if no response within 20 minutes

Pediatric Dosage:
Not used

Routes of Administration:
IV

Onset of Action:
1 minute

Peak Effects:
30 minutes

Duration of Action:
Variable

Dosage Forms/Packaging:
1 mg ampule

Special Notes:
Ineffective if glycogen stores are depleted
Should always be used in conjunction with 50% Dextrose

(continued)

APPENDIX D.
EMERGENCY DRUGS (continued)

Generic Name: glucose (oral)
Brand Name: Glucola, Insta-glucose
Class: hyperglycemic

Mechanism of Action:
Provides a quickly absorbed form of glucose to increase blood glucose levels

Indications and Field Use:
Conscious patients with suspected hypoglycemia

Contraindications:
Decreased level of consciousness
Nausea/vomiting

Adverse Reactions:
Nausea/vomiting

NOTES ON ADMINISTRATION
Incompatibilities/Drug Interactions:
None

Adult Dosage:
Should be sipped slowly by the patient until a feeling of improvement is noted

Pediatric Dosage:
Same as adult

Routes of Administration:
Oral

Onset of Action:
Minutes

Peak Effects:
Variable

Duration of Action:
Variable

Dosage Forms/Packaging:
Glucola—300 ml bottles
Glucose pastes and gels also available in various forms

Special Notes:
Not applicable

Generic Name: haloperidol
Brand Name: Haldol
Class: antipsychotic

Mechanism of Action:
Acts on CNS to depress subcortical areas, midbrain, and ascending reticular activating system (interrupts articulation between diencephalon and cortex)
Inhibits CNS catecholamine receptors
Strong CNS antidopaminergic and weak CNS anticholinergic properties

(continued)

APPENDIX D.
EMERGENCY DRUGS (continued)

Indications and Field Use:
Rarely used in the field

Used more often in-hospital for agitated patients with chronic or acute psychosis or severe behavioral problems

Contraindications:
Agitation secondary to shock or hypoxia

Adverse Reactions:
Extrapyramidal signs and symptoms (rare with single dose—more common with long-term use)—restlessness, Parkinson-like symptoms, spasms, drooling, involuntary fixation of the eyes upward, stiff neck due to spasm

Tardive dyskinesia—rhythmic, repetitive, involuntary movements of mouth or jaw, with occasional movements of trunk and extremities; may be permanent despite discontinuing the drug

Hypotension

Dry mouth

CNS depression

NOTES ON ADMINISTRATION

Incompatibilities/Drug Interactions:
Enhanced CNS depression and possible hypotension in combination with alcohol

Antagonizes amphetamines

Antagonizes epinephrine—blocks α sites so β effects predominate (can lead to hypotension)

Adult Dosage:
2–5 mg IM every 30–60 minutes until sedation achieved

Pediatric Dosage:
0.5–1.0 mg IM every 4 hours

Routes of Administration:
IM

Onset of Action:
10 minutes

Peak Effects:
30–45 minutes

Duration of Action:
Variable

Dosage Forms/Packaging:
5 mg/ml ampule

Special Notes:
Do not use epinephrine to treat hypotension that may result from use of haloperidol—treat with fluids and norepinephrine

If patient is on long-term therapy, he may also be taking benztropine mesylate (Cogentin) to control extrapyramidal effects

(continued)

APPENDIX D.
EMERGENCY DRUGS (continued)

Generic Name: heparin sodium
Brand Name: None
Class: anticoagulant

Mechanism of Action:
Prevents conversion of fibrinogen to fibrin
Also affects coagulation factors IX, XI, XII, and plasmin
Does not lyse existing clots

Indications and Field Use:
Rarely used in the field
Used in-hospital for prophylaxis and treatment of: venous thrombosis, pulmonary embolus, coronary occlusion, disseminated intravascular coagulation (DIC), post-operative thrombosis

Contraindications:
Known hypersensitivity
Patients on antiplatelet drugs
Patients currently on streptokinase therapy

Adverse Reactions:
Hemorrhage
Thrombocytopenia
Allergic reactions

NOTES ON ADMINISTRATION

Incompatibilities/Drug Interactions:
Incompatible with all other drugs

Adult Dosage:
IV: loading dose—70 u/kg; maintenance dose—14–17 u/kg/hr
SQ: loading dose—70 u/kg IV and 140 u/kg SQ; follow with—140 u/kg every 8 hours

Pediatric Dosage:
IV: loading dose—50 u/kg; maintenance dose—75 u/kg/hr

Routes of Administration:
IV, SQ

Onset of Action:
IV—immediate; SQ—20–60 minutes

Peak Effects:
Not available

Duration of Action:
4 hours after continuous infusion is discontinued

Dosage Forms/Packaging:
1000 to 40,000 u/ml

Special Notes:
May be neutralized with protamine sulfate at 1 mg protamine/100 u heparin; give slow IV over 1–3 minutes

(continued)

APPENDIX D.
EMERGENCY DRUGS (continued)

Generic Name: hydralazine
Brand Name: Apresoline
Class: vasodilator

Mechanism of Action:
Vasodilator—decreases systemic vascular resistance; has a direct effect on vascular smooth muscle, more pronounced on arterioles than venules

Decreases diastolic blood pressure more than systolic

Increases heart rate, cardiac output, stroke volume

Increases blood flow to heart, brain, and kidneys

Indications and Field Use:
Moderate to severe hypertension (rarely used in the field)
Pre-eclampsia

Contraindications:
Hypotension
Elevated intracranial pressure

Adverse Reactions:
Hypotension
Headache
Palpitations
Tachycardia
Angina
Nasal congestion
May precipitate myocardial infarction

NOTES ON ADMINISTRATION

Incompatibilities/Drug Interactions:
Hydrocortisone
Aminophylline
Ampicillin
Chlorothiazide
May decompose in D_5W

Adult Dosage:
20–40 mg slow IV push over 1–2 minutes; titrate to effect; may repeat in 4–6 hrs; or
10–40 mg IM

Pediatric Dosage:
1.7–3.5 mg/kg daily; do not exceed 20 mg

Routes of Administration:
IV slow push; or IM
May also be taken orally

Onset of Action:
5–10 minutes

Peak Effects:
10–80 minutes

(continued)

APPENDIX D.
EMERGENCY DRUGS (continued)

Duration of Action:
2–6 hours

Dosage Forms/Packaging:
20 mg/ml, 2 ml ampule

Special Notes:
Hepatic or renal failure may prolong drug action

Generic Name: hydrocortisone sodium succinate
Brand Name: Solu-Cortef
Class: corticosteroid

Mechanism of Action:
Enters target cells and binds to cytoplasmic receptors thereby initiating many complex reactions that are responsible for its anti-inflammatory and immunosuppressive, and salt-retaining actions

Indications and Field Use:
Status asthmaticus
Shock due to acute adrenocortical insufficiency (abrupt cessation of cortisone therapy)

Contraindications:
None for a single dose

Adverse Reactions:
None with a single dose; side effects come from long-term use or repeated doses

NOTES ON ADMINISTRATION

Incompatibilities/Drug Interactions:
Heparin
Metaraminol

Adult Dosage:
4 mg/kg slow IV bolus
In anaphylaxis—500 mg bolus to prevent recurrence of symptoms (not a first-line drug)

Pediatric Dosage:
0.16–1.0 mg/kg slow to IV bolus

Routes of Administration:
IV bolus

Onset of Action:
1 hour

Peak Effects:
Variable

Duration of Action:
8–12 hours

Dosage Forms/Packaging:
Vials, also containing diluent, with 100, 250, or 500 mg

Special Notes:
Not applicable

(continued)

APPENDIX D.
EMERGENCY DRUGS (continued)

Generic Name: insulin
Brand Name: (Regular Insulin, Humulin R, others)
Class: antidiabetic

Mechanism of Action:
Necessary for carbohydrate, fat, and protein metabolism
Allows glucose transport into cells of muscle, cardiac, CNS, and all other tissue
Converts glycogen to fat
Allows glucose storage in the liver
Promotes fat and protein synthesis while antagonizing fat breakdown
Produces intracellular shift of potassium and magnesium to reduce elevated serum levels of those electrolytes

Indications and Field Use:
Not used in field—blood glucose levels are necessary before administering in an emergency situation
In-hospital use—diabetic ketoacidosis or other hyperglycemic state
Hyperkalemia

Contraindications:
Hypoglycemia
Hypokalemia

Adverse Reactions:
Hypokalemia
Hypoglycemia

NOTES ON ADMINISTRATION

Incompatibilities/Drug Interactions:
Incompatible in solution with all other drugs
Antagonizes actions of epinephrine, steroids, estrogens, thyroid hormones, diazoxide, dilantin

Adult Dosage:
Dosage adjusted relative to blood sugar levels

Pediatric Dosage:
Dosage adjusted relative to blood sugar levels

Routes of Administration:
SQ or IV
(As a protein, insulin is rapidly degraded by GI tract if given orally)
If given IV bolus, give as close to hub of needle as possible; if given as infusion, prime tubing with approximately 100 ml of infusion solution—insulin binds to plastic tubing and drug delivery to the patient will be erratic unless tubing is first "coated" with insulin

Onset of Action:
Within minutes

Peak Effects:
Approximately 1 hour

Duration of Action:
Up to 12 hours

Dosage Forms/Packaging:
Vials of 100 units/ml, 10 ml

(continued)

APPENDIX D.
EMERGENCY DRUGS (continued)

Special Notes:
Usually refrigerated

Oral hypoglycemics, such as Orinase, Diabinese, and Dymelor, are not substitutes for insulin; they stimulate the release of insulin from a "sluggish" pancreas

Generic Name: isoetharine
Brand Name: Bronkosol, Bronkometer
Class: sympathomimetic

Mechanism of Action:
β_2 agonist: relaxes smooth muscle of bronchioles, vasculature, uterus

Indications and Field Use:
Acute bronchial asthma

Bronchospasm

Contraindications:
Use with caution in patients with diabetes, hyperthyroidism, cardiovascular and cerebrovascular disease

Adverse Reactions:
Dose-related tachycardia, palpitations, tremors, nervousness, peripheral vasodilation, nausea, transient hyperglycemia life-threatening arrhythmias; multiple successive doses can cause paradoxical bronchoconstriction

Use with caution in patients with hyperthyroidism, diabetes, cerebrovascular and cardiovascular disorders

NOTES ON ADMINISTRATION
Incompatibilities/Drug Interactions:
Additive adverse effects with other β agonists

Adult Dosage:
1–2 inhalations with metered-dose inhaler

Pediatric Dosage:
Not recommended in children less than 12 years

Routes of Administration:
Nebulized

Metered-dose inhaler

Onset of Action:
Immediate

Peak Effects:
5–15 minutes

Duration of Action:
1–4 hours

Dosage Forms/Packaging:
Metered-dose inhaler

2 ml unit-dose of 1% solution

Special Notes:
Not applicable

(continued)

APPENDIX D.
EMERGENCY DRUGS (continued)

Generic Name: isoproterenol
Brand Name: Isuprel
Class: sympathomimetic

Mechanism of Action:
β agonist, especially β_1—positive inotropy and chronotropy

Bronchodilation

Relaxes GI, vascular, and uterine smooth muscle

Stimulates insulin secretion

Indications and Field Use:
Atropine-refractory bradycardia, including complete heart block

Refractory bronchospasm

Contraindications:
Digitalis toxicity

Adverse Reactions:
Tachycardia

Increased myocardial oxygen consumption (may increase infarct size or cause ventricular arrhythmias)

Tremors, anxiety

Hypertension

NOTES ON ADMINISTRATION

Incompatibilities/Drug Interactions:
Lidocaine

Alkaline solutions

Adult Dosage:
2–10 mcg/minute IV infusion and titrate for effect

Pediatric Dosage:
0.1 mcg/kg/minute

Routes of Administration:
IV infusion

IV boluses are rarely given

Onset of Action:
Immediate

Peak Effects:
Minutes

Duration of Action:
Minutes after infusion is discontinued

Dosage Forms/Packaging:
1 mg/5ml, 5 ml vials

May also be given via nebulization but rarely used by this route in the field

Special Notes:
Serious toxicity may result in patients with acidosis, hypoxia, hyper- or hypokalemia

Carefully monitor the patient for tachycardia and ventricular arrhythmias during isoproterenol infusion

(continued)

APPENDIX D.
EMERGENCY DRUGS (continued)

Generic Name: lidocaine HCl (2%)
Brand Name: Xylocaine
Class: antiarrhythmic

Mechanism of Action:
Decreases automaticity by slowing the rate of spontaneous phase 4 depolarization

Terminates re-entry by decreasing conduction in re-entrant pathways (by slowing conduction in ischemic tissue, equalizes conduction speed among fibers)

Increases ventricular fibrillation threshold

No effect on supraventricular automaticity

Indications and Field Use:
Suppression of ventricular arrhythmias (ventricular tachycardia, ventricular fibrillation, PVC's)

Prophylaxis against ectopy in suspected acute myocardial infarction

Prophylaxis against recurrence after conversion from ventricular tachycardia or ventricular fibrillation

Frequent PVC's (more than 6 per minute, 2 or more PVC's in a row, multiform PVC's, or R-on-T phenomenon)

Contraindications:
Known hypersensitivity/allergy

Use extreme caution in patients with conduction disturbance (second or third degree block)

Do not treat ectopic beats if heart rate is <60—they are probably compensating for the bradycardia; instead, treat the bradycardia!

Adverse Reactions:
CNS depression in large doses: Drowsiness, disorientation, paresthesias, decreased hearing acuity, muscle twitching, agitation, focal or generalized seizures

May also cause SA depression or conduction problems and hypotension in large doses, or if given too rapidly

NOTES ON ADMINISTRATION

Incompatibilities/Drug Interactions:
None known

Adult Dosage:
1 mg/kg IV bolus no faster than 50 mg/minute (may also be given IM, ET) followed by infusion of 1–4 mg/minute if bolus has been successful at terminating the arrhythmia

Pediatric Dosage:
Same as adult (rarely used)
Followed by infusion of 20–50 mcg/kg/minute

Routes of Administration:
IV bolus, followed by IV infusion
May be given ET if IV access is delayed

Onset of Action:
1–5 minutes

Peak Effects:
5–10 minutes

Duration of Action:
Bolus only—20 minutes

(continued)

APPENDIX D.
EMERGENCY DRUGS (continued)

Dosage Forms/Packaging:
100 mg/5 ml prefilled syringe
2 g in 500 ml D$_5$W pre-mixed bags
2 g in 20 ml vials

Special Notes:
Decrease dose by 50% in cases of congestive heart failure, shock, liver disease

Cross-allergenicity between local anesthetic –caine drugs is controversial, but it is advisable to withhold lidocaine from those patients who report allergies to local anesthetics

Generic Name: mannitol 20%
Brand Name: Osmitrol
Class: osmotic diuretic

Mechanism of Action:
Promotes rapid diuresis by increasing osmotic pressure in renal glomeruli–hinders water reabsorption in the renal tubules

Indications and Field Use:
Cerebral edema

Contraindications:
Hypovolemia
Renal failure
Pulmonary edema
Intracranial hemorrhage

Adverse Reactions:
Hypernatremia
Hyperkalemia
Rebound cerebral edema may occur approximately 12 hours after administration

NOTES ON ADMINISTRATION

Incompatibilities/Drug Interactions:
Incompatible with most other drugs
May crystallize in low temperatures

Adult Dosage:
1.5–2 g/kg IV infusion

Pediatric Dosage:
2 g/kg IV infusion

Routes of Administration:
IV infusion over 20–60 minutes, with filter

Onset of Action:
15 minutes

Peak Effects:
1–3 hours

Duration of Action:
3–8 hours

(continued)

APPENDIX D.
EMERGENCY DRUGS (continued)

Dosage Forms/Packaging:
Premixed 500 ml bag of 20% solution (20 g per 100 ml)

Special Notes:
Must be used with filter, due to potential of crystal formation
If possible, catheterize patient when administering mannitol

Generic Name: meperidine
Brand Name: Demerol, Pethadol
Class: narcotic agonist

Mechanism of Action:
Acts on opiate receptors in the sensory cortex of frontal lobes and deincephalon
Interferes with perception of pain

Indications and Field Use:
Moderate to severe pain

Contraindications:
Hypovolemia
Hypersensitivity
Patients taking monoamine oxidase (MAO) inhibitors

Adverse Reactions:
Respiratory depression
Peripheral vasodilation
Nausea/vomiting
Excessive sedation
Agitation
Dizziness
Dysphoria—exaggerated depression or euphoria
Tachy- or bradycardia
Bronchospasm

NOTES ON ADMINISTRATION

Incompatibilities/Drug Interactions:
Heparin
Alkaline solutions

Adult Dosage:
50–150 mg IM every 3–4 hours when required
10–50 mg slow IV push

Pediatric Dosage:
1–1.8 mg/kg every 4 hours to maximum of 100 mg IM

Routes of Administration:
IM or slow IV push

Onset of Action:
Approximately 15–20 minutes IM

Peak Effects:
30–60 minutes

(continued)

APPENDIX D.
EMERGENCY DRUGS (continued)

Duration of Action:
2–4 hours

Dosage Forms/Packaging:
25, 50, 75, or 100 mg vials or prefilled syringe

Special Notes:
Schedule II narcotic
Tolerance may occur with prolonged use

Generic Name: metaproterenol sulfate
Brand Name: Alupent, Metaprel
Class: sympathomimetic

Mechanism of Action:
β_2 agonist—acts directly on bronchial smooth muscle

Indications and Field Use:
Bronchospasm of COPD and asthma

Contraindications:
Diabetes
Hyperthyroidism
Cerebrovascular or cardiovascular disorders

Adverse Reactions:
Dose-related tachycardia
Palpitations
Nervousness
Peripheral vasodilation
With excessive use—lethal arrhythmias, paradoxical bronchospasm

NOTES ON ADMINISTRATION

Incompatibilities/Drug Interactions:
beta blockers
MAO inhibitors, tricyclic antidepressants
Potentiates other β agonists

Adult Dosage:
2.5 ml of an 0.4% or 0.6% unit dose (10 or 15 mg of drug, respectively) in nebulizer over 10–15 minutes

Pediatric Dosage:
Not recommended in children under 12 years

Routes of Administration:
Nebulized
Metered-dose inhaler

Onset of Action:
1 minute

Peak Effects:
1 hour

(continued)

APPENDIX D.
EMERGENCY DRUGS (continued)

Duration of Action:
1–5 hours with single dose; up to 2.5 hours with repeated doses

Dosage Forms/Packaging:
Vial with measuring dropper; used with nebulizer and oxygen metered-dose inhaler

Special Notes:
Use caution when administering epinephrine with metaproterenol sulfate
Antagonist—propranolol

Generic Name: metaraminol bitartrate
Brand Name: Aramine
Class: sympathomimetic

Mechanism of Action:
Direct effects: α and β stimulator, increases chronotropy, inotropy, peripheral vascular resistance
Indirect effects: Causes release of norepinephrine from nerve endings
Results in severe vasoconstriction

Indications and Field Use:
Hypotension not due to hypovolemia
Not a drug of choice in the field

Contraindications:
hypovolemia
Diabetics, hyperthyroid patients on MAO inhibitors or tricyclic antidepressants may be very sensitive to drug's effects

Adverse Reactions:
Severe vascular and peripheral vasoconstriction; decreased blood flow to vital organs
Extravasation leads to local necrosis
Toxicity—apprehension, tremors, weakness, headache, diaphoresis
Greatly increases cardiac workload (and oxygen demand)
May lead to arrhythmias, congestive heart failure, renal failure, metabolic acidosis, cerebral hemorrhage, seizures

NOTES ON ADMINISTRATION
Incompatibilities/Drug Interactions:
Barbiturates
Ringer's lactate
Steroids

Adult Dosage:
0.5–5 mg IV push, then titrated to effect

Pediatric Dosage:
Same as adult

Routes of Administration:
IV infusion

Onset of Action:
Immediate

Peak Effects:
Minutes

(continued)

APPENDIX D.
EMERGENCY DRUGS (continued)

Duration of Action:
Within minutes after discontinued

Dosage Forms/Packaging:
10 mg/ml, 10 ml vial

Special Notes:
Not applicable

Generic Name: methylprednisolone sodium succinate
Brand Name: Solu-Medrol
Class: corticosteroid

Mechanism of Action:
Enters target cells and binds to cytoplasmic receptors, thereby initiating many complex reactions that are responsible for its anti-inflammatory and immunosuppressive effects

Indications and Field Use:
Adjunct in treatment of:
   Hypovolemic shock
   Anaphylaxis
   Esophageal and airway burns
   Cerebral edema
   Septic shock

Contraindications:
None for single dose

Adverse Reactions:
None from single dose; side effects result from long-term, repeated doses

NOTES ON ADMINISTRATION

Incompatibilities/Drug Interactions:
None

Adult Dosage:
15–30 mg/kg, up to 1 g slow IV bolus

Pediatric Dosage:
30–200 mcg/kg slow IV bolus

Routes of Administration:
IV bolus

Onset of Action:
Hours

Peak Effects:
8 hours

Duration of Action:
18–36 hours

Dosage Forms/Packaging:
Mix-a-vials with 40, 125, 500, and 1000 mg or 20 mg/1 ml vials

Special Notes:
Not applicable

(continued)

APPENDIX D.
EMERGENCY DRUGS (continued)

Generic Name: morphine sulfate
Brand Name: None
Class: narcotic agonist

Mechanism of Action:
Alleviates pain by acting on the sensory cortex of frontal lobes and the diencephalon
Depresses fear and anxiety centers
Depresses brainstem respiratory centers—decreases responsiveness to changes in $PaCO_2$; also depresses pons and medulla centers of respiratory rhythmicity
Elevates pain threshold
Increases venous capacitance (venous pooling); and vasodilates arterioles, reducing afterload
Direct stimulus on chemoreceptor trigger zone in the medulla, causing emesis
Suppresses adrenergic tone
Decreases GI motility

Indications and Field Use:
Analgesia, especially in patients with burns, myocardial infarction, or renal colic
Pulmonary edema

Contraindications:
Respiratory depression—use caution in patients with emphysema
Head injuries
Elevated intracranial pressure
Asthma
Use caution in liver or renal disease

Adverse Reactions:
Excess sedation
GI spasm
Vomiting
Brady- or tachycardia
Orthostatic hypotension
Respiratory depression or arrest
Seizures

NOTES ON ADMINISTRATION

Incompatibilities/Drug Interactions:
Heparin, meperidine
Phenothiazines (potentiates sedative effect)

Adult Dosage:
2–20 mg slow IV push; repeat as required; patient response is variable—use lowest effective dose

Pediatric Dosage:
100–200 mcg/kg slow IV push

Routes of Administration:
Usually given IV in the field

Onset of Action:
Immediate

Peak Effects:
20 minutes

(continued)

APPENDIX D.
EMERGENCY DRUGS (continued)

Duration of Action:
2–4 hours

Dosage Forms/Packaging:
10 mg/ml and 15 mg/ml pre-filled syringes or vials

Special Notes:
Schedule II narcotic

Beware of allergies—watch for wheals or urticaria proximal to IV site and discontinue drug if noted

Correct hypotension before administration

Maximum respiratory depression 7–10 minutes after administration; can be reversed with naloxone

Generic Name: nalbuphine HCl
Brand Name: Nubain
Class: narcotic agonist/antagonist

Mechanism of Action:
Synthetic narcotic agonist/antagonist—analgesia occurs due to activation of an opiate receptor in the limbic system of the CNS; also acts as opiate antagonist due to competitive inhibition at receptors

Indications and Field Use:
Moderate to severe pain—has less respiratory depressant effect than opiate-derivatives

Contraindications:
Pulmonary insufficiency
Head injury—elevated intracranial pressure (causes vasodilation)
Narcotic dependence
Myocardial infarction
Renal or hepatic disease

Adverse Reactions:
Sedation
Nausea/vomiting
Dizziness
Agitation, euphoria
Hallucinations
Change in blood pressure and heart rate
Respiratory depression

NOTES ON ADMINISTRATION

Incompatibilities/Drug Interactions:
Diazepam

Adult Dosage:
10–20 mg slow IV push or IM

Pediatric Dosage:
Not recommended

(continued)

APPENDIX D.
EMERGENCY DRUGS (continued)

Routes of Administration:
IV
IM

Onset of Action:
IV: 2–3 minutes
IM: 15 minutes

Peak Effects:
30 minutes

Duration of Action:
3–6 hours

Dosage Forms/Packaging:
10 mg/ml, 1 and 2 ml ampules

Special Notes:
Immediate morphine-like effects without severe respiratory depression
Overdose may be treated with naloxone

Generic Name: naloxone
Brand Name: Narcan
Class: narcotic antagonist

Mechanism of Action:
Competitive inhibition at narcotic receptor sites
Reverses respiratory depression secondary to depressant drugs

Indications and Field Use:
Antidote for:
   Narcotics
   Lomotil
   Talwin
   Darvon
Occasionally given for diazepam overdose
Differentiates drug-induced coma from other causes

Contraindications:
Hypersensitivity

Adverse Reactions:
Withdrawal symptoms, especially in neonates (nausea, vomiting, diaphoresis, increased heart rate, falling blood pressure, tremors)
Be prepared for a combative patient after administration

NOTES ON ADMINISTRATION

Incompatibilities/Drug Interactions:
Should not be mixed with other drugs

Adult Dosage:
0.4–2.0 mg IV, IM, SQ, SL, ET
Titrate to respiratory effort and rate

Pediatric Dosage:
0.01 mg/kg

(continued)

APPENDIX D.
EMERGENCY DRUGS (continued)

Routes of Administration:
IV, ET, IM, SQ, SL

Onset of Action:
IV—within 2 minutes

Peak Effects:
Variable

Duration of Action:
Approximately 45 minutes

Dosage Forms/Packaging:
0.4 mg/ml ampules
2.0 mg/5 ml ampules
2 mg/5 ml prefilled syringe

Generic Name: nifedipine
Brand Name: Procardia
Class: calcium channel blocker

Mechanism of Action:
Arterial and venous vasodilator; both actions reduce cardiac work and oxygen demand (reduced afterload and preload)

Indications and Field Use:
Hypertensive crisis
Congestive heart failure
Angina

Contraindications:
Hypotension
Hypovolemia

Adverse Reactions:
Palpitations
Hypotension
Flushing
Dizziness
Edema (with prolonged use)

NOTES ON ADMINISTRATION
Incompatibilities/Drug Interactions:
Potentiates other calcium channel blockers

Adult Dosage:
10–20 mg sublingual

Pediatric Dosage:
Not used

Routes of Administration:
Sublingual (pierce capsule and squirt under tongue)
As home medication, may be swallowed (sometimes after biting)

(continued)

APPENDIX D.
EMERGENCY DRUGS (continued)

Onset of Action:
Minutes

Peak Effects:
1–3 hours

Duration of Action:
3–4 hours

Dosage Forms/Packaging:
10 mg gelatin capsules

Special Notes:
Not applicable

Generic Name: nitroglycerin
Brand Name: Nitrostat, Tridil
Class: vasodilator

Mechanism of Action:
Smooth muscle relaxant acting on vascular, uterine, bronchial, and intestinal smooth muscle
Exact mechanism of action unknown
Reduces workload on the heart by causing blood pooling (decreased preload) and peripheral vasodilation (decreased afterload)
Coronary artery vasodilation

Indications and Field Use:
Angina
Congestive heart failure

Contraindications:
Hypolvolemia
Increased intracranial pressure
Severe hepatic or renal disease

Adverse Reactions:
Hypotension
Reflex tachycardia
Bradycardia
Decreased coronary perfusion at high doses (secondary to hypotension)
Headache

NOTES ON ADMINISTRATION

Incompatibilities/Drug Interactions:
IV: all other drugs

Adult Dosage:
IV (Tri-dil): 5 mcg/minute; increase in increments of 5 mcg, monitoring pain and blood pressure
Sublingual (Nitro-stat): 1/150 gr (0.4 mg) tablet
Topical: 1 inch of paste
Aerosol: Spray preparation delivers 0.4 mg/metered dose. Spray 1–2 metered doses onto oral mucosa; no more than 3 doses/15 minutes should be used

Pediatric Dosage:
Not used

(continued)

APPENDIX D.
EMERGENCY DRUGS (continued)

Routes of Administration:
IV
SL
Topical/transdermal
Aerosol

Onset of Action:
Immediate

Peak Effects:
5–10 minutes

Duration of Action:
1–10 minutes after IV discontinued

Dosage Forms/Packaging:
IV: 50 mg/10 ml ampules

Special Notes:
SL: Should have IV in place before giving nitroglycerine to a patient who has never received it before
IV: Special nitroglycerine tubing and glass bottle is needed—variable drug delivery in regular IV tubing due to drug absorption into plastic
Closely monitor vital signs, cardiac rhythm

Generic Name: nitrous oxide, N₂0, dinitrous monoxide
Brand Name: None
Class: analgesic gas

Mechanism of Action:
Exact mechanism unknown; affects phospholipids in CNS

Indications and Field Use:
Moderate to severe pain
Surgical or diagnostic procedures such as burn or abrasion debridement, fracture reduction, dental procedures
Childbirth
Renal colic

Contraindications:
Patients who require constant evaluation of their neurologic status, or anyone who can't self-administer the drug
Pneumothorax, perforated viscus, otitis, air embolism, decompression sickness—expands pockets of air and can exacerbate these problems
Nitrogen narcosis

Adverse Reactions:
Administration of greater than 50% nitrogen gas may lead to hypoxia, dyspnea, dizziness, drowsiness
No effect on pupils, respiratory drive, or gag reflex
Minimal cardiovascular effects

NOTES ON ADMINISTRATION
Incompatibilities/Drug Interactions:
None

(continued)

APPENDIX D.
EMERGENCY DRUGS (continued)

Adult Dosage:
Less than 30 minutes/episode, mixed with oxygen (at least 50% oxygen is required to prevent hypoxia)

Pediatric Dosage:
Same

Routes of Administration:
Self-administered with mask held over face
Absorbed by pulmonary circulation and excreted unchanged by lungs

Onset of Action:
2–6 minutes

Peak Effects:
Variable

Duration of Action:
2–5 minutes after discontinued

Dosage Forms/Packaging:
Blue tanks with blenders and mask with demand valve
Scavenger system needed to prevent exhalation into environment (not generally available prehospital

Special Notes:
Not flammable or combustible
Ineffective for 20% of population

Generic Name: norepinephrine
Brand Name: Levophed, Levarterenol
Class: sympathomimetic

Mechanism of Action:
Potent α agonist (90% α, 10% β_1 effects), causing intense vasoconstriction
Positive chronotropic action (can be overcome by vagal response to increasing arterial pressure)
Increased inotropism (from β_1 effects) and increased cardiac output, if bradycardia is not present

Indications and Field Use:
Second-line pressor for cardiogenic shock, other forms of shock with low or normal peripheral vascular resistance (for example, spinal shock)

Contraindications:
Pregnancy (relative contraindication)

Adverse Reactions:
Increases myocardial oxygen consumption—ventricular arrhythmias may be increased
Decreased blood flow to kidneys, gut, skeletal muscle, and skin can lead to renal shutdown, necrotic bowel, necrotic limbs
Hypertension
Reflex bradycardia
Cerebral hemorrhage
Severe tissue necrosis in infiltration

(continued)

APPENDIX D.
EMERGENCY DRUGS (continued)

NOTES ON ADMINISTRATION

Incompatibilities/Drug Interactions:
Alkaline solutions, barbiturates, aminophylline, phenytoin

Prior use of MAO inhibitors or cocaine may increase reaction to catecholamines

Adult Dosage:
2–4 mcg/minute, up to 20 ug/minute IV infusion and titrate to desired blood pressure (usually 80–100 systolic)

Mix in D_5W, not 0.9% NaCl

Pediatric Dosage:
0.1 mcg/kg/minute IV infusion

Routes of Administration:
IV infusion

Onset of Action:
Immediate

Peak Effects:
Not available

Duration of Action:
Lasts only approximately 1 minute after infusion discontinued

Dosage Forms/Packaging:
1 mg/ml / 4 ml ampule

Special Notes:
Best administered via through-the-needle catheter or central line

Local necrosis may be partially counteracted by transdermal injection of phentolamine (Regitine), an α blocker

May be used in conjunction with other pressors, especially low-dose dopamine, to spare renal and mesenteric blood flow

Generic Name: Oxygen
Brand Name: None
Class: gas

Mechanism of Action:
Required for normal physiological processes of all cells

Indications and Field Use:
Any suspected hypoxic state

Cardiac or pulmonary complaints

Anesthesia

Shock

CNS injuries

Decreased level of consciousness

Sickle cell crisis

Cardiac arrest

Contraindications:
Emphysema—deliver less than 35% oxygen unless severely hypoxic

Hyperventilation

(continued)

APPENDIX D.
EMERGENCY DRUGS (continued)

Adverse Reactions:
Respiratory arrest in patients with hypoxic drive
Drying of respiratory mucosa
Possible bronchospasm if oxygen is extremely cold and dry

NOTES ON ADMINISTRATION

Incompatibilities/Drug Interactions:
None

Adult Dosage:
24%–100% based on patient status

Pediatric Dosage:
24%–100% based on patient status

Routes of Administration:
Be familiar with appropriate liter flow and amount of oxygen delivered with each type of delivery device

Onset of Action:
Immediate

Peak Effects:
Not applicable

Duration of Action:
20 minutes

Dosage Forms/Packaging:
Green cylinders labeled "Oxygen" with pin-index safety system

Special Notes:
Patient needs an airway and needs to be breathing before oxygen is effective!
Humidify if possible to prevent drying of mucosa and subsequent respiratory infections
Supports combustion

Generic Name: oxytocin
Brand Name: Pitocin, Syntocin
Class: pituitary hormone

Mechanism of Action:
Increases amplitude and frequency of uterine contractions
Dilation of vascular smooth muscle (increases renal, coronary, and cerebral blood flow)

Indications and Field Use:
Postpartum hemorrhage
Used in-hospital for induction of labor

Contraindications:
Hypersensitivity
Unfavorable fetal position

Adverse Reactions:
Shock
Tachycardia
Arrhythmias

(continued)

APPENDIX D.
EMERGENCY DRUGS (continued)

Anaphylaxis

Clotting disorders

Electrolyte disturbances

If used prior to delivery, can cause uterine rupture, uterine spasm, lacerations, and fetal damage

NOTES ON ADMINISTRATION

Incompatibilities/Drug Interactions:
Norepinephrine

Heparin

Adult Dosage:
10–20 USP units/liter at rate of 1–4 ml/minute

Pediatric Dosage:
Not applicable

Routes of Administration:
IV

Onset of Action:
Immediate

Peak Effects:
Variable

Duration of Action:
1 hour after discontinued

Dosage Forms/Packaging:
1 ml ampule

10 USP units (20 mg)/ml

Special Notes:
Must be diluted in: normal saline, lactated Ringer's or D_5W

Generic Name: phenobarbital sodium
Brand Name: Luminal Sodium
Class: anticonvulsant

Mechanism of Action:
Not well understood—cerebral depression by interference with transmission of impulses at the cerebral cortex

Also interferes with the reticular activating system

Indications and Field Use:
Seizures

Status epilepticus

Contraindications:
Respiratory depression

Severe pain (paradoxical excitement may occur)

Pregnancy, pneumonia, pulmonary insufficiency, hypersensitivity

Use with caution in the elderly—confusion or excitement may occur

(continued)

APPENDIX D.
EMERGENCY DRUGS (continued)

Adverse Reactions:
Asthma, bronchospasm
Hypotension
Respiratory depression
Pulmonary edema
Renal failure
Confusion, coma
May cause paradoxical CNS stimulation in children
Decreased GI motility
Decreased tissue oxygen consumption
Euphoria if inhibitory centers depressed

NOTES ON ADMINISTRATION
Incompatibilities/Drug Interactions:
Incompatible with all other drugs—flush line before and after use

Adult Dosage:
200–600 mg slow IV bolus at 25–50 mg/minute

Pediatric Dosage:
10–20 mg/kg slow IV push over 5–10 minutes

Routes of Administration:
Slow IV push

Onset of Action:
5 minutes

Peak Effects:
30 minutes

Duration of Action:
4–6 hours (single dose)

Dosage Forms/Packaging:
130 mg/ml vial or prefilled syringe

Special Notes:
Support respirations if diazepam is used concurrently
Monitor vital signs frequently
Use caution in patients with liver damage
Diluent is propylene glycol (cardiotoxic)

Generic Name: **phenytoin sodium**
Brand Name: **Dilantin**
Class: **hydantoin anticonvulsant**

Mechanism of Action:
Inhibits cerebral seizure focus from spreading into adjacent areas
Depresses pacemaker automaticity
Improves AV conduction by decreasing AV node refractory period, especially in digitalis toxicity
Negative inotropy

(continued)

APPENDIX D.
EMERGENCY DRUGS (continued)

Indications and Field Use:
Prophylaxis and treatment of recurrent seizures, in conjunction with more rapid-acting drugs such as diazepam

Not a first-line cardiac drug, except rarely in cases of digitalis toxicity

Ventricular arrhythmias

Contraindications:
Bradycardia

AV block

CHF

Adverse Reactions:
With rapid administration:
 hypotension, cardiovascular collapse, CNS depression, diplopia, nystagmus, lethargy, ataxia, nausea, vomiting

NOTES ON ADMINISTRATION

Incompatibilities/Drug Interactions:
All drugs and solutions

Give only in 0.9% NaCl

Adult Dosage:
16–18 mg/kg (700–1000 mg) slow IV push at 25–50 mg/minutes or less; flush with saline

Pediatric Dosage:
Same as adult

Routes of Administration:
Slow IV push

Onset of Action:
2–30 minutes

Peak Effects:
1–3 hours

Duration of Action:
18–24 hours

Dosage Forms/Packaging:
50 mg/ml, 5 ml ampule

100 mg prefilled syringe

Special Notes:
Diluent is propylene glycol (cardiotoxic)

Use cardiac monitor when administering—discontinue administration if widening QRS complex is noted

May be taken orally

Generic Name: physostigmine salicylate
Brand Name: Antilirium
Class: acetylcholinesterase inhibitor

Mechanism of Action:
Acetylcholinesterase inhibitor—increases concentration of acetylcholine at receptor sites by preventing its breakdown (parasympathetic stimulator)

(continued)

APPENDIX D.
EMERGENCY DRUGS (continued)

Indications and Field Use:
Reverses atropine-like drugs (for example, street drugs, jimsonweed)

May inhibit CNS depressant effects of Valium, tricyclic antidepressants, antihistamines, phenothiazines

Contraindications:
Asthma
Diabetes
Benign prostatic hypertrophy
Cardiovascular disease

Adverse Reactions:
Seizures (with rapid administration)
Excessive salivation
Emesis
Urination
Lacrimation
Bradycardia

NOTES ON ADMINISTRATION

Incompatibilities/Drug Interactions:
None

Adult Dosage:
1–4 mg slow IV push over 1–2 minutes (no faster than 1 mg/minute)
May repeat a 1–2 mg dose in 20 minutes if needed

Pediatric Dosage:
0.5 mg over 1 minute
May be repeated every 5–10 minutes to maximum of 2 mg

Routes of Administration:
Slow IV push

Onset of Action:
Minutes

Peak Effects:
5 minutes

Duration of Action:
30 minutes–5 hours

Dosage Forms/Packaging:
2 mg/2 ml ampules

Special Notes:
Monitor EKG while administering the drug
Antidote: atropine

(continued)

APPENDIX D.
EMERGENCY DRUGS (continued)

Generic Name: potassium chloride (KCl)
Brand Name:
Class: electrolyte

Mechanism of Action:
Essential for normal cell function and impulse formation/conduction
Also essential for acid–base balance and carbohydrate metabolism

Indications and Field Use:
Not used in the field
Patient may be taking oral KCl; may also be used in the hospital setting for treatment/prophylaxis of hypokalemia (serum potassium levels lower than 3.6 mEq/L)

Contraindications:
Hyperkalemia

Adverse Reactions:
Too-rapid administration can cause immediate cardiac arrest that is refractory to treatment
Very irritating to veins—patient may complain of unbearable burning
Hyperkalemia may result (watch for peaked T-waves, depressed S–T segments, flattened P-waves, wide QRS complex)

NOTES ON ADMINISTRATION
Incompatibilities/Drug Interactions:
Mannitol, valium, dilantin, penicillin, other antibiotics

Adult Dosage:
10–20 mEq KCl in at least 50 ml IV fluid; may also be mixed into maintenance IV fluid
Give no faster than 10 mEq/hour (20–40 mEq/hour if potassium level under 2 mEq/L)

Pediatric Dosage:
Rarely given

Routes of Administration:
IV infusion; NEVER GIVE IV BOLUS

Onset of Action:
Immediate

Peak Effects:
Not applicable

Duration of Action:
Not applicable

Dosage Forms/Packaging:
2 mEq/ml; vials of 10 and 20 ml

Special Notes:
Patients taking furosemide or digitalis preparations are usually on potassium supplements
Arrhythmias may result from hypokalemia, especially in the patient taking digitalis

(continued)

APPENDIX D.
EMERGENCY DRUGS (continued)

Generic Name: procainamide
Brand Name: Pronestyl
Class: antiarrhythmic

Mechanism of Action:
Decreases automaticity by suppressing phase 4 depolarization, especially in the His–Purkinje system
Slows conduction velocity by depressing the rate of rise of phase 0
Prolongs effective refractory period and action potential duration in the His–Purkinje system
Shortens effective refractory period of AV node
Some anticholinergic properties that may affect SA and AV nodes to increase heart rate

Indications and Field Use:
Ventricular tachycardia
May also be used to treat PVC's, supraventricular tachycardia, atrial fibrillation with rapid ventricular response

Contraindications:
Any degree of heart block
Myasthenia gravis (a condition of muscle fatigability, caused either by lack of acetylcholine or increase of cholinesterase at the neuromuscular junction)
Known hypersensitivity (history of allergy to local anesthetics)

Adverse Reactions:
Potentiates the effects of skeletal muscle relaxants and neuromuscular blockers
Vasodilation and hypotension with rapid administration, with resulting reflex tachycardia
Complete heart block
Idioventricular rhythm
PVC's and ventricular tachycardia

NOTES ON ADMINISTRATION

Incompatibilities/Drug Interactions:
Phenytoin
Theophylline
Barbiturates
Sodium bicarbonate
Magnesium sulfate

Adult Dosage:
100 mg every 5 minutes (or 20 mg/minute) until ectopy is suppressed, to a maximum of 1 g
If successful, follow with infusion of 1–4 mg/minute

Pediatric Dosage:
Not given

Routes of Administration:
Slow IV push

Onset of Action:
1–4 minutes

Peak Effects:
5–10 minutes

Duration of Action:
Approximately 3.5 hours

(continued)

APPENDIX D.
EMERGENCY DRUGS (continued)

Dosage Forms/Packaging:
100 mg/ml, 10 ml vial

Special Notes:
Use caution in patients with renal failure
Stop infusion if the following are noted:
  50% widening of QRS complex
  Prolonged P–R interval
  Decrease in blood pressure over 15 mm Hg

Generic Name: propranolol
Brand Name: Inderal
Class: beta blocker

Mechanism of Action:
Blocks β receptor sites, causing the following:
  Decreased heart rate, cardiac output, contractility, and conduction
  Decreased myocardial oxygen consumption
Stabilizes myocardial cell membrane

Indications and Field Use:
Rarely used in the field
May be used for:
  Paroxysmal supraventricular tachycardia
  β agonist or digitalis-induced ventricular arrhythmias
  Hyperthyroid crisis

Contraindications:
Bradycardia
Heart blocks
Decreased cardiac output

Adverse Reactions:
Severe bradycardia
Bronchospasm
Congestive heart failure
Cardiogenic shock

NOTES ON ADMINISTRATION

Incompatibilities/Drug Interactions:
Any alkaline solution
Potentiates hypotensive actions of beta blockers, calcium channel blockers

Adult Dosage:
0.5–3.0 mg slow IVP; may repeat in 2 minutes; give smallest effective dose
Patients may also be taking Inderal orally for hypertension, history of tachycardias, or as an adjunct to rehabilitation postmyocardial infarction

Pediatric Dosage:
10–20 mcg/kg IV over 10 minutes

Routes of Administration:
Slow IV push, not to exceed 1 mg/minute

(continued)

APPENDIX D.
EMERGENCY DRUGS (continued)

Onset of Action:
Immediate

Peak Effects:
Within minutes

Duration of Action:
2–3 hours

Dosage Forms/Packaging:
1 mg/ml, 1 ml ampule

Special Notes:
Inderal is also used to prevent migraines, and may be used to minimize tremors in competitive sharpshooters

Generic Name: quinidine gluconate
Brand Name: Quinaglute, Quinidex
Class: antiarrhythmic

Mechanism of Action:

Decreases conduction velocity

Decreases AV node refractory period (improves AV conduction)

Decreases automaticity in His–Purkinje system by prolonging effective refractory period (phase 4) and action potential duration (phase 2) in His–Purkinje system, atria, and ventricular muscle
Negative inotropy
α-adrenergic blocker, which contributes to hypotension and reflex tachycardia

Strong vagal blocking properties

Indications and Field Use:
Rarely used in the field
May be taken orally by patients for:
    Atrial fibrillation or atrial flutter
    Paroxysmal supraventricular tachycardia
    Premature atrial and ventricular complexes

Contraindications:
Digitalis toxicity

AV block

Myasthenia gravis

Concurrent use of skeletal muscle relaxants or neuromuscular blockers

Sick sinus syndrome

Adverse Reactions:
One third of patients on quinidine have immediate adverse reactions:
   Nausea/vomiting, headache, confusion, tinnitus, visual disturbances, diarrhea, blood disorders, hepatotoxicity, paradoxical tachycardia

NOTES ON ADMINISTRATION
Incompatibilities/Drug Interactions:
Cholinergic drugs

Diazepam, warfarin, heparin

Anticonvulsants

Phenothiazines (depress myocardium)

(continued)

APPENDIX D.
EMERGENCY DRUGS (continued)

Similar antiarrhythmics (lidocaine)

Nitroglycerine and quinidine use may result in hypotension

Increases digitalis concentration in blood

Adult Dosage:
324 mg every 8–12 hours orally

Pediatric Dosage:
Not given

Routes of Administration:
Oral–may be given IV but rarely used in the field

Onset of Action:
Within one-half hour

Peak Effects:
1.5 hour

Duration of Action:
Approximately 6 hours

Dosage Forms/Packaging:
Sustained-acting tablets

Special Notes:
Not given in liver failure

Generic Name: racemic epinephrine
Brand Name: Vaponefrin
Class: sympathomimetic

Mechanism of Action:
α and β agonist: arteriole constriction; positive inotropic, positive chronotropic; bronchial smooth muscle relaxer (bronchodilator)

Also blocks histamine release, inhibits insulin secretion (can lead to hyperglycemia), relaxes GI smooth muscle

Indications and Field Use:
Croup

Post extubation edema

Laryngeal angioneurotic edema

Bronchospasm (as a second-line drug)

Contraindications:
Hypersensitivity

Adverse Reactions:
Palpitations

Anxiety

Headache

Hypertension

Nausea/vomiting

Arrhythmias

Rebound edema 15–30 minutes postadministration

(continued)

APPENDIX D.
EMERGENCY DRUGS (continued)

NOTES ON ADMINISTRATION

Incompatibilities/Drug Interactions:
Should not be mixed with other drugs

Adult Dosage:
0.5–0.8 ml in 4 ml normal saline by nebulizer over 10–15 minutes

Pediatric Dosage:
0.3–0.5 ml in 4 ml normal saline by updraft nebulizer over 10–15 minutes

Routes of Administration:
Nebulized

Onset of Action:
1 minute

Peak Effects:
3–5 minutes

Duration of Action:
15–30 minutes

Dosage Forms/Packaging:
7.5 ml, 15 ml, 30 ml

Special Notes:
Not applicable

Generic Name: sodium bicarbonate
Brand Name: None
Class: buffer

Mechanism of Action:
Buffers H^+ in metabolic acidosis, lactic acid is the major source of H^+ in metabolic acidosis in cardiac arrest

Indications and Field Use:
Cardiac arrest

Overdose of aspirin, tricyclic antidepressants

With available blood gas results used in acidosis secondary to shock or other causes

Contraindications:
Alkalosis

Adverse Reactions:
Carbon dioxide formation my exacerbate venous acidemia and tissue acidosis in cardiac arrest

Hyperosmolarity

Metabolic alkalosis

Congestive heart failure, edema secondary to sodium overload, hypernatremia

Excessive sodium bicarbonate can displace the oxyhemoglobin dissociation curve and decrease the oxygen released at the tissue level

NOTES ON ADMINISTRATION

Incompatibilities/Drug Interactions:
Incompatible with all other drugs

(continued)

APPENDIX D.
EMERGENCY DRUGS (continued)

Adult Dosage:
1 mEq/kg IV bolus
First dose usually 1 mEq/kg, with subsequent doses of 0.5 mEq/kg every 10 minutes in cardiac arrest; generally used in cardiac arrest after other standard treatment (defibrillation, intubation, epinephrine injection) has been used

Pediatric Dosage:
Same as adult; used less liberally in children—can actually contribute to acidosis and cause fluid overload

Routes of Administration:
IV bolus

Onset of Action:
Immediate

Peak Effects:
1–2 minutes

Duration of Action:
10 minutes

Dosage Forms/Packaging:
10 mEq/50 ml prefilled syringes
25 mEq/25 ml prefilled syringes (pediatric size)

Special Notes:
Flush tubing before and after administration

Generic Name: sodium nitroprusside
Brand Name: Nipride
Class: vasodilator

Mechanism of Action:
Potent vasodilator—direct action on smooth muscle of arterioles and veins

Indications and Field Use:
Not used in the field; may be used in-hospital for hypertensive crisis, and for reduction of cardiac afterload

Contraindications:
Hypotension
Inadequate cerebral circulation
Hypovolemia

Adverse Reactions:
Severe hypotension, reflex tachycardia
Cyanide toxicity—degrades to thiocyanate (high doses in renal failure may lead to cyanide toxicity; high doses are considered to be: administration for longer than 2 days; doses over 8 mcg/kg/minute); half-life of thiocyanate is 7 days; symptoms—metabolic acidosis, delirium, headache, vomiting, blurred vision, hypotension, dyspnea, tinnitus, coma

NOTES ON ADMINISTRATION
Incompatibilities/Drug Interactions:
All other drugs
Must be given in D_5W

(continued)

APPENDIX D.
EMERGENCY DRUGS (continued)

Adult Dosage:
0.5 mcg/kg/minute IV infusion to start; titrate to desired blood pressure

Pediatric Dosage:
Same as adult

Routes of Administration:
IV infusion

Onset of Action:
Immediate

Peak Effects:
1 minute

Duration of Action:
Within minutes after discontinued

Dosage Forms/Packaging:
50 mg powder vial

Special Notes:
Solution may hang no longer than 24 hours

Must be protected from light—wrap bag and tubing with foil provided in packaging

Often used with pressors to maintain blood pressure while decreasing preload and afterload

Generic Name: **Streptokinase, r-TPA (tissue plasminogen activator)**
Brand Name: **Kabikinase; Activase**
Class: **thrombolytic**

Mechanism of Action:
Promotes dissolution of thrombi by disrupting clotting mechanisms

Streptokinase acts systemically to break up clots by converting plasminogen to the enzyme plasmin; r-TPA acts specifically on the clot itself, affecting only plasminogen bound to fibrin

Indications and Field Use:
Not currently used in the field except in trials

Used in-hospital (and during transport) for myocardial infarction—with EKG evidence; and within 6 hours of onset of symptoms

Contraindications:
Allergy

Current anticoagulant therapy (heparin)

Active bleeding

History of stroke

Recent head or CNS trauma or surgery

Intracranial tumor or aneurysm

Uncontrolled hypertension

Adverse Reactions:
Bleeding problems

Allergy

Fever

Arrhythmias—PVC's, ventricular tachycardia when reperfusion occurs

(continued)

APPENDIX D.
EMERGENCY DRUGS (continued)

NOTES ON ADMINISTRATION

Incompatibilities/Drug Interactions:
Heparin
Vitamin K
Aspirin
Not mixed in same line with any other drug

Adult Dosage:
Streptokinase: 250,000 u over 30 minutes, followed by infusion of 100,000 u per hour (often administered intracoronary during cardiac catheterization).
r-TPA: 60 mg over first hour, 20 mg over second hour, and 20 mg over the third hour

Pediatric Dosage:
Not used

Routes of Administration:
IV

Onset of Action:
Within minutes

Peak Effects:
Not applicable

Duration of Action:
25 minutes to several hours

Dosage Forms/Packaging:
Streptokinase: 100,000 u, 250,000 u, 600,000 u, and 750,000 u vials r-TPA: 50 mg vials

Special Notes:
May give prophylactic lidocaine to control reperfusion arrhythmias
Often followed up with heparin to reduce chances of clot recurrence
If therapy is begun within 4 hrs of onset of symptoms, reperfusion successful in approximately 70% of patients
Patients receiving thrombolytic therapy must be monitored with serial laboratory studies and EKGs

Generic Name: succinylcholine chloride
Brand Name: Anectine
Class: depolarizing blocker

Mechanism of Action:
β_2 agonist—has an affinity for β_2 receptors of bronchial, vascular, and uterine smooth muscle
At increased doses, β_1 effects may occur

Indications and Field Use:
Bronchospasm (more prevalent in patients over the age of 40 or with coronary artery disease)
Used in-hospital to stop preterm labor

Contraindications:
Use with caution in patients on other sypathomimetics

Adverse Reactions:
Tachycardia, tremors, palpitations, nervousness, dizziness—usually dose-related
Tachycardia may persist due to β_1 stimulus or to peripheral vasodilation

(continued)

APPENDIX D.
EMERGENCY DRUGS (continued)

Cardiovascular collapse
Malignant hyperthermia
Hypotension
Bradycardia

NOTES ON ADMINISTRATION

Incompatibilities/Drug Interactions:

Adult Dosage:
1 mg/kg IV

Pediatric Dosage:
1 mg/kg IV

Routes of Administration:
Slow IV push

Onset of Action:
1 minute

Peak Effects:
2 minutes

Duration of Action:
8 minutes

Dosage Forms/Packaging:
10 ml vials containing 20 mg/ml

Special Notes:
No decrease in level of consciousness, pain, tearing, cardiac rhythm, vision, or blood pressure

Blocked with neostigmine

Brief period of excitation (fasciculations), followed by neuromuscular block

Used in combination with other drugs such as Tracrium, Pavulon to provide optimal paralysis, with atropine to prevent bradycardia, and with sedatives (so that the patient is not awake and aware while paralyzed)

Generic Name: syrup of ipecac
Brand Name: None
Class: emetic

Mechanism of Action:
Acts on brain stem and gastric mucosa to produce vomiting

Indications and Field Use:
Oral poisoning and overdose

Contraindications:
Decreased level of consciousness
Ingestion of caustic or petroleum-based substances
Stroke
Heart disease
Seizures

Adverse Reactions:
Myocardial irritant in excessive dosages

(continued)

APPENDIX D.
EMERGENCY DRUGS (continued)

NOTES ON ADMINISTRATION
Incompatibilities/Drug Interactions:
None

Adult Dosage:
12 years or older: 30 ml (6 teaspoons or 2 tablespoons) with 8–16 ounces of clear fluid
Repeat once if there is no emesis within 30 minutes

Pediatric Dosage:
Less than 6 months: do not give
6 months–1 year: 10 ml (2 teaspoons) with 2–4 ounces of clear fluid
1 year–5 years: 15 ml (3 teaspoons or 1–2 tablespoons) with 4–8 ounces of clear fluid
5 years–12 years: 15–30 ml (3–6 teaspoons or 1–2 tablespoons) with 8–16 ounces of clear fluid
Repeat once if there is no emesis within 30 minutes
Note: 5 ml = 1 teaspoon, 15 ml = 1 tablespoon, 1 tablespoon = 3 teaspoons

Routes of Administration:
Oral

Onset of Action:
15–30 minutes

Peak Effects:
Not applicable

Duration of Action:
25 minutes to several hours

Dosage Forms/Packaging:
30 ml bottles

Special Notes:
In lesser concentrations, may be found as an ingredient in pediatric cough syrups
More effective if patient ambulates
May see overdose of ipecac in anorexic/bulimic patients
Effective in 90% of patients with first dose and 98% with second dose

---

Generic Name: terbutaline sulfate
Brand Name: Bricanyl, Brethine
Class: sympathomimetic

Mechanism of Action:
β_2 agonist—has an affinity for β_2 receptors of bronchial, vascular, and uterine smooth muscle
At increased doses, β_1 effects may occur

Indications and Field Use:
Bronchospasm (more prevalent in patients over the age of 40 or with coronary artery disease)
Used in-hospital to stop preterm labor

Contraindications:
Use with caution in patients on other sypathomimetics

Adverse Reactions:
Tachycardia, tremors, palpitations, nervousness, dizziness—usually dose-related
Tachycardia may persist due to β_1 stimulus or to peripheral vasodilation

(continued)

APPENDIX D.
EMERGENCY DRUGS (continued)

NOTES ON ADMINISTRATION

Incompatibilities/Drug Interactions:
Alkaline solutions
Degrades when exposed to light for long periods of time

Adult Dosage:
0.25 mg SQ; repeat in 15–20 minutes
2 inhalations separated by a 60-second interval with a metered dose inhaler

Pediatric Dosage:
Not recommended for patients under the age of 12 years

Routes of Administration:
SQ

Onset of Action:
15 minutes

Peak Effects:
30–60 minutes

Duration of Action:
90 minutes–4 hours

Dosage Forms/Packaging:
1 mg/ml, 1 ml, 2 ml ampules

Special Notes:
Use caution in patients with cardiac disease, arrhythmias, hypertension, diabetes, and hyperthyroidism
Also available in oral tablets and syrup for at-home use

Generic Name: theophylline ethylenediamine
Brand Name: Aminophylline
Class: methylxanthine

Mechanism of Action:
β_2 agonist: Directly relaxes bronchial smooth muscle
Dilates pulmonary and coronary arterioles, decreasing pulmonary hypertension and increasing coronary blood flow
Increases inotropy and chronotropy in higher doses
Strengthens diaphragmatic contractions by affecting intracellular calcium
Stimulates CNS vomiting centers
Diuretic: Increases renal blood flow and decreases renal tubule sodium reabsorption
Stimulates CNS respiratory centers
Stimulates vagal and vasomotor centers in the brain—can lead to decreased HR, vasoconstriction in the brain—depends on CNS or peripheral predominance

Indications and Field Use:
Asthma or bronchospasm
Bronchospasm secondary to asthma, COPD, or anaphylaxis
Pulmonary edema

(continued)

APPENDIX D.
EMERGENCY DRUGS (continued)

Contraindications:
Use caution if patient is already taking theophylline-containing medications, or has a history of cardiac arrhythmias

Reduced dosage may be given in patients with heart failure, liver disease, hypotension, or suspected myocardial infarction

Adverse Reactions:
Vomiting
Cardiac arrhythmias
Hypotension
Tremors
Irritability
Seizures

NOTES ON ADMINISTRATION

Incompatibilities/Drug Interactions:
Incompatible with most drugs

Adult Dosage:
Loading dose of 6 mg/kg IV infusion diluted in 100 ml D_5W or normal saline over 20 minutes if patient has had no theophylline products in the last 36 hours

Loading dose of 1 mg/kg IV infusion diluted in 100 ml D_5W or normal saline over 20 minutes if patient has had theophylline products in the last 36 hours

Pediatric Dosage:
Over 1 year, same loading dose; in $D_5 0.9\%NaCl$

Routes of Administration:
IV infusion—loading dose may be followed with maintenance dose
Several forms of oral theophylline are also available

Onset of Action:
15 minutes

Peak Effects:
30 minutes–1 hour

Duration of Action:
Averages 5 hours

Dosage Forms/Packaging:
25 mg/ml, 10 ml ampules

Special Notes:
Patient must be on cardiac monitor when receiving IV theophylline

Smoking shortens duration of action

Patients with liver failure may become toxic

Common forms of oral aminophylline include: Marax, Primatene, Quibron, Slo-Phyllin, Slobid, Somophyllin, Tedral, Theo-Dur

(continued)

APPENDIX D.
EMERGENCY DRUGS (continued)

Generic Name: thiamine (vitamin B)
Brand Name: Betalin
Class: vitamin

Mechanism of Action:
Required for carbohydrate metabolism

Deficiency leads to anemia, polyneuritis, Wernicke's encephalopathy, cardiomyopathy

Administration may reverse symptoms of deficiency, but effects are dependent upon duration of illness and severity of disease

Indications and Field Use:
Alcoholism, delirium tremens
Other thiamine deficiency syndromes

Contraindications:
Known hypersensitivity
Usually nontoxic even in high doses

Adverse Reactions:
Rare

NOTES ON ADMINISTRATION

Incompatibilities/Drug Interactions:
Alkaline solutions, barbiturates, bicarbonate, cephalosporins, other antibiotics

Adult Dosage:
100 mg

Pediatric Dosage:
Rarely used

Routes of Administration:
IM
IV over several minutes

Onset of Action:
Hours

Peak Effects:
3–5 days

Duration of Action:
Unavailable

Dosage Forms/Packaging:
100 mg/ml; 1 ml ampule

Special Notes:
Not applicable

Generic Name: verapamil HCl
Brand Name: Isoptin, Calan, Verelan
Class: calcium channel blocker

Mechanism of Action:
Blocks calcium influx into cardiac and smooth muscle cells, causing a depressant effect on the contractile mechanism and resulting in negative inotropy

(continued)

APPENDIX D.
EMERGENCY DRUGS (continued)

Reduces contractile tone in vascular smooth muscle resulting in coronary and peripheral vasodilation

Slows conduction and prolongs refractory period in the AV node due to calcium channel blocking

Slows SA node discharge

In summary, decreases myocardial contractile force, and slows AV conduction

Indications and Field Use:
Supraventricular tachycardia

Atrial fibrillation and atrial flutter with rapid ventricular response

Contraindications:
Wolff–Parkinson–White syndrome with atrial fibrillation or flutter (check to see if patient knows he/she has a history of this syndrome; in-hospital records may reveal delta waves and a short PR interval on a previous EKG)

Shock

AV block

Sick sinus syndrome

Severe CHF

Any wide QRS complex tachycardia without certainty of supraventricular origin

Adverse Reactions:
Extreme bradycardia

AV block

Hypotension

Congestive heart failure

Dizziness

Headache

Nausea

Abdominal discomfort

NOTES ON ADMINISTRATION

Incompatibilities/Drug Interactions:
Caffeine

Theophylline

beta-blockers

Adult Dosage:
0.075–0.15 mg/kg (5–10 mg) IV over 2–3 minutes (maximum of 10–15 mg)

Pediatric Dosage:
0.1–0.3 mg/kg over 2–3 minutes

Maximum 5 mg

Routes of Administration:
IV slow push

Onset of Action:
1–10 minutes

Peak Effects:
3–5 minutes

Duration of Action:
2–5 hours

(continued)

APPENDIX D.
EMERGENCY DRUGS (continued)

Dosage Forms/Packaging:
2–5 mg/ml, 2 ml ampule

Special Notes:

May be used in conjunction with cardioversion

Vagal maneuvers may be tried first (carotid massage, Valsalva maneuver, diving reflex)

Monitor closely for hypotension and AV block during administration

Hypotension may be treated with fluids and supine position

May be taken orally; other oral calcium channel blockers include nifedipine (Procardia) and diltiazem (Cardizem), which patients may be taking for angina

APPENDIX E.
COMMON HOME MEDICATIONS

A key component of the medical history is a patient's *past* medical history. Sometimes the paramedic is confronted with unconscious patients or those who are unable to communicate much useful information about themselves. In the process of trying to clarify the patient's problem, a variety of prescription medications is often detected. Some basic knowledge of different prescription medications and why a patient may be taking them can often provide considerable insight into the patient's history.

The following is an overview of drugs categorized by body system followed by a listing of drugs currently used for therapy. The drug listing is not intended to be all-inclusive, as new drugs are constantly being introduced.

NERVOUS SYSTEM

Analgesics
Prescribed to lessen pain; considered for use only after some attempt has been made to identify and treat the problem causing the pain. These are generally categorized as narcotic and non-narcotic analgesics.

Narcotic	Non-Narcotic
butalbital (Fiorinal)	acetaminophen (Tylenol, Datril)
hydrocodone (Vicodin)	aspirin (Bayer, Anacin, Bufferin)
hydromorphine (Dilaudid)	butorphanol (Stadol)
meperidine (Demerol)	ibuprofen (Motrin, Advil, Nuprin, Medipren)
oxycodone (Percodan/Percocet, Tylox)	nalbuphine (Nubain)
pentazocine (Talwin)	naproxen (Anaprox)
propoxyphene (Darvocet, Darvon, Wygesic)	
acetaminophen (Tylenol with codeine)	

Antidepressants
Prescribed to treat depression and frequently encountered in the field. Depressed patients may be suicidal and take intentional overdoses of their medications. Physicians usually attempt to limit the problem by not allowing refills or by prescribing limited amounts. There are two common types of antidepressants: "tricyclics" and "monoamine oxidase (MAO) inhibitors." Tricyclics prevent the reuptake of norepinephrine at synapse sites and overdose often results in severe cardiac arrhythmias, seizures, and profound hypotension. MAO inhibitors interfere with transmission at synapse sites and inhibit the breakdown of norepinephrine and, in some circumstances, in cardiac arrhythmias.

Tricyclics	MAO Inhibitors
amoxapine (Asendin)	isocarboxazid (Marplan)
amitriptyline (Elavil, Endep)	phenelzine (Nardil)
desipramine (Norpramin)	tranylcypromine (Parnate)
doxepin (Sinequan, Adapin)	
imipramine (Tofranil)	
maprotiline (Ludiomil)	
nortriptyline (Pamelor)	
protriptyline (Vivactil)	
trimipramine (Surmontil)	

Anticonvulsants
Prescribed to raise the seizure threshold in patients; may limit some fine motor coordination. The drug prescribed depends on the nature of the seizure and patient suitability.

carbamazepine (Tegretol)

(continued)

APPENDIX E.
COMMON HOME MEDICATIONS (continued)

diazepam (Valium)
mephenytoin (Mesantoin)
mephobarbital (Mebaral)
paramethadione (Paradione)
phenobarbital (Donnatal, Antrocol)
phenytoin (Dilantin)

Antipsychotics
A group of drugs prescribed to treat schizophrenia and other types of psychosis. They are also sometimes called "major tranquilizers." The drug lithium is a "mood stabilizing agent" and is used primarily to treat manic-depressive conditions. Many of these drugs are phenothiazine derivatives; they may cause extrapyramidal reactions, which may be treated with diphenhydramine.

Antipsychotics	Mood Stabilizers
chlorpromazine (Thorazine)	Lithium derivatives:
fluphenazine (Permitil, Prolixin)	Cibalith
haloperidol (Haldol)	Eskalith
prochlorperazine (Compazine)	Lithobid
promazine (Sparine)	
thioridazine (Mellaril)	
thiothixene (Navane)	
trifluoperazine (Stelazine)	

Sedative/Hypnotics
These drugs sedate, relieve anxiety, and may cause central nervous system (CNS) and respiratory depression. Hypnotics induce sleep and drowsiness. They are used to treat anxiety and insomnia, and are sometimes used in the management of seizure disorders. Most are potentiated when combined with alcohol and may result in respiratory depression or arrest.

alprazolam (Xanax)
aprobarbital (Alurate)
butabarbital (Butisol)
clorazepate (Tranxene)
chlordiazepoxide (Librium)
diazepam (Valium)
flurazepam (Dalmane)
hydroxyzine (Atarax, Vistaril)
lorazepam (Ativan)
oxazepam (Serax)
pentobarbital (Nembutal)
phenobarbital (Donnatal, Antrocol)
prazepam (Centrax)
secobarbital
temazepam (Restoril)
triazolam (Halcion)

CARDIOVASCULAR SYSTEM
Antiarrhythmics
Commonly used to treat patients with chronic arrhythmias, atrial or ventricular. Therapy is instituted for rhythms that cause poor cardiac output or might predispose the patient to a more lethal arrhythmia. Some of the medications have more than one intended use and may be prescribed for

(continued)

APPENDIX E.
COMMON HOME MEDICATIONS (continued)

other conditions as well as for arrhythmias. Inderal, for example, is a "beta blocker" and is used for hypertension and angina.

digoxin (Lanoxin)
disopyramide (Norpace)
phenytoin (Dilantin)
procainamide (Procan, Pronestyl)
propranolol (Inderal)
quinidine (Quinaglute, Quinidex)
verapamil (Calan, Isoptin, Verelan)

Antianginal Agents

Prescribed to treat the pain of angina pectoris. Some are "short-acting" drugs taken for pain during an episode of chest pain; but most listed here are for long-term management of coronary artery disease. The "nitrates" act to relax smooth muscle and dilate blood vessels in the myocardium and peripheral blood vessels, thus relieving the cardiac workload. Calcium channel blockers relax smooth muscle to some degree, but also decrease myocardial contractility. The beta blockers help minimize the inotropic and chronotropic effects of catecholamines on the heart.

Nitrates

erythrityl (Cardilate)
isosorbide (Isordil, Dilatrate, Sorbitrate)
nitroglycerine (Nitro-Bid, Nitrodisc, Nitro-Dur, Nitrol, Nitrostat)
pentaerythritol (Peritrate)

Calcium Blockers

diltiazem (Cardizem)
nifedipine (Procardia)
verapamil (Calan, Isoptin, Verelan)

Beta Blockers

atenolol (Tenormin)
metoprolol (Lopressor)
nadolol (Corgard)
pindolol (Visken)
propranolol (Inderal)
timolol (Blocadren)

Cardiac Glycosides

Prescribed for patients who have congestive heart failure or chronic atrial arrhythmias requiring control. Their basic actions are increasing myocardial contractility to improve cardiac output, and causing an increased conduction delay at the AV node. Digitalis can also cause severe arrhythmias when toxic levels are reached, which is fairly common because therapeutic blood levels are relatively close to toxic levels. Many elderly congestive heart failure (CHF) patients are prescribed digitalis products in addition to diuretics to control their condition. Diuretic therapy is apt to cause hypokalemia, which greatly contributes to toxicity; therefore, most patients taking this combination are also prescribed potassium supplements.

deslanoside (Cedilanid)
digitoxin (Crystodigin)
digoxin (Lanoxin)

Antihypertensives

Chronic hypertension damages blood vessels in the heart, kidney, and brain. Accordingly, it can be a precursor to renal failure, stroke, and coronary artery disease. Lowering blood pressure has been shown to reduce mortality from cardiovascular events such as cerebrovascular accidents. The drugs used in treatment often affect the cardiac output or vascular resistance in some manner. Many patients are on two drugs affecting different aspects of regulation because homeostatic mechanisms may overcome the effects of one individual drug and maintain the hypertensive state.

(continued)

APPENDIX E.
COMMON HOME MEDICATIONS (continued)

Alpha Agents
clonidine (Catapres)
guanabenz (Wytensin)
methyldopa (Aldomet)

Beta Blockers
atenolol (Tenormin)
metoprolol (Lopressor)
nadolol (Corgard)
pindolol (Visken)
propranolol (Inderal)
timolol (Blocadren)

Vasodilators
hydralazine (Apresoline)
minoxidil (Loniten)
prazosin (Minipress)

Antihypertensives with Diuretics
chlorthalidone and clonidine (Combipres)
chlorthalidone and reserpine (Regroton)
chlorothiazide and reserpine (Diupres)
chlorothiazide and methyldopa (Aldoclor)
hydrochlorothiazide and guanethidine (Esimil)
hydrochlorothiazide and hydralazine (Apresazide)
hydrochlorothiazide and hydralazine and reserpine (Ser-Ap-Es)
hydrochlorothiazide and methyldopa (Aldoril)
hydrochlorothiazide and reserpine (Hydropres)
hydroflumethiazide and reserpine (Salutensin)
methyclothiazide and cryptenamine (Diutensen)
methyclothiazide and deserpidine (Enduronyl)
propranolol and hydrochlorothiazide (Inderide)
polythiazide and prazosin (Minizide)
timolol and hydrochlorothiazide (Timolide)

RESPIRATORY SYSTEM
Bronchodilators
Prescribed to patients with asthma or chronic obstructive pulmonary disease (COPD) to relieve bronchospasm and dilate the bronchioles, thus improving air flow and oxygenation. Patients with mild asthma may require only inhaled β-selective bronchodilators, PRN. If they have more frequent attacks, theophylline preparations are usually prescribed on a regular basis with inhaled bronchodilators, PRN.

Inhaled Bronchodilators
albuterol (Proventil, Ventolin)
cromolyn sodium (Intal)
isoproterenol (Isuprel)
isoetharine (Bronkometer, Bronkosol)
metaproterenol (Metaprel, Alupent)

Systemic Bronchodilators
albuterol (Ventolin, Proventil)
metaproterenol (Metaprel, Alupent)
terbutaline (Berthine, Bricanyl)

Inhaled Glucocorticoids
beclomethasone (Beclovent, Vanceril)

Theophylline Products
Bronkodyl
Choledyl
Elixophyllin
Lufyllin
Marax

(continued)

APPENDIX E.
COMMON HOME MEDICATIONS (continued)

Quadrinal
Quibron
Slo-Bid
Slo-Phyllin
Somophyllin
Theo-Dur
Theolair

MUSCULOSKELETAL

Anti-inflammatory Agents

Inflammation is the body's mechanism for protection against invading organisms. It is also the cause of some disorders such as arthritis, which results in limited joint function and the destruction of bone and cartilage within the joints. The medications listed suppress the signs and symptoms of inflammation and provide some analgesic effects.

aspirin (acetylsalicylic acid)

fenoprofen (Nalfon)

ibuprofen (Motrin, Advil, Nuprin)

indomethacin (Indocin)

meclofenamate (Meclomen)

mefenamic acid (Ponstel)

naproxen (Naprosyn, Anaprox)

piroxicam (Feldene)

sulindac (Clinoril)

tolmetin (Tolectin)

Muscle Relaxants

Prescribed to patients who have muscle spasm often associated with stroke, multiple sclerosis, or cerebral palsy. Another application is to patients with painful musculoskeletal conditions such as low back pain and sports injuries.

baclofen (Lioresal)

carisoprodol (Soma)

chlorphenesin carbamate (Maolate)

chlorzoxazone (Paraflex)

chlorzoxazone + acetaminophen (Parafon Forte)

cyclobenzaprine (Flexeril)

dantrolene (Dantrium)

diazepam (Valium)

methocarbamol (Robaxin)

orphenadrine citrate (Norflex)

orphenadrine + aspirin + caffeine (Norgesic)

quinine sulfate (Quinamm)

URINARY TRACT

Diuretics

Widely used to treat a variety of conditions that include hypertension, heart failure, liver and renal disease, pulmonary edema, elevated intracranial pressure, and some ophthalmic conditions. Most diuretics prevent the reabsorption of sodium by the kidneys and subsequently cause the loss of water. They also cause the loss of potassium, resulting in hypokalemia, so many patients may be on some sort of potassium supplement. Hypokalemia causes serious arrhythmias in patients that can lead to sudden death.

(continued)

APPENDIX E.
COMMON HOME MEDICATIONS (continued)

Thiazide + Loop Diuretics
chlorothiazide (Diuril)
chlorthalidone (Hygroton)
furosemide (Lasix)
hydrochlorothiazide (Esidrix, Hydrodiuril)
methyclothiazide (Enduron)
metolazone (Zaroxolyn, Diulo)

Potassium Sparing Diuretics
amiloride (Moduretic, Midamor)
spironolactone (Aldactone)
spironolactone + hydrochlorothiazide (Aldactazide)
triamterene (Dyrenium)
triamterene + hydrochlorothiazide (Dyazide)

Urinary Tract Anti-infectives/Analgesics/Antispasmodics
Anti-infective drugs are used to treat urinary tract infections. The others listed have analgesic or antispasmodic actions targeted to the urinary tract.

Anti-infectives
carbenicillin (Geocillin)
cinoxacin (Cinobac)
methenamine (Hiprex)
methenamine mandelate (Mandelamine)
nalidixic acid (NegGram)
nitrofurantoin (Furadantin, Macrodantin)
sulfamethoxazole + phenazopyridine (Azo Gantanol)
sulfasalazine (Azulfidine)
sulfisoxazole (Gantrisin)
trimethoprim (Trimpex, Proloprim)
trimethoprim + sulfamethoxazole (Bactrim, Septra)

Analgesics
flavoxate (Urispas)
L-hyoscyamine (Cystospaz)
oxybutynin (Ditropan)

Antispasmodics
phenazopyridine (Pyridium)

GASTROINTESTINAL TRACT DRUGS
Antacids/Adsorbents
Antacids are used to treat hyperacidity and peptic ulcers. They reduce the acid load in the gastrointestinal (GI) tract and elevate pH. Often patients on salt-restricted diets don't realize their antacids contain sodium chloride (salt). Sometimes this causes water retention and exacerbates their heart failure or hypertension. Adsorbents inhibit the GI absorption of some, but not all, harmful substances. Activated charcoal does not adsorb cyanide, ethanol, methanol, iron, sodium chloride, alkalies, mineral acids, and organic solvents.

Antacids
aluminum hydroxide (AlternaGel, Dialume, Amphojel)
aluminum hydroxide + magnesium trisilicate (Gaviscon)
aluminum hydroxide + magnesium hydroxide (Kolantyl, Maalox)
aluminum hydroxide + magnesium hydroxide + calcium carbonate (Camalox)
aluminum hydroxide + magnesium hydroxide + simethicone (Mylanta)
magaldrate (Riopan)
calcium carbonate (Titralac)
simethicone + aluminum hydroxide + magnesium hydroxide (Mylanta, Gelusil, Simeco)

Adsorbents
activated charcoal

(continued)

APPENDIX E.
COMMON HOME MEDICATIONS (continued)

Antidiarrheals
Given to increase the viscosity of stool, often by decreasing gut motility. Most are designed to treat acute, mild, or chronic cases of diarrhea.

diphenoxylate (Lomotil)

kaolin + pectin (Kaopectate)

Kaolin + pectin + atropine + hyoscine + hyoscyamine + alcohol (Donnagel)

lactobacillus acidophilus (Bacid)

loperamide (Imodium)

tincture of opium (Paregoric)

Laxatives
Used to alleviate or prevent constipation by a variety of different mechanisms.

bisacodyl (Dulcolax)

castor oil

docusate + casanthranol (Peri-Colace)

docusate calcium (Surfak)

docusate sodium (Colace)

glycerine suppositories

Milk of Magnesia

mineral oil

phenolphthalein (Modane)

psyllium (Metamucil)

senna (Senokot)

Antiemetics
Prescribed to prevent or stop nausea and vomiting. Some are also employed to prevent motion sickness. Often chemotherapy patients are prescribed antiemetics to minimize the side effects of cancer chemotherapy. They also act as sedatives and tend to make patients drowsy. A number of them are phenothiazines and cause extrapyramidal reactions when overdoses are taken. Scopolamine is now being used by the transdermal route. Some are also given as suppositories.

benzquinamide (Emete-con)

cyclizine 2 (Marezine)

dimenhydrinate (Dramamine)

diphenhydramine (Benadryl)

meclizine (Antivert, Bonine)

metoclopramide (Reglan)

prochlorperazine (Compazine)

promethazine (Phenergan)

scopolamine (Transderm-Scop)

trimethobenzamide (Tigan)

thiethylperazine (Torecan)

GI Anticholinergics/Antiulcer Agents
Block vagal stimulation to the GI tract, reduce the secretion of gastric juices, and enhance the action of antacids. They are given to patients with peptic ulcers, irritable or spastic colons, and other GI disturbances.

(continued)

APPENDIX E.
COMMON HOME MEDICATIONS (continued)

Anticholinergics
anisotropine methylbromide (Valpin 50)
atropine
clidinium (Quarzan)
dicyclomine (Bentyl)
hyoscyamine (Levsin)
isopropamide (Darbid)
mepenzolate (Cantil)
methantheline (Banthine)

Antiulcer
cimetidine (Tagamet)
sucralfate (Carafate)
ranitidine (Zantac)

ENDOCRINE SYSTEM
Hypoglycemic Agents
Diabetics whose homeostasis cannot be controlled by diet alone are prescribed either oral agents or insulin by injection. Oral agents stimulate the pancreas to secrete insulin and are used in patients with pancreatic function. Patients using injectable insulin do not secrete insulin from their pancreas. Insulin is essential to permit glucose transport across cell membranes.

Insulins
Humulin
Lente Iletin
Novolin
NPH Iletin
Protamine, Zinc + Iletin
Regular Iletin
Semilente
Ultralente

Oral Hypoglycemics
chlorpropamide (Diabinese)
acetohexamide (Dymelor)
tolbutamide (Orinase)
tolazamide (Tolinase)
glyburide (DiaBeta)

Hormones
These are complex agents manufactured by endocrine glands to control growth, sexual development, metabolism, and electrolyte balance. When deficiencies occur, they are treated with natural or synthetic hormones discussed below.

Androgens: Stimulate growth of male accessory sexual organs and promote the development of secondary sex characteristics such as face and body hair, deep voice, and skeletal muscle. Testosterone is the primary androgen in humans.

danazol (Danocrine)
fluoxymesterone (Halotestin)
testosterone cypionate (Depo-Testosterone)

Estrogens: Promote growth and development of the vagina, uterus, and fallopian tubes. They also enlarge the breasts and mold body contours and produce changes in the genital tract and mammary glands during pregnancy. Given to treat symptoms in menopausal women.

chlorotrianisene (Tace)
estradiol (Estrace)
estrogenic substances (Premarin)
estropipate (Ogen)
quinestrol (Estrovis)

Progestogens: Promote endometrial swelling to facilitate the implantation of the fertilized ovum. During pregnancy they prevent uterine contractions and allow the pregnancy to continue to full term.

norethindrone (Norlutin)
norethindrone acetate (Norlutate)
medroxyprogesterone (Provera)

(continued)

APPENDIX E.
COMMON HOME MEDICATIONS (continued)

Thyroid Hormones: Stimulate the rate of metabolism of body tissues by accelerating the rate of cellular oxidation and enhancing carbohydrate and protein synthesis. They are actually prescribed to patients with diminished or absent thyroid function.

Armour Thyroid

levothyroxine (L_4) (Synthroid, Levothroid)

liothyronine (L_3) (Cytomel)

liotrix (Thyrolar, Euthroid)

thyroglobulin (Proloid)

Oral Contraceptives: A popular and effective form of hormonal birth control. Oral contraceptives predispose women to complications due to increased risk of thrombosis.

Brevicon

Demulen

Loestrin

Modicon

Lo/Ovral

Nordette

Norinyl

Norlestrin

Ortho-Novum

Ovcon

Steroids

Used to treat inflammation, allergic reactions, collagen disorders, and adrenocortical insufficiency. Patients on steroid therapy are more susceptible to infections and sometimes have minor GI bleeding. Steroidal actions are complex and their effect on inflammation is not well understood; however, they play a role in suppressing immune response and stabilizing white blood cell (WBC) lysosome membranes.

beclomethasone (Beclovent)

betamethasone (Celestone)

dexamethasone (Decadron, Hexadrol)

hydrocortisone (Solu-Cortef)

methylprednisolone (Solu-Medrol)

prednisone

triamcinolone acetonide (Aristocort, Kenalog)

THE EYES

Ophthalmic Agents

There are a variety of drugs used to treat infections and inflammation and to anesthetise the eye. Each will be listed separately.

Anti-infectives: Used to treat bacterial, viral, or fungal infections of the cornea or conjunctiva.

chloramphenicol (Chloromycetin)

erythromycin (Ilotycin)

gentamycin (Garamycin)

polymyxin + bacitracin (Polysporin)

sulfacetamide (Sulamyd)

sulfisoxazole (Gantrisin)

tobramycin (Tobrex)

vidarabine (Vira-A)

(continued)

APPENDIX E.
COMMON HOME MEDICATIONS (continued)

Anti-inflammatory Agents: Steroids used to treat inflammatory disorders of the eyelids, conjunctiva, cornea, and anterior globe. They are also used to treat corneal injury from burns.

dexamethasone (Decadron-Ophthalmic)

hydrocortisone (Hydrocortone)

Miotics: Used to constrict the pupil for patients with glaucoma; also used for eye surgery.

demecarium (Humorosol)

Mydriatics: Used to dilate the pupil in patients with glaucoma and for diagnostic purposes to examine the retina and optic disc.

epinephrine (Epifrin, Epitrate)

epinephryl (Epinal)

naphazoline (Naphcon)

SKIN AND MUCOUS MEMBRANES

Local Anti-infectives

Widely used to treat local bacterial and fungal infections that are responsive to local treatment. They come in the form of creams, ointments, and lotions.

bacitracin

gramicidin + neomycin (Mycolog)

neomycin + polymyxin B + hydrocortisone (Cortisporin)

polymyxin + bacitracin (Polysporin)

polymyxin + neomycin + bacitracin (Mycitracin)

tetracycline (Terramycin)

Scabicides/Pediculicides

Used to eradicate infestations of head and body lice; also used on crab lice.

crotamiton (Eurax)

lindane (Kwell, Scabene)

pyrethrins (Rid)

Topical Corticosteroids

Used to reduce local inflammation, constrict blood vessels, and relieve itching. They are used to treat psoriasis, eczemas, dermatitis, and other skin disorders.

amcinonide (Cyclocort)

betamethasone dipropionate (Celestone)

betamethasone valerate (Valisone)

desonide (Tridesilon)

desoximetasone (Topicort)

dexamethasone (Decadron)

diflorasone (Florone)

hydrocortisone (Cortaid, Diprosone)

Antipruritics/Topical Anesthetics

Used to relieve discomfort caused by minor burns, cuts, rashes, and insect bites.

Aerocaine

benzocaine (Dermoplast, Solarcaine)

dibucaine (Nupercainal)

lidocaine

tetracaine (Pontocaine)

(continued)

APPENDIX E.
COMMON HOME MEDICATIONS (continued)

Antiseptics/Disinfectants
Antiseptics inhibit the growth of micro-organisms and disinfectants destroy them. Antiseptics are usually used on living tissue and disinfectants are used on inanimate objects. Povidone-iodine is an antiseptic that may be used on the skin and is excellent to prepare the skin prior to IV therapy or surgical procedures.

Disinfectants	Antiseptics
alcohol	benzalkonium chloride (Mercurochrome II, Bactine)
iodine	chlorhexidine gluconate (Hibiclens, Roma-Nol)
hexachlorophene (pHisoHex)	povidone-iodine (betadine)

ANTIHISTAMINES
Act to block the effects of histamine, which causes most of the symptoms associated with allergic reactions. They are commonly used in "over the counter" medications used to treat common cold symptoms. They are also used in the treatment of local and systemic allergic reactions. They tend to cause drowsiness and are also used as sedatives. Some are also used to prevent motion sickness. Most drug interactions with antihistamines are not serious, but if used in combination with alcohol, anticonvulsants, or CNS depressants, the patient may have severe drowsiness and impaired judgment.

brompheniramine maleate (Dimetane)
brompheniramine maleate + phenylpropanolamine (Dimetapp)
carbinoxamine maleate + pseudoephedrine hydrochloride (Rondec)
chlorpheniramine maleate (Chlor-Trimeton)
phenylpropanolamine + chlorpheniramine maleate (Allerest, Novahistine, Ornade)
phenylpropanolamine pheniramine maleate + pyrilamine maleate (Triaminic)
promethazine (Phenergan)
pseudoephedrine + triprolidine (Actifed)

ANTIBIOTICS/ANTI-INFECTIVES
Aminoglycosides
"Broad spectrum" antibiotics used against both gram positive and gram negative bacteria. Because of the risk of serious kidney and inner ear damage their use is usually limited to gram negative infections that are resistant to less toxic agents.

amikacin (Amikin)
gentamycin (Garamycin)
kanamycin (Kantrex)
neomycin (Mycitracin)
tobramycin (Nebcin)

Penicillins
Penicillins have been a popular type of antibiotic for 50 years. They are highly effective against gram positive organisms and will work on some types of gram negative organisms. They are not effective against viruses, yeast, fungi, rickettsiae, or mycobacteria infections. The drug erythromycin (E-mycin, Erye, EES, Ilotycin) is often prescribed instead to individuals with penicillin allergy.

amoxicillin (Amoxil)
ampicillin
carbenicillin (Geocillin)

(continued)

APPENDIX E.
COMMON HOME MEDICATIONS (continued)

cyclacillin (Cyclapen-W)

penicillin G benzathine (Bicillin)

penicillin V potassium (Pen-Vee-K, V-Cillin K)

Cephalosporins

Antibiotics that are structurally related to penicillins are "broad spectrum" antibiotics, and are effective against both gram positive and gram negative organisms. They may also be used in many patients who are allergic to penicillin.

cefaclor (Ceclor)

cefadroxil (Duricef, Ultracef)

cefamandole (Mandol)

cefazolin (Ancef, Kefzol)

cefoperazone (Cefobid)

cefotaxime (Claforan)

cefoxitin (Mefoxin)

ceftriaxone (Rocephin)

cefuroxime (Zinacef)

cephalexin (Keflex)

cephalothin (Seffin)

cephradine (Anspor, Velocef)

Tetracyclines

Used in the prevention and treatment of bacterial diseases. They are the drug of choice in the treatment of the bubonic plague, brucellosis, cholera, and Rocky Mountain Spotted Fever. They are often prescribed to COPD patients to prevent respiratory infections.

demeclocycline (Declomycin)

doxycycline (Vibramycin)

minocycline (Minocin)

oxytetracycline (Terramycin)

tetracycline (Achromycin, Sumycin)

Sulfonamides

Sulfas were the first drugs to be used systemically in the treatment of human bacterial infections. Increased resistance has reduced their usefulness over the years but they are still the drugs of choice for urinary tract infections, otitis media, conjunctivitis, and toxoplasmosis.

trimethoprim + sulfamethoxazole (Bactrim)

sulfamethoxazole (Gantanol)

sulfisoxazole (Gantrisin)

Glossary

abandonment: The paramedic's unilateral termination of the relationship with the patient when care and treatment are still needed so that, as a result of the lack of provision for continued care, the patient is injured

abduction: Movement away from the midline of the body

abortion: Termination of pregnancy before the fetus is viable

abrasion: A scratching of the skin surface without penetration of all layers of the skin

abruptio placenta: Premature separation of the placenta from its uterine attachment

absorption: Manner by which substances can enter the body through the skin

abstinence syndrome: Syndrome that results when a habitual drug user cannot get another dose or elects to stop the drug use

accelerated idioventricular rhythm: Cardiac arrhythmia that results from ventricular pacemaker sites that discharge faster than the inherent ventricular rate; fusion beats are common, and, as the ventricular rate is usually 40 to 100, the ventricles often compete with the SA node for control of the heart

accelerated junctional rhythm: Cardiac arrhythmia that results from increased automaticity of the AV junction, which causes it to discharge faster than its inherent rate and override the SA node; atria commonly are controlled independently by the SA node

acceleration: Change in velocity

acceptance: The final stage of the grieving process in which one disengages or disassociates and accepts the inevitable without fear or despair

accessory muscles: The groups of muscles innervated by the spinal accessory nerve that play a role in respiratory distress

acetylcholine: Parasympathetic chemical mediator; when released, heart rate and conduction are slowed

acid: A chemical compound that gives up or donates a hydrogen [H+] ion

acquired immunodeficiency syndrome (AIDS): Infection with the human immunodeficiency virus, which affects the immune system and can produce opportunistic infections and malignancies

activated charcoal: Substance used to prevent the absorption of an ingested drug or chemical in the small intestine

active transport: The crossing of electrolytes against the diffusion gradient or osmotic gradient (i.e., against pressure)

acute abdomen: Abdominal disorder that develops quickly and is severe in nature

acute arterial occlusion: Sudden blockage of arterial flow in an extremity or the abdomen as a result of trauma, clot formation, or an embolus

acute stress reaction: Reaction that occurs after an individual's exposure to any situation that has a powerful emotional impact

adduction: Movement toward the midline of the body

adenohypophysis: The anterior lobe of the pituitary gland

administrative law: Civil law that pertains to the government's authority to enforce rules, regulations, and pertinent statutes of governmental agencies

adolescence: Teen-age years

adrenal cortex: The outer portion of the adrenal gland that secretes mineralocorticoids and glucocorticoids

adrenal glands: Small, pyramidal-shaped organs located retroperitoneally in close association with the upper part of each kidney; the overall job of the adrenal glands is an adaptive one, in which homeostasis is maintained despite day-to-day stresses

adrenal medulla: Part of the adrenal gland, it secretes as its primary hormones the catecholamines epinephrine and norepinephrine; although not important in the fine regulation of body functions, it serves an important homeostatic function in the face of stress

adrenocorticotropin (ACTH): Hormone secreted by the anterior pituitary gland that modulates function of the adrenal cortex

Adult Glasgow Coma Scale: Scale that evaluates level of consciousness, assigning numeric values to the categories of eyes opening, motor response, and verbal response

Adult Trauma Score: Score that places a numerical value on the assessment of the patient in the categories of respiratory rate, respiratory expansion, systolic blood pressure, and capillary refill

adventitia: The tough outermost layer of fibrous tissue that covers an organ, structure, or blood vessel

aerobic: In the presence of oxygen

aeromedical transport: Air transportation of ill or injured people to special care facilities, either by airplane or helicopter

afferent neuron: Sensory neuron

agonist: Drug that causes a direct change in cellular function when inserted into a receptor

airborne transmission: The transfer of infection from one individual to another through droplets of moisture that contain the infectious agent

air embolism: The obstruction of a blood vessel by an air bubble

air trapping: The increase in the volume of air that remains in the lungs at the end of a maximum expiration

alcoholism: Addiction to alcohol; the most common prehospital toxicologic problem and the largest drug abuse problem in the United States

alkali: The class of compounds that form soluble soaps with fatty acids, turn red litmus blue, and form soluble carbonates

allergic reaction: An oversensitive and harmful response against foreign substances that may actually be harmless

allergy: An abnormal and individual hypersensitivity to substances that are ordinarily harmless

α-adrenergic receptor: One of two types of receptors in the sympathetic division of the autonomic nervous system; stimulation causes vasoconstriction

α particles: One of three principal types of ionizing radiation emitted by radioactive sources

alveolar–capillary interface: System that facilitates gas exchange between the lungs and the circulatory system

alveolar ventilation (V_A): Volume of air, about 350 mL, that comes into contact with the alveolar–capillary interface

alveoli: Delicate, thin-walled chambers within the lungs where the exchange of oxygen and carbon dioxide between the air and blood takes place

Alzheimer's disease: Progressive and degenerative disease process of the brain that affects memory and mental capacity

amnesia: Memory deficit

amniotic fluid: Fluid that the fetus drinks and excretes

amniotic sac: Sac in which the fetus develops

ampule: Breakable glass container from which medication is drawn up with a syringe

amputation: The removal of a limb or any appendage of the body (see *complete, degloving,* and partial amputation

anaerobic: In the absence of oxygen

anaphylactic reaction: An acute generalized allergic reaction that has systemic signs and symptoms that are exaggerated from a simple allergic reaction

anaphylaxis: An acute generalized allergic reaction that occurs after exposure to a foreign substance to which the body is overly sensitive

anastomoses: Communication or interconnection between two vessels

androgen: Chemical substance (i.e., testosterone) that is required for masculinization

anger: The second stage of the grieving process that can be projected toward anything or anyone

angina, angina pectoris: Chest pain that is the result of coronary artery spasm or occlusion

anion: Negatively charged ion

antagonist: Substance that occupies a receptor site but causes no physiologic response

antegrade amnesia: Inability to remember events after a traumatic injury (see retrograde amnesia)

anterior: Front surface of the body

anterior chamber: Space filled with aqueous humor that lies between the cornea and the iris in the eye

antibody: Protective protein substance formed in the body as a result of contact with an antigen

antidiuretic hormone (ADH): Hormone secreted by the posterior pituitary that acts primarily in the kidney, where it stimulates increased water reabsorption (also called vasopressin)

antigen: Foreign substance that induces the formation of antibodies

antipsychotic: A drug that lessens the symptoms of a severe mental illness (psychosis)

anuria: Cessation of urine output

Apgar score: Index for determining a newborn's physiologic status

apnea: Cessation of breathing

apothecary system: A system of units and weights used chiefly in compounding and dispensing drugs

appendicitis: Inflammation of the vermiform appendix

appendicular skeleton: 126 bones that form the appendages to the axial skeleton: the shoulder girdles, arms, wrists, hands, and the hip girdles, legs, ankles, and feet

appendix: Hollow narrow tube with a closed end, located at the lower end of the colon where it joins with the ileum, projecting downward into the right lower quadrant; it has no known digestive function but is susceptible to inflammation, which may result in appendicitis

aqueous humor: Watery fluid that fills the anterior chamber of the eye

aqueous solution: Drug or combination of drugs dissolved in water

aqueous suspension: Preparation of finely divided solid drugs added to sterile distilled water

arachnoid: Delicate membrane that lies between the dura and pia mater; the second of the three meninges that protect the brain

arousability: Condition described according to the patient's response to various types of verbal or painful stimuli

arousal: Awakening from deep sleep

arrhythmia: Abnormal heart rhythm

arterioles: The smallest arteries; they usually lead into capillaries

arteriosclerosis: Primary etiology of coronary artery disease; a chronic disease of arteries that involves thickening and hardening of vessel walls, resulting in a loss of elasticity

articular cartilage: Thin layer of cartilage that covers the joint or articular surfaces of the epiphyses and acts as a cushion

articulation: Joint

artificial cardiac pacemaker: Implantable device used to electronically stimulate the heart in place of the heart's natural pacemaker or conduction system

aspiration: Ingestion or emesis of foreign bodies into the respiratory tract; also applied to the withdrawing of fluid from a body cavity by means of suction

assault: Situation in which a patient has a reasonable apprehension of immediate bodily harm without giving consent, such as with a threat of restraints or a hypodermic injection

asthma: Sudden, periodic dyspnea usually accompanied with wheezing and caused by swollen mucous membranes or bronchial tube spasms

asystole: Absence of electrical activity of the heart

atelectasis: Collapse of the alveoli

atherosclerosis: Localized deposits of lipid material within the intimal surface of blood vessels

atherosclerotic heart disease: Heart disease caused by atherosclerosis

atria: The two superior chambers of the heart; the right atrium receives deoxygenated blood from the body, the left atrium, oxygenated blood from the lungs

atrial fibrillation: Rapid, erratic electrical discharge from multiple atrial foci or from multiple reentry circuits within the atria, generating 350 to 600 impulses per minute

atrial flutter: Cardiac arrhythmia in which the atrial impulses occur at a rate of 250 to 350 per minute; since the AV node cannot physiologically conduct impulses at this rapid a rate, it conducts impulses to the ventricles at a 1:1, 3:1, 4:1, or greater ratio

atrioventricular (AV) block: Condition in which the passage of electrical impulses from the atrium to the AV junction is delayed or interrupted

atrioventricular (AV) node: Part of the AV junctional tissue, which includes some surrounding tissue plus the connected bundle of His; it slows conduction, creating a slight delay before electrical impulses are carried to the ventricles

attitude: The degree of flexion of the fetus when it is delivered

auricle: The skin-covered cartilaginous framework that projects from the head and is part of the outer ear

auscultation: Process of listening, especially with a stethoscope, to the lungs and abdomen to assess respiratory and gastrointestinal status; the second phase of a physical examination

automaticity: Ability to generate an electrical impulse independent of outside stimulation; a property of select myocardial cells called pacemaker cells

autonomic nervous system: The system that plays an essential role in maintaining homeostatic levels; it has sympathetic and parasympathetic divisions

AVPU system: An acronym for responsiveness that represents (A) awake and alert, (V) responds to voice, (P) responds only to pain, and (U) unresponsive or unconscious

avulsion: The tearing loose of a flap of skin, which may either remain hanging or tear off altogether

avulsion fracture: A twisting motion causes part of the bone to be pulled away by a ligament or tendon

axial skeleton: The 80 bones that form the upright axis of the body—the head, the neck, and the thorax—and the tiny middle ear bones

axon: Process of a neuron that carries the impulse away from the cell body

bactericidals: Organisms that engulf and kill bacteria that enter through the nose

bag-valve-mask device: Hand-held external device used to assist or control ventilation; it can deliver 100% oxygen

bargaining: The third stage of the grieving process in which the patient enters into some type of agreement in an attempt to postpone the inevitable

barotrauma: Pressure-related injury

Bartholin's glands: Glands located on either side of the vaginal opening that secrete an alkaline lubricant that supports sperm survival

base: A chemical compound that accepts or receives a hydrogen [H^+] ion

base station: A fixed location that contains a transmitter and a receiver

basilar skull fracture: Fracture that results from the extension of linear fractures onto the floor of the skull

battery: Touching a patient without consent

Battle's sign: Discoloration behind the ears

β_1-adrenergic receptor: One of two types of receptors in the sympathetic division of the autonomic nervous system; stimulation causes an increase in the heart's contractility and force, rate and automaticity, and conduction of impulses

β_2-adrenergic receptor: One of two types of receptors in the sympathetic division of the autonomic nervous system; stimulation results in bronchodilation

β particles: One of three principle types of ionizing radiation emitted by radioactive sources

blast: An explosive force

blood: Thick fluid that lies within the intravascular space

blood–brain barrier: Physiologic barrier that prevents many drugs from leaving the blood and crossing the cerebrospinal fluid into the brain

blood pressure: Measurement that provides information about the patient's blood volume, heart, peripheral vascular integrity, and arterial elasticity

blunt trauma: Type of impact to tissue that causes it to move in an anterior–posterior direction consistent with the angle of impact

B lymphocytes: Agents responsible for the transformation of plasma cells that secrete antibodies into the circulatory system

body surface area (BSA): Determines precent of body that is burned

bone: Tissue that consists of living cells and nonliving intercellular substance

bottom time: Amount of time a diver is at a certain depth

Boyle's law: The volume of a gas varies inversely with the external pressure applied to it

bradypnea: Respiratory rate less than 12 breaths per minute in the adult

brain stem: The portion of the brain inferior to the cerebrum and anterior to the cerebellum; it controls motor, sensory, and reflex functions

braking distance: The distance at which energy is exchanged; it includes the distance from the first brake pedal movement to the point at which the vehicle comes to a full stop

breath sounds: The sound of air passing in and out of the lungs as heard with a stethoscope

breech: Presentation that occurs during delivery when the buttocks, lower extremity, or extremities are the presenting part

bronchi: Airways of the lungs; the two primary bronchi divide into secondary bronchi, which further divide into tertiary bronchi, which finally divide into bronchioles

bronchioles: The final generation of airways before the alveoli are reached *bronchiolitis:* Respiratory infection characterized by wheezing; it affects young children

bruit: A pulse-related blowing sound heard over arteries, usually the result of atherosclerosis

buffer: A chemical system set up in the body to respond to changes in the hydrogen ion concentration to maintain a normal pH

bundle branches: Two conduction paths that split from the bundle of His; they carry electrical impulses at high speed to the tissue of the interventricular septum and to each ventricle simultaneously

bundle of His: Electrical conduction system in the interventricular septum that conducts impulses from the AV junction to the right and left bundle branches

bunker coat: The coat worn for structural fire fighting

burn: See superficial, partial-thickness, and full-thickness burn

calcitonin: Hormone secreted by the thyroid gland and involved in calcium metabolism

capillaries: Structures found at the termination of arterioles that connect the arterial and venous systems

capillary refill test: A noninvasive test to judge the rate of blood flow through peripheral capillary beds; the nail beds of the hands or feet are momentarily compressed, and, in an individual with normal circulation, blanching should disappear and normal color return in less than 2 seconds

capsule: Made from gelatin containers designed to dissolve quickly in the stomach

carbon dioxide: The gas that makes up most of the waste diffused from the bloodstream into the airways, where it is pumped back out into the environment

carbon monoxide: A colorless, odorless, tasteless gas

cardiac contusion: A bruise to the heart

cardiac muscle: Muscle found only in the heart; it has the unique property of generating its own electrical impulses

cardiac output: Stroke volume times heart rate per minute; the amount of blood pumped by the heart each minute

cardiac tamponade: Condition that occurs when extensive pericardial fluid restricts diastolic filling of the heart, compromising cardiac output

cardiogenic shock: Extreme form of pump failure, usually due to myocardial infarction, in which the left ventricle cannot adequately perfuse body tissue

carina: Point at the end of the trachea at which it bifurcates into the bronchi

carotid sinus massage: Technique used to increase vagal tone to convert a paroxysmal supraventricular tachycardia to a sinus rhythm; with the patient's head tilted to one side, the index and middle fingers are placed over the carotid artery below the angle of the jaw and the artery is firmly massaged; the EKG should be monitored closely during this procedure

carpopedal spasm: Spasm of the hands and feet

cartilaginous joint: Slightly movable joint; no synovial cavity; bones held together by cartilage

cataract: Condition in which the lens of the eye becomes cloudy

catecholamine: A group of chemical substances, including epinephrine and norepinephrine

cation: Positively charged ion

causation: The cause or link between a breach of duty in a malpractice claim

caustic: Corrosive; capable of burning

cavitation: A cavity created by the acceleration of tissue particles away from the missile, away from the point of impact

cellular immunity: Body mechanism that defends against infections caused by viruses, fungi, and some bacteria; its action is regulated by lymphocyte production

central cyanosis: Discoloration around the mouth or in the cheek mucosa (see *cyanosis*)

central nervous system (CNS): The system composed of the brain and spinal cord; it functions as the body's communication control center and is directly responsible for all aspects of cognitive and voluntary nervous function

cephalic: Normal head-first position of the fetus during delivery

cerebellum: Portion of the brain posterior and inferior to the cerebrum; it is primarily involved in regulating voluntary muscle activity

cerebral concussion: Transient episode of neuronal dysfunction after a violent jar or shock to the brain with a rapid return to normal neurologic activity

cerebral contusion: Bruising and bleeding of the brain

cerebral cortex: Surface of the cerebrum; it contains millions of neurons and nerve fibers, enabling an immense amount of potential information to be processed by the human brain

cerebral herniation: Protrusion of a portion of the brain through an opening in the wall of the cranial cavity

cerebral perfusion pressure: Equal to the mean arterial pressure minus the intracranial pressure

cerebrospinal fluid (CSF): Thin, watery liquid found in the subarachnoid space and spinal column; by absorbing shock, it protects the brain and spinal cord against blunt trauma

cerebrovascular accident: Technical name for stroke

cerebrum: The largest portion of the brain; it controls sensory and motor functions and houses centers for memory, speech, emotions, and thought processes

certification: Indication of satisfactory completion of an accepted training program

cerumen: Earwax

cervical spine: Top seven bones of the spinal column and the origin of eight pairs of spinal nerves (also called cervical vertebrae)

chemical burn: Burn that results when wet or dry corrosive substances come in contact with the skin

chief complaint: The patient's answer to the question, "Why did you call us today?"

child abuse: Form of domestic violence in which a child or adolescent is maltreated by a parent, guardian, or other caretaker

child neglect: Inadequate parenting of children that can result in failure to thrive

chokes: A type of decompression sickness that originates with bubbles in the pulmonary vasculature

cholecystitis: Inflammation of the gallbladder

chordae tendineae: Small tendinous chords that connect the atrioventricular valves to the papillary muscles

chronic obstructive pulmonary disease (COPD): Disease processes that cause decreased ability of ventilatory function of the lungs, including chronic bronchitis, emphysema, and chronic asthma

ciliated epithelium: The presence of cilia on the surface of the epithelium

circle of Willis: Area at the base of the brain in which the vertebral and carotid arteries communicate with each other

circumduction: The swinging of a part in a circle; it involves displacement of the axis

civil law: Private law between two persons or parties

clitoris: Part of the female genitalia composed of erectile tissue; it is situated between the anterior ends of the labia minora

closed wound: Tissue beneath the skin is crushed when a blunt object strikes the body

clubbing: Enlargement and change in shape of the tip of one or more fingers or toes

coccyx: Small bone at the base of the spinal column; it consists of four or five fused bones and one pair of nerve roots

code of ethics: Ethical considerations and guidelines that serve as a persuasive example for uniformity and expectation of members of a profession

cold zone: Area close to a hazardous materials incident that is safe for agencies directly involved in the intervention (see warm and hot zone)

colic: Spasm of the smooth muscle lining of the intestinal tract

collateral circulation: Process that allows the blood from occluded areas to be diverted to distal myocardial tissues

coma: Abnormally deep state of unconsciousness from which a patient cannot be aroused by external stimuli

combining form: Word root followed by a vowel that facilitates pronunciation; it combines a word root with a suffix or other root

combining vowel: Vowel that links the root to the suffix or to another root to ease pronunciation

comminuted fracture: Produced by a severe direct force; there are three or more fragments

communicable disease: Disease that can be transmitted directly or indirectly from one individual to another

compensated shock: Increase in the strength and rate of cardiac contractions and increase in peripheral resistance; when successful, these mechanisms temporarily compensate for the hypovolemic effects of shock by providing adequate vital organ perfusion

competent: Value judgment by a health care provider that renders a patient capable of giving consent to treatment

complete amputation: Amputation in which the body part is completely severed

complete breech: Fetal delivery in which the legs are flexed at the hips, but one or both knees instead of being extended are also flexed

compression fracture: Damage to the bones with force from both ends

conduction: Mechanism of heat loss in which direct transfer of heat between materials of unequal temperature occurs

conductivity: Ability to pass or propagate an electrical impulse from cell to cell through the heart

confidentiality: Patient's right to expect that the communications made in a relationship of trust will not be disclosed

congenital rubella syndrome: Rubella transmitted by pregnant women that gives rise to fetal anomalies or mental retardation

congestive heart failure: Circulatory congestion that occurs in heart failure with resulting fluid retention and edema formation

conjunctiva: Paper-thin covering to the exposed portion of the white part of the eye

conjunctivitis: Infection that produces a red eye with a variable amount of pus, mucus, or watery discharge

consciousness: General wakefulness

consent: Verbal or written acceptance of medical treatment

Conservation of Energy law: Law that states that energy can neither be created nor destroyed, but the form can be changed

content of consciousness: Evaluation of the patient's ability to respond to simple commands, general orientation, and mental ability

continuing education: Training and study beyond minimum requirements for a license and, at times, mandatory for license retention

Controlled Substance Act: Act that classifies drugs according to their usefulness and abuse potential

contusion: Bruise

convection: Transport of heat away from the skin by air movement

coping: Any behavior that protects an individual from both internal and external stressors

cornea: Clear front portion of the eye

coronary artery disease: Disease caused primarily by arteriosclerosis

cor pulmonale: Hypertrophy or failure of the right ventricle secondary to lung, pulmonary vessel, or chest wall disorders that is independent of left ventricular function

cough, coughing: Modified form of respiration that serves to remove foreign bodies that inadvertently enter the larynx

CRAMS scale: Scale concerned with the measurement of respiratory rate, respiratory expansion, systolic blood pressure, and capillary return

cranial nerves: Twelve pairs of nerves that arise from the undersurface of the brain

crepitus: Grating sound heard on palpation of an extremity

cribriform plate: Portion of the ethmoid bone that separates the roof of the nose from the cranial cavity

cricothyroidotomy: Placement of an airway through the cricothyroid space just below the larynx

criminal law: Conduct or offenses that legally have been classified as "public wrongs" or crimes "against the state"

crisis: When a person or group of people enter a sudden state of emotional turmoil regardless of the cause

crisis intervention: Set of temporary, action-oriented strategies designed to reduce the negative impact of a distressing event (or state of mental distress) on an individual or group of individuals and to restore those affected to as normal a level of function as possible

critical incident: Event that has a powerful emotional impact and results in an acute stress reaction

Critical Incident Stress Debriefing (CISD): Group support that is provided for extremely distressing events

croup: Laryngotracheobronchitis, a viral infection; it usually occurs during late fall or early winter and is seen in children of 3 months to 3 years

crowning: Appearance of the presenting part of the fetus at the vaginal opening

cumulative stress reaction: Destructive stress process that occurs over many years and is not associated with a recognized critical incident

Cushing's reflex, Cushing's triad: Threefold phenomenon associated with increasing intracranial pressure: rising blood pressure, slowing pulse rate, and changes in respiratory pattern

Cushing's syndrome: Disease that results from oversecretion of glucocorticoids from the adrenal cortex, which results from pituitary hypersecretion of ACTH

cutaneous membrane: The skin, both the epidermis and dermis collectively

cyanide: An extremely poisonous compound

cyanosis: Slightly bluish or purplish discoloration of the skin and mucous membranes as a result of hypoxia

cytomegalovirus: Virus common in immune-compromised people; a member of the herpesvirus family

deceleration: Force applied to a moving body to stop or reduce its motion (also called drag)

decerebrate, decerebrate posturing: Type of posture in which the upper extremities extend and rotate inward with palms facing lateral and the lower extremities extend and are rigid

decompression sickness: Nitrogen bubble formation in the tissues or blood that can occur when diving (also called "the bends")

decontamination: Making safe by eliminating or neutralizing harmful agents; removal of contamination

decorticate, decorticate posturing: Flexion of the upper extremities with the lower extremities rigid and extended

deep frostbite: Frostbite that affects deep tissue

defense mechanisms: Coping efforts that may be internal, unnoticed, and sometimes unconscious and automatic efforts to adjust to stressful situations

defibrillation: Passage of electrical current through the heart to depolarize fibrillating cells and allow them to repolarize uniformly; it is reserved for the treatment of ventricular fibrillation

degloving amputation: Amputation in which skin and adipose tissue are torn away, but underlying tissue is left intact

degradation: Loss in the beneficial physical properties of gloves, protective clothing, and other material because of exposure to various liquid chemicals

dehydration: Loss or lack of water from the body or tissues

delayed stress reaction: Acute stress reaction that occurs days or weeks after the critical event

delirium tremens: The most severe phase of abstinence in which tremulousness, visual hallucinations, agitation, confusion, and disorientation occur

delta wave: A "slurring" effect at the beginning of the QRS complex; seen in Wolff–Parkinson–White syndrome

delusion: False belief that results from no appropriate external cause and is contrary to the individual's own knowledge base; differs from hallucination in that the latter involves false excitement of one or more of the senses

dementia: Deterioration in mental capacity that is irrecoverable and the end result of various physical and mental disease processes

dendrites: Fibers that extend from the cell body of the neuron, composed of many branching fibers that carry impulses to the soma

denial: Psychological defense mechanism by which an individual blocks out or refuses to acknowledge stressful circumstances

density: Number of particles per volume

depolarization: Destruction of polarity that stimulates muscle fibers to contract

depressed fracture: A fragment is driven below the surface of the bone

depressed skull fracture: Fracture in which bone fragments are driven into the brain

depression: The fourth stage of the grieving process where a great sense of loss becomes evident

dermatomes: "Zones" created by the 31 pairs of spinal nerves around the body

dermis: Thick layer of dense fibrous connective tissue that lies beneath the epidermis

developmental stages: A child's development based on intellectual growth, social environment, and emotional experiences

diabetes mellitus: Disorder of carbohydrate, fat, and protein metabolism that results from a relative or absolute deficiency of insulin

diabetic ketoacidosis: Complication of diabetes mellitus in which hyperglycemia, ketonemia, and acidosis occur

diaphoresis: Excessive perspiration

diaphragm: Muscular structure that separates the thoracic and abdominal cavities

diaphysis: The main shaftlike portion of a bone

diastole: Relaxation phase of the cardiac cycle when the ventricles are filling

diastolic pressure: Constant force of blood on the arteries when the heart is resting and, as such, an estimate of systemic vascular resistance

diencephalon: Division of the brain that contains the thalamus and the hypothalamus

diffusion: Absorption of a liquid, or the passage of a liquid or solid through a membrane

direct questions: Questions with "yes" or "no" answers used when the patient has an altered level of consciousness or when time does not permit open-ended responses (see open-ended questions)

disaster: Any event that overwhelms the existing manpower, facilities, equipment, and capabilities of a responding agency or institution

disentanglement: To extricate or become free from entanglement

dislocation: Displacement of a bone end from its articular surface, sometimes with associated tearing of the ligaments that normally hold the bone end in place

dissecting aortic aneurysm: Critical hemorrhage into the media of the thoracic aorta, which creates a false passage for blood and hematoma

distal: Away from the point of origin or attachment

distribution: Transport of an absorbed drug to its target site

diverticulitis: Inflammation of a diverticula in the intestinal tract, especially in the colon

domestic violence: Use of physical force in a family setting

Do Not Resuscitate: A physician's order to *not* give cardiopulmonary resuscitation to patients who have cardiopulmonary or respiratory arrests; the exact nature of the treatment that the patient should receive, if any, should be clearly specified (also referred to as "no-cor" or "no heroic measures")

dopplers: Small, effective noise amplifiers available for prehospital personnel that make blood pressure measurement easy and accurate under difficult circumstances

dose: In terms of radiation incidents, the amount of radiation absorbed by the body

drag: See *deceleration*

drowning: Death from asphyxia during an immersion episode with or without inhalation of the surrounding medium

drug: Any chemical agent that affects living processes

Drug Enforcement Agency: Federal agency responsible for the enforcement of drug legislation

duodenal ulcer: Lesion or sore of the duodenal mucosa due to the action of gastric juice

duplex system: Ability to receive and transmit at the same time; similar to telephone operation

dura mater: Outermost and toughest of the three meninges that protect the brain

dyspnea: Shortness of breath

dysuria: Painful urination

ecchymosis: Characteristic black and blue mark

eclampsia: Serious toxic disorder that occurs during pregnancy or shortly after delivery and is characterized by high blood pressure, albuminuria, oliguria, and convulsions; etiology is unknown

ectopic pregnancy: Condition that occurs when a fertilized ovum implants itself outside the uterus

ectopy: An ectopic beat, or one from outside the SA node

edema: Collection of fluid between the cells of the tissue

efferent neuron: Motor neuron

EKG monitoring: Recording and interpreting of the electrical activity of the heart

elasticity: The property of tissue to change its shape in direct response to a force and to recover its original form upon removal of the force

elastic recoil: Property that allows the intercostal muscles and diaphragm to relax and the walls of the alveoli to rebound after inspiration

electrical burn: Burn caused from contact with low- or high-voltage electricity

electrocardiogram (EKG, ECG): Record of the electrical activity of the heart

electrolyte: Substance composed of charged particles or ions when placed in water; any solution that conducts electricity

electromechanical dissociation: Any organized EKG rhythm that has an adequate rate but produces no palpable pulse

elixir: Alcoholic preparations that have been sweetened and are used to act as a vehicle for other medications

emergency: Situation that could not have been reasonably foreseen, threatens public health, welfare, or safety, and requires immediate action

emotional abuse: Abuse that results from withholding or depriving a child of normal emotional and psychological nurturing

emotional crisis: Similar to a psychiatric emergency but less intense and not likely to produce deleterious results if immediate treatment is withheld

EMS communications operator: The person responsible for knowing the capabilities of the various components of the EMS system so that the proper units can be dispatched and for monitoring the status of the units directly under the control of the EMS communications center

EMT-Ambulance (EMT-A): Recognized by the National Standard Curriculum as personnel capable of performing CPR, basic airway and ventilation maneuvers, hemorrhage control, fracture stabilization, emergency childbirth, basic extrication, noninvasive patient diagnosis and management, and some specialized rescue skills

EMT-Intermediate (EMT-I): In addition to the skills of the EMT-A, EMT-I personnel are qualified to insert esophageal obturator airways, perform ventilation techniques, and administer intravenous fluid; in some programs, endotracheal intubation and defibrillation are allowed

EMT-Paramedic (EMT-P): In addition to the skills of an EMT-A and EMT-I, EMT-P personnel are trained in advanced airway management and the treatment of cardiac arrest, diabetes, seizures, coma, respiratory compromise, geriatrics, behavior conditions, and pediatrics; they also have some specialized rescue skills

emulsion: Suspensions of fats or oils in water with an emulsifying agent to remain in solution

endocardium: Smooth layer of connective tissue that lines the inside of the heart

endocrine: Complex and integrated network that functions to maintain homeostasis, promote growth and sexual development, and allow adaptation to the physiologic stresses placed on the organism

endometrium: Made of mucous membrane, the inner-most layer of the uterus; it contains the uterine glands

endotracheal intubation: Placement of a hollow tube through the glottis into the larynx for the entrance of air

endotracheal tube: Tube passed through the nose or mouth into the trachea

energy exchange: The loss of velocity or energy by one body to another

engagement: During delivery, when the fetus is at the midpoint of the pelvis at the ischial tuberosities

enhanced 911: System that offers such capabilities as immediate display of the caller's telephone number (automatic number identification) and identification of the caller's location (automatic location identification)

epicardium: Outermost layer of the walls of the heart

epidermis: The outer, thinner layer of skin; the body's first line of defense against the external environment

epididymis: Tightly coiled, threadlike tube that emerges from the top of the testes to become the vas deferens; it houses the sperm cells until they are ready for fertilization

epidural hematoma: Bleeding that occurs because the meningeal arteries are torn

epidural space: Space above or on the dura

epiglottis: Thin leaf-shaped structure located within the larynx at the juncture of the larynx and esophagus that protects the lower airways from foreign bodies

epiglottitis: Inflammation of the epiglottis; it may cause respiratory obstruction, especially in children

epilepsy: Recurrent seizures from an unknown cause thought to be irreversible

epinephrine: Adrenaline; hormone and drug with vasoconstrictive properties; it also increases heart rate and contractility and relaxes the bronchioles

epiphyses: Part of a long bone found at each end

epistaxis: Nosebleed

erect: Standing upright

erythrocyte: Red blood cell

esophageal gastric tube airway (EGTA)/esophageal obturator airway (EOA)): Airway that prevents air from entering the stomach and vomitus from entering the trachea

ethanol: Ethyl alcohol

ethics: System of principles that identifies behavior deemed morally desirable

eupnea: Normal respiratory rate; in the adult between 12 and 20 breaths per minute

eustachian tube: Tube that allows air to pass into or out of the middle ear and leads to the upper part of the throat

evaporation: Absorption of heat, by water, through the process of vaporization

excitability: Ability of cells to respond to electrical stimulation, resulting in fiber contraction; a property of myocardial fibers (also called contractility)

expiration: Passive activities of elastic recoil that create an increase in intrathoracic pressure, causing air to exit the thorax through the nose or mouth

expiratory reserve volume (ERV): Maximum volume of air that can be exhaled after a normal exhalation

expressed consent: Written or verbal statement by a patient that expresses a desire and willingness to receive medical treatment

exsanguinate: To bleed to death

extension: In a straight position, or the movement of the limbs into a straight position

external or transcutaneous pacing: Temporary noninvasive method of cardiac pacing in which electrical impulses to the heart are delivered via large body surface electrodes

extracellular: Outside of the cells

extract: Active ingredients of animal or vegetable drugs; may be liquids or powders

extravascular: Outside of the vascular space (blood vessels)

extrication: To free from entanglement; a label for tools used for this purpose

fallopian tubes: In females, a passageway for egg cells from the ovaries to the uterus

false imprisonment: Claim based on an intentional and unjustifiable detention of an unwilling, conscious person

fascia: Layers of dense, fibrous tissue that cover the muscle and through which tendons run

febrile illness: Infectious illness in which pyrogens reset the body's hypothalamic thermostat to a higher temperature

febrile seizures: Seizures caused by a high body temperature; seen mostly in children

Federal Communications Commission (FCC): Regulatory agency for radio communications that licenses communications systems and assigns radio frequencies, among other things

Federal Trade Commission: Agency that regulates drug advertising

fibrous joint: Immovable joint, no synovial cavity; bones held together by fibrous tissue

Fick principle: Because shock is anaerobic metabolism at the cellular level, the amount of oxygen delivered to each cell is directly related to oxygen exchange in the lungs, the circulation of oxygen to the cells, and the presence of red blood cells

fight or flight syndrome: See *general adaptation syndrome*

finger sweep: Removal of a foreign body from a patient's mouth with gloved fingers; performed only on the unconscious patient

FiO_2: Fraction of inspired oxygen

first degree AV block: Condition characterized by a delay in conduction of impulses through the AV junction; the PR interval is greater than .2 seconds

flail chest: Two or more adjacent ribs each fractured in at least two places

flexion: The act of bending or the condition of being bent

flowmeter: Permanent attachment to oxygen pressure regulator to permit the regulated release of oxygen in liters per minute

fluid extracts: Most concentrated of any fluid preparation

follicle-stimulating hormone (FSH): Hormone secreted by the anterior pituitary gland

fontanelle: Any of the membrane-covered spaces between the incompletely ossified cranial bones of an infant; commonly called soft spot

Food and Drug Administration: Agency that regulates the manufacturing, research, and testing of drugs and monitors adverse effects of new drugs on the market

footling breech: Presentation during delivery when one or both feet of the baby are folded under the buttocks

foramen magnum: Opening for the spinal cord in the tightly closed box around the brain formed by the skull

force: Equal to an object's mass (weight) multiplied by its acceleration (change in velocity)

fracture: Break in the continuity of a bone that may be either closed, in which the overlying skin is intact, or open, in which the skin over the fracture site has been broken

fragmentation: When a bullet breaks into several parts

frank breech: Most common breech presentation; the legs are flexed at the hips but extended at the knees so that the feet and head are close together

fraternal twins: Twins that result from the fertilization of two ova by two spermatozoa

frequency: Unit of measurement for the number of cycles per unit of time

frontal: Plane that passes vertically through the body at a right angle to the sagittal plane and divides the body into anterior and posterior portions

frontal collision, down and under: Type of frontal collision pattern in which the unrestrained occupant's body travels down into and slides over the edge of the car seat; the knees or feet are the lead points

frontal collision, up and over: Type of frontal collision pattern in which the head of the unrestrained occupant is the lead point; it hits the windshield without any previous dissipation of energy

frostbite: Condition that occurs when small body parts with a high ratio of surface area to tissue mass (fingers, toes, ears, and nose) are exposed to extreme cold (see superficial and deep frostbite)

full-thickness (third-degree) burn: Burn characterized by destruction of both the epidermis and dermis

τ *rays:* One of three principle types of ionizing radiation emitted by radioactive sources

ganglia: Groups of nerves located outside of the central nervous system

general adaptation syndrome: Universal reaction to a

stressor that is regulated by the sympathetic nervous system; by increasing blood pressure, blood sugar, and heart rate and by providing bronchodilatation, it prepares the body for "fight or flight" (also called *fight or flight syndrome*)
geriatric: Elderly
Glasgow Coma Scale: Guide to assess the baseline degree of brain dysfunction from one point in time to another
glottis: Opening between the vocal cords
glucagon: Hormone secreted by the pancreas; it stimulates the breakdown of glycogen and the release of glucose in the liver
glucocorticoids: Group of hormones secreted by the adrenal cortex
gonorrhea: Common sexually transmitted disease caused by the bacterium *Neisseria gonorrhoeae*
Good Samaritan law: Statutes of immunity for emergency medical providers; they vary from state to state
gravida: Pregnant woman
greenstick fracture: An incomplete fracture by a compression force in the long axis of the bone; common among children
growth hormone (GH): Hormone secreted by the anterior pituitary that plays important roles in growth (also called *somatotropin*)
guarding: Contraction of the abdominal wall musculature, either reflexively (involuntary guarding) or consciously (voluntary guarding)
hallucination: Any false perception (e.g., visual, tactile, auditory) that has no relation to reality and no exterior manifestation to others
hallucinogen: Any agent that induces hallucinations
Harrison Narcotic Act of 1914: The Act that regulates the manufacture, import, sale, and use of opium and cocaine and their derivatives
hazardous material: Any substance that jumps out of its container when something goes wrong and hurts or harms the things it touches
hazardous materials incident: The release, or potential release, of a hazardous material from its container into the environment
hazards: The many dangers present in the line of duty
head-tilt/chin-lift: Method of opening the airway that involves tilting back the patient's head by placing one hand on the forehead and applying firm backward pressure; the other hand should be placed with the fingers under the bony part of the patient's lower jaw, near the chin, thus lifting the mandible and helping to tilt the head back
head-to-toe survey: Survey of a patient that begins with the head and neck and proceeds to the chest and back, abdomen, and extremities
heat cramps: Chemical disruption that results from profuse sweating
heat exhaustion: A more advanced stage of the homeostatic imbalance that sometimes begins with heat cramps
heat stroke: A true emergency in which the body's compensatory mechanisms such as vasodilation and sweating are exhausted, or actually cause further trouble through shock and dehydration, and hypothalamic control weakens, then collapses.
hematocrit: Volume percentage of red blood cells in whole blood
hematoma: Blood clot that forms at a site of injury
hematuria: Blood-tinged urine

hemiparesis: Muscular weakness or partial paralysis that affects one side of the body
hemoglobin: Protein that contains iron
hemopoiesis: Process of blood cell formation carried on by red bone marrow
hemoptysis: Expectoration of blood due to hemorrhage of the larynx, trachea, bronchi, or lungs
hemothorax: Condition in which blood accumulates in the pleural space
Henry's law: The amount of gas that dissolves in a fluid is directly proportional to the pressure of that gas as it contacts the fluid
hepatitis: Inflammation of the liver, from toxic or viral origin
hepatitis A: Hepatitis that is transmitted through direct contact with infected stool and urine
hepatitis B: Hepatitis that is caused by the hepatitis B virus and has a more insidious onset than hepatitis A
hepatitis C: Non-A, non-B hepatitis; transfusion-related hepatitis
herpes simplex type 1: Infectious disease caused by herpes simplex virus that results in cold sores or fever blisters
herpes simplex type 2: Commonly referred to as genital herpes; infectious disease caused by herpes simplex type 2 virus that affects the genital area
herpes zoster: Herpes viral infection that presents as a unilateral rash and progresses to pustules; its lesions contain live chickenpox virus that is contagious through direct contact (also called *shingles*)
herpetic whitlow: Herpes viral infection of the finger or fingers; an occupational health risk for health care workers
hiccup: Sudden inspiration against a closed glottis, caused by spasmodic contraction of the diaphragm
histamine: Substance normally present in the body that exerts a pharmacologic action when tissue damage occurs
homeostasis: Body processes and mechanisms that keep the body in an internal state of equilibrium
hormone: Chemical substance that is released into the blood and carried to a distant site where it brings about its action
Hospital Formulary: Published by the American Society of Hospital Pharmacists, a loose-leaf book that provides drug information and is continuously updated as new information is published
hot zone: Area surrounding a hazardous materials incident that is dangerous to life and health (see *cold* and *warm zone*)
human immunodeficiency virus (HIV): Viral agent responsible for acquired immunodeficiency syndrome (AIDS)
humor: Defense mechanism that can reduce tension by providing an outlet for the person faced with a distressing situation
humoral immunity: Through the circulation of antibodies, the body's primary defense against bacterial infections
hydrofluoric acid: A strong acid
hydrostatic pressure: Pressure of fluids at rest
hypercapnia, hypercarbia: The presence of abnormally high concentration of carbon dioxide in the blood
hyperglycemia: Elevated blood glucose concentration
hyperosmolar hyperglycemic nonketotic coma: Clinical entity principally characterized by severe hyperosmolality, often secondary to extreme hyperglycemia
hyperparathyroidism: Condition caused by excessive se-

cretion of parathyroid hormone resulting in a high plasma calcium level and decreased plasma phosphate level

hyperpnea: Deep breathing or increased respiratory rate

hypertension: Abnormally high blood pressure

hyperthermia: The general condition of excess body heat

hyperthyroidism: Excess secretion of thyroid hormone that results in a hypermetabolic state

hypertonic: A fluid with a higher osmotic pressure than another fluid

hyperventilation: Increased alveolar ventilation

hyperventilation syndrome: A number of physiologic effects produced by "anxiety attacks" during which people hyperventilate

hypnotic: Any agent that induces sleep

hypoglycemia: Low blood glucose concentration

hypoparathyroidism: Condition caused by lack of parathyroid secretion, resulting in reduced plasma calcium level and increased plasma phosphate level

hypotension: Abnormally low blood pressure

hypothalamus: Portion of the diencephalon functionally related to the pituitary gland

hypothermia: The general condition of deficient body heat

hypothyroidism: Deficiency of thyroid hormone that results in a hypometabolic state

hypotonic: A fluid with a lower osmotic pressure than another fluid

hypoventilation: Decreased alveolar ventilation associated with acute respiratory acidosis

hypoxemia: Decreased partial pressure of oxygen in arterial blood

hypoxia: Inadequate oxygenation of the blood

identical twins: Twins that result from fertilization of a single ovum

IgA: Immunoglobulin; this antibody appears in the serum within a few days to a week after onset of certain viral illnesses

IgE: Immunoglobulin; this antibody induces the cell to release a number of pharmacologically active agents

IgG: Immunoglobulin; the presence of this antibody signifies past exposure to a disease

IgM: Immunoglobulin; this antibody is the first to respond to the presence of a new antigen

illusion: Misinterpretation of actual stimuli

immersion hypothermia: Chain of events associated with prolonged exposure, shivering, and loss of body temperature caused by immersion in cold water

immune response: Response that occurs when protective cells of the body recognize and fight against foreign substances that can harm the body

immune system: The body's protective mechanism, made up of separate cells and molecules

immunity: Exemption from legal liability; also, the body's natural resistance to poisons and foreign substances

immunoglobulin: Protein capable of acting as an antibody

impacted fracture: The bone ends are violently jammed together so that they telescope into each other

impaled object: Wound in which the instrument that caused the injury remains impacted in the wound

implied consent: Situation in which a patient is unable to communicate consent to treatment and a life-threatening injury or illness requires prompt medical attention

Incident Command System (ICS): System in which the highest ranking officer for each agency is designated as the incident commander (IC), and each shares responsibility for scene management

incompetent: Value judgment by a health care provider that renders a patient incapable of giving consent to treatment

incubation period: Interval between exposure to infection and the appearance of the first symptom

infant: Younger than one year old

infectious disease: An illness caused by invasion of an organism, be it a virus, bacterium or fungus

inferior: On the bottom or toward the feet

informed consent: Patient's agreement to medical treatment after adequate information of the treatment, its risks and consequences, and any alternative methods of treatment have been explained

ingestion: Manner by which substances can enter the body through the mouth

inhalation: Manner by which substances can enter the body through the lungs

injection: Manner by which substances can enter the body through the blood stream

inspection: Close visualization of a patient; the first phase of the physical examination

inspiration: Process by which air enters the lungs through the nose or mouth

inspiratory reserve volume (IRV): Maximum volume of air that can be inhaled after a normal inhalation

insulin: Hormone secreted by the pancreas that is essential for the proper regulation of blood sugar

intercostal muscles: Muscles between the ribs

interneuron: Connecting neuron

internodal and interatrial tracts: Pathways thought to route electrical impulses between the SA and AV nodes and the ones thought to spread impulses across the atrial muscle

intima: Smooth layer of single cells that lines the inside of blood vessels

interstitial: Between the cells

interstitial space: Space between the wall of the capillary and the wall of the alveolus

intervertebral disc: Fluid-filled pad of tough cartilage between each two vertebrae that acts as a shock absorber

intracellular: Within cell membranes

intracerebral hemorrhage: Condition that occurs from bleeding within the brain itself

intracranial pressure: Equals the mean arterial pressure minus the cerebral perfusion pressure

intradermal: Route of administration of a drug that involves injecting it directly into the skin

intramuscular (IM): Route of administration of a drug that involves the injection of small quantities into a muscle

intraosseous, intraosseous infusion: Placement of a rigid needle into a bone and the infusion of fluid and medications directly into the bone marrow

intravascular: Within blood vessels (the vascular space)

intravenous (IV): Administration route that injects the drug directly into the bloodstream

invasion of privacy (breach of confidentiality): Claim based on unauthorized release of confidential or private information that causes the plaintiff damages; differs from libel and slander in that the plaintiff need not show malicious intent or falsity

involuntary consent: Permission to treat a patient granted by the authority of the law, regardless of the patient's desire

iris: Colored portion of the eye

irreversible shock: Shock-related organ failure as the result of irreversible ischemic damage; effects on affected organs may not be apparent for a few days

ischemic colitis: Inflammation of the large intestine caused by poor blood supply

isolation: The act of separating infected individuals from those not infected as a means to prevent the spread of a disease; also stage one of the grieving process which aids in the partial acceptance of the death

isotonic: A fluid with the same osmotic pressure as another fluid

jacksonian seizure: Partial complex seizure that progresses into a general complex attack

jaw-thrust: Method of opening the airway that requires forward displacement of the jaw without any tilting of the head

joule: Work done in one second by current of one ampere against a resistance of one ohm

junctional escape complexes and rhythms: Cardiac complexes or rhythms as a result of the AV junction that function as the heart's pacemaker for one or more cardiac cycles; they occur when impulses from the SA node cannot penetrate the AV node or when the sinus rate drops to less than the AV junction rate (40 to 60 per minute)

Kaposi's sarcoma: Purplish lesions on the skin or mucous membranes

Koplik's spots: White spots on the buccal mucosa seen in people who have rubeola

Kehr's sign: Pain in the shoulder caused by the phrenic nerve being in contact with blood

kinematics: The science of motion that involves the transfer of energy from an external source to a victim's body

kinetic energy: The energy of motion

KKK standards: Federal design specifications by which ambulances are manufactured

Korotkoff's sounds: Series of sounds sometimes used to record blood pressure

kyphosis: Spinal changes

labia majora: Larger, longitudinal outer lips over the vaginal and urethral orifices

labia minora: Smaller, inner lips that cover the vaginal and urethral openings

labor: Process of expelling the fetus and placenta from the uterus and the vagina

laceration: Jagged wound that bleeds freely and is the result of snagging or tearing of tissues

lacrimal gland: Tear gland

laryngeal edema: Swelling in and around the larynx

laryngeal spasm: Acute, involuntary, transitory contraction of the larynx

laryngopharynx: Subdivision of the pharynx that leads to the larynx and esophagus

laryngoscope: Instrument for visualizing the larynx

larynx: Upper end of the trachea that lies below the root of the tongue and contains the vocal cords

lateral: Away from the midline; opposite of medial

lateral collision: Occurs most often at intersections when a vehicle is hit in the side by another vehicle (also called a T-bone collision)

laterally recumbent: Side lying position of the body

lead II: Common lead for prehospital EKG monitoring; negative electrode is on the right arm and the positive one on the left leg

Le Fort's fractures: Midface fractures

left ventricular failure: Inability of the left ventricle to adequately pump blood into the systemic circulation; if severe enough, it can result in pulmonary edema

lens: Structure behind the iris that changes shape to focus light rays on the back of the eye

leukocytes: White blood cells

level of consciousness: One of the four key areas evaluated in a neurologic exam during the secondary survey

libel: Tort action based on a written defamatory statement, falsely or inaccurately made, that damages a person's character, name, or reputation

lice: Small wingless insects that live as parasites on the outer surface of the body

licensure: Process by which a governmental agency grants individuals permission to practice a specific profession

ligaments: Substance that connects bone to bone and helps hold together the bony framework of the body

liniment: Suspensions that contain oil, soap, water, or alcohol, designed for external application to the skin by rubbing

living will: Document in which patients express their desire not to be kept alive through "extraordinary" treatment, such as respirators, when the chance of recovery is minimal

lotion: A liquid preparation designed for external application

lower airway: Route for air transmission from the larynx to the small airways just adjacent to the alveoli

lumbar spine: Five bones of the spinal column (vertebrae) and five pairs of corresponding nerves located between the sacrum and thoracic vertebrae; also, that region of the lower back

Lund–Brower chart: Special table for the most accurate assessment of the extent of a burn

lungs: Organs in which external respiration takes place

luteinizing hormone (LH): Hormone secreted by the anterior pituitary

lymphatic system: Vital component in the overall functioning of the immune system; sometimes described as a "middle man" between the blood and the tissues of the body

lymphocytes: Lymph cells

Magill forceps: Pincer-type instrument used to remove foreign matter or to assist in intubation

magma: Bulky suspensions of insoluble preparations in water

major incident: Event that causes injury or death and damage to property or environment to a degree greater than that which occurs on a routine basis

malleability: The ability of a projectile to change shape

Mallory–Weiss syndrome: Condition in which tears occur in the mucosa just below the gastroesophageal junction secondary to vomiting; the condition usually heals itself

malpractice: Negligent conduct of a professional person; its claim is a common basis for civil liability

mammalian diving reflex: Reflex that is triggered by immersing the face in cold water; blood is diverted from the arms and legs and circulates at a heart rate as low as 5 to 6 beats per minute; a small sufficient supply of oxygen is very slowly circulated among the lungs, heart, and brain

manubrium: Upper handle part of the sternum

mass: Weight

mastoiditis: Inflammation of the mastoid process

mean arterial pressure: More accurate indication of organ perfusion than blood pressure alone; equal to diastolic pressure plus one third of pulse pressure

mechanism of injury: Key aspect of the initial scene survey in a trauma call; its evaluation enables the paramedic, and eventually the physician, to anticipate potential injuries, particularly those that are not readily apparent

meconium: Dark green or black substance found in the large intestine of the fetus

media: Middle layer of a blood vessel wall composed of elastic fibers and muscle

medial: Toward the midline; opposite of lateral

mediastinal shift: Excessive pressure in one lung that causes the mediastinal structures to push over into the opposite hemothorax and put pressure on the other lung, creating a profound compromise of ventilation and reducing cardiac output

medical control (medical direction): Physician's role and responsibility for supervising and monitoring all medical aspects and decisions in the EMS system

medical history: Survey taken to identify a patient's past health problems that may affect the current illness or injury

medical practices act: Legislation that governs the practice of medicine

medulla oblongata: With the pons and the midbrain, it constitutes the brain stem, which is the inferior portion of the brain and also the upper aspect of the spinal cord; it contains important reflex centers

medullary cavity: A tubelike hollow in the diaphysis; serves to manufacture blood cells

melanin: Agent responsible for skin pigmentation

melanocytes: Cells in the deeper aspects of the epidermis that synthesize melanin

melena: Black, sticky, tarry-looking stools that are stained with blood pigment and digested blood

meninges: Membranes

meningitis: Inflammation of the membranes of the spinal cord or brain

menopause: Permanent cessation of ovulation and menstrual activity

menstrual cycle: Changes that occur in the ovaries and uterus between puberty (12 to 14 years of age) and the end of child-bearing potential

mental derangement: State that produces an inability to care for one's basic needs

mental status examination: Short organized format for emergency interviewing developed by psychiatrists to help gather information about a patient's behavioral, psychological, and intellectual functioning

metabolic acidosis: Excess amount of acids in the body

metabolic alkalosis: Excess amount of alkaline in the body

metered dose inhaler: Alternative form of inhalation administration; it contains a canister of liquid medication that does not require dilution or mixing

metric system: System of measurement based on decimals, with all basic units being multiples of 10

midbrain: With the pons and the medulla oblongata, it constitutes the brain stem, which is the inferior portion of the brain and also the upper aspect of the spinal cord; it contains many reflex centers

mineralocorticoids: Chemical substances secreted by the adrenal cortex and involved in regulation of sodium and potassium balance

mitral valve: Bicuspid valve located between the left atrium and the left ventricle of the heart

mobile repeater: Vehicle unit that receives radio communications and rebroadcasts the communications (also called vehicle repeater)

Mobitz I: Type I second degree AV block

Mobitz II: Type II second degree AV block

modified chest lead 1 (MCL$_1$): Selective modified chest electrode; positive electrode is placed between the fourth and fifth intercostal space on the right sternal border, the negative electrode just below the left midclavicle

momentum: Motion

multifocal atrial tachycardia (MAT): Disorder of automaticity characterized by atrial rates greater than 100 per minute, P waves of at least three different morphologies in the same lead, and irregular P-to-P, PR, and R-to-R intervals

mumps: Viral disease caused by the mumps virus, Myxovirus parotiditis; it is less common than other childhood diseases

myelin sheath: Segmented cover that wraps around the axon fiber

myocardial infarction: Heart attack; tissue necrosis of a portion of the heart, usually from thrombus formation in the coronary arteries

myocardial ischemia: Temporary anemia due to obstruction of circulation in the heart; can lead to myocardial infarction

myocardium: Thick muscular middle layer of the walls of the heart

myometrium: Middle layer of the uterus

narcotic: A drug that in moderate doses depresses the central nervous system, thus relieving pain and producing sleep, but that in excessive doses produces unconsciousness, stupor, coma, and possibly death

nasal cannula: An apparatus capable of delivering up to 44% oxygen when operated at a maximum of 6 L/min

nasal flaring: Widening of the nostrils on inspiration

nasal intubation: Technique in which an endotracheal tube is passed through the nose and pharynx into the trachea without using a laryngoscope to directly visualize the vocal cords

nasopharyngeal airway: Device used to maintain an open upper airway by preventing the tongue from obstructing the posterior pharynx

nasopharynx: Subdivision of the pharynx, located posterior to the nose

near drowning: Submersion incident in which recovery occurs

needle chest decompression: See *thoracentesis*

neurilemma: Continuous sheath that covers the myelinated nerve fiber (also called the sheath of Schwann)

neurohypophysis: Posterior lobe of the pituitary gland

neuron: Individual nerve cell

Newton's first law of motion: Law that states that a body, whether in motion or at rest, remains in that state until acted on by an outside force

Newton's second law of motion: Law that states that the force of an object is equal to its mass multiplied by its acceleration

911: Nationally recognized emergency telephone number by which an EMS system can quickly respond to a call

nitrogen narcosis: Syndrome of disorientation and other mental changes related to the use of nitrogen when diving

nitrous oxide: Analgesic gas commonly used in combination with other drugs in general anesthesia

nocturia: Excessive urination at night

nodes of Ranvier: Spaces between each segment of the myelinated axon

nonrebreathing mask: Breathing mask that delivers close to 100% oxygen with the flow at 10 to 15 L/min

norepinephrine: Levophed; parasympathetic chemical mediator and drug with chiefly vasoconstrictive properties, frequently used in the treatment of shock

normothermic: Normal body temperature

nose: Conduit for inspired air, moving the air from the outside into the posterior pharynx

oblique fracture: Fracture line extends obliquely across the bone; usually caused by a twisting force

obstructive lung disease: Disease processes that obstruct the lower airway

O'Donohue's triad: Complex characterized by severe localized pain, joint deformity and dysfunction, and ecchymosis

off-line medical control: The basic administrative framework, standards, and capabilities of on-line medical control

ointment: Semisolid medication in a petroleum or lanolin base for prolonged contact with the skin

oliguria: Decrease in urine output

on-line medical control: The physician advisor who directly supervises and has primary responsibility for the EMT-P, the emergency room staff, and other designated physicians at the base hospital

open-ended questions: Questions that allow patients to tell the story in their own words; the responses are usually more accurate and complete than with direct questioning (see *direct questions*)

open pneumothorax: Pneumothorax in which an open wound connects the pleural space to the outside

open wound: Wound in which the skin is broken and the patient is susceptible to external hemorrhage and wound contamination

oral intubation: Technique in which an endotracheal tube is passed through the mouth into the trachea using a laryngoscope to directly visualize the vocal cords; most secure and reliable airway control without surgical techniques

oropharyngeal airway: Device that essentially serves as a tongue hook, holding the tongue at its base to prevent it from falling back against the posterior pharyngeal wall

oropharynx: Portion of the pharynx that lies between the soft palate and the upper portion of the epiglottis

orthopaedic: Referring to bone

orthopnea: Breathing discomfort or shortness of breath that occurs in all positions except the upright one

Osborne wave (J wave): Wave seen after the QRS complex on EKG monitoring during severe hypothermia

osmosis: The passage of solvents through a semipermeable membrane that separates solutions of different concentrations

osmotic pressure: Pressure that develops in a solution as a result of net osmosis into that solution

ossicles: Three tiny movable bones in the middle ear

osteoarthritis: Condition that causes degeneration of the joints, particularly the weight-bearing joints of the hip, knee, and spine

osteoblasts: Bone-forming cells that compose the inner layer of the periosteum

osteoporosis: Disease that causes a decrease in actual bone mass, which causes the bones to become more fragile

ovaries: In females, two almond-shaped glands on either side of the pelvic cavity that produce and release eggs and secrete female hormones

ovulation: Rupturing of the mature graafian follicle onto the surface of the ovary

oxygen: An odorless, tasteless gas necessary for all cellular life and proper metabolism

oxygen-powered demand valve: Device that delivers both large volumes and 100% oxygen

oxygen pressure regulator: Device used to reduce oxygen pressure to a level suitable for administration under medical conditions, usually 40 to 70 psi

oxytocin: Hormone secreted by the posterior pituitary that effects both the breast, where it stimulates milk ejection, and the uterus, where it causes muscular contraction

PaCO$_2$: Partial pressure of arterial carbon dioxide

palpation: Assessment of a patient by touch or feel; the third phase of a physical examination

pancreas: Soft, oblong gland behind the stomach that secretes digestive enzymes, glucagon, and insulin

PaO$_2$: Partial pressure of oxygen in arterial blood

para: Previous live births

paradoxical motion: Condition that occurs when the flail segment of the chest moves in a direction opposite to that of the rest of the chest wall during respiration

parasympathetic division: Division of the autonomic nervous system; operating without conscious control, it is involved with maintaining and regulating bodily functions such as insulin release, pupil constriction, and salivary and digestive gland secretion

parathyroid glands: Four pea-shaped glands situated in the neck in close proximity to the thyroid gland; they are largely responsible for maintaining proper calcium levels in the bloodstream through the secretion of parathyroid hormone

parathyroid hormone (PTH): Hormone secreted by the parathyroid glands that increases blood calcium levels at the kidney, the bone, and the intestine

parens patriae: Legal doctrine that gives authority to the State, for various reasons, to act in lieu of the parents to protect the welfare and health of a minor

parenteral drugs: Liquid drugs administered into the body by a subcutaneous, intramuscular, or intravenous route

paresis: Weakness

parity: Condition of a woman in relation to the number of children she has borne

paroxysmal junctional tachycardia: Cardiac arrhythmia that occurs when the AV junction stimulates the ventricles at a rate of 100 to 180 per minute; treatment and EKG characteristics are the same as for paroxysmal supraventricular tachycardia

paroxysmal nocturnal dyspnea: Form of transient pulmonary edema that usually occurs at night when the patient is reclining

paroxysmal supraventricular tachycardia (PSVT or SVT): Sudden appearance and cessation of rapid atrial rhythm with a rate between 150 and 250 beats per minute; it is initiated by a premature discharge from the atria or AV junction

partial amputation: Amputation in which more than 50% of the body part is severed

partial rebreathing mask: Device that delivers a high concentration of oxygen at 10 L/min

partial-thickness (second-degree) burn: A superficial partial-thickness burn involves the deep epidermal layers of the skin and always causes injury to the upper layers of the dermis; a deep partial-thickness burn involves the entire epidermis and extends deep into the dermis

patella: Kneecap

peak flow meter: Portable device using a flow gauge that measures how rapidly the patient can exhale

Pediatric Glasgow Coma Scale: Similar to the Adult Glasgow Coma Scale except that the pediatric patient is evaluated by age ranges; categories include eyes opening, motor response, and verbal response

pediatrics: A branch of medicine concerned with the care and development of children and the treatment of their diseases

Pediatric Trauma Score: An assessment of six components commonly evaluated in pediatric trauma graded into three categories; the six components are weight, airway, level of consciousness, systolic blood pressure, open wounds, and fractures

pelvic inflammatory disease (PID): Infective process that leads to inflammation of the pelvic organs

penetrating trauma: Type of impact to tissue that causes it to move in a lateral direction away from the penetrating instrument, creating a cavity in the tissue

penetration: Flow of a hazardous chemical through zippers, stitched seams, pores, or other imperfections in clothing material

percussion: Evaluation tool that involves striking or tapping the patient's skin to determine the size, location, and density of an underlying structure

percutaneous: Intravenous, intramuscular, subcutaneous, or intradermal

pericardial sac: Sac that surrounds the heart

pericardiocentesis: Only effective emergency treatment for life-threatening cardiac tamponade; it involves insertion of a needle into the pericardial sac and aspiration of the accumulating blood

pericarditis: Inflammation of the pericardial sac that surrounds the heart

pericardium: Double-walled fibroserous sac that surrounds the heart

perimetrium: Outer layer of the uterus

periosteum: Dense, white, fibrous membrane that covers the entire outer surface of the bone, except at joint surfaces

peripheral cyanosis: Discoloration in the extremities (see *cyanosis*)

peripheral nervous system: System that includes all nerve fibers outside of the brain and spinal cord; it sends messages in the form of nerve impulses, which it receives from tissues and organs, to the central nervous system

peripheral vascular resistance: Resistance or inability of blood to flow normally in the systemic circulation due to constriction of peripheral blood vessels (also called systemic vascular resistance)

peristalsis: Wavelike muscular movements along the wall of a hollow muscular structure

peritoneum: Membrane that lines the abdominal cavity, which covers the abdominal organs

peritonitis: Inflammation of the peritoneum

permanent cavity: A permanent hole; its size depends on the elasticity of the damaged tissue

permeation: Process by which hazardous chemicals move through protective clothing

permucosal: Around mucous membranes

petroleum distillate: Petroleum products that have a low resistance to flow and a high tendency to evaporate rapidly, making pulmonary toxicity the primary risk

pH: Inverse logarithm of the hydrogen ion concentration

phagocytosis: Process by which the body's defense system activates and increases the production of white blood cells that seek out, attack, and destroy certain antigens

pharmacodynamics: Study of the effects of drugs on the body

pharmacokinetics: Study of the movement of drugs in the body as they are absorbed, distributed, metabolized, and excreted

pharyngeo-tracheal lumen (PtL) airway: Device that consists of a long, cuffed tube, which may pass into either the trachea or the esophagus, and a short, cuffed tube, which is positioned just above the epiglottis

pharynx: Throat; that portion of the airway between the nasal cavity and the larynx

phonation: Ability to speak

Physicians' Desk Reference: Common resource for drug information

physics: Study of space, time, and matter and their interaction with one another

pia mater: Innermost layer of the meninges that directly covers the brain; it is thin and highly vascular

pill: Mixture of a drug with some cohesive material, which is then molded into a form convenient for swallowing

pin-indexing system: Safety mechanism on an oxygen cylinder that allows only the attachment of an oxygen pressure regulator

pituitary gland: Organ located at the base of the brain that secretes a number of hormones to regulate many bodily processes including growth, reproduction, and diverse metabolic activities

placenta: Structure that provides nutrition, excretion, and circulation to the fetus

placenta previa: Condition in which the placenta implants itself in a lower portion of the uterus than is normal

plasma: Fluid outside the cells

platelets: Fragments of cells

pleurae: Membranes that cover the thoracic musculature and the lungs

pleural friction rub: Described as the creaking sound of old leather, it often accompanies pleuritis

pleuritis: An inflammation of the pleura

pneumatic anti-shock garment (PASG): Garment used to establish adequate perfusion

pneumothorax: Presence of air in the pleural space between the visceral pleura and the parietal pleura (see *simple, tension,* and *open pneumothorax*)

pocket face mask: External device used to assist or control ventilation; it delivers adequate volumes but cannot deliver more than 40% oxygen

poison control center: Center designed to answer questions from health care professionals and the public; it often can evaluate a nontoxic or mildly toxic exposure by telephone

polydipsia: Increased thirst

polyphagia: Large intake of food; increased eating and appetite

polyuria: Increased urination, often with voiding of several liters per day

pons: With the midbrain and the medulla oblongata, it constitutes the brain stem, which is the inferior portion of the brain and also the upper aspect of the spinal cord; it accommodates the pneumotaxic centers, which help regulate respiratory rhythms

positive-pressure ventilation: Respiratory assistance through positive pressure

posterior: Dorsal or back surface

postganglionic neurons: Neurons that conduct the impulses to the visceral effectors

postpartum hemorrhage: A woman's loss of more than 500 mL of blood in the 24-hour period after childbirth

potassium: Chief intracellular ion in the blood plasma

potentiation: Process by which the administration of one drug enhances the effects of another

powder: Finely divided or ground drug mixtures that are solid and dry

precipitous delivery: Delivery that occurs within 3 hours of the onset of labor

precordial thump: Sharp blow to the midsternum with the fist from a height of 10 to 12 inches; the blow generates a small amount of electrical current and may interrupt a tachyarrhythmia or restart an asystolic heart; for prehospital use it is recommended only when the patient is monitored by EKG

preeclampsia: Hypertensive disorder specific to pregnancy

prefix: First part of a word or the beginning of a word

preganglionic neurons: Groups of neurons that conduct impulses from the central nervous system to autonomic ganglia

preloaded syringes: Syringes used for administration of intravenous, intramuscular, or subcutaneous medications

premature atrial complex (PAC): Early or premature discharge of an ectopic focus located somewhere in the atria other than the SA node; it frequently depolarizes the SA node and causes a pause in the EKG

premature junctional complex (PJC): Single complex that occurs during sinus rhythm earlier than the next expected sinus beat and is created by premature discharge of an ectopic focus in the AV junctional tissue; the resulting pause may be compensatory or noncompensatory

premature ventricular complex (PVC): Complex that occurs when an ectopic focus in either ventricle creates an impulse before the next expected sinus beat; they are abnormally wide and often bizarre in appearance, and the pause after them is usually compensatory

preschool: 3–5 years old; very active with growth spurts

presentation: Presenting part of the fetus when it is delivered

present illness: Determination of the chronology, nature, and severity of the patient's current illness or injury

pressure waves: Waves that radiate outward from a blast

priapism: Continuing erection of the penis

primary survey: First step once the paramedic is at the patient's side; a rapid evaluation, less than 45 seconds, to determine the patient's status regarding responsiveness, airway, breathing, and circulation

PR interval: Distance between the beginning of the P wave and the beginning of the QRS complex on an EKG

privilege: Legal principle that refers to a statutory restriction on testimony

profession: An occupation, usually one that requires specialized training and knowledge

professionalism: A position in which integrity and diligence are assumed in the fulfillment of its responsibilities

profile: Frontal area

prolactin: Hormone that during pregnancy enhances milk production and, in conjunction with other hormones, stimulates breast development

prolapsed umbilical cord: During labor, premature expulsion or compression of the umbilical cord

prone: Lying on the stomach with the face down; also the position of the hand or foot when facing down; opposite of supine

protocols: Guidelines for the management of patients with specific medical conditions

proximal: Nearest point of origin or attachment

pseudoaneurysm: Partial disruption of the aortic wall, with the adventitia containing the hemorrhage

psychiatric emergency: Any situation in which a patient's moods, thoughts, or actions have the potential to produce death or harm to himself or herself or to others

psychosis: Any type of behavior that is deemed psychotic; any class of serious mental disorders in which the mind does not function normally and the ability to distinguish and cope with reality is impaired

Public Health Service: Federal agency that inspects and licenses establishments that manufacture drugs

pulmonary contusion: Bruise on the lung that frequently accompanies rib fractures and flail chest

pulmonary edema: Serous fluid in the alveoli and interstitial tissue of the lungs

pulmonary embolism: A serious condition that is caused by a foreign body that lodges in the pulmonary capillary bed

pulse: The effect on an artery caused by the movement of blood from the heart as it contracts

pulse deficit: Difference between the apical and peripheral pulse rates

pulsus paradoxus: During inspiration, a weakening of the pulse and a blood pressure drop of greater than 10 mm Hg

pulvule: A gelatin capsule that has a dose of a drug in powder form

puncture wound: An injury caused by a narrow object, such as a knife or nail, cutting the skin

Pure Food and Drug Act of 1906: First major federal drug law; it mandated labelling of preparations that contained certain habit-forming drugs, and it prohibited making false claims about a drug's actions

Purkinje system: Branching terminal network of fibers that receives electrical impulses from the bundle of His and distributes them throughout the ventricular myocardium

P$\bar{v}$CO$_2$: Partial pressure of venous carbon dioxide

P$\bar{v}$O$_2$: Partial pressure of venous oxygen

P wave: First electrical wave seen on an EKG; it is small and roundish and indicates depolarization of the atria

QRS complex: Portion of an EKG tracing that represents depolarization of the ventricles; it usually contains separate Q, R, and S waves, though its configuration varies

Q wave: On an EKG, the first downward (negative) deflection after the P wave

raccoon's eyes: Typical appearance when blood travels into the periorbital subcutaneous tissue

radiation: The process of warmer materials radiating or emitting heat to cooler ones; whether the body emits radiant heat or absorbs it depends on the relation of skin temperature to that of other surfaces in the environment

radiation burn: Burn that occurs from overexposure to ultraviolet light (sunburn) or from the heat of an atomic explosion

radioactive substance: Substance that emits ionizing radiation, so named for its ability to damage organic matter by breaking loose the ions, electrically charged particles, that make up atoms

rales: Abnormal breath sound heard both on inspiration and expiration that is caused by secretions, fluid, or exudate in the bronchial airways or spasms or thickening of their walls

rapport: Harmonious or sympathetic relationship

rationalization: Justification of one's actions or lack of actions

reaction distance: Distance a vehicle travels from the time the driver recognizes the need to stop until brake pedal movement begins

rear-end collision: Vehicle hit from behind by another vehicle

rebound: Pain that occurs when the peritoneal surfaces are rubbed together

receptor: Sites in the body to which a drug binds; determines the quantity of drug necessary to effect a response

reciprocity: Practice by which a state recognizes another state's certification or licensure

re-evaluation: An important assessment tool; patients should be evaluated periodically

repression: Psychological defense mechanism by which individuals attempt to suppress distressing thoughts or ideas

residual volume (RV): Volume of air that remains in the lungs at the end of a maximum expiration

respiration: Breathing

respiratory acidosis: Acidosis as a result of impaired respiration

respiratory alkalosis: Alkalosis as a result of excessive ventilation

restraints: A device used to prevent the movement of patients to protect them from injury

reticular activating system: System that functions in general wakefulness and causes awakening from deep sleep

retina: Innermost layer of the eye that has specialized nerve cells sensitive to light and color

retractions: Shortening or drawing in of the intercostal and clavicle muscles; an indication of respiratory distress

retrograde amnesia: Inability to remember events before a traumatic injury (see *antegrade amnesia*)

retroperitoneal space: Area behind the peritoneum

Reye's syndrome: Rare, acute life-threatening disease that affects all age groups; peak incidence is between 4 and 15 years; the etiology is unclear

rhonchi: Abnormal coarse, rattling breath sound caused by fluid in the large airways

right ventricular failure: Inability of the right side of the heart to effectively pump blood, resulting in back-pressure of blood into the systemic venous circulation

roentgen: Common unit of radiation measurement

rollover collision: Vehicle flips over after being hit

rotation: Turning of a part on its own axis

rotational collisions: Vehicle is hit at an angle and spins

rubella: Viral disease transmitted by direct contact with nasopharyngeal secretions from an infected individual

rubeola: Red measles

rule of nines: Method to estimate the extent of injury to a burn patient in which areas of the body are given percentages related to 9 and totaled to estimate the total burned body surface area

rule of palms: Method to estimate the extent of injury to a burn patient; assuming that the palm size of the burn patient is about 1% of the total body surface area, it estimates the number of "palms" that are burned to approximate the percentage of the total burned area

run report: A factual, complete testimonial of the condition of the patient, emergency management, and the results of the interaction between the patient and the paramedic

run reviews: Reviews of the entire run that can be used to expose gaps or identify needed additions to operational and treatment protocols

R wave: First positive deflection after the P wave

sacral spine: Four to five bones fused together and five nerve roots located between the lumbar and coccyx vertebrae

sagittal: An imaginary line that divides the body into right and left halves

satellite receiver system: Strategically placed remote receivers that receive signals from a mobile radio

scabies: Highly communicable skin disease caused by arachnids, especially mites

scene control: Paramedic's control of the scene to insure personal safety and to be able to properly assess and manage the patient

scene survey: Quick, yet observant, evaluation of potential hazards, mechanism of injury, and clues to medical illness that are provided by the patient's environment

Schedule I drugs: Drugs that do not have a medical use, such as heroin, LSD, peyote, mescaline, and marijuana

Schedule II drugs: Drugs that have a medical use but a high abuse potential, such as morphine, codeine, cocaine, meperidine, and several amphetamines and barbiturates

Schedule III drugs: Drugs used in medical care but that have less abuse potential than Schedule II drugs, including combinations of codeine and other drugs, such as aspirin with codeine and Tylenol with codeine

Schedule IV drugs: Drugs similar to Schedule III but for which the penalties of illegal possession are less severe; drugs in this schedule include Valium, Librium, Talwin, and Darvon

Schedule V drugs: Drugs that have a low potential for abuse and in many states may be dispensed without a prescription, including several cough preparations that contain codeine

school age: 5–12 years old

sclera: Tough outer coat of the eye

sebaceous glands: Oil-secreting glands of the skin

secondary survey: Assessment tool that includes a patient interview, is a more thorough physical evaluation, and proposes to find less obvious and less acute problems than those evaluated in the primary survey

second degree AV block: Cardiac arrhythmia in which atrial impulses are not conducted to the ventricles, resulting in nonconducted P waves on EKG; generally classified into type I (Wenckebach or Mobitz Type I) and type II (Mobitz Type II)

sedative: An agent that exerts a soothing or tranquilizing effect

seizure: Manifestation of a massive electrical discharge of one or more groups of neurons in the brain

self-contained breathing apparatus (SCBA): Respiratory protection device that provides a totally enclosed system of air; used by the fire service

self-contained underwater breathing apparatus (SCUBA): Respiratory protection device that provides a totally enclosed system of air; used by divers

sella turcica: An indentation of the sphenoid bone in which rests the pituitary gland

semilunar valves: Aortic valve located between the left ventricle and aorta, and the pulmonic valve located between the right ventricle and pulmonary artery

semipermeable membrane: A membrane that allows some molecules in a solution to pass through, but not others

sensitization: Exposure to allergens and the resulting production of antibodies

septicemia: Pathogenic bacteria in the blood; if left untreated, the organisms multiply, causing serious infections

sexual abuse: Molestation, touching, or fondling of a child's genitals or asking the child to do so to the adult

sexual assault: Violent and forced sexual attack on a person

shock: Lack of oxygen at the cellular level, leading to anaerobic metabolism; inadequate tissue perfusion or oxygenation (see *compensated, uncompensated, cardiogenic,* and *irreversible shock*)

shoulder lie: The position in which the fetus lies perpendicular to the mother in a transverse lie during delivery; the shoulder may become wedged in the pelvic canal

sickle cell anemia: A hereditary chronic form of anemia in which abnormal or crescent-shaped erythrocytes are present

sighing: Slow, deep inspiration followed by prolonged expiration

signature of release: Witnessed statement in writing from a patient who refuses treatment or transport

simple mask: A breathing device that can deliver as much as 60% oxygen at 7 to 8 L/min

simple pneumothorax: Pneumothorax that results from a fractured rib that punctures lung tissue, allowing air into the pleural space, or from a blunt force to the chest that simply ruptures a weak portion of the lung tissue, allowing air leakage into the pleural space; it is also possible for a simple pneumothorax to occur spontaneously in an otherwise normal patient for no apparent reason

simplex system: Ability to transmit or receive, but not both simultaneously

sinoatrial (SA) or sinus node: Located in the right atrium, it is the normal dominant pacemaker of the heart

sinus arrest: Failure of the SA node to discharge, manifested by the absence of an electrical activity on EKG

sinus arrhythmia: Rhythm that results from an irregular discharge rate of the SA node; frequently a normal phenomenon in young and aged patients

sinus bradycardia: Rhythm that results when the discharge rate of the SA node decreases to less than 60 per minute

sinus tachycardia: An increase in the discharge rate of the SA node to greater than 100 per minute

skeletal muscle: All muscle that is predominantly under voluntary control (also called striated muscle)

slander: Similar to libel, it pertains to verbal defamatory statements about one person to another

smooth muscle: All muscle that is primarily involuntary and that makes up most of the muscular tissue of the digestive tract, bronchi, urinary bladder, and blood vessels (also called visceral muscle)

sneeze: Forceful exhalation from the nose, usually caused by nasal irritation

sodium: Chief extracellular ion in the blood plasma

soma: Cell body that composes each neuron

sovereign immunity: If allowed, it relieves governmental employees from liability for certain types of negligent acts

spinal cord: Two-way path for conducting impulses to and from the brain; it is also a reflex center

spinal nerves: Nerves that extend from each of the 31 spinal nerve roots and branch to the skin to transmit signals of pain, temperature, and touch to the spinal cord

spinal shock: Shock secondary to spinal injury

spiral fracture: Usually results from twisting injuries; the fracture line has the appearance of a spiral or S shape

spirits: Concentrated alcoholic solutions of volatile substances, also called essences

sprain: Injury in which ligaments are stretched or even partially torn

squelch: Special receiver circuit that suppresses the unwanted radio noise, which would otherwise be heard between transmissions

standard of care: Basis for evaluating a claim of negligence

standing orders: Authorizations for specific patient treatments to be administered without the presence of a physician

station: Presenting part of the fetus and its relationship to the mother's ischial spines

status asthmaticus: Severe prolonged asthmatic attack that does not respond to therapy

status epilepticus: Epileptic attacks in rapid succession with no regaining of consciousness

sternum: Dagger-shaped structure that supports the medial part of the anterior chest wall

stopping distance: Reaction distance plus braking distance

strain: Soft tissue injury or muscle spasm that occurs around a joint anywhere in the musculature (also called a muscle pull)

stress: State of physical and psychological arousal that appears as a response to some external stimulus

stressor: External stimulus that results in stress

stretch: To draw out or extend to full length

stridor: Harsh sounding respirations due to airway obstruction

stroke: Sudden interruption in blood flow to the brain with resultant neurologic deficits

stroke volume: Amount of blood ejected by the left ventricle with each contraction of the heart

ST segment: Distance between the S wave of the QRS complex and the beginning of the T wave on an EKG

stylet: Soft metal wire placed inside the endotracheal tube to help guide it into the trachea

subarachnoid hemorrhage: Bleeding that occurs between the arachnoid membrane and the pia mater

subarachnoid space: Area below the arachnoid membrane but above the pia mater that contains cerebrospinal fluid *subcutaneous (SQ, SC):* Administration of a drug by injection into the fatty tissue beneath the skin

subcutaneous connective tissue: Adherent layer of adipose tissue just below the dermal layer

subcutaneous emphysema: Dilatation of the subcutaneous space due to the presence of air

subdural hematoma: Bleeding that occurs between the dura mater and arachnoid membrane, usually as a result of injury

subdural space: Space between the dura mater and arachnoid

suction: Procedure that uses negative pressure to withdraw foreign material from the posterior pharynx

suction catheter: Flexible, narrow plastic tube that uses air pressure to remove blood, mucous, or other body fluids

sudden infant death syndrome (SIDS): Sudden and unexpected death of an infant or young child; the etiology is uncertain

suffix: Last part of a word

suicide: Taking of one's own life

superficial (first-degree) burn: Burn confined to the epidermal layers of the skin

superficial frostbite: Frostbite that affects superficial tissue

superior: On top or toward the head

supine: Lying on the back face upward; also the position of the hand or foot facing upward; opposite of prone

suppository: A mixture of a drug in a firm base that melts at body temperature

surfactant: Fluid that prevents the alveoli from collapsing by lowering fluid surface tension along the alveolar walls

surgical cricothyroidotomy: An incision through the cricothyroid space (see *cricothyroidotomy*)

surname: A person's last name

S wave: First negative deflection after the R wave

sweat glands: Route for evaporative heat loss

sympathetic division: Division of the autonomic nervous system; operating without conscious control, it provides systemic effects that result in the "fight or flight" phenomenon that prepares the body for physical and mental emergencies (see *general adaptation syndrome*)

synapse: Area between two neurons in which the connecting impulse travels

synchronized cardioversion: Defibrillation in which the shock is set to deliver during the down slope of the R wave or within the S wave and thus avoids stimulation during the heart's relative refractory period

syncope: Temporary loss of consciousness due to transient inadequate blood flow to the brain

synergistic: In reference to drugs, having a greater effect when combined with other drugs than when administered alone

synovial joint: Freely movable joint; synovial cavity and articular cartilage present

syphilis: Sexually transmitted disease present throughout the world; causative organism is the spirochete *Treponema pallidum*

syrup: Aqueous solution of 85% sucrose

syrup of ipecac: Most effective way to induce emesis; its components are absorbed in the small intestine and act on the region of the brain stem that triggers vomiting

systemic vascular resistance: See *peripheral vascular resistance*

systole: Portion of the cardiac cycle during which the heart is contracting; it usually occurs between the first and second heart sound when blood is being ejected through the aorta and pulmonary artery

systolic pressure: Maximum pressure against the arteries when the heart contracts

tablet: Powdered drug formed into small disks

tachyphylaxis: State in which a person's tolerance for a drug develops so rapidly that it can have no pharmacologic effect

tachypnea: Rapid respirations; in an adult, more than 25 breaths per minute

telemetry: In EMS communications systems, the use of the communications system to transmit patient data, typically an EKG

temporary cavity: Shortly after impact tissues move back to their original position

tenderness: Demonstrating an increased sensitivity to touch

tendon: Tough, whitish cord at the end of most voluntary muscles, by which they are attached to the bones that they move

tension pneumothorax: Pneumothorax that may result from the same mechanisms that cause a simple pneumothorax except that the leakage of air into the pleural space continues to occur, with no avenue of escape from the pleural space for the accumulating air and pressure

testes: Paired oval glands in males located outside the body and suspended in the scrotum; they function in the production and secretion of testosterone

tetanus: Disease caused by a soil bacterium introduced into open wounds

thalamus: With the hypothalamus, it forms the diencephalon

thermal burn: Burn that results from heat conducted by hot liquids, solids, and super-heated gases, as well as a flame burn that result from fire

thermostasis: The body's control of temperature

third degree AV block: Complete heart block; total absence of conduction between atria and ventricles due to complete electrical block at or below the AV node

thoracentesis: The fastest and easiest treatment for a tension pneumothorax; a needle is inserted into the wall of the affected chest to relieve the accumulating pressure (also called a needle chest decompression)

thoracic spine: Twelve thoracic vertebrae below the cervical spine that correspond to twelve nerve roots

thrombophlebitis: Inflammation in veins, particularly in the lower extremities

thyroid gland: Highly vascular endocrine gland that plays a major role in the regulation of metabolism, growth and development, and calcium balance; it secretes the hormones triiodothyronine, thyroxine, and calcitonin

thyroid-stimulating hormone (TSH): Hormone that acts on the thyroid gland, promoting growth of the gland as well as increased synthesis and release of thyroid hormones

thyroxine (T_4): Hormone released by the thyroid gland

tidal volume (V_T): Volume of air normally inhaled or exhaled during each respiratory cycle

tilt test: An assessment tool to measure vital signs

tincture: Chemical or plant substance dissolved in an alcoholic solution

GLOSSARY

T lymphocytes: Agents responsible for antibody production

toddler: 1–3 years old

tongue: Located in the oropharynx, it assists with speech and the swallowing of food

tonsil tip: See *yankauer*

topical: Administration of a drug through a surface membrane, such as the skin and mucous membranes

torsades de pointes: Condition in which the polarity of the complexes on the EKG constantly shifts, giving the rhythm strip a twisted appearance; may be caused by several disorders, including electrolyte imbalances and acute ischemia, and commonly is an effect of certain antiarrhythmic agents that increase the QT interval

tort: Any wrongful act that does not involve a breach of contract and from which a civil suit can be brought

total lung capacity (TLC): Volume of air in the lungs after a maximum inhalation

trachea: Tube, 1.5 to 2.5 cm in diameter, that runs from the larynx to the carina, where it splits into the left and right primary bronchi

tracheal tugging: Pulling inward on tissue at the neck

transient ischemic attacks: Temporary interference of blood supply to the brain, usually the result of carotid artery disease; symptoms of cerebral dysfunction last from minutes to several hours

translaryngeal jet ventilation: Placement of a catheter through the cricothyroid space (see *cricothyroidotomy*)

transtentorial herniation: Condition that occurs when the falx cerebri is displaced

transverse: Plane that divides the body or any of its parts horizontally into superior and inferior portions; sometimes referred to as a cross section

transverse fracture: The fracture line is more or less at right angles to the long axis of the bone

triage: Process of prioritization of medical care, treatment, and transportation

tricuspid valve: Three-cuspid valve between the right atrium and ventricle of the heart

tricyclic antidepressant: Effective antidepressant medication prescribed to suicidal patients

triiodothyronine (T₃): Hormone released by the thyroid gland

tuberculosis: Airborne communicable disease caused by the tubercle bacillus *Mycobacterium tuberculosis*

turnout gear: Protective clothing designed for structural fire fighting

T wave: Rounded wave that follows and is usually in the same direction as the QRS complex; it indicates ventricular repolarization

tympanic membrane: Eardrum

type I second degree AV block: An intermittent block in which the AV junction becomes progressively slower in transmitting the sinus impulse over a series of cycles, until it finally blocks an impulse completely (also called *Mobitz I* or *Wenckebach*)

type II second degree AV block: An intermittent block producing P-waves that are not conducted, but it does not have any prolongation of the P–R interval before the dropped QRS complex (also called *Mobitz II*)

ultra-high frequency (UHF): Frequency band that extends from about 300 MHz to 3000 MHz; in EMS communications, typically refers to frequencies in the 450- to 470-MHz range

umbilical cord: Cord that carries oxygen and nutrients from the mother to the fetus and blood with waste products from the fetus

uncompensated shock: Shock that occurs when the compensatory mechanisms in compensated shock are unsuccessful; a systolic blood pressure cannot be maintained and perfusion to ischemia-sensitive organs is inadequate

United States Pharmacopeia: Government publication that lists the official name of a drug

universal precautions: Concept that the blood and body fluids of all persons should be considered potentially infectious for HIV, hepatitis B virus, and other blood-borne pathogens

upper airway: One of the four subsystems of the respiratory system

uterine inversion: Rare event in which the uterus turns inside out after birth

uterine rupture: Rare event in which the wall of the uterus ruptures when it is unable to withstand the strain placed on it

uterus: An organ of the female reproductive system for containing and nourishing the embryo and fetus from the time the fertilized egg is implanted to the time of birth of the fetus

vagina: In females, a muscular tube extending from the uterus to the vulva; it serves as a passageway for menstrual flow and a receptacle for the penis during sexual intercourse

vaginal show: One sign of labor; vaginal discharge that occurs when the presenting fetal part ruptures maternal capillaries; it is pinkish in color and contains some cervical mucus

vagus nerve: Tenth cranial nerve; it has both motor and sensory functions and is responsible for parasympathetic innervation to the heart

vallecula: A depression or crevice; the depression between the epiglottis and the root of the tongue, on either side of the median glossoepiglottic fold

Valsalva's maneuver: Action in which a person strains and bears down as if having a bowel movement

valvular heart disease: Problems with the mechanical functioning of heart valves; stenosis, regurgitation, and prolapse are the three most common problems

varicella: Member of the herpesvirus family and the cause of chickenpox

vehicle transmission: Transmission of disease through the ingestion of infected food or matter

velocity: Speed

ventricles: Two thick-muscled lower chambers of the heart

ventricular escape complexes and rhythms: Idioventricular rhythm that occurs when the ventricle takes over as pacemaker for the heart and creates an escape complex or rhythm at a rate of 20 to 40 per minute, the inherent rate of the ventricles

ventricular fibrillation: Quivering and twitching of the heart due to disorganized electrical activity in the ventricles; ventricular contractions are aberrant and ineffectual

ventricular tachycardia: Continuous broad, rapid ventricular contractions on EKG; a life-threatening arrhythmia

Venturi mask: Specialized mask that enables delivery of precise concentrations of oxygen between 24% and 50%

vertebrae: 24 irregularly shaped bones that are part of the spinal column

vertebral foramen: Central opening to the vertebrae that serves as a protective casing or tunnel through which the spinal cord passes

very-high frequency (VHF): Frequency band that extends from about 30 MHz to 300 MHz; in EMS communications, typically refers to frequencies either in the 30- to 50-MHz range ("low band") or the 150- to 175-MHz range ("high band")

vial: Glass or plastic container that has a self-sealing rubber stopper in the top, from which multiple doses may be drawn

vial of life: Container that lists a patient's medical history and medications

vital capacity (VC): Largest volume measured during complete expiration after the deepest inspiration

vital signs: Important to the secondary survey, vital signs to be assessed include respiration, pulse, and blood pressure

vitreous body: Cavity behind the lens of the eye filled with the vitreous humor

vitreous humor: Clear jelly that fills the vitreous body

vocal cords: Two thin reedlike folds of tissue within the larynx that vibrate as air passes between them producing sounds that are the basis of speech

volume of dead space gas (V_D): The volume, approximately 150 mL, that does not participate in pulmonary gas exchange

vulva: External structures of the female genitalia

wandering atrial pacemaker: Cardiac arrhythmia that occurs when the pacemaker site shifts from the SA node to other foci in the atria and AV junction and then moves back to the SA node; often a normal phenomenon in young and aged patients

warm zone: In a hazardous materials incident, the area outside of the hot zone, where personal protection is not required (see *cold* and *hot zones*)

Wenckebach: A form of incomplete heart block in which there is progressive lengthening of the P–R interval until there is not a ventricular response, and then the cycle of increasing P–R intervals begins again (see *Type I second degree AV block*)

wheezes: High-pitched musical sounds that indicate narrowing of the airways from any cause

whiplash: Severe cervical strains

Wolff–Parkinson–White syndrome: Preexcitation syndrome that occurs when the atria uses accessory conduction pathways to stimulate the ventricles earlier than is expected from the normal conduction syndrome; paroxysmal tachycardia frequently occurs in these patients

word root: Part of a medical term that usually indicates the tissue, organ, or body system that is involved, such as derma- (skin), nephro- (kidney), and neuro- (nerve)

written record: Legal medical record of the incident that should include complete, accurate, and legible information pertinent to the call

xiphoid process: Small cartilaginous projection located on the lowest portion of the sternum

yankauer: Rigid-tipped suction device used to remove secretions and foreign matter from the oropharynx (also called tonsil tip)

Index

Page numbers followed by *f* indicate figures; those followed by *t* indicate tabular material.

A

Abandonment, as basis of liability, 26–27
Abbreviations, 80, 124
 list of, 81
Abdomen. *See also specific organs and organ systems*
 acute, 563–566
  assessment of, 564–565
  management of, 566
  pathophysiology of, 563–564
  physical examination in, 565–566
 anatomy and physiology of, 560f, 560–561
 examination of, 118–119, 563–564
 inspection and palpation of, procedure for, 100, 100f
 muscles of, 351t, 353f
 pain in
  assessment of, 565, 565f, 698–699
  conditions causing, 563–564
  in pelvic inflammatory disease, 699
 quadrants of, 342, 560, 560f
 trauma to, 341–347
  assessment of, 344–346
  in children, 681
  closed and open, 342
  complications of, 342–343, 343t
  large intestine injury and, 344
  liver injury and, 343–344
  management of, 346
  mechanisms of, 342
  patient approach and, 345
  penetrating, 272
  small intestine injury and, 344
  splenic injury and, 343
  sports injuries and, 281
  stomach injury and, 344
Abdominal distention, 563
Abdominopelvic cavity, 82, 85f, 560
Abduction, 82, 84f, 365
Aberrant conduction, 491, 492f, 494–495
Abortion, 702–703
 types of, 702
Abrasion, 288, 289f
Abruptio placentae, 704, 704f
Absorption, of hazardous materials, 641
Abstinence syndromes
 alcoholism and, 599
 drug abuse and, 597–598
Abuse
 of children. *See* Child abuse
 of elders, 664–665, 726–727
  risk factors for, 664
 emotional, of children, 681
 sexual, of children, 681, 682, 683
 of spouse, 726–727
Abuse laws, 21–22
Accelerated idioventricular rhythm, 470
Accelerated junctional rhythm, 467, 502t–503t
Accelerated ventricular rhythm, 502t–503t
Acceleration, 265
Acceptance, in grieving process, 71–72
Access, to patient, gaining, 47–48, 48f
Accessory muscles, respiratory, 383, 383f
Accidents
 in children, 672–673
 vehicular. *See* Vehicular accidents
Acetaminophen, overdose of, 592
Acetylcholine, 547, 548
 cardiac function and, 414
Acetylcholinesterase inhibition, 587
Achilles tendon, 352t, 354f
Acid(s), 187
 ingestion of, 584–585
Acid-base balance, 187f, 187–191
 clinical abnormalities of, 189f, 189–190
 management of, 191
 compensation mechanisms and, 188–189
 buffer systems and, 188
 kidney function and, 189, 189t
 respiration and, 188–189
Acidosis, 188
 metabolic, 190f, 190–191, 530
 respiratory, 189, 189f

INDEX

Acquired immunodeficiency syndrome (AIDS), 609f, 609–611, 610t
ACTH (adrenocorticotropin; corticotropin), 525
Activase (tissue plasminogen activator; r-TPA), 820–821
Activated charcoal (Charcola), 766
 in poisoning and overdose, 584, 766
Active transport, 181
Acute abdomen. See Abdomen, acute
Adduction, 82, 84f, 365
Adenohypophysis, 525
Adenosine (Adenocard), 766–767
Adenosine (Adeoncard), in paroxysmal supraventricular tachycardia, 453
Adenosine triphosphate, 355
ADH (antidiuretic hormone; vasopressin), 525
Adipose (fatty) tissue, 287
 insulin and, 529
Administrative law, 20–21
Adolescents, developmental approach to, 672t
Adrenal glands, 527–528
 adrenal cortex and, 528
  hormones of, 524t, 528
 adrenal medulla and, 528
  heat transfer and, 622
  hormones of, 524t, 528
Adrenalin. See Epinephrine
Adrenocorticotropin (ACTH; corticotropin), 525
Adsorbents, 766, 834
Adult Glasgow Coma Scale, 119, 121, 762, 763
Adult Trauma Score, 119, 763
Advanced cardiac life support protocols
 for asystole, 481, 481f
 for bradycardia, 483, 484f
Adventitia, 407
AEIOU TIPS, coma and, 551
Aerobic metabolism, 176
Aeromedical transport, 14f, 14–15, 49
 application of, 14
 of divers, 633
 helicopter safety and, 15, 15f
 indications for use of, 14
 landing zone and, 14–15, 15f
Affective disorders. See also Behavioral and psychiatric disorders; Depression
 in geriatric patients, 659

Afferent (sensory) neurons, 538, 539f
Age. See also specific age groups
 burn injuries and, 296
Aging. See also Geriatric patients
 anatomy and physiology of, 651–653
  cardiovascular system and, 651–652
  gastrointestinal system and, 653
  musculoskeletal system and, 653
  nervous system and, 652–653
  renal system and, 652
  respiratory system and, 651
Agonal rhythm, 506t–507t
AICDs (automatic implantable cardioverter-defibrillators), 512
AIDS (acquired immunodeficiency syndrome), 609f, 609–611, 610t
Air bags, 273
Airborne transmission, 603
Air embolism, 318–319
 in decompression sickness, 632f, 632–633
 management of, 632f, 632–633632–633
Air trapping, 384
 in chronic obstructive pulmonary disease, 394, 394f, 395f
Airway (of respiratory system). See also Airway obstruction; Lower airway; Upper airway
 allergic reactions and, 574
 checking, 103
  in burn injuries, 298
  in poisoning and overdose, 582
 procedure for, 94, 94f
 in shock, 194
 in children, 671
 management of. See Airway management
 of newborn, 714
Airway management
 in children, 684–685
  cricothyroidotomy and, 685
  endotracheal intubation and, 684–685, 685t
  nasopharyngeal airway and, 684
  oropharyngeal airway and, 684
  resuscitation bags and, 684
  resuscitation mask and, 684

 coma and, 551
 drowning and, 629
 stroke and, 555
Airway obstruction, 128–129, 393
 assessment of, 393
 in children, 676–677
  anaphylaxis and, 677
  face and neck injuries and, 677
  foreign bodies and, 676–677
 finger sweeps in, 130
 foreign bodies and, performance sheets for, 129, 676–677, 750–751, 753–754, 756–757, 761
 foreign body aspiration and, 129
 fractures larynx and airway trauma and, 129
 laryngeal edema and, 129
 laryngeal spasm and, 129
 management of, 393
 pathophysiology of, 393
 by tongue, 128–129
Airways (devices)
 esophageal gastric tube, 139, 155, 155f
  procedure for, 160–164, 161f–164f
 esophageal obturator, 139, 155, 155f
  equipment for, 155, 160
  procedure for, 160–164, 161f–164f
 nasopharyngeal, 136, 136f, 141, 393
  pediatric, 684
 oropharyngeal, 135f, 135–136, 393
  pediatric, 684
 pharyngo-tracheal lumen, 139, 149, 149f, 154–155
  equipment for, 154–155
  procedure for, 156–160, 156f–160f
Albuterol (Proventil; Ventolin), 767–768
 in bronchospasm, in children, 679
 in chronic obstructive pulmonary disease, 398, 399t
Alcohol ingestion
 cautions regarding management of intoxicated patient and, 27
 hypothermia and, 624
 management of, 585
  ethanol (ethyl alcohol) and, 585
  ethylene glycol and, 585

isopropanol (isopropyl alcohol) and, 585
methanol (methyl alcohol) and, 585
Alcoholism, 598–599
abstinence syndromes and, 599
acute intoxication and, 598
Antabuse and, 598–599
chronic, 598
Alkali, 188
ingestions of, 584
Alkalosis, 188
metabolic, 191
respiratory, 190
Allergens, 573f, 573–574
inhaled, 574
Allergic reactions, 571–577
allergens and, 573f, 573–574
anaphylactic, 573, 575–577
assessment of, 575–576
in children, 677
management of, 576–577
insect bites and stings and, 590
management of, 576–577
to marine animals, 590–591
pathophysiology of, 574t, 574–575, 575f
prevention and education and, 576–577
Allergy(ies), 573. *See also* Allergic reactions
asking questions about, 107
Alpha agents, 832
α particles, 642
Alupent (metaproterenol sulfate), 797–798
in chronic obstructive pulmonary disease, 397f, 397–398, 399t
Alveolar-capillary interface, 381
Alveolar ventilation (V_A), 384
Alveoli, 381
hyperinflated, in chronic obstructive pulmonary disease, 394, 395f
Alzheimer's disease, 659
Ambulances. *See* Transportation; Vehicle(s)
American Ambulance Association, 8
American Association of Poison Control Centers, 581
American Hospital Association, accreditation requirements of, 13
American Society of Hospital Based Emergency Air Medical Services (ASH-BEAMS), 8

Aminoglycosides, 839
Aminophylline. *See* Theophylline ethylenediamine
Ammonia
anhydrous, poisoning and, 586–587
aromatic (smelling salts), hysterical seizures and, 553
Amnesia, 313–314
antegrade, 313
retrograde, 110, 313
Amniotic fluid, 694
meconium in, 717
Amniotic sac, 694
Amphetamines, 594t–595t
abuse of, 596–597
Ampulla, of fallopian tube, 690
Amputation, 290, 290f, 291f
complete, 290
degloving, 290
management of, 291
partial, 290
Amyl nitrate, 768–769
in cyanide poisoning, 586
Anaerobic metabolism, 176
Analgesics
allergic reaction to, 573
common home medications and, 834, 839
gaseous, 805–806
narcotic, 829
non-narcotic, 829
over-the-counter, overdose of, 592
for urinary tract, 834
Anaphylactic reaction, 573
airway obstruction and, in children, 677
assessment of, 575–576
management of, 576–577
Anaphylaxis, 573
Anastomoses, 413
Anatomical directions, 82, 83f
Anatomical planes, 82, 83f
Androgens, 528, 836
Anectine (succinylcholine chloride), 821–822
Anemia, sickle cell, 185
Anesthetics
local, allergic reaction to, 573
topical, 838–839
Aneurysm, 428–429
aortic
abdominal, 428–429, 429f, 564
dissecting, 429f, 429–430, 430f
thoracic, 429f, 429–430, 430f
of arteriovenous fistula, 567

Anger, in grieving process, 71
Angina pectoris, 419–420
stable and unstable, 420
Angular pattern, of motorcycle injuries, 279
Anions, 183
Ankle, bones of, 362, 363, 363f
Anorexia, in diabetic ketoacidosis, 531
Antabuse (disulfiram), 598–599
Antacids, 834–835
Anterior chamber, 306, 307f
Anterior (ventral) direction, 82, 83f
Anterior nares (nostrils), 309
Antianginal drugs, 831
Antiarrhythmic drugs, 766–767, 771, 794–795, 814–815, 816–817, 830–831
Antibody, 186, 572
Anticholinergics, 779–780
gastrointestinal, 835–836
Anticholinesterase inhibiting drugs, 811–812
Anticoagulant drugs, 788
Anticonvulsant drugs, 553
list of, 592
Antidepressant drugs
monoamine oxidase inhibitors, 829
tricyclic, 829
list of, 592
overdose of, 592
Antidiabetic drugs. *See* Insulin
Antidiarrheal drugs, 835
Antidiuretic hormone (ADH; vasopressin), 525
Antidotes, in cyanide poisoning, 586, 768–769
Antiemetic drugs, 835
Antigens, 186, 572, 603
Antihistamines, 779–780, 839
Antihypertensive drugs, 831–832
with diuretics, 832
Anti-infective drugs, 839–840
ophthalmic, 837–838
for skin and mucous membranes, 838
for urinary tract, 834
Anti-inflammatory drugs
for musculoskeletal system, 833
ophthalmic, 838
Antilirium (physostigmine salicylate), 811–812
Antipruritic drugs, 838–839
Antipsychotic drugs, 786–787, 830
list of, 593
overdose of, 593
Antiseptics, 839

Antispasmodic drugs, for urinary tract, 834
Antiulcer drugs, 835–836
Antivenins, for snake bites, 590
Ants, allergic reaction to, 574, 590
Anuria, 566
Anvil (incus), 304
Anxiety
  parental, 669
  separation, children and, 669
Anxiety attacks. See Hyperventilation syndrome
Anxiety states, 721t, 722t
Aorta, aneurysms of. See Aneurysm, aortic
Aortic dissection, 429f, 429–430, 430f
Aortic valve sclerosis, in geriatric patients, 656
APCO (Associated Public-Safety Communication Officers, Inc.), code sysem developed by, 38
Apgar score, 715, 716t
Aphasia, 658
Apnea, 385, 388f
Apneustic breathing, 388f
Appendicitis, 564
Appendicular skeleton, 85, 357, 359–365
Appendix, 559f, 560, 564
Apresoline (hydralazine), 789–780
Aqueous humor, 306, 307f
Aqueous solutions, 210
Aqueous suspensions, 210
Arachnoid membrane, 538
Aramine (metaraminol bitartrate), 798–799
Arc injuries, 292, 293f
Arms. See Extremities
Aromatic ammonia (smelling salts), hysterical seizures and, 553
Arousability, 109
Arousal, reticular activating system and, 311
Arrhythmias, 434–519, 502t–507t
  in acute renal failure, 566
  allergic reactions and, 574
  artificial pacemaker rhythms and, 495f, 495–501
  cardiac arrest and, 424–425, 425f
  conduction disorders and, 483f, 483–495, 484f
  electrocardiographic monitoring and, 434f–437f, 434–440, 438t, 439f, 440f, 501, 506
  etiology and mechanism of, 441f, 441–442, 442f
  in geriatric patients, 657
  management of, drugs for, 422
  myocardial infarction and, 420, 421, 422
  originating in atria, 448–461
  originating in atrioventricular junction, 462f, 462–468
  originating in sinoatrial node, 443–447
  originating in ventricles, 468–482
  resulting from decreased automaticity or conduction disturbances, prehospital interventions for, 518–519
  resulting from increased automaticity or reentry, prehospital interventions for, 506–518
  sinus, 445–446, 502t–503t
  stroke and, 555–556
Arterial blood gases, 187
Arterial occlusion, acute, 428
Arterioles, 408
Arteriosclerosis, 418
  renal circulation and, 652
Arteriovenous fistula, hemodialysis and, 567, 567f
Artery(ies), 407–408, 409f. See also Blood vessels; Circulation
  coronary, 412f, 412–413
  major, laceration of, 288, 289f
Articular cartilage, 356, 356f
Articulations. See Joints
Artifacts, electrocardiogram and, 436–437, 437f
Artificial cardiac pacemaker, 495
  heart rhythms and, 495f, 495–501
Ascending colon, 344, 559f, 560
Ascites, 118, 423
ASHBEAMS (American Society of Hospital Based Emergency Air Medical Services), 8
Aspirin, allergic reaction to, 573
Assault
  as basis of liability, 27
  sexual, 699–700, 726–727
Associated Public-Safety Communication Officers, Inc. (APCO), code system developed by, 38
Association of American Railroads Hazardous Materials System, 638
Asthma, 395
  in children, 679
  in geriatric patients, 655
Asystole, 481f, 481–482, 506t–507t
  management of, 425–426
Ataxia, 658
  in alcoholism, 598
Ataxic (Biot's) breathing, 312, 388f
Atelectasis, 399
Atherosclerosis, 418–419, 419f
  dizziness and, 658
  intimal, 418
  peripheral vascular disease and, 428
  risk factors for, 419
  stroke and, 555
  sudden death and, 424
Atria, 411, 411f
  arrhythmias originating in, 448–461
Atrial fibrillation, 457–459, 506t–507t
Atrial flutter, 455–456, 506t–507t
Atrial tachycardia (paroxysmal supraventricular tachycardia; PSVT; SVT), 452f, 452–454, 454f, 502t–503t
  multifocal, 460–461, 502t–503t
Atrioventricular (AV) blocks, 483–490
  first degree, 483–484, 504t–505t
  second degree, 485–487
    type I (Mobitz I; Wenckebach), 485, 504t–505t
    type II (Mobitz II), 487, 504t–505t
  third degree (complete heart block), 488–490, 504t–505t
Atrioventricular (AV) junction, arrhythmias originating in, 462f, 462–468
Atrioventricular (AV) node, 415
Atrioventricular (AV) valves, 411–412, 412f
Atropine sulfate, 769–770
  in arrhythmias, 518
  in insecticide poisoning, 587–588
Attitude, labor and, 705
Auricle (pinna), 304
Auscultation, 107
  abdominal trauma and, 345
  acute abdomen and, 566
  of bowel sounds, 118

INDEX **865**

of breath sounds. *See* Breath
sounds
of heart, 118, 418
cardiac-related problems and, 418
Automatic implantable cardioverter-defibrillators (AICDs), 512
Automaticity, cardiac, 415
aging and, 652
disorders of, arrhythmias and, 441, 506–519
Automobile accidents. *See* Vehicular accidents
Autonomic nervous system, 85
anatomy and physiology of, 545–548, 546f
parasympathetic division of, 546–547
anatomy and physiology of, 547–548
sympathetic division of, 546–547
anatomy and physiology of, 547
AV blocks. *See* Atrioventricular (AV) blocks
AV (atrioventricular) bundle (bundle of His; common bundle), 415
AV (atrioventricular) junction, arrhythmias originating in, 462f, 462–468
AV (atrioventricular) node, 415
AV (atrioventricular) valves, 411–412, 412f
AVPU system, 109
neurologic evaluation and, 549
Avulsion, 289f, 289–290
of tip of nose, 310
Avulsion fractures, 368, 369f
Axial loading, spinal injuries and, 319
Axial skeleton, 85, 357–359
Axons, 537, 537f

B

Back
inspection and palpation of, procedure for, 102, 102f
muscles of, 351t, 354f
Bactericidals, nasal, 127
Bag-valve-mask device, 138, 138f, 139f
in upper airway obstruction, 393
Ball-and-socket joints, 364t

Barbiturates, 591, 594t–595t
list of, 592
overdose of, 591–592
Bargaining, in grieving process, 71
Baroreceptors, 191
aging and, 652
Barotrauma, 629–633, 630f
air evacuation and, 633
gas expansion and air embolism and, 632f, 632–633
management of, 632–633
nitrogen and decompression sickness and, 630–632
management of, 631f, 631–632
Barrier protection, 45
Bartholin's glands, 692
Base (chemical), 187, 188. *See also* Acid-base balance
Base station
communicating patient data to, 122
for radio communication, 30
Basic life support skills, ability to perform, 28
Basilar skull fracture, 314–315, 315f
Battery, as basis of liability, 27
Battle's sign, basilar skull fracture and, 315
Beclomethasone dipropionate, respiratory distress and, 387t
Bee stings, allergic reaction to, 573f, 573–574, 590
Behavioral and psychiatric disorders, 596, 598, 719–732
assessment of, 723–726
emergency interview and, 723–724
factors affecting emotional states and, 725–726
information sources for, 723
mental status examination in, 724–725
transporting patient and, 725
characteristics of, 722t, 722–723
psychiatric emergency versus emotional crisis and, 722–723
child, spouse, or elder abuse and, 726–727
crisis intervention and, 728–732
controlling violent situations and, 730f, 730–732, 731f
emotional reactions to crisis and, 729
general strategies for, 729
legal ramifications of, 732

outline for, 729
severe mental disturbances and, 729–730
domestic violence and, 726
forms of, 721, 721t
in geriatric patients, 659–660
management of, 660
misconceptions about, 720–721
sexual assault and, 727
substance abuse and, 726
suicide and, 727–728, 728t
Benadryl (diphenhydramine), 779–780
in allergic and anaphylactic reactions, 576
in antipsychotic overdose, 593
Bends. *See* Decompression sickness
Benner, Ludwig, Jr., 633–634
Benzodiazepines, 591, 594t–595t
list of, 592
overdose of, 591–592
Benzoic acid, allergic reaction to, 574
Beta agonists, in chronic obstructive pulmonary disease, 398
Beta antagonists, in chronic obstructive pulmonary disease, 397
Beta blockers, 815–816, 831, 832
Betalin (thiamine; vitamin B), 826
β particles, 642
Bicarbonate-carbonic acid buffer system, 188
Biceps, 351t, 353f
Biot's (ataxic) breathing, 312, 388f
Bipolar lead, 434
Birth. *See* Delivery; Labor
Black widow spider bites, 590
Bladder, 86, 561f, 562
Blanching, 116
Blast, 281
Blast injuries, 281–282, 282f
heat and, 281–282
light and, 281
pressure and, 282
Blastocyst, 694
Blebs, in chronic obstructive pulmonary disease, 394, 394f
Bleeding. *See also* Hemorrhage
abdominal injuries and, 346
arterial, 318
gastrointestinal, conditions causing, 564
intrathoracic, 339f, 340

Bleeding (continued)
  from nose, 309
    management of, 310
  in pregnancy, third trimester, 703–704
  from scalp, control of, 317
  vaginal, traumatic and nontraumatic, 699
  venous, 318
Blindness, communicating with patient and, 105
Blood, 184–187, 185f, 186f
  blood preparations and substitutes and, 186–187
  color of, arterial versus venous bleeding and, 318
  exposure to, follow-up and, 604
  gas exchange and, 382f, 382–382
  heat transfer and, 622
  hemopoiesis and, 356–357
  loss of
    in children, 680
    exsanguination and, 318
    in geriatric patients, 662
    during labor, 705
    in pregnancy, 700
  pH of, 187
  spilled, cleaning, 613–614
  in sputum, 386
  typing of, 186, 186t
  in urine (hematuria), 567
  virus in, 607
  volume of, 178, 179f
    thoracic injuries and, 339f, 340
  vomiting, 564
Blood exposure, follow-up for, 614
Blood gases, arterial, 187
Blood glucose, hypoglycemia and hyperglycemia and, 528
Blood pressure, 111–114, 112f, 113f, 113t, 114t
  aging and, 652
  cerebral perfusion pressure and, 311
  diastolic, 111, 112
    normal, 114
    in shock, 192, 195
  elevated. See Hypertension
  head injuries and, 312
  of infant, newborn, 715
  intracranial, 311, 312
    decreasing, 317–318
  low. See Hypotension
  mean arterial pressure and, 311
  measuring, 112, 113f
    common errors in, 113, 113t

  in infants and children, 114, 670, 670t
  during pregnancy, 695
  shock and, 191, 192, 195
  systolic, 111, 112
    normal, 114
    pulsus paradoxus and, 131
    in shock, 195
  tilt test and, 114–115
Blood samples, laws regarding, 22
Blood vessels, 86, 178, 178f, 179, 180f, 407f–410f, 407–408. See also Artery(ies); Circulation; Veins
  abdominal, 343
  aging and, 652
  auscultation of, cardiac-related problems and, 418
  of brain, 539–540, 541f
  coronary, 412f, 412–413
  laceration of major and artery, 288, 289f
  of pelvic cavity, 361–362
  peripheral vascular disease and, 428–430, 429f, 430f
  thoracic, injuries of, 339f, 340
Blunt trauma. See Trauma, blunt
B lymphocytes, 603
Body cavities, 82, 84, 85f
Body language, 105
Body orientation, 82, 82f, 84
Body surface area (BSA), burn injuries and, 295–296
  Lund-Brower chart and, 296, 296f, 297f
  rule of nines and, 295f, 295–296
  rule of palms and, 295
Body systems, 84–87. See also specific systems
Body temperature, 115, 115f. See also Frostbite; Hyperthermia; Hypothermia; Thermoregulation
  in children, 670
  core, 619, 624
  of newborn, maintaining warmth and, 716
  peripheral, 619
  rectal, oral, and axillary, 115, 115f
Bone(s). See also Joints; Musculoskeletal system; Skeletal system; Skeleton
  of ear, 304
  facial, 357
  functions of, 356–357
  injuries of, 366–373. See also Dislocation(s); Fracture(s)
  metatarsal, 363, 363f

  of nose, 309
  of skull, 357, 358f
  tarsal, 362, 363, 363f
  types of, 356, 356f
Bone marrow
  hemopoiesis and, 356–357
  medullary cavity and, 356, 356f
  red, 356–357
  yellow, 357
Bottom time, 630
Botulism, 588
Bowel sounds, 118
  abdominal trauma and, 345
Boyle's law, 632
Bradycardia, 111, 502t–503t
  head injuries and, 312, 317
  management of, 425–426
  sinus, 443, 502t–503t
Bradypnea, 388f, 389
Brain
  anatomy and physiology of, 538–543
    blood supply and, 311, 539–540, 541f
    divisions and, 540–543, 541f, 542f
    meninges and, 538–539, 540f
  injuries of. See Head injuries
  meningitis and, in children, 675
  stroke and. See Stroke
Brain stem, anatomy and physiology of, 543
Braking distance, 265
Braxton-Hicks contractions, 705
Breathing, 86. See also Hyperventilation; Hyperventilation syndrome; Respiration(s); headings beginning with term Respiratory
  ataxic, 312
  checking, 103
  in burn injuries, 298–299
  in poisoning and overdose, 582
  procedure for, 94, 94f
  flail chest and, 328, 328f, 329f
  head injuries and, 312
  hemothorax and, 336, 336f
  neurologic control of, 384–385
  of newborn, 714f, 714–715
  paradoxical
    in children, 671
    flail chest and, 328
  pneumothorax and
    open, 332f, 335–336
    simple, 330–331, 331f
    tension, 331–335, 332f
  pulmonary contusion and, 328–329, 329f

rib fractures and, 327–328
ruptured diaphragm and, 329–330, 330f
Breath sounds, 117–118, 131
cardiac-related problems and, 418
in children, 671
evaluating, procedure for, 100, 100f
pneumothorax and, 327
in respiratory distress, 390f–392f, 390–391
thoracic injuries and, 327
upper airway disorders and, 131
Breech presentation, 705, 710–711, 711f
Brethine (terbutaline sulfate), 823–824
in chronic obstructive pulmonary disease, 397
Bretylium tosylate (Bretylol), 771
in arrhythmias, 510–511
Bricanyl (terbutaline sulfate), 823–824
in chronic obstructive pulmonary disease, 397
Bronchi, 380, 380f
Bronchioles, 380f, 380–381
Bronchiolitis, in children, 678f, 678–679
Bronchoconstriction, in chronic obstructive pulmonary disease, 395–396, 396f
Bronchodilators, 399t, 832–833
inhaled and systemic, 832
Bronchospasm
allergic reactions and, 574
in children, 677
bronchiolitis and, in children, 679
management of, 585
Bronkometer (isoetharine), 792
in chronic obstructive pulmonary disease, 398, 399t
Bronkosol (isoetharine), 792
in chronic obstructive pulmonary disease, 398, 399t
Brown recluse spider bites, 590
Brow presentation, 711
Bruises. See Contusion; Ecchymosis
Bruit, 418
BSA. See Body surface area
Buccinator muscle, 352t
Buffer(s), 818–819
Buffer systems, acid-base balance and, 188
Bundle branch(es), 415

Bundle-branch block, 491–493, 492f, 495
Bundle of His (AV bundle; common bundle), 415
Bunker coat, 43
Burn injuries, 292–302
body surface area calculation and, 295–296
Lund-Brower chart for, 296, 296f, 297f
rule of nines for, 295f, 295–296
rule of palms for, 295
chemical, 292, 292t
management of, 300–301
child abuse and, 682, 683, 683f
electrical, 292, 292t
arc injuries and, 292
contact burns and, 292
flame or flash burns and, 292
lightning injuries and, 292, 293f
management of, 299–300
to eye, 298, 308
management of, 301
fluid resuscitation and, 301
full-thickness (third-degree), 294t, 295, 295f
history of, 299
in infants, 681
inhalation, 297–298, 400
management of, 301
management of, 299–301
partial-thickness (second-degree), 204–295, 294f, 294t
deep, 295
superficial, 294–295
pathophysiology of, 293
local, 293
systemic, 293
patient assessment and, 298–299
prevention and patient education about, 301
radiation, 292, 292t
management of, 301
severity of, 296–297
categories of, 297, 298t
factors affecting, 296–297
sources of, 292t, 292–293
superficial (first-degree), 293–294, 294t
thermal (heat), 292, 292t, 298
management of, 299, 300t
Burnout, 68–69
Buttocks, muscles of, 351t, 354f
Bystanders
disaster management and, 61
providing roles for, 46, 92

C

Caisson disease. See Decompression sickness
Calan. See Verapamil hydrochloride
Calcaneus, 362, 363, 363f
Calcitonin, 526
Calcium
bones and, 357
in hypocalcemia and hypercalcemia, 527
osteoporosis and, 660
Calcium channel blockers, 803–804, 826–828, 831
Calcium chloride, 772
Calcium gluconate, 772
Canadian Transportation Emergency Center (CANUTEC), 638
Cancer, of intestine and rectum, in geriatric patients, 661
Cannabis, 596t–597t
CANUTEC (Canadian Transportation Emergency Center), 638
Capillaries, 178, 178f, 408, 409f
alveolar-capillary interface and, 381
Capillary refill test, 116
dislocations and, 370
in shock, 194
Capsules, 210
Carbamate insecticide poisoning, 587–588
Carbolic acid (phenol), burn injuries and, 300
Carbon dioxide
acid-base balance and, 187
arterial partial pressure of ($PaCO_2$), 381
during pregnancy, 695
gas exchange and, 381–382, 382f
inhalation of, 586
venous partial pressure of ($PvCO_2$), 381
Carbonic acid, acid-base balance and, 187, 188–189
Carbon monoxide, 400
poisoning and, 297, 585–586
Carboxyhemoglobin, 297
Cardiac arrest, 424–426, 425f, 426f
management of, 424–425, 425f
Cardiac arrhythmias. See Arrhythmias
Cardiac contusion, 336

Cardiac glycosides, 778–779, 831
Cardiac muscle, 85, 352, 355, 355f, 411, 411f
Cardiac output, 179, 414
 aging and, 651
 cardiac contusion and, 336
 cardiac tamponade and, 336–339, 339f
 during pregnancy, 695
Cardiac pacing, 495
 heart rhythms and, 495f, 495–501
 noninvasive, 519
Cardiac syncope, 417
Cardiac tamponade, 336–339, 339f, 427
 pericardiocentesis and, 339
 skill procedure for, 337–338, 337–338f
Cardiogenic shock, 424
Cardiopulmonary arrest, in children, 679–680
Cardiopulmonary resuscitation, performance sheets for, 749, 752, 755, 758–760
Cardiovascular disorders. See also Arrhythmias
 common home medications for, 830–832
 in geriatric patients, 656–658
 management of, 657–658
 patient assessment for, 416–418
 history taking in, 417
 physical examination in, 417–418
 prehospital interventions for, 430–434
 dopamine and, 432–433
 epinephrine and, 433
 furosemide and, 432
 morphine sulfate and, 431
 nitroglycerin and, 430–431
 nitrous oxide and, 431–432
 oxygen and, 430
 sodium bicarbonate and, 433–434
 theophylline ethylenediamine and, 432
Cardiovascular system, 85–86, 405–519, Color Plates 8–12. See also Artery(ies); Blood vessels; Cardiovascular disorders; Circulation; Heart; Veins
 allergic reactions and, 574
 anatomy and physiology of, 407–416
 aging and, 651–652

pulmonary circulation and, 408, 411f
 systemic circulation and, 407f–410f, 407–408
 disorders of. See Cardiovascular disorders
Cardioversion
 synchronized
 emergency, 517–518
 skill procedure for, 514–517, 514f–517f
 in ventricular tachycardia, 476, 477f
Carina, 379
Carotid sinus massage, 506–507, 507f
 contraindication to, 506
 in paroxysmal supraventricular tachycardia, 453
Carpal bones, 359, 361f
Carpopedal spasms, 402
 in hypoparathyroidism, 527
Cartilage, 356, 356f
Cartilaginous joints, 363, 364t
Cataract, 306, 307f
Catastrophic stress, 66–67
Catecholamines, 528
Catheters, for airway suctioning, 137, 137f
Cations, 183
Caudal (inferior) direction, 82, 83f
Causation, malpractice claims and, 25
Caustic ingestions, 584–585
Cavitation, penetrating trauma and, 269
 energy and, 270, 271f
 permanent cavity and, 268, 268f, 269f
 temporary cavity and, 268, 268f, 269f
Cellular immunity, 602–603
Cellular telephones, 31, 31f, 36
Central cyanosis, 131, 389
Central line placement
 femoral, procedure for, 239–241, 239f–241f
 internal jugular
 anterior approach, procedure for, 242–244, 242f–244f
 middle approach, procedure for, 245–247, 245f–247f
 posterior approach, procedure for, 248–251, 248f–251f
 subclavian approach, procedure for, 252–255, 252f–255f
Central nervous system (CNS), 85, 536. See also Brain;

Nervous system; Spinal cord
 disorders of. See also Coma; Seizures; Status epilepticus; Stroke
 in geriatric patients, 658–659
 poisoning and overdose and, 582
 respiratory disorders and, 401–402
 assessment of, 402
 management of, 402
 pathophysiology of, 401–402
Central neurogenic hyperventilation, 388f
Central syndrome, 312, 313f
Cephalic presentation, 705
Cephalopelvic disproportion, 712
Cephalosporins, 840
Cerebellum, anatomy and physiology of, 542–543
Cerebral concussion, 313–314
Cerebral contusion, 314, 314f
 contrecoup, 314
Cerebral cortex, 540
 coma and, 550–551
Cerebral edema, in children, 681
Cerebral herniation, 312, 313f
 transtentorial, 312
Cerebral perfusion pressure, 311
Cerebrospinal fluid (CSF), 305, 539
 leakage of
 from ears, 305, 306
 from nose, 309–310
Cerebrovascular accident. See Stroke
Cerebrum, 103
 anatomy and physiology of, 540, 542f
Certification, 7
 EMT-A, 16
 EMT-I, 16
 EMT-P, 16
 reciprocity and, 7
Cerumen (earwax), 304
Cervical collars, 323
Cervical spine, 357, 359f, 543
Chancre, in syphilis, 607
Charcola (activated charcoal), 766
 in poisoning and overdose, 584, 766
Charts, hazardous materials, front end paper, back end paper
Chemical(s). See Burn injuries, chemical; Hazardous materials
Chemical hazards, 46
Chemical Transportation Emergency Center (CHEMTREC), 638

Chest. *See also* Thorax
  anterior, muscles of, 351t, 353f
  examination of, 117–118
  flail, in children, 681
  injuries of. *See also* Thorax, injuries of
    in children, 681
    sucking, 332f, 335–336
  inspection and palpation of, procedure for, 99, 99f
  pain in
    angina pectoris and, 419, 420
    cardiac-related problems and, 417
    in myocardial infarction, 420–421, 657
    in pulmonary edema, 422–423
    respiratory distress and, 386
  paradoxical movement of, 118
  posterior, muscles of, 351t, 354f
Chest wall
  anatomy and physiology of, 380–382
  palpation of, in respiratory distress, 390
Cheyne-Stokes respirations, 312, 388f
Chickenpox (varicella), 606, 606f, 610t
Chief complaint, 106
Child abuse, 681–684, 726–727
  assessment of, 682f, 682–683, 683f
  characteristics of abused children and, 681–682
  characteristics of child abusers and, 682
  laws regarding, 21–22
  management of abused children and, 683–684
Child neglect, 681
Children, 667–687. *See also* Infant(s); Newborn
  accidents in, 672–673
  airway management in, 684–685
  airway obstruction in, 676–677
  approach to, 668–671, 669f
    physical examination and, 670t, 670–671
  asthma in, 679
  blood pressure measurement in, 114
  body temperature variations in, 115
  bronchiolitis in, 678f, 678–679
  cardiopulmonary arrest in, 679–680
  consent and, 26

croup in, 677f, 677–678
dehydration in, 674–675
developmental stages and, 671–672, 672t
epiglottitis in, 678, 678f
hypothermia and, 624
intraosseous insertion in, 687
intravenous fluid administration rate for, 686
intravenous insertion in, 685–687, 686f
  fluids and, 685–687
  needles and cannulas for, 685
  veins for, 687, 687f
meningitis in, 675
pedestrian injuries of, 278, 278f
problems common in, 672–673
Reye's syndrome in, 675–676, 676t
seizures in, 674
septicemia in, 675
shock in, 680
sudden infant death syndrome and, 673–674
trauma in, 680–681
Chloral hydrate, 594t–595t
Chlorine poisoning, 586–587
Chokes, 630–631
Cholecystitis (gallstones), 563
Chordae tendineae, 412, 412f
Choreoathetosis, 593
Chronic obstructive pulmonary disease (COPD), 393–399
  assessment of, 395–396, 396f
  cor pulmonale and, 427
  in geriatric patients, 655
  management of, 396–399, 397f, 398f, 399t
  pathophysiology of, 393–395, 394f, 395f
Cigarette smoking, chronic obstructive pulmonary disease and, 395
Cilia, tracheal, 379
Ciliary escalator, 379
Ciliated epithelium, of nose, 127
Circle of Willis, 540, 541f
Circulation. *See also* Artery(ies); Blood vessels; Heart; Veins
  of brain, 311, 539–540, 541f
  checking, 103, 116
    in anaphylactic reactions, 576
    in burn injuries, 299
    in poisoning and overdose, 582
  procedure for, 95, 95f
  respiratory distress and, 385

collateral, 418
  aging and, 652
fetal, 694, 696f
fractures and, 370
of newborn, 715
pulmonary, 408, 411f
systemic, 407f–410f, 407–408
Circumduction, 82, 84f, 365
CISD (Critical Incident Stress Debriefing), 62
Civil law, 20
Claudication, intermittent, 428
Clitoris, 692
Closed wounds, 288
Clubbing, of digits, 389
CMV (cytomegalovirus), 607
CNS. *See* Central nervous system
Cocaine, 594t–595t
  abuse of, 597
Coccyx (tail bone), 357, 359f, 543
Codeine, 594t–595t, 773–774
  allergic reaction to, 573
Code of ethics, 4–5
Code system, radio communication and, 37–38
Cold. *See* Frostbite; Hypothermia
Cold sores (fever blisters), 605
Cold zone, hazardous materials incidents and, 640, 641f
Colic, intestinal, 563
Colitis, ischemic, in geriatric patients, 661
Collagen fibers, 356
Collateral circulation, 418
  aging and, 652
Colles' fracture, 366
Colon (large intestine), 558, 559f, 560
  ascending, 344, 559f, 560
  cancer of, in geriatric patients, 661
  descending, 344, 559f, 560
  injuries of, 344
  sigmoid, 559f, 560
  transverse, 344, 559f, 560
Coma, 550–552. *See also* Consciousness level; Glasgow Coma Scale; Unconsciousness
  assessment of, 551
  in geriatric patients, 658
  hyperosmolar hyperglycemia nonketotic coma, 532
  hypoglycemic, 533
  management of, 551–552
  pathophysiology of, 550–551
Combining forms, of medical terms, 80
Combining vowels, in medical terms, 80

Command, disaster management and, 58, 61
Command post, for disaster management, 58, 59
Comminuted fractures, 368, 369f
Common bundle (AV bundle; bundle of His), 415
Communicable diseases, 603–611. *See also* Infectious diseases; *specific diseases*
  definition of, 603
Communication (interpersonal)
  barriers to, 105
  body language and, 105
  with geriatric patients, 653, 654f
  history taking and, 104–105
  of patient data, to patient and family, 121–122
  touching and, 105
Communication links, establishing, 35
Communications center, 33f, 33–34
Communications operator, 34f, 34–35
  assessment of scene and, 46
  communications links established by, 35
  medical instructions provided to callers by, 35
  requests for response received by, 35
  system resources allocation and monitoring by, 32, 35
  training of, 32
Communication system, 13, 29–39
  access to, 32
  communication of patient data and, 121–124
    to base station or hospital, 122
    written record and, 122, 123f, 124
  communications center and, 33f, 33–34
  communication with medical facilities and, 32
  disaster management and, 61
  duplex system of, 17
  Federal Communications Commission and, 33
  frequencies assigned to emergency medical services for, 17, 31, 33
  hazardous materials incidents and, 639, 640f, 641
  incident sequence and, 35–37
  mobile radio and, 34

911 emergency telephone number and, 16, 32, 35
  operator and. *See* Communications operator
  radio communication and, 30–31, 31f
    mobile radio and, 34
    portable radio equipment and, 34
    technique for, 37–38
    repeaters and remote receivers and, 31, 34
  resource coordination and allocation and, 32
  simplex system of, 17
  training of personnel for, 32
Compensated shock, 191–192
Competence, consent and, 25
Complete breech presentation, 705
Complete heart block (third degree AV block), 488–490
Compound presentations, 711–712
Compression, spinal injuries and, 319
Compression fractures, 368, 369f
Computers, communication and, 31, 31f
Conceptus, 702
Concussion
  cardiac, 280, 281f
  cerebral, 313–314
Conduction, cardiac, 415
  aberrant, 491, 492f, 494–495
  disorders of, arrhythmias and, 483f, 483–495, 484f, 518–519
Conduction (process), heat transfer and, 619, 621f, 716
Condyloid joints, 364t
Confidentiality
  breach of, as basis of liability, 27
  legal principle of, 24
Congenital rubella syndrome, 608
Congestion, disaster management and, 61
Congestive heart failure, 422
  in geriatric patients, 657
Conjunctiva, 306, 307f
Conjunctivitis, 306
Connective tissue, subcutaneous, 287
Consciousness, content of, 109–110
Consciousness level. *See also* Coma; Glasgow Coma Scale; Unconsciousness

  in children, 671
  evaluating, 109–110
  in poisoning and overdose, 582–583
  reticular activating system and, 311
  in shock, 194–195
Consent, 25–26
  competence and, 25
  expressed, 26
  implied, 26
  informed, 25
  involuntary, 26
  minors and, 26
Conservation of Energy law, 264–265, 265f
Consumers. *See* Patient(s)
Containers, for hazardous materials
  bulk, 636
  fixed facilities and, 635f, 635–636
  markings and colors of, 635f, 635–636
  nunbulk, 636
  shapes of, 634, 634f
Contaminated articles, disposal of, 613
Continuing education, 8
Contraceptive drugs, oral, 837
Contrecoup contusions, 314
Control, disaster management and, 61
Controller. *See* Communications operator
Contusion
  cardiac, 336
  cerebral, 314, 314f
    contrecoup, 314
  pulmonary, 328–329, 329f
    in children, 681
Contusion (bruise), 288. *See also* Ecchymosis
  cardiac, 280, 281f
  child abuse and, 682, 682f
Convection, heat transfer and, 619, 621f, 716
COPD. *See* Chronic obstructive pulmonary disease
Coping, with stress, 69–71
Coping strategies, 70–71
Copperhead bites, 590
Coral stings, 590
Corium (dermis), 86–87, 286
Cornea, 306, 307f
Coronary artery(ies), 412f, 412–413
Coronary artery disease, 418. *See also* Atherosclerosis
  arrhythmias caused by, 657

Coronary veins, 413
Cor pulmonale, 427
Corticosteroids, 774, 790, 799
    respiratory distress and, 387, 387t
    topical, 838
Corticotropin (ACTH; adrenocorticotropin), 525
Cottonmouth (water moccasin) bites, 590
Coughing, 127, 383, 386
    allergic reactions and, 574
    in croup, 677
    hemoptysis and, 386
CRAMS Scale, 121, 762
Cranial cavity, 84, 85f
Cranial (superior) direction, 82, 83f
Cranial nerves, 543, 544f
Craniosacral division. *See* Parasympathetic nervous system
Cranium, 357, 358f. *See also* Skull
    sutures of, 538
Crepitus, fractures and, 370
Crib death (SIDS; sudden infant death syndrome), 673–674
    diagnosis of, 673
    management of, 673–674
Cribriform plate, 309, 309f
Cricothyroid membrane, 164, 164f, 169
Cricothyroidotomy, 160, 164, 164f, 169, 173–174
    in children, 685
    needle, 174
        procedure for, 170–173, 170f–173f
    surgical, 173–174
        procedure for, 165–169, 165f–169f
Criminal law, 20
Crisis, 728
    emotional reactions to, 729
Crisis intervention, in behavioral and psychiatric emergencies. *See* Behavioral and psychiatric disorders, crisis intervention in
Critical care units, 13
    patient transfer between, 13
Critical incidents, disaster management and, 61–62
Critical incident stress, 66–67
Critical Incident Stress Debriefing (CISD), 62
Cromolyn sodium, respiratory distress and, 387, 387t

Croup (laryngotracheobronchitis), 677f, 677–678
Crowning, 706
Crush injuries, 288
Crying, in newborn, 715
CSF. *See* Cerebrospinal fluid
Cushing's reflex, nervous system emergencies and, 549
Cushing's syndrome, 529
Cushing's triad, 312, 317
Cutaneous membrane, 287
Cyanide poisoning, 586
    Cyanide Antidote Package and, 586, 768–769
Cyanmethemoglobin, 586
Cyanosis, 116, 131, 389
    central, 131, 389
    peripheral, 131, 389
    in shock, 194
Cysts, ovarian, 568–569
Cytomegalovirus (CMV), 607

D

Darvon (propoxyphene), overdose of, 591
Deafness, communicating with patient and, 105
Death and dying
    appearance of, in hypothermia, 626
    dealing with, 72
    exsanguination and, 318
    grieving process and, 71–72
    irreversible shock and, 193
    management of, 72
    myocardial infarction and, 420
    sudden death and, cardiac arrest and, 424–426, 425f, 426f
    sudden infant death syndrome and, 673–674
Decadron (dexamethasone sodium phosphate, 774
Deceleration (drag), 265
Deceleration injuries, 280, 281f
Decerebrate posturing (extensor response), 119, 312, 550
D.E.C.I.D.E., hazardous materials and, 638
Decompression sickness (the bends; caisson disease), 630–632
    management of, 631f, 631–632
        fluid and drug therapy in, 631–632
        recompression in, 631
    nitrogen and, 630–632

Decontamination
    hazardous materials and, 643–644
    poisoning and, 583–584
        activated charcoal in, 584
        syrup of ipecac and, 583–584
Decorticate posturing (flexor response), 119, 312, 550
Deep vein thrombophlebitis, 428
Defense mechanisms, 70
Defibrillation
    automated, 513, 517
    manual, 511–513, 512f
        skill procedure for, 514–517, 514f–517f
    in ventricular fibrillation, 480
Degloving amputation, 290
    management of, 291–292
Degradation, chemicals and, 642
Dehydration
    in children, 674–675
    heat transfer and, 622
Delirium tremens (DT's), 599
Delivery, 706t, 706–707, 708f–711f, 710. *See also* Labor
    abnormal, 710–713
        breech, 710–711, 711f
        precipitous, 713
        prolapsed umbilical cord and, 712f, 712–713
    multiple births and, 712
    postpartum hemorrhage and, 713
    premature, 694–695, 716–717
    procedure for, 706–707, 708f–711f, 710
        breech presentation and, 711
    statistics on conditions of, 706t
    uterine inversion and, 714
    uterine rupture and, 713–714
Delta wave, 452, 452f
Deltoid muscle, 351t, 353f, 354f
Delusions, 725
Dementia, 659
Demerol (meperidine), 796–797
Dendrites, 537, 537f
Denial, 70
    in grieving process, 71
Density, energy exchange and, 266
    body tissue and, 267, 267f
Depolarization, cardiac, 415–416, 416f
Depolarizing blockers, 821–822
Depressants, list of, 594t–595t
Depressed fractures, 368, 369f
    of skull, 314, 314f
Depression
    in geriatric patients, 659
    in grieving process, 71

Dermatomes, 454, 545f
Dermis (corium), 86–87, 286
DERM method, 109
Descending colon, 344, 559f, 560
Development, 671–672
Developmental stages, 671–672, 672t
Dexamethasone, respiratory distress and, 387t
Dexamethasone sodium phosphate (Decadron; Hexadrol), 774
Dextrose, 775
　in alcoholism, 598
　in coma, 552
　in diabetic ketoacidosis, 532
　in hyperosmolar hyperglycemia nonketotic coma, 532
　in hypoglycemia, 582
　　in children, 674
　in seizures, 553
Diabetes mellitus, 529
　emergencies associated with, 530–533, 531t
　types I and II, 529
Diabetic ketoacidosis, 530–532, 531t
　assessment of, 531
　management of, 532
Diagnostic signs, 109–116
Diaphoresis (profuse sweating), 389
Diaphragm, 351t
　anatomy and physiology of, 382–384, 383f
　ruptured, 329–330, 330f
Diaphysis, 356, 356f
Diastole, 413
Diastolic pressure. See Blood pressure, diastolic
Diazepam (Valium), 776–777
　in hypoglycemia, in children, 674
　in seizures, 553, 582
　　eclamptic, 703
　in status epilepticus, 554
Diazoxide (Hyperstat), 777–778
Diencephalon, anatomy and physiology of, 540, 542
Diffusion, 181, 181f, 381
Digestive system, 86, Color Plate 14, Color Plate 15. See also Gastrointestinal system; specific organs
Digital clubbing, 389
Digoxin (Lanoxin), 778–779
Dilantin (phenytoin sodium), 810–811

Dinitrous monoxide (nitrous oxide; NO$_2$), 805–806
Diphenhydramine (Benadryl), 779–780
　in allergic and anaphylactic reactions, 576
　in antipsychotic overdose, 593
Diplopia, 658
Directions, anatomical, 82, 83f
Disaster, 51–62, 52, 54f, 54–55
　common problems of, 59, 61
　emergency medical services organization for, 60f
　levels of intensity of, 52–55
　scene management and, 59–60
Disaster linkage, 13
Disaster plan, 55–62
　postdisaster phase of, 61–62
　preplan phase of, 55–56
　response plan phase of, 56–59, 61
Disc, intervertebral, 357
Disentanglement, 48, 49f
Disinfectants, 839
Dislocations, 370–373, 372f–373f
　assessment of, 370–373
　management of, 371t, 373
Dispatch, of emergency units, 36, 36f
Dispatcher. See Communications operator
Disposal
　of contaminated articles, 613
　of needles, 613
Dissecting aortic aneurysm, 429f, 429–430, 430f
Distal direction, 82, 83f
Distraction, spinal injuries and, 319
Distractions, removing from scene, 92
Disulfiram (Antabuse), 598–599
Diuresis, reflex, 622
Diuretics, 832, 833–834
　antihypertensives with, 832
　loop, 784, 834
　osmotic, 795–796
　potassium sparing, 834
　thiazide, 834
Divers. See Barotrauma
Diverticula, in geriatric patients, 661
Diverticulitis, 563–564
Dizziness (vertigo), 658
　in geriatric patients, 658–659
　trauma and, 662
DNR (do not resuscitate; no-code; no heroic measures) orders, 22

Dobutamine (Dobutrex), 780–781
Documentation. See Record keeping
Doll's eye exam, 117
Domestic violence, 726
Do not resuscitate (DNR; no-code; no heroic measures) orders, 22
Dopamine (Intropin), 781–782
　in cardiac disorders, 432–433
　in cardiogenic shock, 424
Dopplers, 114
Dorsal cavity, 82, 84, 85f
Dorsal (posterior) direction, 82, 83f
Dose, of radiation, 642
Down-and-under frontal collisions, 274–275, 275f
Drag (deceleration), 265
Drowning, 627–629, 628f
　cold water, 629
　　management of, 629
　dry, 628
　management of, 629
　near, 628
　salt versus fresh water, 628–629
　wet, 628
Drug(s), 205–260. See also specific drugs
　abuse of. See Drug abuse; Drug overdose
　administration routes and. See Drug administration
　adsorbent, 766, 834
　amphetamine, 594t–595t
　　abuse of, 596–597
　　in amphetamine abuse, 597
　analgesic, 829, 834
　　allergic reaction to, 573
　　gaseous, 805–806
　　narcotic, 773–774, 829
　　non-narcotic, 829
　　over-the-counter, overdose of, 592
　　for urinary tract, 834
　anesthetic
　　local, allergic reaction to, 573
　　topical, 838–839
　antacid, 834–835
　antianginal, 831
　antiarrhythmic, 766–767, 771, 794–795, 814–815, 816–817, 830–831
　antibiotic, 839–840
　anticholinergic, 779–780
　　gastrointestinal, 835–836
　anticholinesterase inhibiting, 811–812
　anticoagulant, 788

anticonvulsant, 553, 809–811, 829–830
  list of, 592
antidepressant, 829
  monoamine oxidase inhibitors, 829
  tricyclic, 592, 829
antidiabetic, 791–792
antidiarrheal, 835
antiemetic, 835
antihistamine, 779–780, 839
antihypertensive, 831–832
anti-infective, 834, 837–838, 839–840
anti-inflammatory, 833, 838
antipruritic, 838–839
antipsychotic, 786–787, 830
  list of, 593
  overdose of, 593
antiseptic, 839
antispasmodic, 834
antiulcer, 835–836
asking questions about, 107
in asystole, 481
in atrial fibrillation, 457
in atrial flutter, 455
in atrioventricular blocks
  third degree, 488
  type II second degree, 487
  type I second degree, 485
bactericidal, nasal, 127
barbiturate, 591, 594t–595t
  list of, 592
  overdose of, 591–592
benzodiazepine, 591, 594t–595t, 776–777
  list of, 592
  overdose of, 591–592
beta blocker, 815–816, 831, 832
bronchodilator, 399t, 832–833
  inhaled and systemic, 832
buffering, 818–819
calcium channel blocker, 803–804, 826–828, 831
calculating dosages of, 219–222
  decimals and, 220
  intravenous infusion rate calculation and, 221–222, 222f
  metric system and, 219–220
in cardiac disorders, 430–434
cardiac glycoside, 778–779, 831
central nervous system and, respiratory disorders and, 401–402
in coma, 552
contraceptive, oral, 837
controlled, uses and effects of, 594t–597t

corticosteroid, 387, 387t, 774, 790, 799, 838
cyanide poisoning antidotes and, 586, 768–769
in decompression sickness, 631–632
decreasing intracranial pressure, 318
definition of, 207
depolarizing blockers, 821–822
depressant, list of, 594t–595t
disinfectant, 839
diuretic, 832, 833–834
  antihypertensives with, 832
  loop, 784, 834
  osmotic, 795–796
  thiazide, 834
electrolytes and, 772, 813
emergency, list of, 765–828
emetic, 583–584, 822–823
features of, 207
forms of, 209, 209f, 210, 211f
in geriatric patients, 663
  drug-induced illness and, 663
  toxicity and, 663
hallucinogenic
  abuse of, 597
  list of, 594t–595t
home medications and, 829–840
hormones, 836–837
hyperglycemic, 775, 785–786
hypoglycemic, 836
laxative, 835
legislation affecting, 207–208
methylxanthine, 824–825
miotic, 838
mood stabilizing, 830
muscle relaxant, 833
mydriatic, 838
in myocardial infarction, 422
names of, 208–209
narcotic agonist, 796–797, 800–802
narcotic antagonist, 801–803
ophthalmic, 837–838
overdose of. See Drug overdose
parasympatholytic, 769–770
in paroxysmal supraventricular tachycardia, 453
pediculocidal, 838
pharmacodynamics of, 215–219
  autonomic nervous system and, 215–219, 216t
pharmacokinetics of, 209, 211–215, 212f
  absorption and, 211–214
  biotransformation and elimination and, 215

distribution and, 214f, 214–215
pituitary hormones and, 808–809
in premature ventricular complex, 472, 472f
in pulmonary edema, 423
references and resources for, 209
scabicidal, 838
sedative/hypnotic, 830
in seizures, 553
in sinus arrest, 447
in sinus bradycardia, 443
sources of, 207
stimulant
  abuse of, 596–597
  list of, 594t–595t
sympathomimetic, 767–768, 780–784, 792–793, 797–799, 806–807, 817–818, 823–824
  in chronic obstructive pulmonary disease, 396–397, 397f, 397–398
  respiratory distress and, 387, 387t
in tachycardia, 422
thrombolytic, 820–821
torsades de pointes and, 479
urinary tract anti-infectives/analgesics/antispasmodics, 834
vasodilator, 777–778, 789–790, 804–805, 819–820, 832
in ventricular escape complexes and rhythms, 468
in ventricular fibrillation, 480
in ventricular tachycardia, 476
vitamins and, 826
Drug abuse, 593–598. See also Drug overdose
abstinence syndromes and, 597–598
behavioral emergencies and, 726
narcotics and, 593, 596
reactions to substances and, 726
solvents and, 597
stimulants and, 596–597
Drug administration, 222–259
endotracheal, 255, 259
  in chronic obstructive pulmonary disease, 397f, 397–398
  epinephrine and, 397
intradermal, 224–226
  absorption and, 213

Drug administration, intradermal (*continued*)
　　procedure for, 225–226, 225f–226f
　intramuscular, 227, 230f
　　absorption and, 213
　　procedure for, 231–232, 231f–232f
　intraosseous, 234, 247, 251, 255–259
　　in children, 687
　　procedure for, 256–259, 256f–259f
　intravenous, 203, 230, 233–234, 237
　　absorption and, 213, 213f
　　central, 233–234, 234f, 239–255, 239f–255f
　　peripheral, 230, 233, 233f, 235–238, 235f–238f
　oral, absorption and, 212
　packaging and preparations and, 222–224
　parenteral, 224–259
　　absorption and, 213–214
　subcutaneous, 227f, 227–229
　　absorption and, 213
　　epinephrine and, 397
　　procedure for, 228–229, 228f–229f
　sublingual, 255
　topical, absorption and, 213
　tracheal, absorption and, 213–214
Drug overdose, 583–584, 591–593
　antipsychotics and, 593
　exposure and absorption routes and, 581
　over-the-counter analgesics and, 592
　poison control centers and, 580–581
　prescription narcotics and, 591
　primary survey and, 581–582
　scene survey and, 581
　secondary survey and, 582–583
　sedatives and hypnotics and, 591–592
　tricyclic antidepressants and, 592–593
Dry drowning, 628
Dry lime, burn injuries and, 300
DT's (delirium tremens), 599
Duodenal ulcers, 563
Duodenum, 344, 558, 559f
Duplex communication system, 17
Dura mater, 538
Dying. *See* Death and dying
Dyspnea, 129, 385
　allergic reactions and, 574
　cardiac-related problems and, 417
　paroxysmal nocturnal, 422
Dystonia, antipsychotic overdose and, 593
Dysuria, 567

E

Ear(s)
　anatomy and physiology of, 304, 305f
　discoloration behind (Battle's sign), basilar skull fracture and, 315
　injuries to, 304–306
　　assessment of, 305
　　management of, 306
　　pathophysiology of, 305
　inspection and palpation of, procedure for, 98, 98f
　vertigo and, 658–659, 662
Eardrum (tympanic membrane), 304
Earwax (cerumen), 304
Ecchymosis (bruising), 288. *See also* Contusion
　of eyes, 307
ECG. *See* Electrocardiogram
Eclampsia, 703
Ectopic pregnancy, 563, 568, 701f, 701–702
Ectopy, 437–438
Edema, 180
　allergic reactions and, 574
　laryngeal, 129
　peripheral, testing for, 119
　pitting, 119
　in pregnancy, 703
　pulmonary. *See* Pulmonary edema
Efferent (motor) neurons, 538
Effusions, pericardial and pleural, 423
Eggs (ova), 690
EGTA (esophageal gastric tube airway), 139, 155, 155f
　equipment for, 155, 160
　procedure for, 160–164, 161f–164f
Ejection pattern, of motorcycle injuries, 279
EKG. *See* Electrocardiogram
Elasticity, of damaged tissue, 268
Elastic recoil, 383, 383f
Elbow joint, 359, 361f
Elder abuse, 664–665, 726–727
　risk factors for, 664

Elderly patients. *See* Geriatric patients
Electrical burns. *See* Burn injuries, electrical
Electrical hazards, 46
Electrocardiogram (ECG; EKG), 416
　in arrhythmias, 443–501, 506
　　conduction disorders and, 483f, 483–495, 484f
　　originating in atria, 448–461
　　originating in atrioventricular junction, 462f, 462–468
　　originating in sinoatrial node, 443–447
　　originating in ventricles, 468–482
　artifacts and, 436–437, 437f
　artificial pacemaker rhythms and, 495f, 495–501
　monitoring, 434f, 434–440, 435f, 501, 506
　　P wave, QRS complex, and T wave and, 436f, 436–438, 437f
　　rhythm strip analysis and, 438t, 438–440, 439f, 440f
　telemetry and, 31
Electrolytes, 183–184, 184t, 772, 813. *See also* Fluid and electrolytes
Electromechanical dissociation, 426
Elixirs, 210
Embolism
　air, 318–319
　pulmonary. *See* Pulmonary embolism
　stroke and, 555
Emergency, 52
Emergency care, 49
Emergency management, as responsibility of paramedic, 6
Emergency medical care facilities, patient transfer between, 13
Emergency medical dispatcher. *See* Communications operator
Emergency medical services system, 9–18, 11f
　aeromedical transport and, 14f, 14–15
　citizen access to, 16
　communications and, 17
　components of, 12f, 12–13
　definition of, 12
　medical control and, 10–11

medical standards and, 17
operation of, 17–18
organization for disasters, 60f
personnel and, 16
retrospective review of, 18
systems management and, 13
vehicles and equipment and, 13–14
Emergency medical technician-ambulance (EMT-A), 16
Emergency medical technician-intermediate (EMT-I), 16
Emergency medical technician-paramedic (EMT-P), 16
Emergency transport, as responsibility of paramedic, 6
Emetics, 583–584, 882–823
Emotional abuse, of children, 681
Emotional crisis, psychiatric emergency versus, 722–723
Emotional disturbances. *See* Behavioral and psychiatric disorders
Emphysema
 in geriatric patients, 655
 subcutaneous, 117, 131
EMT-A, 16
EMT-I, 16
EMT-P, 16
Emulsions, 210
Endocardium, 411, 411f
Endocrine system, 86, 521–533, Color Plate 19
 anatomy and physiology of, 522–529
  endocrine glands and, 523f, 523–529, 524t
  hormones and, 522–523
 disorders of
  assessment of, 529–530
  diabetic, 530–533, 531t
  medications for, 836–837
Endometrium, 692
Endotracheal intubation, 139–149, 140f
 in children, 684–685, 685t
 identifying landmarks for, 128, 128f
 nasal, 139, 143, 148–149
  procedure for, 149, 150–154, 150f–154f
 oral, 139, 140–142
  equipment for, 140–142, 141f, 142f
  procedure for, 142–148, 143f–148f
 in upper airway obstruction, 393

Endotracheal tube, 139, 140, 141f
Energy
 Conservation of Energy law and, 264–265, 265f
 exchange of, 266–268
  density of body tissue and, 267, 267f
  particle motion and, 267f–269f, 267–268
 kinetic, 265–266
 penetrating trauma and, 269–270, 270t, 271f
 production of, muscles and, 355
Engagement, labor and, 705
Enhanced 911 emergency telephone number, 32
Enterotoxins, 588
Environment, assessment of, anaphylactic reactions and, 575–576
Environmental emergencies. *See also* Frostbite; Hyperthermia; Hypothermia
 in geriatric patients, 663–664
EOA (esophageal obturator airway), 139, 155, 155f
 equipment for, 155, 160
 procedure for, 160–164, 161f–164f
Epicardium, 411, 411f
Epidermis, 86–87, 286
Epididymis, 562, 562f
Epididymitis, 568
Epidural hematoma, 315–316
Epidural space, 538
Epiglottis, 127, 127f, 558, 559f
 cherry-red, in epiglottitis, 678
Epiglottitis, in children, 678, 678f
Epinephrine (Adrenalin), 782–784
 in allergic and anaphylactic reactions, 576
 in anaphylactic reactions, 575–576
 in asthma, in children, 679
 in bronchospasm, in children, 677, 679
 in cardiac disorders, 433
 in chronic obstructive pulmonary disease, 397, 399t
 racemic (Vaponephrin), 817–818
 in respiratory distress and, 387t
 in respiratory emergencies, in geriatric patients, 656
 in ventricular fibrillation, 480
Epinephrine (physiologic), 528, 547
 heat transfer and, 622
Epi Pens, 575–576

Epiphyses, 356, 356f
 fractures of, 368
Epistaxis (nosebleeds), 309
 management of, 310
Equipment, 14
 communication, maintenance of, 38
 for hazardous materials incidents, 639
 maintenance of, as responsibility of paramedic, 7
 for primary survey, 93, 93f
 for secondary survey, 107–109, 108f
Erect posture, 82
ERV (expiratory reserve volume), 383–384
Erythema (redness), burn injuries and, 294
Erythrocytes (red blood cells), 185f, 185–186, 186f
 formation of, 356–357
 for transfusion, 186–187
Escape complexes, 504t–505t
 junctional and ventricular, 504t–505t
Esophageal gastric tube airway (EGTA), 139, 155, 155f
 equipment for, 155, 160
 procedure for, 160–164, 161f–164f
Esophageal obturator airway (EOA), 139, 155, 155f
 equipment for, 155, 160
 procedure for, 160–164, 161f–164f
Esophageal tracheal comitube (ETC), 139
Esophagus, 558, 559f
 varices of, 564, 598
 in geriatric patients, 661
Estimated time of arrival (ETA), communicating to hospital, 122
Estrogens, 690, 836
 menstrual cycle and, 693
ETA (estimated time of arrival), communicating to hospital, 122
ETC (esophageal tracheal comitube), 139
Ethanol (ethyl alcohol). *See* Alcohol ingestion; Alcoholism
Ethics, 4–6
 code of, 4–5
 medical, 4
Ethmoid bone, 309
Ethylene glycol ingestion, 598
 management of, 585

Eupnea, 385, 388f
Eustachian tube, 128, 305
Evaporation, heat transfer and, 619–620, 621f, 716
Excitability, cardiac, 415
Exocrine glands, 523
Exothermic reactions, 584
Expiration, 383, 383f
Expiratory reserve volume (ERV), 383–384
Explosion hazards, 46
Expressed consent, 26
Exsanguination, 318
Extension, 82, 84f, 365
Extensor carpi radialis brevis muscle, 352t
Extensor response (decerebrate posturing), 119, 312, 550
External (transcutaneous) cardiac pacing, 519
Extracellular fluid, 182, 183
Extracts, 210
Extravascular fluid, 182
Extremities
  examination of, 119
  inspection and palpation of, procedure for, 101, 101f, 102f
  lower
    bones of, 361–362, 362f, 363f
    muscles of, 351t–352t, 353f, 354f
  penetrating injuries of, 272–273
  sports injuries of, 281
  upper
    bones of, 359, 361, 361f
    muscles of, 351t, 353f, 354f
Extrication, 49
Eye(s)
  anatomy and physiology of, 306, 307f
  disorders of, common home medications for, 837–838
  examination of, 117
  injuries to, 306–308
    assessment of, 307–308
    burns and, 298, 301
    management of, 301, 308
    pathophysiology of, 307
  inspection of, procedure for, 97, 97f
  movements of, neurologic emergencies and, 550
  nystagmus and, phencyclidine abuse and, 596
  oculogyric crisis and, 593
  ophthalmic drugs and, 837–838

  raccoon's eyes appearance and, basilar skull fracture and, 315
Eyeball (globe), 307
Eyelids, 306, 307f
  laceration of, 308
Eye protection
  for rescue operations, 43
  universal precautions and, 109
Eye sockets (orbits), 307

F

Face
  injuries of, airway obstruction and, in children, 677
  inspection and palpation of, procedure for, 97, 97f
Face masks
  for infection control, 109, 613
  for oxygen delivery, 133–134, 134f
Face presentation, 711
Face shields, 611, 611f
Facial bones, 357
Facial fractures, 366, 368f, 369
Facilities component, of emergency medical services system, 13
Fainting (syncope), cardiac-related problems and, 417
Fallopian tubes, 563
  anatomy and physiology of, 690, 692
Falls, geriatric patients and, 662
False imprisonment, as basis of liability, 27
Falx cerebri, 312
Family. See also Parents
  amount of information given to, 121–122
  at scene, dealing with, 92
Fascia, 352
Fatty (adipose) tissue, 287
FCC (Federal Communications Commission), 33
Febrile illness, 623
  management of, 623
Febrile seizures, 623
  in children, 674
Federal Communications Commission (FCC), 33
Feet
  bones of, 362–363, 363f
  muscles of, 352t
Femur, 362, 363f
Fertilization, 694
Fetus
  assessment of, 698

  growth of, 694–695, 695t, 696f
  heart rate of, 698
Fever. See Body temperature; Febrile illness; Febrile seizures
Fever blisters (cold sores), 605
Fibrillation
  atrial, 457–459, 506t–507t
  ventricular, 424–425, 425f, 480, 506t–507t
Fibrous joints, 363, 364t
Fibula, 362, 363f
Fick principle, 176
Fight or flight response, 65, 528, 547. See also Stress reactions
Fimbria, ovarian, 692
Fingers, clubbing of, 389
Finger sweep, 130
FiO_2 (fraction of inspired oxygen), 132
Fire ants, allergic reaction to, 574
Fire hazards, 46
First-degree (superficial) burns, 293–294, 294t
First responders
  dealing with, 92
  hazardous materials incidents and, 633
Fistula, arteriovenous, hemodialysis and, 567, 567f
Flail chest, 328, 328f, 329f
  in children, 681
Flame burns, 292, 293f
Flash burns, 292, 293f
Flexion, 82, 84f, 365
Flexor carpi radialis muscle, 352t
Flexor response (decorticate posturing), 119, 312, 550
Flowmeters, 132
Fluid and electrolytes, 172, 180–191, 183f, 184t, 813. See also Blood; Intravenous fluids
  acid-base balance and, 187f, 187–191
  active transport and, 181
  diffusion and, 181, 181f
  evaluation of, 180, 180t
  osmosis and, 181
  osmotic pressure and, 181–182, 182f, 183t
Fluid extracts, 210
Flutter, atrial, 455–456, 506t–507t
Follicle-stimulating hormone (FSH), 525
  menstrual cycle and, 693
Fontanelle (soft spot), 670–671
Food(s), allergic reaction to, 574

Food additives, allergic reaction to, 574
Food poisoning, 588
Foot
  bones of, 362–363, 363f
  muscles of, 352t
Footling breech presentation, 705, 710, 711f
Footwear, for rescue operations, 45, 45f
Foramen magnum, 311
Force, 265. *See also* Restraints
  laws regarding use of, 22
Foreign object(s)
  airway obstruction and, 129
    in children, 676–677
  in ear, 306
  in eye, 308
  in nose, 310
Four-digit identification system, for hazardous materials, 636, 636f, 637t
Four-quadrant system, 342, 560, 560f
Fracture(s), 366–370, 367f–369f
  avulsion, 368, 369f
  basilar, of skull, 314–315, 315f
  Colles', 366
  comminuted, 368, 369f
  compression, 368, 369f
  depressed, 368, 369f
    of skull, 314, 314f
  epiphyseal, 368
  greenstick, 368, 369f
  impacted, 368, 369f
  of larynx, 318
  Le Fort's, 366, 368f, 369
  management of, 371t
  of nose, 310
  oblique, 368, 369f
  pathologic, 368
  of ribs, 327–328
    in geriatric patients, 662
  of skull, 314–315
    basilar, 314–315, 315f
    depressed, 314, 314f
  spiral, 368, 369f
  transverse, 368, 369f
  vertebral, 320
    compression, 320
  x-ray appearance of, 366, 367f
Fragmentation, penetrating trauma and, 269, 270f
Frank breech presentation, 705, 710, 711f
Frederick, Calvin, 720
Frontal collisions, 274–275
  down-and-under pattern of, 274–275, 275f
  up-and-over pattern of, 275

Frontal plane, 82, 83f
Frostbite, 626–627
  deep, 626, 627f
  management of, 626–627
  superficial, 626
FSH (follicle-stimulating hormone), 525
  menstrual cycle and, 693
Full-thickness (third-degree) burns, 295, 295f
Furosemide (Lasix), 784
  in cardiac disorders, 432
  in pulmonary edema, 423
    in geriatric patients, 656
Fusion complexes, 504t–505t

G

Gallbladder, 559f, 560
Gallstones (cholecystitis), 563
[gamma] rays, 642
Ganglia, 536
  sympathetic and parasympathetic, 547
Gas exchange, 381–382, 382f
Gas expansion, in decompression sickness, 632f, 632–633
Gastrocnemius muscle, 352t, 353f, 354f
Gastroenteritis, 564
Gastrointestinal system. *See also* Digestive system; *specific organs*
  allergic reactions and, 574
  anatomy and physiology of, 558–560, 559f
    aging and, 653
  bleeding from
    conditions causing, 564
    in geriatric patients, 661
  disorders of
    common home medications for, 834–836
    in geriatric patients, 660–662
  food poisoning and, 588
General adaptation syndrome, 65, 65f. *See also* Stress reactions
General appearance, evaluating, 109
Genitalia
  examination of, 119
  female, anatomy and physiology of, 692, 693f
Geriatric patients, 649–665, 651f
  abuse of, 664–665, 726–727
    risk factors for, 664

aging process and, anatomy and physiology of, 651–653
  assessment of, 653–655
    communication and, 653, 654f
    history taking and, 653–654
    physical examination and, 654–655
  cardiovascular emergencies and, 656–658
  environmental emergencies and, 663–664
  gastrointestinal emergencies and, 660–662
  hypothermia and, 624
  musculoskeletal problems in, 660
  neurologic emergencies and, 658–659
  pharmacology and, 663
  psychiatric disorders in, 659–660
  respiratory emergencies and, 655–656
  rights of, 650, 651f
  trauma in, 662–663
GH (growth hormone; somatotropin), 525
Glasgow Coma Scale, 109, 317, 550
  Adult, 119, 121, 762, 763
  Pediatric, 121, 764
  in poisoning and overdose, 582–583
Gliding joints, 364t
Gliding movements, 365
Globe (eyeball), 307
Glottis, 127
Gloves
  gloving technique and, 613
  for rescue operations, 43
  universal precautions and, 109
Glucagon, 528, 785
Glucocorticoids, 528
  inhaled, 832
Glucose (Glucola; Insta-glucose), 786
  in status epilepticus, 554
Glucose, blood, hypoglycemia and hyperglycemia and, 528
Glutethimide, 594t–595t
Gluteus maximus muscle, 351t, 354f
Gluteus medius muscle, 351t
Gluteus minimus muscle, 351t
Glycosuria, 530
Gonadotropins, 525

Gonorrhea, 607–608, 610t
Good Samaritan Law, 22, 24
Goose flesh (piloerection), narcotic withdrawal and, 596
Governmental immunity, 24
Gowns
 for infection control, 613
 universal precautions and, 109
Gracilis muscle, 351t
Gravida, 697
Gray matter, 540
Greenstick fractures, 368, 369f
Grieving process, 71–72
Growth, 671–672
 fetal, 694–695, 695t, 696f
Growth hormone (GH; somatotropin), 525
Guarding, abdominal injuries and, 118, 345
Gynecologic emergencies, 698–700
 patient assessment in, 696–698

H

Hallucinations, 725
Hallucinogens
 abuse of, 597
 list of, 594t–595t
Haloperidol (Haldol), 786–787
Hammer (malleus), 304
Hamstring muscle, 351t
Hand(s)
 bones of, 359, 361, 361f
 muscles of, 352t
Hand washing, 612–613
 universal precautions and, 109
Hashish, 596t–597t
Hashish oil, 596t–597t
Hazard(s)
 analysis of, disaster plan and, 55
 electrical, 46
 on-scene, 45–46
 scene survey and, 90–91
Hazardous materials, 633–645
 classes of, 636, 637t
 decontamination and, 643–644
 definition of, 634
 emergency numbers for, 638
 exposure to, 641–642
  acute versus chronic, 642
  ionizing radiation and, 641–642
  patient management and, 644
  postevent considerations and, 645
  routes of entry and, 641
  transport and, 644–645
  triage and, 644
 planning and preparedness for, 639–641
  communications and, 639, 640f
  rescue considerations and, 639–641, 641f
  responding to calls and, 641
  vehicle equipment and, 639
 protection from, 642–643
  ambulance protection and, 643
  forms of chemical intrusion and, 642
  levels of, 643
  self-care precautions and, 642–643
 recognition of, 633–638
  container shapes and, 634, 634f
  markings and colors and, 635f, 635–636
  occupancy and location and, 634
  placards and labels and, 636, 636f, 637t, 638f
  senses and, 636, 638
  shipping papers and, 636
Hazardous materials charts, front end paper, back end paper
Hazardous materials incident, 634
Hazardous substance, definition of, 634
Hazardous waste, definition of, 634
Head. See also specific organs
 bones of, 357, 358f. See also Skull
 examination of, 116–117
 muscles of, 352t, 353f
Head injuries, 304–318, 550. See also Ear(s), injuries to; Eye(s), injuries to; Nose, injuries to
 blood flow to brain and, 311
 cerebral concussion and, 313–314
 cerebral contusion and, 314, 314f
 cerebral herniation and, 312, 313f
 in children, 681
 intracranial hematomas and and hemorrhage and, 315–318
 pathophysiology of, 311f, 311–312
 penetrating, 271–272
 skull fracture and, 314–315
 sports-related, 280
Head-on pattern, of motorcycle injuries, 279
Head-tilt/chin-lift method, 94, 94f, 103, 130, 130f
Head-to-toe survey, 104, 116–119
Hearing impairment
 access to emergency medical services communications system and, 32
 communicating with patient and, 105
Heart. See also headings beginning with terms Cardiac; Cardiopulmonary; Cardiovascular
 aging and, 652
 anatomy of, 410–413, 411f, 412f
 arrhythmias and. See Arrhythmias
 artificial pacemaker and, 495f, 495–501
 atherosclerosis and. See Atherosclerosis
 auscultation of, 118
 concussion of, 280, 281f
 contusion of, 280, 281f
 physiology of, 413f, 413–416
  electrophysiology and, 415f, 415–416, 416f
  regulation of cardiac function and, 414f, 414–415
 pulmonary function and, 381
 shock and, 177f–179f, 177–179
Heart block, complete (third degree AV block), 488–490
Heartburn, aging and, 653
Heart disease, valvular, 426–427
Heart failure, 422–423
 congestive, 422
  in geriatric patients, 657
 left-sided, 381
  in geriatric patients, 656
 left ventricular, pulmonary edema and, 422–423
 right ventricular, 423
Heart rate
 aging and, 652
 bradycardia and, management of, 425–426
 fetal, 698
 of infant, newborn, 715
 irregularities in, 417. See also Arrhythmias
 tachycardia and, 422
Heart rhythm, irregularities in, 417
Heart sounds, 118
 cardiac-related problems and, 418

Heart valves, 411–412, 412f
    aging and, 652
    valvular heart disease and, 426–427
Heat. *See also* Hyperthermia
    blast injuries and, 281–282
Heat cramps, 622
    management of, 622
Heat exhaustion, 622–623
    in geriatric patients, 664
Heat stroke, 46, 623
    in geriatric patients, 664
    management of, 623
Heat transfer
    organ mediation of, 620–622
    physical principles of, 619–620, 621f, 716
Helicopters, 49
    rotor wash and, 14–15
    safety and, 15, 15f
Helmets
    motorcycle injuries and, 279
    for rescue operations, 44, 44f
Help, requesting, 46–47
Hematemesis, 564
Hematocrit, 186
Hematoma, 288
    epidural, 315–316
    subdural, 316, 316f, 538–539
Hematuria, 567
Hemiparesis, 119, 316, 549
Hemiplegia, 549
Hemodialysis, 567f, 567–568
    patient management and, 568
Hemoglobin, 185–186
    carbon monoxide poisoning and, 400
Hemopoiesis, 356–357
Hemoptysis, 386
    allergic reactions and, 574
    in geriatric patients, 655
Hemorrhage. *See also* Bleeding
    checking for, 103
        procedure for, 95, 95f
    intracerebral, 316
    intravenous fluids and, 196
    postpartum, 713
    stroke and, 555
    subarachnoid, 316
        stroke and, 658
Hemothorax, 336, 336f
Henry's law, 630
Heparin sodium, 788
Hepatitis, 603–605
    type A, 604, 610t
    type B, 604, 610t
    type C, 604–605, 610t
Herbicide poisoning, 587

Herniation, cerebral, 312, 313f
    transtentorial, 312
Heroin, 594t–595t
Herpes, 605–607, 610t
    cytomegalovirus and, 607
    genital, 605
    herpes simplex types 1 and 2 and, 605–606
    herpes zoster (shingles) and, 606f, 606–607
    herpetic whitlow and, 606
    varicella and, 606, 606f
Herpetic whitlow, 606
Hexadrol (dexamethasone sodium phosphate), 774
Hiccup, 383
Highway Safety Act of 1966, 10
Hinge joints, 364t
Histamine, 574
History taking, 104–107
    acute abdomen and, 564–565, 565f
    anaphylaxis and, 575
    burn injuries and, 299
    cardiac-related problems and, 417
    from children, 669
    communication principles and, 104–105
    components of, 106–107, 108t
    endocrine emergencies and, 530
    geriatric patients and, 653–654
    gynecologic and obstetric patient and, 697–698
    interview techniques and, 105t, 105–106
    nervous system emergencies and, 548–549
    in poisoning and overdose, 582
    respiratory distress and, 385–389, 387t
    upper airway disorders and, 130
HIV (human immunodeficiency virus), 609, 610t
Hives (urticaria), 574
Hollow organs, 343, 561
Homeostasis, 536, 619
Hormones, 522–523, 524t
    effector, 522
    negative feedback system and, 523, 523f
    regulation of, 522–523, 523f
    secretion of, 86
    tropic, 522, 523
    vaginal bleeding and, 699
Hornet stings, allergic reaction to, 573f, 573–574
Horse serum, allergic reaction to, 573

Hospital. *See* Medical facilities
Hostile situations, 46. *See also* Violence
Hot zone, hazardous materials incidents and, 640, 641f
Human immunodeficiency virus (HIV), 609, 610t
Humerus, 359, 361f
Humor, 70
Humoral immunity, 602
Humulin R (insulin), 791–792
Hydralazine (Apresoline), 789–780
Hydrocarbon poisoning, 584, 585
Hydrocortisone sodium succinate (Solu-Cortef), 790
    respiratory distress and, 387t
Hydrofluoric acid ingestion, 300, 584–585
Hydrogen sulfide inhalation, 586
Hydromorphone, 594t–595t
Hydrostatic pressure, 184
Hydrostatic (water) pressure, 630
Hypercalcemia, 527
Hypercapnia, 389
Hypercarbia, 131
Hyperglycemia, 528
Hyperglycemic drugs, 775, 785–786
Hyperosmolar hyperglycemia nonketotic coma, 531t, 532
    assessment of, 532
    management of, 532
Hyperparathyroidism, 527
Hyperpnea, 389
    in diabetic ketoacidosis, 530
Hyperstat (diazoxide), 777–778
Hypertension, 114, 427–428
    acute hypertensive emergency and, 428
    aging and, 652
    in pregnancy, 703
Hyperthermia, 622–623
    febrile illness and, 623
    in geriatric patients, 664
    heat cramps and, 622
    heat exhaustion and, 622–623
    heat stroke and, 623
    preventing, 45, 46
    signs and symptoms of, 623t
Hyperthyroidism (thyrotoxicosis), 526–527
Hypertonic solutions, 182, 183t
Hyperventilation, 384
    central neurogenic, 388f
    head injuries and, 317–318
Hyperventilation syndrome, 402–403
    assessment of, 402
    management of, 402–403
    pathophysiology of, 402

Hypnotics, 830
  overdose of, 591–592
Hypocalcemia, 527
Hypochondriasis, in geriatric patients, 660
Hypoglycemia, 528, 532–533
  in alcoholism, 598
  assessment of, 533
  in children, management of, 674
  management of, 533, 582
Hypoglycemic coma (insulin shock), 533
Hypoglycemic drugs, 836
Hypoparathyroidism, 527
Hypotension, 114
  orthostatic (postural)
    aging and, 652
    dizziness and, 659
  in pregnancy, 700
  supine-induced, during pregnancy, 695
Hypothalamus, 542
  heat transfer and, 620–621, 622
  hormones of, 523, 524t
  thermostasis and, 619, 620f
Hypothermia, 623–626
  in geriatric patients, 664
  high-risk groups and, 624
  immersion, 629
  intoxicants and, 624
  management of, 625–626
  medical conditions and, 624
  moderate, 624, 625
  pathophysiology of, 624–625
  preventing, 45, 46
  rate of onset of, 624
  severe, 624–625, 625f
  trauma and, 624
Hypothyroidism (myxedema), 526–527
Hypotonic solutions, 182, 183t
Hypoventilation, 384
Hypovolemia, 178, 179f
  in hypothermia, 626
Hypovolemic shock, allergic reactions and, 574
Hypoxemia, 131, 381
  in children, 671
Hypoxia, 381
Hysterical seizures, 553

I

IC (incident commander), disaster management and, 58
ICS (Incident Command System), 58

Idioventricular rhythm, 502t–503t
  accelerated, 470
IgA, 603
IgE, 603
IgG, 603
IgM, 603
Ileum, 344, 558, 559f
Ileus, 345
Ilium, 361, 362f
Illness, drug-induced, in geriatric patients, 663
Illusions, 725
Imipramine, overdose of, 592
Immersion hypothermia, 629
Immobilization
  fractures and, 370, 371t, 372f–373f
    spinal, 321–323, 322f
  indications for, 317
Immune system, 602–603
  immune response and, 602–603
  infectious and communicable diseases and, 603
Immunity, 572
Immunization (vaccination), 602
Immunoglobulins, 603
Impacted fractures, 368, 369f
Impaled object wound, 289f, 290
Implied consent, 26
Imprisonment, false, as basis of liability, 27
Incident
  critical
    critical incident stress and, 66–67
    disaster management and, 61–62
  hazardous materials, 634
  major, 53f, 53–54, 54f
Incident commander (IC), disaster management and, 58
Incident Command Post, 59
Incident Command System (ICS), 58
Incident scene. *See also* Scene survey
  assessment of, 46–47
Incisions, 288
Incompetence, consent and, 25
Incomplete breech presentation, 710, 711f
Incontinence, 549
Incubation period, 603
Incus (anvil), 304
Inderal (propranolol), 815–816
Inert gas, 630
Infant(s). *See also* Newborn
  blood pressure measurement in, 114

burn injuries in, 681
developmental approach to, 672t
genital herpes and, 605
intravenous fluid administration rate for, 686
maternal narcotic addiction and, 596
respiratory rate in, 670
veins for intravenous infusions in, 687, 687f
Infection(s). *See also* Infection control; Infectious diseases; *specific infections*
  respiratory
    aging and, 652
    signs of, 386
  of urinary tract, 566
Infection control, 611–614
  blood exposure follow-up and, 614
  cleaning blood spills and, 613–614
  disposal of contaminated articles and, 613
  face mask and, 613
  gloving technique and, 613
  gowns and, 613
  handling and disposal of needles and, 613
  hand washing and, 612–613
  protective eye wear and, 613
  universal precautions and, 611f, 611–612, 612t
  vehicle cleaning and, 614
Infectious diseases, 601–614. *See also* Infection control; *specific diseases*
  definition of, 603
  immune system and, 602–603
Inferior (caudal) direction, 82, 83f
Informed consent, 25
Infundibulum, of fallopian tube, 690
Ingestion. *See also* Drug overdose; Poisoning; *specific substances*
  of hazardous materials, 641
Inhalation injuries, 297–298, 400–401, 581
  assessment of, 400–401
  carbon monoxide and, 297
  hazardous materials and, 641
  management of, 301, 401, 585–587
    carbon monoxide and, 585–586
  pathophysiology of, 400
  smoke inhalation and, 297–298

Inhalers, metered dose, 398, 398f
Injection, of hazardous materials, 641
Injuries. *See* Mechanism of injury; Trauma; *specific sites of injuries*
Inotropin (dopamine)
  in cardiac disorders, 432–433
  in cardiogenic shock, 424
Insecticide poisoning, 587–588
Insect stings and bites, allergic reaction to, 573f, 573–574, 590
Inspection, 107
  of abdomen, 118
    acute abdomen and, 565–566
    cardiac-related problems and, 418
  in respiratory distress, 388f, 389
  upper airway disorders and, 130–131
Inspiration, 383, 383f
Inspiratory reserve volume (IRV), 383, 384
Insta-glucose (glucose), 786
Insulin (Humulin R; Regular Insulin), 791–792, 836
Insulin (physiologic), 528–529
  hypoglycemia and, 532
Insulin shock (hypoglycemic coma), 532
Insurance, liability, 28
Integumentary system, 86–87, Color Plate 20. *See also* Skin
Interatrial tracts, 415
Intercostal muscles, 351t, 353f, 382–383, 383f
Intermittent claudication, 428
Interneurons, 538
Internodal tracts, 415
Interstitial fluid, 182
Interstitial pneumonitis, 381
Interstitial space, 381
Intervertebral disc, 357
Interview techniques, 105t, 105–106
  direct questions and, 105, 105t, 106
  open-ended questions and, 105, 105t, 106
Intestine
  appendicitis and, 563, 564
  colitis and, ischemic, 661
  diverticulitis and, 563–564
  duodenal ulcers and, 563
  gastroenteritis and, 564
  large. *See* Colon

obstruction of, 563
  in geriatric patients, 662
  small, 558, 559f
    cancer of, 661
    injuries of, 344
Intima, 407
Intoxication. *See also* Alcohol ingestion; Alcoholism
  cautions regarding patient treatment and, 27
Intracellular fluid, 182–183
Intracerebral hemorrhage, 316
Intracranial pressure, 311, 312
  decreasing, 317–318
  nervous system emergencies and, 549
Intraosseous drug administration, in children, 687
Intravascular fluid, 182
Intravenous fluids, 197, 201–203, 202t, 202–203. *See also* Central line placement; Drug administration, intravenous
  in abdominal injuries, 346
  in burn injuries, 300t, 301
  in children, 685–687, 686f
    in bronchospasm, 677
    fluids for, 685–687
    needles and cannulas for, 685
    in seizures, 674
    in shock, 680
  in chronic obstructive pulmonary disease, 396
  in coma, 552
  in decompression sickness, 631–632
  in ectopic pregnancy, 702
  in head injuries, 317
  in heat cramps, 622
  in heat exhaustion, 622–623
  in heat stroke, 623
  in hyperosmolar hyperglycemia nonketotic coma, 532
  in hypothermia, 626
  intravenous access and, 201
  medication administration and, 203
  in neurologic emergencies, in geriatric patients, 659
  in preeclampsia and eclampsia, 703
  in pregnancy, trauma and, 700
  in pulmonary edema, 423
  rate of administration of, 203
  in status epilepticus, 554
  types of, 202t
Intropin (dopamine), 781–782
  in cardiac disorders, 432–433
  in cardiogenic shock, 424

Invasion of privacy, as basis of liability, 27
Involuntary consent, 26
Involuntary guarding, abdominal injuries and, 345
Involuntary (smooth; visceral) muscle, 85, 350, 352, 355f
Ionizing radiation, 641–642
Iris, 306, 307f
Irreversible shock, 192–193
  ischemic phase of, 193
  staged death and, 193
  stagnant phase of, 193
  washout phase of, 193
IRV (inspiratory reserve volume), 383, 384
Ischemia, myocardial, 419, 419f
Ischemic colitis, in geriatric patients, 661
Ischium, 361, 362f
Islets of Langerhans, 528
Isoelectric line, 434
Isoetharine (Bronkometer; Bronkosol), 792
  in chronic obstructive pulmonary disease, 398, 399t
  respiratory distress and, 387t
Isolation, in grieving process, 71
Isopropanol (isopropyl alcohol) ingestion, 598
  management of, 585
Isoproterenol, in arrhythmias, 518–519
Isoproterenol hydrochloride (Isuprel), 793
  respiratory distress and, 387t
Isoproterenol sulfate, respiratory distress and, 387t
Isoptin. *See* Verapamil hydrochloride
Isotonic solutions, 182, 183t, 203
  for children, 686–687
Isthmus, of fallopian tube, 690
  ectopic pregnancy and, 702
Isuprel (isoproterenol hydrochloride), 793
  respiratory distress and, 387t

J

Jacksonian seizure, 553
Jaundice, 116, 604
Jaw-thrust method, 94, 94f, 103, 130, 130f
Jejunum, 344, 558, 559f
Jellyfish stings, 590
Joints (articulations), 363, 364t, 365, 365f

Joints (articulations) (continued)
   cartilaginous, 363, 364t
   elbow, 359, 361f
   fibrous, 363, 364t
   knee, 362, 363f
   movement of, 365
   synovial, 363, 364t
Joules, 511
Jugular venous distension, 389
Junctional escape complexes and rhythms, 462–464, 504t–505t
Junctional rhythm, 502t–503t
Junctional tachycardia, 502t–503t
   paroxysmal, 468
J wave (Osborne wave), 624, 625f

K

Kabikinase (streptokinase), 820–821
Kaposi's sarcoma, 610
Keep vein open (KVO) fluid administration rate, 202
Kehr's sign, splenic injuries and, 343
Kernig's sign, in meningitis, 675
Kerosene ingestion, 585
Ketoacidosis, diabetic, 530–532, 531t
   assessment of, 531
   management of, 532
Ketone bodies, 530
Kidney(s), 86, 561, 561f
   acid-base balance and, 189, 189t
   anatomy and physiology of, aging and, 652
   failure of
     acute and chronic, 566
       hemodialysis and, 567f, 567–568
Kidney stones (renal calculi), 566
Kinetic energy, 265–266
KKK standards, 13
Kneecap (patella), 362, 363f
Knee joint, 362, 363f
Koplik's spots, 609, 609f
Korotkoff's sounds, 112, 113f
Korsakoff's psychosis, 598
Kussmaul's respiration, 388f
   in acute renal failure, 566
   in diabetic ketoacidosis, 530
KVO (keep vein open) fluid administration rate, 202
Kyphosis, 323, 651, 653

L

Labels, for hazardous materials, 636
Labia majora, 692
Labia minora, 692
Labor, 705. See also Delivery
   stages of, 705
Laceration, 288, 289f, 290f
   arterial, 288, 289f
   of eyelid, 308
Lacrimal gland, 306, 307f
Lactated Ringer's, 203
Landing zones, 14–15, 15f
Lanoxin (digoxin), 778–779
Large intestine. See Colon
Laryngopharynx, 128
Laryngoscope, 139, 141, 141f
Laryngoscope blades, 141, 142f
Laryngotracheobronchitis (croup), 677f, 677–678
Larynx, 128, 128f
   edema of, 129
   fractures of, 129, 318
   spasm of, 129
Lasix. See Furosemide
Lateral bending, spinal injuries and, 319
Lateral (T-bone) collisions, 276–277
Lateral direction, 82, 83f
Laterally recumbent posture, 82
Lateral (uncal) syndrome, 312, 313f
Latissimus dorsi muscle, 351t, 354f
Law(s). See Legal issues; *specific laws*
Laxatives, 835
Laying the bike down pattern, of motorcycle injuries, 279
Leaders (tendons), 352
Lead II, electrocardiogram and, 434, 435f, 501
Leaky capillary syndrome, 193
Le Fort, Renée, 366
Le Fort fractures, 366, 368f, 369
Left-sided heart failure, 381
   in geriatric patients, 656
Left ventricular failure, pulmonary edema and, 422–423
Legal issues, 19–28
   administrative law and, 20–21
   bases of liability and, 26–27
   blood samples and, 22
   child and adult abuse and, 21–22
   civil law and, 20
   consent and, 25–26
      minors and, 26
   criminal law and, 20
   in crisis care, 732
   do not resuscitate orders and, 22
   force and, 22
   Good Samaritan Law and, 22, 24
   governmental immunity and, 24
   insurance and liability protection and, 28
   living wills and, 22
   malpractice actions and, 24–25
      claim of malpractice and, 24–25
      standard of care and, 24–25
   medical practices act and, 21
   motor vehicle laws and, 21
   organ donation and, 22, 23f
   patient refusal and, 26
   privilege and, 24
   problems areas for paramedics and, 27–28
   state emergency medical services laws and, 21
Legs. See Extremities
Lens, of eye, 306, 307f
Leukocytes (white blood cells), 186
   formation of, 356–357
   immune response and, 603
Levarterenol (norepinephrine), 806–807
Level A protection, 643
Level B protection, 643
Level C protection, 643
Level D protection, 643
Levophed (norepinephrine), 806–807
LH (luteinizing hormone), 525
   menstrual cycle and, 693–694
Liability, 26–27
   abandonment as basis of, 26–27
   battery as basis of, 27
   false imprisonment as basis of, 27
   insurance and, 28
   invasion of privacy as basis of, 27
   libel as basis of, 27
   slander as basis of, 27
Libel, as basis of liability, 27
Lice, 608
Licensure, 7
   reciprocity and, 7
Lidocaine
   allergic reaction to, 573
   in arrhythmias, 509–510

Lidocaine (*continued*)
  in myocardial infarction, 422
  in premature ventricular complex, 472, 472f
  in ventricular fibrillation, 480
  in ventricular tachycardia, 476
Lidocaine hydrochloride (Xylocaine), 794–795
Ligaments, 356
Light injuries
  blast injuries and, 281
  to eye, 308
Lightning injuries, 292, 293f
Lime, dry, burn injuries and, 300
Lindane poisoning, 587
Liniments, 210
Lipids (triglycerides), insulin and, 529
Listening skills, history taking and, 104–105
Litters, 48, 48f
Liver, 559f, 560
  hepatitis and, 603–604
  injuries of, 343–344
    in children, 681
Living will, 22
Lotions, 210
Lower airway
  anatomy and physiology of, 378–382, 379f
  central nervous system disorders and, 401–402
  obstructive lung disease and, 393–399
  pneumonia and, 399–400
  pulmonary embolism and, 401
  smoke and toxic product inhalation and, 400–401
LSD, 594t–595t
Lumbar spine, 357, 359f, 543
Luminal Sodium (phenobarbital sodium), 809–810
Lund-Brower chart, 296, 296f, 297f
Lung(s). *See also* Breathing; Chronic obstructive pulmonary disease; Respiration(s); *headings beginning with terms* Pulmonary *and* Respiratory
  aging and, 651
  anatomy and physiology of, 380–382
  disorders of, affecting heart, 427
  drowning and, 628
    management of, 629
    salt versus fresh water, 628

pulmonary circulation and, 408, 411f
respiratory volumes and capacities and, 383–384, 384f
Lutein, 692
Luteinizing hormone (LH), 525
  menstrual cycle and, 693–694
Lye, burn injuries and, 300
Lymphatic system, 602
  pharyngeal, 128
Lymphocyte, 186

M

McBurney's point, 564
MacIntosh blade, 141
Magill blade, 141
Magill forceps, 141, 142f
Magmas, 210
Magnesium sulfate, in seizures, eclamptic, 703
Mainlining, 593
Major incident, 53f, 53–54, 54f
Malleability, penetrating trauma and, 269
Malleus (hammer), 304
Mallory-Weiss syndrome, in geriatric patients, 661
Malpractice, 24–25
  claim of, 25
  standard of care and, 24–25
Mammalian diving reflex, 629
Mania, in geriatric patients, 659
Mannitol (Osmitrol), 795–796
Manpower. *See also* Paramedic(s)
  disaster management and, staging and canteen and, 59
Manpower component, of emergency medical services system, 12
Manubrium, 359, 360f
MAO (monoamine oxidase) inhibitors, 829
Marijuana, 596t–597t
  abuse of, 597
Marine animals, allergic reactions to, 590–591
Marrow (medullary) cavity, 356, 356f
Masks
  for oxygen delivery, 133–134, 134f
  universal precautions and, 109
Mass, 265
Masseter muscle, 352t
Mastoiditis, 305
MAT (multifocal atrial tachycardia), 460–461, 502t–503t
  in geriatric patients, 655

MCL_1 (modified chest lead 1), electrocardiogram and, 434, 435f, 501
Mean arterial pressure, 311
Measles, 608–609, 609f, 610t
  rubella and, 608
  rubeola and, 608–609, 609f
Mechanism of injury
  penetrating trauma and, 270–271, 271f
  scene survey and, 91–92
  spinal injuries and, 319–320
  upper airway and, 129
Meconium, 717
Media, 407
Medial direction, 82, 83f
Mediastinal shift, 331
Medical care, access to, 13
Medical commander, disaster management and, 58
Medical Command Post, 59
Medical control (medical direction), 10–11
  medical director and, 10–11
  off-line, 11
  on-line, 11
  protocols and, 11
  standing orders and, 11
Medical director, 10–11
Medical ethics, 4
Medical facilities
  communicating patient data to, 122
  communication with, 32, 37
  medical standards and, 17
  radio communication with, 38
Medical history, 107
  burn injuries and, 299
  gynecologic and obstetric patient and, 697–698
  respiratory distress and, 386–387, 387t, 389
Medical instructions, provided by communications operator, 35
Medical practices act, 21
Medical standards, 17
  hospital care and, 17
Medical supply pool, disaster management and, 59
Medical terminology, 78–80
  abbreviations and, 80, 81
  avoiding use with patient, 105
  pronunciation and spelling of, 78
  word building and, 79–80
Medications. *See* Drug(s); *specific drugs*
Medihaler-Epi, 575–576

Medulla oblongata, 543
Medullary (marrow) cavity, 356, 356f
Melanin, 286
Melanocytes, 286
Melena, 118, 564
Memory deficits
　antegrade amnesia and, 313
　retrograde amnesia and, 110
Meninges, 538–539, 540f
Meningitis, 605, 610t
　in children, 675
　viral, 605
Menopause, 694
Menstrual cycle, 692–694, 693f
　history of, 697–698
　menstrual phase of, 694
　premenstrual phase of, 694
　proliferative phase of, 693
　secretory phase of, 693–694
Mental problems. See Behavioral and psychiatric disorders
Mental status examination, 724–725
Meperidine (Demerol; Pethadol), 796–797
Meperidine (pethidine), 594t–595t
Mescaline, 594t–595t
Metabolic acidosis, 190f, 190–191
　in diabetic ketoacidosis, 530
Metabolic alkalosis, 191
Metabolism, aerobic and anaerobic, 176
Metaproterenol sulfate (Alupent; Metaprel), 797–798
　in chronic obstructive pulmonary disease, 397f, 397–398, 399t
Metaraminol bitartrate (Aramine), 798–799
Metatarsal bones, 363, 363f
Metered dose inhaler, 398, 398f
Methadone, 594t–595t
　overdose of, 591
Methane inhalation, 586
Methanol (methyl alcohol) ingestion, 598
　management of, 585
Methaqualone, 594t–595t
Methemoglobin, cyanide poisoning and, 586
Methylphenidate, 594t–595t
Methylprednisolone sodium succinate (Solu-Medrol), 799
　respiratory distress and, 387t
Methylxanthines, 824–825
　in chronic obstructive pulmonary disease, 396

respiratory distress and, 387, 387t
Mettag triage tagging system, 57, 58f
Midbrain, 543
Miller blade, 141
Mineralocorticoids, 528
Minors, consent and, 26
Minute volume, 381, 383
Miotics, 838
Mitchell, Jeffrey T., 61–62
Mitral valve, 411
Mobile radio, 34, 36, 36f
Mobile repeater, for radio communication, 31, 34
Mobility, health status and, aging and, 653
Mobitz I block (type I second degree AV block; Wenckebach block), 485
Mobitz II block (type II second degree AV block), 487
Modified chest lead 1 (MCL$_1$), electrocardiogram and, 434, 435f, 501
Momentum, 265
Monoamine oxidase (MAO) inhibitors, 829
Mood stabilizing drugs, 830
Morgue, disaster management and, 59
Morphine sulfate, 594t–595t, 800–801
　allergic reaction to, 573
　in cardiac disorders, 431
　in myocardial infarction, 421–422
　in pulmonary edema, 423
　in geriatric patients, 656
Motorcycle injuries, 279
　angular pattern of, 279
　ejection pattern of, 279
　head-on pattern of, 279
　laying the bike down pattern of, 279
Motor (efferent) neurons, 538
Motor vehicle laws, 21
Mountain search and rescue, 49f
Mouth (oral cavity), 558, 559f
　inspection and palpation of, procedure for, 97, 98f
Movement(s)
　neurologic emergencies and, 550
　terms for, 82, 84f, 365
Mucous glands, tracheal, 379
Mucous membranes, disorders of, common home medications for, 838–839

Multifocal atrial tachycardia (MAT), 460–461, 502t–503t
　in geriatric patients, 655
Multiple births, 712
Mumps, 608
Muscle(s). See also Musculoskeletal system
　bipennate, 350
　cardiac, 85, 352, 355, 355f, 411, 411f
　energy production and, 355
　injuries of, 365–366
　　assessment of, 366
　　management of, 366
　　sprains and, 365, 366
　　strains and, 365, 366
　neuromuscular diseases and, respiratory disorders and, 402
　of respiration, 382–384, 383f
　respiratory, innervation of, 384
　skeletal (striated; voluntary), 85, 350, 352, 355f
　smooth (involuntary; visceral), 85, 352, 355, 355f
　stretching of, 268
Muscle guarding, 118, 345
Muscle relaxants, 833
Musculoskeletal system, 85, Color Plate 2, Color Plate 3. See also Bone(s); Muscle(s); headings beginning with term Skeletal
　anatomy and physiology of, 350, 351t–352t, 352–355, 353f–355f
　aging and, 653
　disorders of
　　common home medications for, 833
　　in geriatric patients, 660
　　management of, 660
　　respiratory disorders and, 402
Mushroom poisoning, 589, 589f
Mutual aid agreements, 13, 46–47
Mydriatics, 838
Myelin sheath, 537f, 538
Myocardial infarction, 420f, 420–422
　in geriatric patients, 657
　silent, 421
Myocardial ischemia, 419, 419f
Myocardium, 411, 411f
Myometrium, 692
Myxedema (hypothyroidism), 526–527
Myxedema crisis, 526–527

N

NAEMT (National Association of Emergency Medical Technicians), 8
Nagel, Eugene, 10
Nalbuphine hydrochloride (Nubain), 801–802
Naloxone (Narcan), 802–803
　in alcoholism, 598
　in coma, 552
　in diabetic ketoacidosis, 532
　in hyperosmolar hyperglycemia nonketotic coma, 532
　in narcotic abuse, 596
　in narcotic overdose, 582, 591, 593, 596
　in neurologic emergencies, in geriatric patients, 659
　in poisoning and overdose, 582
　in seizures, 553
Narcosis, nitrogen, 630
Narcotics, 773–774, 829
　abuse of, 593, 596
　agonists of, 796–797, 800–802
　antagonists of, 801–803
　list of, 594t–595t
　prescription
　　list of, 591
　　overdose of, 591
Nasal cannula, 133, 133f
Nasal flaring, 389
　in children, 671
Nasal intubation, 139, 143, 148–149
　procedure for, 149, 150–154, 150f–154f
Nasopharyngeal airway (nasal trumpet), 136, 136f, 393
　pediatric, 684
Nasopharynx, 128
　obstruction of, in upper airway obstruction, 393
National Association of Emergency Medical Technicians (NAEMT), 8
National Association of Emergency Medical Technicians, code of ethics established by, 5
National Council of Instructors and Coordinators, 8
National Fire Protection Association (NFPA), marking system of, for hazardous materials, 635f, 635–636
National organizations, for paramedics, 8

National Registry of Emergency Medical Technicians (NREMT), 7, 8
　advanced level practical examination of, 733–735, 738, 740–747
　paramedic level practical examination of, 733, 736–737, 739
National Ski Patrol, 49f
NAVEL mnemonic, endotracheal drug administration and, 259
Near drowning, 628
Nebulizers, 397f, 397–398
Neck
　examination of, 116–117
　injuries of, airway obstruction and, in children, 677
　inspection and palpation of, procedure for, 99, 99f
　muscles of, 351t, 353f, 354f
　penetrating injuries of, 272
　soft-tissue injuries to, 318–319
　　assessment of, 318
　　management of, 318–319
　　pathophysiology of, 318
　sports injuries of, 280
Needle(s)
　handling and disposal of, 613
　universal precautions and, 109
Needle chest decompression (thoracentesis), 331–332, 335
　skill procedure for, 333–335, 333–335f
Needle stick injury, 610–611
Negative feedback system, 523, 523f
Nematocysts, 590
Nervous system, 85, 535–556, Color Plates 4–7
　anatomy and physiology of, 536–548
　　aging and, 652–653
　　neurons and, 537–538
　　spinal cord and, 543
　autonomic, anatomy and physiology of, 545–548, 546f
　central. See Brain; Central nervous system; Spinal cord
　disorders of. See also Coma; Seizures; Status epilepticus; Stroke; Unconsciousness
　　common home medications for, 829–830
　neuromuscular, respiratory disorders and, 402
　primary survey and, 548

　secondary survey and, 548–550
　parasympathetic, anatomy and physiology of, 547–548
　peripheral, anatomy and physiology of, 543, 544f, 544t, 545f, 545–548
　sympathetic, anatomy and physiology of, 547
Neurilemma (sheath of Schwann), 538, 539f
Neurohypophysis, 525
Neurologic evaluation, 549
Neuromuscular diseases, respiratory disorders and, 402
Neurons, 537–538
　afferent (sensory), 538, 539f
　axons and, 537, 537f
　connecting (interneurons), 538
　dendrites and, 537, 537f
　efferent (motor), 538
　myelin sheath and, 537f, 538
　neurilemma and, 538, 539f
　postganglionic, 546
　preganglionic, 546, 547
　soma of, 536
Neurotransmitters, 547
Newborn, 714–717
　airway of, 714
　breathing and circulation of, 714f, 714–715
　characteristics of, 715t
　distressed, management of, 717
　initial evaluation of, 715, 715t, 716t
　maintaining warmth of, 716
　premature, 694–695, 716–717
　reflexes and other characteristics of, 716t
Newton's laws of motion
　first, 265
　second, 265, 266f
NFPA (National Fire Protection Association), marking system of, for hazardous materials, 635f, 635–636
Nifedipine (Procardia), 803–804
911 emergency telephone number, 16, 32, 35
Nipride (sodium nitroprusside), 819–820
Nitrates, 831
Nitrogen, decompression sickness and, 630–632
Nitrogen narcosis, 630
Nitroglycerin
　in cardiac disorders, 421–422, 430–431
　in pulmonary edema, 423

Nitroglycerin (Nitrostat; Tridil), 804–805
Nitrous oxide (dinitrous monoxide; NO$_2$), 805–806
  in cardiac disorders, 431–432
No-code (DNR; do not resuscitate; no heroic measures) orders, 22
Nocturia, aging and, 652
Nodes of Ranvier, 538
No heroic measures (DNR; do not resuscitate; no-code) orders, 22
Nonrebreathing mask, for oxygen delivery, 134, 134f
Norepinephrine (Levarterenol; Levophed), 806–807
Norepinephrine (physiologic), 528, 547
  cardiac function and, 414
Normal anatomical position, 82, 82f
Normal sinus rhythm, 502t–503t
Normothermic patients, 625–626
Nose, 127. *See also headings beginning with term* Nasal
  anatomy and physiology of, 309, 309f
  injuries to, 309–310
    assessment of, 310
    management of, 310
    pathophysiology of, 309–310
  inspection and palpation of, procedure for, 97, 97f
  nasal flaring and, 389
  in children, 671, 714, 714f
Nosebleeds (epistaxis), 309
  management of, 310
Nostrils (anterior nares), 309
Novocaine (procaine), allergic reaction to, 573
NREMT (National Registry of Emergency Medical Technicians), 7, 8
  advanced level practical examination of, 733–735, 738, 740–747
  paramedic level practical examination of, 733, 736–737, 739
Nubain (nalbuphine hydrochloride), 801–802
Nystagmus, phencyclidine abuse and, 596

O

Oblique fractures, 368, 369f
Oblique muscles, internal and external, 351t, 353f
Obstetric emergencies. *See also* Delivery; Labor; Pregnancy
  patient assessment in, 696–698
Obstetric history, 697–698
Obstructive respiration, 388f
Occupational Safety and Health Administration (OSHA), 633
Oculogyric crisis, 593
O'Donohue's triad, 277
Off-line medical control, 11
Oil (sebaceous) glands, 286
  of nose, 309
Ointments, 210
Old age. *See* Geriatric patients
Olecranon process, 359, 361f
Olfactory nerve, 309
Oliguria, 566
On-line medical control, 11
On-site treatment, 36, 36f
Open pneumothorax, 332f, 335–336
Opium, 594t–595t
Oral cavity (mouth), 558, 559f
  inspection and palpation of, procedure for, 97, 98f
Oral contraceptives, 837
Oral hypoglycemic drugs, 836
Oral intubation, 139, 140–142
  equipment for, 140–142, 141f, 142f
  procedure for, 142–148, 143f–148f
Orbicularis oculi muscle, 352t, 353f
Orbicularis oris muscle, 352t, 353f
Orbits (eye sockets), 307
Orchitis, mumps and, 608
Organ donation, laws regarding, 22, 23f
Organophosphate insecticide poisoning, 587–588
Oropharyngeal airways, 135f, 135–136, 141
  pediatric, 684
  in upper airway obstruction, 393
Oropharynx, 128
Orthopaedic injuries. *See* Bone(s), injuries of; Dislocations; Fracture(s)
Orthopnea, 385
Orthostatic changes, endocrine emergencies and, 530
Orthostatic (postural) hypotension
  aging and, 652
  dizziness and, 659

Osborne wave (J wave), 624, 625f
OSHA (Occupational Safety and Health Administration), 633
Osmitrol (mannitol), 795–796
Osmosis, 181
Osmotic pressure, 181–182, 182f, 183t
Ossicles, 304
Osteoarthritis, in geriatric patients, 660
Osteoblasts, 356
Osteoporosis, in geriatric patients, 660
Ova (eggs), 690
Ovaries, 529, 563
  anatomy and physiology of, 690, 691f
  cysts of, 568–569
  hormones of, 524t
Overpressure injuries, 632
  blasts and, 282
Ovulation, 690, 692
Oxtriphylline, respiratory distress and, 387t
Oxygen, 132f, 132–134
  gas exchange and, 381–382, 382f
  inspired, fraction of, 132
  partial pressure of
    in arterial blood (PaO$_2$), 381
    in venous blood (PvO$_2$), 381
Oxygen (therapeutic), 47–48, 807–808
  in asthma, in children, 679
  in cardiac disorders, 430
  in chronic obstructive pulmonary disease, 396
  in distressed newborn, 717
  oxygen delivery devices and, 132–134, 133f, 134f
  in preeclampsia and eclampsia, 703
  in respiratory emergencies, in geriatric patients, 656
  in shock, in children, 680
Oxygen-powered demand valve, 138, 138f
Oxygen pressure regulator, 132
Oxytocin (Pitocin; Syntocin), 808–809
  in postpartum hemorrhage, 713
Oxytocin (physiologic), 525

P

PAC (premature atrial complex), 449–451, 504t–505t

Pacemaker
 artificial, 495
  heart rhythms and, 495f, 495–501
  noninvasive, 519
 atrial, wandering, 448, 502t–503t
Pacemaker cardioverter-defibrillators (PCDs), 512
Pacemaker cells, 416
PaCO₂ (partial pressure of carbon dioxide in arterial blood), 381, 695
Pain
 abdominal
  assessment of, 565, 565f
  conditions causing, 563–564
  in pelvic inflammatory disease, 699
 cardiac-related problems and, 417
 in chest. See Chest, pain in
 pleuritic, in pneumonia, in geriatric patients, 656
 PQRST method for evaluating, 106, 106t
 on urination (dysuria), 567
Palatine bones, 309
Palpation, 107
 of abdomen, 118
  abdominal injuries and, 345–346
  acute abdomen and, 566
 of chest, 118
  cardiac-related problems and, 418
  in respiratory distress, 389–390
  upper airway disorders and, 131
 for pulse, locations for, 110, 111f
Pancreas, 528–529, 559f, 560
 hormones of, 524t, 528–529
PaO₂ (partial pressure of oxygen in arterial blood), 381
Paper bag effect, injuries to thorax and, 280, 281f
Para, definition of, 697
Paradoxical breathing motion
 in children, 671
 flail chest and, 328
Paramedic(s)
 certification of, 7, 16
  reciprocity and, 7
 continuing education and, 8
 ethics and, 4–5
 licensure and, 7
  reciprocity and, 7

national organizations for, 8
professionalism and, 4
responsibilities of, 6–7
 for assessment at the scene, 6
 for emergency management, 6
 for emergency transport, 6
 for equipment maintenance, 7
 for record keeping, 6–7
 for vehicle maintenance, 7
safety of. See Personal safety
stress on, disaster management and, 61–62
Paranoid disorders, in geriatric patients, 659–660
Parasympathetic nervous system, 85, 546–547
 anatomy and physiology of, 547–548
Parasympatholytic drugs, 769–770
Parathyroid glands, 526f, 527
 hormones of, 524t
Parathyroid hormone (PTH), 527
Parens patriae doctrine, 26
Parents
 anxiety in, 669
 sudden infant death syndrome and, 673–674
Paresis, spinal injuries and, 321
Paresthesia, in hypoparathyroidism, 527
Parity, 704
Paroxysmal junctional tachycardia, 468
Paroxysmal nocturnal dyspnea, 422
Paroxysmal supraventricular tachycardia (PSVT; SVT), 452f, 452–454, 454f, 502t–503t
Partial rebreathing mask, for oxygen delivery, 133–134, 134f
Partial-thickness (second-degree) burns, 294f, 294t, 294–295
 deep, 295
 superficial, 294–295
PASG (pneumatic anti-shock garment), 195–201, 197f–201f
 deflation of, 196
Patella (kneecap), 362, 363f
Pathologic fractures, 368
Patient(s)
 amount of information given to, 121
 calling by name, 104

confidentiality and
 breach of, as basis of liability, 27
 legal principle of, 24
disentanglement of, 48, 49f
emergency care and transportation of, 49
gaining access to, 47–48, 48f
geriatric. See Geriatric patients
information and education provided to, 13
intoxicated, 27
911 emergency telephone number and, 16
pediatric. See Children; Infant(s); Newborn
removal of, 48–49
Patient assessment, 89–124, 91f. See also Primary survey; Secondary survey; specific body sites
 abdominal trauma and, 344–346
 acute abdomen and, 564–565
 anaphylaxis and, 575–576
 behavioral emergencies and, 723–726
  emergency interview and, 723–724
  factors affecting emotional states and, 725–726
  information sources for, 723
  mental status examination in, 724–725
  transporting patient and, 725
 burn injuries and, 298–299
 cardiac-related problems and, 416–418
  history taking in, 417
  physical examination in, 417–418
 central nervous system disorders and, respiratory disorders and, 402
 chronic obstructive pulmonary disease and, 395–396, 396f
 coma and, 551
 communicating patient data and, 121–124
 dislocations and, 370, 373
 ear injuries and, 305
 endocrine emergencies and, 529–530
  diabetic, 531, 532, 533
 eye injuries and, 307–308
 fractures and, 368–370
 geriatric patients and, 653–655
  communication and, 653, 654f

Patient assessment, geriatric patients and (continued)
  history taking and, 653–654
  physical examination and, 654–655
  of gynecologic and obstetric patients, 696–698
    fetal assessment in, 698
    history in, 697–698
    physical examination in, 698
  head injuries and, 316–317
  inhalation injuries and, 400–401
  muscle injuries and, 366
  pneumonia and, 399–400
  pulmonary embolism and, 401
  re-evaluation in, 121
  respiratory distress and, 385–393
  at scene, as responsibility of paramedic, 6
  scene control and, 92
  scene survey and, 90–92
  shock and, 193–195
  soft-tissue injuries and, 290–291
    to neck, 318
  status epilepticus and, 554
  stroke and, 555
  suicide victim and, 728t
  trauma scoring systems and, 119–121, 120f
  upper airway and, 129–131
  upper airway obstruction and, 393
  urinary system disorders and, 566–567
Patient care areas, disaster management and, 59
Patient education
  allergic and anaphylactic reactions and, 577
  burn injury prevention and, 301
Patient history. See History taking
Patient refusal, 26
Patient safety, 45
Patient transfer, 13
Payment, ability to pay and, access to care and, 13
PCDs (pacemaker cardioverter-defibrillators), 512
Peak flow
  in asthma, in children, 679
  in chronic obstructive pulmonary disease, 395–396, 396f
Peak flow meter, 396, 396f
Pectoralis major muscle, 351t, 353f
Pectoralis minor muscle, 351t
Pedestrian congestion, disaster management and, 61
Pedestrian injuries, 277–279, 278f

Pediatric(s), 668. See also Children; Infant(s); Newborn
Pediatric Glasgow Coma Scale, 121, 764
Pediatric Trauma Score, 119–120, 764
Pediculocidal agents, 838
Pelvic cavity, 82, 85f
Pelvic girdle, 361, 362f
Pelvic inflammatory disease (PID), 568, 699
Pelvic region, inspection and palpation of, procedure for, 101, 101f
Penetrating trauma. See Trauma, penetrating
Penetration, by chemicals, 642
Penicillins, 839–840
  allergic reaction to, 573
Penis, priapism and, 119
  spinal injuries and, 321
Peptic ulcers, in geriatric patients, 661
Percussion, of chest, 118
Percutaneous exposure, 604
Perfusion, 103
  in shock, 195–203
    evaluation of, 194
    intravenous fluids and, 197, 201–203
    pneumatic anti-shock garment and, 195–201, 197f–201f
Pericardial effusion, 423
Pericardial sac, 339, 339f
Pericardiocentesis, 339
  skill procedure for, 337–338, 337–338f
Pericarditis, 427
Pericardium, 411, 411f
Perimetrium, 692
Periosteum, 356, 356f, 538
Peripheral cyanosis, 131, 389
Peripheral edema, testing for, 119
Peripheral nervous system, 85, 536. See also Autonomic nervous system
  anatomy and physiology of, 543, 544f, 544t, 545f, 545–548
Peripheral vascular disease, 428–430, 429f, 430f
Peripheral (systemic) vascular resistance, 178
  aging and, 651
  during pregnancy, 695
Peripheral vasoconstriction, 622
Peristalsis, 558
Peritoneum, 561

Peritonitis, 344, 563
Permanent cavity, 268, 268f, 269f
Permeation, by chemicals, 642
Permucosal exposure, 604
Peroneus longus muscle, 352t, 353f
Personal safety, 42–44
  acquired immunodeficiency syndrome and, 610–611
  eye protection and, 43
  footwear and, 45, 45f
  gloves and, 43
  hazardous materials and, 642–643
    levels of protection and, 643
  hepatitis and, 604, 605
  herpes and, 606
  as professional responsibility, 42, 45
  respiratory protection and, 43–45, 44f
  rubella and, 608
  turnout gear and, 43, 43f, 44f
  varicella and, 606
Pertinent negatives, 122
  documenting, 124
Pertinent positives, 122
Pesticide poisoning, 587–588
  organophosphate and carbamate insecticides and, 587–588
Pethadol (meperidine), 796–797
Pethidine (meperidine), 594t–595t
Petroleum distillate ingestion, 585
Peyote, 594t–595t
pH, 187, 187f
Phagocytosis, 603
Pharyngo-tracheal lumen (PtL) airway, 139, 149, 149f, 154–155
  equipment for, 154–155
  procedure for, 156–160, 156f–160f
Pharynx (throat), 128, 558, 559f
  alignment of planes of, for endotracheal intubation, 139, 140f
Phencyclidine (angel dust; crystal; PCP), 594t–595t
  abuse of, 596
  analogs of, 594t–595t
Phenmetrazine, 594t–595t
Phenobarbital, in seizures, in children, 674
Phenobarbital sodium (Luminal Sodium), 809–810
Phenol (carbolic acid), burn injuries and, 300
Phenothiazines, overdose of, 593

Phenylephrine hydrochloride, respiratory distress and, 387t
Phenylpropanolamine, abuse of, 597
Phenytoin sodium (Dilantin), 810–811
Phonation, 127
Physical examination, 116–119
　of abdomen, 118–119
　　acute abdomen and, 565–566
　in anaphylactic reactions, 576
　cardiac-related problems and, 417–418
　of chest and back, 117–118
　in children, 669, 670t, 670–671
　in diabetic ketoacidosis, 531
　of extremities, 119
　geriatric patients and, 654–655
　gynecologic and obstetric patient and, 698
　of head and neck, 116–117
　nervous system emergencies and, 549–550, 550f
　in poisoning and overdose, 583
　in respiratory distress, 389–393
　upper airway disorders and, 130–131
Physics, 264–268
　Conservation of Energy law and, 264–265, 265f
　energy exchange and, 266–268
　　density of body tissue and, 267, 267f
　　particle motion and, 267f–268f, 267–268
　kinetic energy and, 265–266
　Newton's first law of motion and, 265
　Newton's second law of motion and, 265, 266f
Physostigmine salicylate (Antilirium), 811–812
Pia mater, 538
PID (pelvic inflammatory disease), 699
Pills, 210
Piloerection (goose flesh), narcotic withdrawal and, 596
Pin-indexing system, 132
Pinna (auricle), 304
Pitocin (oxytocin), 808–809
　in postpartum hemorrhage, 713
Pitting edema, 119
Pituitary gland, 523, 524–525, 525f
　hormones of, 524t, 808–809
Pivot joints, 364t

PJC (premature junctional complex), 465–466, 504t–505t
Placards, hazardous materials and, 636, 636f, 637t, 638f
Placenta, 694
　abruptio placentae and, 704, 704f
Placenta previa, 703–704, 704f
Planes, anatomical, 82, 83f
Plants, poisonous, 588–589
Plasma, 182, 185
　for transfusion, 186
Platelets, 186
　aggregation of, in decompression sickness, 630
　formation of, 356–357
Pleurae, 382
Pleural effusion, 423
Pleural friction rub, 386
Pleuritic pain, in pneumonia, in geriatric patients, 656
Pleuritis, 399
Pneumatic anti-shock garment (PASG), 195–201, 197f–201f
　deflation of, 196
Pneumonia, 399–400
　assessment of, 399–400
　in geriatric patients, 656
　management of, 400
　pathophysiology of, 399
Pneumonitis, interstitial, 381
Pneumothorax, 280, 330–336
　auscultation and, 327
　open, 332f, 335–336
　simple, 330–331, 331f
　tension, 331–335, 332f
　　thoracentesis and, 331–335, 333–335f
Pocket face mask, 138, 138f
　in upper airway obstruction, 393
Poison control center, 580–581
Poisoning, 580–593. See also Drug overdose
　alcohols and, 585
　bites and stings and, 590–591
　caustics and, 584–585
　exposure and absorption routes and, 581
　food poisoning and, 588
　inhalation injuries and, 585–587. See also Inhalation injuries; Smoke inhalation
　management of, 581–584
　　decontamination in, 583–584
　　primary survey in, 581–582
　　scene survey in, 581
　　secondary survey in, 582–583

　pesticides and, 587–588
　petroleum distillates and, 585
　poison control centers and, 580–581
　poisonous plants and, 588–589
Polydipsia, 529
Polymorphous ventricular tachycardia, 479
Polyphagia, 529
Polyuria, 529
Pons, 543
Portable radio equipment, 34
Portuguese man-of-war stings, 590
Positive-pressure ventilation, 138, 138f, 139f
Postdisaster plan, 61–62
Postganglionic neurons, 546
Postpartum hemorrhage, 713
Post-traumatic stress disorders, 65–66, 67
Postural (orthostatic) hypotension
　aging and, 652
　dizziness and, 659
Postures, terms for, 82
Potassium, 184
Potassium chloride, 813
Powders, 210
PQRST method, 106, 106t
Precipitous delivery, 713
Precordial thump, 511
Prednisone, respiratory distress and, 387t
Preeclampsia, 703
Prefixes, of medical terms, 79
Preganglionic neurons, 546, 547
Pregnancy, 694–696, 700–704
　abortion and, 702–703
　delivery and. See Delivery; Labor
　eclampsia and, 703
　ectopic, 563, 568, 701f, 701–702
　fertilization and, 694
　fetal growth during, 694–695, 695t, 696f
　labor and, 705
　maternal changes during, 695–696
　medical conditions in, 701
　narcotic addiction in, 596
　normal signs of, 697
　patient assessment in, 696–698
　　fetal assessment in, 698
　　history taking in, 697–698
　　physical examination in, 698
　preeclampsia and, 703
　premature birth and, 694–695
　statistics on conditions of, 706t

Pregnancy (*continued*)
    third trimester bleeding and, 703–704
        abruptio placentae and, 704, 704f
        placenta previa and, 703–704, 704f
    trauma in, 700
    uterine rupture during, 713–714
    vaginal bleeding during, 699
Premature atrial complex (PAC), 449–451, 504t–505t
Premature infants, 694–695, 716–717
Premature junctional complex (PJC), 465–466, 504t–505t
Premature ventricular complex (PVC), 471–475, 472f
Presentation, labor and, 705
Present illness, history of, 106, 106t
Pressure. *See also* Blood pressure
    hydrostatic (water), 184, 630
    intracranial, 311, 312
        decreasing, 317–318
        nervous system emergencies and, 549
    osmotic, 181–182, 182f, 183t
Pressure-related injury. *See* Barotrauma
Pressure waves, blast injuries and, 282
Priapism, 119
    spinal injuries and, 321
Primary survey, 92–103
    abdominal trauma and, 344
    acute abdomen and, 565
    burn injuries and, 298–299
    cardiac-related problems and, 417
    endocrine emergencies and, 530
    nervous system emergencies and, 548
    poisoning and overdose and, 581–582
    respiratory distress and, 385
    shock and, 193–194
    simultaneous evaluation in, 103
    skill procedure for, 93f–102f, 93–102
    thoracic injuries and, 326
    upper airway and, 129–130
Primary ventricular standstill, 506t–507t
PR interval, 436
Privacy, invasion of, as basis of liability, 27
Privilege, legal principle of, 24
Procainamide (Pronestyl), 814–815

Procaine (Novocaine), allergic reaction to, 573
Procardia (nifedipine), 803–804
Prodrome, coma and, 551
Profession, 4
Professionalism, 4
    personal safety and, 42, 45
Professional organizations, for paramedics, 8
Profile, penetrating trauma and, 269, 269f
Progesterone, 690
    menstrual cycle and, 694
Progestogens, 836–837
Prolactin, 525
Prolapse, of heart valves, 426
Prolapsed umbilical cord, 712f, 712–713
Pronation, 365
Prone posture, 82
Pronestyl (procainamide), 814–815
Pronunciation, of medical terms, 78
Propoxyphene (Darvon), overdose of, 591
Propranolol (Inderal), 815–816
Prostaglandins, 623
Prostate gland, 562, 562f
Protective barriers, 611, 611f
Protective eye wear, 611, 611f, 613
Protein, 184
Proteinaceous matter, 613
Protocols, 11
Proventil (albuterol), 767–768
    in bronchospasm, in children, 679
    in chronic obstructive pulmonary disease, 398, 399t
Proximal direction, 82, 83f
Pseudoaneurysm, 276
PSVT (paroxysmal supraventricular tachycardia; SVT), 452f, 452–454, 454f, 502t–503t
Psychiatric disorders. *See* Behavioral and psychiatric disorders
Psychiatric emergency, emotional crisis versus, 722–723
Psychogenic disorders, in geriatric patients, 660
Psychological reaction, to sexual assault, 699
Psychoses, 721t, 722t, 725
    Korsakoff's, 598
    phencyclidine abuse and, 596
PTH (parathyroid hormone), 527

PtL (pharyngo-tracheal lumen) airway, 139, 149, 149f, 154–155
    equipment for, 154–155
    procedure for, 156–160, 156f–160f
Pubis, 361, 362f
Public education, 13
Public safety agencies, 13
Pulmonary circulation, 408, 411f
Pulmonary contusions, 328–329, 329f
    in children, 681
Pulmonary edema
    allergic reactions and, 574
    in geriatric patients, 656
    left ventricular failure and, 422–423
    in narcotic abuse, 596
Pulmonary embolism, 427
    assessment of, 401
    in geriatric patients, 655–656
    management of, 401
    pathophysiology of, 401
Pulse, 110–111, 111f, 111t
    checking, procedure for, 95, 95f
    of infant, newborn, 715
    locations to palpate for, 110, 111f
    rhythm of, 110
        normal and abnormal deviations in, 111
    in shock, 194
    strength of, 110
    tilt test and, 114–115
Pulse deficit, 418
Pulse pressure, 111
    in compensated shock, 192
Pulse rate, 110
    abnormal, causes of, 111, 111t
    in respiratory distress, 389
Pulsus paradoxus, 131, 427
    in chronic obstructive pulmonary disease, 394–395, 395
    in respiratory distress, 391–393
Puncture wound, 288–289, 289f
Pupils
    examination of, 117
    fixed and dilated, 312, 549
        in coma, 658
        head injuries and, 317
        narcotic overdose and, 591
Purkinje system, 415
Purulent exudate (pus), 399
PVC (premature ventricular complex), 471–475, 472f

PvCO₂ (partial pressure of carbon dioxide in venous blood), 381
P wave, 436, 436f
Pyrogens, 623
Pyrolysis, 585

Q

QRS complex, 436, 436f
Quadriceps femoris muscle, 351t, 353f
Questions
  direct, 105, 105t, 106
  open-ended, 105, 105t, 106
Quinidine gluconate (Quinaglute; Quinidex), 816–817
Q wave, 436, 436f

R

R (roentgen), 642
Raccoon's eyes, basilar skull fracture and, 315
Racemic epinephrine (Vaponephrin), 817–818
Radiation (process), heat transfer and, 619, 621f, 716
Radiation, ionizing, 46, 641–642
  burns and, 292
    management of, 301
Radiation hazards, 46
Radioactive substances, 641–642
Radio communication, 30–31, 31f
  equipment maintenance and, 38
  frequencies for, 17, 30, 33
  with medical facilities, 38
  mobile equipment for, 34, 36, 36f
  repeaters and remote receivers for, 34
  technique for
    codes used in, 37–38
    medical facilities and, 38
    transmitting techniques and, 37
Radiographic contrast material, allergic reaction to, 573
Radius (bone), 359, 361f
Rales, 117, 391
  in pulmonary edema, 422
Rape, 699–700, 726–727
Rapport, 104
Rationalization, 70
Rattlesnake bites, 590
Reaction distance, 265
Rear-end collisions, 275f, 275–276, 276f

Reasonable force, in violent situations, 730
Rebound, abdominal injuries and, 345
Reciprocity, certification and licensure and, 7
Recompression, in decompression sickness, 631
Record keeping
  communicating patient data and, 122, 123f, 124
  coordinated, 13
  faulty, dangers of, 28
  as responsibility of paramedic, 6–7
Rectum, 344, 559f, 560
  cancer of, in geriatric patients, 661
Rectus abdominis muscle, 351t, 353f
Red blood cells (erythrocytes), 185f, 185–186, 186f
  formation of, 356–357
  for transfusion, 186–187
Reentry, arrhythmias and, 441f, 441–442, 442f
  prehospital intervention for, 506–518
Re-evaluation, of patient, 121
Reflex(es)
  Cushing's, nervous system emergencies and, 549
  diving, mammalian, 629
  of newborn, 716t
Reflex diuresis, 622
Refractory period, cardiac, 436, 437f
  relative, 436
Regular Insulin (insulin), 791–792
Regurgitation (insufficiency), of heart valves, 426
Relative refractory period, cardiac, 436
Release, signature of, 26
Remote receivers, for radio communication, 34
Removal, 48–49
Renal calculi (kidney stones), 566
Repression, 70
Reproductive system, 86, Color Plate 17, Color Plate 18
  female. *See also* Pregnancy
    anatomy and physiology of, 563, 690–692
    disorders of, 568–569
  male
    anatomy and physiology of, 562, 562f
    disorders of, 568

Rescue litters, 48, 48f
Rescue management, 41–50
  assessment of scene and, 46–47
  disentanglement and, 48, 49f
  emergency care and transportation and, 49
  gaining access and, 47–48, 48f
  hazardous materials incidents and, 639–641, 641f
  removal and, 48–49
  safety and, 42–46
    on-scene hazards and, 45–46
    of patient, 45
    personal, 42–44
Residual volume (RV), 384
Resource(s), coordination and allocation of
  communications system and, 32
  disaster management and, 61
Resource inventory, disaster plan and, 55
Respiration(s), 86. *See also* Breathing; Hyperventilation; Hyperventilation syndrome; Lung(s); *headings beginning with terms* Pulmonary *and* Respiratory
  acid-base balance and, 188–189
  Cheyne-Stokes, 312, 388f
  depth of, 110
  evaluating, 110, 110t
  hypoventilation and, 384
  Kussmaul's, 388f
    in acute renal failure, 566
    in diabetic ketoacidosis, 566
  modified forms of, 383
  muscles of, 351t, 353f, 382–384, 383f
    innervation of, 384
  nervous system emergencies and, 549
  obstructive, 388f
  respiratory volumes and capacities and, 383–384, 384f
Respiratory acidosis, 189, 189f
Respiratory alkalosis, 190
Respiratory distress, patient assessment in, 385–393
  primary survey and, 385
  secondary survey and, 385–393
Respiratory protection, for rescue operations, 43–45, 44f
Respiratory rate, 110, 110t
  in children, 670
  respiratory distress and, 385
Respiratory rhythm, 110

Respiratory system, 86, 126, Color Plate 13. *See also* Lower airway; Upper airway; Upper airway disorders; *specific organs*
  allergic reactions and, 574
  anatomy and physiology of, 378–385
    aging and, 651
  disorders of, 377–403
    in children, 671
    common home medications for, 832–833
    in geriatric patients, 655–656
      management of, 656
  fetal, 694–695
  during pregnancy, 695
Response plan, for disasters, 56–59, 61
Responsiveness, checking, 103
  in burn injuries, 298
  in poisoning and overdose, 581
  procedure for, 93, 93f
  in shock, 193–194
Restraints, in violent situations, 730f, 730–732
  methods of, 730f, 730–731, 731f
  procedures for, 731–732
Resuscitation
  cardiopulmonary, performance sheets for, 749, 752, 755, 758–766
  in shock, 195
Resuscitation bags, pediatric, 684
Resuscitation mask, pediatric, 684
Reticular activating system, 311
  coma and, 551
Retina, 306, 307f
Retractions, 131, 389
  in chronic obstructive pulmonary disease, 395
Retriage, 59
Retrograde amnesia, 110
Retroperitoneal space, 561
Rewarming
  in frostbite, 626
  in hypothermia, 625
Reye's syndrome, in children, 675–676, 676t
Rh antigen, 186
Rhinorrhea, drug withdrawal and, 598
Rhonchi, 117–118, 391
Ribs, 359, 360f
  fractures of, 327–328
    in geriatric patients, 662
RICE care, sprains and, 366
Right ventricular failure, 423
Rodenticide poisoning, 587

Roentgen (R), 642
Rollover collisions, 277, 278f
Rotation, 82, 84f
  penetrating trauma and, 269, 270f
Rotational collisions, 277, 277f
Rotor wash, 14–15
Rouleaux formation, 193
r-TPA (Activase; tissue plasminogen activator), 820–821
Rubella, 608
Rubeola, 608–609, 609f
Rule of nines, 295f, 295–296
Rule of palms, 295
Run report, 6–7
Run reviews, 18
RV (residual volume), 384
R wave, 436, 436f

S

Sacral spine, 357, 359f, 543
Saddle joints, 364t
Safety
  burn injury prevention and, 301
  helicopters and, 15, 15f
  of patient, rescue management and, 45
  personal. *See* Personal safety
Safety belts, 273
Sagittal plane, 82, 83f
Salicylates, overdose of, 592
Salivary glands, 559f, 560
Salt water drowning, 628–629
SA (sinoatrial; sinus) node, 415
  arrhythmias originating in, 443–447
Sartorius muscle, 351t
Satellite receiver system, 31
Scabicidal agents, 838
Scabies, 608
Scalp
  bleeding from, control of, 317
  inspection and palpation of, procedure for, 96, 96f
SCBA (self-contained breathing apparatus), 43–45, 44f
Scene control, 92
  dealing with people on the scene and, 92
  distractions and, removing, 92
Scene survey, 90–92
  burn injuries and, 298
  clues to medical illness in, 92
  mechanism of injury and, 91–92
  poisoning and overdose and, 581
  potential hazards and, 90–91

Schizophrenia, in geriatric patients, 659–660
Sclera, 306, 307f
Scorpion stings, 590
SCUBA (self-contained underwater breathing apparatus), 44, 44f
SEA-3, mental status examination and, 725
Seat belts, spinal injuries and, 320
Sea wasp stings, 590
Sebaceous (oil) glands, 286
  of nose, 309
Secondary survey, 103–119
  abdominal trauma and, 344–346
  acute abdomen and, 565–566
  burn injuries and, 299
  cardiac-related problems and, 417–418
  data collection in, 107–109
  diagnostic signs in, 109–116
  head-to-toe direction for, 104
  nervous system emergencies and, 548–550
    history in, 548–549
    neurologic evaluation in, 549
    physical examination in, 549–550, 550f
    vital signs in, 549
  patient history in, 104–107
    communication principles and, 104–105
    components of, 106–107
    interview techniques and, 105t, 105–106
  physical examination in, 117–119
  poisoning and overdose and, 582–583
  respiratory distress and, 385–393
    history in, 385–389
    physical examination in, 389–393
  in shock, 194–195
  thoracic injuries and, 326–327
  toe-to-head direction for, 104
  upper airway and, 130–131
Second-degree (partial-thickness) burns, 294f, 294t, 294–295
  deep, 295
  superficial, 294–295
Sedatives, 830
  overdose of, 591–592
Seizures, 552–553
  assessment of, 552–553

in children, 674
  assessment of, 674
  management of, 674
clonic, 553
eclamptic, 703
epileptogenic foci (seizure foci) and, 552
febrile, 623
  in children, 674
focal motor, 553
general complex (focal), 552, 553
in geriatric patients, 658
grand mal, 553
hysterical, 553
Jacksonian, 553
management of, 553
partial complex, 552
pathophysiology of, 552
petit mal, 553
in poisoning and overdose, 582
psychomotor, 553
status epilepticus and, 553–554
  in children, 674
tonic, 553
Self-contained breathing apparatus (SCBA), 43–45, 44f
Self-contained underwater breathing apparatus (SCUBA), 44, 44f
Sella turcica, 524
Selye, Hans, 65
Semilunar valves, 412
Semipermeable membrane, 180
Sensation, checking, dislocations and, 370, 373
Senses, detection of hazardous materials by, 636, 638
Sensitization, 573
Sensory (afferent) neurons, 538, 539f
Separation anxiety, children and, 669
Septicemia, in children, 675
Septum, nasal, 309
Serratus anterior muscle, 351t, 353f
Sewer gas, 586
Sexual abuse, of children, 681, 682, 683
Sexual assault, 699–700, 726–727
Sexually transmitted diseases, 605, 607–608, 609–611
Sharp instruments, universal precautions and, 109
Sheath of Schwann (neurilemma), 538, 539f
Shingles (herpes zoster), 606f, 606–607

Shipping papers, for hazardous materials, 636
Shivering, 620–621
Shock, 175–203
  aerobic and anaerobic metabolism and, 176
  assessment of, 193–195
    primary survey in, 193–194
    secondary survey in, 194–195
  cardiogenic, 424
    in children, 680
  compensated, 191–192
  Fick principle and, 176
  head injuries and, management of, 317
  hypovolemic, allergic reactions and, 574
  insulin, 532, 533
  irreversible, 192–193
    cellular pathophysiology of, 193
  management of, 195–203
    head injuries and, 317
    perfusion in, 195–203
    resuscitation in, 195
  pathophysiology of, 177–191
    blood vessels and, 179, 180f
    fluid and electrolytes and. See Blood; Fluid and electrolytes
    heart and, 177–179, 177f–179f
    pressure changes and, 191
  in pregnancy, trauma and, 700
  spinal, 320
  uncompensated, 192
Shoulder(s), muscles of, 351t, 353f, 354f
Shoulder (transverse) lie presentation, 705, 711
Sickle cell anemia, 185
Sick sinus syndrome, 495
SIDS (crib death; sudden infant death syndrome), 673–674
  diagnosis of, 673
  management of, 673–674
Sighing, 383
Sigmoid colon, 559f, 560
Sigmoid flexure, 344
Signature of release, 26
Silence, as breath sound, 131
Silo gas, 586
Simple mask, for oxygen delivery, 133, 134f
Simple Triage and Rapid Treatment (START), 56, 57f
Simplex communication system, 17, 30

Sinoatrial (SA; sinus) node, 415
  arrhythmias originating in, 443–447
Sinus arrest, 447, 502t–503t
Sinus arrhythmia, 445–446, 502t–503t
Sinus bradycardia, 443, 502t–503t
Sinus (SA; sinoatrial) node, 415
  arrhythmias originating in, 443–447
Sinus rhythm, normal, 502t–503t
Sinus tachycardia, 444, 502t–503t
Skeletal (striated; voluntary) muscle, 85, 350, 352, 355f
Skeletal system, 85, Color Plate 1. See also Bone(s); Musculoskeletal system; Skeleton
  anatomy and physiology of, 355–365, 356f
Skeleton. See also Bone(s); Skeletal system
  appendicular, 85, 357, 359–365
  axial, 85, 357–359
Skin, 86–87, 115–116, 116t. See also Integumentary system
  allergic reactions and, 574
  burn injuries of. See Burn injuries
  color of, 116
    in shock, 194
  cyanosis of, 389
  disorders of, common home medications for, 838–839
  function of, 287
  in respiratory distress, 389
  soft-tissue injuries and. See Soft-tissue injuries
  structure of, 286–287, 287f
  temperature of, in shock, 194
  turgor of, 116
    in respiratory distress, 389
Skin popping, 593
Skull, 357, 358f
  fracture of, 314–315
    basilar, 314–315, 315f
    closed and open, 314
    depressed, 314, 314f
Slander, as basis of liability, 27
SLUD, in acetylcholinesterase inhibition, 587
Small intestine, 558, 559f
  cancer of, in geriatric patients, 661
  injuries of, 344
Smell, during secondary survey, 107

Smelling salts (aromatic ammonia), hysterical seizures and, 553
Smoke hazards, 46
Smoke inhalation, 297–298, 400–401
 assessment of, 400–401
 management of, 401, 585–586
 pathophysiology of, 400
Smoking, chronic obstructive pulmonary disease and, 395
Smooth (involuntary; visceral) muscle, 85, 350, 352, 355f
Snake bites, 590
 antivenins and, 590
Sneeze, 383
Sniffing position, 139
 endotracheal intubation and, in children, 684
Sodium, 184
Sodium bicarbonate, 818–819
 in acid-base disorders, cautions regarding use of, 191
 in cardiac disorders, 433–434
 in coma, 552
 in drowning victims, 629
Sodium chloride solution, 203
Sodium nitrite, 768–769
 in cyanide poisoning, 586
Sodium nitroprusside (Nipride), 819–820
Sodium thiosulfate, 768–769
 in cyanide poisoning, 586
Soft spot (fontanelle), 670–671
Soft-tissue injuries, 287–292
 amputation and, 290, 290f, 291f
  management of, 291
 assessment of, 290–291
 closed wounds and, 288
  management of, 291
 impaled objects and, 290, 290f
  management of, 291–292
 management of, 291–292
 to neck, 318–319
  assessment of, 318
  management of, 318–319
  pathophysiology of, 318
 open wounds and, 288–290
  management of, 291
Soleus muscle, 352t, 353f, 354f
Solid organs, 561
 abdominal, 343
Solu-Cortef (hydrocortisone sodium succinate), 790
Solu-Medrol (methylprednisolone sodium succinate), 799
 respiratory distress and, 387t
Solvent abuse, 597

Soma, of neuron, 536
Somatotropin (GH; growth hormone), 525
Sovereign immunity, 24
Spasms
 carpopedal, 402
  in hypoparathyroidism, 527
 laryngeal, 129
Speech, 127
 aphasia and, 658
 neurologic emergencies and, 549–550
Spelling, of medical terms, 78
Spermatogenesis, 525
Spider bites, 590
Spinal cavity, 84, 85f
Spinal column. *See* Spinal injuries; Vertebrae
Spinal cord
 anatomy and physiology of, 543
 meningitis and, in children, 675
Spinal injuries, 319–323
 assessment of, 320–321
 cervical, aggravation of, 318
 immobilization and, indications for, 317
 indications of, 320
 management of, 321–323, 322f
 mechanism of injury and, 319–320
 pathophysiology of, 320
 respiratory disorders and, 402
Spinal nerves, 543, 545
Spinal shock, 320
Spiral fractures, 368, 369f
Spirits, 210
Spleen, 86
 injuries of, 343
Sports injuries, 280–281
 of abdomen, 281
 of extremities, 281
 of head, 280
 of neck, 280
 of thorax, 280, 281f
Spouse abuse, 726–727
Sprain, 365
 management of, 366
Squelch control, radio communication and, 34
Staging areas, for disaster management, 58
Standard of care, malpractice and, 24–25
Standing orders, 11
Stapes (stirrup), 304
START (Simple Triage and Rapid Treatment), 56, 57f
State laws, 21
Station, labor and, 705

Status asthmaticus, 395
 in children, 679
  management of, 679
Status epilepticus, 553–554
 assessment of, 554
 in children, 674
 management of, 554
 pathophysiology of, 554
Stenosis, of heart valves, 426
Sternocleidomastoid muscle, 351t, 353f, 354f
Sternum, 359, 360f
Steroids, 837
Stethoscope, 108, 108f. *See also* Auscultation
Stimulants
 abuse of, 596–597
 list of, 594t–595t
Stingray stings, 591
Stirrup (stapes), 304
Stokes-Adams syndrome, 488
Stomach, 558, 559f
 gastroenteritis and, 564
 injuries of, 344
Stools, gastrointestinal bleeding and, 118, 564
Stopping distance, 265
Strain (muscle pull), 365
 management of, 366
Streptokinase (Kabikinase), 820–821
Stress, 63–73
 causes of, 66
 coping with, 69–71
 death and dying and, 71–72
 fight or flight response and, 65, 65f
 on rescuers, 61
  cumulative, 62
Stressors, 64
 paramedics and, 69
Stress reactions, 64–69, 65f. *See also* Fight or flight response
 acute, 66–67
 cumulative, 68–69
 delayed, 65–66, 67
Stretch, of muscles, 268
Striated (skeletal; voluntary) muscle, 85, 350, 352, 355f
Stridor, 131, 391
 allergic reactions and, 574
Stroke (cerebrovascular accident), 554–556
 assessment of, 555
 in geriatric patients, 658
 management of, 555–556
 pathophysiology of, 555
 thrombotic, 555

Stroke volume, 178–179, 413–414
Structures, stabilization of, 46
Strychnine ingestion, 587
ST segment, 436
Stylet, for endotracheal intubation, 141
Subarachnoid hemorrhage, 316
  stroke and, in geriatric patients, 658
Subarachnoid space, 539
Subcutaneous connective tissue, 287
Subcutaneous emphysema, 117, 131
Subdural hematoma, 316, 316f, 538–539
Subdural space, 538–539
Subluxation, vertebral, 320
Succinylcholine chloride (Anectine), 821–822
Sucking chest wound, 332f, 335–336
Suction, 141
  catheters for, 137, 137f
  of upper airway, 136f, 136–137, 137f
Sudden infant death syndrome (crib death; SIDS), 673–674
  diagnosis of, 673
  management of, 673–674
Sudoriferous (sweat) glands, 286
  heat transfer and, 621–622
Suffixes, of medical terms, 80
Suicide, 727–728, 728t
  emergency assessment scheme for, 728t
Sulfite, allergic reaction to, 574
Sulfonamides, 840
Sulfuric acid, burn injuries and, 300
Sunburn, 292
Superficial (first-degree) burns, 293–294, 294t
Superior (cranial) direction, 82, 83f
Supination, 365
Supine hypotensive syndrome, during pregnancy, 695
Supine posture, 82
Suppositories, 210
Surfactant, 381
  drowning and, salt versus fresh water, 628
Surname, 104
Survey. See Primary survey; Secondary survey
Sutures, cranial, 538

SVT (paroxysmal supraventricular tachycardia; PSVT), 452f, 452–454, 454f, 502t–503t
S wave, 436, 436f
Sweat (sudoriferous) glands, 286
  heat transfer and, 621–622
Sweating, profuse (diaphoresis), 389
Swimming muscle, 351t
Sympathetic nervous system, 85, 546–547
  anatomy and physiology of, 547
Sympathomimetics, 767–768, 780–784, 792–793, 797–799, 806–807, 817–818, 823–824
  in chronic obstructive pulmonary disease, 396–397, 397f, 397–398
  respiratory distress and, 387, 387t
Synapses, 546
Synchronized cardioversion
  emergency, 517–518
  skill procedure for, 514–517, 514f–517f
Syncope (fainting)
  cardiac-related problems and, 417
  in geriatric patients, 657
Synergistic effect, 328
Synovial cavity, 363
Synovial joints, 363, 364t
Syntocin (oxytocin), 808–809
  in postpartum hemorrhage, 713
Syphilis, 607, 610t
Syrup(s), 210
Syrup of ipecac, 822–823
  in poisoning and overdose, 583–584
Systemic (peripheral) vascular resistance, 178
Systems management, 13
System status manager. See Communications operator
Systole, 413
Systolic pressure. See Blood pressure, systolic

T

T_3 (triiodothyronine), 526
T_4 (thyroxine), 526
  heat transfer and, 622
Tablets, 210
Tachycardia, 111, 502t–503t
  atrial, 452f, 452–454, 454f, 502t–503t

  multifocal, 460–461, 502t–503t
  in chronic obstructive pulmonary disease, 395
  junctional, 502t–503t
    paroxysmal, 468
  management of, drugs in, 422
  in respiratory distress, 389
  sinus, 444, 502t–503t
  supraventricular, paroxysmal, 452f, 452–454, 454f, 502t–503t
  ventricular, 476, 477f, 478–479, 502t–503t
    polymorphous, 479
Tachyphylaxis, 656
Tachypnea, 131, 194, 388f, 389
  in diabetic ketoacidosis, 530
Tail bone (coccyx), 357, 359f, 543
Tailor's muscle, 351t
Talus, 362, 363, 363f
Talwin, overdose of, 591
Tarsal bones, 362, 363, 363f
Tartrazine yellow, allergic reaction to, 574
T-bone (lateral) collisions, 276–277
TDY (telephone device for the deaf), 32
Tear gas, 587
Teeth, 560
Telecommunicator. See Communications operator
Telemetry, 31
Telephone(s), cellular, 31, 31f, 36
Telephone device for the deaf (TDY), 32
Teletype (TTY), 32
Temperature. See Body temperature; Frostbite; Hyperthermia; Hypothermia
Temporary cavity, 268, 268f, 269f
10-Code systems, 37–38
Tenderness, abdominal injuries and, 345
Tendons (leaders), 352
Tension pneumothorax, 331–335, 332f
  thoracentesis and, 331–335, 333–335f
Terbutaline sulfate (Brethine; Bricanyl), 823–824
  in chronic obstructive pulmonary disease, 397, 399t
  respiratory distress and, 387t
Terminal rhythms, 506t–507t
Terminology. See Medical terminology

Testes, 529, 562, 562f
  hormones of, 524t
  mumps and, 608
  torsion of, 568
Testosterone, 562
Tetanus, 289
Tetracyclines, 840
Tetrahydrocannabinol, 596t–597t
Texas Tech University Pesticide Hotline, 638
Thalamus, 542
Theophylline, 832–833
  respiratory distress and, 387, 387t
Theophylline ethylenediamine (Aminophylline), 824–825
  in allergic and anaphylactic reactions, 576–577
  in asthma, in children, 679
  in cardiac disorders, 432
  in chronic obstructive pulmonary disease, 398–399, 399t
  in pulmonary edema, 423
  respiratory distress and, 387t
  in respiratory emergencies, in geriatric patients, 656
Thermal (heat) burns, 292, 292t, 298
  management of, 299, 300t
Thermometers
  electric, 115
  low reading, 624
  rectal, oral, and axillary, 115, 115f
Thermoregulation, 619–622. *See also* Frostbite; Hyperthermia; Hypothermia
  disruptions of, 622–627
  hypothalamus and thermostasis and, 619, 620f
  organ mediation of heat transfer and, 620–622
  physical principles of heat transfer and, 619–620, 621f
Thermostasis, hypothalamus and, 619, 620f
Thiamine (Betalin; vitamin B), 826
  in alcoholism, 598
  in coma, 552
  in diabetic ketoacidosis, 532
  in hyperosmolar hyperglycemia nonketotic coma, 532
  in neurologic emergencies, in geriatric patients, 659
Thigh
  bones of, 362, 363f
  muscles of, 351t, 353f

Third-degree (full-thickness) burns, 295, 295f
Thoracentesis (needle chest decompression), 331–332, 335
  skill procedure for, 333–335, 333–335f
Thoracic cavity, 82, 85f
Thoracic spine, 357, 359f, 543
Thorax, 359. *See also* Chest
  injuries of, 325–340
    assessment of, 326–327
    inadequate cardiac output and, 336–339
    inadequate circulating blood volume and, 339f, 340
    inadequate ventilation and, 327–336
    pathophysiology of, 327
  penetrating injuries of, 272
  sports injuries of, 280, 281f
Throat (pharynx), 128, 558, 559f
  alignment of planes of, for endotracheal intubation, 139, 140f
Thrombolytic drugs, 820–821
Thrombophlebitis, 119, 427
  deep vein, 428
Thrombosis
  hemodialysis and, 567–568
  stroke and, 555
Thyroid gland, 526f, 526–527
  heat transfer and, 622
  hormones of, 524t, 526, 837
Thyroid-stimulating hormone (thyrotropin; TSH), 525
Thyroid storm (thyrotoxic crisis), 526–527
Thyrotoxicosis (hyperthyroidism), 526–527
Thyrotropin (thyroid-stimulating hormone; TSH), 525
Thyroxine (T$_4$), 526
  heat transfer and, 622
Tibia, 362, 363f
Tibialis anterior muscle, 351t, 353f
Tick bites, 590
Tidal volume (V$_T$), 383
Tilt test, 114–115
Tinctures, 210
Tinnitus, 658
Tissue plasminogen activator (Activase; r-TPA), 820–821
TKO (to keep open) fluid administration rate, 202
TLC (total lung capacity), 383
T lymphocytes, 603

Toddler, developmental approach to, 672t
Toe-to-head survey, 104
  in children, 670
To keep open (TKO) fluid administration rate, 202
Tongue, 128
  upper airway obstruction by, 128–129
Tonsil tip (Yankauer), 136–137, 137f
Torsades de pointes, 479
Tort, 20
Torticollis, 351t, 593
Total lung capacity (TLC), 383
Touching
  anxiety about, 104
  children and, 669
  communication and, 105
Trachea
  alignment of planes of, for endotracheal intubation, 139, 140f
  anatomy and physiology of, 379fm 379–380
  injuries of, 318
Tracheal deviation, 390
Tracheal tugging, 389
Training, levels of, 16
Training component, of emergency medical services system, 12
Transcutaneous (external) cardiac pacing, 519
Transient ischemic attacks, in geriatric patients, 658
Transient states, emotional disturbance and, 721, 721t, 722t
Translaryngeal jet ventilation, 174
  procedure for, 170–173, 170f–173f
Transportation, 49. *See also* Aeromedical transport
  assessing need for specialized vehicles and, 47
  behavioral emergencies and, 725
  communication and, 37
  coordination of, disaster management and, 61
  disaster management and ambulance loading zone and, 59
  staging of, 59
  emergency care provided during, 49
  hazardous material exposure and, 644–645
  patient transfer and, 13

Transportation component, of emergency medical services system, 12
Transtentorial herniation, 312
Transverse colon, 344, 559f, 560
Transverse fractures, 368, 369f
Transverse (shoulder) lie presentation, 705, 711
Transverse plane, 82, 83f
Transversus abdominis muscle, 351t
Trapezius dorsi muscle, 351t
Trauma, 263–283. *See also specific injuries and sites of injuries*
  adult trauma score, 763
  blunt, 273f, 273–283
    abdominal, 342
    automotive injuries and, 273–277, 274f
    blast injuries and, 281–282, 282f
    to eye, 308
    motorcycle injuries and, 279
    particle motion and, 267
    pedestrian injuries and, 277–279, 278f
    sports injuries and, 280–281
    thoracic, 327
  in children, 680–681
  in geriatric patients, 662–663
    contributing factors and, 662
    management of, 662–663
    pathophysiology of, 662
  hypothermia and, 624
  pediatric trauma score, 764
  penetrating, 268–273
    to abdomen, 272
    abdominal, 342
    cavitation and, 269
    energy and, 269–270, 270t, 271f
    to extremities, 272–273
    fragmentation and, 269, 270f
    to head, 271–272
    mechanism of injury and, 270–271, 271f
    to neck, 272
    particle motion and, 267
    profile and, 269, 269f
    thoracic, 327
    to thorax, 272
    tumble or rotation and, 269, 270f
  physics and, 264–268
  in pregnancy, 700
  vaginal bleeding and, 699
Trauma scoring systems, 119–121, 120f

Triage
  color-coded systems for, 56
  common language systems for, 56
  coordination of, disaster management and, 61
  disaster plan and, 55–56, 57f, 58f
  hazardous material exposure and, 644
  numeric systems for, 56
  retriage and, 59
  tagging system for, 57, 58f
Triage decision scheme, 119, 120f
Triceps, 351t, 354f
Tricuspid valve, 411
Tridil (nitroglycerin), 804–805
Triglycerides (lipids), insulin and, 529
Triiodothyronine (T_3), 526
Trophoblast, 694
TSH (thyroid-stimulating hormone; thyrotropin), 525
TTY (Teletype), 32
Tuberculosis, 603, 610t
Tumble, penetrating trauma and, 269, 270f
Tumors, vaginal bleeding and, 699
Turgor, of skin, 116
  in respiratory distress, 389
Turnout gear, 43, 43f, 44f
T wave, 436, 436f
Twins
  fraternal, 712
  identical, 712
Tympanic membrane (eardrum), 304

U

UHF (ultra-high) radio frequencies, 33
  for radio communication, 31
Ulcers
  duodenal, 563
  peptic, in geriatric patients, 661
Ulna, 359, 361f
Ultra-high frequency (UHF) radio frequencies, 31, 33
Umbilical cord, 694
  prolapsed, 712f, 712–713
Uncal (lateral) syndrome, 312, 313f
Uncompensated shock, 192
Unconsciousness. *See also* Coma; Consciousness level; Glasgow Coma Scale
  duration of, cerebral concussion and, 314

examination of extremities and, 119
  in geriatric patients, 658
United Nations (UN) hazard class number, 636
U.S. Coast Guard National Response Center, 638
U.S. Department of Transportation
  Emergency Response Guidebook published by, 636, 641
  hazardous materials markings and, 636, 638f
U.S. Department of Transportation National Response Center, 638
Universal precautions, 108–109, 126, 132, 611f, 611–612, 612t
  open wounds and, 288
Up-and-over frontal collisions, 275
Upper airway
  anatomy and physiology of, 378
  assessment of, 129–131
    mechanism of injury and, 129
    primary survey and, 129–130
    secondary survey and, 130–131
  disorders of. *See* Airway obstruction; Upper airway disorders
  structures and functions of, 126–128, 127f
Upper airway disorders, 131–174. *See also* Airway obstruction
  cricothyroidotomy in, 160, 160f, 164, 169, 173
    needle, 170–173, 174
    surgical, 165–169, 173–174
  endotracheal intubation in. *See* Endotracheal intubation
  esophageal airways in, 139, 155, 155f, 160–164
  nasopharyngeal airways in, 136, 136f, 684
  oropharyngeal airways in, 135f, 135–136, 141, 393, 684
  oxygen in, 132f, 132–134. *See also* Oxygen (therapeutic)
  pharyngo-tracheal lumen airways in, 139, 149, 149f, 154–160
  positive-pressure ventilation in, 138, 138f, 139f
  suction in, 136f, 136–137, 137f
  traumatic, 129

Uremia, 566
Uremic frost, 566
Ureters, 561f, 561-562
Urethra, 86, 561f, 562
Urinary bladder, 86, 561f, 562
Urinary system, 86, Color Plate 16
  anatomy and physiology of, 561f, 561-562
  disorders of, 566-568
    acute, 566
    assessment of, 566-567
    chronic, 566
    common home medications for, 833-834
    management of, 567-568
Urinary tract infections, 566
Urticaria (hives), 574
Uterus, 563
  anatomy and physiology of, 692
  inversion of, postpartum, 714
  rupture of, pregnancy and, 713-714

V

V_A (alveolar ventilation), 384
Vaccination (immunization), 602
Vagina, 563
  anatomy and physiology of, 692
  bleeding from
    nontraumatic, 699
    traumatic, 699
  discharge from, gynecologic and obstetric patient and, 697-698
Vaginal show, 705
Vagus nerve, 414, 547-548
Valium. See Diazepam
Vallecula, 141
Valsalva's maneuver, 111
  in arrhythmias, 507
  in paroxysmal supraventricular tachycardia, 453
Valvular heart disease, 426-427
Vaponephrin (racemic epinephrine), 817-818
Varicella (chickenpox), 606, 606f, 610t
Varices, esophageal, 564, 598
  in geriatric patients, 661
Vas deferens, 562, 562f
Vasoconstriction, peripheral, 622
Vasodilators, 777-778, 789-790, 804-805, 819-820, 832
Vasopressin (ADH; antidiuretic hormone), 525
VC (vital capacity), 384

v_D (volume of dead space gas), 384
Vehicle(s), 13
  cleaning, 614
  extrication from, 49
  hazardous materials and contamination by, 644
    protection from, 643
  hazardous materials incident materials for, 639
  KKK standards for, 13
  maintenance of, as responsibility of paramedic, 7
  stabilization of, 46
Vehicle transmission, 603
Vehicular accidents
  air bags and, 273
  assessment of damage to car and, 264
  blunt trauma and, 273-274, 274f
  distance required to stop and, 265
  fracture of larynx and, 129
  frontal collisions and, 274-275
    down-and-under pattern of, 274-275, 275f
    up-and-over pattern of, 275
  lateral collisions and, 276-277
  in pregnancy, 700
  rear-end collisions and, 275f, 275-276, 276f
  rollover collisions and, 277, 278f
  rotational collisions and, 277, 277f
  safety belts and, 273
Vehicular congestion, disaster management and, 61
Veins, 408, 410f
  coronary, 413
  for intravenous infusions, in children, 687, 687f
  peripheral venipuncture and, procedure for, 235-238, 235f-238f
Velocity, 266
Venipuncture, peripheral, procedure for, 235-238, 235f-238f
Ventolin (albuterol), 767-768
  in chronic obstructive pulmonary disease, 398, 399t
Ventral cavity, 82, 85f
Ventral (anterior) direction, 82, 83f
Ventricles, 411, 411f
  arrhythmias originating in, 468-482

Ventricular escape complexes and rhythms, 468-469, 504t-505t
Ventricular fibrillation, 424-425, 425f, 480, 506t-507t
Ventricular standstill, primary, 506t-507t
Ventricular tachycardia, 476, 477f, 478-479, 502t-503t
  polymorphous, 479
Venturi mask, 134, 134f
Verapamil hydrochloride (Calan; Isoptic; Verelan), 826-828
  in arrhythmias, 508-509
  in atrial fibrillation, 457
  in atrial flutter, 455
  in multifocal atrial tachycardia, 655
Vertebrae, 357, 359, 359f, 360f, 543. See also Spinal injuries
  cervical, 357, 359f, 543
  coccygeal, 357, 359f
  fractures of, 320
    compression, 320
  lumbar, 357, 359f, 543
  sacral, 357, 359f, 543
  subluxation of, 320
  thoracic, 357, 359f, 543
Vertebral foramen, 357
Vertigo (dizziness), 658
  in geriatric patients, 658-659
  trauma and, 662
Very-high frequency (VHF) radio frequencies, 33
Vial of life, 654
Vibrissae, 309
Violence
  controlling violent situations and, 730f, 730-732, 731f
  domestic, 726
  hostile situations and, 46
Viral meningitis, 605
Viremia, 607
Visceral (involuntary; smooth) muscle, 85, 350, 352, 355f
Viscosity, of petroleum distillates, 584, 585
Vision
  double (diplopia), 658
  in geriatric patients, trauma and, 662
  impairment of, communicating with patient and, 105
Vital capacity (VC), 384
  aging and, 651

Vital signs, 110–114. *See also* Body temperature; Breathing; Pulse; Pupils; Respiration(s)
  acute abdomen and, 565
  in children, 670
  evaluating, procedure for, 96, 96f
  myocardial infarction and, 421
  nervous system emergencies and, 549
  in pulmonary edema, 422
Vitamin B (Betalin; thiamine), 826
Vitreous body, 306, 307f
Vitreous humor, 306, 307f
Vocal cords, 128
Volatility, of petroleum distillates, 585
Volume of dead space gas (V_D), 384
Voluntary guarding, abdominal injuries and, 345
Voluntary (skeletal; striated) muscle, 85, 350, 352, 355f
V_T (tidal volume), 383
Vulva, 692

W

Wandering atrial pacemaker (WAP), 448, 502t–503t
Warm zone, hazardous materials incidents and, 640, 641f
Wasp stings, 590
Waste, hazardous, definition of, 634
Water, loss of, routes of, 182, 183t
Water emergencies. *See* Barotrauma; Drowning
Water moccasin (cottonmouth) bites, 590
Water (hydrostatic) pressure, 184, 630
Wenckebach block (Mobitz I block; type I second degree AV block), 485
Wernicke's encephalopathy, 598
Wet drowning, 628
Wharton's jelly, 694
Wheezing, 118, 386, 391
  allergic reactions and, 574
  in pulmonary edema, 422
Whiplash, 276
White blood cells (leukocytes), 186
  formation of, 356–357
  immune response and, 603
White matter, 540
Will, living, 22
Wind chill, 627
Wisconsin blade, 141
Wolff-Parkinson-White syndrome, 452, 452f
  drugs in, 457, 508–509
Word roots, for medical terms, 79
Wounds
  closed, 288
    management of, 291
  open, 288–390
    abrasion, 288, 289f
    amputation, 290, 290f, 291, 291f
    avulsion, 289f, 289–290
    impaled objects and, 289f, 290, 291–292
    laceration, 288, 289f, 290f
    management of, 291
    puncture, 288–289, 289f
Wrist, bones of, 359, 361f

X

Xiphoid process, 359, 360f
Xylocaine. *See* Lidocaine hydrochloride

Y

Yankauer (tonsil tip), 136–137, 137f
Yellow jacket stings, allergic reaction to, 573f, 573–574

Z

Zygote, 694